BONTRAGER'S TEXTBOOK OF

Radiographic Positioning and Related Anatomy

TENTH EDITION **10**

BONTRAGER'S TEXTBOOK OF

Radiographic Positioning and Related Anatomy

JOHN P. LAMPIGNANO, MEd, RT(R)(CT)

LESLIE E. KENDRICK, MS, RT(R)(CT)(MR)

ELSEVIER

Elsevier
3251 Riverport Lane
St. Louis, Missouri 63043

BONTRAGER'S TEXTBOOK OF RADIOGRAPHIC POSITIONING AND
RELATED ANATOMY, 10TH EDITION

ISBN: 978-0-323-65367-1

Notice

Previous edition copyrighted 2018 Elsevier Inc.
Previous edition copyrighted 2014 by Mosby, an affiliate of Elsevier Inc.
Previous editions copyrighted 2010, 2005, 2001, 1997, 1993, 1987, and 1982 by Mosby, Inc., an affiliate of Else-
vier Inc.

International Standard Book Number: 978-0-323-65367-1

Executive Content Strategist: Sonya Seigafuse
Senior Content Development Manager: Lisa P. Newton
Senior Content Development Specialist: Tina Kaemmerer
Publishing Services Manager: Julie Eddy
Senior Project Manager: Richard Barber
Design Direction: Amy Buxton

Printed in China

Last digit is the print number: 9 8 7 6 5 4 3 2

Working together
to grow libraries in
developing countries

www.elsevier.com • www.bookaid.org

Acknowledgments and Dedication

John P. Lampignano

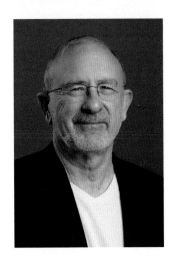

First, I must acknowledge the contributions from students and imaging faculty throughout the United States and various aspects of the world, including Puerto Rico and South America. We hear frequently from them, as they provide feedback on the text and ancillaries. They have provided us with fresh ideas and perspectives for the text and how to improve it. A special thank you to Chris Wertz, with Idaho State University, for being so instrumental in this edition. Chris and his brother, Dr. Joss Wertz, provided many of the images for the tenth edition. Chris is an excellent writer and the contributor for Chapters 5 and 6.

The Radiologic Sciences faculty and staff at Boise State University are outstanding role models for their students and the profession—Joie Burns, Leslie Kendrick, Cathy Masters, Travis Armstrong, Natalie Mourant, and Sue Antonich. They have made my transition to Boise State a positive and supportive experience. Special recognition to Michele Patrícia Müller Mansur Vieira, who is a lecturer at Federal Institute of Paraná - Campus Curitiba in Brazil. Michele is a valued colleague and good friend. Michele contributed to Chapters 12 and 13.

The contributing authors for the tenth edition did an outstanding job in researching and writing the content for numerous chapters. My heartfelt gratitude to each of them for making this edition truly reflective of the current practice in medical imaging. Special thanks to Andrew Woodward and the faculty at GateWay Community College, Bradley Johnson, Nicole Hightower, Janelle Black, and Michelle Wilt. Andrew redesigned Chapters 1 and 18 in this edition, served as consultant for all of the digital imaging concepts, and provided numerous photographs and images. The GateWay faculty and their students helped us secure many of the new images for this edition.

Ken Bontrager was dedicated to this text and other instructional media in radiologic technology for more than 48 years. Ken gave of himself fully to this text and its ancillaries. We hope our profession never forgets Ken Bontrager and his contributions.

Leslie E. Kendrick formally became co-author for the ninth edition. Leslie is a driven, detailed, and outstanding writer. She took on this huge endeavor while maintaining her program responsibilities at Boise State University, completing her research for a doctorate, and taking care of her family. You can't measure the character of a writer until they are tested by long hours, pressing deadlines, and personal sacrifice. Leslie has the character and heart of a writer. I am privileged to work with her.

More than 250 photographs were taken for the tenth edition. This feat would not have been possible without the special talents of KJ Filmworks, including Jack Quirk, Renee Settlemires, and Ken Helms.

Our gratitude to photography models Jamie Blum, Tina Kaemmerer, Misti Walker, Livia Kendrick, Travis Kendrick, Atticus Rosenkoetter, Aubrie Rosenkoetter, Robyn Pedraza, Carlos Pedraza, Calliope Pedraza, and Deborah Lampignano, who served as models for this edition. They maintained a high degree of professionalism and tremendous patience throughout the long photo shoots.

We were honored to have Jamie Blum and Sonya Seigafuse as our Executive Content Strategists. Jaime was our editor for the tenth edition from inception to near completion. Sonya helped us navigate through the final stages of the tenth edition. Both of these individuals made the process of creating the tenth edition seamless.

Our Senior Content Development Specialist, Tina Kaemmerer, was simply incredible. She is a perfectionist who challenged us to bring forth our best effort in a loving way. Her support was ongoing, professional, and always positive. We shall always treasure our friendship with Tina.

Rich Barber is the Senior Project Manager who led us through the production phase. We couldn't have produced this edition without his expertise.

Most importantly, a thank you to Elsevier Publishing for allowing us to continue to be part of this wonderful reference for the past 46 years.

Finally, my thanks to my family for their ongoing support. My wife Deborah, son Daniel, daughter Molly, and granddaughter, Tatum. I'm especially proud that Daniel and Molly have entered the medical profession. They are both excellent professionals and they understand the importance of treating their patients with dignity and compassion. They have always been important to me, even though I don't express it adequately. My true inspiration is my granddaughter, Tatum. Now 14 years old, she has turned into a loving, bright, and caring young person. When things got difficult and overwhelming, I only needed to see her picture or spend a few minutes with her and my spirit was renewed. Tatum will always own my heart. Finally, to Buddy and Segen—the family dogs—and the joy (and occasional challenge) they provide us.

Deborah has been at my side for more than 42 years. She has been the compassionate anchor that provides our family with the stability and encouragement to be successful in all our professional and personal endeavors. My life changed in so many positive ways since I first met her. Meeting the demands of a new edition of the text would not have been possible if it wasn't for her enduring love and support.

Our world has faced a great challenge with the coronavirus pandemic that struck at the end of 2019/beginning of 2020. We wish to recognize the dedication and sacrifice of the many imaging technologists and students who continue to serve their patients and those facing this potentially life-threatening condition. This service is often at risk of their own health and the health of their families. To each of you, we dedicate this tenth edition.

JPL

Acknowledgments and Dedication

Leslie E. Kendrick

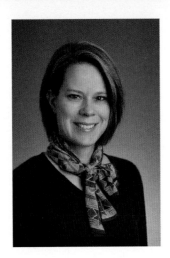

John Lampignano has eloquently acknowledged many outstanding individuals from the worlds of medical imaging and publishing. I sincerely echo his appreciation and recognition that this tenth edition has been made possible with the time and talents of many. Special thanks to Dr. José Rafael Moscoso-Alvarez, of the Universidad Central de Caribe, Puerto Rico for serving as technical advisor for this edition. José is a cherished colleague and friend. We respect and appreciate his contributions to this edition. Working alongside and with so many amazing professionals is an incredible honor. Your tireless dedication, compassion for patients, and tremendous respect for each other are what makes this profession such a joy to be part of. I genuinely appreciate the opportunity to give back to the profession as the co-author of this textbook and ancillaries with utmost gratitude.

I am especially grateful to Darlene Travis, O. Scott Staley, Duane McCrorie (rest in peace), Lorrie Kelley, Joie Burns, Cathy Masters, Travis Armstrong, Natalie Mourant, and Sue Antonich of Boise State University for freely sharing your vast knowledge and expertise in the field of radiologic sciences. Thank you for fostering in me the passion and drive for life-long learning. You each stand as a pillar of greatness in the field. It is truly an honor to be your colleague.

I also thank my loving family for their unfailing patience. My youngest, Livia, has sat by patiently many times waiting for mommy to proofread a paragraph just one more time. My incredible husband, Travis, recognizes the honor of my participation in this project and continues to support my insatiable desire to get it right. Words cannot express the pride I feel when I reflect on my family: seven beautiful children—each talented, kind, and a blessing to those around them: CJ, Ren, Robyn, Kade, Atticus, Aubrie, and Livia; seven lovely grandchildren—each filled with wonder and delight: Fox, Killian, Kellen, Charlotte, Haydin, Addison, and Calliope; one amazing husband who loves me unconditionally and makes my life complete. There aren't enough words to express the joy you each bring to me. Thank you for sharing so much of yourselves.

Lastly, I thank John P. Lampignano for opening a whole new world by extending me the invitation of co-authorship. This project continually presents opportunities for collaboration across the United States and around the globe. The professional growth from exposure to new ideas, concepts, and intellects has been exponential. The first time I met John, I was impressed by his professionalism and poise. To now be his colleague is an incredible privilege. I will work hard to uphold the high standards set for this textbook and ancillaries by Kenneth Bontrager and now John. I will continue to recognize the value of collaboration with professionals across the United States and the world to ensure quality and accuracy. I encourage communication from all readers of these materials on how to improve and better meet the needs of the users. It is our goal to be a continued invaluable resource for educators, students, and imaging professionals.

LEK

Contributors

Janelle M. Black, BS(DMIT), RT(R) (ARRT)
Chapter 4
Faculty
Medical Radiography
GateWay Community College
Phoenix, Arizona
Radiologic Technologist
Scottsdale Medical Imaging Ltd.
Scottsdale, Arizona

Joie Burns, MS, RT(R)(S), RDMS, RVT
Chapter 20
Diagnostic Medical Sonography Program
Director/Chair
Radiologic Sciences
Boise State University
Boise, Idaho

Shaun T. Caldwell, MS, RT (R)(T)
Chapter 20
Associate Professor
School of Health Professions
The University of Texas MD Anderson
Cancer Center,
Houston, Texas

Jeanne M. Dial, MED, CNMT, NMTCB(CT)
Chapter 20
Program Director
Nuclear Medicine Technology
GateWay Community College
Phoenix, Arizona

Cheryl DuBose, EDD, RT(R)(MR)(CT) (QM)
Chapter 2
Department Chair
Medical Imaging and Radiologic
Sciences
Arkansas State University
Jonesboro, Arkansas

Frank Goerner, PHD
Chapter 1
Medical Physicist
Medical Physics
The Queens Medical Center
Honolulu, Hawaii

Michele Gray-Murphy, MEd, RT(R)(M), ARRT
Chapter 11
Faculty
Associate of Science in Radiography
Program
Allen College
Waterloo, Iowa

Kelli Welch Haynes, Ed.D, RT(R)
Chapter 3
Program Director
Allied Health
Northwestern State University
Shreveport, Louisiana

Chad Hensley, PhD, RT(R)(MR)
Chapters 14 and 16
Clinical Coordinator
Radiography
University of Nevada Las Vegas
Las Vegas, Nevada

Nicolle Hightower, MEd, RT(R)(VI)
Chapter 17
Medical Radiography Faculty and Director
of Clinical Education
Health Sciences
Gateway Community College
Phoenix, Arizona

Bradley Johnson, MEd, RT(R)
Chapters 15 and 19
Faculty
Medical Radiography
GateWay Community College
Phoenix, Arizona

Derek Lee, BS, CNMT, PET
Chapter 20
Supervisor Nuclear Medicine, PET/CT &
PET/MRI
Nuclear Medicine
Phoenix VA Medical Center
Phoenix, Arizona
Adjunct Faculty
Nuclear Medicine Technology Program
Gateway Community College
Phoenix, Arizona

Michele Patricia Müller Mansur Vieira, MSc TCNL-CRTR-PR (BRAZIL)
Chapters 12 and 13
Professora e Coordenadora do Curso
Técnico em Radiologia
Instituto Federal do Paraná
Curitiba, Brazil

Katrina L. Steinsultz, RT(R)(M), MAdm, MPH
Chapter 10
Clinical Assistant Professor
University of North Carolina at Chapel Hill
Chapel Hill, North Carolina

Beth L. Veale, PhD, RT(R)(QM)
Chapter 7
Professor/Interim Chair– The Shimadzu
School of Radiologic Sciences
Midwestern State University
Wichita Falls, Texas

Patti Ward, PHD, (RT)(R)
Chapters 8 and 9
Instructor of Radiologic Sciences
Health Sciences
Colorado Mesa University
Grand Junction, Colorado

Sharon Wartenbee, RTR, BD, CBDT, FASRT
Chapter 20
Senior Bone Densitometry Technologist
Radiology
Avera Medical Group McGreevy Clinic
Sioux Falls, South Dakota

Christopher Wertz, MSRS, RT(R)
Chapters 5 and 6
Program Director
Radiographic Science
Idaho State University
Pocatello, Idaho

Michelle A. Wilt, MHA, RT (R)(M) (ARRT)
Chapter 20
Faculty
Medical Radiography
GateWay Community College
Phoenix, Arizona

Kathryn Wissink, AAS, RT(R), (MR)
MR Education Development Specialist
Chapter 20
MRI
Siemens Healthineers
Cary, North Carolina

Andrew Woodward, MA, RT(R)(CT) (QM)
Chapters 1 and 18
Assistant Professor (retired)
Radiologic Sciences
The University of North Carolina at Chapel Hill
Chapel Hill, North Carolina

Contributors to Past Editions

Barry T. Anthony, RT(R)
Englewood, Colorado

Patrick Apfel, MED, RT(R)
Las Vegas, Nevada

April Apple, RT(R)
Durham, North Carolina

Alex Backus, MS, RT(R)
Phoenix, Arizona

Daniel J. Bandy, MS, CNMT
Phoenix, Arizona

Kristi Blackhurst, BS, RT(R)(MR)
Gilbert, Arizona

Karen Brown, RT(R)
Phoenix, Arizona

Claudia Calandrino, MPA, RT(R)
Los Angeles, California

Mary J. Carrillo, MBA/HCM, RT(R)(M), CDT
Phoenix, Arizona

Timothy C. Chapman, RT(R)(CT)
Phoenix, Arizona

Donna Davis, MED, RT(R)(CV)
Little Rock, Arkansas

Nancy L. Dickerson, RT(R)(M)
Rochester, Minnesota

Eugene D. Frank, MA, RT(R), FASRT, FAERS
Rochester, Minnesota

Richard Geise, PHD, FACR, FAAPM
Minneapolis, Minnesota

Cecilie Godderidge, BS, RT(R)
Boston, Massachusetts

Jeannean Hall-Rollins, MRC, BS, RT(R)(CV)
Jonesboro, Arkansas

Jessie R. Harris, RT(R)
Los Angeles, California

W.R. Hedrick, PHD, FACR
Canton, Ohio

Dan L. Hobbs, MSRS, RT(R)(CT)(MR)
Pocatello, Idaho

Brenda K. Hoopingarner, MS, RT(R)(CT)
Hays, Kansas

Julia Jacobs, MBA, RT(R)(T)
Phoenix, Arizona

Nancy Johnson, MED, RT(R)(CV)(CT)(QM)(ARRT), FASRT
Phoenix, Arizona

Jenny A. Kellstrom, MED, RT(R)
Klamath Falls, Oregon

Leslie E. Kendrick, MS, RT(R)(CT)(MR)
Boise, Idaho

Molly E. Lampignano, CNMT, PET
Phoenix, Arizona

Linda S. Lingar, MED, RT(R)(M)
Little Rock, Arkansas

James D. Lipcamon, RT(R)
Torrance, California

Kathy M. Martensen, BS, RT(R)
Iowa City, Iowa

Cindy Murphy, BHSC, RT(R), ACR
Halifax, Nova Scotia, Canada

Kathleen Murphy, MBA, RDMS, RT(R)
Apache Junction, Arizona

Manjusha Namjoshi, BS, RDMS, RT(R)
Phoenix, Arizona

Sandra J. Nauman, RT(R)(M)
Austin, Minnesota

Joseph Popovitch, RT(R), ACR, DHSA
Halifax, Nova Scotia, Canada

E. Russel Ritenour, PHD
Minneapolis, Minnesota

Bette Schans, PHD, RT(R)
Grand Junction, Colorado

Mindy S. Shapiro, RT(R)(CT)
Tucson, Arizona

Marianne Tortorici, EDD, RT(R)
San Diego, California

Renee F. Tossell, PHD, RT(R)(M)(CV)
Phoenix, Arizona

Charles R. Wilson, PHD, FAAPM, FACR
Milwaukee, Wisconsin

Donna L. Wright, EDD, RT(R)
Wichita Falls, Texas

Linda Wright, MHSA, RT(R)
Denver, Colorado

Preface

Purpose and Goal of the Tenth Edition

The tenth edition of *Bontrager's Textbook of Radiographic Position-ing and Related Anatomy* is a one-volume reference that provides the essential knowledge for the student in radiographic positioning. Positioning remains as one of the critical variables in medical radi-ography that is solely in the hands of the technologist. Proper positioning displays anatomy and pathology correctly to enable the radiologist and other physicians to make an accurate diagnosis. In many respects, the patient's health and well-being is in the hands of the technologist. The authors and contributors had this goal in mind as we made the revisions for the tenth edition. Each position and procedure were carefully evaluated to provide the most accu-rate information for the student and practicing technologist. Our goals were to be accurate, use language that was easy to follow, and observe current practices for reducing dose to the patient and technologist. Our aim was to continue this format in the *Workbook*, *Handbook*, and web-based resources.

We hope we have met these goals. We continue to be open to your feedback and suggestions to make this text and its ancillaries more accurate and valuable resources.

Methodology

We apply the principle of presenting information from simple to complex, from known to unknown, and we provide diagrams and images to illustrate these concepts. The chapters are arranged to first describe the more basic radiographic procedures and proceed to the more complex ones in later chapters. This method is con-tinued in the format of the *Workbook* and *Handbook* as well.

New to This Latest Edition

- Chapter 1, *Terminology, Positioning, and Imaging Principles* contains examples of terminology, basic principles, both analog and digital system imaging, grids, radiographic quality factors, and radiation protection that provide a central resource for these principles and concepts. Information on digital imaging concepts has been updated and reflects current practices. The information on analog imaging has been reduced due to the predominance of digital imaging. The chapter on radiation protection reinforces the recommendations and practices promoted by the Image-Gently® and ImageWisely® initiatives.
- Chapter 4, *Upper Limb* added the AP axial-Brewerton method, which demonstrates early signs of rheumatoid arthritis in the joints of the hands.
- Chapter 5, *Shoulder Girdle and Humerus* added PA axial-Bernageau method for the scapulohumeral joint space and the AP axial-Zanca method for assessment of the acromioclavicular (AC) joints.
- Chapter 15, *Trauma, Mobile, and Surgical Radiography* was revised extensively to focus on key concepts of mobile, trauma, and surgical radiography. In doing so, we retained key concepts while eliminating procedures no longer performed.

- Chapter 16, *Pediatric Radiography* has been updated to reflect best practices in reducing dose to young patients. Image-Gently® principles are stressed in this chapter and Chapter 1. Photographs of pediatric immobilization devices have been updated.
- Chapter 17, *Angiography and Interventional Procedures* has new art and photographs added to illustrate current procedures and angiographic devices currently seen in clinical practice.
- Chapter 18, *Computed Tomography* was revised to reflect the newest technology available. New procedures and current CT technology were added in this chapter.
- Chapter 19, *Special Radiographic Procedures* was updated to reflect new procedures and imaging modalities including Digital Tomosynthesis (DTS).
- Chapter 20 *Diagnostic and Therapeutic Procedures.* Each of the modalities were updated to reflect current imaging systems and procedures. Mammography has new digital images and the Magnetic Resonance Imaging (MRI) section was revised to include current technology, current protocols, and high quality images.
- The tenth edition follows closely the procedures and positioning concepts required by the American Registry of Radiologic Tech-nologists (ARRT) Content Specifications for the Radiography Examination.
- More than **250 positioning photographs** have been replaced in the tenth edition. A different perspective was used with these photos. They demonstrate close-ups of the positioning model so students and technologists can better view positioning land-marks, CR centering points, and collimation. Erect versions of positions are now included for many positions to reflect current clinical practice.
- **New images** have been added throughout the tenth edition. We replaced many analog film-based images with digital ver-sions. Several of the commercial medical imaging companies graciously allowed us to use their images for this edition.
- **Revised Radiographic Critique.** At the end of Chapters 2-11 and 18, the radiographic critique section has been revised to provide students a method to compare an ideal image to others than demonstrate common positioning and technical errors. Solutions for these critique assessments are provided in the faculty Evolve site.
- **Digital imaging** continues to be emphasized in the tenth edition. Terminology, technical factors, part centering, and kVp ranges are described with a primary focus on digital systems.
- kVp ranges have been reviewed by experts in the field to ensure they are consistent with current practice and will provide the most diagnostic images while reducing patient dose.
- **Consistent positioning terminology** is used throughout the *Textbook*, *Workbook*, and *Handbook*. Projection names are used that are formally recognized in the profession. All projections match those stated in the ARRT Content Specifications in Radiography.

- **Twenty chapters.** The number of chapters for the tenth edition **remains 20 chapters.** To keep the size and page count of the text to a reasonable size, we kept this edition to the relative size of the previous edition. The body of knowledge in medical imaging continues to grow exponentially. This edition provides the most essential concepts in radiographic anatomy and positioning while keeping the size and weight of this text consistent with past editions.
- The authors and contributors believe the changes and improvements in this latest edition will enhance learning and reflect current clinical practice.

Ancillaries
WORKBOOK
This edition contains new learning-exercise and self-test questions, including more situation-based questions and new questions on digital imaging. All questions have been reviewed by a team of educators and students to ensure the accuracy of the content and answers. The radiographic critique section was expanded to include images in the workbook pages.

EVOLVE INSTRUCTOR RESOURCES
A computerized test bank is available on Evolve to instructors who use this textbook in their classrooms. The test bank features more than 1200 questions. They include registry-type questions, which can be used as final evaluation exams for each chapter, or they can be put into custom exams that educators create. These tests can be administered as either computer- or print-based assessments, and are available in ExamView® format.

Also available on Evolve is an electronic image collection featuring more than 2700 images that are fully coordinated with the tenth edition *Textbook* and *Workbook*. Instructors can create their own customized classroom presentations using these electronic images, which closely follow the *Textbook* and *Workbook*, chapter by chapter.

The Evolve Instructor Resources also provide a complete Power-Point presentation that correlates with the *Textbook*.

EVOLVE STUDENT RESOURCES
New to the tenth edition, students will have access to 400 additional review questions (20 questions per chapter) to help them review important concepts. Each question will include detailed rationales.

HANDBOOK
The new tenth edition revised pocket *Handbook*, also authored by John P. Lampignano and Leslie E. Kendrick, is now available from Elsevier as one of the ancillary components along with student workbooks and an electronic image collection for a complete current student resource on radiographic positioning.

MOSBY'S® RADIOGRAPHY ONLINE
Mosby's® Radiography Online for Bontrager's Textbook of Radiographic Positioning and Related Anatomy is a unique online courseware program promoting problem-based learning with the goal of developing critical thinking skills needed in the clinical setting. Developed to be used in conjunction with the Lampignano/Kendrick *Textbook* and *Workbook*, the online course enhances learning with animations and interactive exercises and offers application opportunities that can accommodate multiple learning styles and circumstances.

How to Use the Positioning Pages

1 **PROJECTION TITLE BARS** describe the specific position/projection to be radiographed, including the proper name of the position, if such applies.

2 **CLINICAL INDICATIONS** section summarizes conditions or pathologies that may be demonstrated by the examination and/or projection. This brief review helps the technologist understand the purpose of the examination and which structures or tissues should be most clearly demonstrated.

3 **PROJECTION SUMMARY BOXES** list all the specific routine or special projections most commonly performed for that body part.

4 **TECHNICAL FACTORS** section includes the image receptor (IR) size recommended for the average adult; whether the IR should be placed portrait or landscape in relation to the patient; a grid, if one is needed; and recommended kVp ranges. The minimum SID (source-to-image receptor distance) is listed.

5 **IMAGE RECEPTOR ICONS** give a visual display of the IR relative size (cm) and orientation (portrait or landscape), relative collimated field size, location of R and L markers, and the recommended AEC cell location (if AEC is used).

6 **SHIELDING** section describes shielding that is recommended for the projection.

7 **PATIENT POSITION** section indicates the general body position required for the projection.

8 **PART POSITION** section gives a clear, step-by-step description of how the body part should be positioned in relation to the IR and/or tabletop. The CR icon is included for all those projections in which the CR is of primary importance to remind the technologist to pay special attention to the CR during the positioning process for that projection.

9 **CENTRAL RAY (CR)** section describes the precise location of the CR in relation to both the IR and the body part.

10 **RECOMMENDED COLLIMATION** section describes the collimation of the x-ray field recommended for that projection.

11 **RESPIRATION** section lists the breathing requirements for that projection.

12 **EVALUATION CRITERIA** boxes describe evaluation/critique process that should be completed for each processed radiographic image. This process is divided into the following three broad categories: (1) anatomy demonstrated, (2) position, (3) exposure.

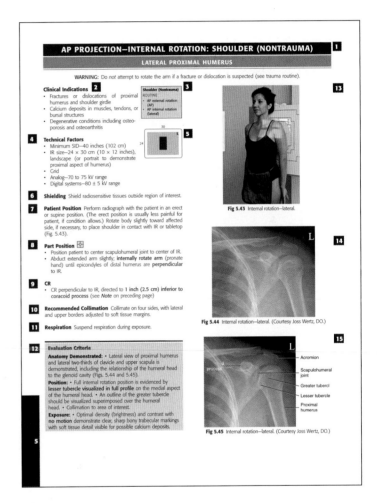

13 **POSITIONING PHOTOGRAPHS** show a correctly positioned patient and part in relation to the CR and IR.

14 **RADIOGRAPHIC IMAGES** provide an example of a correctly positioned and correctly exposed radiographic image of the featured projection.

15 **ANATOMY LABELED IMAGES** identify specific anatomy that should be demonstrated on the radiographic image shown. The labeled image, in most cases, matches the radiographic image example on the same page.

Contents

CHAPTER 1

Terminology, Positioning, and Imaging Principles

CONTRIBUTIONS BY **Andrew Woodward,** MA, RT(R)(CT)(QM)

RADIATION PROTECTION CONTRIBUTOR **Frank Goerner,** PhD, DABR

CONTRIBUTORS TO PAST EDITIONS   W. R. Hedrick, PhD, FACR, Cindy Murphy, BHSc, RT(R), ACR, Joseph Popovitch, RT(R), ACR, DHSA, Kathy M. Martensen, BS, RT(R), Barry T. Anthony, RT(R), Katrina Lynn Steinsultz, BS, RT(R)(M)

RADIATION PROTECTION PAST CONTRIBUTORS   Richard Geise, PhD, FACR, FAAPM, E. Russel Ritenour, PhD

CONTENTS

PART ONE ▪ TERMINOLOGY AND POSITIONING

GENERAL, SYSTEMIC, AND SKELETAL ANATOMY AND ARTHROLOGY

1

General Anatomy

Anatomy is the study, classification, and description of the structure and organs of the human body, whereas **physiology** deals with the processes and functions of the body, or how the body parts work. In the living subject, it is almost impossible to study anatomy without also studying some physiology. However, radiographic study of the human body is primarily a study of the anatomy of the various systems, with less emphasis on the physiology. Consequently, anatomy of the human system is emphasized in this radiographic anatomy and positioning textbook.

NOTE: Phonetic respelling[1] of anatomic and positioning terms is included throughout this text to facilitate correct pronunciation of the terms commonly used in medical radiography.

STRUCTURAL ORGANIZATION

Several levels of structural organization make up the human body. The lowest level of organization is the **chemical level.** All chemicals necessary for maintaining life are composed of **atoms,** which are joined in various ways to form **molecules.** Various chemicals in the form of molecules are organized to form **cells.**

Cells

The cell is the basic structural and functional unit of all living tissue. Every single part of the body, whether muscle, bone, cartilage, fat, nerve, skin, or blood, is composed of cells.

Tissues

Tissues are cohesive groups of similar cells that, together with their intercellular material, perform a specific function. The four basic types of tissue are as follows:

1. *Epithelial (ep″-i-the′le-al):* Tissues that cover internal and external surfaces of the body, including the lining of vessels and organs, such as the stomach and the intestines
2. *Connective:* Supportive tissues that bind together and support various structures
3. *Muscular:* Tissues that make up the substance of a muscle
4. *Nervous:* Tissues that make up the substance of nerves and nerve centers

Organs

When complex assemblies of tissues are joined to perform a specific function, the result is an organ. Organs usually have a specific shape. Examples of organs of the human body are the kidneys, heart, liver, lungs, stomach, and brain.

System

A system consists of a group or an association of organs that have a similar or common function. The urinary system, consisting of the kidneys, ureters, bladder, and urethra, is an example of a body system. The total body comprises **10 individual body systems.**

Organism

The 10 systems of the body when functioning together make up the total organism—one living being (Fig. 1.1).

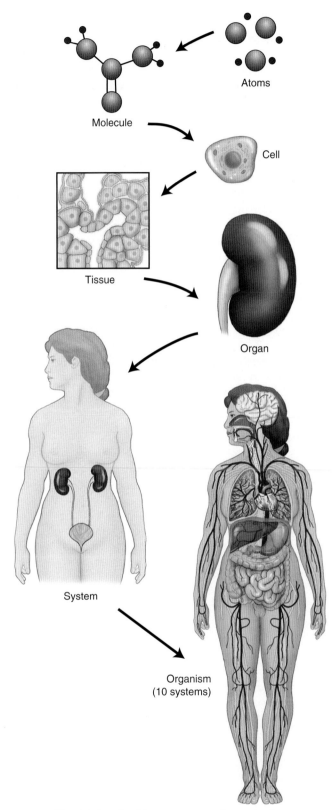

Atoms

Molecule

Cell

Tissue

Organ

System

Organism
(10 systems)

Fig. 1.1 Levels of human structural organization.

Systemic Anatomy
BODY SYSTEMS

The human body is a structural and functional unit made up of 10 lesser units called *systems.* These 10 systems are the (1) skeletal, (2) circulatory, (3) digestive, (4) respiratory, (5) urinary, (6) reproductive, (7) nervous, (8) muscular, (9) endocrine, and (10) integumentary *(in-teg″-u-men′-tar-e)* systems.

Skeletal System

The skeletal system (Fig. 1.2) is important for the technologist to learn. The skeletal system includes the **206 separate bones** of the body and their associated cartilages and joints. The study of bones is termed **osteology,** whereas the study of joints is called **arthrology.**

The four functions of the skeletal system are as follows:
1. Support and protect many soft tissues of the body
2. Allow movement through interaction with the muscles to form a system of levers
3. Produce blood cells
4. Store calcium

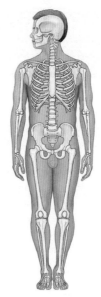

Fig. 1.2 Skeletal system.

Circulatory System

The circulatory system (Fig. 1.3) is composed of the following:
- The **cardiovascular organs**—heart, blood, and blood vessels
- The **lymphatic system**—lymph nodes, lymph vessels, lymph glands, and spleen

The six functions of the circulatory system are as follows:
1. Distribute oxygen and nutrients to the cells of the body
2. Transport cell waste and carbon dioxide from the cells
3. Transport water, electrolytes, hormones, and enzymes
4. Protect against disease
5. Prevent hemorrhage by forming blood clots
6. Assist in regulating body temperature

Digestive System

The digestive system includes the alimentary canal and certain accessory organs (Fig. 1.4). The alimentary canal is made up of the mouth, pharynx, esophagus, stomach, small intestine, large intestine, and anus. Accessory organs of digestion include the salivary glands, liver, gallbladder, and pancreas.

The twofold function of the digestive system is as follows:
1. Prepare food for absorption by the cells through numerous physical and chemical breakdown processes
2. Eliminate solid wastes from the body

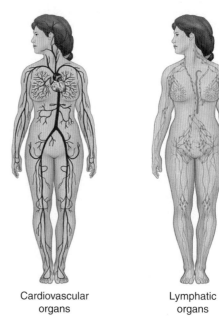

Cardiovascular organs   Lymphatic organs

Fig. 1.3 Circulatory system.

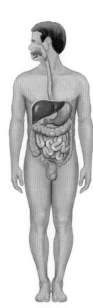

Fig. 1.4 Digestive system.

Respiratory System

The respiratory system is composed of two lungs and a series of passages that connect the lungs to the outside atmosphere (Fig. 1.5). The structures that make up the passageway from the exterior to the alveoli of the lung interior include the nose, mouth, pharynx, larynx, trachea, and bronchial tree.

The three primary functions of the respiratory system are as follows:

1. Supply oxygen to the blood and eventually to the cells
2. Eliminate carbon dioxide from the blood
3. Assist in regulating the acid-base balance of the blood

Urinary System

The urinary system includes the organs that produce, collect, and eliminate urine. The organs of the urinary system consist of the kidneys, ureters, bladder, and urethra (Fig. 1.6).

The four functions of the urinary system are as follows:

1. Regulate the chemical composition of the blood
2. Eliminate many waste products
3. Regulate fluid and electrolyte balance and volume
4. Maintain the acid-base balance of the body

Reproductive System

The reproductive system is made up of organs that produce, transport, and store the germ cells (Fig. 1.7). The testes in the male and the ovaries in the female produce mature germ cells. Transport and storage organs of the male include the vas deferens, prostate gland, and penis. The organs of reproduction in the female are the ovaries, uterine (fallopian) tubes, uterus, and vagina (Fig. 1.7).

The function of the reproductive system is to reproduce the organism.

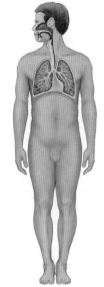

Fig. 1.5 Respiratory system.

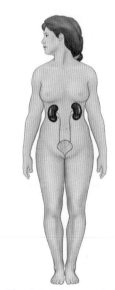

Fig. 1.6 Urinary system.

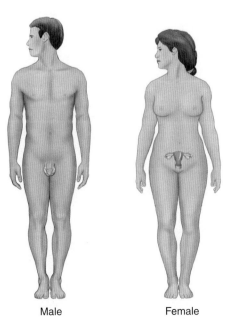

Male   Female

Fig. 1.7 Reproductive system.

Nervous System

The nervous system is composed of the brain, spinal cord, nerves, ganglia, and special sense organs such as the eyes and ears (Fig. 1.8).

The function of the nervous system is to coordinate voluntary and involuntary body activities and transmit electrical impulses to various parts of the body and the brain.

Muscular System

The muscular system (Fig. 1.9), which includes all muscle tissues of the body, is subdivided into three types of muscles: (1) **skeletal,** (2) **smooth,** and (3) **cardiac.**

Most of the muscle mass of the body is skeletal muscle, which is striated and under voluntary control. The voluntary muscles act in conjunction with the skeleton to allow body movement. About 43% of the weight of the human body is accounted for by voluntary or striated skeletal muscle.

Smooth muscle, which is involuntary, is located in the walls of hollow internal organs such as blood vessels, the stomach, and intestines. These muscles are called *involuntary* because their contraction usually is not under voluntary or conscious control.

Cardiac muscle is found only in the walls of the heart and is involuntary but striated.

The three functions of muscle tissue are as follows:
1. Allow movement, such as locomotion of the body or movement of substances through the alimentary canal
2. Maintain posture
3. Produce body heat

Endocrine System

The endocrine system includes **all the ductless glands** of the body (Fig. 1.10). These glands include the testes, ovaries, pancreas, adrenals, thymus, thyroid, parathyroid, pineal, and pituitary. The placenta acts as a temporary endocrine gland.

Hormones, which are the secretions of the endocrine glands, are released directly into the bloodstream.

The function of the endocrine system is to regulate bodily activities through the various hormones carried by the cardiovascular system.

Integumentary System

The tenth and final body system is the **integumentary** *(in-teg"-u-men'-tar-e)* system, which is composed of the **skin** and **all structures derived from the skin** (Fig. 1.11). These derived structures include hair, nails, and sweat and oil glands.

The skin is an organ that is essential to life. The skin is the **largest organ of the body,** covering a surface area of approximately 3000 in^2 (7620 cm^2) and constituting 8% of total body mass in the average adult.

The five functions of the integumentary system are as follows:
1. Regulate body temperature
2. Protect the body, within limits, against microbial invasion and mechanical, chemical, and ultraviolet (UV) radiation damage
3. Eliminate waste products through perspiration
4. Receive certain stimuli such as temperature, pressure, and pain
5. Synthesize certain vitamins and biochemicals such as vitamin D

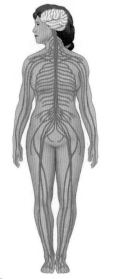

Fig. 1.8 Nervous system.

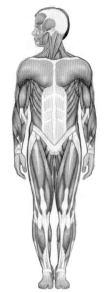

Fig. 1.9 Muscular system.

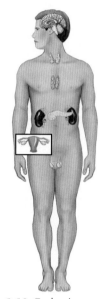

Fig. 1.10 Endocrine system.

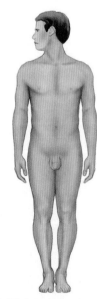

Fig. 1.11 Integumentary system.

Skeletal Anatomy

Because a large part of general diagnostic radiography involves examination of the bones and joints, **osteology** *(os″-te-ol′-o-je)* (the study of bones) and **arthrology** *(ar-throl′-o-je)* (the study of joints) are important subjects for the technologist.

OSTEOLOGY

The adult skeletal system is composed of **206 separate bones,** which form the framework of the entire body. Certain cartilages, such as those at the ends of long bones, are included in the skeletal system. These bones and cartilages are united by ligaments and provide surfaces to which the muscles attach. Because muscles and bones must combine to allow body movement, these two systems sometimes are collectively referred to as the *locomotor system.*

   The adult human skeleton is divided into the **axial skeleton** and the **appendicular skeleton.**

Axial Skeleton

The **axial** *(ak′-se-al)* skeleton includes all bones that lie on or near the central axis of the body (Table 1.1). The adult axial skeleton consists of **80 bones** and includes the skull, vertebral column, ribs, and sternum (the dark-shaded regions of the body skeleton in Fig. 1.12).

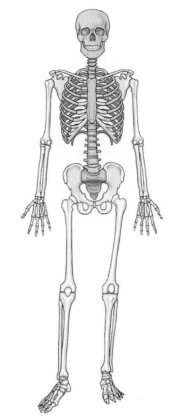

Fig. 1.12 Axial skeleton—80 bones.

TABLE 1.1 **ADULT AXIAL SKELETON**		
Skull	Cranium	8
	Facial bones	14
Hyoid		1
Auditory ossicles (3 small bones in each ear)		6
Vertebral column	Cervical	7
	Thoracic	12
	Lumbar	5
	Sacral	1
	Coccyx	1
Thorax	Sternum	1
	Ribs	24
Total bones in adult axial skeleton		*80*

Appendicular Skeleton

The second division of the skeleton is the **appendicular** *(ap″-en-dik′-u-lar)* portion. This division consists of all bones of the upper and lower limbs (extremities) and the shoulder and pelvic girdles (the dark-shaded regions in Fig. 1.13). The appendicular skeleton attaches to the axial skeleton. The adult appendicular skeleton comprises **126 separate bones** (Table 1.2).

TABLE 1.2 **ADULT APPENDICULAR SKELETON**		
Shoulder girdles	Clavicles	2
	Scapula (scapulae)	2
Upper limbs	Humerus (humeri)	2
	Ulna (ulnae)	2
	Radius (radii)	2
	Carpals	16
	Metacarpals	10
	Phalanges	28
Pelvic girdle	Hip bones **(innominate bones)**	2
Lower limbs	Femur (femora)	2
	Tibia	2
	Fibula (fibulae)	2
	Patella (patellae)	2
	Tarsals	14
	Metatarsals	10
	Phalanges	28
Total bones in adult appendicular skeleton		*126*
Entire number of separate bones in adult skeleton[a]		*206*

[a]This includes the two sesamoid bones anterior to the knees: the right and left patellae.

Sesamoid Bones

A sesamoid bone is a special type of small, oval-shaped bone that is embedded in certain tendons (most often near joints). Although sesamoid bones are present even in a developing fetus, they are not counted as part of the normal axial or appendicular skeleton except for the two patellae, the largest sesamoid bones. The other most common sesamoid bones are located in the posterior foot at the base of the first toe (Figs. 1.14 and 1.15).

In the upper limb, sesamoid bones are found most commonly in tendons near the anterior (palmar) surface of the hand at the base of the thumb. Others may be found in tendons of other upper or lower limb joints.

Sesamoid bone may be fractured by trauma; sesamoid bones can be demonstrated radiographically or by computed tomography (CT).

CLASSIFICATION OF BONES

Each of the 206 bones of the body can be classified according to shape as follows:

- Long bones
- Short bones
- Flat bones
- Irregular bones

Long Bones

Long bones consist of a **body** and **two ends** or **extremities**. Long bones are found only in the appendicular skeleton. (Fig. 1.16 is a radiograph of a humerus, a typical long bone of the upper arm.)

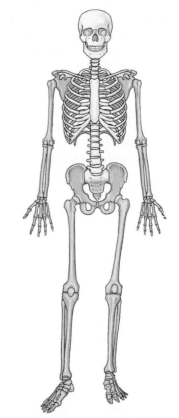

Fig. 1.13 Appendicular skeleton—126 bones.

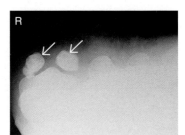

Fig. 1.15 Sesamoid bones. Tangential projection (base of first toe).

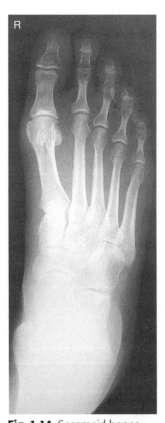

Fig. 1.14 Sesamoid bones on the posterior base of the first toe.

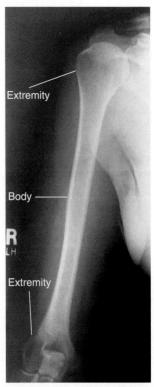

Fig. 1.16 Long bone (humerus).

Composition The outer shell of most bones is composed of hard or dense bone tissue known as **compact bone,** or **cortex,** meaning an external layer. Compact bone has few intercellular empty spaces and serves to protect and support the entire bone.

The **body** (older term is **shaft**) contains a thicker layer of compact bone than is found at the ends, to help resist the stress of the weight placed on them.

Inside the shell of compact bone and especially at both ends of each long bone is found **spongy,** or **cancellous, bone.** Cancellous bone is highly porous and usually contains red bone marrow, which is responsible for the production of red blood cells.

The body of a long bone is hollow. This hollow portion is known as the **medullary** *(med'-u-lar"-e)* **cavity.** In adults, the medullary cavity usually contains fatty yellow marrow. A dense fibrous membrane, the **periosteum** *(per"-e-os'-te-am),* covers bone except at the articulating surfaces. The articulating surfaces are covered by a layer of **hyaline cartilage** (Fig. 1.17).

Hyaline *(hi'-ah-lin),* meaning glassy or clear, is a common type of cartilage or connecting tissue. Its name comes from the fact that it is not visible with ordinary staining techniques, and it appears "clear" or glassy in laboratory studies. It is present in many places, including within the covering over ends of bones, where it is called **articular cartilage.**

The **periosteum** is essential for bone growth, repair, and nutrition. Bones are richly supplied with blood vessels that pass into them from the periosteum. Near the center of the body of long bones, a **nutrient artery** passes obliquely through the compact bone via a **nutrient foramen** into the medullary cavity.

Short Bones
Short bones are roughly cuboidal and are found only in the wrists and ankles. Short bones consist mainly of cancellous tissue with a thin outer covering of compact bone. The eight **carpal bones** of each wrist (Fig. 1.18) and the seven **tarsal bones** of each foot are short bones.

Flat Bones
Flat bones consist of two plates of compact bone with cancellous bone and bone marrow between them. Examples of flat bones are the bones that make up the **calvaria** (skull cap) (Fig. 1.19), **sternum, ribs,** and **scapulae.**

The narrow space between the two layers of compact bone of flat bones within the cranium is known as the **diploe** *(dip'-lo-e).* Flat bones provide protection for interior contents and broad surfaces for muscle attachment.

Irregular Bones
Bones that have peculiar shapes are lumped into one final category—irregular bones. **Vertebrae** (Fig. 1.20), **facial bones, bones of the base of the cranium,** and **bones of the pelvis** are examples of irregular bones.

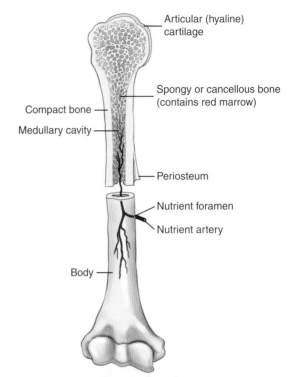

Articular (hyaline) cartilage

Spongy or cancellous bone (contains red marrow)

Compact bone

Medullary cavity

Periosteum

Nutrient foramen

Nutrient artery

Body

Fig. 1.17 Long bone.

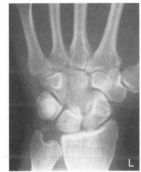

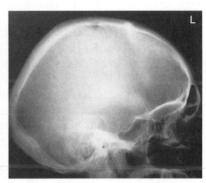

Fig. 1.18 Short bones (carpals).

Fig. 1.19 Flat bones (calvaria).

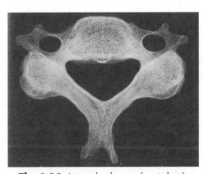

Fig. 1.20 Irregular bone (vertebra).

DEVELOPMENT OF BONES

The process by which bones form within the body is known as **ossification** *(os″-i-fi-ka′-shun).* The embryonic skeleton is composed of fibrous membranes and hyaline cartilage. Ossification begins at about the sixth embryonic week and continues until adulthood.

Blood Cell Production

In adults, **red blood cells (RBCs)** are produced by the red bone marrow of certain flat and irregular bones such as the **sternum, ribs, vertebrae,** and **pelvis,** as well as the ends of the long bones.

Bone Formation

Two types of bone formation are known. When bone replaces membranes, the ossification is called **intramembranous** *(in″-trah-mem′-brah-nus).* When bone replaces cartilage, the result is **endochondral** *(en″-do-kon′-dral)* (intracartilaginous) ossification.

Intramembranous Ossification Intramembranous ossification occurs rapidly and takes place in bones that are needed for protection, such as sutures of the flat bones of the calvaria (skullcap), which are centers of growth in early bone development.

Endochondral Ossification Endochondral ossification, which is much slower than intramembranous ossification, occurs in most parts of the skeleton, especially in the long bones.

Primary and Secondary Centers of Endochondral Ossification (Fig. 1.21)

The first center of ossification, which is called the **primary center,** occurs in the midbody area. This primary center of ossification in growing bones is called the **diaphysis** *(di-af′-i-sis).* This becomes the **body** in a fully developed bone.

Secondary centers of ossification appear near the ends of the limbs of long bones. Most secondary centers appear after birth, whereas most primary centers appear before birth. Each secondary center of ossification is called an **epiphysis** *(e-pif′-i-sis).* Epiphyses of the distal femur and the proximal tibia are the first to appear and may be present at birth in a term newborn. Cartilaginous plates, called **epiphyseal plates,** are found between the metaphysis and each epiphysis until skeletal growth is complete. The **metaphysis** is the wider portion of a long bone adjacent to the epiphyseal plate. The metaphysis is the area where bone growth in length occurs. Growth in the length of bones results from a longitudinal increase in these epiphyseal cartilaginous plates. This is followed by progressive ossification through endochondral bone development until all the cartilage has been replaced by bone, at which time growth of the skeleton is complete. This process of epiphyseal fusion of the long bones occurs progressively from the age of puberty to **full maturity,** which is **between the ages of 20 and 25 years.**[1] However, the time for each bone to complete growth varies for different regions of the body. On average, the female skeleton matures more quickly than the male skeleton. Also, geography, socioeconomic, genetic factors, and disease affect epiphyseal fusion.[1]

Fig. 1.22 shows a radiograph of the knee region of a 6-year-old child. Primary and secondary centers of endochondral ossification or bone growth are well demonstrated and labeled.

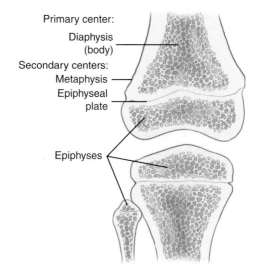

Primary center:
Diaphysis (body)
Secondary centers:
Metaphysis
Epiphyseal plate
Epiphyses

Fig. 1.21 Endochondral ossification.

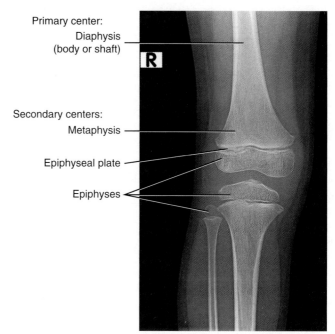

Primary center:
Diaphysis (body or shaft)
Secondary centers:
Metaphysis
Epiphyseal plate
Epiphyses

Fig. 1.22 Knee region (6-year-old child).

Arthrology (Joints)

The study of joints or articulations is called **arthrology.** It is important to understand that movement does not occur in all joints. The first two types of joints to be described are immovable joints and only slightly movable joints, which are held together by several fibrous layers, or cartilage. These joints are adapted for growth rather than for movement.

CLASSIFICATION OF JOINTS

Functional

Joints may be classified according to their function in relation to their mobility or lack of mobility as follows:

- **Synarthrosis** *(sin″-ar-thro′-sis)*—immovable joint
- **Amphiarthrosis** *(am″-fe-ar-thro′-sis)*—joint with limited movement
- **Diarthrosis** *(di″-ar-thro′-sis)*—freely movable joint

Structural

The primary classification system of joints, described in *Gray's Anatomy*[2] and used in this textbook, is a **structural classification** based on the **three types of tissue that separate the ends of bones** in the different joints. These three classifications by tissue type, along with their subclasses, are as follows:

1. Fibrous *(fi′-brus)* joints
   - Syndesmosis *(sin″-des-mo′-sis)*
   - Suture *(su′-tur)*
   - Gomphosis *(gom-fo′-sis)*
2. Cartilaginous *(kar″-ti-laj′-i-nus)* joints
   - Symphysis *(sim′-fi-sis)*
   - Synchondrosis *(sin″-kon-dro′-sis)*
3. Synovial *(si-no′-ve-al)* joints

Fibrous Joints

Fibrous joints lack a joint cavity. The adjoining bones, which are nearly in direct contact with each other, are held together by fibrous connective tissue. Three types of fibrous joints are syndesmoses, which are slightly movable; sutures, which are immovable; and gomphoses, a unique type of joint with only very limited movement (Fig. 1.23).

Syndesmoses[1] Syndesmoses are fibrous types of articulations that are held together by interosseous ligaments and slender fibrous cords that allow slight movement at these joints. Some earlier references restricted the fibrous syndesmosis classification to the inferior tibiofibular joint. However, fibrous-type connections also may occur in other joints, such as the sacroiliac junction with its massive interosseous ligaments that in later life become almost totally fibrous articulations. The carpal and tarsal joints of the wrist and foot also include interosseous membranes that can be classified as syndesmosis-type joints that are only slightly movable, or amphiarthrodial.

Sutures Sutures are found only between bones in the skull. These bones make contact with one another along interlocking or serrated edges and are held together by layers of fibrous tissue, or sutural ligaments. Movement is very limited at these articulations; in adults, these are considered **immovable, or synarthrodial, joints.**

Limited expansion- or compression-type movement at these sutures can occur in the infant skull (e.g., during the birth process). However, by adulthood, active bone deposition partially or completely obliterates these suture lines.

Gomphoses A **gomphosis** joint is the third unique type of fibrous joint, in which a conical process is inserted into a socket-like portion of bone. This joint or fibrous union—which, strictly speaking, does not occur between bones but between the roots of the teeth and the alveolar sockets of the mandible and the maxillae—is a specialized type of articulation that allows only very limited movement.

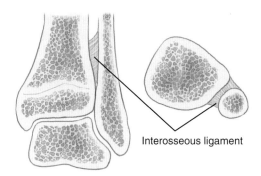

Distal tibiofibular joint
1. Syndesmosis–Amphiarthrodial (slightly movable)

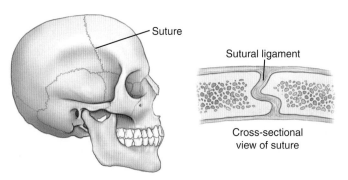

Skull suture
2. Suture–Synarthrodial (immovable)

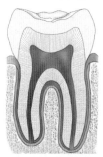

Roots of teeth
3. Gomphosis–Amphiarthrodial (only limited movement)
Fig. 1.23 Fibrous joints—three types.

Cartilaginous Joints

Cartilaginous joints also lack a joint cavity, and the articulating bones are held together tightly by cartilage. Similar to fibrous joints, cartilaginous joints allow little or no movement. These joints are synarthrodial or amphiarthrodial and are held together by two types of cartilage: symphyses and synchondroses (Fig. 1.24).

Symphyses The essential feature of a symphysis is the **presence of a broad, flattened disk of fibrocartilage** between two contiguous bony surfaces. These fibrocartilage disks form relatively thick pads that are capable of being compressed or displaced, allowing some movement of these bones, which makes these joints **amphiarthrodial** (slightly movable).

Examples of such symphyses are the intervertebral disks (between bodies of the vertebrae), between the manubrium (upper portion) and body of the sternum, and the symphysis pubis (between the two pubic bones of the pelvis).

Synchondroses A typical synchondrosis is a **temporary form of joint** wherein the connecting **hyaline cartilage** (which on long bones is called an *epiphyseal plate*) is converted into bone at adulthood. These temporary types of growth joints are considered **synarthrodial** or immovable.

Examples of such joints are the epiphyseal plates between the epiphyses and the metaphysis of long bones and at the three-part union of the pelvis, which forms a cup-shaped acetabulum for the hip joint.

Synovial Joints

Synovial joints are freely movable joints, most often found in the upper and lower limbs, which are characterized by a **fibrous capsule that contains synovial fluid** (Fig. 1.25). The ends of the bones that make up a synovial joint may make contact but are completely separate and contain a joint space or cavity, which allows for a wide range of movement at these joints. Synovial joints are generally **diarthrodial,** or freely movable. (Exceptions include the sacroiliac joints of the pelvis, which are amphiarthrodial, or slightly movable.)

The exposed ends of these bones contain thin protective coverings of **articular cartilage**. The **joint cavity,** which contains a viscous lubricating **synovial fluid,** is enclosed and surrounded by a **fibrous capsule** that is reinforced by strengthening **accessory ligaments**. These ligaments limit motion in undesirable directions. The inner surface of this fibrous capsule is thought to secrete the lubricating synovial fluid.

Movement Types of Synovial Joints There are a considerable number and variety of synovial joints, and they are grouped according to the **seven types of movement** that they permit. These are listed in order from the least to the greatest permitted movement.

NOTE: The preferred name is listed first, followed by a synonym in parentheses. (This practice is followed throughout this textbook.)

Plane (gliding) joints This type of synovial joint permits the least movement, which, as the name implies, is a **sliding or gliding motion between the articulating surfaces.**

Examples of plane joints are the **intermetacarpal, carpometacarpal,** and **intercarpal** joints of the hand and wrist (Fig. 1.26). The right and left lateral **atlantoaxial joints** between C1 and C2 vertebrae are also classified as plane, or gliding, joints; they permit some rotational movement between these vertebrae, as is described in Chapter 8.

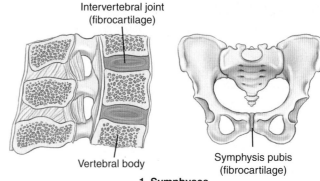

1. Symphyses
Amphiarthrodial (slightly movable)

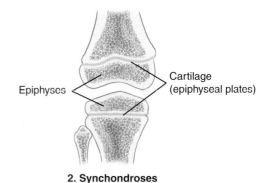

2. Synchondroses
Synarthrodial (immovable)

Fig. 1.24 Cartilaginous joints—two types.

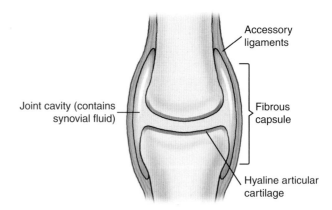

Fig. 1.25 Synovial joints—diarthrodial (freely movable).

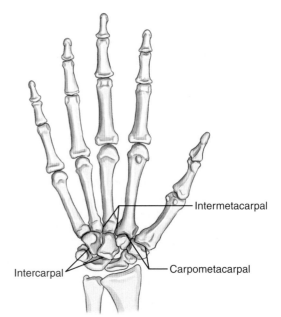

Fig. 1.26 Plane (gliding) joints.

Ginglymus (hinge) joints The articular surfaces of ginglymi, or ginglymus *(jin'-gli-mus)* joints, are molded to each other in such a way that they permit **flexion and extension movements** only. The articular fibrous capsule on this type of joint is thin on surfaces where bending takes place, but strong collateral ligaments firmly secure the bones at the lateral margins of the fibrous capsule.

Examples of ginglymi include the **interphalangeal joints** of fingers and toes and the **elbow joint** (Fig. 1.27).

Pivot (trochoid) joints The pivot or trochoid *(tro'-koid)* joint is formed by a bony, pivot-like process that is surrounded by a ring of ligaments or a bony structure or both. This type of joint allows **rotational movement** around a single axis.

Examples of pivot joints are the **proximal** and **distal radioulnar joints** of the forearm, which demonstrate this pivot movement during rotation of the hand and wrist.

Another example is the joint **between the first and second cervical vertebrae.** The odontoid process (dens) of the axis (C2) forms the pivot, and the anterior arch of the atlas (C1), combined with ligaments, forms the ring (Fig. 1.28).

Ellipsoid (condylar) joints In the ellipsoid *(e-lip'-soid)* joint, movement occurs primarily in one plane and is combined with a slight degree of rotation at an axis at right angles to the primary plane of movement. The rotational movement is limited by associated ligaments and tendons.

This type of joint allows primarily four directional movements: **flexion and extension** and **abduction and adduction. Circumduction** movement also occurs; this results from conelike sequential movements of flexion, abduction, extension, and adduction.

Examples of ellipsoidal joints include the metacarpophalangeal joints of the fingers, the radiocarpal (wrist joint), and the metatarsophalangeal joints of the toes (Fig. 1.29).

Saddle (sellar) joints The term saddle, or *sellar (sel'-ar)*, describes this joint structure well in that the ends of the bones are shaped concave-convex and are positioned opposite each other (Fig. 1.30). (Two saddle-like structures fit into each other.)

Movements of this biaxial type of saddle joint are the same as for ellipsoidal joints—**flexion, extension, adduction, abduction, and circumduction.**

The best example of a true *saddle* joint is the **first carpometacarpal joint** of the thumb. Other sellar joints include the ankle and the calcaneocuboid joints. Although the ankle joint was classified as a ginglymus in earlier references, current references classify it as a saddle joint.[3]

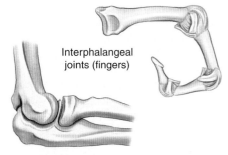

Interphalangeal joints (fingers)

Elbow joint

Fig. 1.27 Ginglymus (hinge) joints.

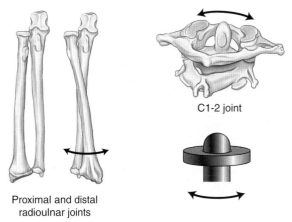

C1-2 joint

Proximal and distal radioulnar joints

Fig. 1.28 Pivot (trochoid) joints.

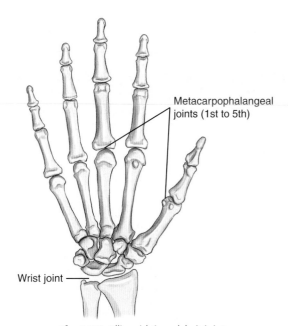

Metacarpophalangeal joints (1st to 5th)

Wrist joint

Fig. 1.29 Ellipsoid (condylar) joints.

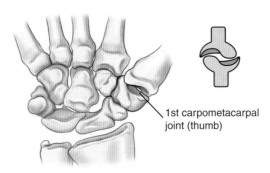

1st carpometacarpal joint (thumb)

Fig. 1.30 Saddle (sellar) joints.

Ball-and-socket (spheroidal) joints The ball-and-socket or sphe-roidal *(sfe′-roid-el)* joint allows for the greatest freedom of motion. The distal bone (humerus) that makes up the joint is capable of motion around an almost indefinite number of axes, with one common center.

The greater the depth of the socket, the more limited is the movement. However, the deeper joint is stronger and more stable. For example, the hip joint is a much stronger and more stable joint than the shoulder joint, but the range of movement is more limited in the hip.

Movements of ball-and-socket joints include flexion, extension, abduction, adduction, circumduction, and medial and lateral rotation.

Two examples of ball-and-socket joints are the **hip joint** and the **shoulder joint** (Fig. 1.31).

Bicondylar joints[3] Bicondylar joints usually provide movement in a single axis, such as flexion and extension. They can permit limited rotation. Bicondylar joints are formed by two convex condyles, which may be encased by a fibrous capsule.

Two examples of bicondylar joints are the knee (formerly classified as ginglymus) and the temporomandibular joint (TMJ) (Fig. 1.32).

See Table 1.3 for a summary of joint classification.

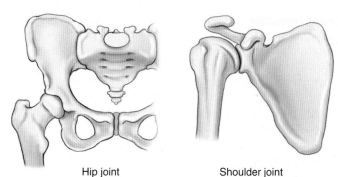

Hip joint   Shoulder joint

Fig. 1.31 Ball-and-socket (spheroidal) joints.

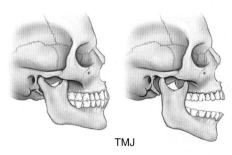

TMJ

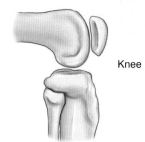

Knee

Fig. 1.32 Bicondylar joints.

TABLE 1.3 **SUMMARY OF JOINT CLASSIFICATION**				
JOINT CLASSIFICATION	**MOBILITY CLASSIFICATION**	**MOVEMENT TYPES**	**MOVEMENT DESCRIPTION**	**EXAMPLES**
Fibrous Joints				
Syndesmoses	Amphiarthrodial (slightly movable)	—	—	Distal tibiofibular, sacroiliac, carpal, and tarsal joints
Sutures	Synarthrodial (immovable)	—	—	Skull sutures
Gomphoses	Very limited movement	—	—	Areas around roots of teeth
Cartilaginous Joints				
Symphyses	Amphiarthrodial (slightly movable)	—	—	Intervertebral disks Symphysis pubis
Synchondroses	Synarthrodial (immovable)	—	—	Epiphyseal plates of long bones and between the three parts of the pelvis
Synovial joints	Diarthrodial (freely movable) except for the sacroiliac joints (synovial joints with only very limited motion [amphiarthrodial])	Plane (gliding)	Sliding or gliding	Intermetacarpal, intercarpal, and carpometacarpal joints, C1 on C2 vertebrae
		Ginglymi (hinge)	Flexion and extension	Interphalangeal joints of fingers, toes, and elbow joints
		Pivot (trochoid)	Rotational	Proximal and distal radioulnar and between C1 and C2 vertebrae (atlantoaxial joint)
		Ellipsoid (condylar)	Flexion and extension Abduction and adduction Circumduction	Metacarpophalangeal and wrist joints
		Saddle (sellar)	Flexion and extension Abduction and adduction Circumduction	First carpometacarpal joint (thumb), ankle, and calcaneocuboid joints
		Ball and socket (spheroidal)	Flexion and extension Abduction and adduction Circumduction Medial and lateral rotation	Hip and shoulder joints
		Bicondylar	Movement primarily along one axis with some limited rotation	Knee and temporomandibular joints

NOTE: Arthrology is the study of joints. The nomenclature for joints described in this chapter will be used in subsequent chapters throughout the text.

Body Habitus

Body habitus is generally defined as the build, physique, and general shape of the human body. The size, dimensions, and shape of the patient's body affect the positioning of specific regions of the body such as the respiratory, gastrointestinal, and biliary systems.

Body habitus is classified into four general body styles:

1. **Sthenic:** Approximately **50%** of the population falls into this category. For the purpose of radiographic positioning, sthenic body styles are considered average in shape and internal organ location (Fig. 1.33).
2. **Hyposthenic:** A body style which is more slender than the sthenic body habitus. Approximately **35%** of the population is classified as hyposthenic (Fig. 1.34).
3. **Hypersthenic:** A body style which has a broad frame as compared to the sthenic body habitus. Approximately **5%** of the population is classified as hypersthenic (Fig. 1.35).
4. **Asthenic:** Approximately **10%** of the population is very thin or slender with a long and narrow body build. More slight in stature than the hyposthenic patient.

IMPACT OF BODY HABITUS ON RADIOGRAPHIC POSITIONING

The technologist must consider the patient's body habitus and alter centering and image receptor (IR) placement accordingly. This is especially true during adult chest radiography (described in Chapter 2). For the hyposthenic and asthenic patient, the image receptor is typically placed in **portrait** (lengthwise) alignment because the lungs are generally longer than those of the hypersthenic patient (Fig. 1.36). For the hypersthenic patient, the image receptor is typically placed in **landscape** (crosswise) alignment because the lungs are generally shorter in length and more broad in width than those of the hyposthenic or asthenic patient (Fig. 1.37). IR placement for the sthenic adult patient may be portrait or landscape, depending on the person's age, height, and even pathology. Other anatomic regions also are affected by body habitus. This will be discussed further in Chapter 12, Biliary Tract and Upper Gastrointestinal System.

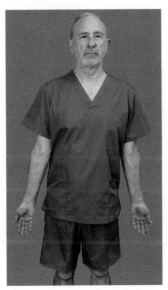

Fig. 1.33 Sthenic body habitus.

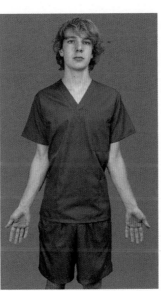

Fig. 1.34 Hyposthenic body habitus.

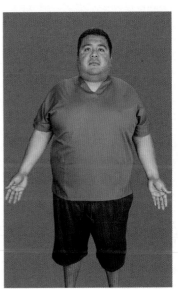

Fig. 1.35 Hypersthenic body habitus.

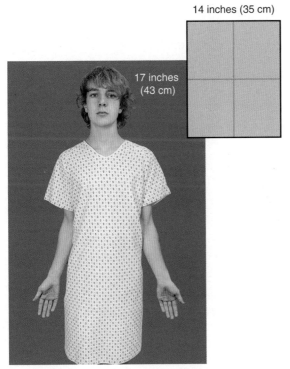

Fig. 1.36 Portrait alignment of image receptor.

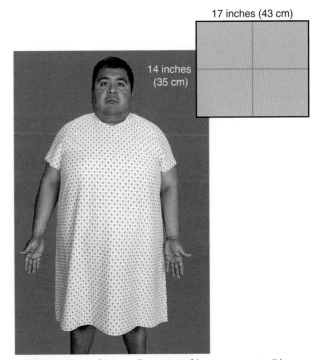

Fig. 1.37 Landscape alignment of image receptor Ditto.

POSITIONING TERMINOLOGY

Radiographic positioning refers to the study of patient positioning performed for **radiographic demonstration or visualization of specific body parts on image receptors.** The radiologic technologist must clearly understand the correct use of positioning terminology. This section lists, describes, and illustrates the commonly used terms consistent with the positioning and projection terminology as approved and published by the American Registry of Radiologic Technologists (ARRT).[4]

Throughout this text, named positions (i.e., with the proper name of the person who first described a specific position or procedure) are referred to as **methods,** such as the Towne, Waters, and Caldwell methods. The ARRT concurs regarding the use of the named method in parentheses after the projection or position term. The description of radiographic positions by the proper name method is becoming less common.

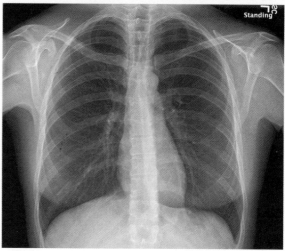

Fig. 1.38 Chest radiograph.

General Terms

Radiograph *(ra'-de-o-graf):* (1) An image of a patient's anatomic part(s), as produced by the action of x-rays on an image receptor (Fig. 1.38). If the radiograph is produced with the use of traditional film-screen (analog) technology, the image is captured and displayed on film; if the radiograph is produced via digital technology, the image is viewed and stored on display monitors. (2) The term *radiograph* refers to the recording medium *and* the image.

Radiography *(ra"-de-og'-rah-fe):* The process and procedures of producing a radiograph.

Image receptor (IR): The device that responds to the ionizing radiation to create the radiographic image after it exits the patient; refers to both analog (film-based) cassettes and digital acquisition devices.

Central ray (CR): Refers to the centermost portion of the x-ray beam emitted from the x-ray tube—the portion of the x-ray beam that has the least divergence.

Radiographic Examination or Procedure A radiologic technologist is shown positioning a patient for a routine chest examination or procedure (Fig. 1.39). A radiographic examination involves five general functions:

1. Positioning of body part and alignment with the IR and CR
2. Application of radiation protection measures and devices
3. Selection of exposure factors (radiographic technique)
4. Instructions to the patient related to respiration (breathing) and initiation of the x-ray exposure
5. Processing of the IR (analog) [chemical processing] or digital processing systems

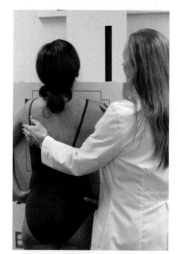

Fig. 1.39 Radiographic examination.

Anatomic Position The *anatomic (an"-ah-tom'-ik) position* is a reference position that defines specific surfaces and planes of the body. It also defines anatomic directional terms such as anterior, posterior, medial, lateral, superior, and inferior regions of the body. The anatomic position is an upright position with arms abducted slightly (down), hands by sides with palms forward, and head and feet together and directed straight ahead (Fig. 1.40).

Viewing Radiographs A general rule in viewing radiographs is to display them so that the **patient is facing the viewer,** with the patient in the **anatomic position.**

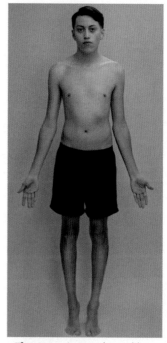

Fig. 1.40 Anatomic position.

Body Planes, Sections, and Lines (Fig. 1.41)

Positioning terms that describe CR angles or relationships between body parts often are related to **imaginary planes** that pass through the body in the **anatomic position.** The study of CT, MRI (magnetic resonance imaging), and sonography (diagnostic medical ultrasound) emphasizes sectional anatomy, which also involves the primary body planes and sections as described subsequently.

PLANE: STRAIGHT LINE SURFACE CONNECTING TWO POINTS

Four common planes used in medical imaging are the sagittal plane, coronal plane, horizontal (axial) plane, and oblique plane.

Sagittal Plane

A sagittal *(saj'-i-tal)* plane is any **longitudinal** plane that divides the body into **right and left parts.**

The **midsagittal plane,** sometimes called the **median plane,** is a midline sagittal plane that divides the body into **equal right and left parts.** It passes approximately through the sagittal suture of the skull. Any plane parallel to the midsagittal or median plane is called a **sagittal plane.**

Coronal Plane

A coronal *(ko-ro'-nal)* plane is any **longitudinal** plane that divides the body into **anterior and posterior parts.**

The **midcoronal plane** divides the body into approximately **equal anterior and posterior parts.** It is called a coronal plane because it passes approximately through the coronal suture of the skull. Any plane parallel to the midcoronal or frontal plane is called a **coronal plane.**

Horizontal (Axial) Plane

A horizontal (axial) plane is any **transverse** plane that passes through the body at **right angles to a longitudinal plane,** dividing the body into superior and inferior portions.

Oblique Plane

An oblique plane is a **longitudinal** or **transverse** plane that is at an angle or slant and is **not parallel** to the sagittal, coronal, or horizontal plane.

SECTIONAL IMAGE OF BODY PART

Longitudinal Sections—Sagittal, Coronal, and Oblique

These sections or images run **lengthwise** in the direction of the long axis of the body or any of its parts, regardless of the position of the body (erect or recumbent). Longitudinal sections or images may be taken in the **sagittal, coronal,** or **oblique plane.**

Transverse or Axial Sections (Cross-Sections)

Sectional images are at right angles along any point of the longitudinal axis of the body or its parts (Fig. 1.42)

Sagittal, Coronal, and Axial Images

CT, magnetic resonance imaging (MRI), and sonography images are obtained in these three common orientations or views. These common orientations are sagittal, coronal, and transverse (axial). (MRI sectional images are shown in Figs. 1.43 through 1.45.)

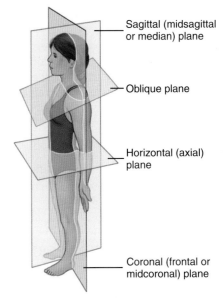

Sagittal (midsagittal or median) plane

Oblique plane

Horizontal (axial) plane

Coronal (frontal or midcoronal) plane

Fig. 1.41 Sagittal, coronal, oblique, and horizontal body planes.

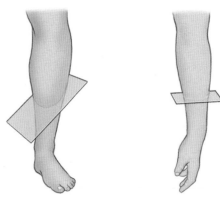

Oblique transverse plane or section of leg

Transverse (axial or cross-sectional) plane or section of arm

Fig. 1.42 Transverse and oblique sections of body parts.

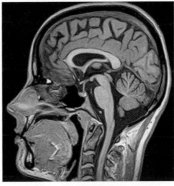

Fig. 1.43 Sagittal image.

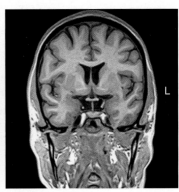

Fig. 1.44 Coronal image.

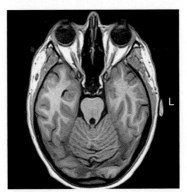

Fig. 1.45 Transverse (axial) image.

PLANES OF THE SKULL (FIG. 1.46)

Base Plane of Skull

This precise transverse plane is formed by connecting the lines from the infraorbital margins (inferior edge of bony orbits) to the superior margin of the external auditory meatus (EAM), the external opening of the ear. This sometimes is called the **Frankfort horizontal plane,**[1] as used in orthodontics and cranial topography to measure and locate specific cranial points or structures.

Occlusal Plane

This horizontal plane is formed by the biting surfaces of the upper and lower teeth with jaws closed (used as a reference plane of the head for cervical spine and skull radiography).

Body Surfaces and Parts

TERMS FOR THE BACK AND FRONT PORTIONS OF THE BODY

Posterior or Dorsal (FIG. 1.47)

Posterior *(pos-te'-re-or)* or dorsal *(dor'-sal)* refers to the **back half** of the patient, or the part of the body seen when the person is viewed from the back; includes the bottoms of the feet and the backs of the hands as demonstrated in the anatomic position.

Anterior or Ventral

Anterior *(an-te'-re-or)* or ventral *(ven'-tral)* refers to the **front half** of the patient, or the part seen when viewed from the front; includes the tops of the feet and the fronts or palms of the hands in the anatomic position.

TERMS FOR SURFACES OF THE HANDS AND FEET

Three terms are used in radiography to describe specific surfaces of the upper and lower limbs.

Plantar

Plantar *(plan'-tar)* refers to the **sole** or **posterior** surface of the foot.

Dorsal

Foot Dorsal *(dor'-sal)* refers to the **top** or **anterior** surface of the foot (dorsum pedis).

Hand Dorsal also refers to the **back** or **posterior** aspect of the hand (dorsum manus) (Fig. 1.48).

NOTE: The term **dorsum** (or **dorsal**) in general refers to the vertebral or posterior part of the body. However, when used in relationship with the foot, *dorsum* (dorsum pedis) specifically refers to the **upper surface,** or **anterior aspect,** of the foot opposite the sole, whereas for the hand (dorsum manus), it refers to the back or posterior surface opposite the palm.[1]

Palmar

Palmar *(pal'-mar)* refers to the **palm of the hand;** in the anatomic position, the same as the **anterior or ventral** surface of the hand.[1]

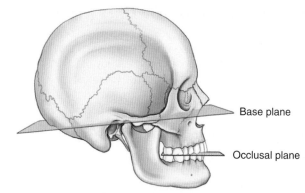

Fig. 1.46 Planes of skull.

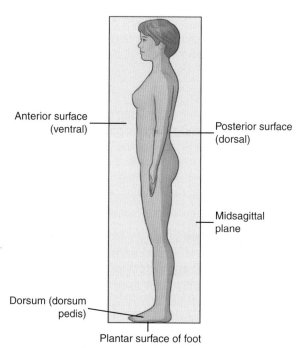

Fig. 1.47 Posterior vs. anterior.

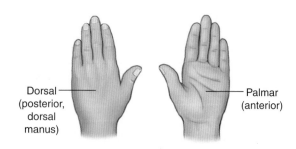

Fig. 1.48 Dorsal and palmar surfaces of hand.

Radiographic Projections

Projection is a positioning term that describes the **direction or path of the CR of the x-ray beam** as it passes through the patient, projecting an image onto the IR. Although the term *position* is used in the clinical setting, the term *projection* is considered to be the most accurate term for describing how the procedure is performed. Therefore, the term **projection** is used most frequently throughout this text.

COMMON PROJECTION TERMS

Posteroanterior (PA) Projection

Posteroanterior *(pos″-ter-o-an-te′-re-or)* (PA) projection refers to a projection of the CR from **posterior to anterior.**

The term *posteroanterior* combines the two terms *posterior* and *anterior* into one word, abbreviated as PA. The CR enters at the posterior surface and exits at the anterior surface **(PA projection)** (Fig. 1.49).

This projection assumes a **true PA** without intentional rotation, which requires the CR to be perpendicular to the coronal body plane and parallel to the sagittal plane, unless some qualifying oblique or rotational term is used to indicate otherwise.

Anteroposterior (AP) Projection

Anteroposterior *(an″-ter-o-pos-te′-re-or)* (AP) projection refers to a projection of the CR from **anterior to posterior,** the opposite of PA. *Anteroposterior* combines the two terms *anterior* and *posterior* into one word.

Anteroposterior describes the direction of travel of the CR, which enters at an anterior surface and exits at a posterior surface **(AP projection)** (Fig. 1.50).

The term assumes a **true AP** without rotation unless a qualifier term also is used, indicating it to be an oblique projection.

AP Oblique Projection

An AP projection of the upper or lower limb that is rotated is called *oblique.* This is not a true AP projection and **must also include a qualifying term** that indicates which way it is rotated, such as medial or lateral rotation (Fig. 1.51). (For an oblique projection of the whole body, see **oblique position** descriptions later in this chapter.) With an AP oblique projection, the CR enters the anterior surface and exits the posterior surface of the body or body part.

PA Oblique Projection

A PA projection of the upper limb with lateral rotation (from PA) is shown in Fig. 1.52. (This is applicable to both upper and lower limbs.) This projection is described as a PA oblique. It **must also include a qualifying term** that indicates which way it is rotated. With a PA oblique projection, the CR enters the posterior surface and exits the anterior surface of the body or body part.

Mediolateral and Lateromedial Projections

A **lateral** projection is described by the **path of the CR.** Two examples are the **mediolateral** projection of the ankle (Fig. 1.53) and the **lateromedial** projection of the wrist (Fig. 1.54). The medial and lateral sides are determined with the patient in the anatomic position. In the case of the mediolateral ankle projection, the CR enters the medial aspect and exits the lateral aspect of the ankle.

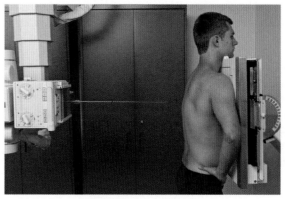
Fig. 1.49 PA projection.

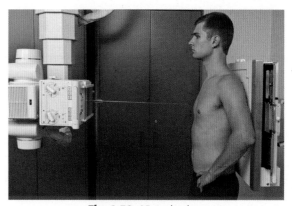
Fig. 1.50 AP projection.

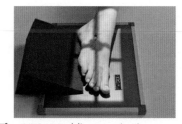
Fig. 1.51 AP oblique projection—medial rotation (from AP).

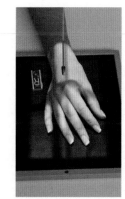
Fig. 1.52 PA oblique projection—lateral rotation (from PA).

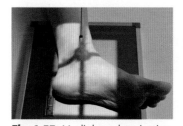
Fig. 1.53 Mediolateral projection (ankle).

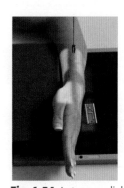
Fig. 1.54 Lateromedial projection (wrist).

Body Positions

In radiography, the term *position* is used in two ways, first as **general body positions,** as described next, and second as **specific body positions,** which are described in the pages that follow.

GENERAL BODY POSITIONS

The eight most commonly used general body positions in medical imaging are as follows:

1. **Supine** *(soo'-pine):* **Lying on back,** facing upward (Fig. 1.55)
2. **Prone** *(prohn):* **Lying on abdomen,** facing downward (head may be turned to one side) (Fig. 1.56)
3. **Erect** *(e-reckt')* (upright): An **upright position,** to stand or sit erect
4. **Recumbent** *(re-kum'-bent)* (reclining): **Lying down in any position** (prone, supine, or on side)
   - **Dorsal recumbent:** Lying on back (supine)
   - **Ventral recumbent:** Lying face down (prone)
   - **Lateral recumbent:** Lying on side (right or left lateral)
5. **Trendelenburg**[5] *(tren-del'-en-berg)* position: A recumbent position with the body tilted with the **head lower than the feet** (Fig. 1.57)
6. **Fowler**[6] *(fow'-ler)* position: A recumbent position with the body tilted with the **head higher than the feet** (Fig. 1.58)
7. **Sims position** (semiprone position): A recumbent oblique position with the patient lying on the **left anterior side,** with the right knee and thigh flexed and the left arm extended down behind the back. A **modified Sims** position as used for insertion of the rectal tube for a barium enema is shown in Fig. 1.59 (demonstrated in Chapter 13).
8. **Lithotomy** *(li-thot'-o-me)* position: A **recumbent** (supine) position with knees and hip flexed and thighs abducted and rotated externally, supported by ankle supports (Fig. 1.60). This position is seen frequently in the surgical suite for certain urinary studies.

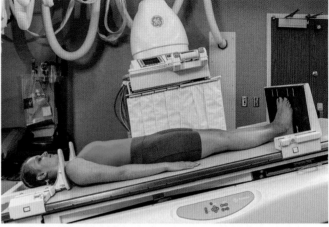

Fig. 1.57 Trendelenburg position—head lower than feet.

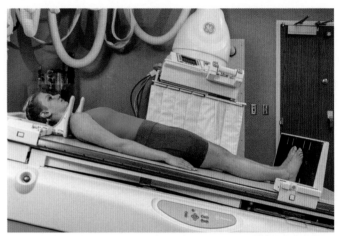

Fig. 1.58 Fowler position—feet lower than head.

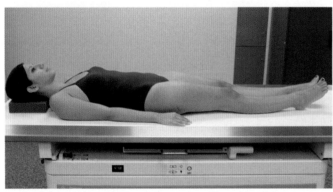

Fig. 1.55 Supine position.

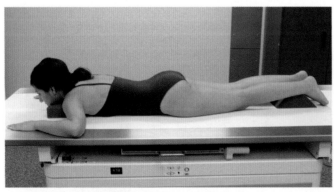

Fig. 1.56 Prone position.

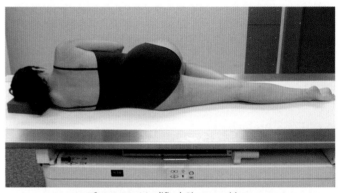

Fig. 1.59 Modified Sims position.

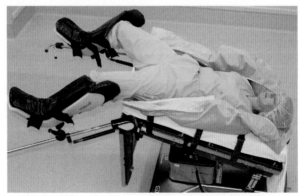

Fig. 1.60 Lithotomy position. (From Chitlik A: Safe positioning for robotic-assisted laparoscopic prostatectomy, *AORN J* 90[1]:39, 2011.)

SPECIFIC BODY POSITIONS

In addition to identifying general body positions, the term *position* is used in radiography to refer to a specific body position described by the body part closest to the IR (oblique and lateral) or by the surface on which the patient is lying (decubitus).

Lateral Position

Lateral *(lat'-er-al)* position refers to the side of, or a side view.

Specific lateral positions are described by the **side of the body closest to the IR** or the **body part from which the CR exits.** A **right lateral** position is shown with the right side of the body closest to the IR in the erect position (Fig. 1.61). Fig. 1.62 demonstrates a recumbent **left lateral** position.

A true lateral position is always 90°, or perpendicular, or at a right angle, to a true AP or PA projection. If it is not a true lateral, it is an oblique position.

Oblique Position[5]

Oblique *(ob-lek', or ob-lik')*[7] *(oh bleek', or oh blike')* position refers to an angled position in which neither the sagittal nor the coronal body plane is perpendicular or at a right angle to the IR.

Oblique body positions of the thorax, abdomen, or pelvis are described by the **side of the body closest to the IR** or the **body part from which the CR exits.**

Left and Right Posterior Oblique (LPO and RPO) Positions

LPO and RPO describe the specific oblique positions in which the **left or right posterior** aspect of the body is closest to the IR. A left posterior oblique (LPO) is demonstrated in both the erect (Fig. 1.63 and recumbent (Fig. 1.64) positions.

The CR exits from the left or right posterior aspect of the body.

NOTE: These also can be referred to as **AP oblique projections** because the CR enters an anterior surface and exits posteriorly. However, this **is not a complete description** and requires a specific position clarifier such as **LPO or RPO position.** Therefore, throughout this text, these body obliques are referred to as **positions** and not projections.

Obliques of upper and lower limbs are described correctly as AP and PA oblique but require the use of either **medial** or **lateral rotation** as a qualifier (see Figs. 1.51 and 1.52).

Right and Left Anterior Oblique (RAO and LAO) Positions

RAO and LAO refer to oblique positions in which the **right or left anterior** aspect of the body is closest to the IR and can be erect or recumbent general body positions. (A right anterior oblique [RAO] is shown in both examples (Figs. 1.65 and 1.66).

NOTE: These also can be described as **PA oblique projections** if a position clarifier is added, such as an RAO or LAO **position.**

It is *not* correct to use these oblique terms or the abbreviations LPO, RPO, RAO, or LAO as projections because they do not describe the direction or path of the CR; rather, these are **positions.**

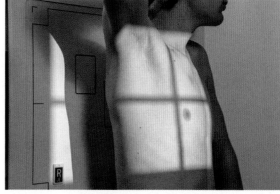

Fig. 1.63 Erect LPO position.

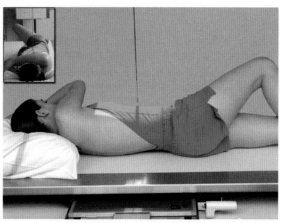

Fig. 1.64 Recumbent LPO position.

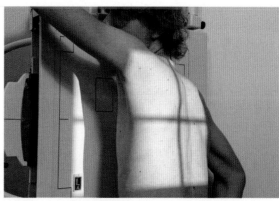

Fig. 1.65 Erect RAO position.

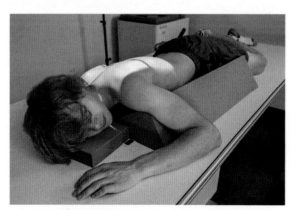

Fig. 1.66 Recumbent RAO position.

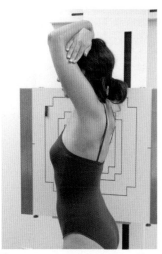

Fig. 1.61 Erect R lateral position.

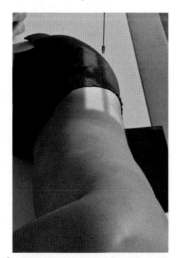

Fig. 1.62 Recumbent L lateral position.

Decubitus (Decub) Position

The word **decubitus** *(de-ku'bi-tus)* literally means to lie down, or the position assumed in lying down.

This body position, meaning to **lie on a horizontal surface**, is designated according to the **surface on which the body is resting**. This term describes a patient who is lying on one of the following body surfaces: **back** (dorsal), **front** (ventral), or **side** (right or left lateral).

In radiographic positioning, decubitus is *always* performed with the CR **horizontal**.

Decubitus positions are essential for detecting air-fluid levels or free air in a body cavity such as the chest or abdomen, where the air rises to the uppermost part of the body cavity. Decubitus positions are often performed if the patient cannot assume erect position.

Right or Left Lateral Decubitus Position—AP or PA Projection

In this position, the patient lies on the side, and the x-ray beam is directed horizontally from anterior to posterior (AP) (Fig. 1.67) or from posterior to anterior (PA) (Fig. 1.68).

The AP or PA projection is important as a qualifying term with decubitus positions to denote the direction of the CR.

This position is either a **left lateral decubitus** (see Fig. 1.67) or a **right lateral decubitus** (see Fig. 1.68).

NOTE: The decubitus position is identified according to the dependent side (side down) and the AP or PA projection indication. Example: Left lateral decubitus (PA projection) is with the patient lying on left side facing the image receptor. The CR enters the posterior side and exits the anterior side.

Dorsal Decubitus Position—Left or Right Lateral

In this position, the patient is **lying on the dorsal** (posterior) surface with the **x-ray beam directed horizontally,** exiting from the side closest to the IR (Fig. 1.69).

The position is named according to the surface on which the patient is lying (dorsal or ventral) and by the side closest to the IR (right or left).

Ventral Decubitus Position—Right or Left Lateral

In this position, the patient is lying on the ventral (anterior) surface with the x-ray beam directed horizontally, exiting from the side closest to the IR (Fig. 1.70).

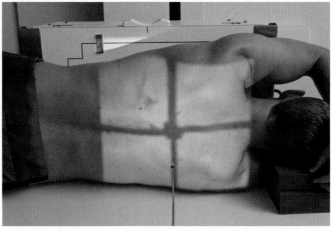

Fig. 1.68 Right lateral decubitus position (PA projection).

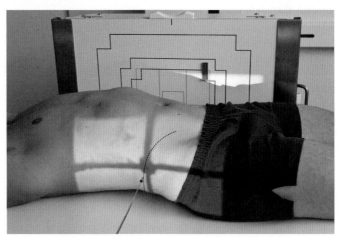

Fig. 1.69 Dorsal decubitus position (L lateral).

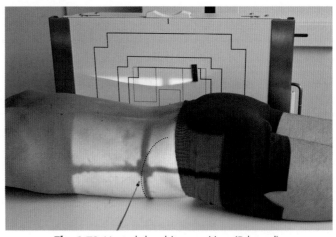

Fig. 1.70 Ventral decubitus position (R lateral).

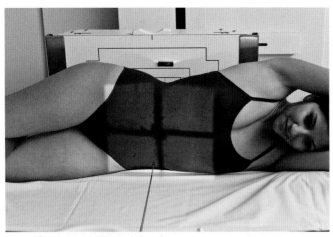

Fig. 1.67 Left lateral decubitus position (AP projection).

Additional Special-Use Projection Terms

Following are some additional terms commonly used to describe projections. These terms, as shown by their definitions, also refer to the path or projection of the CR and are projections rather than positions.

Axial Projection

Axial (ak'-se-al) refers to the **long axis** of a structure or part (around which a rotating body turns or is arranged).

Special application—AP or PA axial: In radiographic positioning, the term *axial* is used to describe **any angle of the CR of 10° or more along the long axis of the body or body part.**[7] However, in a true sense, an axial projection would be directed along, or parallel to, the long axis of the body or part. The term *semiaxial,* or "partly" axial, more accurately describes any angle along the axis that is not truly perpendicular or parallel to the long axis. However, for the sake of consistency with other references, the term **axial projection** is used throughout this text to describe both axial and semiaxial projections, as defined earlier and as illustrated in Figs. 1.71 through 1.73.

Inferosuperior and Superoinferior Axial Projections **Inferosuperior** axial projections are frequently performed for the shoulder and hip, where the CR enters below or inferiorly and exits above or superiorly (see Fig. 1.73).

The opposite of this is the **superoinferior** axial projection, such as a special nasal bone projection (see Fig. 1.71).

Tangential Projection

Tangential (ta"-jen'-shal) means touching a curve or surface at only one point.

This is a special use of the term *projection* to describe the CR that skims a body part to project the anatomy into profile and free of superimposition of surrounding body structures.

Examples Following are two examples or applications of the term *tangential projection*:
- Tangential projection of zygomatic arch (Fig. 1.74)
- Tangential projection of patella (Fig. 1.75)

AP Axial Projection—Lordotic Position

This is a **specific AP axial chest projection** for demonstrating the apices of the lungs. It also is called the **AP lordotic position.** In this case, the long axis of the body rather than the CR is angled.

The term **lordotic** comes from **lordosis,** a term that denotes curvature of the cervical and lumbar spine (see Chapters 8 and 9). As the patient assumes this position (Fig. 1.76), the lumbar lordotic curvature is exaggerated, making this a descriptive term for this special chest projection.

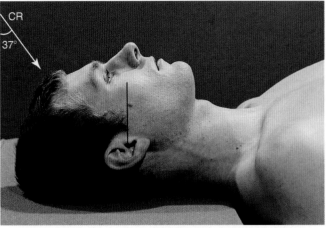

Fig. 1.72 AP axial (semiaxial) projection (CR 37° caudal).

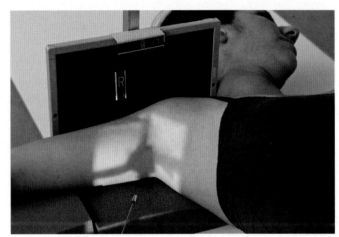

Fig. 1.73 Inferosuperior axial projection.

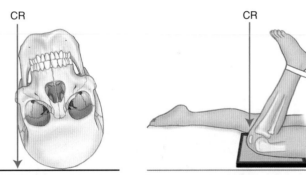

Fig. 1.74 Tangential projection (zygomatic arch).   **Fig. 1.75** Tangential projection (patella).

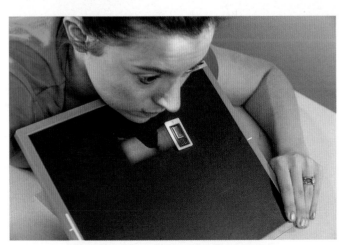

Fig. 1.71 Superoinferior (axial) projection.

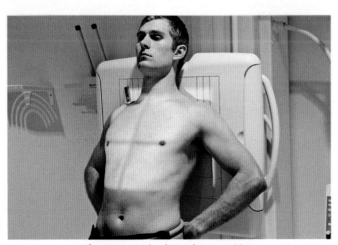

Fig. 1.76 AP lordotic chest position.

Transthoracic Lateral Projection (Right Lateral Position)

This is a lateral projection through the thorax. It requires a qualifying positioning term (right or left lateral position) to indicate which shoulder is closest to the IR and is being examined (Fig. 1.77).

NOTE: This is a special adaptation of the projection term, indicating that the CR passes through the thorax even though it does not include an entrance or exit site. In practice, this is a common lateral shoulder projection and is referred to as a **right** or **left transthoracic lateral shoulder.**

Dorsoplantar and Plantodorsal Projections

These are secondary terms for AP or PA projections of the foot.

  Dorsoplantar (DP) describes the path of the CR from the **dorsal** (anterior) surface to the **plantar** (posterior) surface of the foot (Fig. 1.78).

  A special plantodorsal projection of the heel bone (calcaneus) is called an **axial plantodorsal projection** (PD) because the angled CR enters the plantar surface of the foot and exits the dorsal surface (Fig. 1.79).

NOTE: The term **dorsum** for the **foot** refers to the anterior surface, dorsum pedis (see Fig. 1.47).

Parietoacanthial and Acanthioparietal Projections

The CR enters at the cranial **parietal** bone and exits at the **acanthion** (junction of nose and upper lip) for the **parietoacanthial projection** (Fig. 1.80).

  The opposite CR direction would describe the **acanthioparietal projection** (Fig. 1.81).

  These are also known as **PA Waters** and **AP reverse Waters** methods and are used to visualize the facial bones.

Submentovertical (SMV) and Verticosubmental (VSM) Projections

These projections are used for the **skull** and **mandible.**

  The CR enters below the chin, or mentum, and exits at the vertex or top of the skull for the **submentovertical (SMV) projection** (Fig. 1.82).

  The less common, opposite projection of this would be the **verticosubmental (VSM) projection,** entering at the top of the skull and exiting below the mandible (not shown).

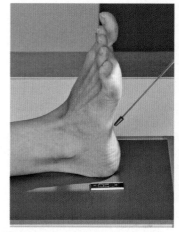
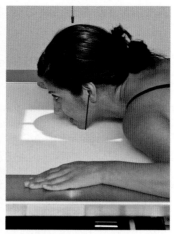

Fig. 1.79 Axial plantodorsal (PD) projection of calcaneus.

Fig. 1.80 Parietoacanthial projection (PA Waters position).

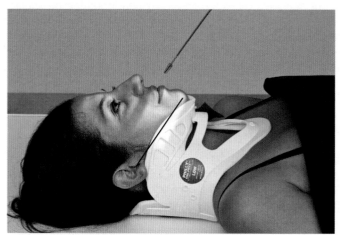

Fig. 1.81 Acanthioparietal projection.

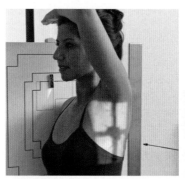
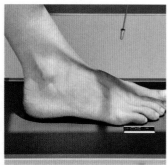

Fig. 1.77 Transthoracic lateral shoulder projection (R lateral shoulder position).

Fig. 1.78 AP or dorsoplantar (DP) projection of foot.

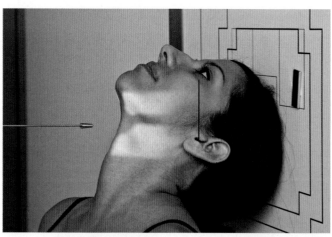

Fig. 1.82 Submentovertical (SMV) projection.

Relationship Terms

Following are paired positioning or anatomic terms that are used to describe relationships to parts of the body with opposite meanings.

Medial Versus Lateral

Medial *(me'-de-al)* versus lateral refers to **toward** versus **away from** the center, or median plane.

In the anatomic position, the medial aspect of any body part is the "inside" part closest to the median plane, and the lateral part is away from the center, or away from the median plane or midline of the body (Fig. 1.83).

Examples In the anatomic position, the thumb is on the lateral aspect of the hand. The lateral part of the abdomen and thorax is the part away from the median plane.

Proximal Versus Distal

Proximal *(prok'-si-mal)* is **near the source** or beginning, and **distal** *(dis'-tal)* is **away from.** In regard to the upper and lower limbs, proximal and distal would be the part closest to or away from the trunk, the source or beginning of that limb (see Fig. 1.83).

Examples The elbow is proximal to the wrist. The finger joint closest to the palm of the hand is called the *proximal interphalangeal (PIP) joint,* and the joint near the distal end of the finger is the *distal interphalangeal (DIP) joint* (see Chapter 4).

Cephalad Versus Caudad

Cephalad *(sef'-ah-lad)* means **toward** the head end of the body; caudad *(kaw'-dad)* means **away from** the head end of the body.

A **cephalad angle** is any angle toward the head end of the body (Fig. 1.84; also see Fig. 1.86). (*Cephalad,* or *cephalic,* literally means "head" or "toward the head.")

A **caudad angle** is any angle toward the feet or away from the head end (Fig. 1.85). (*Caudad* or *caudal* comes from *cauda,* literally meaning "tail.")

In human anatomy, cephalad and caudad also can be described as **superior** (toward the head) or **inferior** (toward the feet).

NOTE: As is shown in Figs. 1.84, 1.85, and 1.86, these terms are correctly used to describe the direction of the CR angle for axial projections along the entire length of the body, not just projections of the head.

Interior (Internal, Inside) Versus Exterior (External, Outer)

Interior is inside of something, nearer to the center, and exterior is situated on or near the outside.

The prefix **intra-** means **within** or **inside** (e.g., intravenous: inside a vein).

The prefix **inter-** means situated **between things** (e.g., intercostal: located between the ribs).

The prefix **exo-** means **outside** or **outward** (e.g., exocardial: something that develops or is situated outside the heart).

Superficial Versus Deep

Superficial is nearer the skin surface; deep is farther away.

Example The cross-sectional drawing in Fig. 1.87 shows that the humerus is deep compared with the skin of the arm, which is superficial.

Another example would be a superficial tumor or lesion, which is located near the surface, compared with a deep tumor or lesion, which is located deeper within the body or part.

Ipsilateral Versus Contralateral

Ipsilateral *(ip"-si-lat'-er-al)* is on the same side of the body or part; contralateral *(kon"-trah-lat'-er-al)* is on the opposite side.

Example The right thumb and the right great toe are ipsilateral; the right knee and the left hand are contralateral.

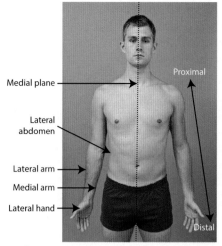

Fig. 1.83 Medial vs. lateral, proximal vs. distal.

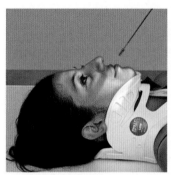
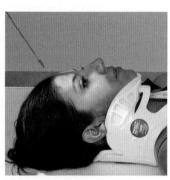

Fig. 1.84 Cephalad CR angle (toward head).

Fig. 1.85 Caudad CR angle (away from head).

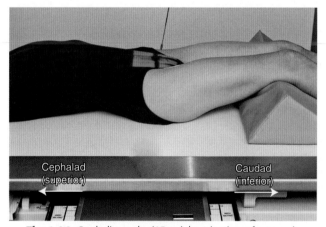

Fig. 1.86 Cephalic angle (AP axial projection of sacrum).

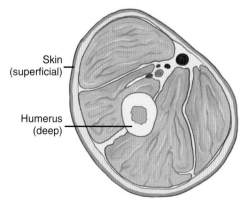

Fig. 1.87 Cross-section of arm.

Terms Related to Movement

The final group of positioning and related terms that every technologist should know relates to various movements. Most of these are listed as paired terms that describe movements in opposite directions.

Flexion Versus Extension

When a joint is flexed or extended, the **angle** between parts is **decreased** or **increased.**

Flexion decreases the angle of the joint (see examples of knee, elbow, and wrist flexions in Fig. 1.88).

Extension increases the angle as the body part moves from a flexed to a straightened position. This is true for the knee, elbow, and wrist joints, as is shown in Fig. 1.88.

Hyperextension

Hyperextension is extending a joint beyond the straight or neutral position.

Abnormal Hyperextension

A hyperextended elbow or knee results when the joint is extended beyond the straightened or neutral position. This is not a natural movement for these two joints and results in injury or trauma.

Normal Flexion and Hyperextension of the Spine

Flexion is bending forward, and extension is returning to the straight or neutral position. A backward bending **beyond the neutral position is hyperextension.** In practice, however, the terms *flexion* and *extension* are commonly used for these two extreme flexion and hyperextension projections of the spine (Fig. 1.89).

Normal Hyperextension of the Wrist

A second example of a special use of the term *hyperextension* concerns the wrist, where the carpal canal (tangential, inferosuperior) projection of the carpals is visualized by a special **hyperextended wrist movement** in which the wrist is extended beyond the neutral position. This specific wrist movement is also called **dorsiflexion** (backward or posterior flexion) (Fig. 1.90A).

Acute Flexion of the Wrist

An acute or full flexion of the wrist is required for a special tangential projection for a carpal bridge projection of the posterior aspect of the wrist (see Fig. 1.90B).

Ulnar Deviation Versus Radial Deviation of the Wrist

Deviation literally means "to turn aside" or "to turn away from the standard or course."[8]

Ulnar deviation (Fig. 1.91A) is to turn or bend the hand and wrist from the natural position toward the ulnar side, and **radial deviation** (Fig. 1.91B) is toward the radial side of the wrist.

NOTE: Earlier editions of this textbook and other positioning references have defined these wrist movements as ulnar and radial flexion movements because they describe specific flexion movements toward either the ulna or the radius.[9] However, because practitioners in the medical community, including orthopedic physicians, commonly use the terms *ulnar* and *radial deviation* for these wrist movements, this text also has changed this terminology to *ulnar* and *radial deviation movements* to prevent confusion and to ensure consistency with other medical references.

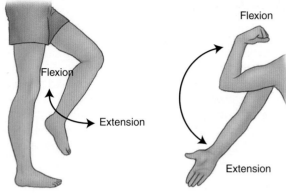

Fig. 1.88 Flexion vs. extension.

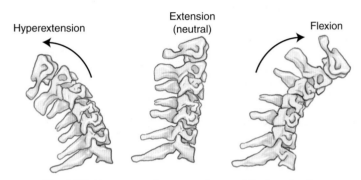

Fig. 1.89 Hyperextension, extension, and flexion of spine.

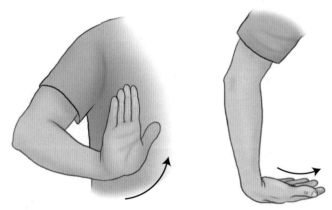

A   Hyperextension or dorsiflexion   B   Acute flexion

Fig. 1.90 Wrist extension and flexion movements. A, Hyperextension. B, Acute flexion.

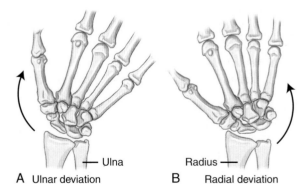

A Ulnar deviation   B   Radial deviation

Fig. 1.91 Deviation wrist movements. A, Ulnar deviation. B, Radial deviation.

Dorsiflexion Versus Plantar Flexion of the Foot and Ankle

Dorsiflexion of the Foot This term means to **decrease the angle** (flex) between the dorsum (top of foot) and the lower leg, moving foot and toes upward (Fig. 1.92A).

Plantar Flexion of the Foot **Extending the ankle joint,** moving foot and toes downward from the normal position; flexing or decreasing the angle toward the plantar (posterior) surface of the foot (see Fig. 1.92B).

NOTE: See preceding page for dorsiflexion of the wrist (see Fig. 1.90A) compared with dorsiflexion of the foot (see Fig. 1.92A).

Eversion Versus Inversion

Eversion *(e-ver'-zhun)* is an **outward stress movement** of the foot at the ankle joint (Fig. 1.93).

Inversion *(in-ver'-zhun)* is **inward stress** movement of the foot as applied to the foot without rotation of the leg (Fig. 1.94).

The plantar surface (sole) of the foot is turned or rotated away from the median plane of the body (the sole faces in a more lateral direction) for eversion and toward the median plane for inversion.

The leg does not rotate, and stress is applied to the medial and lateral aspects of the ankle joint for evaluation of possible widening of the joint space (ankle mortise).

Valgus Versus Varus[1]

Valgus *(val'-gus)* describes an abnormal position in which a part or limb is forced outward from the midline of the body. *Valgus* sometimes is used to describe **eversion stress** of the ankle joint.

Varus *(va'-rus)* describes an abnormal position in which a part or limb is forced inward toward the midline of the body. The term *varus stress* sometimes is used to describe **inversion stress** applied at the ankle joint.

NOTE: The terms *valgus* and *varus* are also used to describe the loss of normal alignment of bones due to fracture (see Chapter 15).

Medial (Internal) Rotation Versus Lateral (External) Rotation

Medial rotation is a rotation or turning of a body part with movement of the **anterior** aspect of the part **toward the inside,** or median, plane (Fig. 1.95A).

Lateral rotation is a rotation of an **anterior** body part **toward the outside,** or away from the median plane (Fig. 1.95B).

NOTE: In radiographic positioning, these terms describe movement of the **anterior** aspect of the part that is being rotated. In the forearm movements (see Fig. 1.95A and B), the anterior aspect of the forearm moves medially or internally on medial rotation and laterally or externally on lateral rotation. Another example is the medial and lateral oblique projections of the knee, in which the **anterior** part of the knee is rotated medially and laterally in **either the AP or PA** projections (see Chapter 6).

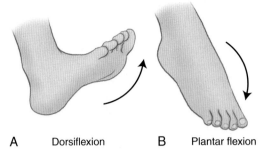

A   Dorsiflexion   B   Plantar flexion

Fig. 1.92 Movements of ankle and foot. A, Dorsiflexion. B, Plantar flexion.

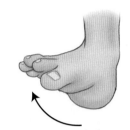

Fig. 1.93 Eversion (valgus stress).

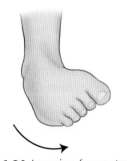

Fig. 1.94 Inversion (varus stress).

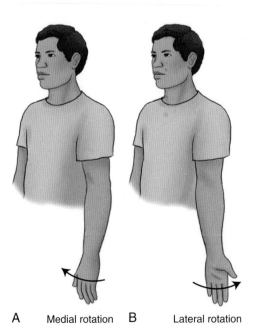

A   Medial rotation   B   Lateral rotation

Fig. 1.95 Rotational movements of upper limb. A, Medial (internal) rotation. B, Lateral (external) rotation.

Abduction Versus Adduction

Abduction *(ab-duk'-shun)* is the lateral movement of the arm or leg **away** from the body.

Another application of this term is the abduction of the fingers or toes, which means spreading them apart (Fig. 1.96A).

Adduction *(ah-duk'-shun)* is a movement of the arm or leg **toward** the body, to draw toward a center or medial line (Fig. 1.96B).

Adduction of the fingers or toes means moving them together or toward each other.

Supination Versus Pronation

Supination *(su"-pi-na'-shun)* is a rotational movement of the hand into the anatomic position (palm up in supine position or forward in erect position) (Fig. 1.97A). This movement rotates the radius of the forearm laterally along its long axis.

Pronation *(pro-na'-shun)* is a rotation of the hand into the opposite of the anatomic position (palm down or back) (Fig. 1.97B).

NOTE: To help remember these terms, relate them to the body positions of supine and prone. *Supine* or *supination* means face up or palm up, and *prone* or *pronation* means face down or palm down.

Protraction Versus Retraction

Protraction *(pro-trak'-shun)* is a **movement forward** from a normal position (Fig. 1.98A).

Retraction *(re-trak'-shun)* is a **movement backward** or the condition of being drawn back (Fig. 1.98B).

Example Protraction is moving the jaw forward (sticking the chin out) or drawing the shoulders forward. Retraction is the opposite of this—that is, moving the jaw backward or squaring the shoulders, as in a military stance.

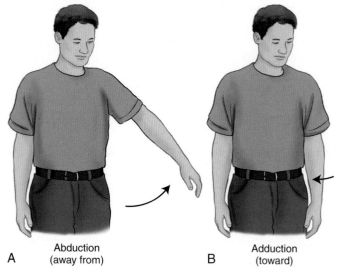

A Abduction (away from) B Adduction (toward)

Fig. 1.96 Movements of upper limbs. A, Abduction. B, Adduction.

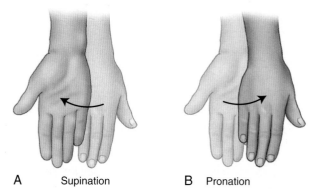

A Supination B Pronation

Fig. 1.97 Movements of hand. A, Supination. B, Pronation.

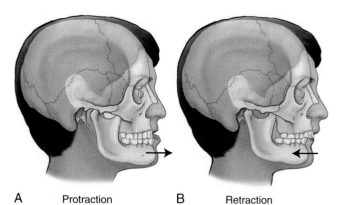

A Protraction B Retraction

Fig. 1.98 Movements of mandible. A, Protraction. B, Retraction.

Elevation Versus Depression

Elevation is a **lifting, raising,** or **moving of a part superiorly** (Fig. 1.99A).

Depression is a **letting down, lowering,** or **moving of a part inferiorly** (Fig. 1.99B).

Example Shoulders are elevated when they are raised, as when shrugging the shoulders. Depressing the shoulders is lowering them.

Circumduction

Circumduction *(ser″-kum-duk′-shun)* means **to move around in the form of a circle** (Fig. 1.100). This term describes sequential movements of flexion, abduction, extension, and adduction, resulting in a cone-type movement at any joint where the four movements are possible (e.g., fingers, wrist, arm, leg).

Rotation Versus Tilt

Rotate is to turn or rotate a body part on its axis. In Fig. 1.101, the midsagittal plane of the entire body, including the head, is **rotated.**

Tilt is a slanting or tilting movement with respect to the long axis. Fig. 1.102 demonstrates no rotation of the head but a **tilting** (slanting) of the midsagittal plane of the head, which therefore is not parallel to the tabletop.

Understanding the difference between these two terms is important in cranial and facial bone positioning (see Chapter 11).

See Table 1.4 for a summary of positioning-related terminology.

Summary of Projections and Positions

The three terms **position, projection,** and **view** are sometimes confusing and may be used incorrectly in practice. These terms should be understood and used correctly (Table 1.5).

Position

Position is a term that is used to indicate the patient's general physical position, such as supine, prone, recumbent, erect, or Trendelenburg.

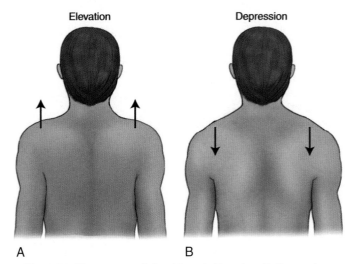

Fig. 1.99 Movements of shoulders. A, Elevation. B, Depression.

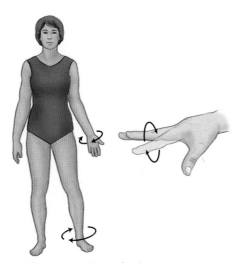

Fig. 1.100 Circumduction movements.

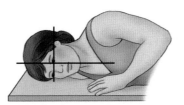

Fig. 1.101 Rotation—midsagittal plane rotated.

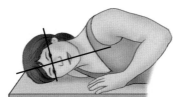

Fig. 1.102 Tilt—midsagittal plane of head tilted.

TABLE 1.4 SUMMARY OF POSITIONING-RELATED TERMS

Body Planes, Sections, and Lines	Relationship Terms
Longitudinal planes or sections	Medial vs. lateral
• Sagittal	Proximal vs. distal
• Coronal	Cephalad vs. caudad
• Oblique	Ipsilateral vs. contralateral
Transverse planes or sections	Internal vs. external
• Horizontal, axial, or cross-section	Superficial vs. deep
• Oblique	Lordosis vs. kyphosis (scoliosis)
Base plane	**Movement Terms**
Occlusal plane	Flexion vs. extension (acute flexion
Infraorbitomeatal line (IOML)	vs. hyperextension)
Body Surfaces	Ulnar vs. radial deviation
Posterior	Dorsiflexion vs. plantar flexion
Anterior	Eversion vs. inversion
Plantar	Valgus vs. varus
Dorsum	Medial vs. lateral rotation
Palmar	Abduction vs. adduction
	Supination vs. pronation
	Protraction vs. retraction
	Elevation vs. depression
	Tilt vs. rotation
	Circumduction
	Cephalad vs. caudad

TABLE 1.5 SUMMARY OF PROJECTIONS AND POSITIONS

PROJECTIONS (PATH OF CR)	GENERAL BODY POSITIONS	SPECIFIC BODY POSITIONS
Posteroanterior (PA)	Anatomic	R or L lateral
Anteroposterior (AP)	Supine	Oblique
Mediolateral	Prone	Left posterior oblique
Lateromedial	Erect (upright)	(LPO)
AP or PA oblique	Recumbent	Right posterior oblique
AP or PA axial	Trendelenburg	(RPO)
Tangential	Sims	Left anterior oblique
Transthoracic	Fowler	(LAO)
Dorsoplantar (DP)	Lithotomy	Right anterior oblique
Plantodorsal (PD)		(RAO)
Inferosuperior axial		Decubitus
Superoinferior axial		Left lateral decubitus
Axiolateral		Right lateral decubitus
Submentovertex (SMV)		Ventral decubitus
Verticosubmental (VSM)		Dorsal decubitus
Parietoacanthial		Lordotic
Acanthioparietal		
Craniocaudal		

1

Position also is used to describe **specific body positions** by the anatomy closest to the IR, such as **lateral** and **oblique positions.**

The term *position* should be "restricted to discussion of the patient's physical position."[11]

Projection

Projection is a correct positioning term that describes or refers to the **path or direction of the central ray,** projecting an image onto an IR.

The term *projection* should be "restricted to discussion of the path of the central ray."[10]

View

View is *not* a correct positioning term in the United States.

View describes the anatomy or body part as seen by the IR or other recording medium, such as a fluoroscopic screen. In the United States, the term *view* should be **"restricted to discussion of a radiograph or image."**[10]

POSITIONING PRINCIPLES

Evaluation Criteria

The goal of every technologist should be to take not just a "passable" radiograph but rather an optimal one that can be evaluated by a **definable standard,** as described under **evaluation criteria** (Fig. 1.103).

An example of a three-part radiographic image evaluation as used in this text for a lateral forearm is shown on the right. The positioning photo and the resulting optimal radiograph (Figs. 1.104 and 1.105) are shown for this lateral forearm, as described in Chapter 4.

EVALUATION CRITERIA FORMAT

The technologist should review and compare radiographs using this standard to determine how close to an optimal image was achieved. A systematic method of learning how to critique radiographs is to break the evaluation down into these **three parts.**

1. **Anatomy demonstrated:** Describes precisely what anatomic parts and structures should be clearly visualized on that image (radiograph).
2. **Position:** Generally evaluates four issues: (1) placement of body part in relationship to the IR, (2) positioning factors that are important for the projection, (3) correct centering of anatomy, and (4) collimation.
3. **Exposure:** Describes how exposure factors or technique (kilovoltage [kVp], milliamperage [mA], and time [milliseconds]) can be evaluated for optimum exposure for that body part. **No motion** is a first priority, and a description of how the presence or absence of motion can be determined is listed. (Motion is included with exposure criteria because exposure time is the primary controlling factor for motion.)

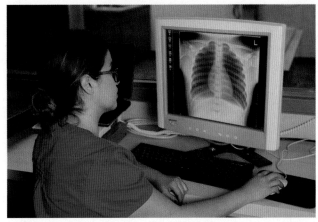
Fig. 1.103 Technologist viewing digital images on monitor.

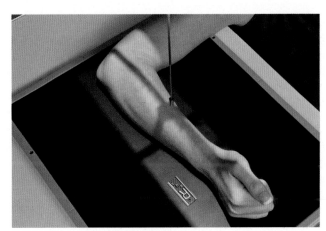
Fig. 1.104 Accurate positioning for lateral forearm.

Sample Lateral Forearm Evaluation Criteria

Anatomy Demonstrated: • Lateral projection of entire radius and ulna; proximal row of carpals, elbow, and distal end of humerus; and pertinent soft tissues such as fat pads and stripes of wrist and elbow joints.

Position: • Long axis of forearm aligned with long axis of IR. • Elbow flexed 90°. • No rotation from true lateral as evidenced by the following: • Head of the ulna should be superimposed over the radius. • Humeral epicondyles should be superimposed. • Radial head should superimpose the coronoid process with radial tuberosity seen in profile. • Collimation to **area of interest.**

Exposure: • Optimum density (brightness) and contrast with no motion will reveal sharp cortical margins and clear, bony trabecular markings and fat pads and stripes of the wrist and elbow joints.

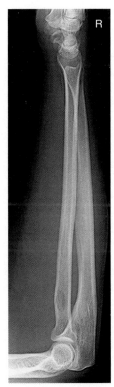
Fig. 1.105 Lateral forearm.

Image Markers and Patient Identification

A **minimum** of two types of markers should be imprinted on every radiographic image. These are (1) **patient identification and date** and (2) **anatomic side markers.**

PATIENT IDENTIFICATION AND DATE (FILM-SCREEN CASSETTE [ANALOG] SYSTEMS)

With analog (film) systems, patient information, which includes data such as name, date, case number, and institution, are photoflashed on the film in the space provided by a lead block in the film cassette (Fig. 1.106A). Each IR has a marker on the exterior indicating this area where the patient ID, including the date, should be placed. A general rule for most chest studies is to place the patient ID information at the top margin of the IR on chests. The patient ID marker is always placed where it is least likely to cover essential anatomy. The anatomic side markers are and should still be placed in a manner on the IR so that they are legible and esthetically correct (Fig. 1.106B). They must be within the collimation field so that they provide a permanent indicator of the correct side of the body or anatomic part.

Digital Systems

With photostimulable storage phosphor (PSP) cassette-based systems, often a bar code system imprints the patient information before or after exposure (Fig. 1.107). With digital imaging systems, patient identification is entered during registration and prior to exposure.

ANATOMIC SIDE MARKER

A right or left marker must also appear on every radiographic image correctly indicating the patient's right or left side or which limb is being radiographed, the right or the left. This may be provided as the word "Right" or "Left" or just the initials "R" or "L." This side marker preferably should be placed directly on the IR inside the lateral portion of the collimated border of the side being identified, with the placement such that the marker will not be superimposed over essential anatomy.

These radiopaque markers must be placed just within the collimation field so that they will be exposed by the x-ray beam and included on the image.

The two markers, the patient ID, and the anatomic side marker must be placed correctly on *all* radiographic images **including digitally produced images.** Generally, it is an unacceptable practice to write or annotate digitally this information on the image after it is processed because of legal and liability problems caused by potential mis-markings. A **radiograph taken without these two markers often has to be repeated,** which results in unnecessary radiation to the patient, making this a serious error. In the case of digital images, annotating the image to indicate side markers is an unacceptable practice. The exposure should be repeated to ensure the correct anatomy was imaged.

ADDITIONAL MARKERS OR IDENTIFICATION

Certain other markers or identifiers also may be used, such as **technologist initials,** which generally are placed on the R or L marker to identify the specific technologist responsible for the examination. Sometimes the examination room number is also included.

Time indicators are also commonly used; these note the minutes of elapsed time in a series, such as the 20-minute, 30-minute, 1-hour, and 2-hour series of radiographs taken in a small bowel series (SBS) procedure (see Chapter 13).

Another important marker on all decubitus positions is a decubitus marker or some type of indicator such as an **arrow identifying which side is up.** An **"upright"** or **"erect"** marker must also

be used to identify erect chest or abdomen positions compared with recumbent, in addition to an arrow indicating which side is up.

Inspiration (INSP) and **expiration** (EXP) markers are used for special comparison PA projections of the chest. **Internal** (INT) and **external** (EXT) markers may be used for rotation projections, such as for the proximal humerus and shoulder. Sample markers are shown in Fig. 1.108.

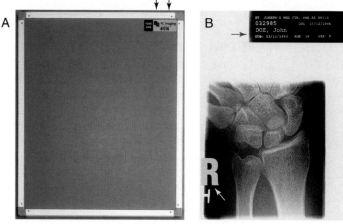

Fig. 1.106 A, Film cassette with patient information in block *(arrows)*. B, Radiograph *(blue arrow,* Patient identification information; *yellow arrow,* Anatomic side marker to indicate right wrist).

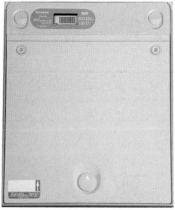

Fig. 1.107 PSP cassette with bar coding for patient information

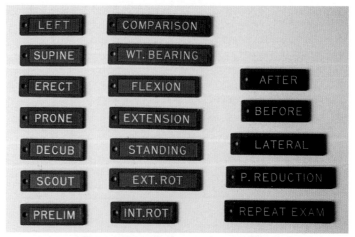

Fig. 1.108 Sample procedure markers.

Professional Ethics and Patient Care

The radiologic technologist is an important member of the health care team who is responsible in general for radiologic examination of patients. This includes being responsible for one's actions under a specific **code of ethics.**

Code of ethics describes the rules of acceptable conduct toward patients and other health care team members as well as personal actions and behaviors as defined within the profession. The ARRT code of ethics[11] is provided in Box 1.1. The **announce, communicate, and explain (ACE)** campaign of the American Society of Radiologic Technologists (ASRT)is an initiative to educate patients about the role of the radiologic technologist. ACE is an acronym to help you remember to share and gain important information with and from your patients (Box 1.2).

Patient Assessment and Clinical History[12]

Once in the radiology imaging suite, the patient will interact directly with the radiologic technologist. Key responsibilities of the technologist are to introduce yourself, ensure you are performing the correct procedure on the correct patient, ask questions and acquire clinical history pertinent to the procedure, and explain the imaging procedure briefly. This protocol must be followed for every patient and for every radiologic procedure. The ASRT recommends the following initial communication with the patient:

- **Introduce yourself:** By name and role as the radiologic technologist performing the procedure.
- **Patient identification by two means:** Ask patient their name and verify by reviewing the patient arm band, patient chart, and/ or examination requisition.
- **Verification of procedure(s) ordered:** Make sure it is the correct procedure for the correct patient by examining the patient chart or examination requisition.

- **Acquire clinical history:** Interview patient to determine chief complaints, allergy history, symptoms, duration and frequency of symptoms.
- **Pregnancy status:** Ask females if there is any possibility they might be pregnant. If the response of the patient, is "yes," "maybe," or "I don't know," inform supervisor or physician before proceeding with procedure. Age range for this type of questioning is often determined by the medical facility.
- **Explain procedure:** Explain the radiologic procedure that will be performed. Use terms and language the patient can understand.
- **Provide opportunity for patient to ask questions:** Encourage patient to ask questions about the procedure or other concerns before beginning the procedure.

BOX 1.2 ACE CAMPAIGN

In addition to performing medical imaging procedures, radiologic technologists must also communicate with patients. It is important for patients to understand that radiologic technologists are highly qualified medical imaging professionals who are educated in patient positioning, radiation safety, radiation protection, and equipment protocols. Furthermore, patients should have an understanding of the medical imaging procedure they are undergoing.

To communicate these points to patients, the American Society of Radiologic Technologists (ASRT) recommends that medical imaging professionals use the ACE initiative. The easy-to-remember acronym reminds radiologic technologists to:

- **A**nnounce your name.
- **C**ommunicate your credentials.
- **E**xplain what you're going to do.

The ACE acronym provides medical imaging professionals with a unique and simple tool to educate patients about the radiologic technologist's role on the health care team.

BOX 1.1 AMERICAN REGISTRY OF RADIOLOGIC TECHNOLOGISTS CODE OF ETHICS

The Code of Ethics forms the first part of the *Standards of Ethics.* The Code of Ethics shall serve as a guide by which Certificate Holders and Candidates may evaluate their professional conduct as it relates to patients, healthcare consumers, employers, colleagues, and other members of the healthcare team. The Code of Ethics is intended to assist Certificate Holders and Candidates in maintaining a high level of ethical conduct and in providing for the protection, safety, and comfort of patients. The Code of Ethics is aspirational.

1. The radiologic technologist acts in a professional manner, responds to patient needs, and supports colleagues and associates in providing quality patient care.
2. The radiologic technologist acts to advance the principal objective of the profession to provide services to humanity with full respect for the dignity of mankind.
3. The radiologic technologist delivers patient care and service unrestricted by the concerns of personal attributes or the nature of the disease or illness, and without discrimination on the basis of sex, race, creed, religion, or socio-economic status.
4. The radiologic technologist practices technology founded upon theoretical knowledge and concepts, uses equipment and accessories consistent with the purposes for which they were designed, and employs procedures and techniques appropriately.
5. The radiologic technologist assesses situations; exercises care, discretion, and judgment; assumes responsibility for professional decisions; and acts in the best interest of the patient.

6. The radiologic technologist acts as an agent through observation and communication to obtain pertinent information for the physician to aid in the diagnosis and treatment of the patient and recognizes that interpretation and diagnosis are outside the scope of practice for the profession.
7. The radiologic technologist uses equipment and accessories, employs techniques and procedures, performs services in accordance with an accepted standard of practice, and demonstrates expertise in minimizing radiation exposure to the patient, self, and other members of the healthcare team.
8. The radiologic technologist practices ethical conduct appropriate to the profession and protects the patient's right to quality radiologic technology care.
9. The radiologic technologist respects confidences entrusted in the course of professional practice, respects the patient's right to privacy, and reveals confidential information only as required by law or to protect the welfare of the individual or the community.
10. The radiologic technologist continually strives to improve knowledge and skills by participating in continuing education and professional activities, sharing knowledge with colleagues, and investigating new aspects of professional practice.
11. The radiologic technologist refrains from the use of illegal drugs and/ or any legally controlled substances which result in impairment of professional judgment and/or ability to practice radiologic technology with reasonable skill and safety to patients.

Essential Projections

ROUTINE PROJECTIONS

Certain basic projections are listed and described in this text for each radiographic examination or procedure commonly performed throughout the United States and Canada. Routine projections are defined as **projections commonly taken on patients who can cooperate fully.** This varies depending on radiologist and department preference and on geographic differences.

SPECIAL PROJECTIONS

In addition to routine projections, certain special projections are included for each examination or procedure described in this text. These are defined as **projections most commonly taken to demonstrate better specific anatomic parts or certain pathologic conditions or projections that may be necessary for patients who cannot cooperate fully.**

The authors recommend (on the basis of recent survey results) that all students learn and demonstrate proficiency in all essential projections as listed in this text. This includes all routine projections and all special projections as listed and described in each chapter. The following are examples of these routine projection and special projection boxes for Chapter 2. Becoming competent in these projections helps to ensure students are prepared to function as imaging technologists in any part of the United States.

General Principles for Determining Positioning Routines

Two general rules or principles are helpful for remembering and understanding the reasons certain minimum projections are performed for various radiographic examinations.

MINIMUM OF TWO PROJECTIONS (90° FROM EACH OTHER)

The first general rule in diagnostic radiology suggests that a **minimum of two projections** taken as near as possible to 90° from each other are required for most radiographic procedures. Exceptions include an AP mobile (portable) chest, a single AP abdomen (called a KUB—**k**idneys, **u**reter, and **b**ladder), and an AP of the pelvis, in which only one projection usually provides adequate information.

Three reasons for this general rule of a minimum of two projections are as follows:

1. **Superimposition of anatomic structures**
   Certain pathologic conditions (e.g., some fractures, small tumors) may not be visualized on one projection only.
2. **Localization of lesions or foreign bodies**
   A minimum of two projections, taken at 90° or as near as possible to right angles of each other, are essential in determining the location of any lesion or foreign body (Fig. 1.109).

Example

Foreign bodies embedded in tissues of the knee. Both AP/PA and lateral projections are necessary to determine the exact location of this "nail."
3. **Determination of alignment of fractures**
   All fractures require a minimum of two projections, taken at 90° or as near as possible to right angles of each other. This is both to fully visualize the fracture site and to determine alignment of the fractured parts following surgery (Figs. 1.110 and 1.111).

Chest	
ROUTINE	
• PA, p. XXX	
• Lateral, p. XXX	

Upper Airway	
ROUTINE	
• Lateral, p. XXX	
• AP, p. XXX	

Chest	
SPECIAL	
• AP supine or semierect, p. XXX	
• Lateral decubitus, p. XXX	
• AP lordotic, p. XXX	
• Anterior oblique, p. XXX	
• Posterior oblique, p. XXX	

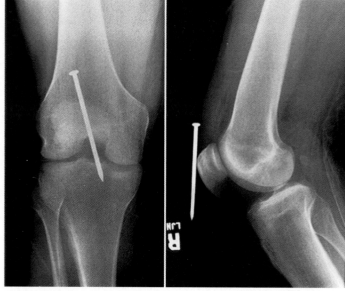

Fig. 1.109 AP and lateral projection for foreign body (nail through anterior knee).

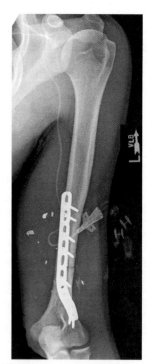

Fig. 1.110 AP humerus projection for postoperative fracture alignment.

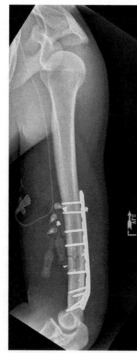

Fig. 1.111 Lateral humerus projection for postoperative fracture alignment.

MINIMUM OF THREE PROJECTIONS WHEN JOINTS ARE IN AREA OF INTEREST

This second general rule or principle suggests that all radiographic procedures of the skeletal system involving joints require a minimum of **three** projections rather than only two. These are **AP** or **PA**, lateral, and **oblique projections.**

The reason for this rule is that more information is needed than can be provided on only two projections. For example, with multiple surfaces and angles of the bones making up the joint, a small oblique chip fracture or other abnormality within the joint space may not be visualized on either frontal or lateral views but may be well demonstrated in the oblique position.

Following are examples of examinations that generally require three projections as routine (joint is in prime interest area):

- Fingers
- Toes
- Hand
- Wrist (Fig. 1.112)
- Elbow
- Ankle
- Foot
- Knee

Examples of examinations that require two projections as routine include the following:

- Forearm
- Humerus
- Femur
- Hips
- Tibia-fibula (Figs. 1.113 and 1.114)
- Chest

Exceptions to Rules

- Postreduction upper and lower limbs generally require only two projections for checking fracture alignment.
- **A pelvis study requires only a single AP projection unless a hip injury is suspected.**

Palpation of Topographic Positioning Landmarks

Radiographic positioning requires the location of specific structures or organs within the body, many of which are not visible to the eye from the exterior. Therefore, the technologist must rely on bony landmarks to indicate their location. These bony structures are referred to as **topographic landmarks.** Fig. 1.115 shows examples of topographic landmarks of the pelvis. (see Chapter 2, Chest, p. 70, and Chapter 3, Abdomen, p. 103, for topographic landmarks for chest, abdomen, and pelvis). Topographic landmarks can be located by a process referred to as *palpation*.

PALPATION

Palpation refers to the process of applying light pressure with the fingertips directly on the patient to locate positioning landmarks. **This must be done gently,** because the area being palpated may be painful or sensitive for the patient. Also, **the patient should always be informed of the purpose of this palpation before this process is begun, and patient permission should be obtained.**

NOTE: Palpation of certain landmarks, such as the ischial tuberosity and the symphysis pubis, may be embarrassing for the patient and **may not be permitted by institutional policy.** Technologists should use alternative landmarks as described in later chapters.

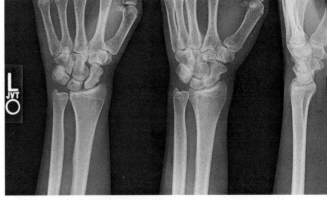

Fig. 1.112 Wrist—requires three projections.

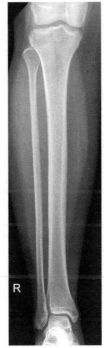

Fig. 1.113 AP lower leg projection.

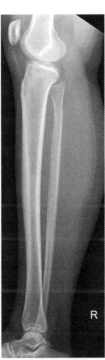

Fig. 1.114 Lateral lower leg projection (same patient as Fig. 1.113).

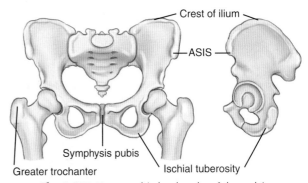

Fig. 1.115 Topographic landmarks of the pelvis.

Image Receptor Alignment

The alignment of the IR to the anatomy is an important consideration. In most cases, the long axis of the anatomic part is aligned to the longest dimension of the IR. This allows for the majority of an anatomic structure to be demonstrated and permits closer collimation of the x-ray field to the anatomy. The example in Fig. 1.116 is an image of a smaller adult chest. The IR is in the **portrait (lengthwise)** alignment in which the long axis of the lungs is aligned to the longest dimension of the IR. In another case, the hypersthenic adult PA chest often requires the IR to be placed in the **landscape (crosswise)** alignment. This permits the broader lateral borders of the lung to be demonstrated (Fig. 1.117). For each position in the text, the terms **landscape** or **portrait** will be listed following the recommended size of IR to indicate how the IR should be aligned to the anatomic part.

Viewing Radiographic Images

The manner in which **PA** and **AP projection** radiographic images are placed for viewing depends on the radiologist's preference and the most common practice in that part of the United States. However, in the United States and Canada, a common and accepted way to place radiographic images for viewing is to display them so that **the patient is facing the viewer,** with the patient in the anatomic position (Fig. 1.118). **This always places the patient's left to the viewer's right.** This is true for **either AP or PA projections** (Figs. 1.119 and 1.120).

Lateral positions are marked R or L by the side of the patient closest to the IR. Placement of lateral radiographic images for viewing varies depending on the radiologist's preference. One common method is to place the image so that the viewer is seeing the image from the same perspective as the x-ray tube. If the left marker is placed anteriorly to the patient, the L would be on the viewer's right (Fig. 1.121). However, some radiologists prefer to view laterals turned 90° and with the anteriorly placed L marker on the viewer's left. Technologists should determine the preferred method for viewing laterals in their department.

PA or AP oblique projections are placed for viewing the same way that a PA or AP projection is placed, with the patient's right to the viewer's left.

Decubitus chest and abdomen projections are generally viewed the way the x-ray tube "sees" them, placed in a portrait alignment with the upside of the patient also on the upper part of the view box (Fig. 1.122).

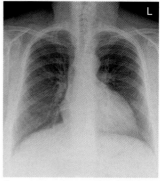
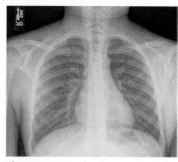

Fig. 1.116 Portrait (lengthwise) IR alignment of PA chest.

Fig. 1.117 Landscape (crosswise) IR alignment of PA chest.

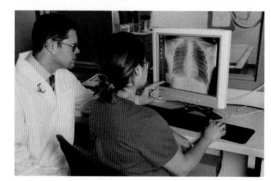

Fig. 1.118 Viewing digital chest radiographs (patient's right always to viewer's left, both PA and AP).

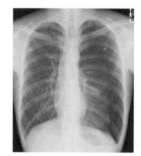
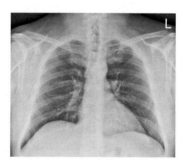

Fig. 1.119 PA chest projection.

Fig. 1.120 AP chest projection.

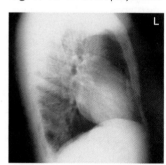
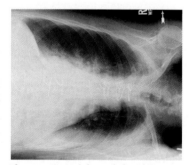

Fig. 1.121 Left lateral chest.

Fig. 1.122 Left lateral decubitus chest.

Upper and lower limb projections are viewed as projected by the x-ray beam onto the IR; the R or L lead marker appears right-side-up if it has been placed on the IR correctly.

Images that include the digits (hands and feet) generally are placed with the **digits up.** However, other images of the limbs are viewed in the anatomic position with the **limbs hanging down** (Fig. 1.123).

Viewing CT or MRI Images

The generally accepted way of viewing all CT and MRI axial images is similar to that used for conventional radiographs, even though the image represents a thin "slice" or sectional view of anatomic structures. In general, these images are placed **so the patient's right is to the viewer's left** (Fig. 1.124).

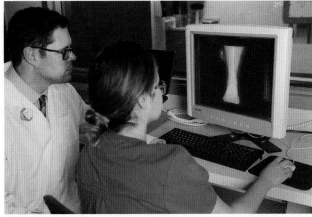

Fig. 1.123 Viewing digital upper or lower limb images.

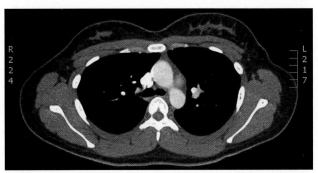

Fig. 1.124 Axial (cross-sectional) image (mid thorax level of T5) (patient's right to viewer's left).

PART TWO ▪ IMAGING PRINCIPLES

Contributor **Andrew Woodward,** MA, RT(R)(CT)(QM)

This period of technologic transition necessitates that students have an understanding of all image acquisition technologies, because they will find themselves working in imaging departments that acquire images by using only digital technology, only film-screen technology, or a combination of both.

This part provides an introduction to radiographic technique and image quality for both film-screen imaging and digital imaging. The study of radiographic technique and image quality includes factors that determine the accuracy with which structures that are being imaged are reproduced in the image. Each of these factors has a specific effect on the final image, and the technologist must strive to maximize these factors to produce the best image possible at the lowest achievable dose.

This part also describes methods of digital image acquisition, discusses the application of digital imaging, and provides an introduction to the important principles of radiation safety.

Technical considerations for both analog and digital imaging technology are discussed in the following sections.

Exposure Factors

For each radiographic image obtained, the radiographer must select *exposure factors* on the control panel of the imaging equipment. The exposure factors required for each examination are determined by numerous variables, including the density/atomic number and thickness of the anatomic part, any pathology present, and image acquisition technology. Fig. 1.125 is an example of a more current radiographic control console.

Exposure factors, sometimes referred to as *technique factors,* include the following:

- **Kilovoltage (kVp)**—controls the energy (penetrating power) of the x-ray beam. This can also be referred to as **kilovoltage peak (kVp)**—the maximum electrical potential used to create the x-ray photons within the x-ray tube.
- **Milliamperage (mA)**—controls the quantity or number of x-rays produced.
- **Exposure time (ms)**—controls the duration of the exposure, usually expressed in milliseconds.

Each of these exposure factors has a specific effect on the signal collected to produce the radiographic image. When performing radiographic procedures, technologists must apply their knowledge of exposure factors and imaging principles to ensure that images obtained are of the **highest quality possible** while exposing patients to the **lowest radiation dose possible.**

Image Quality

- Spatial resolution
- Distortion
- Scatter radiation and grids

SPATIAL RESOLUTION

Spatial resolution is defined as the **recorded sharpness of structures on the image.** Resolution on a radiographic image is demonstrated by the clarity or sharpness of fine structural lines and borders of tissues or structures on the image. Resolution is also known as **detail, recorded detail, image sharpness,** or **definition.** Resolution of images generally is measured and expressed as line pairs per millimeter (lp/mm), in which a line pair is seen as a single line and an interspace of equal width. The higher the line pair measure, the greater is the resolution; it is typically 5 to 6 lp/mm for general imaging. Lack of visible sharpness or resolution is known as **blur** or **unsharpness.**

Geometric Factors Affecting Spatial Resolution

Geometric factors that control or influence resolution consist of **focal spot size, source–image receptor distance (SID),** and **object–image receptor distance (OID).** The effect of OID is explained and illustrated in Fig. 1.131.

The use of the **small focal spot** results in **less geometric unsharpness** (Fig. 1.126). To illustrate, a point source is used commonly as the source of x-rays in the x-ray tube; however, the actual source of x-rays is an area on the anode known as the *focal spot.* Most x-ray tubes exhibit dual focus; that is, they have two focal spots: large and small. Use of the small focal spot results in less unsharpness of the image, or an image with a decreased *penumbra.* Penumbra refers to the **unsharp edges of objects in the projected image.** However, even with the use of the small focal spot, some penumbra is present.

Motion The greatest deterrent to image sharpness as related to positioning is *motion.* Two types of motion influence radiographic detail: **voluntary** and **involuntary.**

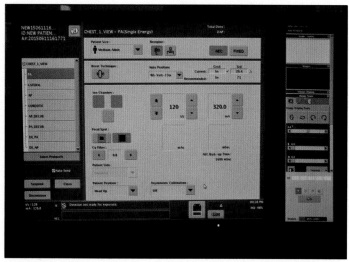

Fig. 1.125 Example of radiographic console (selecting kVp, mA, and mAs factors).

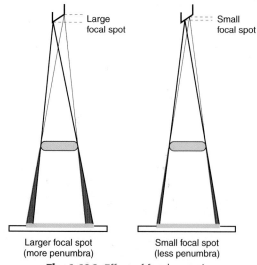

Fig. 1.126 Effect of focal spot size.

Voluntary motion is that which the patient can control. Motion from breathing or movement of body parts during exposure can be prevented or at least minimized by **controlled breathing** and **patient immobilization.** Support blocks, sandbags, or other immobilization devices can be used to reduce motion effectively. These devices are most effective for examination of upper or lower limbs, as will be demonstrated throughout this text.

Involuntary motion cannot be controlled by the patient at will. Therefore, involuntary motion, such as peristaltic action of abdominal organs, tremors, or chills, is more difficult, if not impossible, to control.

If motion unsharpness is apparent on the image, the technologist must determine whether this blurring or unsharpness is due to voluntary or involuntary motion. This determination is important, because these two types of motion can be controlled in various ways.

Difference between voluntary and involuntary motion Voluntary motion is visualized as **generalized blurring of linked structures,** such as blurring of the thoracic bony and soft tissue structures as evident in Fig. 1.127. Voluntary motion can be minimized through the use of high mA and short exposure times. Increased patient cooperation is another factor that may contribute to decreased voluntary motion; a thorough explanation of the procedure and clear breathing instructions may prove helpful.

Involuntary motion is identified by **localized unsharpness or blurring**. This type of motion is less obvious but can be visualized on abdominal images as localized blurring of the edges of the bowel, with other bowel outlines appearing sharp (gas in the bowel appears as dark areas). Study Fig. 1.128 carefully to see this slight blurring in the left upper abdomen, indicated by *arrows.* The remaining edges of the bowel throughout the abdomen appear sharp. Fig. 1.127, by comparison, demonstrates overall blurring of the heart, ribs, and diaphragm. A clear explanation of the procedure by the technologist may aid in reducing voluntary motion; however, a decrease in exposure time with an associated increase in mA is the best and sometimes the only way to minimize motion unsharpness caused by involuntary motion.

Summary of Spatial Resolution Factors

Use of a **small focal spot,** an **increase in SID,** and a **decrease in OID** result in less geometric unsharpness and increased resolution. Patient motion also affects image quality; **short exposure times** and **increased patient cooperation** help to minimize voluntary motion unsharpness. Involuntary motion unsharpness is controlled only by short exposure times.

DISTORTION

The second image quality factor is *distortion,* which is defined as the **misrepresentation of object size or shape** as projected onto radiographic recording media. Two types of distortion have been identified: size distortion (magnification) and shape distortion.

No radiographic image reproduces the exact size of the body part that is being radiographed. This is impossible to do because a degree of magnification or distortion or both always exists as a result of OID and divergence of the x-ray beam. Nevertheless, distortion can be minimized and controlled if some basic principles are used as a guide.

X-Ray Beam Divergence

X-ray beam divergence is a basic but important concept in the study of radiographic positioning. It occurs because x-rays originate from a small source in the x-ray tube (the focal spot) and diverge as they travel to the IR (Fig. 1.129). The field size of the x-ray beam is limited by a collimator that consists of adjustable lead attenuators

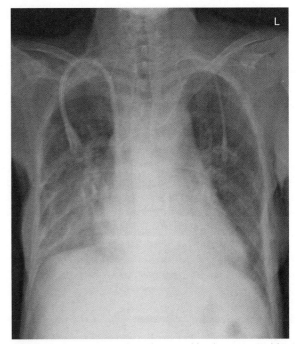

Fig. 1.127 Voluntary motion (breathing and body motion)—blurring of entire chest and overall unsharpness.

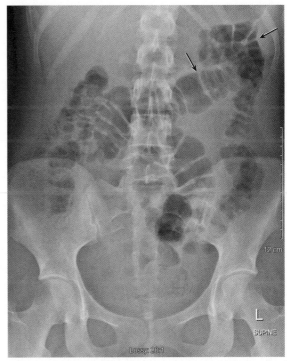

Fig. 1.128 Involuntary motion (from peristaltic action)—localized blurring in upper left abdomen *(arrows).*

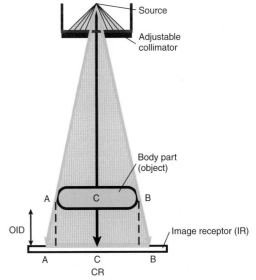

Fig. 1.129 X-ray beam divergence.

or shutters. The collimator and shutters absorb the x-rays on the periphery, controlling the size of the x-ray beam.

The **center point of the x-ray beam,** which is called the *central ray (CR),* theoretically has no divergence; the **least amount of distortion** is seen at this point on the image. All other aspects of the x-ray beam strike the IR at some angle, with the angle of divergence increasing to the outermost portions of the x-ray beam. The potential for distortion at these outer margins is increased.

Fig. 1.129 demonstrates three points on a body part (marked A, B, and C) as projected onto the IR. Greater magnification is demonstrated at the periphery (A and B) than at the point of the central ray (C). Because of the effect of the divergent x-ray beam, combined with at least some OID, this type of size distortion is inevitable. It is important for technologists to control closely and minimize distortion as much as possible.

Controlling Factors

Following are **four** primary controlling factors of distortion:
1. SID
2. OID
3. Object–image receptor alignment
4. CR alignment/centering

SID The first controlling factor for distortion is SID. The effect of SID on size distortion (magnification) is demonstrated in Fig. 1.130. Note that **less magnification occurs at a greater SID than at a shorter SID.** This is the reason that chest radiographs are obtained at a minimum SID of 72 inches (180 cm) rather than of 40 to 48 inches (100 to 120 cm), which is commonly used for most other examinations. A 72-inch (180-cm) SID results in less magnification of the heart and other structures within the thorax.

Minimum 40-inch (100-cm) SID It has been a long-standing common practice to use 40 inches (100 cm) as the standard SID for most skeletal radiographic examinations. However, in the interest of improving image resolution by decreasing magnification and distortion, it is becoming more common to increase the standard SID to 44 inches or 48 inches (110 cm or 120 cm). Additionally, it has been shown that increasing the SID from 40 to 48 inches reduces the entrance or skin dose even when the requirement for increased mAs is considered. In this textbook, the suggested SID listed on each skeletal positioning page is a **minimum of 40 inches,** with 44 inches or 48 inches recommended if the equipment and departmental protocol allow.

OID The second controlling factor for distortion is OID. The effect of OID on magnification or size distortion is illustrated clearly in Fig. 1.131. **The closer the object being radiographed is to the IR, the less are the magnification and shape distortion and the better is the resolution.**

Object–Image Receptor Alignment A third important controlling factor of distortion is *object–IR alignment.* This refers to the alignment or plane of the object that is being radiographed in relation to the plane of the image receptor. If the object plane is not parallel to the plane of the IR, distortion occurs. The greater the angle of inclination of the object or the IR, the greater the amount of distortion. For example, if a finger being radiographed is not parallel to the IR, the interphalangeal joint spaces will not be open because of the overlapping of bones, as is demonstrated in Fig. 1.132.

Effect of improper object-IR alignment In Fig. 1.133, the digits (fingers) are supported and aligned **parallel to the image receptor,** resulting in open interphalangeal joints and undistorted phalanges.

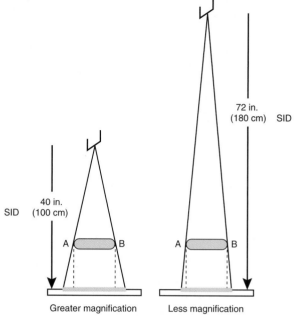
Greater magnification   Less magnification
Fig. 1.130 Effect of SID.

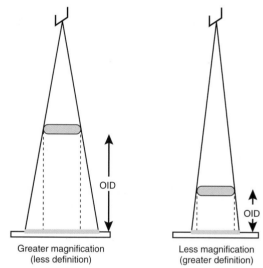
Greater magnification
(less definition)   Less magnification
                                (greater definition)
Fig. 1.131 Effect of OID.

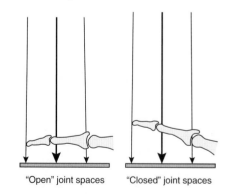
"Open" joint spaces   "Closed" joint spaces
Fig. 1.132 Object alignment and distortion.

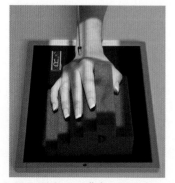
Fig. 1.133 Digits parallel to IR—joints open.

In Fig. 1.134, in which the digits are not parallel to the IR, the interphalangeal joints of the digits are not open, and possible pathology within these joint regions may not be visible. Note the open joints of the digits in Fig. 1.135 compared with Fig. 1.136 (see arrows). Additionally, the phalanges will be either foreshortened or elongated.

These examples demonstrate the important principle of correct object-IR alignment. **The plane of the body part that is being imaged must be as near parallel to the plane of the IR as possible** to produce an image of minimal distortion.

CR Alignment The fourth and final controlling factor for distortion is *central ray alignment* (centering), an important principle in positioning. As was previously stated, only the center of the x-ray beam, the CR, has no divergence because it projects that part of the object at 90°, or perpendicular to the plane of the IR (refer to Fig. 1.129). Therefore, the **least possible distortion occurs at the CR.** Distortion increases as the angle of divergence increases from the center of the x-ray beam to the outer edges. For this reason, correct centering or correct central ray alignment and placement is important in minimizing image distortion.

Examples of correct CR placement for an AP knee are shown in Figs. 1.137 and 1.138. The CR passes through the knee joint space with minimal distortion, and the joint space should appear open.

Fig. 1.139 demonstrates correct centering for an AP distal femur, in which the CR is correctly directed perpendicular to the IR and centered to the mid distal femur. However, the knee joint is now exposed to divergent rays (as shown by the arrow), and this causes the knee joint to appear closed (Fig. 1.140).

CR angle For most projections, the CR is aligned **perpendicular,** or 90°, to the plane of the IR. For certain body parts, however, a specific angle of the CR is required, as is indicated by the positioning descriptions in this text as the *CR angle*. This means that the CR is angled from the vertical in a cephalic or caudad direction so as to use distortion intentionally without superimposing anatomic structures.

Summary of Factors That May Affect Distortion

Use of the correct SID while minimizing OID, ensuring the object and IR are aligned, and correctly aligning or centering the CR to the part can minimize distortion on a radiographic image (Table 1.6).

SCATTER RADIATION AND GRIDS
Grids

Because the amount of scatter increases with the thickness of the tissue irradiated, it generally is recommended that a grid should be used for radiography of any body part that is thicker than 10 cm. Depending on the examination, the grid may be portable or may be built into the x-ray equipment. It is positioned between the patient and the IR and absorbs much of the scatter radiation before it hits the IR. Absorption of scatter is a key event that increases image contrast.

Correct Use of Grids An in-depth discussion of grid construction and characteristics is beyond the scope of this text. However,

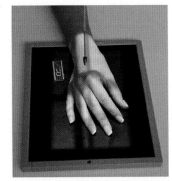

Fig. 1.134 Digits not parallel to IR—joints not open.

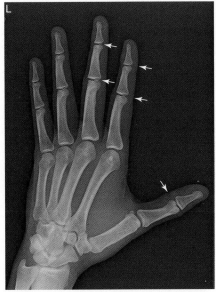

Fig. 1.135 Digits parallel—joints open.

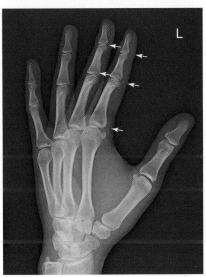

Fig. 1.136 Digits not parallel—joints not open.

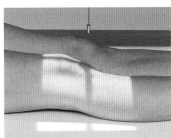
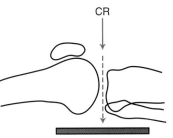

Fig. 1.137 Correct CR centering for AP knee.

Fig. 1.138 Correct CR centering for knee.

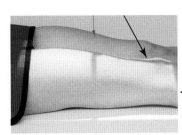
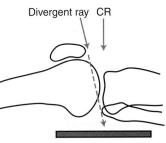

Fig. 1.139 Correct CR centering for AP femur (distortion occurs at knee).

Fig. 1.140 Incorrect CR centering for knee.

TABLE 1.6 **SUMMARY OF FACTORS CONTRIBUTING TO DISTORTION**	
QUALITY FACTOR	**PRIMARY CONTRIBUTING FACTORS**
Distortion	SID (Source-Image receptor Distance)
	OID (Object-Image receptor Distance)
	Object IR alignment
	CR alignment or centering

several rules must be followed to ensure optimal image quality when grids are used. Incorrect use of grids results in loss of optical density across all or part of the radiographic image; this feature is called *grid cutoff*. Grid cutoff occurs in various degrees and has several causes. Causes of grid cutoff include the following:
1. Off-center grid
2. Off-level grid
3. Off-focus grid
4. Upside-down grid

Off-center grid The CR must be centered along the center axis of the grid. If it is not, lateral decentering is said to occur. The more the CR is off center from the **cen**terline of the grid, the greater is the cutoff that results (Fig. 1.141).

In certain clinical situations in which it is difficult to position the area of interest in the center of the grid, the grid may have to be turned so that the lead strips run perpendicular to the length of the patient to allow accurate centering (e.g., horizontal beam lateral lumbar spine).

Exception: decubitus–short dimension (SD)–type linear grids An exception to the more common lengthwise focused grid with the lead strips and center axis running lengthwise with the grid is the **decubitus-type** crosswise linear grid. This grid, in which the lead strips and center axis are running crosswise along the shorter dimension of the grid, is useful for horizontal beam decubitus-type projections. For these projections, the grid is placed lengthwise with the patient, but the CR is centered along the crosswise axis of the grid to prevent grid cutoff.

Off-level grid With angling, the CR must be angled along the long axis of the lead strips. Angling across the grid lines results in grid cutoff. Off-level grid cutoff also occurs if the grid is tilted; the CR hits the lead lines at an angle (Fig. 1.142).

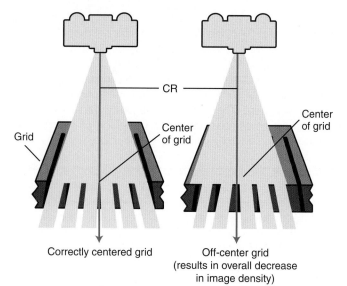

Correctly centered grid   Off-center grid (results in overall decrease in image density)

Fig. 1.141 Off-center grid cutoff.

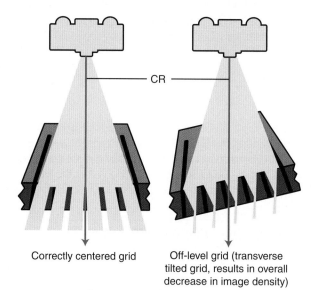

Correctly centered grid   Off-level grid (transverse tilted grid, results in overall decrease in image density)

Fig. 1.142 Off-level grid cutoff.

Off-focus grid A focused grid must be used at a specified SID if grid cutoff is to be prevented. Grids typically have a minimum and a maximum usable SID; this is called the *focal range*. The focal range is determined by the **grid frequency** (number of grid strips per inch or centimeter) and the **grid ratio** (height of lead strips compared with the space between them). Portable grids generally have a lower grid frequency and a lower grid ratio than fixed grids or bucky-type grids. A common grid ratio for portable grids is **6:1** or **8:1** compared with **12:1** for bucky grids. This indicates a greater focal range for portable grids, but SID limitations still exist to prevent grid cutoff (Fig. 1.143). Each technologist should know which types of portable grids are available and should know the focal range of each.

Upside-down focused grid Each grid is labeled to indicate the side that must be positioned to face the x-ray tube. The lead strips are tilted or focused to allow the x-ray beam to pass through unimpeded (if the SID is within the focal range and the grid is correctly placed). If the grid is positioned upside-down, the image will show severe cutoff (Fig. 1.144).

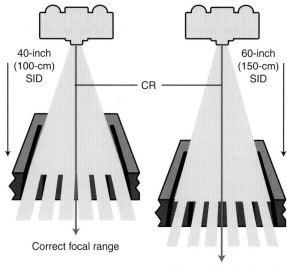

40-inch
(100-cm)
SID

CR

60-inch
(150-cm)
SID

Correct focal range

Off-focus grid, excessive SID
(results in overall decrease
in image density)

Fig. 1.143 Off-focus grid cutoff.

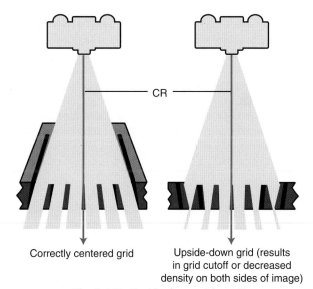

CR

Correctly centered grid

Upside-down grid (results
in grid cutoff or decreased
density on both sides of image)

Fig. 1.144 Upside-down grid cutoff.

1

IMAGE QUALITY IN FILM-SCREEN (ANALOG) RADIOGRAPHY

Since the discovery of x-rays in 1895, methods of acquiring and storing x-ray images have evolved. Conventional film-screen technology with the associated chemical processing and film libraries is being replaced rapidly by digital technology. Digital technology uses computers and x-ray receptors to acquire and process images; specialized digital communication networks are used to transmit and store the x-ray images.

Analog Images

Analog (film) images provide a two-dimensional image of anatomic structures. The image acquisition device is a film-screen system that consists of a pair of intensifying screens with a film between them. The screens and film are housed in an x-ray cassette that protects the film from light and ensures that screens are in close contact with the film. When screens receive the remnant radiation from the patient, they fluoresce; this light exposes the film, which must be chemically processed so the image can be viewed. Chemical processing includes several steps (developing, fixing, washing, and drying) and typically takes 60 to 90 seconds.

The film image (radiograph), which actually is composed of a deposit of metallic silver on a polyester base, is permanent; it cannot be altered. The various shades of gray displayed on the image are representative of the densities and atomic numbers of the tissues being examined. The film image is often referred to as a *hard-copy image*.

Analog image receptors are best described as self-regulating systems with a limited dynamic range. Analog image receptors are also described using the term *exposure latitude*. Exposure latitude is the range of exposure over which a film produces an acceptable image. An image produced with a level of exposure outside of the exposure latitude is an unacceptable image. Figs. 1.145 and 1.146 illustrate the dynamic range and exposure latitude of an analog IR. Note the impact of doubling the mAs on the diagnostic quality of the images of the elbow. Analog images have relatively narrow exposure latitude.

Image Quality Factors

Film-based radiographic images are evaluated on the basis of **four quality factors.** These four primary image quality factors are:
- Density
- Contrast
- Spatial resolution (discussed earlier)
- Distortion (discussed earlier)

Each of these factors has specific parameters by which it is controlled.

DENSITY
Definition

Radiographic film density is defined as the **amount of "blackness" on the processed radiograph.** When a radiograph with high density is viewed, less light is transmitted through the image.

Controlling Factors

The **primary controlling factor** of film density is **mAs.** mAs controls density by controlling the quantity of x-rays emitted from the x-ray tube and the duration of the exposure. The relationship for our purpose can be described as linear; doubling the mAs doubles the quantity or duration of x-rays emitted, thus doubling the density on the film.

The distance of the x-ray source from the IR, or the **source–image receptor distance,** also has an effect on radiographic density according to the inverse square law. If the SID is doubled, at the IR, the intensity of the x-ray beam is reduced to one-fourth,

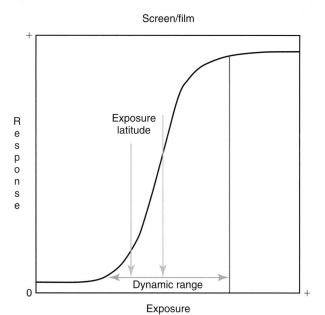

Fig. 1.145 Analog dynamic range.

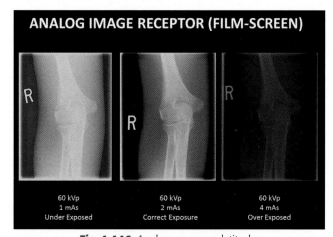

Fig. 1.146 Analog exposure latitude.

which then reduces radiographic density to one-fourth. A standard SID generally is used to reduce this variable.

Other factors that influence the density on a film image include kVp, part thickness, chemical development time/temperature, grid ratio, and film-screen speed.

Adjusting Analog Image Density

When film images (made with manual technique settings) are underexposed or overexposed, a general rule states that a minimum change in mAs of 25% to 30% is required to make a visible difference in radiographic density on the repeat radiograph. Some incorrectly exposed images may require a greater change, frequently 50% to 100%, or sometimes even greater. The radiograph of the elbow obtained with the use of 1 mAs shown in Fig. 1.147 was underexposed; the repeat radiograph was obtained with the use of 2 mAs (Fig. 1.148). Doubling the mAs in this example resulted in doubling of the density on the radiograph. kVp should not require an adjustment, provided that the optimal kVp for the part thickness was used. SID also should not require adjustment; it is a constant.

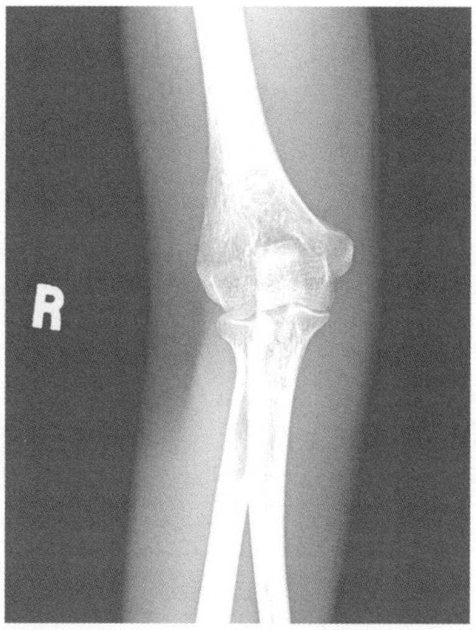

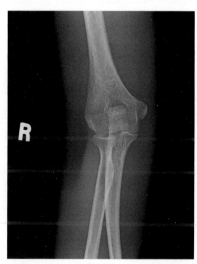

Fig. 1.147 1 mAs (60 kVp)—underexposed.

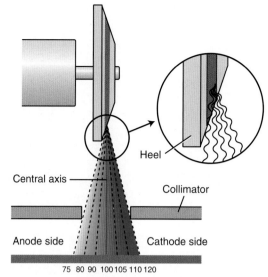

Percent intensity of x-ray beam
(more pronounced at shorter SID and larger IR)
Fig. 1.149 Anode heel effect.

Fig. 1.148 2 mAs (60 kVp)—repeated, double mAs.

TABLE 1.7 **SUMMARY OF ANODE HEEL EFFECT APPLICATIONS**		
PROJECTION	**ANODE END**	**CATHODE END**
Thoracic Spine		
AP	Head	Feet
Femur		
AP and lateral (see Fig. 1.123)	Feet	Head
Humerus		
AP and lateral	Elbow	Shoulder
Leg (Tibia/Fibula)		
AP and lateral	Ankle	Knee
Forearm		
AP and lateral	Wrist	Elbow

Density and Anode Heel Effect

The intensity of radiation emitted from the cathode end of the x-ray tube is greater than that emitted at the anode end; this phenomenon is known as the *anode heel effect.* Greater attenuation or absorption of x-rays occurs at the anode end because of the angle of the anode; x-rays emitted from deeper within the anode must travel through more anode material before exiting; thus, they are attenuated more.

Studies show that the difference in intensity from the cathode to the anode end of the x-ray field when a 17-inch (43-cm) IR is used at 40-inch (100-cm) SID can vary by 45%, depending on the anode angle[13] (Fig. 1.149). The anode heel effect is more pronounced when a short SID and a large field size are used.

Applying the anode heel effect to clinical practice assists the technologist in obtaining quality images of body parts that exhibit significant variation in thickness along the longitudinal axis of the x-ray field. The patient should be positioned so that the **thicker portion of the part is at the cathode end** of the x-ray tube and the **thinner part is under the anode** (the cathode and anode ends of the x-ray tube usually are marked on the protective housing). The abdomen, thoracic spine, and long bones of the limbs (e.g., the femur and tibia/fibula) are examples of structures that vary enough in thickness to warrant correct use of the anode heel effect.

A summary chart of body parts and projections for which the anode heel effect can be applied is provided in Table 1.7; this information is also noted in the positioning pages for each of these projections throughout the text. In practice, the most common application of the anode heel effect is for AP projections of the thoracic spine.

It may not always be practical or even possible to take advantage of the anode heel effect; this depends on the patient's condition or the arrangement of specific x-ray equipment within a room.

Compensating Filters

As was discussed in the previous section, body parts of varying anatomic density may result in an image that is partially overexposed or underexposed because the anatomic parts attenuate the beam differently. This problem can be overcome through the use of *compensating filters,* which filter out a portion of the primary beam toward the thin or less dense part of the body that is being imaged. Several types of compensating filters are in use; most are made of aluminum; however, some include plastic as well. The type of compensating filter used by the technologist depends on the clinical application (Fig. 1.150).

Compensating filters in common use include the following:
- Wedge filter (Fig. 1.151A): Mounts on the collimator; the thicker portion of the wedge is placed toward the least dense part of the anatomy to even out the densities. This filter has numerous applications; the most common include AP foot, AP thoracic spine, and axiolateral projection of the hip.
- Trough filter: Mounts on the collimator and is used for chest imaging. The thicker peripheral portions of the filter are placed

1

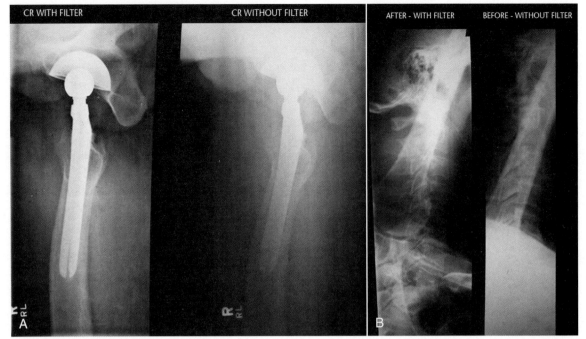

Fig. 1.150 Radiographic applications of compensating filters: hip (A) and upper thoracic spine (B). (Courtesy Ferlic Filters, Ferlic Filter Co, LLC.)

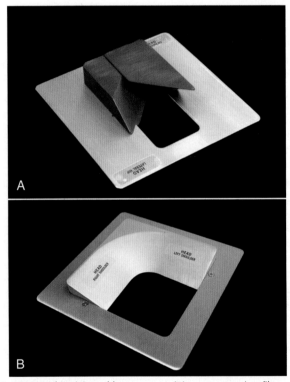

Fig. 1.151 Wedge (A) and boomerang (B) compensating filters (for use for upper thoracic spine and lateral hip projections). (Courtesy Ferlic Filters, Ferlic Filter Co, LLC.)

to correspond to the anatomically less dense lungs; the thinner portion of the filter corresponds to the mediastinum.
- Boomerang filter (Fig. 1.151B): Placed behind the patient and used primarily for shoulder and upper thoracic spine radiography; it provides improved visualization of soft tissues on the superior aspect of the shoulder and upper thoracic spine.

Summary of Density Factors
Adequate density, as **primarily controlled by mAs,** must be visible on processed film if the structures being radiographed are to be accurately represented. Too little density (underexposed) or too

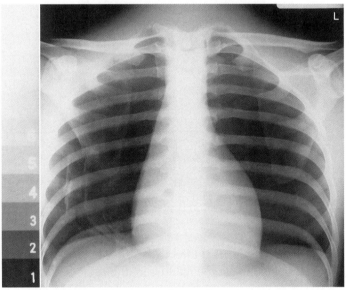

Fig. 1.152 High-contrast, short-scale 50 kVp, 800 mAs.

much density (overexposed) does not adequately demonstrate the required structures. Correct use of the anode heel effect and compensating filters helps to demonstrate optimal film density on anatomic parts that vary significantly in thickness.

CONTRAST
Definition
Radiographic contrast is defined as the **difference in density between adjacent areas of a radiographic image.** When the density difference is large, the contrast is high, and when the density difference is small, the contrast is low. This is demonstrated by the step wedge and by the chest radiograph in Fig. 1.152, which shows greater differences in density between adjacent areas; thus, this would be **high contrast.** Fig. 1.153 shows **low contrast** with less difference in density on adjacent areas of the step wedge and the associated radiograph.

Contrast can be described as **long-scale** or **short-scale contrast,** referring to the total range of optical densities from the lightest to the darkest part of the radiographic image. This is also demonstrated in Fig. 1.152, which shows short-scale/high-contrast (greater

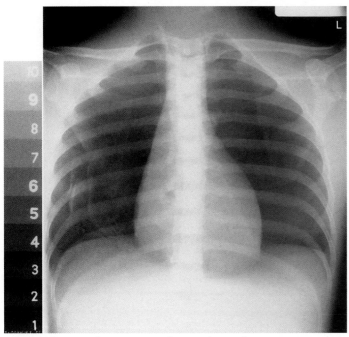

Fig. 1.153 Low-contrast, long-scale 110 kVp, 10 mAs.

differences in adjacent densities and fewer visible density steps), compared with Fig. 1.153, which illustrates long-scale/low-contrast.

Contrast allows the anatomic detail on a radiographic image to be visualized. Optimum radiographic contrast is important, and an understanding of contrast is essential for evaluating image quality.

Low or high contrast is not good or bad by itself. For example, low contrast (long-scale contrast) is desirable on radiographic images of the chest. Many shades of gray are required for visualization of fine lung markings, as is illustrated by the two chest radiographs in Figs. 1.152 and 1.153. The low-contrast (long-scale contrast) image in Fig. 1.153 reveals more shades of gray, as evident by the faint outlines of vertebrae that are visible through the heart and the mediastinal structures. The shades of gray that outline the vertebrae are less visible through the heart and the mediastinum on the high-contrast chest radiograph shown in Fig. 1.152.

Adjusting Analog Image Contrast

Contrast in film-based imaging may be adjusted in a variety of ways. The radiographer may choose to alter the kVp using the 15% rule; change the amount of beam restriction; or change grid ratio. In each of those circumstances, the technologist will need to make changes in the mAs settings in order to compensate for adjustment made for the change in contrast.

Controlling Factors

The **primary controlling factor** for contrast in film-based imaging is kilovolts peak **(kVp).** kVp controls the energy or penetrating power of the primary x-ray beam. The higher the kVp, the greater the energy and the more uniformly the x-ray beam penetrates the various mass densities of all tissues. Therefore, **higher kVp produces** less variation in attenuation (differential absorption), resulting in **lower contrast.**

kVp is also a **secondary controlling factor** of density. Higher kVp, resulting in both more numerous x-rays and greater energy x-rays, causes more x-ray energy to reach the IR, with a corresponding increase in overall density. A general rule of thumb states that a **15% increase in kVp will increase film density, similar to doubling the mAs.** In the lower kVp range, such as 50 to 70 kVp, an 8- to 10-kVp increase would double the density (equivalent to doubling the mAs). In the 80- to 100-kVp range, a 12- to 15-kVp increase is required to double the density. The importance of this relates to radiation protection, because as kVp is increased, mAs can be significantly reduced, resulting in absorption of less radiation by the patient.

Other factors may affect radiographic contrast. The amount of *scatter* radiation the film-screen receives influences the radiographic contrast. Scatter radiation is radiation that has been changed in direction and intensity as a result of interaction with patient tissue. The amount of scatter produced depends on the intensity of the x-ray beam, the amount of tissue irradiated, and the type and thickness of the tissue. Close collimation of the x-ray field reduces the amount of tissue irradiated, reducing the amount of scatter produced and increasing contrast. Close collimation also reduces the radiation dose to the patient and the technologist.

Irradiation of thick body parts produces a considerable amount of scatter radiation, which decreases image contrast. A device called a *grid* is used to absorb much of the scatter radiation before it hits the IR.

Summary of Contrast Factors

Selection of the appropriate kVp is a balance between optimal image contrast and lowest possible patient dose. A general rule states that the **highest kVp and the lowest mAs that yield sufficient diagnostic information should be used on each radiographic examination.**[13] Close collimation and correct use of grids also ensure the processed radiographic image displays optimal contrast.

SPATIAL RESOLUTION

Controlling Factors Specific to Analog

Film-screen system With film-screen imaging systems, the *film-screen speed* used for an examination affects the detail shown on the resultant film. A faster film-screen system allows shorter exposure times, which are helpful in preventing patient motion and reducing dose; however, the image is less sharp than when a slower system is used.

IMAGE QUALITY IN DIGITAL RADIOGRAPHY

Digital imaging in radiologic technology involves application of the analog-to-digital conversion theory and computer software and hardware. Although digital imaging differs from film-screen imaging in terms of the method of image acquisition, factors that may affect x-ray production, attenuation, and geometry of the x-ray beam still apply. This section provides a brief practical introduction to a very complex topic.

Digital Images

Digital radiographic images also provide a two-dimensional image of anatomic structures; however, they are viewed on a computer monitor and are referred to as **soft-copy images.** These images are a **numeric representation of the x-ray intensities that are transmitted through the patient.** Each digital image is two-dimensional and is formed by a *matrix* of picture elements called *pixels* (Fig. 1.154). In diagnostic imaging, each pixel represents the smallest unit in the image; columns and rows of pixels make up the matrix. For illustrative purposes, consider a sheet of graph paper. The series of squares on the sheet can be compared with the matrix, and each individual square can be compared with a pixel.

Digital imaging requires the use of computer hardware and software applications to view images (Fig. 1.155), whereas film-based images use chemical processing to visualize anatomic structures. Digital processing involves the **systematic application of highly complex mathematical formulas** called *algorithms.* Numerous mathematical manipulations are performed on image data to enhance image appearance and to optimize quality. Algorithms are applied by the computer to every data set obtained before the technologist sees the image.

Digital imaging systems are capable of producing a radiographic image across a large range of exposure values and are described as having a wide dynamic range (Fig. 1.156). Because of this wide dynamic range, it is essential that an institution define the exposure latitude for the digital imaging systems within its department. The exposure latitude for a digital imaging system is defined as the acceptable level of exposure that produces the desired image quality for the department. Fig. 1.157 demonstrates the dynamic range and exposure latitude of a digital imaging system. Note that the increase from 1 to 8 mAs still produces a diagnostic image of the elbow.

Exposure Factors for Digital Imaging

Although kVp and mA and time (mAs) must be selected if radiographic images are to be digitally acquired (see Fig. 1.157), they do not have the same direct effect on image quality as they do in film-screen imaging. It must be remembered, however, that the kVp and mAs used for the exposure affect patient dose.

Display matrix

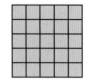

Pixel

Fig. 1.154 Two-dimensional matrix display—pixel.

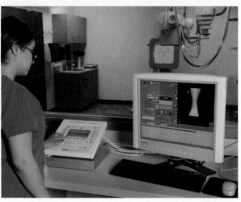

Fig. 1.155 Processing digital image.

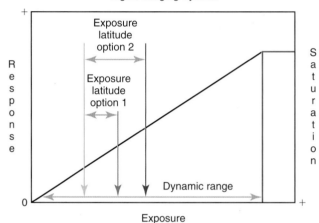

Fig. 1.156 Digital imaging systems.

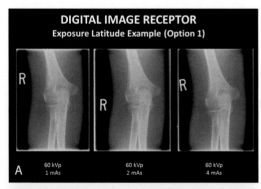

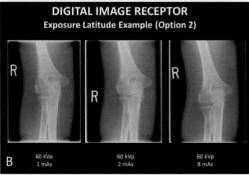

Fig. 1.157 Digital exposure latitudes. A, Option 1. B, Option 2.

Image Quality Factors

The factors used to evaluate digital image quality include the following:

- Brightness
- Contrast resolution
- Spatial resolution (discussed earlier)
- Distortion (discussed earlier)
- Exposure indicator
- Noise

BRIGHTNESS

Brightness is defined as the intensity of light that represents the individual pixels in the image on the monitor. In digital imaging, the term *brightness* replaces the film-based term *density* (Figs. 1.158 and 1.159).

Controlling Factors

Digital imaging systems are designed to display electronically the optimal image brightness under a wide range of exposure factors. Brightness is controlled by the processing software through the application of predetermined digital processing algorithms. In contrast to the linear relationship between mAs and density in film-screen imaging, changes in mAs do not have a controlling effect on digital image brightness. Although the density of a film image cannot be altered once it is exposed and chemically processed, the user can adjust the brightness of the digital image after exposure (see section on postprocessing later in this chapter).

CONTRAST RESOLUTION

In digital imaging, *contrast* is defined as the **difference in brightness between light and dark areas of an image.** This definition is similar to the definition used in film-based imaging, where contrast is the difference in density of adjacent areas on the film (Figs. 1.160 and 1.161 show examples of different contrast images). *Contrast resolution* refers to the ability of an imaging system to distinguish between similar tissues.

Controlling Factors

Digital imaging systems are designed to display electronically optimal image contrast under a wide range of exposure factors. Radiographic contrast is affected by the digital processing computer through the application of predetermined algorithms, in contrast to film-screen imaging, in which kVp is the controlling factor for image contrast. Although the contrast of a film image cannot be altered after exposure and processing, the user can manipulate the contrast of the digital image (see later section on postprocessing).

The ability of the image processing software to display a desired image contrast provides the radiographer with a potential opportunity to reduce entrance skin exposure to the patient through the use of higher kVp levels. Figs. 1.162 to 1.164 represent the ability to use the 15% rule and decrease patient entrance skin dose by approximately 22%. It is critical that the radiographer consult with the interpreting radiologist and medical physicist prior to implementing across-the-board kVp increases in order to ensure that acceptable image quality is maintained.

Pixels and Bit Depth

Each pixel in an image matrix demonstrates a single shade of gray when viewed on a monitor; this is representative of the physical properties of the anatomic structure. The range of possible shades of gray demonstrated is related to the *bit depth* of the pixel, which is determined by the manufacturer. Although a comprehensive description of bit depth is beyond the scope of this text, it is important to note that the **greater the bit depth of a system, the greater the contrast resolution (i.e., the greater the number of possible shades of gray that a pixel can have).**

Because computer theory is based on the binary system, a 14-bit system, for example, is represented as 2^{14}; the 14-bit-deep pixel could represent any one of 16,384 possible shades of gray, from black to white. Bit depth is determined by the manufacturer's system design and is closely related to the imaging procedures for which the equipment is designed. The most common bit depths available are 10, 12, and 16. For example, a digital system for chest imaging should have a bit depth greater than 10 bits (2^{10}) if it is to capture all required information; the x-ray beam that exits a patient who is having a chest x-ray can have a range of more than 1024 intensities.

Pixel size Two pixel sizes are used in medical imaging. These are *acquisition pixel size*, which is the minimum size that is inherent to the acquisition system, and *display pixel size*, which is the minimum pixel size that can be displayed by a monitor. A general radiography acquisition matrix may be 3000 × 3000 pixels—more than 9 million pixels (9 megapixels)—in a 17 × 17-inch (43 × 43-cm) image.

Scatter Radiation Control

Because digital receptors are more sensitive to low-energy radiation, controlling scatter radiation is an important factor in obtaining the appropriate image contrast. This is accomplished by the correct use of grids, by close collimation, and by selection of the optimal kVp. Grid cutoff occurring with digital image receptors will result in an image that has decreased contrast and has an exposure indicator reflecting a decrease in exposure. The change in exposure indicator is due to the decrease in amount of exit radiation striking the receptor.

Postprocessing software has been developed to minimize the presentation of scatter radiation on the final displayed image. It is important to recognize; however, that it does not prevent scatter radiation from reaching the image receptor, it simply minimizes to display of scatter on the final image.

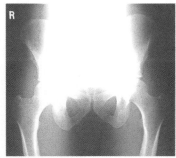

Fig. 1.158 AP pelvis—high brightness (light).

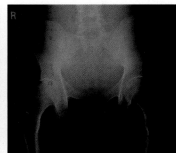

Fig. 1.159 AP pelvis—less brightness (dark).

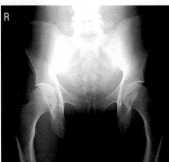

Fig. 1.160 AP pelvis—higher contrast.

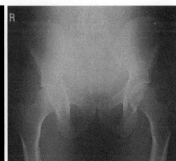

Fig. 1.161 AP pelvis—lower contrast.

SPATIAL RESOLUTION

Spatial resolution in digital imaging is defined as the **recorded sharpness or detail of structures on the image**—the same as defined for film-screen imaging.

Resolution in a digital image represents a combination of the traditional factors explained previously for film-screen imaging (focal spot size, geometric factors, and motion) and, just as important, the **acquisition pixel size.** This pixel size is inherent to the digital imaging receptor. The smaller the acquisition pixel size, the greater the spatial resolution. Spatial resolution is measured in line pairs per millimeter. Current digital imaging systems employed for general radiography have spatial resolution capabilities ranging from approximately 2.5 lp/mm to 5 lp/mm.

Controlling Factors

In addition to acquisition **pixel size,** resolution is controlled by the **display matrix.** The perceived resolution of the image depends on the display capabilities of the monitor. Monitors with a larger display matrix can display images with higher resolution.

EXPOSURE INDICATOR

The *exposure indicator* in digital imaging is a **numeric value that is representative of the exposure that the IR has received.** Depending on the manufacturer of the system, the exposure indicator may also be called the *sensitivity (S) number; Exposure Index (EI, EXI); Reached Exposure Value (REX);* or possibly *Detector Exposure Index (DEI).*

Deviation Index

In addition to the *Exposure Index,* there is also a *Deviation Index (DI).* The DI provides feedback to the operator regarding receptor exposure. The DI ranges from −3 to +3. A DI value of 0 indicates that the level of exposure was appropriate. A positive DI value indicates overexposure and a negative DI value indicates underexposure. A DI value of +1 indicates a 26% overexposure whereas a value of −1 indicates a 20% underexposure. The DI values of +3 and −3 represent exposure levels that are two times greater and less than the defined target exposure index.

Controlling Factors

The exposure indicator depends on the dose of radiation that strikes the receptor. It is a value that is calculated from the effect of mAs, the kVp, the total receptor area irradiated, and the objects exposed (e.g., air, metal implants, patient anatomy). Depending on the manufacturer and the technique used to calculate this value, the exposure indicator is displayed for each exposure.

An exposure indicator, as used by certain manufacturers, is **inversely related** to the radiation that strikes the receptor. For example, if the range for an acceptable image for certain examinations is 150 to 250, a value greater than 250 would indicate underexposure, and a value less than 150 would indicate overexposure.

An **exposure indicator** as used by other manufacturers is **directly related** to the radiation striking the IR, as determined by logarithmic calculations. For example, if an acceptable exposure indicator is typically 2.0 to 2.4, an indicator value less than 2.0 would indicate underexposure, whereas an indicator value greater than 2.4 would indicate overexposure.

This text uses the term **exposure indicator** when referring to this variable.

It has been stated previously that digital imaging systems are able to display images that have been obtained through the use of a wide range of exposure factors. Despite this wide dynamic range, there are limitations, and the technologist must ensure that the exposure factors used are acceptable and within the institution's defined exposure latitude (similar to reviewing an analog [film] image to confirm that adequate contrast and density are present) (see Figs. 1.162 to 1.164). Checking the exposure indicator is key in verifying that acceptable **quality digital radiographic images have been obtained with the least possible dose to the patient.**

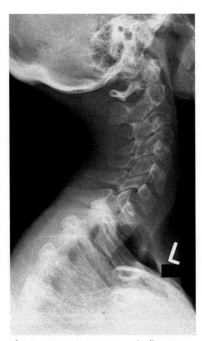

Fig. 1.162 Low exposure indicator indicates underexposure with "noisy" undesirable image.

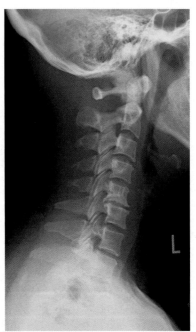

Fig. 1.163 Example of desirable exposure with acceptable exposure indicator.

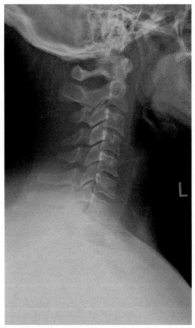

Fig. 1.164 High exposure indicator indicates overexposure.

If the exposure indicator is outside the recommended range for the digital system, the image may still appear acceptable when viewed on the monitor of the technologist's workstation. The monitor the technologist uses to view the image typically provides lower resolution than is provided by the radiologist's reporting workstation. The technologist's workstation is intended to allow verification of positioning and general image quality; however, this image is typically not of diagnostic quality. The monitor of a radiologist's reporting workstation typically provides superior spatial and contrast resolution caused by an increased display matrix with smaller pixels and superior brightness characteristics.

NOISE

Noise is defined as a **random disturbance that obscures or reduces clarity.** In a radiographic image, this translates into a grainy or mottled appearance of the image.

Signal-to-Noise Ratio

One way to describe noise in digital image acquisition is the concept of *signal-to-noise ratio* (SNR). The number of x-ray photons that strike the receptor (mAs) can be considered the *"signal."* Other factors that negatively affect the final image are classified as *"noise."* A **high SNR is desirable** in imaging, in which the signal (mAs) is greater than the noise, so that low-contrast soft tissue structures can be demonstrated. A **low SNR is undesirable;** a low signal (low mAs) with accompanying high noise obscures soft tissue detail and produces a grainy or mottled image.

High SNR Although a high SNR is favorable (Fig. 1.165), technologists must ensure exposure factors used are not beyond what is required for the projection so as not to overexpose the patient needlessly. Overexposed images are not readily evident with digital processing and display, so checking the exposure indicator as described on the previous page is the best way to determine this.

Low SNR When insufficient mAs is selected for a projection, the receptor does not receive the appropriate number of x-ray photons, resulting in a low SNR and a *noisy* image (Fig. 1.166). This insufficient signal may not be readily visible on the lower resolution monitor of the technologist's workstation, but the exposure indicator, as checked for each projection, can aid in determining this. The technologist may check for noise at the workstation by using the magnify feature and magnifying the image to determine the level of noise present within the image. In the event that noise is clearly visible in the image without any magnification, the image should be reviewed by the radiologist to determine if the image needs to be repeated.

Scatter radiation leads to a degradation of image contrast that can be controlled by the use of grids and correct collimation, as was described previously.

A secondary factor related to noise in a radiographic image is *electronic noise*. Although a comprehensive discussion of electronic noise is beyond the scope of this text, electronic noise typically results from inherent noise in the electronic system, nonuniformity of the image receptor, or power fluctuations.

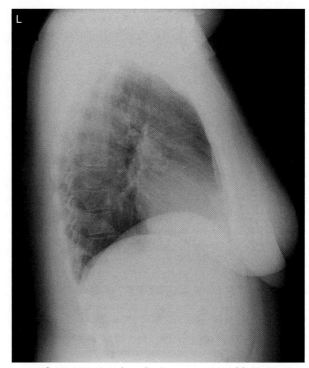

Fig. 1.165 Good-quality image—acceptable SNR.

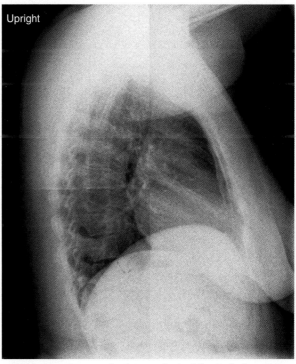

Fig. 1.166 Poor-quality image, "noisy" (grainy)—low SNR.

POSTPROCESSING

One of the advantages of digital imaging technology over film-screen technology is the ability to *postprocess* the image at the technologist's workstation. Postprocessing refers to **changing or enhancing the electronic image for the purpose of improving its diagnostic quality.** In postprocessing, algorithms are applied to the image to modify pixel values. Once viewed, the changes made may be saved, or the image default settings may be reapplied to enhance the diagnostic quality of the image. It is important to note that an image modified at the technologist's workstation and sent to the picture archiving and communication system (PACS) cannot be unmodified on the PACS. As a result of this inability to undo changes made at the technologist's workstation once the image is sent to the PACS, postprocessing of images at the technologist's workstation should be avoided.

Postprocessing and Exposure Indicator Range

After an acceptable exposure indicator range for the system has been established, it is important to determine whether the image is inside or outside this range. If the exposure indicator is below this range (indicating low SNR), postprocessing would not be effective in minimizing noise; more "signal" cannot be created through postprocessing. Theoretically, if the algorithms are correct, the image should display with the optimal contrast and brightness. However, even if the algorithms used are correct and exposure factors are within an acceptable range, as indicated by the exposure indicator, certain postprocessing options may still be applied for specific image effects.

POSTPROCESSING OPTIONS

Various postprocessing options are available in medical imaging (Figs. 1.167 through 1.170). The most common of these options include the following:

Windowing and Leveling: The user can adjust image contrast and brightness on the monitor. Two types of adjustment are possible: *window width (windowing)* which controls the **contrast** of the image (within a certain range), and *window level (leveling)* which controls the **brightness** of the image, also within a certain range. It is important to note that when adjusting the display window for a digital radiograph, the manner in which the values assigned for each characteristic vary is dependent on the viewing system software. In some PACS, increasing the window level results in a darker image, and in others, it results in a brighter image.

Smoothing: Specific image processing is applied to reduce the display of noise in an image. The process of smoothing the image data does not eliminate the noise present in the image at the time of acquisition.

Magnification: All or part of an image can be magnified.

Edge enhancement: Specific image processing that alters pixel values in the image is applied to make the edges of structures appear more prominent compared with images with less or no edge enhancement. The spatial resolution of the image does not change when edge enhancement is applied.

Equalization: Specific image processing that alters the pixel values across the image is applied to present a more uniform image appearance. The pixel values representing low brightness are made brighter, and pixel values with high brightness are made to appear less bright.

Subtraction: Background anatomy can be removed to allow visualization of contrast media–filled vessels (used in angiography).

Image reversal: The dark and light pixel values of an image are reversed—the x-ray image reverses from a negative to a positive.

Annotation: Text may be added to images.

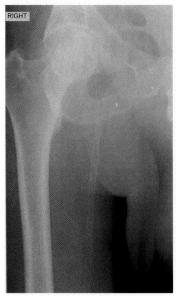

Fig. 1.167 AP hip image applied to create angiographic mask.

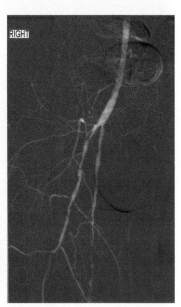

Fig. 1.168 AP hip image with subtraction.

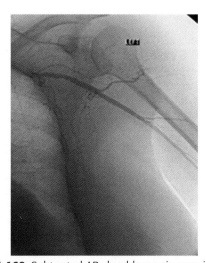

Fig. 1.169 Subtracted AP shoulder angiogram image.

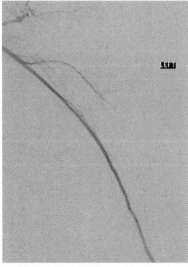

Fig. 1.170 Subtracted and magnified option of shoulder angiogram.

APPLICATIONS OF DIGITAL TECHNOLOGY

Although digital technology has been used for years in digital fluoroscopy and CT (further information on these modalities is available in Chapters 12 and 18), its widespread application to general imaging is more recent. This section introduces and briefly describes the digital imaging technology used in general radiography. Each of the systems described starts the imaging process using an x-ray beam that is captured and converted into a digital signal.

DIGITAL IMAGING SYSTEMS

The many acronyms associated with digital imaging have created a plethora of misconceptions regarding digital imaging systems, and these misconceptions have resulted in technologists not having a thorough understanding of how various digital imaging systems work. The following sections describe the current digital imaging systems, based first on how the image data are captured and extracted, and second on their appearance. Regardless of appearance and how the image data are captured and extracted, each of the digital imaging systems described has a wide dynamic range that requires a defined set of exposure indices to enable the technologist to adhere to the ALARA principle—as low as reasonably achievable.

Computed Radiography (CR) (Photostimulable Storage Phosphor Plate [PSP])

PSP technology was the first widely implemented digital imaging system for general radiography. It is most commonly called *computed radiography (CR)*. A CR digital imaging system relies on the use of a storage phosphor plate that serves the purpose of capturing and storing the x-ray beam exiting the patient. When the plate is exposed to radiation, electrons migrate to electron traps within the phosphor material. The greater the exposure to the plate, the more electrons move to the electron traps. The exposed plate containing the latent image undergoes a reading process following the exposure (Fig. 1.171). The reading of the plate involves scanning the entire plate from side to side using a laser beam. As the laser moves across the plate, the trapped electrons in the phosphor are released from the electron traps and migrate back to their resting location. This migration results in the emission of light from the phosphor. The greater the exposure to the plate, the greater the intensity of the light emitted from the plate during the reading process. The light released is collected by an optical system that sends the light to a device responsible for converting the light into an analog electrical signal. The device may be a photomultiplier tube or charge-coupled device (CCD). The analog electrical signal is sent to an analog-to-digital converter (ADC) so that the image data may be processed by the computer to create the desired digital image. Depending on the manufacturer, the image may be viewed on the technologist's workstation as quickly as 5 seconds after plate reading. After the reading process, the PSP plate is exposed to bright white light so that any remaining latent image is erased from the plate and the plate may be used for the next exposure.

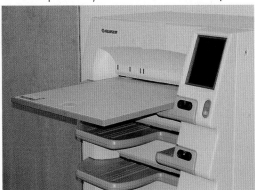

Fig. 1.171 PSP cassette and reader.

A CR digital imaging system may be cassette based or cassette-less. A cassette-based system allows the technologist to place the IR physically in a variety of locations. The cassette-less system (Figs. 1.172 and 1.173) provides the technologist with a larger device that encloses the IR. The IR in a cassette-less system has a limited amount of movement to align with the x-ray beam and anatomic structure owing to its design. The appearance of the device is not an indication of what is happening inside of the device after exposure to the x-ray beam. Therefore, it is critical that technologists recognize and understand what is inside the equipment with which they work.

Technologist Workstation

The workstation includes a bar-code reader (optional), a monitor for image display, and a keyboard with a mouse or trackball for entering commands for postprocessing. The technologist verifies the patient position and checks the exposure indicator at this workstation.

IMAGE ARCHIVING

After the image quality has been verified and any needed adjustments have been made, the image can be transmitted to the digital archive for viewing and reading by the referring physician or radiologist. Images also may be printed onto film by a laser printer.

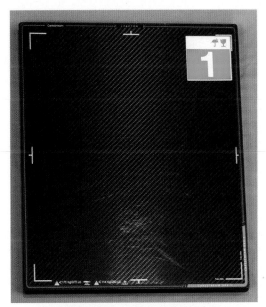

Fig. 1.172 Cassette-less imaging system.

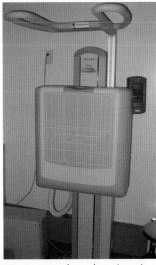

Fig. 1.173 Cassette-less chest imaging system.

APPLICATION OF CR DIGITAL SYSTEMS

Regardless of the technology used to acquire radiographic images, accurate positioning and attention to technical details are important. However, when digital technology is used, attention to these details becomes more important because of the following factors.

COLLIMATION

In addition to the benefit of reducing radiation dose to the patient, collimation that is closely restricted to the part that is being examined is key to ensuring optimal image quality. The software processes the entire x-ray field as a data set; any unexpected attenuation of the beam may be included in the calculations for brightness, contrast, and exposure indicator. If the collimation is not closely restricted, the exposure indicator may be misrepresented, and the image may exhibit lower contrast or possibly incorrect brightness.

ACCURATE CENTERING OF PART AND IR

Because of the way the extracted image data are analyzed, the body part and collimated exposure field should be centered to the IR to ensure proper image display. Failure to align the part to the receptor accurately and collimate the exposure field properly may result in poor image quality on initial image display.

USE OF LEAD MASKS

Use of lead masks or a blocker for multiple images on a single IR is recommended when a cassette-based CR or analog system is used (Fig. 1.174). This recommendation is due to the hypersensitivity of the PSP plate to lower energy scatter radiation; even small amounts may affect the image.

NOTE: Some manufacturers recommend that only one image be centered and placed per IR. Check with your department to find out whether multiple images can be placed on a single IR.

USE OF GRIDS

Use of grids (as explained in an earlier section of this chapter) for body parts larger (thicker) than 10 cm is especially important when images are acquired with the use of PSP image receptors because of the hypersensitivity of the image plate phosphors to scatter radiation.

EXPOSURE FACTORS

Because of their wide dynamic range, CR systems are able to display an acceptable image from a broad range of exposure factors (kVp, mAs). It is important to remember, however, that the ALARA principle (exposure to patient as low as reasonably achievable) must be followed, and the lowest exposure factors required to obtain a diagnostic image must be used. When the image is available for viewing, the technologist must check the exposure indicator to verify that the exposure factors used are consistent with the ALARA principle and diagnostic image quality. In some circumstances it is possible to increase kVp by 5 to 10 while decreasing mAs by the equivalent ratio with digital imaging equipment to maintain image quality while significantly reducing entrance skin exposure dose to the patient (refer to Figs. 1.162 to 1.164).

EVALUATION OF EXPOSURE INDICATOR

As soon as the image is available for viewing at the workstation, it is critiqued for positioning and exposure accuracy. The technologist must check the exposure indicator to verify the exposure factors used were in the correct range for optimum quality with the lowest radiation dose to the patient.

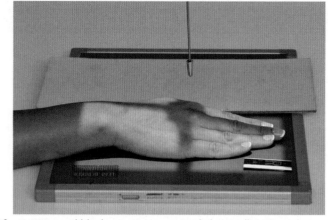

Fig. 1.174 Lead blockers on cassette and close collimation are important with the use of cassette-based PSP systems.

Direct Radiography (DR) (Flat-Panel Detector with Thin-Film Transistor)

The **direct radiography** imaging system for general radiography is a second type of digital imaging system. The flat-panel detector with thin-film transistor (FPD-TFT) system is commonly referred to as **digital radiography (DR) or direct digital radiography (DDR).**

The DR unit may be constructed using amorphous selenium or amorphous silicon. The purpose of those two materials is to provide a source of electrons to the thin-film transistor that collects the electrons during the exposure. The creation of the electrons for the TFT is different with the two materials. The exposure of amorphous selenium to x-ray photons causes electrons to move through the material and into the electron collection portion of the TFT. Amorphous silicon requires the use of a scintillator, which produces light when struck by x-ray photons. The light exiting the scintillator causes the movement of electrons through the amorphous silicon and into the electron collection centers of the TFT. The TFT collects the electrons in an ordered manner and then sends the analog electrical signal to an ADC. The signal from the ADC is sent to the computer to create the digital image. The display of the radiographic image on the technologist's workstation with the DR system occurs within seconds after the exposure ends.

A DR imaging system may be cassette-less (Fig. 1.175) or cassette based (Fig. 1.176). The appearance of the IR does not indicate how the device captures and produces the image. Therefore, it is important for the technologist to know what type of IR is being used.

ADVANTAGES OF DR SYSTEMS

One advantage of DR-based systems compared with CR systems is that the DR system is capable of displaying the image faster. The faster image display applies to both the cassette-less and the cassette-based DR systems. One other advantage is the potential to produce diagnostic radiographs with lower levels of exposure. However, the ability to produce these images using a lower level of exposure depends on the manufacturer's choice of materials used to construct the system.

DR and CR systems both give the technologist the advantage of being able to view a *preview image* to evaluate for positioning errors and confirm the exposure indicator. The projection may be repeated immediately if necessary. Also, the operator is able to postprocess and manipulate the image.

As with CR systems and film-screen acquisition, DR-based systems can be used for both grid and nongrid examinations. In reality, however, when cassette-less DR-based systems are used for traditional nongrid examinations, the grid often is not removed for practical reasons: It is expensive and fragile and may be damaged easily. Because of the high efficiency of the receptor, the increase in exposure that is required when a grid is used is less of an issue; the exception to this would be pediatric examinations (because of the greater sensitivity of pediatric patients to radiation exposure).

APPLICATION OF DR-BASED SYSTEMS

Regardless of the digital technology used to acquire radiographic images, accurate positioning and attention to certain technical details are important, as described previously for CR systems. For

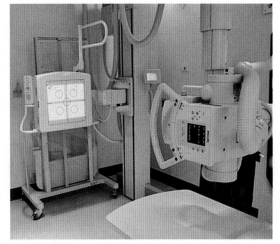

Fig. 1.175 FPD-TFT cassette-less imaging system.

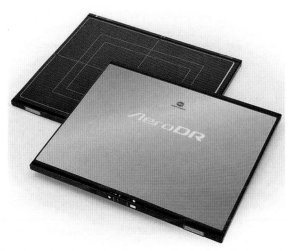

Fig. 1.176 FPD-TFT cassette. (Courtesy Konica Minolta Medical Imaging, Inc.)

DR-based systems, these details include **careful collimation,** correct use of **grids,** and careful attention to **exposure factors and evaluation of exposure indicator values,** combined with adherence to the ALARA principle. When either CR or DR technology is used, attention to these details is essential.

The most current FPD-TFT–based receptors are cassette based with wireless capability. The wireless connectivity allows the radiographer to easily move the DR detector from the conventional table bucky to the upright bucky. Furthermore, the wireless DR detectors are routinely adapted to mobile radiographic units.

It is highly recommended that a department that mixes vendors and CR and DR technology develop standardized protocols to ensure image quality regardless of the method of image capture. Specifically, the department needs to establish exposure field sizes; projections per receptor, if permitted; and uniform processing parameters on all technologist workstations.

Image Receptor Sizes and Orientation

As noted previously, the term *image receptor,* or *IR,* applies to the device that captures the radiation that exits the patient; IR refers to the film cassette and to the digital acquisition device. Use of metric Système Internationale (SI) units to describe the size of analog cassettes and image receptors in CR has primarily replaced use of the English units. See Tables 1.8, 1.9, and 1.10 for a list of available IR size options for analog, CR, and DR.

TABLE 1.8 AVAILABLE IR SIZES IN ANALOG (FILM-SCREEN) IMAGING

METRIC (SI) SIZE (CM)	ENGLISH UNIT REFERENCE (INCHES)	CLINICAL APPLICATION
18 × 24	8 × 10	General imaging, mammography
24 × 24	9 × 9	Fluoroscopic spot imaging
18 × 43	7 × 17	General imaging
24 × 30	10 × 12	General imaging, mammography
30 × 35; 35 × 35; 30 × 40	11 × 14	General imaging
NA	14 × 36; 14 × 51	Full spine/lower limbs
35 × 43	14 × 17	General imaging
NA	5 × 12; 6 × 12	Mandible/orthopantomography

TABLE 1.9 AVAILABLE IR SIZES IN CR SYSTEMS

METRIC (SI) SIZE (CM)	ENGLISH UNIT REFERENCE (INCHES)	CLINICAL APPLICATION
18 × 24	8 × 10	General imaging, mammography
24 × 30	10 × 12	General imaging, mammography
35 × 35	14 × 14	General imaging
35 × 43	14 × 17	General imaging

TABLE 1.10 AVAILABLE IR SIZES IN DR SYSTEMS

METRIC (SI) SIZE (CM)	ENGLISH UNIT REFERENCE (INCHES)	CLINICAL APPLICATION
18 × 24	8 × 10	General imaging, mammography
24 × 30	10 × 12	General imaging, mammography
35 × 43	14 × 17	General imaging
43 × 43	17 × 17	General imaging

The selection of IR size depends primarily on the body part that is to be examined. The size and shape of the body part being examined also determine the orientation of the IR. If the IR is positioned with the longer dimension of the IR parallel to the long axis of the body part, the orientation is **portrait;** if the IR is positioned with the shorter dimension of the IR parallel to the long axis of the body part, the orientation is **landscape.** A common example applied to clinical practice relates to chest radiography. Patients who are hypersthenic are imaged with the IR in landscape orientation, so the lateral aspects of the chest may be included in the image (Fig. 1.177).

Students also may hear the terms *lengthwise* and *crosswise* used to describe IR orientation. These correspond to *portrait* and *landscape,* respectively.

The size of the image displayed will be affected by the size of the CR imaging plate chosen or the size of the collimated exposure field for DR systems. The change in image size is based on the number of pixels in the image matrix that in turn must be displayed on the technologist workstation or radiologist's reading station.

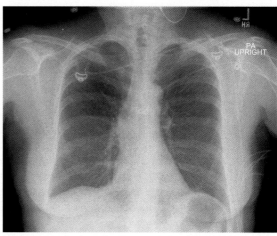

Fig. 1.177 PA chest landscape (crosswise) IR alignment.

Picture Archiving and Communication System

As imaging departments move from film-based acquisition and archiving (hard-copy film and document storage) to digital acquisition and archiving (soft-copy storage), a complex computer network has been created to manage images. This network, called a *picture archiving and communication system,* can be likened to a virtual film library. Images stored on digital media are housed in PACS archives.

PACS is a sophisticated array of hardware and software that can connect all modalities with digital output (nuclear medicine, ultrasound, CT, MRI, angiography, mammography, and radiography), as illustrated in Fig. 1.178. The acronym PACS can best be defined as follows:

P	Picture	Digital medical image(s)
A	Archiving	"Electronic" storage of images
C	Communication	Routing (retrieval/sending) and displaying of images
S	System	Specialized computer network that manages the complete system

The connection of various equipment types and modalities to a PACS is complex. Standards have been developed to ensure that all manufacturers and types of equipment are able to communicate and transmit images and information effectively. Current standards include **DICOM** (**D**igital **I**maging and **C**ommunications in **M**edicine) and **HL7** (**h**ealth **l**evel **7**). Although standards may not always provide for an instantaneous functionality between devices, they do allow for resolution of connectivity problems.

For optimum efficiency, PACS should be integrated with the radiology information system (**RIS**) or the hospital information system (**HIS**). Because these information systems support the operations of an imaging department through examination scheduling, patient registration, report archiving, and film tracking, integration with PACS maintains integrity of patient data and records and promotes overall efficiency.

When PACS is used, instead of hard-copy radiographs that must be processed, handled, viewed, transported, and stored, the soft-copy digital images are processed with the use of a computer, viewed on a monitor, and stored electronically. Most PACS use web browsers to enable easy access to the images by users from any location. Physicians may view these radiologic images from a personal computer at virtually any location, including their homes.

ADVANTAGES OF PACS

Advantages of PACS include the following:
- Elimination of less efficient traditional film libraries and their inherent problem of physical space requirements for hard-copy images.
- Convenient search for and retrieval of images.
- Rapid (electronic) transfer of images within the hospital (e.g., clinics, operating rooms, treatment units).
- Ease in consulting outside specialists—teleradiology. Teleradiography is the electronic transmission of diagnostic images from one location to another for purposes of interpretation or consultation.
- Simultaneous viewing of images at multiple locations.
- Elimination of misplaced, damaged, or missing films.
- Increase in efficiency of reporting examinations with soft-copy images (compared with hard-copy images).
- Reduction of the health and environmental impact associated with chemical processing as a result of decreased use.

The growth of computer applications in radiologic technology has led to new career paths for radiologic technologists. PACS Administrator and the Diagnostic Imaging Information Technologist are new positions that many radiologic technologists are pursuing.

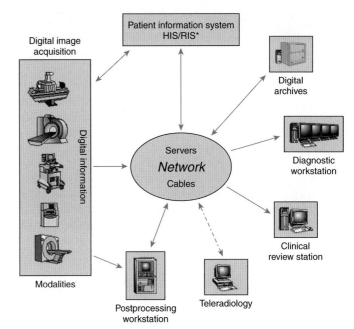

Fig. 1.178 A full PACS network that includes digital acquisition, communication, reporting, and archiving. *HIS/RIS,* Hospital information system/radiology information system. (Modification of diagram from Philips Medical Systems.)

PART THREE ▪ RADIATION PROTECTION

Contributor **Frank Goerner**, PhD, DABR

As professionals, radiologic technologists have the important responsibility to protect their patients, themselves, and fellow workers from unnecessary radiation. A complete understanding of radiation protection is essential for every technologist, but a comprehensive review[13] is beyond the scope of this anatomy and positioning text. The basic principles and applied aspects of radiation protection, as described in this part, should be an essential component of a course in radiographic positioning. Every technologist has the obligation **to ensure that the radiation dose to both the patient and other health care professionals is kept as low as reasonably achievable (ALARA).**

Radiologic technologists are the last line of defense between patients and unnecessary radiation exposure, making radiation protection awareness of primary importance.

It is important to keep in mind that the three most effective ways to protect patients and staff from ionizing radiation are:

1. **Time**—Minimize radiation beam-on time
2. **Distance**—Maximize distance from the radiation source of both patients and staff
3. **Shielding**—Use shielding on staff and patients

Radiation Units

Determining the amount of radiation is a critical element in protecting patients and staff. The most important quantities for a radiographic technologist to be familiar with are absorbed dose (Gy/rad) and equivalent dose (Sv/rem). Personnel badge reports typically use equivalent dose to quantify radiation, whereas radiography and fluoroscopy equipment tends to display absorbed dose to help estimate patient dose during procedures. Additional terms used to quantify radiation are defined next and include exposure, air kerma, absorbed dose, equivalent dose, and effective dose.

Exposure (C/Kg or **R)**—measures the amount of ionization created in air by x-rays. Roentgen (R) or coulomb per kilogram (C/Kg) are the units of exposure. X-ray tube output, patient entrance exposure, and scattered radiation levels are usually indicated by measurements of exposure.

Air kerma (Gy or **rad)**—indicates the amount of energy transferred to a mass of air by the photons; this has replaced exposure as the preferred quantity for the applications listed above. The unit of measurement for air kerma is the gray **(Gy)** or **rad.**

Absorbed dose (Gy or **rad)** is the amount of energy deposited per unit mass by the interactions of ionizing radiation with tissue and has units of **gray (Gy)** or **rad.**

Equivalent dose (Sv or **rem)** quantifies the risk for different types of radiation using the same relative scale; the units are **sieverts (Sv)** or **rem.** The product of the absorbed dose and the radiation-weighting factor yields the equivalent dose. The radiation-weighting factor depends on the type and energy of the radiation. In radiography, the radiation-weighting factor is always one. When a patient is x-rayed, air kerma, absorbed dose, and equivalent dose all are considered numerically equal but have different conceptual meanings.

Effective dose (Sv or **rem)** indicates the risk from a partial body exposure by multiplying the equivalent dose by the tissue-weighting factor that corresponds to the area of the body that is exposed. Effective dose allows comparisons of the relative risk from various imaging procedures and exposure of different areas of the body.

Traditional and SI Units

The SI system has been the international standard for units of radiation measurement since 1958. However, just as the United States has been slow to convert to the metric system for other applications, traditional units of radiation measurement such as the roentgen, rad, and rem are still in common use in the United States. Dose limits and patient doses in this section are designated in both SI and traditional units (1 gray = 100 rads and 1 rad = 10 mGy) (Table 1.11). The gray is an extremely large unit for most dose considerations in medicine. A smaller unit of milligray is often used (1000 mGy = 1 Gy).

DOSE LIMITS

High doses of radiation are harmful. Scientists have established dose limits to help eliminate the risk of adverse effects (Table 1.12). The rationale for the dose limits is to make risk from occupational exposure comparable to the risks for workers in other safe industries (excluding mining and agriculture). The annual dose limit for occupationally exposed workers is **50 mSv (5000 mrem)** whole-body effective dose equivalent. Higher annual dose limits are applied for partial body exposure: 150 mSv (15,000 mrem) for the lens of the eye and 500 mSv (50,000 mrem) for the skin, hands, and feet. Medical radiation received as a patient and background radiation are not included in these occupational dose limits.

The annual dose limit for the general public is 1 mSv (100 mrem) for frequent exposure and 5 mSv (500 mrem) for infrequent exposure. For practical purposes, the shielding design for x-ray facilities is based on the lower limit. In essence, the facility must demonstrate that x-ray operation is unlikely to deliver a dose greater than 1 mSv to any member of the public over a period of 1 year.

The recommended cumulative lifetime dose for the occupationally exposed worker is 10 mSv (1 rem) times the age in years. For example,

TABLE 1.11 **CONVERSION TABLE—TRADITIONAL TO SI UNITS**		
TO CONVERT FROM (TRADITIONAL UNITS)	**TO (SI UNITS)**	**MULTIPLY BY**
Roentgen (R)	C/kg	2.58×10^{-4} (0.000258)
Rad	Gray (Gy)	10^{-2} (1 rad = 0.01 Gy)
Rem	Sievert (Sv)	10^{-2} (1 rem = 0.01 Sv)

TABLE 1.12 **SUMMARY OF DOSE-LIMITING RECOMMENDATIONS**							
OCCUPATIONAL WORKERS[a]		**GENERAL PUBLIC**		**INDIVIDUALS <18 YEARS OLD**		**PREGNANT WORKERS**	
Annual	50 mSv (5 rem)	Annual	1 mSv (100 mrem)	Annual	1 mSv (100 mrem)	Month	0.5 mSv (50 mrem)
Lifetime accumulation	10 mSv (1 rem) × years of age					Gestation period	5 mSv (500 mrem)

[a]Whole-body effective dose equivalent.

a 50-year-old technologist has a recommended accumulated dose of no more than 500 mSv (50 rem). However, the principle of ALARA should be practiced so that the occupational dose is accrued at a rate that is very much less than the dose limit of 50 mSv (5 rem) per year.

Individuals younger than 18 years of age should not be employed in situations in which they are occupationally exposed. The dose limit for minors is the same as that for the general public—1 mSv (0.1 rem) per year.

PERSONNEL MONITORING

Personnel monitoring refers to the measurement of the amount of radiation dose received by occupationally exposed individuals. The monitor offers no protection but simply provides an indication of radiation dose received by the wearer of the monitoring device. On a periodic basis (monthly or quarterly), the personnel monitor (film badge, thermoluminescent dosimeter [TLD], or optically stimulated luminescence dosimeter [OSL]) is exchanged for a new one. A commercial personnel dosimetry company processes the dosimeter, and the radiation dose for the period is determined. Measurement of occupational dose is an essential aspect of radiation safety as a means to ensure that workers do not exceed the dose limit and to assess that the dose received is reasonable for the work activities.

Each worker who is likely to receive 10% of the dose limit must be issued a personnel monitor. Generally, health care professionals, including emergency department and operating room nursing personnel, who are occasionally present when mobile x-ray equipment is in operation, do not require personnel monitoring devices. The radiation dose received by nursing personnel (with the exception of some angiography and cath lab nursing staff) is typically less than 10% of the annual dose limit. Clerical and support staff working near the x-ray room do not need and should not be monitored with a personnel dosimeter.

The personnel dosimeter is worn at the level of the chest or waist during radiography (Fig. 1.179). If an individual is involved in fluoroscopic procedures, the dose under the apron is known to be a small fraction of the dose to the head and neck.[14,15] The dosimeter should be positioned on the collar outside the protective apron (or outside the thyroid collar) during fluoroscopy. The personnel dosimeter should not be worn on the sleeve. The collar reading greatly overestimates the dose to the total body. To account for the protective effect of the apron and determine an effective whole-body dose (called the *effective dose equivalent*), the collar reading is multiplied by a factor of 0.3. A measured value of 3 mSv (300 mrem) for the collar dosimeter is equivalent to a whole-body dose of 0.9 mSv (90 mrem). The annual dose limit of 50 mSv (5000 mrem) applies to the effective dose equivalent.

When not in use, personnel monitoring devices should remain at the place of employment in a low-background area, such as a locker or office. Personnel monitoring devices should not be stored in areas of x-ray use.

ALARA

In recent years, radiation protection measures have been devised according to the principle of ALARA. Radiation exposure should be maintained at the lowest practicable level and very much below the dose limits. All technologists should practice the ALARA principle so that patients and other health care professionals do not receive unnecessary radiation. Following is a summary of four important ways that ALARA can be achieved:

1. **Always wear a personnel monitoring device.** Although the device does not reduce the dose to the wearer, exposure history has an important impact on protection practices. Radiologic technologists should ensure that individuals present during x-ray operation wear personnel monitors as appropriate.
2. **Mechanical holding devices** (e.g., compression bands, sponges, sandbags, and 2-inch-wide tape) are effective tools for the

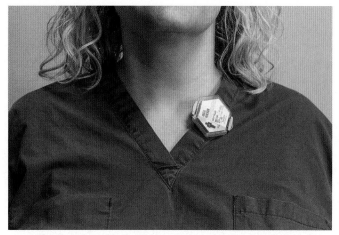

Fig. 1.179 Technologist wearing a personnel dosimeter.

immobilization of patients and should be used if the procedure permits. Only as a last resort should someone hold the patient. The following criteria are applicable for the selection of someone to hold a patient during a radiographic procedure:
- No individual shall be regularly used to hold patients.
- An individual who is pregnant shall not hold patients.
- An individual younger than 18 years of age shall not hold patients.
- Whenever possible, an individual occupationally exposed to radiation shall not hold patients during exposures.
- A parent or family member should be used to hold the patient if necessary.
- A hospital employee who is not occupationally exposed may be used to hold the patient if necessary.
- If an individual holds the patient, he or she is provided with a protective apron and gloves. The individual is positioned so that the primary beam exposes no part of his or her body except hands and arms. Only individuals required for the radiographic procedure should be in the room during exposure. All persons in the room except the patient are provided protective devices.

3. Close collimation, filtration of the primary beam, optimum kVp technique, high-speed IRs, and avoidance of repeat projections reduce the dose to the patient.
4. Practice the three cardinal principles of radiation protection: time, distance, and shielding. The technologist should minimize the time in the radiation field, stand as far away from the source as possible, and use shielding (protective devices or control booth barrier). For individuals not shielded by a protective barrier during x-ray operation, the radiologic technologist should ensure that these persons wear lead aprons and gloves as appropriate.

Exposure to persons outside a shielded barrier is due primarily to scattered radiation from the patient. Therefore, a reduction in patient exposure results in decreased dose to workers in unshielded locations. Protection from scatter radiation is an important consideration during mobile C-arm fluoroscopy, as described in detail in Chapter 15 in the discussion of trauma and mobile radiography.

In the absence of a radiologist during an x-ray examination, the radiologic technologist generally has the highest level of training in radiation protection in a patient care setting. An essential component of a radiation safety program is that individuals present during x-ray operation wear protective lead aprons and personnel monitors as appropriate. Management must have a clearly defined and enforced radiation safety policy, which includes the use of protective apparel and designates who can hold patients. Individuals who do not follow radiation safety policy of the institution should be subject to disciplinary action.

PREGNANT TECHNOLOGISTS

Studies have shown that the fetus is sensitive to high doses of ionizing radiation, especially during the first 3 months of gestation. A small risk of harmful effects from low doses of radiation is assumed, but not proven, to exist. That is, any radiation dose, however small, is considered to increase probability of harm to the fetus.

Effective, fair management of pregnant employees exposed to radiation requires the balancing of three factors: (1) the rights of the expectant mother to pursue her career without discrimination based on gender, (2) the protection of the fetus, and (3) the needs of the employer. Each health care organization should establish a realistic policy that addresses these three concerns by clearly articulating the expectations of the employer and the options available to the employee. A sample pregnancy policy for radiation workers has been published in the literature.[16] The pregnant technologist should review the institutional policy and other professional references and consult with the radiation safety officer (if available) to determine expectations and the best practices to protect her unborn child.

The recommended equivalent dose limits to the embryo/fetus is 0.5 mSv (50 mrem) during any 1 month and 5 mSv (500 mrem) for the gestation period. To recognize the increased radiosensitivity of the fetus, the total fetal dose is restricted to a level that is much less than that allowed for the occupationally exposed mother. However, the expectant mother's exposure from other sources, such as medical procedures, is excluded from the fetus dose limit. The fetal dose limit can be applied only if the employer is informed of the pregnancy. The regulations define the declared pregnant woman as one who voluntarily informed her employer, in writing, of her pregnancy and the estimated date of conception.

In recent years, radiation protection measures have been devised according to the principle of ALARA. Radiation exposure should be maintained at the lowest practicable level. **Radiation protection practices do not change because the worker becomes pregnant.** The measures that reduce the dose to the worker also reduce the dose to the fetus. The major ways to decrease the dose further are to restrict the type of tasks performed or to limit the number of times a particular task is performed.

When an employee first discovers she is pregnant, an individualized review of her exposure history and work assignments should be conducted. If she averaged 0.3 mSv (30 mrem) per month for the last several months, a reasonable projection is that this individual, and her unborn child, will not receive more than 5 mSv (500 mrem) during the period of gestation. This radiologic technologist could continue to work in her current capacity during her pregnancy. However, she should monitor her dosimeter readings and report any unusual reading to the radiation safety officer. Contrary to general belief, fluoroscopy procedures do not cause high exposures to the fetus. In fluoroscopy, attenuation by the lead apron and by overlying maternal tissues reduces the dose to the fetus. Personnel dosimeter readings totaling

5 mSv (500 mrem) at the collar correspond to a fetal dose of 0.075 mSv (7.5 mrem). Therefore, radiologic technologists can continue their work assignments in fluoroscopy throughout pregnancy.

A declared pregnant radiation worker may monitor the dose to the fetus by placing a second dosimeter at waist level under the protective apron. This monitoring method generally produces readings below the detectable limit of the dosimeter and is useful only in demonstrating that the fetus received no measurable radiation exposure. The fetal badge must be clearly marked to distinguish the device worn under the apron from that worn at the collar.

RADIOGRAPHIC PATIENT DOSE

For a particular radiographic examination, several different "doses" may be used to characterize patient dose. The most common descriptor is the exposure to the skin in the region where the x-rays enter the body, called the *entrance skin exposure*. Air kerma is rapidly replacing exposure because it is easily converted to skin dose with the application of the backscatter factor. The backscatter factor takes into account the additional dose at the surface caused by scattering from tissue within the irradiated volume. As the x-rays directed toward the IR pass through the body, attenuation causes a dramatic reduction in dose (Fig. 1.180). Exit dose is often a small percentage of the entrance dose. Specific organ dose varies depending on depth and radiation quality. If the organ is located outside the primary beam, dose is from scattered radiation only and is a small fraction of the in-beam dose. Entrance air kerma and organ doses from common radiographic examinations are shown in Table 1.13. These values represent multiple facilities but vary according to technique factors, type of IR, field size, and patient size.

The **effective dose (ED)** takes into account the respective dose to each organ and the cumulated relative risk from all organs that received dose. This dose metric essentially specifies a whole-body dose that yields the same overall risk as incurred by the nonuniform dose distribution in the patient. Effective dose becomes a means to compare different imaging procedures with respect to potential for harm (Table 1.14).

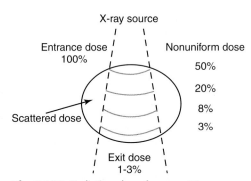

Fig. 1.180 Radiation dose from an AP abdomen decreases markedly from the entrance side to the exit side of the patient.

TABLE 1.13 PATIENT DOSE CHART

PROJECTION	ENTRANCE AIR KERMA (MGY)	ORGAN DOSE (MGY)				
		TESTES	OVARIES	THYROID	MARROW	UTERUS
Chest PA	0.2	<0.001	<0.001	0.008	0.02	<0.001
Skull (lateral)	1.7	<0.001	<0.001	0.05	0.06	<0.001
Abdomen AP	4.0	0.09	1.0	<0.001	0.19	1.3
Retrogram pyelogram	6.0	0.13	1.5	<0.001	0.29	2.0
Cervical spine AP	1.1	<0.001	<0.001	0.9	0.02	<0.001
Thoracic spine AP	4.0	<0.001	0.003	0.5	0.16	0.002
Lumbar spine AP	3.4	0.02	0.52	0.002	0.16	1.0

TABLE 1.14 EFFECTIVE DOSE (ED)

EXAMINATION	EFFECTIVE DOSE (MSV)	EXAMINATION	EFFECTIVE DOSE (MSV)
Skull	0.07	Cerebral angiography	2.0
Chest	0.14	Cardiac angiography	7.3
Abdomen	0.53		
Lumbar spine	1.8	PTCA	22
Thoracic spine	1.4	Barium enema	20
Cervical spine	0.27	CT head	2.3
Extremities	0.06	CT abdomen	13
Mammography	0.22	CT coronary angiography	20
Upper GI	3.6		
Small bowel	6.4		

PTCA, Percutaneous transluminal coronary angiography.

Patient Protection in Radiography

Radiologic technologists subscribe to a code of ethics that includes responsibility to control the radiation dose to all patients under their care. This is a serious responsibility, and each of the following seven ways of reducing patient exposure must be understood and put into practice as described in the next sections:

1. Minimum repeat radiographs
2. Correct filtration
3. Accurate collimation
4. Specific area shielding (gonadal and female breast shielding)
5. Protection of the fetus
6. Optimum imaging system speed
7. Select projections and technique factors appropriate for the examination
   - Use high-kVp and low-mAs techniques
   - Use PA rather than AP projections to reduce dose to anterior upper thoracic region (thyroid and female breasts) (see Chapter 8)
   - Use techniques consistent with system speed for digital radiography as confirmed by exposure indicator values

MINIMUM REPEAT RADIOGRAPHS

The first basic and most important method to prevent unnecessary exposure is to **avoid repeat radiographs.** A primary cause of repeat radiographs is poor communication between the technologist and the patient. Unclear and misunderstood breathing instructions are a common cause of motion, which requires a repeat radiograph.

When the procedures are not explained clearly, the patient can have added anxiety and nervousness from fear of the unknown. Stress often increases the patient's mental confusion and hinders his or her ability to cooperate fully. To engage the patient, the technologist must take the time, even with heavy workloads, to explain carefully and fully the breathing instructions and the procedure in general in simple terms that the patient can understand (Fig. 1.181). Patients must be forewarned of any movements or strange noises by equipment that may occur during the examination. In addition, any burning sensation or other possible effects of injections should be explained to the patient.

Avoid carelessness in positioning and selection of erroneous technique factors, as these are common causes of repeats. Correct and accurate positioning requires a thorough knowledge and understanding of anatomy, which enables the technologist to visualize the size, shape, and location of structures to be radiographed. This is the reason that every chapter in this text combines anatomy with positioning.

CORRECT FILTRATION

Filtration of the primary x-ray beam reduces exposure to the patient by preferentially absorbing low-energy "unusable" x-rays, which mainly expose the patient's skin and superficial tissue without contributing to image formation. The effect of filtration is a "hardening" of the x-ray beam, which shifts the beam to a higher effective energy, resulting in increased penetrability (Fig. 1.182).

Filtration is described in two ways. First is inherent or built-in filtration from components of the x-ray tube itself. For most radiographic tubes, this is approximately 0.5 mm aluminum equivalent. Second, and more important to technologists, is **added filtration,** which is accomplished by placing a metal filter (aluminum or copper or combination of these) in the beam within the collimator housing. The amount of **minimum total filtration** as established by federal regulations depends on the operating kVp range. The manufacturers of x-ray equipment are required to meet these standards. Minimum total filtration (inherent plus added) for diagnostic radiology (excluding mammography) is 2.5 mm aluminum for equipment operating at 70 kVp or higher.

Often, radiographic equipment has variable added filtration, which can be selected by the technologist. Added filtration becomes another component to adapt the acquisition parameters to the patient. Generally, as patient size increases, more added filtration provides skin dose sparing. The technique chart should specify the use of added filtration. The technologist has the responsibility to ensure that proper filtration is in place.

The filtration of each x-ray tube **should be checked annually and after major repair** (x-ray tube or collimator replacement). Qualified personnel, such as the medical physicist, should test the filtration of each tube. The test typically used to ensure adequate filtration is measurement of the half-value layer.

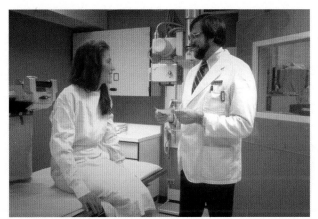

Fig. 1.181 Clear, precise instructions help relieve patient anxieties and prevent unnecessary repeats.

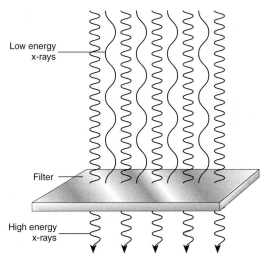

Fig. 1.182 A metal filter preferentially removes low-energy x-rays, shifting the x-ray beam to higher effective energy.

ACCURATE COLLIMATION

Accurate collimation reduces patient exposure by **limiting the size and shape of the x-ray field to the area of clinical interest.** Careful and accurate collimation is emphasized and demonstrated throughout this textbook. The adjustable collimator is used routinely for general diagnostic radiography. The illuminated light field defines the x-ray field on accurately calibrated equipment and can be used effectively to determine the tissue area to be irradiated. Safety standards require light field and x-ray field concurrence within **2% of the selected SID.**

The concept of divergence of the x-ray beam must be considered for accurate collimation. Therefore, the illuminated field size as it appears on the skin surface appears smaller than the actual size of the anatomic area, which would be visualized on the IR. This is most evident on a projection such as lateral thoracic or lumbar spine (Fig. 1.183), in which the distance from the skin surface to the IR is considerable. In such cases, the light field, when collimated correctly to the area of interest, appears too small unless one considers the divergence of the x-ray beam.

Collimation and Tissue Dose

Accurate and close collimation to the area of interest results in a dramatic drop-off in tissue dose as distance from the border of the collimated x-ray field is increased. For example, the dose **3 cm** from the edge of the x-ray field is about **10%** of that within the x-ray field. At a distance of **12 cm** the reduction in dose is about **1%** of that within the x-ray field.

Positive Beam Limitation

All general-purpose x-ray equipment built between 1974 and 1993 in the United States required collimators with positive beam limitation (PBL) that automatically adjusts the useful x-ray beam to the film size (this requirement became optional after May 3, 1993, as a result of a change in U.S. Food and Drug Administration [FDA] regulations). The PBL feature consists of sensors in the cassette holder that, when activated by placing a cassette in the bucky tray, automatically signal the collimator to adjust the x-ray field to that film size. PBL can be deactivated or overridden with a key, but this should be done only under special circumstances, in which collimation by manual control is needed. A red warning light is illuminated to indicate that PBL has been deactivated. The key cannot be removed while PBL is overridden (Fig. 1.184).

Manual Collimation

Even with automatic collimation (PBL), the operator can manually reduce the collimation field size. This adjustment should be made for every projection in which the IR is larger than the critical area to be radiographed. Accurate manual collimation also is required for upper and lower limbs that are radiographed on the tabletop, in which PBL is not engaged. Throughout the positioning pages in this textbook, collimation guidelines are provided to maximize patient protection through careful and accurate collimation.

The practice of close collimation to only the area of interest reduces patient dose in **two ways.** First, the **volume of tissue directly irradiated is diminished,** and second, the **amount of accompanying scattered radiation is decreased.** Scatter radiation produced by additional tissue in the x-ray field from improper collimation or lack of shielding not only adds unnecessary patient dose but also degrades image quality through the "fogging" effect of scatter radiation. (This is especially true in high-volume tissue imaging such as abdomen and chest.)

The practice of visible collimation on all four sides of a radiograph reduces patient exposure, improves image quality, and acts as a method to ensure that appropriate collimation did occur. If no collimation border is visible on the radiograph, evidence does not exist that the primary beam was restricted to the area of clinical interest. An added benefit of showing the extent of collimation on all four sides is the ability to check the final radiograph for correct central ray location. As described previously, this is done by imagining a large X extending from the four corners of the collimation field, the center of which is the CR location.

Collimation Rule

A general rule followed throughout this text indicates that collimation should **limit the x-ray field to only the area of interest, and collimation borders should be visible on the IR on all four sides** if the IR size is large enough to allow four-sided collimation without cutting off essential anatomy.

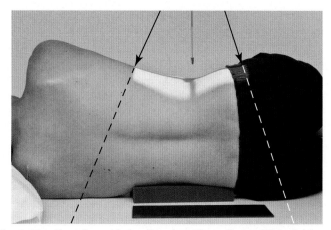

Fig. 1.183 Close four-sided collimation. The collimated light field may appear too small because of divergence of x-rays.

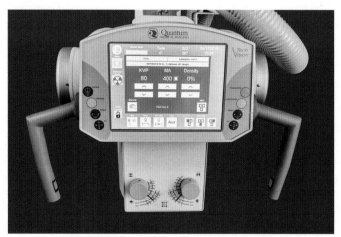

Fig. 1.184 Automatic collimation (PBL).

SPECIFIC AREA SHIELDING

Specific area shielding can be used to protect radiosensitive organs, such as the thyroid gland, breasts, and gonads, when they are in the useful beam and the use of such shielding does not interfere with the objectives of the examination. Historically the most commonly shielded area has been the gonads, which significantly lowers the dose to the reproductive organs. Gonadal shields, if placed correctly, reduce the gonadal dose by 50% to 90% if the gonads are in the primary x-ray field. Recent studies have shown that the breasts are actually more radiosensitive than the gonads and thus the efficacy of gonadal shielding is being brought into question. Additionally, improper placement of gonadal shields is a common and well-documented problem. Furthermore, the use of the same contact shield on different patients can lead to infection control issues, particularly in sensitive patients such as those in the neonatal intensive care unit (NICU). These factors have led some institutions to eliminate or more closely monitor gonadal shielding, because often the benefit does not outweigh the risk. Although there is evidence that gonadal shielding may not offer as much protection as originally anticipated, it is still recommended in many countries and in most states within the U.S.

The two general types of specific area shielding are shadow shields and contact shields.

Shadow Shields

As the name implies, **shadow shields,** which are attached to the collimator, are placed between the x-ray tube and the patient and cast a shadow on the patient when the collimator light is turned on. The position of the shadow shield is adjusted to define the shielded area. One such type of breast shadow shields, as shown in Fig. 1.185, is affixed to the collimator exit surface with Velcro. Another type of shadow shield, as shown in Fig. 1.186, is mounted with magnets directly to the bottom of the collimator. These shields may be combined with clear lead compensating filters to provide more uniform exposure for body parts that vary in thickness or density, such as for a thoracic and lumbar spine scoliosis radiograph (Fig. 1.187).

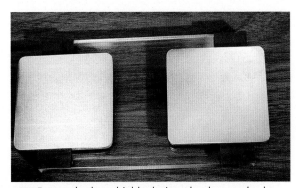

Fig. 1.185 Breast shadow shields designed to be attached to collimator exit surface with Velcro.

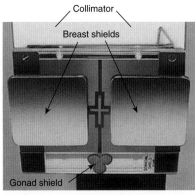

Fig. 1.186 Shadow shields in place under collimator (attached with magnets). (Courtesy Nuclear Associates, Carle, NY.)

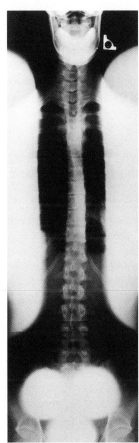

Fig. 1.187 AP spine for scoliosis with compensating filter and breast and gonadal shields in place. (Courtesy Nuclear Associates, Carle, NY.)

Contact Shields

Flat gonadal contact shields are used most commonly for patients in recumbent positions. Vinyl-covered lead shields are placed over the gonadal area to attenuate scatter or leakage radiation or both (Fig. 1.188). These shields usually are made from the same lead-impregnated vinyl materials that compose lead aprons. Gonadal contact shields, 1 mm lead equivalent, absorb 95% to 99% of primary rays in the 50- to 100-kVp range. Examples of these include small vinyl-covered lead material cut into various shapes to be placed directly over the reproductive organs, as shown in Figs. 1.189 and 1.190.

Male

Gonadal shields should be placed distally to the symphysis pubis, covering the area of the testes and scrotum (see Fig. 1.189A). The upper margin of the shield should be at the symphysis pubis. These shields are tapered slightly at the top and are wider at the bottom to cover the testes and scrotum without obscuring pelvic and hip structures. Smaller sizes should be used for smaller males or children.

Female

Gonadal shielding is placed to cover the area of the ovaries, uterine (fallopian) tubes, and uterus but may be more difficult to achieve. A general guideline for women is to shield an area 4½ to 5 inches (11 to 13 cm) proximal or superior to the symphysis pubis extending 3 to 3½ inches (8 to 9 cm) each way from the pelvic midline. The lower border of the shield should be at or slightly above the symphysis pubis, with the upper border extending just above the level of the anterior superior iliac spines (ASIS) (see Fig. 1.190A).

Various-shaped female ovarian shields may be used, but they should be wider in the upper region to cover the area of the ovaries and narrower toward the bottom to offer less obstruction of pelvic or hip structures. The shielded area should be proportionally smaller on children. For example, a 1-year-old girl would require a shield that is only about 2 to 3 inches (6 to 7 cm) wide and 2 inches (5 cm) high placed directly superior to the symphysis pubis.[18]

Summary of Rules for Specific Area Shielding

Proper specific area shielding is a challenge for each technologist because its use requires additional time and equipment. Additionally, improper shielding can lead to repeat examinations, thus defeating their intention:

1. **Gonadal shielding should be considered for all patients.** A common policy of many imaging facilities directs the use of specific area shielding for all children and adults of reproductive age.
2. Placement of gonadal shielding is necessary **when the organ of concern lies within or near (2 inches [5 cm]) the primary beam,** unless such shielding obscures essential diagnostic information or may introduce pathogens to a sensitive patient population.
3. **Accurate beam collimation** and careful positioning are essential. Specific area shielding is an additional protective measure but no substitute for accurate collimation.

PREGNANT PATIENT

All women of childbearing age should be screened for the possibility of pregnancy before x-ray examination of the abdomen or pelvis area. This concern is particularly critical during the first 2 months of pregnancy, when the fetus is most sensitive to radiation and the mother may not yet be aware of the pregnancy. Posters or signs (Figs. 1.191 and 1.192) should be prominently displayed in examination rooms and waiting room areas, reminding the

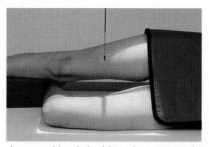

Fig. 1.188 Vinyl-covered lead shield in place over pelvis for lateral mid and distal femur.

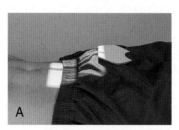
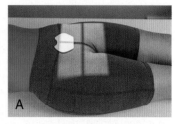
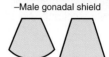

−Male gonadal shield

−Female ovarian shield

Possible shapes

Possible shapes

Fig. 1.189 A, AP pelvis with flat contact shield (1 mm lead equivalent). B, Male gonadal shield shapes.

Fig. 1.190 A, AP right hip with flat contact shield (1 mm lead equivalent). B, Female ovarian shield shapes.

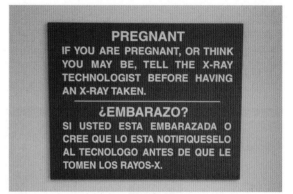

PREGNANT

IF YOU ARE PREGNANT, OR THINK YOU MAY BE, TELL THE X-RAY TECHNOLOGIST BEFORE HAVING AN X-RAY TAKEN.

¿EMBARAZO?

SI USTED ESTA EMBARAZADA O CREE QUE LO ESTA NOTIFIQUESELO AL TECNOLOGO ANTES DE QUE LE TOMEN LOS RAYOS-X.

Fig. 1.191 Warning sign. (From Ehrlich RA, Coakes D: *Patient care in radiography*, ed 9, St. Louis, 2017, Elsevier.)

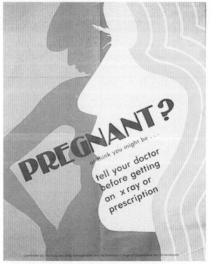

Fig. 1.192 Warning poster.

patient to inform the technologist of any known or potential pregnancy.

If the patient **indicates that she is pregnant or may be pregnant,** the technologist should consult the radiologist before proceeding with the examination. If the mother's health is at risk and clear indications for an imaging study exist, the examination should not be denied or delayed because of the pregnancy. Radiation protection practices already described, especially **careful collimation,** should be used.

For examinations of body parts above the diaphragm or below the hips, the scattered dose to the fetus is very low, and the examination may proceed normally. For examinations in which the fetus is in the direct beam and the estimated fetal dose is less than 10 mGy (1 rad), the radiation dose should be kept as low as possible consistent with obtaining the desired diagnostic information. Shielding of the abdomen and pelvis with a lead apron should be considered. Limiting the number of views should be considered. For examinations in which the fetus is in the direct beam and the estimated fetal dose is greater than 10 mGy (1 rad), the radiologist and referring physician should discuss other options such as sonography and MRI that can provide the needed information.

If the x-ray imaging procedure is deemed appropriate, the patient should be informed of the risks and benefits of the procedure. The clinician responsible for the care of the patient should document in the medical record that the test is indicated for the management of the patient.

In the past, the **10-day** or **LMP rule** (last menstrual period) was applied to prevent exposure to the embryo/fetus early in pregnancy, when the pregnancy is not known. This rule stated that all radiologic examinations involving the pelvis and lower abdomen should be scheduled during the first 10 days following the onset of menstruation because conception will not have occurred during this period. Currently, this rule is considered obsolete because the potential harm associated with canceling essential x-ray procedures may greatly exceed the risk of the fetal radiation dose.

The following examinations deliver a dose of less than 10 mGy (1 rad) to the embryo/fetus:

- Extremities
- Chest
- Skull
- Thoracic spine
- Head CT
- Chest CT

The following examinations have the potential to deliver a dose of more than 10 mGy (1 rad) to the fetus and embryo:

- Lumbar spine series
- Fluoroscopic procedures (abdomen)
- Abdomen or pelvis with three or more views
- Scoliosis: full series
- CT abdomen
- CT pelvis

OPTIMUM SPEED

Analog imaging systems. As a general guideline, the highest-speed film-screen combination that results in diagnostically acceptable radiographs is desirable to manage patient dose. The presence of the screen does result in some loss of spatial resolution and becomes more pronounced as the speed is increased. The radiologist must balance the reduction in patient exposure with the potential loss of detail in the resultant image. A common practice is to select a slow 100-speed (detail) screen with tabletop procedures, such as upper and lower limbs, when a grid is not used and spatial detail is important. A 400-speed screen is commonly preferred for larger body parts when grids and higher-exposure techniques are required. For other applications, a 200-speed screen may be preferred. Departmental protocol generally indicates the film-screen combination for each procedure. This is not a decision that is usually made by individual technologists.

Digital imaging systems have essentially replaced film-screen for most radiographic applications. These digital receptors are more sensitive than film-screen and have the potential to reduce patient dose greatly. In addition, their wide dynamic range can result in fewer repeated "films." Automatic exposure control (AEC) for digital systems is usually set at an exposure indicator level that produces images with an acceptable level of noise. However, the technologist may adjust the AEC density control to change the effective system speed. The wide dynamic range of digital receptors enables this variation in dose while still producing a quality image (although noise becomes more pronounced as the dose is reduced). Because the FPD-TFT is often integrated into the radiographic unit, the variable-speed option is readily available to customize the speed for each imaging protocol.

SELECTION OF PROJECTIONS AND EXPOSURE FACTORS WITH THE LEAST PATIENT DOSE

The seventh and final method to reduce patient dose requires an understanding of the factors that affect patient dose. For example, technologists should know that patient dose is decreased with AEC use when the kVp is increased. For manual technique, an increase in kVp with no change in mAs results in a higher dose to the patient. The goal is to use the combination of technique factors that will provide acceptable image quality and minimize patient dose.

There is a substantial difference in dose to the thyroid and female breasts for the AP projection compared with the PA projection for the head, neck, and upper thorax region. The ovarian dose can be reduced for certain projections, such as a female hip, if a specific area shield is correctly placed. An axiolateral or inferosuperior lateral hip projection compared with a lateral hip projection delivers a higher dose to the testes.

RADIATION SAFETY PRACTICES

Technologists must adhere to ethical and safe practice when using digital technology. The wide dynamic range of digital imaging enables an acceptable image to be obtained with a broad range of exposure factors. During the evaluation of the quality of an image, the technologist must ensure the exposure indicator is within the recommended range. Any attempt to process an image with a different algorithm to correct overexposure is unacceptable; it is vital that patient dose be minimized at the outset and the ALARA principle be upheld.

To maintain dose at a reasonable, consistent dose level, the following practices are recommended:

1. Use protocol-specific kVp and mAs values for all procedures. If no exposure protocol exists, consult with the lead technologist, physicist, or manufacturer to establish one. Increasing kVp by 5 to 10 and decreasing mAs by the equivalent ratio can produce a quality image with digital imaging systems while reducing patient dose.
2. Monitor dose by reviewing all images to ensure radiographs were obtained with the established exposure indicator.
3. If the exposure indicator for a given procedure is outside of the acceptable range, review all factors, including kVp and mAs, to determine the cause of this disparity. Processing of digital images can be adversely affected if the exposure indicator deviates from the manufacturer's acceptable values.

Fluoroscopic Patient Dose

Because fluoroscopy can potentially deliver a **high patient dose,** federal standards have set a limit of 10 R/min for the tabletop exposure rate, which corresponds to an air kerma rate of 88 mGy/min. In **high-level fluoroscopy (HLF) mode,** the exposure rate at tabletop cannot exceed 20 R/min or an air kerma rate of 176 mGy/min. For C-arm fluoroscopic units, the point of measurement is specified as 30 cm from the image receptor. HLF mode should be reserved for instances in which the lack of penetration creates a poor image (large patients). There is no exposure rate limit when the image is recorded, as in digital cine and serial digital spot filming. With most modern equipment, the average tabletop fluoroscopy exposure rate is 1 to 3 R/min (air kerma rate of 8.8 to 26 mGy/min). Use of magnification mode increases the instantaneous exposure rate but decreases the volume of tissue irradiated.

Typical patient doses during gastrointestinal fluoroscopy procedures are shown in Table 1.15, which includes approximate entrance air kerma during fluoroscopy and spot filming. Fluoroscopic procedures generally involve a much higher patient dose than conventional overhead-tube radiographic examinations because of the need to penetrate the contrast medium and the time required to conduct the study. The volume of tissue exposed during fluoroscopy and spot filming is fairly small.

Dose Area Product

The FDA requires fluoroscopic units manufactured after 2006 to provide a means for the operator to monitor radiation output. Two types of readout, **dose area product (DAP)** and **cumulative total dose,** have been developed for this purpose. The total dose in mGy represents the dose to a point at a specific distance from the focal spot. DAP is a quantity that indicates a combination of dose and the amount of tissue irradiated. It is calculated as the product of the air kerma and the cross-sectional area of the beam, expressed in units of $\mu Gy\text{-}m^2$ or $cGy\text{-}cm^2$ or $rad\text{-}cm^2$. Some manufacturers also provide DAP readings for general diagnostic radiography as well.

SKIN INJURY

The FDA has issued a **Public Health Advisory** regarding radiation-induced skin injuries from fluoroscopic procedures. These injuries are usually delayed, so the physician cannot discern damage by observing the patient immediately after the procedure. The radiation dose required to cause skin injury is typically 3 Gy (300 rad) for temporary epilation (onset 2 to 3 weeks after exposure), 6 Gy (600 rad) for main erythema (onset 10 to 14 days after exposure), and 15 to 20 Gy (1500 to 2000 rad) for moist desquamation (onset several weeks after exposure).

The procedures of concern are primarily interventional procedures during which fluoroscopy is used to guide instruments. The risk of skin injury is associated with prolonged fluoroscopy time and multiple digital cine acquisitions **to a single skin site.** At the maximum rate of 10 R/min, the fluoroscopy time must exceed 30 minutes to cause skin injury (see Table 1.15). However, during angiography, the patient may be positioned close to the x-ray tube, where the fluoroscopy exposure rate can exceed 10 R/min. Digital recording may use very high exposure rates. If digital recording is performed, fluoroscopic skin injuries occur much more rapidly. Monitoring of the total dose or DAP during interventional procedures is essential for the prevention of skin injury.

DOSE REDUCTION TECHNIQUES DURING FLUOROSCOPY

Most operators are trained to activate the x-ray beam for a few seconds at a time, long enough to view the current catheter position or the bolus of contrast agent. Total fluoroscopic times can be reduced dramatically with **intermittent fluoroscopy.** This technique is particularly effective when combined with last image hold. Many modern fluoroscopy systems have the capability to retain the last fluoroscopic image on the monitor after x-ray exposure is terminated. This allows the physician to study the most recent acquisition and plan the next task without radiation exposure to the patient.

During pulsed fluoroscopy, the x-ray beam is emitted as a series of short pulses rather than continuously. For conventional fluoroscopy, the image is acquired and displayed at a constant 30 frames per second. Pulsed fluoroscopy at 15 frames per second compared with the usual 30 frames per second demonstrates substantial dose reduction (factor of 2). However, manufacturers may increase the

TABLE 1.15 **TYPICAL PATIENT DOSE DURING FLUOROSCOPY**	
UPPER GI	
DIVISION OF USE	**MAXIMUM IN ONE LOCATION**
17 spot films	5 spot films at 1.75 mGy each
5 minutes of fluoroscopy	1.5 minutes at 26 mGy/min
Total maximum entrance air kerma: 48 mGy	
Total maximum entrance exposure: 5.5 R	
DOUBLE-CONTRAST BARIUM ENEMA	
DIVISION OF USE	**MAXIMUM IN ONE LOCATION**
11 spot films	3 spot films at 1 mGy each
7 minutes of fluoroscopy	1.5 minutes at 35 mGy/min
Total maximum entrance air kerma: 55 mGy	
Total maximum entrance exposure: 6.3 R	

radiation level per frame to achieve a more pleasing visual appearance (less noise), and the dose reduction may be only 25%. Mobile C-arm fluoroscopic units make pulsed fluoroscopy available at low frame rates (e.g., 8 frames per second). **Low frame rates** adversely affect the ability to display rapidly moving structures.

Large field size increases the amount of scatter radiation produced. Additional scatter radiation enters the receptor and degrades the resulting video image. Collimation to the area of interest improves image quality but also reduces the total volume of tissue irradiated by excluding tissue with little diagnostic value.

The design of the fluoroscopy system may incorporate **variable or operator-selectable filtration.** Substantial reductions in skin dose can be achieved by inserting appropriate metal filters (aluminum or copper) into the x-ray beam at the collimator. Filtration reduces skin dose by preferentially removing low-energy x-rays, which generally do not penetrate the patient to contribute to the image.

The presence of a grid improves contrast by absorbing scattered x-rays. However, the dose to the patient is increased by a factor of 2 or more. For pediatric cases, the removal of the grid reduces the dose with little degradation of image quality. Grids should be used with discretion when fluoroscopic studies are performed on children. These systems should have the capability for easy removal and reintroduction of the grid.

In most interventional fluoroscopic procedures, most of the fluoroscopic time the x-ray beam is directed toward a particular anatomic region. Some reduction in maximum skin dose can be achieved by **periodically rotating the fluoroscopic x-ray tube** to image the anatomy of interest from a different direction. This method tends to spread the entry dose over a broader area, reducing the maximum skin dose.

SCATTERED RADIATION

During routine fluoroscopy of the gastrointestinal tract, personnel are exposed to radiation scattered by the patient and other structures in the x-ray beam. Scattered radiation levels depend on entrance exposure rate, field size, beam quality, and patient thickness but decrease rapidly with distance from the patient. The pattern of scattered radiation is shown in Fig. 1.193, in which the tower drape shielding is not in place.

The IR, tower lead drapes, bucky slot shield, x-ray table, foot rest (if present), and radiologist all provide a source of shielding for the technologist. The bucky slot shield covers the gap under the tabletop that allows the bucky to move along the length of the table for radiography. The area behind the radiologist and away from the table has the lowest scattered radiation level (<10 mR/hr) (Fig. 1.194).

When the receptor is lowered as close as possible to the patient, much of the scatter to the worker's eyes and neck is eliminated. The vertical and lateral extents of the scattered radiation field contract dramatically as the distance between patient and receptor is reduced.

Radiation Protection Practices During Fluoroscopy

Even with correct shielding in place and the IR as close to the patient as possible, scatter radiation is still present during fluoroscopy. Radiation levels are highest in the region close to the table on each side of the radiologist (Table 1.16). The presence of tower drapes greatly reduces the dose to the radiologist. Technologists and others in the room can decrease their dose by not standing close to the table on either side of the radiologist.

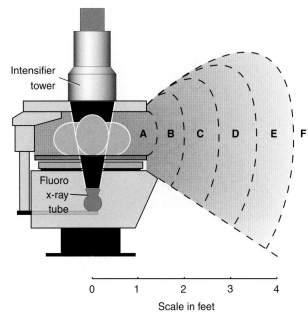

Fig. 1.193 Fluoroscopy scattered radiation pattern without tower drape shields in place.

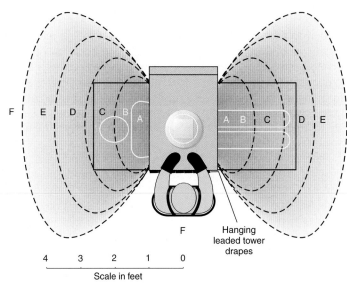

Fig. 1.194 Fluoroscopy scattered radiation pattern with tower drape shields in place and image receptor close to the patient.

TABLE 1.16 EXPOSURE LEVELS

ZONE	EXPOSURE RATE (MR/HR)	AIR KERMA RATE (MGY/HR)
A	>400	>3.5
B	400	3.5
	200	1.75
C	200	1.75
	100	0.88
D	100	0.88
	50	0.44
E	50	0.44
	10	0.088
F	<10	0.088

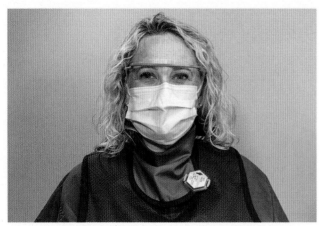

Fig. 1.195 Thyroid shields with regular neck cutout apron.

All individuals participating in fluoroscopic procedures must wear a protective apron. A 0.5 mm lead equivalent apron, which reduces the exposure by a factor 50 over the diagnostic x-ray energy range, is recommended.[1] Typical doses under the apron are below the threshold of detectability for personnel monitors. Dosimeters placed under the apron show readings only for individuals approaching the dose limit, which are typically less than 20 mrem. Aprons of multiple element composition with a 0.5 mm lead equivalence between 80 and 110 kVp offer the advantage of reduced weight. However, some manufacturers of "light" aprons achieve a weight reduction by the removal of lead vinyl layers, sacrificing some protection. Technologists should be cautious about using aprons with large cutouts around the arms and low necklines. These allow greater exposure to the thyroid and breasts. Although some protective aprons have a thyroid shield built into them, most do not. A separate **thyroid shield** can be worn with the apron to protect the neck region (Fig. 1.195).

Although a thyroid shield is not required for an individual participating in fluoroscopic procedures, a thyroid shield should be available (provided by the health care facility) for use at the option of the radiation worker. Wearing the thyroid shield is consistent with the ALARA principle, but the overall reduction in effective dose provided by this device is small. For an individual approaching a significant fraction of the dose limit, the thyroid shield is recommended.

In 2012, the International Commission on Radiological Protection (ICRP) published the modified threshold for a vision-impairing cataract from an acute dose of 5 Gy to an acute dose of 0.5 Gy.[18] This was due to new evidence indicating that the eye is more radiosensitive than originally thought. Most occupationally exposed personnel will not exceed this threshold under normal working conditions if recommended practices are followed. However, very busy **interventionalists** may be at risk to exceed this threshold. There are various ways to protect the eye from unnecessary radiation exposure, including leaded face shields. The use of leaded eyewear is not usually necessary or recommended unless the occupationally exposed worker is consistently participating in long fluoroscopy cases that require very close proximity to the patient. Most interventional radiologists and interventional cardiologists should wear leaded glasses.

Radiation-attenuating surgical gloves offer minimal protection of the operator's hands, provide a false sense of protection, and are not recommended. The instantaneous dose from scatter radiation is reduced when hands covered with **one layer of glove material** are located near the radiation field. However, the total time near the radiation field depends on the speed with which the procedure is performed, as well as the distance from the imaged anatomy when the x-ray beam is activated. The increased thickness of these gloves reduces dexterity and can increase procedure time. The automatic exposure control system in fluoroscopy increases the radiation output to penetrate the glove when the hand is present in the beam. This can be confirmed by noting that anatomy is seen even though the glove is present. The dose to the hand is comparable to the dose when the radiation-attenuating glove is not present. The cost of radiation-attenuating surgical gloves and the minimal dose reduction do not justify the use of these devices according to the ALARA principle.

Image Wisely and Image Gently

Image Wisely[19] is an awareness program, developed jointly by the American College of Radiology, Radiological Society of North America, American Association of Physicists in Medicine, and American Society of Radiologic Technologists, to promote radiation safety in adult medical imaging. The goal is to eliminate unnecessary radiation associated with adult imaging by avoiding non–medically indicated imaging procedures, by conducting the most appropriate imaging procedure, and by using the lowest optimal dose in all imaging practices.

Printed and electronic educational resources have been developed for radiologists, medical physicists, radiologic technologists, referring physicians, patients, and the general public. Topics include dose, dose reduction techniques, appropriateness of imaging procedures, and risks. The information is directed at each respective target audience. A similar campaign, called **Image Gently**[20], is designed to minimize the radiation exposure in children, whose long life expectancy and increased radiosensitivity contribute to higher lifetime cancer risk. More information on the Image Wisely and Image Gently campaigns can be found at www.imagewisely.org and www.imagegently.org.

CHAPTER 2

Chest

CONTRIBUTIONS BY **Cheryl O. DuBose,** Ed.D., RT(R)(MR)(CT)(QM), MRSO

CONTRIBUTORS TO PAST EDITIONS Nancy Johnson, MEd, RT(R)(CV)(CT)(QM)(ARRT), FASRT, Karen Brown, RT(R), Kathy M. Martensen, BS, RT(R)

CONTENTS

RADIOGRAPHIC ANATOMY

Chest

Chest radiographic examinations are the most common of all radiographic procedures. Student radiographers typically begin their clinical experience taking chest radiographs. However, before beginning such clinical experience, it is important to learn and understand chest anatomy, including relative relationships of all anatomy within the chest cavity.

The **chest**, or **thorax**, is the upper portion of the trunk between the neck and the abdomen. Radiographic anatomy of the chest is divided into three sections: **bony thorax, respiratory system proper,** and **mediastinum.**

BONY THORAX

The **bony thorax** is the part of the skeletal system that provides a protective framework for the parts of the chest involved with breathing and blood circulation. **Thoracic viscera** is the term used to describe these parts of the chest, consisting of the lungs and the remaining thoracic organs contained in the mediastinum.

Anteriorly, the bony thorax consists of the **sternum** (breastbone), which has three divisions. The superior portion is the **manubrium** *(mah-nu'-bre-um),* the large center portion is the **body,** and the smaller inferior portion is the **xiphoid process.**

Superiorly, the bony thorax consists of the **2 clavicles** (collarbones) that connect the sternum to the **2 scapulae** (shoulder blades), the **12 pairs of ribs** that circle the thorax, and the **12 thoracic vertebrae** posteriorly (Fig. 2.1). A detailed description of all parts of the bony thorax is presented in Chapter 10.

Topographic Positioning Landmarks

Accurate and consistent radiographic positioning requires certain landmarks, or reference points, that can be used to center the image receptor (IR) correctly to ensure that all essential anatomy is included on that specific projection. These topographic landmarks should be parts of the body that are easily and consistently located on patients, such as parts of the bony thorax. For chest positioning, two of these landmarks are the **vertebra prominens** and the **jugular notch.**

VERTEBRA PROMINENS (SEVENTH CERVICAL VERTEBRA)

The vertebra prominens is an important landmark for determining the central ray (CR) location on a posteroanterior (PA) chest projection. It is the spinous process of the seventh cervical vertebrae (see Chapter 8). It can be palpated readily on most patients by applying light pressure with the fingertips at the base of the neck. The vertebra prominens is the first prominent process felt as you gently but firmly palpate down the back of the neck. With a little practice, this landmark can be located readily on most patients, especially with the neck in a flexed position.

JUGULAR NOTCH (MANUBRIAL OR SUPRASTERNAL NOTCH)

The jugular notch is an important landmark for determining the CR placement on anteroposterior (AP) chest projections. This is palpated easily as a deep notch or depression on the superior portion of the sternum below the thyroid cartilage.

The midthorax, at the level of T7 (seventh thoracic vertebra), can be located easily from these two landmarks, as described later in this chapter.

XIPHOID PROCESS (TIP)

The inferior tip of the sternum, the **xiphoid process,** which corresponds to the level of T9–T10, can also be palpated. The xiphoid process corresponds to the approximate level of the anterior portion of the diaphragm, which separates the chest cavity from the abdominal cavity. However, this is not a reliable landmark for positioning the chest because of variations in body habitus and the variable lower position of the posterior lungs, which may extend as far as T11 or T12 on inspiration, as shown in Fig. 2.2.

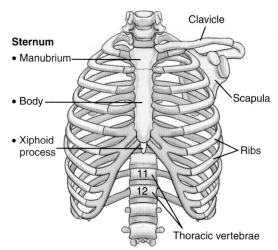

Fig. 2.1 Bony thorax.

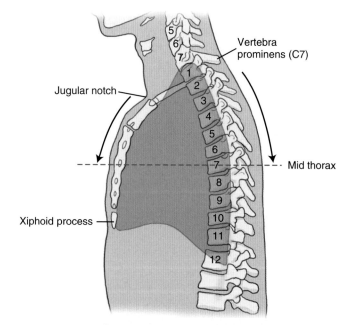

Fig. 2.2 Topographic landmarks.

PARTS OF THE RESPIRATORY SYSTEM

Respiration is the exchange of gaseous substances between the air we breathe and the bloodstream. The respiratory system consists of the parts of the body through which air passes as it travels from the nose and mouth into the lungs. Four general divisions of the respiratory system, shown in Fig. 2.3, are the **pharynx, trachea, bronchi,** and **lungs.**

An important structure of the respiratory system is the dome-shaped **diaphragm,** which is the primary muscle of inspiration. Each half of the diaphragm is called a **hemidiaphragm** ("hemi-" meaning half). As the dome of the diaphragm moves downward, it **increases** the volume of the thoracic cavity. This increase in volume, along with certain other dimensional movements of the thorax described later in this chapter, **decreases** the intrathoracic pressure, creating a "sucking" action or negative pressure effect, resulting in air being drawn into the lungs through the nose and mouth, pharynx, larynx, trachea, and bronchi. This causes the lungs to fill with air, which is known as inspiration.

PHARYNX

The **pharynx** *(far'-inks)* serves as a **passageway for food and fluids as well as air, making it common to the digestive and respiratory systems.** Air must pass through the pharynx before entering the rest of the respiratory system. The pharynx can be found in the posterior area between the nose and mouth above and the larynx and esophagus below.

The pharynx is approximately 5 inches (13 cm) in length and consists of three divisions, as shown in Fig. 2.4: **nasopharynx** *(na"-zo-far'-inks)*, **oropharynx** *(o"-ro-far'-inks)*, and **laryngopharynx** *(lah-ring"-go-far'-inks)*. The superior portion of the pharynx is the nasopharynx, which is located posterior to the nose and houses the opening of the eustachian or auditory tube and the pharyngeal tonsils. The other end of the auditory tube is found in the middle ear and is useful in equalizing air pressure between the middle ear and the outside atmosphere.

The **hard palate** and the **soft palate** make up the roof of the oral cavity, separating the nasal cavity above from the mouth below. The lower posterior aspect of the soft palate is called the **uvula** *(u'-vu-lah);* this marks the boundary between the nasopharynx and the oropharynx. The oropharynx is found posterior to the mouth, with the tongue creating the anterior wall of the oropharynx. This section of the pharynx contains the palatine tonsils and the lingual tonsils.

The laryngopharynx lies above and posterior to the larynx (voice box) and extends from the upper border of the **epiglottis** *(ep"-i-glot'-is)* to where the laryngopharynx narrows to join the esophagus.

The upper portion of the epiglottis projects upward behind the tongue and acts as a lid for the slanted opening of the larynx. During the act of swallowing, the epiglottis flips down and covers the laryngeal opening, preventing food and fluid from entering the larynx and bronchi.

Additional structures shown on this sectional lateral drawing are the **hyoid bone, thyroid cartilage** of the larynx (Adam's apple), **thyroid gland,** and **trachea,** which are described in greater detail in the subsequent sections on the larynx and the trachea.

Esophagus

The **esophagus** is the part of the digestive system that connects the pharynx with the stomach. Note the relationship of the esophagus to both the pharynx and the larynx. It begins at the distal end

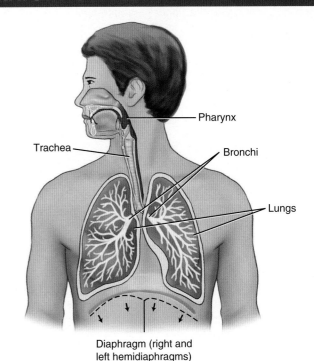

Diaphragm (right and left hemidiaphragms)

Fig. 2.3 Respiratory system.

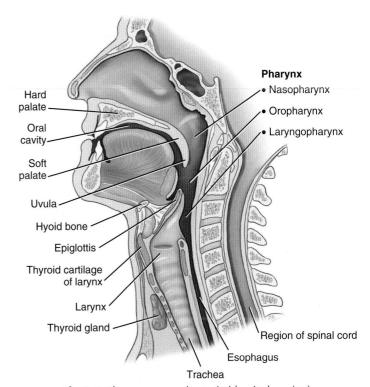

Fig. 2.4 Pharynx, upper airway (midsagittal section).

of the laryngopharynx and continues downward to the stomach, **posterior to the larynx and trachea.** (Chapter 12 describes the esophagus, along with the upper gastrointestinal [UGI] system, in detail.)

Larynx (Voice Box)

The **larynx** is a cagelike, cartilaginous structure that is approximately 1½ to 2 inches (4 to 5 cm) in length in an adult. The larynx is located in the anterior portion of the neck, suspended from a small bone called the **hyoid** (Fig. 2.5). The hyoid bone is found in the upper neck just below the tongue or floor of the mouth (see Fig. 2.4). The hyoid bone is *not* part of the larynx.

The larynx serves as the organ of voice. Sounds are made as air passes between the **vocal cords** located within the larynx (Fig. 2.6). The upper margin of the larynx is at the approximate level of **C3** (third cervical vertebra). Its lower margin, where the larynx joins with the trachea, is at the level of **C6.**

The framework of the larynx consists of cartilages that are connected by ligaments and moved by numerous muscles that assist in the complex sound-making or voice process. The largest and least mobile of these cartilages is the **thyroid cartilage,** which consists of two fused platelike structures that form the anterior wall of the larynx. The prominent anterior projection of the thyroid cartilage is palpated easily and is known as the **laryngeal prominence,** or Adam's apple. This prominent structure is an important positioning landmark because it is easy to locate. Generally larger in males than females, the laryngeal prominence of the thyroid cartilage is located at the level of C4–**C5** and is an excellent topographic reference for locating specific skeletal structures in this region.

The **cricoid** *(kri'-koid)* **cartilage** is a ring of cartilage that forms the inferior and posterior wall of the larynx. It is attached to the first ring of cartilage of the trachea.

One of the cartilages that make up the larynx is the uniquely shaped **epiglottis,** which resembles a leaf with the narrow distal stem portion attached to a part of the thyroid cartilage. As described previously, the epiglottis flips down and covers the trachea during the act of swallowing (see arrow in Fig. 2.6).

Sectional Image of Larynx Because of the wide acceptance of computed tomography (CT) and magnetic resonance imaging (MRI), the technologist must recognize anatomic structures in sectional images. Fig. 2.7 shows an axial CT view of the midportion of the larynx at the approximate level of C5. Only major structures are labeled in this section.

NOTE: CT images such as those seen here often are viewed as though one were standing at the patient's feet, looking toward the head. Thus, the patient's right is to the viewer's left. This is the same way that radiographs are reviewed. (see Chapter 1).

TRACHEA

Connecting the larynx to the main bronchi is the **trachea,** or windpipe. It is a fibrous muscular tube about ¾ inch (2 cm) in diameter and 4½ inches (11 cm) long. Approximately 16 to 20 C-shaped rings of cartilage are embedded in its anterior wall. These rigid rings keep the airway open by preventing the trachea from collapsing during expiration.

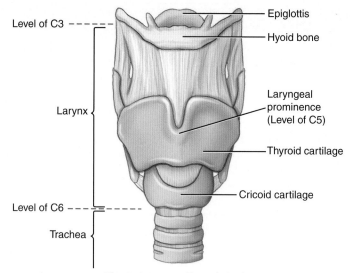

Fig. 2.5 Larynx (frontal view).

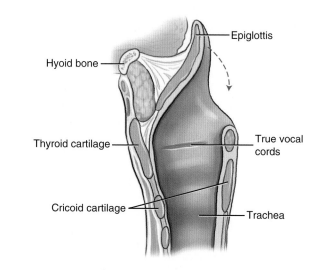

Fig. 2.6 Larynx (lateral view).

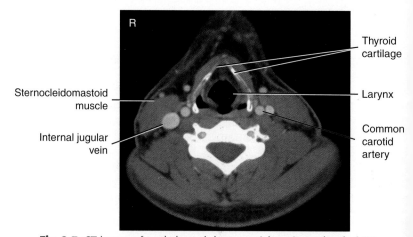

Fig. 2.7 CT image of neck through larynx—axial section at level of C5.

The trachea, located just anterior to the esophagus, extends from its junction with the larynx at the level of **C6** downward to the level of **T4** or **T5** (fourth or fifth thoracic vertebra), where it divides at the **carina** (last tracheal cartilage) into the right and left primary bronchi.

The endocrine system glands typically imaged with the respiratory system include the **thyroid, parathyroid,** and **thymus glands.**

Thyroid Gland

The thyroid gland is located anteriorly in the neck region just below the thyroid cartilage, with its right and left lobes lying on each side of the trachea (Fig. 2.8). In an adult, it weighs about 1 ounce (25 to 30 g) and is more radiosensitive than most body structures or organs. It is important for technologists to reduce exposure to this region as much as possible by shielding and collimation of the x-ray beam.

A unique feature of the thyroid gland is its ability to store certain hormones and release them slowly to aid in the regulation of body metabolism. These hormones also help to regulate body growth and development, especially in children. The thyroid gland serves as a counterweight to the parathyroid glands, stimulating the increased deposition of calcium in the bone, thereby lowering blood calcium levels.

Parathyroid Glands

Parathyroid glands are small, round glands that are embedded in the posterior surface of each lobe of the thyroid gland. Usually, two parathyroids are attached to each lateral thyroid lobe (four total), as shown in Fig. 2.8. These glands store and secrete hormones that aid in specific blood functions, including maintenance of blood calcium levels by stimulating bone breakdown to increase calcium in the blood.

Thymus Gland

The thymus gland is located inferior to the thyroid gland and anterior and superior to the heart (see Fig. 2.8). It is described later in this chapter as part of the mediastinal structures (see Fig. 2.22).

RADIOGRAPHS

AP and lateral radiographs of the upper airway allow visualization of the air-filled trachea and larynx. The AP radiograph in Fig. 2.9 shows a column of air primarily in the upper trachea region, as is seen in the lower half of the radiograph (darkened area, arrows). Certain enlargements or other abnormalities of the thymus or thyroid glands can be demonstrated on such radiographs, as can pathology within the airway system itself.

The lateral radiograph (Fig. 2.10) shows the air-filled trachea and larynx (A) and the region of the esophagus (B) and shows the locations relative to each other. The esophagus is located posteriorly in relation to the trachea. The general locations of the thyroid gland (C) and the thymus gland (D) are identified.

Sectional Image of the Trachea

Fig. 2.11 is a CT image through the upper chest at the approximate level of T3. Observe that the trachea is located anteriorly to the esophagus and that both of these are anterior to the thoracic vertebrae. The upper lungs are located to each side of the trachea and the thoracic vertebrae.

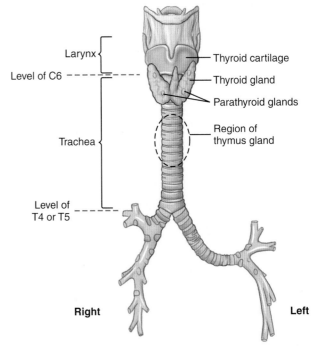

Fig. 2.8 Trachea.

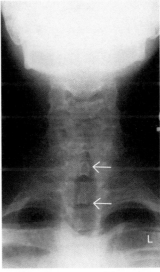

Fig. 2.9 AP upper airway.

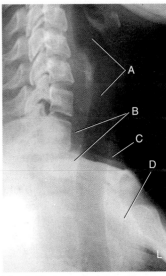

Fig. 2.10 Lateral upper airway. A, Air-filled trachea and larynx. B, Esophagus. C, Region of the thyroid gland. D, Region of the thymus gland.

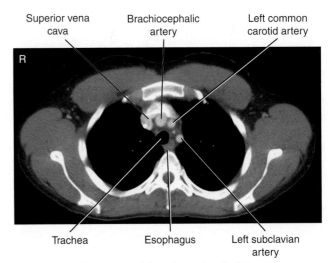

Fig. 2.11 Axial section at level of T3.

Branches of Aortic Arch

The major arterial branches from the aortic arch are identified in Fig. 2.11. The major branches include the brachiocephalic, left common carotid, and left subclavian arteries. The superior vena cava is a large vein draining blood from the head, neck, and upper limbs and returning it to the heart.

RIGHT AND LEFT BRONCHI

The trachea bifurcates at the carina to form the **right** and **left primary bronchi,** also known as the right and left main stem bronchi.

The **right primary bronchus** is **wider** and **shorter** than the left bronchus. The right primary bronchus is also more **vertical;** therefore, the angle of divergence from the distal trachea is less abrupt for the right bronchus than for the left. This **difference in size and shape** between the two primary bronchi is important because food particles or other foreign objects that happen to enter the respiratory system are more likely to enter and lodge in the **right** bronchus.

The **carina** *(kah-ri'-nah)* is a specific prominence, or ridge, of the lowest tracheal cartilage and marks the division of the trachea into the right and left bronchi (Fig. 2.12). As viewed from above through a bronchoscope, the carina is to the left of the midline, and the right bronchus appears more open than the left, demonstrating the likelihood that particles descending the trachea will enter the right bronchus.

Secondary Bronchi, Lobes, and Alveoli

In addition to differences in size and shape between the right and left bronchi, another important difference is that the **right** bronchus divides into **three** secondary bronchi, but the **left** divides into only **two,** with each entering individual lobes of the lungs (Fig. 2.13). The **right lung** contains **three lobes,** and the **left lung** contains **two lobes,** as is demonstrated in Figs. 2.14 and 2.15. These secondary bronchi continue to subdivide into smaller branches, called **bronchioles,** that spread to all parts of each lobe.

Each of these small **terminal bronchioles** terminates in very small air sacs called **alveoli.** The two lungs contain approximately 500 million to 700 million alveoli. Oxygen and carbon dioxide are exchanged in the blood through the thin walls of the alveoli.

Sectional Image of Bronchi and Lungs   Fig. 2.14 presents an axial (sectional) drawing through the heart at the approximate level of T7.

LUNGS

The fourth and last division of the respiratory system comprises the two large, spongy **lungs,** which are located on each side of the thoracic cavity. The lungs fill all of the space not occupied by other structures. The right lung is made up of **three** lobes—the **superior** (upper), **middle,** and **inferior** (lower) lobes—divided by **two deep fissures.** The oblique fissure separates the inferior and middle lobes, whereas the horizontal fissure separates the superior and middle lobes. The left lung has only **two** lobes—the **superior** (upper) and **inferior** (lower)—separated by a **single deep oblique fissure.**

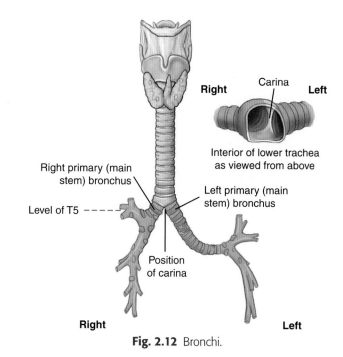

Fig. 2.12 Bronchi.

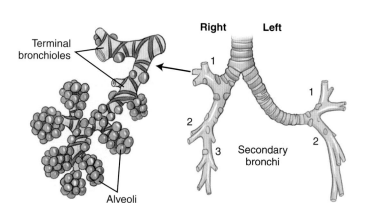

Fig. 2.13 Secondary bronchi and alveoli.

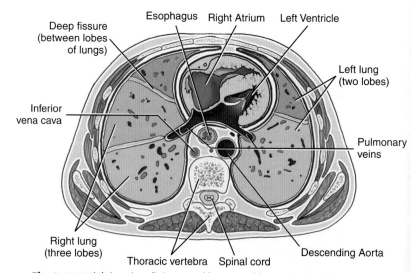

Fig. 2.14 Axial (sectional) image of lungs and heart, level of T7.

The lungs are composed of a light, spongy, highly elastic substance called **parenchyma** *(pah-reng'-ki-mah)*. This substance allows for the breathing mechanism responsible for expansion and contraction of the lungs, which brings oxygen into and removes carbon dioxide from the blood through the thin walls of the alveoli.

Each lung is contained in a delicate double-walled sac, or membrane, called the **pleura,** which can be visualized in both frontal (see Fig. 2.15) and sectional (Fig. 2.16) drawings. The outer layer of this pleural sac lines the inner surface of the chest wall and diaphragm and is called the **parietal pleura.** The inner layer that covers the surface of the lungs, also dipping into the fissures between the lobes, is called the **pulmonary** or **visceral pleura** (Fig. 2.16).

The potential space between the double-walled pleura, called the **pleural cavity,** contains a lubricating fluid that allows movement of one or the other during breathing. When a lung collapses, or when air or fluid collects between these two layers, this space may be visualized radiographically. Air or gas present in this pleural cavity results in a condition called a **pneumothorax,** in which air or gas pressure in the pleural cavity may cause the lung to collapse. Accumulation of blood in the pleural cavity creates a condition called a **hemothorax,** whereas fluid within the cavity is referred to as **pleural effusion.**

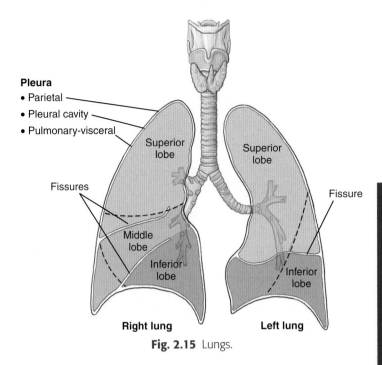

Fig. 2.15 Lungs.

Sectional Drawing of Lungs and Heart

Fig. 2.16 presents an axial sectional drawing through the lower third of the mediastinum and lungs. The double-walled membrane, the **pleura,** which completely encloses the lungs, including around the heart, is clearly shown. The outer membrane, the **parietal pleura,** and the inner membrane, the **pulmonary** (or **visceral**) **pleura,** are clearly visible, as is the potential space between them, the **pleural cavity.**

The double-walled **pericardial sac,** which surrounds the heart, is also identified. This drawing shows the relationship of the pericardial sac surrounding the heart with the pleural sac surrounding the lungs. The pleural and pericardial spaces or cavities are exaggerated on this drawing to show these parts better. Normally, no space exists between the double walls of the pericardial sac or between the parietal and visceral pleura unless pathology is present.

Sectional Image

The CT image in Fig. 2.17 at the approximate level of T10 demonstrates the relationship and relative size of the heart, descending aorta, esophagus, and lungs. The heart is located more to the **left,** as can be seen on a PA chest radiograph. The heart is also shown to be located in the anterior portion of the chest cavity directly behind the sternum and left anterior ribs. The esophagus is posterior to the heart, with the descending aorta between the esophagus and the thoracic vertebrae.

PA Chest Radiograph

An enormous amount of medical information can be obtained from a properly exposed and carefully positioned PA chest radiograph. Although the technical factors are designed for optimal visualization of the lungs and other soft tissues, the bony thorax can also be seen. The clavicles, scapulae, and ribs can be identified through careful study of the chest radiograph in Fig. 2.18. The sternum and thoracic vertebrae are superimposed along with mediastinal structures, such as the heart and great vessels;

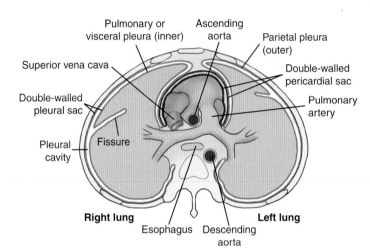

Fig. 2.16 Cross-section of lower mediastinum and lungs.

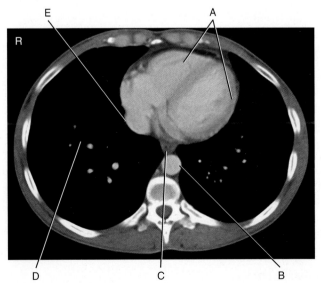

Fig. 2.17 CT image of lower thorax (level of T10). A, Heart. B, Descending aorta. C, Esophagus. D, Right lung. E, Inferior vena cava.

therefore, the sternum and vertebrae are not well visualized on a PA chest radiograph.

The **lungs** and the **trachea** (see Fig. 2.18, dotted outline, A) of the respiratory system are well shown, although usually the primary bronchi are not seen easily. The larynx is usually located above the top border of the radiograph and cannot be seen. The heart, large blood vessels, and diaphragm are well visualized.

The labeled parts of the radiograph are demonstrated in Fig. 2.19, a frontal view of the thorax with the bony structures removed. The thyroid gland, large blood vessels, and thymus gland are shown in relation to the lungs and heart.

Parts of lungs Radiographically important parts of the lungs, most also shown in the accompanying drawing, (see Figs. 2.18 and 2.19) include the following:

The **apex** (B) of each lung is the **rounded upper area above the level of the clavicles.** The apices of the lungs extend up into the lower neck area to the level of T1 (first thoracic vertebra). This important part of the lungs must be included on chest radiographs.

The **carina** (C) is shown as the point of bifurcation, the lowest margin of the separation of the trachea into the right and left bronchi.

The **base** (D) of each lung is the lower concave area of each lung that rests on the **diaphragm** (E). The diaphragm is a muscular partition that separates the thoracic and abdominal cavities.

The **costophrenic angle** (F) refers to the extreme outermost lower corner of each lung, where the diaphragm meets the ribs. When positioning for chest radiographs, you should know the relative locations of the uppermost and lowermost parts of the lungs—the apices and the costophrenic angles, respectively—to ensure that these regions are included on every chest radiograph. Pathology, such as a small amount of fluid collection, would be evident at these costophrenic angles in the erect position.

The **hilum** (hilus) (G), also known as the **root** region, is the central area of each lung, where the bronchi, blood vessels, lymph vessels, and nerves enter and leave the lungs.

Lateral chest view The lateral chest radiograph (Fig. 2.20) is marked to show the same parts as those labeled in the accompanying drawing (Fig. 2.21). This drawing depicts the left lung as seen from the medial aspect. Because this is the left lung, only two lobes are seen. Some of the **lower lobe** (D) extends above the level of the **hilum** (C) posteriorly, whereas some of the **upper lobe** (B) extends below the hilum anteriorly. The posterior portion of the diaphragm is the most inferior part of the **diaphragm**. The single deep **oblique fissure** that divides the two lobes of the left lung is shown again, as is the end-on view of a bronchus in the hilar region.

The right lung is usually about 1 inch (2.5 cm) shorter than the left lung. The reason for this difference is the large space-occupying liver, which is located in the right upper abdomen and which pushes up on the **right hemidiaphragm.** The right and left hemidiaphragms are seen on the lateral chest radiograph (Fig. 2.20F). The more superior of the two is the right hemidiaphragm, which is also seen on the PA chest radiograph (see Fig. 2.18).

Mediastinum

The medial portion of the thoracic cavity between the lungs is called the **mediastinum.** The thyroid and parathyroid glands, as described

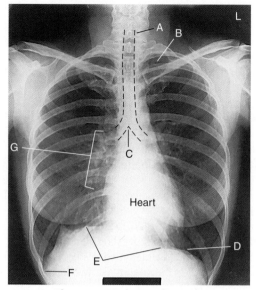
Fig. 2.18 PA chest radiograph.

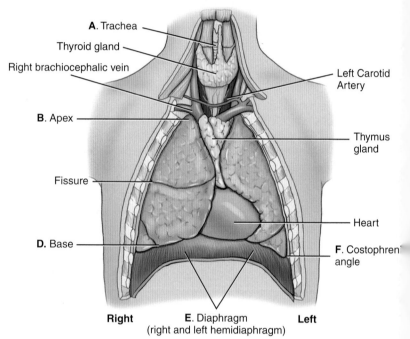
A. Trachea
Thyroid gland
Right brachiocephalic vein
Left Carotid Artery
B. Apex
Thymus gland
Fissure
Heart
D. Base
F. Costophrenic angle
Right   **E. Diaphragm**   **Left**
(right and left hemidiaphragm)
Fig. 2.19 Lungs and mediastinum.

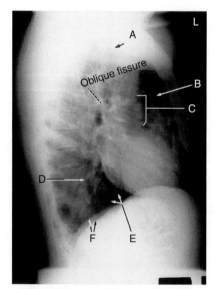
Fig. 2.20 Lateral chest radiograph.

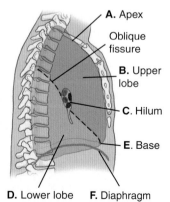
A. Apex
Oblique fissure
B. Upper lobe
C. Hilum
E. Base
D. Lower lobe   F. Diaphragm
Fig. 2.21 Medial left lung.

earlier in this chapter, are *not* considered mediastinal structures because they are located more superiorly and are not within the mediastinum. However, the thymus gland is located within the mediastinum, inferior to the thyroid gland and anterior to the trachea and esophagus (Fig. 2.22).

Four radiographically important structures located in the mediastinum are the (1) **thymus gland,** (2) **heart and great vessels,** (3) **trachea,** and (4) **esophagus.**

Thymus gland The **thymus gland,** located behind the upper sternum, is said to be a temporary organ because it is very prominent in infancy and reaches its maximum size of about 40 g at puberty, then gradually decreases in size until it almost disappears in adulthood. At its maximum size, it would appear much larger than the organ shown in Fig. 2.22. It may be visualized on chest radiographs of children but generally is not seen in adult radiographs because the denser lymphatic tissue has been replaced by less dense fatty tissue. At its maximum development, the thymus gland lies above and anterior to the heart and pericardium.[1]

The thymus gland has a large role in the development of the immune system that helps the body resist disease. It is essential to the growth and development of thymic lymphocytes or T cells, which serve in rejecting things foreign to the body.

Heart and great vessels The **heart** and the roots of the **great vessels** are enclosed in a double-walled sac called the pericardial sac (shown in Fig. 2.16). The heart is located posterior to the body of the sternum and anterior to T5 to T8. It lies obliquely in the mediastinal space, and approximately two-thirds of the heart lies to the left of the median plane.

The **great vessels** in the mediastinum are the inferior vena cava and superior vena cava, aorta, and large pulmonary arteries and veins. The **superior vena cava** is a large vein that returns blood to the heart from the upper half of the body (see Fig. 2.22). The **inferior vena cava** is a large vein that returns blood from the lower half of the body.

The **aorta** is the largest artery in the body (2 to 3 cm in diameter in an average adult). It carries blood to all parts of the body through its various branches. The aorta is divided into three parts: **ascending aorta** (coming up out of the heart); **arch of the aorta;** and **descending aorta,** which passes through the diaphragm into the abdomen, where it becomes the abdominal aorta.

Various **pulmonary arteries and veins** present in the mediastinum are shown in Figs. 2.23 and 2.24. These supply blood and return blood to and from all segments of the lungs. The capillary network surrounds the small air sacs, or alveoli, where oxygen and carbon dioxide are exchanged with the blood through the thin-walled air sacs.

See Chapter 17 for more complete drawings of the heart and great vessels as part of the total-body circulatory system.

Trachea and esophagus The trachea, within the mediastinum, separates into the right and left primary and secondary bronchi, as shown in Fig. 2.23.

The proximal esophagus is located posterior to the trachea and continues down through the mediastinum **anterior to the descending aorta** until it passes through the diaphragm into the stomach.

Note in Fig. 2.24 that the heart is located in the **anterior** aspect of the thoracic cavity, directly behind the sternum.

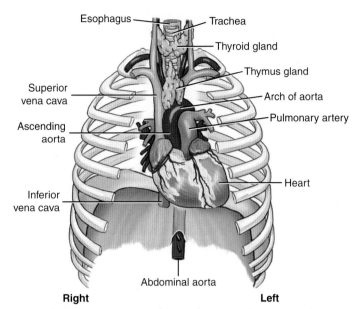

Fig. 2.22 Structures within mediastinum (anterior view).

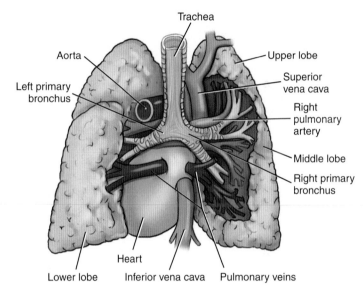

Fig. 2.23 Lungs and structures within mediastinum (posterior view).

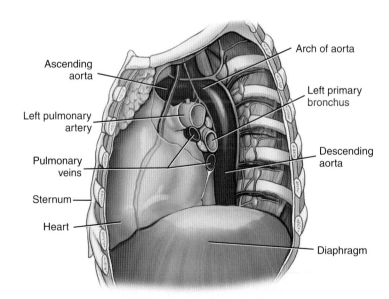

Fig. 2.24 Mediastinal relationships on left side with lung removal.

RADIOGRAPHIC POSITIONING

Body Habitus

Body habitus requires special consideration in chest radiography. There are four different styles of body build or habitus (Fig. 2.25). The four types of body habitus were explained in Chapter 1. A massively built **hypersthenic** patient has a thorax that is very **broad** and very **deep** from front to back but is **shallow** in vertical dimension, as is shown in the PA radiograph in Fig. 2.26. Therefore, care must be taken that the sides or the costophrenic angles are not cut off on a PA chest radiograph. Careful centering is also required on the lateral projection to ensure that the anterior or posterior margins are included on the radiograph.

The other extreme is a slender **asthenic** patient. With this build, the thorax is **narrow** in width and **shallow** from front to back but is very **long** in its vertical dimension. Therefore, in positioning for a chest radiograph, the technologist must ensure that the IR is positioned to include both the upper apex areas, which extend well above the clavicles, and the lower costophrenic angles. A chest PA radiograph in a nearer average **hyposthenic** patient is shown in Fig. 2.27. Care in vertical collimation for such patients must be exercised so that the costophrenic angles are not cut off on the lower margin.

Breathing Movements

Movements of the bony thorax during inspiration (taking air in) and expiration (expelling air) greatly change the dimensions of the thorax and the thoracic volume. To increase the volume of the chest during inspiration (Fig. 2.28), the thoracic cavity increases in diameter in **three dimensions.**

The first of these is the **vertical diameter,** which is increased primarily by contraction and downward movement of the diaphragm, increasing the thoracic volume.

The **transverse diameter** is the second dimension that is increased during inspiration. The ribs swing outward and upward, and this increases the transverse diameter of the thorax.

The third dimension is the **anteroposterior diameter,** which is also increased during inspiration by the raising of the ribs, especially the second through sixth ribs.

During expiration, the elastic recoil of the lungs, along with the weight of the thoracic walls, causes the three diameters of the thorax to return to normal (Fig. 2.29).

DEGREE OF INSPIRATION

To determine the degree of inspiration in chest radiography, one should be able to identify and count the rib pairs on a chest radiograph. The first and second pairs are the most difficult to locate. When a chest radiograph is taken, the patient should take as deep a breath as possible and then hold it to aerate the lungs fully. Taking a second deep breath before holding it allows for a deeper inspiration.

The best method that can be used to determine the degree of inspiration is to observe how far down the diaphragm has moved by counting the pairs of posterior ribs in the lung area above the diaphragm. A general rule for average adult patients is to "show" a **minimum of 10** pairs of ribs on a good PA chest radiograph. To determine this, start at the top with the first rib and count down to the **tenth** or **eleventh** rib posteriorly. The posterior part of each rib, where it joins a thoracic vertebra, is the most superior part of the rib. The diaphragm should always be checked to see that it is below the level of at least the tenth posterior rib (see following NOTE). (Fig. 2.30 shows 11 posterior ribs, which can be expected in many healthy patients.)

NOTE: Patients with pulmonary diseases and trauma may be unable to inspire deeply. Therefore, it may be impossible to demonstrate 10 ribs above the diaphragm for these chest projections.

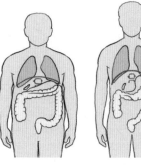
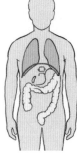
Hypersthenic (5%)　　　Sthenic (50%)

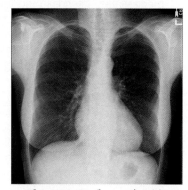
Fig. 2.26 PA (hypersthenic).

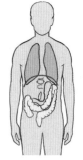
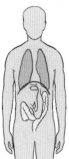
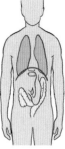
Hyposthenic (35%)　　Asthenic (10%)
Fig. 2.25 Body habitus.

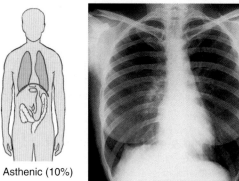
Fig. 2.27 PA (hyposthenic).

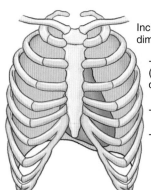
Increases in 3 dimensions:

- Vertical (diaphragm downward)

- Transverse

- AP dimension

Fig. 2.28 Inspiration.

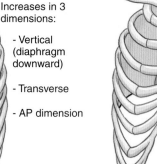
Fig. 2.29 Expiration.

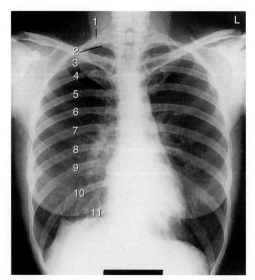
Fig. 2.30 Posterior ribs.

Positioning Considerations

Patient preparation for chest radiography includes the removal of all opaque objects from the chest and neck regions, including clothes with buttons, snaps, hooks, or any objects that would be visualized on the radiograph as a shadow (radiopaque artifact). To ensure that all opaque objects are removed from the chest region, the usual procedure is to ask the patient to remove all clothing, including bras, necklaces, or other objects around the neck. The patient then puts on a hospital gown, which commonly has the opening in the back.

Long hair may be visible as an artifact on chest radiographs taken with digital imaging systems. Long hair should be drawn up or draped across the shoulder to eliminate superimposition within the chest anatomy. Hair that is braided or tied together in bunches with rubber bands or other fasteners may also cause suspicious shadows on the radiograph if left superimposing the chest area. Oxygen lines or electrocardiogram (ECG) monitor leads should be moved carefully to the side of the chest if possible. All radiopaque objects should be moved carefully from the radiographic field of interest to prevent artifacts from interfering with the quality of the diagnostic image.

Radiation Protection

Patients should be protected from unnecessary radiation for all diagnostic radiographic examinations, especially for chest radiographs, because these are the most common of all radiographic examinations.

REPEAT EXPOSURES

Although the chest radiographic examination often is considered the simplest of all radiographic procedures, it also is the examination with the highest number of repeats in many radiology departments. Therefore, unnecessary radiation exposure from repeat exposures should be minimized by taking extra care in positioning, CR centering, and selecting correct exposure factors if automatic exposure control (AEC) systems are not used. Reduce patient dose as much as possible through the use of correct radiation protection practices by close collimation and protective shielding.

COLLIMATION

Careful collimation is important in chest radiography. Restricting the primary x-ray beam by collimation not only reduces patient dose by reducing the volume of tissue irradiated but also improves image quality by reducing scatter radiation.

LEAD SHIELDING

In addition to careful collimation, a lead shield should be used to protect the abdominal area below the lungs. This shielding is especially important for children, pregnant women, and all individuals of childbearing age. However, many departments have a general policy of shielding for all patients undergoing chest radiography.

A common type of shield for chest radiography is a type of freestanding, adjustable mobile shield placed between the patient and the x-ray tube. A vinyl-covered lead shield that ties around the waist can also be used. Both of these types of shields should provide shielding from the level of the iliac crests, or slightly higher, to the midthigh area.

BACKSCATTER PROTECTION

To protect the gonads from scatter and secondary radiation from the IR holder device and the wall behind it, some references suggest that a freestanding shield or a wraparound shield also should be placed over the radiosensitive structures outside the anatomy of interest between the patient and the IR.

TECHNICAL FACTORS
Kilovoltage

Kilovoltage (kVp) should be high enough to result in sufficient contrast to demonstrate the many shades of gray needed to visualize finer lung markings. In general, chest radiography uses **low contrast,** described as **long-scale contrast,** with more shades of gray. This requires a high kVp of 110 to 125.

Lower kVp, yielding high contrast, would not provide sufficient penetration to allow clear visualization of the fine lung markings in the areas behind the heart and lung bases. Too high contrast is evident when the heart and other mediastinal structures appear underexposed, even though the lung fields are sufficiently penetrated.

As a general rule, in chest radiography, the use of high kVp (>100) **requires the use of grids.** Moving grids or fine-line focused fixed grids can be used. Advancements in portable or mobile chest radiography include the use of low-ratio grids (6:1 or 8:1) to reduce scatter radiation and overall improve image quality.

Exposure Time and Milliamperage (mAs—Milliampere Seconds)

Generally, chest radiography requires the use of **high mA and short exposure time** to minimize the chance of motion and resultant loss of sharpness. Sufficient mAs should be used to demonstrate the lungs and mediastinal structures without mottle or noise.

Placement of Image Markers

Throughout the positioning sections of this text, the correct or best placement of patient identification (ID) information and image markers is indicated. The top portion of each positioning page includes a drawing that demonstrates the correct IR size and placement (portrait or landscape) for computed radiography (CR) systems and the location and type of image marker used for that specific projection or position.

Although there is an assumption that the heart is located in the left thorax, there are conditions such as **situs inversus (also known as visceral inversion)**[2] in which the major organs of the body are on the opposite side. With this condition, the heart is located in the right thorax. An anatomic side marker (left or right) must be placed on the image receptor **prior** to exposure. If the marker is not seen radiographically, the exposure should be retaken to ensure the correct side of the thorax is identified.

PEDIATRIC APPLICATIONS
Supine Versus Erect

Generally, with newborns and small infants, for whom head support is required, chest radiographs are taken AP supine. Laterals also may be taken supine with a horizontal beam to demonstrate fluid levels (dorsal decubitus). However, erect PA and laterals are preferred whenever possible, with the use of immobilization devices such as the **Pigg-O-Stat** (Modern Way Immobilizers, Inc, Clifton, Tennessee) (described in Chapter 16).

Technical Factors

Lower kVp (70 to 85) and **less mAs** are required for pediatric patients with the **shortest exposure time possible** (to prevent motion). Higher-speed imaging systems or receptors generally are used with pediatric patients for two reasons: (1) to reduce the chance of motion and (2) to reduce the patient exposure dose (important because of the sensitivity of young tissue to radiation exposure). See Chapter 16 for more detailed information on special positioning considerations required with pediatric patients.

GERIATRIC APPLICATIONS
CR Centering
Frequently, older patients have less inhalation capability with resultant smaller lung fields, and a **higher CR location** is required (CR to T6–T7).

Technical Factors
Certain pathologic conditions are more common in geriatric patients, such as **pneumonia** and **emphysema,** which may require different exposure factor adjustments, as described under Clinical Indications.

Instructions and Patient Handling
More care, time, and patience frequently are required when breathing and positioning requirements are explained to geriatric patients. Help and support provided to these patients during the positioning process are important. Arm supports for keeping the arms raised high for the lateral position are essential for many older patients.

BARIATRIC PATIENT CONSIDERATIONS
A bariatric patient may present positioning and centering challenges. Because of a larger body girth, the technologist may place the top of the IR 1 to 2 inches (2.5 to 5 cm) above the shoulder. Because the lung apices may not reach as high as perceived, center the CR and IR to the level of T7 rather than base centering on the levels of the shoulders. T7 remains your centering point for most chest projections. T7 is generally located at the level of the inferior angle of the scapula. If it cannot be located, the vertebra prominens may serve as a landmark to assist in locating the T7 level. See p. 84 for information on CR centering based on the vertebra prominens.

For the AP chest projection, the jugular notch is a palpable landmark on the bariatric patient. T7 is approximately 3 to 4 inches (8 to 10 cm) inferior to the jugular notch.

Breathing Instructions
Breathing instructions are very important in chest radiography because any chest or lung movement that occurs during the exposure results in blurring of the radiographic image. Chest radiographs must be taken on **full** inspiration to show the lungs fully expanded.

HOLD BREATH ON SECOND INSPIRATION
More air can be inhaled without too much strain on the **second** breath compared with the first. Therefore, the patient should be asked to **hold the second full inspiration** rather than the first. However, the full inspiration should not be forced to the point of strain that causes unsteadiness; this should be explained to the patient before the exposure as the patient is being positioned.

INSPIRATION AND EXPIRATION
Occasional exceptions have been noted to taking chest radiographs on full inspiration only. For certain conditions, comparison radiographs are taken on both **full inspiration** (Fig. 2.31) and **full expiration** (Fig. 2.32). Indicators for this include a possible small **pneumothorax** (air or gas in the pleural cavity), fixation or lack of normal movement of the diaphragm, the presence of a foreign body, and the need to distinguish between an opacity in the rib and one in the lung. When such comparison radiographs are taken, they should be labeled "inspiration" and "expiration."

Note the number of ribs demonstrated above the diaphragm on the expiration projection. There are a greater number of ribs demonstrated above the diaphragm in the full inspiration radiograph. Also note the position of the two opacities in the right lung between inspiration and expiration projections. They shift position, which indicates they are within the lungs or pleura. Note also the number of ribs visible above the diaphragm, indicating the degree of inspiration (10 posterior ribs) and expiration (8 posterior ribs).

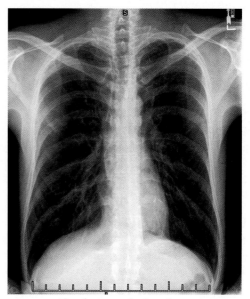

Fig. 2.31 Inspiration chest.

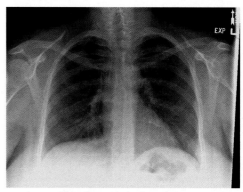

Fig. 2.32 Expiration chest.

ERECT CHEST RADIOGRAPHS

All chest radiographs should be taken in an erect position if the patient's condition allows. Three reasons for this are as follows:

1. **The diaphragm is able to move down farther.** An erect position causes the liver and other abdominal organs to drop, allowing the diaphragm to move farther down (inferior) on full inspiration and allowing the lungs to aerate fully.

2. **Air and fluid levels in the chest may be visualized.** If both air and fluid are present within a lung or within the pleural space, the heavier fluid, such as blood or pleural fluid resulting from infection or trauma, gravitates to the lowest position, whereas the air rises. In the recumbent position, a pleural effusion spreads out over the posterior surface of the lung, producing a hazy appearance of the entire lung. In the upright position, free fluid is located near the base of the lung. The PA erect chest radiograph (Fig. 2.33) shows some fluid in the left lower thoracic cavity near the base of the lung. The supine radiograph taken on a different patient (Fig. 2.34) demonstrates a generalized hazy appearance of the entire right lung, resulting from the presence of fluid now spread throughout the right thorax.

3. **Engorgement and hyperemia of pulmonary vessels may be prevented.** The term **engorgement** literally means "distended or swollen with fluid." **Hyperemia** *(hy″-per-e′-me-ah)* is an excess of blood that results in part from relaxation of the distal small blood vessels or arterioles.[3,4]

An erect position tends to minimize engorgement and hyperemia of pulmonary vessels, whereas a supine position increases these, which can change the radiographic appearance of these vessels and the lungs in general.

PA 72-Inch (180-cm) Source–Image Receptor Distance

Chest radiographs taken AP rather than PA at 72 inches (180 cm) result in **increased magnification of the heart shadow,** which complicates the diagnosis of possible cardiac enlargement. The reason for this increased magnification is the **anterior location** of the heart within the mediastinum; placing it closer to the IR on the PA results in less magnification. A longer source-to-image receptor distance (SID), such as 72 inches (180 cm), magnifies less because the x-ray beam has less divergence.

Evaluation Criteria

The description for each chest projection or position in this chapter includes an evaluation criteria section. This section lists and describes specific criteria by which one can evaluate the resultant radiograph. The goal of every technologist should be to take the optimal radiograph. These criteria provide a **definable standard** by which every chest radiographic image can be evaluated to determine where improvements can be made.

Important evaluation criteria for all routine PA and lateral chest radiographs are described in the following sections.

PA CHEST POSITIONING
True PA, No Rotation

Even a slight amount of rotation on a PA chest projection results in distortion of the size and shape of the heart shadow because the heart is located anteriorly in the thorax. Therefore, it is important that there be *no* rotation (Fig. 2.35). To prevent rotation, ensure that the patient is standing evenly on both feet with both shoulders rolled forward and downward. Also, check the posterior aspect of the shoulders and the lower posterior rib cage and the pelvis to ensure no rotation. **Scoliosis** and excessive **kyphosis** make it more difficult to prevent rotation. Scoliosis is lateral, or side-to-side, curvature of the spine, which frequently is combined with excessive kyphosis, a humpback curvature. Together, these

spinal curvatures frequently result in a "twisting" deformity of the bony thorax, making a true PA without some rotation more difficult or impossible.

Rotation on PA chest radiographs can be determined by examination of both sternal ends of the clavicles for a symmetric appearance in relationship to the spine. On a true PA chest without rotation, **both the right and the left sternal ends of the clavicles are the same distance from the center line of the spine.** Note the rotation evident in Fig. 2.36 by the difference in distance between the center of the spinal column and the sternal end of the right clavicle compared with the left.

The direction of rotation can be determined by noting which sternal end of the clavicle is closest to the spine. For example, in Fig. 2.36, the left side of the thorax is rotated toward the IR (right side moved away from IR), which creates a slight left anterior oblique (LAO) that decreases the distance of the left clavicle from the spine.

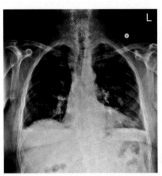

Fig. 2.33 PA erect, some fluid evident in left lower lung. (Note flat line appearance near left hemidiaphragm.)

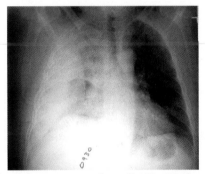

Fig. 2.34 Supine AP chest (fluid in right lung).

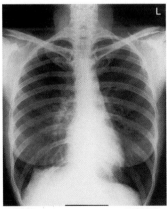
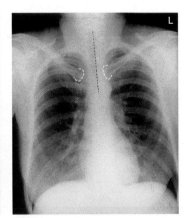

Fig. 2.35 Without rotation.　　**Fig. 2.36** With rotation (slight LAO).

Extending the Chin
Sufficient extension of the patient's neck ensures that the chin and neck are not superimposing the uppermost lung regions, the apices of the lungs. This is demonstrated by the two radiographs in Figs. 2.37 and 2.38. Also, ensure that the upper collimation border is high enough so that the apices are not cut off.

Minimizing Breast Shadows
A patient with large pendulous breasts should be asked to lift them up and outward and then to remove her hands as she leans against the chest board (IR) to keep them in this position. This position lessens the effect of breast shadows over the lower lung fields. However, depending on the size and density of the breasts, breast shadows over the lower lateral lung fields cannot be totally eliminated (Fig. 2.39).

LATERAL CHEST POSITIONINGWW

Side Closest to IR
The patient's side closest to the IR is best demonstrated on the finished radiograph. A **left lateral** (Fig. 2.40) should be performed unless departmental protocol indicates otherwise or unless certain pathology in the right lung indicates the need for a right lateral. A left lateral more accurately demonstrates the heart region (without as much magnification) because the heart is located primarily in the left thoracic cavity.

True Lateral, No Rotation or Tilt
Ensure the patient is standing straight with weight evenly distributed on both feet and arms raised. As a check against rotation, confirm that the posterior surfaces of the shoulder and the pelvis are directly superimposed and perpendicular to the IR. Because of the divergent x-ray beam, the posterior ribs on the side farthest away from the IR are magnified slightly and projected slightly posterior compared with the side closest to the IR on a true lateral chest; this is more noticeable on a broad-shouldered patient. However, this separation of posterior ribs resulting from divergence of the x-ray beam at the commonly used 72-inch (180-cm) SID **should be only ¼ to ½ inch (about 1 cm).** Any greater separation than this indicates rotation of the thorax from a true lateral position.[4]

NOTE: Some references recommend an intentional slight anterior rotation of the side away from the IR so that the posterior ribs are directly superimposed. This rotation may be preferred in some departments, but because the heart and most lung structures are near-midline structures and are not affected by the beam divergence, a straight lateral with respect to the IR is more common; this causes slight separation of the posterior ribs and costophrenic angles, as described earlier.

Fig. 2.41 shows a lateral chest with **excessive rotation,** as indicated by the **amount of separation of the right and left posterior ribs** and **separation of the two costophrenic angles.** This represents a positioning error and generally would require a repeat radiograph.

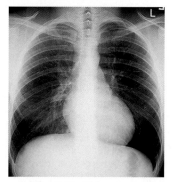

Fig. 2.37 Chin up.

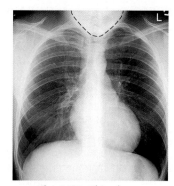

Fig. 2.38 Chin down.

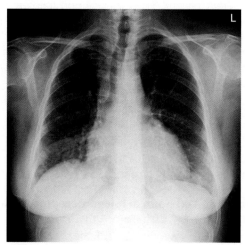

Fig. 2.39 Breast shadows evident—patient has pneumonia.

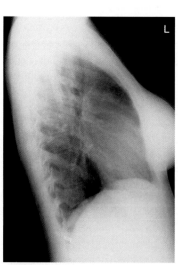

Fig. 2.40 Without excessive rotation (ribs superimposed).

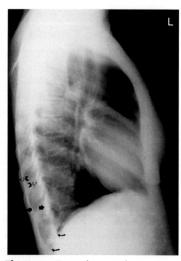

Fig. 2.41 Excessive rotation—positioning error (ribs not superimposed).

Direction of Rotation

The direction of rotation on a lateral chest is sometimes difficult to determine. Frequently, however, this can be done by identifying the left hemidiaphragm by the gastric air bubble in the stomach or by the inferior border of the heart shadow, both of which are associated with the left hemidiaphragm.[3]

No Tilt

There also should be **no tilt,** or leaning "sideways." The **midsagittal plane must be parallel to the IR.** If the patient's shoulders are placed firmly against the chest board (IR) on a lateral chest, the lower lateral thorax or hips or both may be 1 or 2 inches (2.5 to 5 cm) away. This is especially true on broad-shouldered patients. Tilt, if present, may be evident by closed disk spaces in the thoracic vertebra.

Arms Raised High

Ensure the patient raises both arms sufficiently high to prevent superimposition on the upper chest field. Patients who are weak or unstable may need to grasp a support (Fig. 2.42).

When the patient's arms are not raised sufficiently, the soft tissues of the upper arm superimpose portions of the lung field, as is demonstrated in Fig. 2.43. The arrows in this figure show margins of soft tissues of the arms overlying upper lung fields. This would require a repeat and should be avoided.

CR Location

The top of the shoulder traditionally has been used for chest positioning. This method includes placing the top of the IR 1½ to 2 inches (4 to 5 cm) above the shoulders and centering the CR to the center of the IR. However, this positioning method is inconsistent, given variations in lung field dimensions owing to differences in body habitus, as demonstrated by a comparison of Figs. 2.44 and 2.45. The small circle indicates where the CR was placed on these two patients. The center of the lungs (indicated by X) is shown to be near the center of the IR for the male patient in Fig. 2.44 but is above center on the small and older female patient in Fig. 2.45. This centering error unnecessarily exposes a large portion of the upper abdomen.

These variations demonstrate the importance of a chest positioning method that consistently centers the CR to the center of the lung fields on all types of patients with accurate collimation on *both* top and bottom.

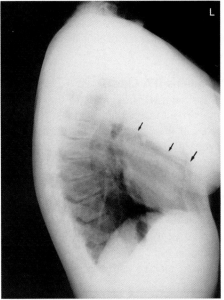

Fig. 2.43 Arms not raised—positioning error.

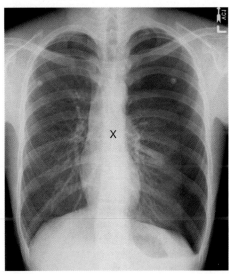

Fig. 2.44 Average sthenic/hyposthenic male patient (correct CR and collimation).

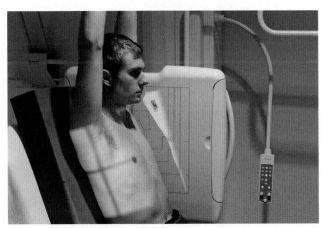

Fig. 2.42 Arms raised high.

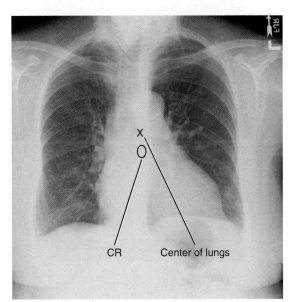

Fig. 2.45 Small and older female patient (incorrect CR and collimation and tilt).

CR CHEST-POSITIONING METHOD

Bony landmarks are consistent and reliable as a means of determining CR locations. Landmarks for locating the center of the lung fields are as follows.

Vertebra Prominens (PA Chest)

The vertebra prominens corresponds to the level of T1 and the uppermost margin of the apex of the lungs. This landmark, which can be palpated at the base of the neck, is the preferred landmark for locating the CR on a PA chest (Figs. 2.46 and 2.47). For an average adult female patient, this is down about 7 inches (18 cm); for an average adult male patient, this is down about 8 inches (20 cm).

One method of determining this distance is by using an average hand spread, as shown in Fig. 2.48. Most hands can reach 7 inches (18 cm). The 8-inch (20-cm) distance can be determined by estimating an additional inch. If the hand spread method is used, the technologist should practice with a ruler to determine these distances consistently.

These differences between male and female are true for near-average body types in the general population, with crossover exceptions in which certain larger athletic women may have longer lung fields and some men may have shorter lungs. However, for purposes of chest positioning for the general population, the average measurements of **7 inches (18 cm) for a woman** and **8 inches (20 cm) for a man** can be used as reliable guidelines (Fig. 2.49).

Exceptions

Other noteworthy exceptions in centering involve variations in body type. For example, the author found that well-developed athletic sthenic/hyposthenic body types require centering nearer to T8, or 9 inches (23 cm) down from the vertebra prominens. The hypersthenic body type requires centering only from 6 to 7 inches (15 to 18 cm) down.

NOTE: For most patients, this CR level for PA chests is near the level of the inferior angle of the scapula, which corresponds to the level of T7 on an average patient.

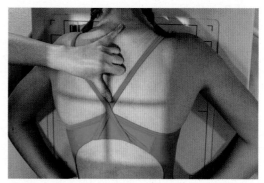
Fig. 2.47 Correct CR using vertebra prominens. Distance on an average female is 7 inches (18 cm).

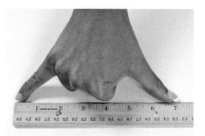
Fig. 2.48 Hand spread method—7 to 8 inches (18 to 20 cm).

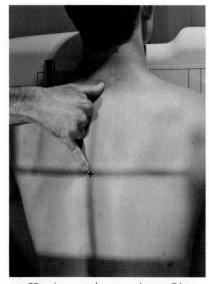
Fig. 2.46 Correct CR using vertebra prominens. Distance on an average male is 8 inches (20 cm).

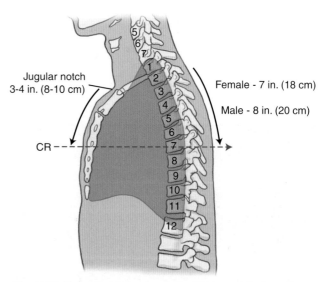

Jugular notch
3-4 in. (8-10 cm)

Female - 7 in. (18 cm)

Male - 8 in. (20 cm)

CR

Fig. 2.49 Topographic landmark for AP chest. *CR,* Central ray.

Jugular Notch (AP Chest)

The easily palpated jugular notch is the recommended landmark for location of the CR for AP chest radiographs. The level of T7 on an average adult is 3 to 4 inches (8 to 10 cm) below the jugular notch. For most older or hypersthenic patients, this is approximately **3 inches (8 cm).** For younger or sthenic/hyposthenic athletic types, this is nearer **4 to 5 inches (10 to 13 cm).**

This distance can be determined by the technologist's hand width. The average-sized hand width with the fingers together is approximately 3 inches (8 cm) as shown in Fig. 2.50.

Lung Dimensions and IR Placement

Contrary to common belief, the **width or horizontal dimension of the average PA or AP chest is greater than the vertical dimension.** If using computed radiography or analog systems, the technologist should use his or her discretion to determine whether the IR should be placed portrait (lengthwise) or landscape (crosswise) for PA or AP projections based on the size and body habitus of the patient, ensuring that the right and left costophrenic angles of the lungs are imaged.

For recumbent AP chest radiographs (usually taken at <72 inches [180 cm], with an accompanying increase in divergence of the x-ray beam), the chance that the side borders of the lungs may be cut off is increased when the IR is placed portrait. It is recommended that for most AP chest radiographs, the 14 × 17-inch (35 × 43-cm) IR should be placed landscape. The IR and CR should be centered to a point 3 to 4 inches (8 to 10 cm) below the jugular notch (see Fig. 2.50).

PA Chest

Some erect PA chests are performed with direct digital chest systems, which have a 17 × 17-inch (43 × 43-cm) IR that will accommodate both long and broad chest dimensions. Proper collimation with these systems is imperative. Ideally, the field is collimated on all four sides to the area of the lung fields. At a minimum, the field should be collimated to 14 × 17 inches (35 × 43 cm) or smaller. As the patient is standing and facing the chest IR, one can determine the amount of collimation by standing behind the patient and placing one's hands squarely on each side of the chest. If there is any doubt that both sides of the chest can be included, the IR should be collimated in a landscape direction, because the height of the average lung field is less than the width.

Collimation Guidelines

Side collimation borders can be determined easily by adjusting the illuminated field margins to the **outer skin margins** on each side of the posterior chest surface (given that lungs expand during deep inspiration). However, the upper and lower collimation borders are more difficult to determine, because these lung margins are not visible externally.

A reliable method for upper and lower chest collimation is to adjust the upper border of the illuminated light field to the **vertebra prominens,** which (with the divergent rays) results

in an upper collimation margin on the IR of about 1½ inches (4 cm) above the vertebra prominens (Fig. 2.51). This also results in a lower collimation border of 1 to 2 inches (2.5 to 5 cm) below the costophrenic angles if the CR was centered correctly. These distances above and below the lungs allow for some margin of error in CR placement without cutting off upper or lower lungs.

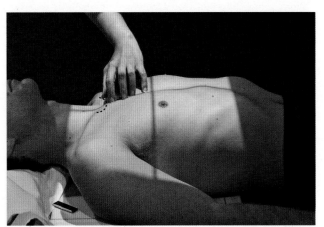

Fig. 2.50 IR landscape, CR 3 to 4 inches (8 to 11 cm) below jugular notch.

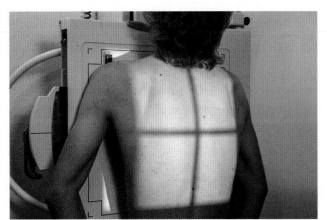

Fig. 2.51 Collimation guidelines, PA chest: CR—T7 or T8; sides—outer skin margins; upper—level of vertebra prominens.

Digital Imaging Considerations

Guidelines as listed next should be followed when chest images are acquired through the use of digital imaging technology. (See Chapter 1 for a discussion of applications of digital technology.)

1. **Collimation.** In addition to the benefit of reducing radiation dose to the patient, collimation that is closely restricted to the part that is being examined is key to ensuring the image processed by the computer is of optimal quality. Close collimation also improves image quality by preventing secondary and scatter radiation from surrounding areas (e.g., the dense abdomen below) from reaching the highly sensitive photostimulable storage phosphor plate (PSP) or digital radiography IR. With the digital IR being larger than other IRs, close collimation is critical for patient dose reduction and improved image quality. Close collimation also allows the computer to provide accurate information regarding the exposure indicator.

2. **Accurate centering.** Because of the exposure factors used for the digital image receptor, it is important that the body part and CR be accurately centered to the IR. In chest imaging, this involves centering the CR to the center of the lung fields, as described previously.

3. **Exposure factors.** Digital imaging systems are known for their wide exposure latitude; they are able to process an acceptable image from a broad range of exposure factors (kVp and mAs). However, the ALARA (as low as reasonably achievable) principle related to patient exposure still must be followed, and the lowest exposure factors required to obtain a diagnostic image must be used. This includes using the highest possible kVp and the lowest mAs consistent with optimal image quality.

4. **Post-processing evaluation of exposure indicator.** When the image is available for viewing, it is critiqued for positioning and exposure accuracy. The technologist must also **check the exposure indicator** to verify that the exposure factors used were in the correct range to ensure optimal quality with the least radiation to the patient. A standardized exposure index (EI) has been established for new digital systems; however, CR and digital systems without recent upgrades may have varying acceptable exposure ranges. It is important to learn the acceptable ranges for the exposure indicator for each digital system.

Alternative Modalities and Procedures

Conventional Tomography and CT

CT is performed frequently to examine and identify pathology of the mediastinum and lungs. Multi-detector computed tomography (MDCT) or **multislice CT** (MSCT) provides for faster scanning due to its ability to acquire numerous slices within one rotation of the gantry, which is especially advantageous in the thoracic region. Multidetector CT scanners can produce high-quality images of the heart and lungs with just one breath hold required of patients. MDCT is now routinely used in cardiac angiography for the demonstration of calcification and/or stenosis of the coronary arteries (see Chapter 18).

Sonography

Sonography (ultrasound) may be used to detect **pleural effusion** (fluid within pleural space) or for guidance when a needle is inserted to aspirate the fluid (thoracentesis).

An **echocardiogram** is an ultrasound examination in which sound waves are used to create an image of the heart. (This is not the same as an electrocardiogram [ECG], which is a completely different type of examination that assesses the electrical activity of the heart.) This imaging modality is valuable to demonstrate the dynamic movement and function of the heart valves.

Nuclear Medicine

Certain nuclear medicine procedures involving radionuclides can be used to evaluate and diagnose pulmonary diffusion conditions or pulmonary emboli. With the use of single-photon emission computed tomography (SPECT), the heart can be evaluated specifically for myocardial infarction.

MRI

Cardiovascular MRI procedures can be performed to demonstrate and evaluate pathology including congenital heart disorders, graft patency, cardiac tumors, thrombi, pericardial masses, and aortic dissection and aneurysm. MRI is unlikely to replace echocardiography for cardiac evaluation. However, MRI is a viable supplement to other imaging modalities, because it can provide multiplanar views of tumors and masses, further assess mediastinal pathology, and evaluate aortic dissection and aneurysm.

Clinical Indications

The **clinical indications** (Table 2.1), as listed subsequently and in each chapter of this textbook, are not intended to be inclusive of all diseases or pathologic conditions of which technologists should be aware or that may be covered in a separate pathology course. However, they do represent conditions that are encountered more commonly, and knowledge and understanding of these clinical indications should be considered **routine** and **essential** for all technologists.

Patient histories in which these clinical indications are noted help the technologist select the optimum exposure factors and ensure that the necessary projections or body positions are being used. When adjusting the exposure factors, the technologist must ensure that a quality diagnostic image is obtained without obscuring or accentuating the disease process.

This information is also important for the technologist in understanding and being prepared to respond to patient needs and reactions during the radiographic procedure. For the chest, these clinical indications are numerous and complex. The more common indications for youth and adults are listed as follows (see Chapter 16 for information on infants and children).

CHEST PATHOLOGY, CONDITIONS, AND TRAUMA[5]

Aspiration *(as-pi-ra'-shun)* (mechanical obstruction) is most common in small children when **foreign objects** are swallowed or aspirated into the air passages of the bronchial tree. In adults, it may occur with food particles, creating coughing and gagging (relieved by the Heimlich maneuver). Aspiration may be evident in the lower airways on frontal and lateral chest radiographs or AP and lateral radiographs of the upper airway.

Atelectasis *(at"-e-lek'-tah-sis)* is a condition rather than a disease, in which collapse of all or a portion of a lung occurs as the result of obstruction of the bronchus or puncture or "blowout" of an air passageway. With less air in the lung than normal, this region appears more radiodense, and this may cause the trachea and heart to shift to the affected side.

Bronchiectasis *(brong"-ke-ek'-tah-sis)* is an irreversible dilation or widening of bronchi or bronchioles that may result from repeated pulmonary infection or obstruction. Areas of bronchial walls are destroyed and become chronically inflamed, resulting in increased production of mucus and causing chronic cough and expectoration (coughing up sputum). Pus can collect in dilated regions, resulting in an increase in regional radiodensity with less air in these regions (most common in the lower lobes).

Bronchitis *(brong-ki'-tis)* is an acute (short-term) or chronic (long-term) condition in which excessive mucus is secreted into the bronchi, causing cough and shortness of breath. The chief cause is cigarette smoking. Infectious bronchitis is caused by viruses or bacteria. Bronchitis generally involves lower lobes and in severe cases is demonstrated on radiographs by hyperinflation and more dominant lung markings.

TABLE 2.1 SUMMARY OF CLINICAL INDICATIONS

CONDITION OR DISEASE	MOST COMMON RADIOGRAPHIC EXAMINATION	POSSIBLE RADIOGRAPHIC APPEARANCE	EXPOSURE FACTOR ADJUSTMENT[a]
Aspiration (mechanical obstruction)	PA and lateral chest and lateral upper airway	Radiodense or radiopaque outline	Soft tissue technique for upper airway (−)
Atelectasis (collapse of all or portion of lung)	PA and lateral chest and PA inspiration/expiration	Radiodense lung regions with shift of heart and trachea in severe cases	Increase (+)
Bronchiectasis	PA and lateral chest with bronchogram or CT	Radiodense lower lungs	Generally none
Bronchitis	PA and lateral chest	Hyperinflation (general radiolucency) and dominant lung markings of lower lungs	Generally none
Chronic obstructive pulmonary disease (COPD)	PA and lateral chest	Depends on underlying cause	Changes in severe cases only
Cystic fibrosis	PA and lateral chest	Increased radiodensities in specific lung regions	Increase with severe condition (+)
Dyspnea (difficult breathing)	PA and lateral chest	Depends on cause of dyspnea	Depends on cause
Emphysema	PA and lateral chest	Increased lung dimensions, barrel chest, flattened diaphragm, radiolucent lungs	Significantly decreased, dependent on severity (−)
Epiglottitis	Soft tissue lateral upper airway	Narrowing of upper airway at epiglottic region	Soft tissue lateral technique (−)
Lung neoplasm			
Benign (hamartoma)	PA and lateral chest	Radiodensities with sharp outlines; mass may be calcified (radiopaque)	Generally none
Malignant types	PA and lateral chest, CT scans	Slight shadows in early stages, larger defined radiopaque masses in advanced stages	Generally none
Pleural effusion (hydrothorax) (in pleural cavity) Empyema (fluid is pus) Hemothorax (fluid is blood)	Erect PA and lateral chest or horizontal beam lateral decubitus with **affected side down**	Increased radiodensity, air-fluid levels, possible mediastinal shift (see Atelectasis)	Increase (+)
Pleurisy	PA and lateral chest	Possible air-fluid levels, or none with "dry" pleurisy	Generally none
Pneumonia (pneumonitis)	PA and lateral chest	Patchy infiltrate with increased radiodensity	Generally none
Aspiration pneumonia			
Bronchopneumonia			
Lobar (pneumococcal)			
Viral (interstitial)			
Pneumothorax	Erect PA and lateral chest or lateral decubitus with **affected side up,** PA inspiration/expiration for small pneumothorax	Lung seen displaced from chest wall, no lung markings	Generally none
Pulmonary edema (fluid within lungs)	PA and lateral chest; horizontal beam projection for air-fluid levels	Increased diffuse radiodensity in hilar regions; air-fluid levels	Increase (+) in severe cases
Pulmonary emboli (sudden blockage of artery in lung)	PA and lateral chest and perfusion scans (nuclear medicine), CT scans	Rarely demonstrated on chest radiographs except for possible wedge-shaped opacity (Hampton's hump)	Generally none
Respiratory distress syndrome (RDS)—commonly called hyaline membrane disease (HMD) in children	PA and lateral erect chest	Granular pattern of increased radiodensity throughout lungs, possible air-fluid levels	Increase (+) without obscuring pathology
Tuberculosis			
Primary tuberculosis	PA and lateral chest	Small opaque spots throughout lungs; enlargement of hilar region in early stages	Generally none
Reactivation (secondary) tuberculosis	PA and lateral chest and AP lordotic chest, tomograms	Regions of calcification with cavitations, frequently in area of upper lobes and apices with upward retraction of hila	None or increase slightly (+)
Occupational lung diseases (forms of pneumoconiosis)			
Anthracosis (black lung)	PA and lateral chest	Small opaque spots throughout lungs	Generally none
Asbestosis	PA and lateral chest	Calcifications (radiodensities) involving the pleura	Generally none
Silicosis	PA and lateral chest	Distinctive pattern of scarring and dense nodules	Generally none

[a]Automatic exposure control (AEC) systems are designed to optimize mAs. Digital radiographic systems will correct exposure brightness automatically for patient size variances and for these pathologic conditions through processing algorithms; manual adjustments generally are not needed when AEC is used if the AEC system is calibrated correctly and used as intended. However, these exposure adjustments may be needed for more extreme cases or for repeats, even with AEC. Manual exposure adjustments are also important when manual exposure techniques such as for tabletop or mobile examinations are set when AEC is not used.

Chronic obstructive pulmonary disease (COPD) is a form of persistent obstruction of the airways that usually causes difficulty in emptying the lungs of air; it may be caused by emphysema or chronic bronchitis (smoking is the predominant cause of COPD). Asthma also is considered a COPD. Mild cases of COPD usually are not detectable on chest radiographs, but more severe conditions are clearly demonstrated (see **emphysema** later in this list).

Cystic fibrosis *(sis'-tik fi-bro'-sis)*, the most common of inherited diseases, is a condition in which secretions of heavy mucus cause progressive "clogging" of bronchi and bronchioles. This may be evident on chest radiographs as increased radiodensities in specific lung regions, along with hyperinflation.

Dyspnea *(disp'-ne-ah)* is a condition of shortness of breath, which creates a sensation of difficulty in breathing; it is most common in older persons. Although generally caused by physical exertion, it may be caused by restrictive or obstructive defects within the lungs or airways. Dyspnea also may be caused by pulmonary edema related to cardiac conditions. PA and lateral chest radiographs are commonly taken as an initial procedure followed by other examinations in an effort to make a diagnosis.

Emphysema *(em"-fi-se'-mah)* is an irreversible and chronic lung disease in which air spaces in the alveoli become greatly enlarged as a result of alveolar wall destruction and loss of alveolar elasticity. Air tends not to be expelled during expiration, resulting in seriously labored breathing with impedance of gas exchange within the lungs. Causes include smoking and long-term dust inhalation. In severe cases, emphysema is evident on chest radiographs by **increased lung dimensions,** barrel chest with depressed and flattened diaphragm obscuring costophrenic angles, and an elongated heart shadow. Lung fields appear very **radiolucent,** requiring a significant **decrease** in exposure factors from a normal chest, even with the increased chest dimensions.

Epiglottitis *(ep"-i-glo-ti'-tis)* is most common in children ages 2 to 5. See Chapter 16 for more information on this serious, **life-threatening condition, which can develop very rapidly.** A soft tissue lateral of the upper airway may demonstrate edema or swelling at the point of the epiglottis.

Lung neoplasm refers to a new growth or tumor. Neoplasms may be benign (noncancerous) or malignant (cancerous).

- **Benign:** A **hamartoma** *(ham"-ahr-to'-ma)* is the most common benign pulmonary mass, and it generally is found in peripheral regions of the lungs. These are seen on chest radiographs as small radiodense masses with sharp outlines.
- **Malignant:** Many types of lung cancers have been identified, and more than 90% start in the bronchi (bronchogenic carcinoma). Less common is alveolar cell carcinoma, which originates in the alveoli of the lungs. Also, many cancers, such as breast, colon, and prostate, start elsewhere in the body before spreading to the lungs as **pulmonary metastases.** Studies have shown that smoking is the primary cause in about 90% of all lung cancers in men. In the past 50 years, a woman's risk of dying from lung cancer from smoking has more than tripled and is nearly equal to men's risk.[6]

Lung cancer may be demonstrated on chest radiography as slight shadows in the early stages and as more sharply defined, larger radiopaque masses in more advanced cases. Malignant lung tumors rarely calcify; therefore, calcified radiopaque masses or nodules are generally benign.

CT scans may reveal small nodules that are not yet seen on chest radiographs. Biopsies usually are required to determine whether these shadows are the result of inflammation or are cancerous.

Occupational lung disease (forms of pneumoconiosis) arises from occupational exposures, including certain types of mine work, sandblasting, and similar professions. Chest x-rays show distinctive patterns of nodules and scarring densities.

- **Anthracosis** *(an"-thre-ko'-sis)*, also called **black lung pneumoconiosis,** is caused by deposits of coal dust. With long-term inhalation ($\geq$10 years), it spreads throughout the lungs and is seen on chest radiographs as small opaque spots or conglomerate masses.
- **Asbestosis** *(as"-bes-to'-sis)* is caused by inhalation of asbestos dust (fibers), which results in pulmonary fibrosis. It may develop into lung cancer, especially in smokers.
- **Silicosis** *(sil"-i-ko'-sis)* is a permanent condition of the lungs that is caused by inhalation of silica (quartz) dust, a form of sand dust. Patients with silicosis are three times more likely to develop TB than are persons without silicosis.[7]

Pleural effusion (an older, outdated term is hydrothorax) is a condition of abnormal accumulation of fluid in the pleural cavity. Types of pleural effusion include the following:

- **Empyema** *(em"-pi-e'-mah),* which occurs when the fluid is pus. Empyema may be caused by chest wounds, obstruction of bronchi, or ruptured lung abscess. It may develop when pneumonia or a lung abscess spreads into the pleural space.
- **Hemothorax** *(he"-mo-thor'-aks),* which occurs when the fluid is blood. A common cause of right-sided or bilateral pleural effusion is congestive heart failure. Causes of left-sided effusion include trauma, pulmonary infarct, pancreatitis, and subphrenic abscess.

Any type of pleural effusion is demonstrated by **fluid levels** on horizontal-beam chest radiographs. Small amounts are best shown by a lateral decubitus position with **affected side down** or with **erect positioning.**

Pleurisy *(ploor'-i-se)* is characterized by inflammation (usually caused by a virus or bacterium) of the pleura surrounding the lungs. The cause is visceral and parietal pleura "rubbing" during respiration, which results in severe pain. It frequently follows pneumonia or trauma to the chest. Pleurisy may be demonstrated radiographically by associated pleural effusion. A condition called "dry pleurisy" does not include fluid accumulation and generally is not visible on radiographs.

Pneumonia *(noo-mon'-ya)* (pneumonitis) is an inflammation of the lungs that results in **accumulation of fluid** within certain sections of the lungs, creating increased radiodensities in these regions. The most common initial diagnostic examination consists of PA and lateral erect horizontal beam radiographs. Types of pneumonia are derived from the location and cause of the inflammation. Normal exposure factors generally are used initially. The radiologist may request secondary images with increased density (brightness) to see through the area of interest to rule out a lesion in the same anatomic region when film-screen imaging methods are being used. The different types of pneumonia include the following:

- **Aspiration pneumonia** is caused by aspiration of a foreign object or food into the lungs, which irritates the bronchi, resulting in edema.
- **Bronchopneumonia** is bronchitis of both lungs that most commonly is caused by *Streptococcus* or *Staphylococcus* bacteria.
- **Lobar pneumonia** generally is confined to one or two lobes of the lungs.
- **Viral (interstitial) pneumonia** causes inflammation of the alveoli and connecting lung structures. It most commonly is evident as increased radiodensities in the region surrounding the hila.

Pneumothorax *(noo"-mo-thor'-aks)* is an accumulation of air in the pleural space that causes partial or complete collapse of the lung and results in immediate and severe shortness of breath and chest pain. It may be caused by trauma or a pathologic condition that causes spontaneous rupture of a weakened area of lung.

Radiographically, the affected lung can be seen displaced away from the chest wall. Most evident on chest radiographs is the fact that **no lung markings** are seen in the region of the collapsed lung. Care should be taken to identify the lung edge or boundary. Chest radiographs for pneumothorax should be taken **erect.** If the patient cannot assume an erect position, a horizontal beam **lateral decubitus** position with the **affected side up** should be taken (not down as with pleural effusion).

Erect PA inspiration/expiration radiographs often are taken to demonstrate a small pneumothorax, which is best seen at the apex of an erect PA radiograph with maximum expiration.

Pulmonary edema is a condition of excess fluid within the lung that most frequently is caused by a backup in pulmonary circulation commonly associated with congestive heart failure. A common cause is coronary artery disease, in which blood flow to the heart muscle is restricted. Coronary artery disease weakens the heart and results in inadequate pulmonary circulation, causing backup of blood in the lungs. The condition is seen on chest radiographs as a diffuse increase in radiodensity in the hilar regions fading toward the periphery of the lung and as increased air-fluid levels with horizontal beam projections in more severe conditions.

Respiratory distress syndrome (RDS) (commonly called **hyaline membrane disease [HMD]** in infants and **adult respiratory distress syndrome [ARDS]** in adults) is an emergent condition in which the alveoli and capillaries of the lung are injured or infected, resulting in leakage of fluid and blood into the spaces between alveoli or into the alveoli themselves with formation of hyaline membranes. (HMD results from a lack of lung development in which the alveoli collapse as the result of lack of internal tension.) This leakage can be detected radiographically as increased density (brightness) throughout the lungs in a granular pattern as the normally air-filled spaces are filled with fluid. The most common radiographic sign is an "air bronchogram."

Tuberculosis *(too-ber"-ku-lo'-sis)* (TB) is a contagious disease (potentially fatal) that is caused by airborne bacteria. At one time, TB resulted in more than 30% of all deaths, but the development of vaccines and antibiotics such as streptomycin in the 1940s and 1950s nearly eliminated the threat of this disease. However, occurrence of TB has begun to increase again with the increased incidence of acquired immunodeficiency syndrome (AIDS) and in the presence of urban overcrowding and unsanitary conditions.

- **Primary tuberculosis** refers to TB that occurs in persons who have never had the disease before. Hilar enlargement, along with enlarged mediastinal lymph nodes, is an important indicator of primary TB. Small focal spot lesions may be found anywhere in the lungs, and unilateral pleural effusion is common, especially in adults.

- **Reactivation (secondary) tuberculosis** usually develops in adults and generally is first evident on radiography bilaterally in the upper lobes as irregular calcifications that are mottled in appearance. Upward retraction of the hila is frequently evident. As healing occurs, fibrous tissue develops, with calcification surrounding the region and leaving a type of cavity that can be seen on tomograms of this region. **AP lordotic projections** are frequently requested for visualization of calcifications and cavitations of the apices and upper lobes.

Routine and Special Projections

The chest projections shown and described on the following pages are suggested routine and special departmental projections that all student technologists should master.

Routine projections are those that are commonly taken on average patients who are helpful and can cooperate in performing the procedure.

Special projections are more common projections that are taken as extra or additional projections to demonstrate better certain pathologic conditions or specific body parts or when the patient is unable to cooperate fully.

PA PROJECTION—CHEST

AMBULATORY PATIENT

Clinical Indications
- When performed erect, PA demonstrates pleural effusion, pneumothorax, atelectasis, and signs of infection

Chest
ROUTINE
• PA
• Lateral

Technical Factors
- Minimum SID—72 inches (180 cm)
- IR size—14 × 17 inches (35 × 43 cm), portrait or landscape (see NOTE 1)
- Grid
- kVp range—110–125

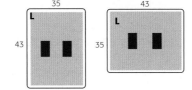

Shielding
Shield radiosensitive tissues outside region of interest

Patient Position
- Patient erect, feet spread slightly, weight equally distributed on both feet
- Chin raised, resting against IR
- Hands on lower hips, palms out, elbows partially flexed (Fig. 2.52)
- Shoulders rotated forward against IR to allow scapulae to move laterally clear of lung fields; shoulders depressed downward to move clavicles below the apices

Part Position ⊹
- Align midsagittal plane with CR and with midline of IR with equal margins between lateral thorax and sides of IR
- Ensure **no rotation** of thorax by placing the midcoronal plane parallel to the IR
- Raise or lower CR and IR as needed to the level of T7 for an average patient (top of IR is approximately 1½ to 2 inches [4 to 5 cm] above shoulders on average patients)

CR
- CR perpendicular to IR and centered to **midsagittal plane at level of T7** (7 to 8 inches [18 to 20 cm] below vertebra prominens, or to the inferior angle of scapula)
- IR centered to CR

Recommended Collimation
Collimate on four sides to area of lung fields (top border of illuminated field should be to the level of vertebra prominens, and lateral border should be to outer skin margins)

Respiration
Exposure is made at end of **second full inspiration.**

NOTE 1: For hypersthenic and broad-chested patients, place 14 × 17 inch (35 × 43 cm) IR landscape (or collimate to at least this size when possible with larger digital plates).

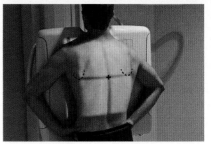

Fig. 2.52 PA chest.

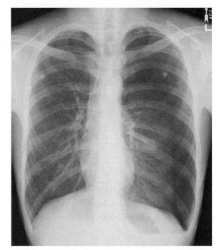

Fig. 2.53 PA chest.

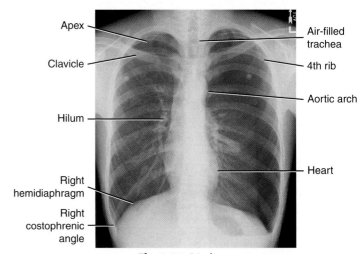

Apex — Clavicle — Hilum — Right hemidiaphragm — Right costophrenic angle — Air-filled trachea — 4th rib — Aortic arch — Heart

Fig. 2.54 PA chest.

Evaluation Criteria
Anatomy Demonstrated: • Included are both lungs from apices to costophrenic angles and the air-filled trachea from T1 down. • Hilum region markings, heart, great vessels, and bony thorax are demonstrated (Figs. 2.53 and 2.54).

Position: • Chin sufficiently elevated to prevent superimposing apices. • Sufficient forward shoulder rotation to prevent superimposition of scapulae over lung fields. • Larger breast shadows (if present) primarily lateral to lung fields. • No rotation: Both sternoclavicular joints the same distance from center line of spine.[4] • Distance from lateral rib margins to vertebral column the same on each side from upper to lower rib cage (see NOTE 2). • Collimation margins near equal on top and bottom with center

of collimation field (CR) to T7 region on most patients. • Full inspiration with no motion. • Visualizes a minimum of 10 posterior ribs above diaphragm (11 on many patients).

NOTE 2: Scoliosis and kyphosis also may cause asymmetry of sternoclavicular joints and rib cage margins, as evidenced by R to L spinal curvature.

Exposure: • No motion, as evidenced by sharp outlines of rib margins, diaphragm, and heart borders and also sharp lung markings in hilar region and throughout lungs. • Sufficient long-scale contrast for visualization of fine vascular markings within lungs. • Faint outlines of at least midthoracic and upper thoracic vertebrae and posterior ribs visible through heart and mediastinal structures.

PA PROJECTION–CHEST

ON STRETCHER IF PATIENT CANNOT STAND

Clinical Indications
- When performed erect, PA demonstrates pleural effusion, pneumothorax, atelectasis, and signs of infection

Chest
ROUTINE
• PA
• Lateral

Technical Factors
- Minimum SID–72 inches (180 cm)
- IR size–14 × 17 inches (35 × 43 cm), portrait or landscape
- Grid
- kVp range–110–125

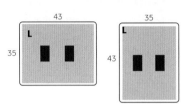

Shielding
Shield radiosensitive tissues outside region of interest.

Patient Position
- Patient erect, seated on cart, legs over the edge (Fig. 2.55)
- Arms around cassette unless a chest IR device is used, then position as for an ambulatory patient
- Shoulders rotated forward and downward

Part Position
- Ensure no rotation of thorax.
- Adjust height of IR so that top of IR is about 1½ to 2 inches (4 to 5 cm) above top of shoulders and CR is at T7.
- If portable image receptor is used because patient cannot be placed up against wall bucky, place pillow or padding on lap to raise and support image receptor as shown, but keep it against chest for minimum object–image receptor distance (OID) (Fig. 2.56).

CR
- CR perpendicular to the IR and centered to the **midsagittal plane at the level of T7** (7 to 8 inches [18 to 20 cm] below vertebra prominens or to the inferior angles of scapulae)
- Cassette centered to level of CR

Recommended Collimation
Collimate to area of lung fields. Upper border of illuminated field should be to the **level of vertebra prominens,** which with divergent rays will result in upper collimation border on IR to about 1½ inches (3.5 cm) above apex of lungs

Respiration
Make exposure on second full inspiration.

NOTE: Use a compression band or other means to ensure that patient is stable and will not waver or move during exposure.

Evaluation Criteria
Radiograph should appear similar to ambulatory PA chest, as described on preceding page. (Fig. 2.57).

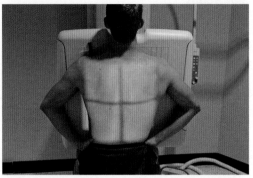

Fig. 2.55 PA chest (patient seated, chest against wall bucky).

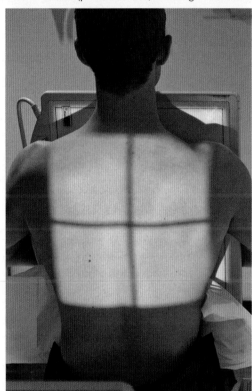

Fig. 2.56 PA chest (patient seated, holding cassette-less detector).

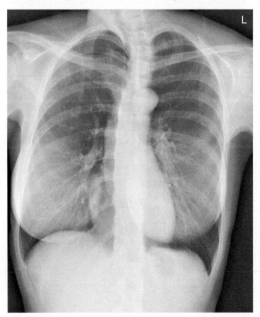

Fig. 2.57 PA chest.

LATERAL POSITION—CHEST

AMBULATORY PATIENT

Clinical Indications
- A 90° perspective from PA projection may demonstrate pathology situated posterior to the heart, great vessels, and sternum

Chest
ROUTINE
• PA
• Lateral

Technical Factors
- Minimum SID—72 inches (180 cm)
- IR size—14 × 17 inches (35 × 43 cm), portrait
- Grid
- kVp range—110–125

Shielding
Shield radiosensitive tissues outside region of interest.

Patient Position
- Patient erect, **left side** against IR unless patient complaint involves right side (in that case, do a right lateral if departmental protocol includes this option)
- Weight evenly distributed on both feet
- Arms raised above head, chin up

Part Position
- Center patient to CR and to IR anteriorly and posteriorly (Fig. 2.58)
- Position in a **true lateral** position (coronal plane is perpendicular and sagittal plane is parallel to IR; see NOTE 1)
- Lower CR and IR slightly from PA if needed (see NOTE 2)

CR
- CR perpendicular, directed to **midthorax at level of T7** (3 to 4 inches [7.5 to 10 cm] below level of jugular notch)

Recommended Collimation
Collimate on four sides to area of lung fields (top border of light field to level of vertebra prominens).

Respiration
Make exposure at end of **second full inspiration.**

NOTE 1: Ensure that **midsagittal plane** is **parallel to IR,** which for slender but broad-shouldered patients results in hips and lower thorax *not* being against IR.

NOTE 2: This increase in OID of the lower chest results in the costophrenic angles of the lungs being projected lower because of divergence of the x-ray beam. Therefore, **CR and IR should be lowered a minimum of 1 inch (2.5 cm) from the PA** on this type of patient to prevent cutoff of costophrenic angles.

Evaluation Criteria
Anatomy Demonstrated: • Included are the entire lungs from apices to the costophrenic angles and from the sternum anteriorly to the posterior ribs and thorax posteriorly (Figs. 2.59 and 2.60).

Position: • Chin and arms elevated sufficiently to prevent excessive soft tissues from superimposing apices. • **No rotation:** Posterior ribs and costophrenic angle on side away from IR projected slightly (¼ to ½ inch [or about 1 cm] posterior because of divergent rays). • The hilar region should be in the approximate center of the IR.

NOTE: To determine direction of rotation and critique radiographs, see p. 14.

Exposure: • No motion, as evidenced by sharp outlines of the diaphragm and lung markings. • Should have sufficient exposure and long-scale contrast for **visualization of rib outlines and lung markings through the heart shadow and upper lung areas** without overexposing other regions of the lungs.

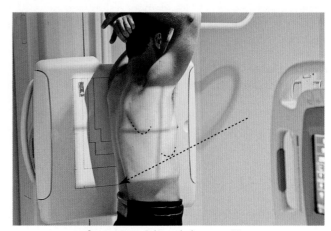

Fig. 2.58 Left lateral chest position.

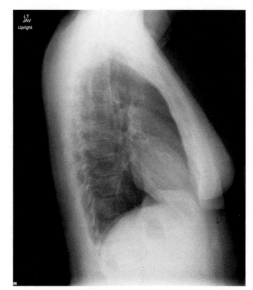

Fig. 2.59 Left lateral chest.

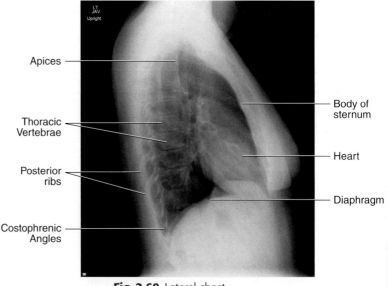

Apices

Thoracic Vertebrae

Posterior ribs

Costophrenic Angles

Body of sternum

Heart

Diaphragm

Fig. 2.60 Lateral chest.

ALTERNATIVE LATERAL POSITIONS—CHEST

WITH WHEELCHAIR OR CART IF PATIENT CANNOT STAND

Clinical Indications
- A 90° perspective from PA may demonstrate pathology situated posterior to the heart, great vessels, and sternum

Chest
ROUTINE
• PA
• Lateral

Technical Factors
- Minimum SID—72 inches (180 cm)
- IR size—14 × 17 inches (35 × 43 cm), portrait
- Grid
- kVp range—110–125

Shielding Shield radiosensitive tissues outside region of interest.

Patient Position on Cart
- Patient seated on cart; legs over the edge if this is easier for patient (ensure that cart is locked and does not move)
- Arms crossed above head or hold on to arm support (Fig. 2.61)
- Chin extended upward

Patient Position in Wheelchair
- Remove armrests, if possible, or place pillow or other support under smaller patients so that armrests of wheelchair do not superimpose lower lungs. (Fig. 2.62).
- Turn patient in wheelchair to lateral position as close to IR as possible.
- Have patient lean forward and place support blocks behind back; raise arms above head and have patient hold on to support bar—**keeping arms high.**

Part Position
- Center patient to CR and to IR by checking anterior and posterior aspects of thorax; adjust CR and IR to level of T7.
- Ensure **no rotation** by viewing patient from tube position.

CR
- CR perpendicular, directed to **level of T7** (3 to 4 inches [8 to 10 cm] below level of jugular notch)
- Top of IR approximately 1 inch (2.5 cm) above vertebra prominens

Recommended Collimation Collimate on four sides to area of lung fields (top border of light field to level of vertebra prominens).

Respiration Make exposure at end of **second full inspiration.**

NOTE: Always attempt to have patient sit completely erect in wheelchair or on cart if possible. However, if the patient's condition does not allow this, the head end of the cart can be raised as nearly erect as possible with a radiolucent support behind the back (Fig. 2.63). All attempts should be made to get patient as nearly erect as possible.

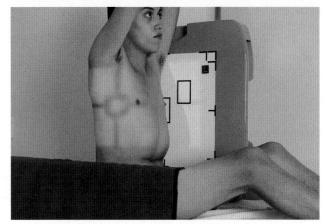
Fig. 2.61 Left lateral chest position on cart.

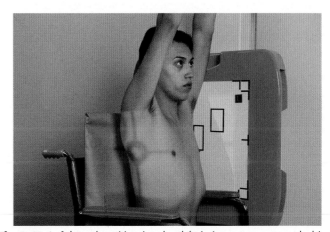
Fig. 2.62 Left lateral position in wheelchair (arms up, support behind back).

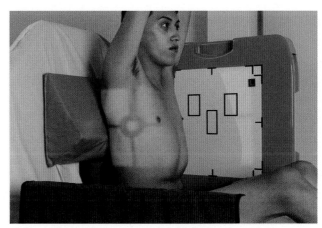
Fig. 2.63 Erect, supported left lateral position.

Evaluation Criteria
Radiograph should appear similar to ambulatory lateral position as described under Evaluation Criteria on preceding page.

AP PROJECTION—CHEST

SUPINE OR SEMIERECT (IN DEPARTMENT OR AS BEDSIDE PORTABLE)

Clinical Indications
- Demonstrates pathology involving the lungs, diaphragm, and mediastinum
- Determining air-fluid levels (pleural effusion) requires a completely erect position with a horizontal CR, as in a PA or decubitus chest projection

Chest
SPECIAL
• AP supine or semierect

Technical Factors
- Minimum SID—72 inches (180 cm) for semierect (see NOTES)
- IR size—14 × 17 inches (35 × 43 cm), portrait or landscape
- Grid (due to higher kVp, the use of a grid is strongly recommended)
- kVp range—110–125

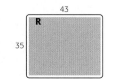

Shielding
Shield radiosensitive tissues outside region of interest.

Patient Position
- Patient is supine on cart; if possible, the head end of the cart or bed should be raised into a semierect position (see NOTES).
- Roll patient's shoulders forward by rotating arms medially or internally.

Part Position
- Place IR under or behind patient; align center of IR to CR (top of IR about 1½ inches [4 to 5 cm] above shoulders) (Fig. 2.64).
- Center patient to CR and to IR; check by viewing patient from the top, near the tube position.

CR
- CR angled **caudad to be perpendicular to long axis of sternum** (generally requires ±5° caudad angle, to prevent clavicles from obscuring the apices)
- CR to **level of T7,** 3 to 4 inches (8 to 10 cm) below jugular notch

Recommended Collimation
Collimate on four sides to area of lung fields (top border of light field to level of vertebra prominens).

Respiration
Make exposure at end of **second full inspiration.**

NOTES: Crosswise IR placement is recommended for large or hypersthenic or broad-chested patients to minimize chance of lateral cutoff. This requires **accurate CR alignment with center of IR** with only minimal caudal angle to prevent grid cutoff if grid is used.

For **semierect position,** use 72-inch (180-cm) SID if possible. **Always** place markers on the IR or label the image to indicate the SID used; also indicate the projections obtained, such as AP supine or AP semierect (Fig. 2.65).

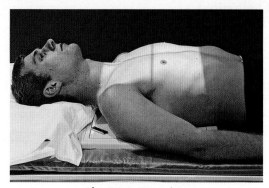

Fig. 2.64 AP supine.

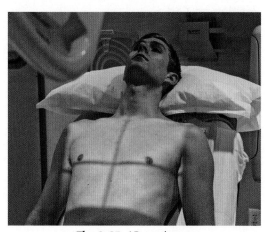

Fig. 2.65 AP semierect.

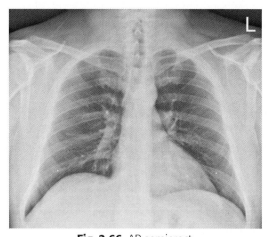

Fig. 2.66 AP semierect.

Evaluation Criteria
- Criteria for chest radiographs taken in supine or semierect positions should be similar to criteria for PA projection described earlier, with three exceptions:
  1. The heart appears larger as a result of increased magnification from a shorter SID and increased OID of the heart.
  2. Possible pleural effusion for this type of patient often obscures vascular lung markings compared with a fully erect PA chest projection. Without a horizontal beam, fluid levels may not be demonstrated.
  3. Usually, inspiration is not as full, and only eight or nine posterior ribs are visualized above the diaphragm. The lungs may appear denser because they are not as fully aerated (Fig. 2.66).
- **Correct CR angle:** The clavicles should be in the same horizontal plane with an unobstructed view of the apical region.[4]

LATERAL DECUBITUS POSITION (AP PROJECTION)—CHEST

Clinical Indications
- Small **pleural effusions** are demonstrated by air-fluid levels in pleural space
- **Small amounts of air** in pleural cavity may demonstrate a possible pneumothorax (see NOTES)

Chest
SPECIAL
• AP supine or semierect
• Lateral decubitus (AP)

Technical Factors
- Minimum SID—72 inches (180 cm)
- IR size—14 × 17 inches (35 × 43 cm), landscape (with respect to patient position)
- Grid
- kVp range—110–125
- Use decubitus (decub) marker

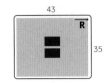

Shielding Shield radiosensitive tissues outside region of interest.

Patient Position
- Cardiac board on the cart or radiolucent pad under patient
- Patient lying on right side for right lateral decubitus and on left side for left lateral decubitus (see NOTES)
- Patient's chin extended and both arms raised above head to clear lung field; back of patient firmly against IR; cart secured to prevent patient from moving forward and possibly falling; pillow under patient's head (Fig. 2.67)
- Knees flexed slightly and coronal plane parallel to IR with **no body rotation**

Part Position
- Adjust height of IR to center thorax to IR (see NOTES)
- Adjust patient and cart to center midsagittal plane and T7 to CR (top of IR is approximately 1 inch [2.5 cm] above vertebra prominens)

CR
- CR horizontal, directed to center of IR, to **level of T7,** 3 to 4 inches (8 to 10 cm) inferior to level of jugular notch. A **horizontal beam must be used** to show air-fluid level or pneumothorax.

Recommended Collimation Collimate on four sides to area of lung fields (top border of light field to level of vertebra prominens) (see NOTES).

Respiration Make exposure at end of **second full inspiration.**

Alternative Positioning Some department protocols state that the head should be 10° lower than the hips to reduce the apical lift caused by the shoulder, allowing the entire chest to remain horizontal (requires support under hips).

NOTES: Place appropriate decubitus marker and R or L to indicate which side of chest is down.

Radiograph may be taken as a right or left lateral decubitus. To produce the most diagnostic images, both lungs should be included on the image. For **possible fluid** in the pleural cavity (pleural effusion), the suspected side should be **down**. Do *not* cut off that side of the chest. The anatomic side marker must correspond with the patient's left or right side of the body. The marker must be placed on the IR before exposure. It is unacceptable practice to indicate the side of the body either digitally or with a marking pen after the exposure.

For possible **small amounts of air** in the pleural cavity (pneumothorax), the affected side should be **up,** and care must be taken *not* to cut off this side of the chest.

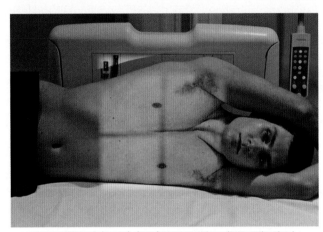

Fig. 2.67 Left lateral decubitus position (AP projection).

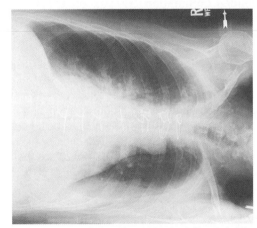

Fig. 2.68 Left lateral decubitus (fluid evident in left lung).

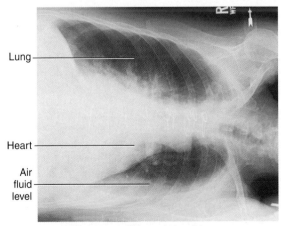

Lung

Heart

Air fluid level

Fig. 2.69 Left lateral decubitus.

AP LORDOTIC PROJECTION—CHEST

Clinical Indications
- Rule out calcifications and masses beneath the clavicles

Chest
SPECIAL
• AP supine or semierect
• Lateral decubitus (AP)
• AP lordotic

Technical Factors
- Minimum SID—72 inches (180 cm)
- IR size—14 × 17 inches (35 × 43 cm), portrait or landscape
- Grid
- kVp range—110–125

Shielding Shield radiosensitive tissues outside region of interest.

Patient Position
- Patient standing about 1 foot (30 cm) away from IR and leaning back with shoulders, neck, and back of head against IR
- Both patient's hands on hips, palms out; shoulders rolled forward (Fig. 2.70)

Part Position
- Center midsagittal plane to CR and to centerline of IR.
- Center cassette to CR (top of IR should be about 3 inches [7 to 8 cm] above shoulders on an average patient).
- Palpate clavicles to ensure they are at level or above shoulders.

CR
- CR **perpendicular** to IR, centered to **midsternum** (3 to 4 inches [9 cm] below jugular notch)

Recommended Collimation Collimate on four sides to area of lung fields (top border of light field to level of vertebra prominens).

Respiration Make exposure at end of **second full inspiration.**

Alternative Lordotic Projection If patient is weak and unstable or is unable to assume the erect lordotic position, an AP semiaxial projection may be taken with the patient in a supine position (Fig. 2.71). Shoulders are rolled forward and arms positioned as for lordotic position. The **CR** is directed **15° to 20° cephalad,** to the midsternum.

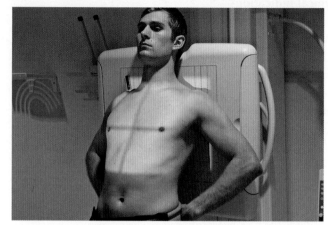

Fig. 2.70 AP lordotic position.

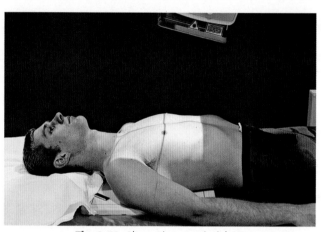

Fig. 2.71 Alternative: semiaxial AP.

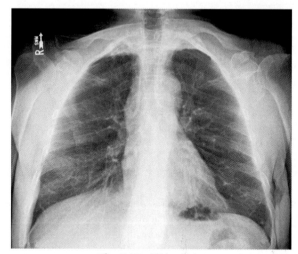

Fig. 2.72 AP lordotic.

Evaluation Criteria
Anatomy Demonstrated: • Entire lung fields and clavicles should be included (Fig. 2.72).
Position: • Clavicles should appear nearly horizontal and **above or superior** to apices, with medial aspects of clavicles superimposed by first ribs. • Ribs appear distorted, with posterior ribs appearing nearly horizontal and superimposing anterior ribs. • **No rotation:** Sternal ends of the clavicles should be the same distance from the vertebral column on each side. The lateral borders of the ribs on both sides should appear to be at nearly equal distances from the vertebral column. • Center of collimation field (CR) should be midsternum with collimation visible on top and bottom.
Exposure: • No motion; diaphragm, heart, and rib outlines should appear sharp. • Optimal contrast scale and exposure should allow visualization of the faint vascular markings of lungs, especially in area of the apices and upper lungs.

ANTERIOR OBLIQUE POSITIONS: RAO AND LAO—CHEST

Clinical Indications
- Investigate pathology involving the lung fields, trachea, and mediastinal structures
- Determine the size and contours of the heart and great vessels

Chest
SPECIAL
- AP supine or semierect
- Lateral decubitus (AP)
- AP lordotic
- Anterior oblique

Technical Factors
- Minimum SID—72 inches (180 cm)
- IR size—14 × 17 inches (35 × 43 cm), portrait
- Grid
- kVp range—110–125

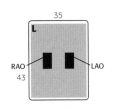

Shielding Shield radiosensitive tissues outside region of interest.

Patient Position
- Patient erect, rotated 45° with right anterior shoulder against IR for RAO (Fig. 2.73) and 45° with left anterior shoulder against IR for LAO (Fig. 2.74) (see NOTES for 60° LAO)
- Patient's arm flexed nearest IR and hand placed on hip, palm out
- Opposite arm raised to clear lung field and hand rested on head or on chest unit for support, keeping arm raised as high as possible
- Patient looking straight ahead; chin raised

Part Position
As viewed from the x-ray tube, center the patient to CR and to IR, with top of IR about 1 inch (2.5 cm) above vertebra prominens.

CR
- CR perpendicular, directed to **level of T7** (7 to 8 inches [8 to 10 cm] below level of vertebra prominens)
- CR midway between midsagittal plane and lateral margin of thorax

Recommended Collimation Collimate on four sides to area of lung fields (top border of light field to level of vertebra prominens).

Respiration Make exposure at end of **second full inspiration.**

NOTES: For **anterior** oblique, the side of interest generally is the side **farthest** from the IR. Thus, the **RAO** provides the best visualization of the **left** lung.

Certain positions for studies of the heart and great vessels require oblique positions with an increase in rotation of 45° to 60° (see Figs. 2.75 and 2.76).

Less rotation (15° to 20°) may be valuable for better visualization of the various areas of the lungs for possible pulmonary disease (Fig. 2.77).

Exception Either erect or recumbent posterior oblique projections can be taken if the patient cannot assume an erect position for anterior oblique, or if supplementary projections are required.

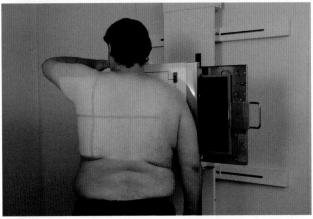
Fig. 2.73 45° RAO position.

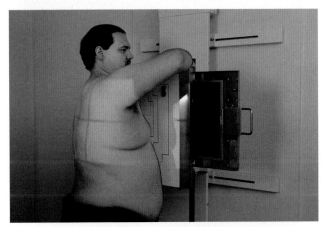
Fig. 2.74 45° LAO position.

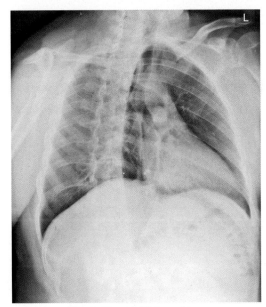
Fig. 2.75 45° RAO position.

Evaluation Criteria
Anatomy Demonstrated: • Both lungs from the apices to the costophrenic angles should be included. • Air-filled trachea, great vessels, and heart outlines are best visualized with 60° LAO position.
Position: • To evaluate for a 45° rotation, the distance from the outer margin of the ribs to the vertebral column on the side farthest from the IR should be approximately two times the distance of the side closest to the IR (Figs. 2.78 and 2.79). • CR centered at level of T7.
Exposure: • No motion; outline of the diaphragm and heart should appear sharp. • Optimal exposure and contrast allow visualization of vascular markings throughout the lungs and rib outlines except through the densest regions of the heart.

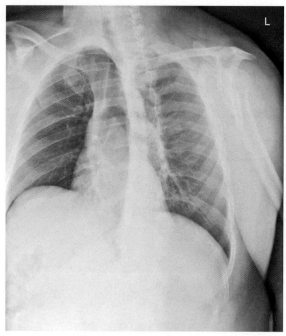

Fig. 2.76 45° LAO position.

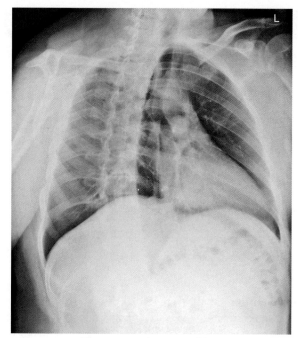

Fig. 2.78 45° RAO position.

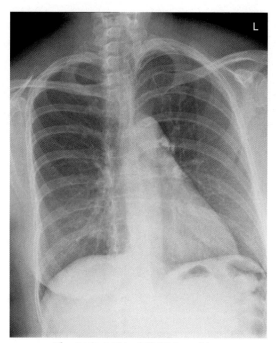

Fig. 2.77 15° to 20° RAO position.

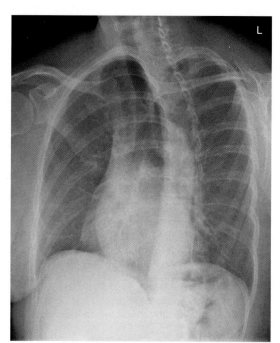

Fig. 2.79 45° LAO position.

POSTERIOR OBLIQUE POSITIONS: RPO AND LPO—CHEST

Clinical Indications
- Investigate pathology involving the lung fields, trachea, and mediastinal structures
- Determine the size and contours of the heart and great vessels

Chest
SPECIAL
- AP supine or semierect
- Lateral decubitus (AP)
- AP lordotic
- Anterior oblique
- Posterior oblique

Technical Factors
- Minimum SID—72 inches (180 cm)
- IR size—14 × 17 inches (35 × 43 cm), portrait
- Grid
- kVp range—110–125

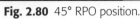

Shielding Shield radiosensitive tissues outside region of interest.

Patient Position (Erect)
- Patient erect, rotated 45° (up to 60°) with right posterior shoulder against IR for RPO (Fig. 2.80) and 45° (up to 60°) with left posterior shoulder against IR for LPO (Fig. 2.81)
- Arm closest to the IR raised, resting on head; other arm placed on hip with palm out
- Patient looking straight ahead

Patient Position (Recumbent)
- If patient cannot stand or sit, perform posterior oblique projections on table.
- Place supports under patient's head and under elevated hip and shoulder.

Part Position
- Top of IR about 1 inch (2 cm) above vertebra prominens or about 5 inches (12 cm) above level of jugular notch (2 inches [5 cm] above shoulders)
- Thorax centered to CR and to IR

CR
- CR perpendicular, to **level of T7**
- CR midway between midsagittal plane and lateral margin of thorax

Recommended Collimation Collimate on four sides to area of lung fields (top border of light field to level of vertebra prominens).

Respiration Make exposure after second full inspiration.

NOTES: Posterior oblique projections provide best visualization of the side **closest** to the IR.

Posterior positions show the same anatomy as the opposite anterior oblique positions. Thus, the RPO (Fig. 2.82) corresponds to the LAO position and the LPO (Fig. 2.83) corresponds to the RAO position.

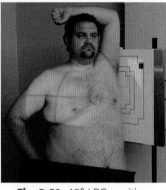

Fig. 2.80 45° RPO position.   **Fig. 2.81** 45° LPO position.

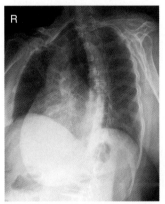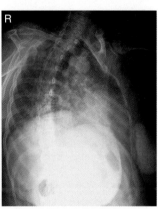

Fig. 2.82 45° to 60° RPO position. **Fig. 2.83** 45° to 60° LPO position.

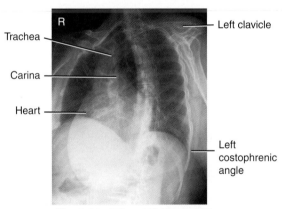

Fig. 2.84 45° to 60° RPO position.

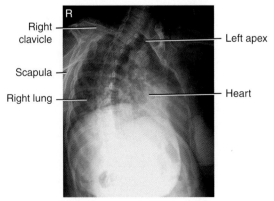

Fig. 2.85 45° to 60° LPO position.

Evaluation Criteria
Evaluation criteria are similar to criteria for anterior oblique positions described earlier. • However, because of increased magnification of the anterior diaphragm, lung fields usually appear shorter on posterior oblique than on anterior oblique projections. • The heart and great vessels also appear larger on posterior oblique because they are farther from the IR (Figs. 2.84 and 2.85).

LATERAL POSITION—UPPER AIRWAY

Clinical Indications
- Investigate pathology of the air-filled larynx and trachea, including the region of thyroid and thymus glands and upper esophagus, for opaque foreign object or if contrast medium is present
- Rule out **epiglottitis,** which may be life-threatening for a young child

Upper Airway
ROUTINE
• Lateral
• AP

Technical Factors
- Minimum SID—72 inches (180 cm) to minimize magnification
- IR size—10 × 12 inches (24 × 30 cm), portrait
- Grid
- kVp range—75–85

Shielding Shield radiosensitive tissues outside region of interest.

Patient Position Patient should be upright if possible, seated, or standing in a lateral position (may be taken in R or L lateral and may be taken recumbent tabletop if necessary).

Part Position
- Position patient to center upper airway to CR and to center of IR (larynx and trachea lie anterior to cervical and thoracic vertebrae).
- Rotate shoulders posteriorly with arms hanging down and hands clasped behind back.
- Raise chin slightly and have patient look directly ahead (Fig. 2.86).
- Adjust IR height to place top of IR at level of external auditory meatus (EAM), which is the opening of the external ear canal (see Respiration if area of primary interest is the trachea rather than the larynx).

CR
- CR perpendicular to center of IR at **level of C6** or **C7,** midway between the laryngeal prominence of the thyroid cartilage and the jugular notch

Recommended Collimation Collimate to region of soft tissue of the neck.

Respiration Make exposure **during a slow, deep inspiration** to ensure filling trachea and upper airway with air.

NOTE (centering and exposure for neck region): Centering should be to laryngeal prominence (C5) with exposure factors for a soft tissue lateral neck if the area of interest is primarily the larynx and upper trachea.

NOTE (centering and exposure for distal larynx and trachea region): If the distal larynx and upper trachea and midtrachea are the primary areas of interest, the IR and CR should be lowered to place the CR at the upper jugular notch (T1–T2) with exposure factors approximately those for a lateral chest.

Evaluation Criteria
Anatomy Demonstrated: • The larynx and trachea should be filled with air and well visualized (Figs. 2.87 and 2.88).
Position: • Centering for the neck region (larynx and proximal trachea) should include the EAM at the upper border of the image and T2 or T3 on the lower border. If the **distal larynx and trachea** is the primary area of interest, centering should be lower to include the area from C3 to T4 or T5 on the image. • The shadows of the shoulders should be primarily posterior to and should not superimpose the area of the trachea. • Collimation borders should appear on both sides with ideally only minimal (≤¼ inch) borders on top and bottom.
Exposure: • Optimal exposure includes a soft tissue technique wherein the air-filled larynx and upper trachea are not overexposed. • Cervical vertebrae appear underexposed.

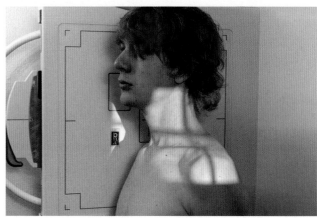
Fig. 2.86 Right lateral position—upper airway.

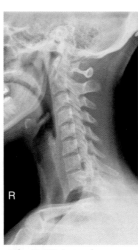
Fig. 2.87 Lateral—upper airway (for distal larynx and trachea region).

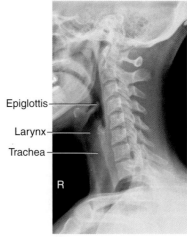
Epiglottis

Larynx

Trachea

Fig. 2.88 Lateral—upper airway.

AP PROJECTION—UPPER AIRWAY

Clinical Indications
- Investigate pathology of the air-filled larynx and trachea, including the region of the thyroid and thymus glands and upper esophagus for opaque foreign object or if contrast medium is present

Upper Airway
ROUTINE
• Lateral
• AP

Technical Factors
- Minimum SID—40 inches (100 cm) if possible, to minimize magnification
- IR size—10 × 12 inches (24 × 30 cm), portrait
- Grid
- kVp range—75–85

Shielding
Shield radiosensitive tissues outside region of interest.

Patient Position
Patient should be upright if possible, seated or standing with back of head and shoulders against IR (may be taken recumbent tabletop if necessary)

Part Position
- Align midsagittal plane with CR and with midline of grid or table.
- Raise chin so that **acanthiomeatal line is perpendicular to the IR** (line from the acanthion or area directly under the nose and the meatus or EAM); have patient look directly ahead (Fig. 2.89)

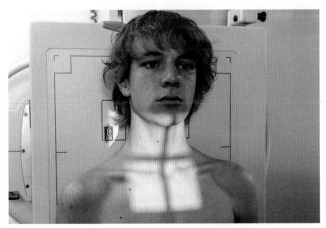

Fig. 2.89 AP—upper airway.

- Adjust the IR height to place top of IR about 1 or 1½ inches (3 to 4 cm) below EAM (see NOTE for explanation of centering)

CR
- CR perpendicular to center of IR at **level of T1–T2**, about 1 inch (2.5 cm) above the jugular notch

Recommended Collimation Collimate to region of soft tissue neck.

Respiration Make exposure **during a slow, deep inspiration** to ensure filling of trachea and upper airway with air.

NOTE (exposure): Exposure for this AP projection should be approximately that of an AP of the cervical or thoracic spine.

NOTE (centering for upper airway and trachea): Centering for this AP projection is similar to that of the lateral distal larynx and upper trachea position described on the previous page because the most proximal area of the larynx is not visualized on the AP as a result of the superimposed base of the skull and mandible. Therefore, more of the trachea can be visualized.

Evaluation Criteria
Anatomy Demonstrated: • The larynx and trachea from C3 to T4 should be filled with air and visualized through the spine. • The area of the proximal cervical vertebrae (the lower margin of the shadow of the superimposed mandible and base of skull) to the midthoracic region should be included (Fig. 2.90).
Position (see previous Notes): • **No rotation** should occur, as evidenced by the symmetric appearance of the sternoclavicular joints. • The mandible should superimpose the base of the skull with the spine aligned with the center of the film. • Collimation borders should appear on both sides with ideally only minimal (≤¼ inch) borders on top and bottom. • The collimation field (CR) should be centered to the area of T1–T2.
Exposure: • Optimal exposure should be just dark enough to allow visualization of the air-filled trachea through the cervical and thoracic vertebrae.

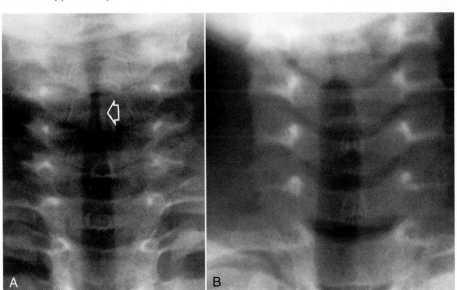

Fig. 2.90 Croup. A, Arrow indicates smooth, tapered narrowing of subglottic portion of trachea (Gothic arch sign). B, Normal trachea with broad shouldering in subglottic region. (From Eisenberg R, Johnson N: Comprehensive radiographic pathology, ed 5, St Louis, 2012, Mosby.)

RADIOGRAPHS FOR CRITIQUE

This section consists of an ideal projection (Image A) along with one or more projections that may demonstrate positioning and/or technical errors. Critique Figs C2.91 through C2.92. Compare Image A to the other projections and identify the errors. While examining each image, consider the following questions:

1. Is all essential anatomy demonstrated on the image?
2. What positioning errors are present that compromise image quality?

3. Are technical factors optimal?
4. Is there evidence of collimation and pre-exposure anatomical side markers visible on the image?
5. Do these errors require a repeat exposure?

Feedback for each set of images is located on the faculty Evolve site.

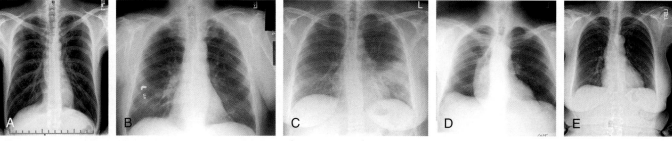

Fig. C2.91 PA chest.

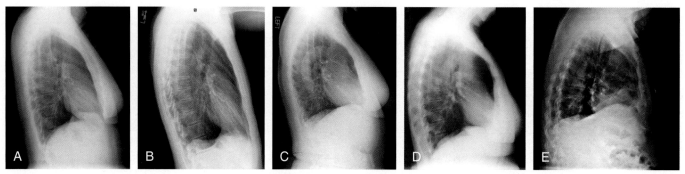

Fig. C2.92 Lateral chest.

Abdomen

CONTRIBUTIONS BY **Kelli Welch Haynes,** ED.D., RT(R)

CONTRIBUTORS TO PAST EDITIONS   Dan L. Hobbs, MSRS, RT(R)(CT)(MR), John P. Lampignano, MEd, RT(R)(CT), Kathy M. Martensen, BS, RT(R), Barry T. Anthony, RT(R)

CONTENTS

RADIOGRAPHIC ANATOMY

Abdominal Radiography

This chapter covers the anatomy and positioning for images of the abdomen. To examine the abdomen radiographically, one or more projections may be performed. The most common image is an anteroposterior (AP) supine abdomen, also sometimes called a *KUB* (*k*idneys, *u*reters, and *b*ladder) because of the regions visualized. These are taken without the use of contrast media. Radiographs of the abdomen (KUB) are commonly performed prior to fluoroscopic abdominal examinations, which are performed with the use of contrast media to rule out certain pathologies.

ACUTE ABDOMINAL SERIES

Certain acute or emergency conditions of the abdomen may develop from conditions such as bowel obstruction, perforations involving free intraperitoneal air (air outside the digestive tract), excessive fluid in the abdomen (ascites), or a possible intra-abdominal mass. These acute or emergency conditions require what is commonly referred to as an "acute abdominal series," wherein several abdominal images are taken in different positions to demonstrate air-fluid levels, free air, or both within the abdominal cavity. Typically, a supine KUB along with an upright AP or decubitus abdomen and a PA or AP chest are performed to complete the series.

Abdominal radiography requires an understanding of anatomy and relationships of the organs and structures within the abdominopelvic cavity.

ABDOMINAL MUSCLES

Many muscles are associated with the abdominopelvic cavity. The most important in abdominal radiography are the right and left hemi-diaphragms and the right and left psoas *(so′-es)* major and minor muscles. The right hemi-diaphragm is attached anteriorly to the fifth rib and posteriorly at the level of the tenth rib. The left hemi-diaphragm is located near the first intercostal space. The psoas major muscles are located laterally to the lumbar vertebrae.

The **diaphragm** is an umbrella-shaped muscle that separates the abdominal cavity from the thoracic cavity. The diaphragm must be perfectly motionless during imaging of the abdomen or the chest. Motion of the patient's diaphragm can be stopped when appropriate breathing instructions are given to the patient.

The two **psoas major** and minor muscles are located on either side of the lumbar vertebral column. The lateral borders of these two muscles should be faintly visible on a diagnostic abdominal image of a small to average-sized patient when correct exposure factors are used (see arrows, Figs. 3.1 and 3.2).

Abdominal Organ Systems

The various organ systems found within the abdominopelvic cavity are presented briefly in this chapter. Each system is described in greater detail in later chapters devoted to the specific systems.

DIGESTIVE SYSTEM

The **digestive system,** along with its accessory organs, the **liver, gallbladder,** and **pancreas,** fills much of the abdominal cavity. The six organs of the digestive system are as follows:

1. Oral cavity   4. Stomach
2. Pharynx   5. Small intestine
3. Esophagus   6. Large intestine

Oral Cavity, Pharynx, and Esophagus

The **oral cavity** (mouth) and the pharynx (oropharynx and laryngopharynx) are common to the respiratory system and the digestive system, as illustrated in Fig. 2.4 (see Chapter 2). The **esophagus** is located in the mediastinum of the thoracic cavity.

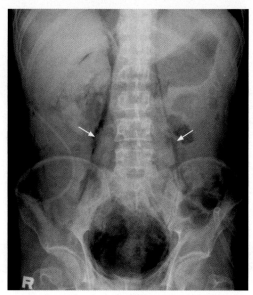

Fig. 3.1 AP abdomen (KUB). Arrows indicate psoas muscles.

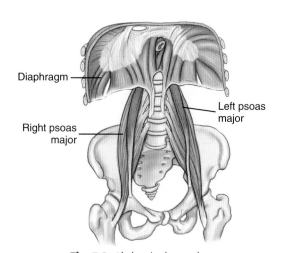

Fig. 3.2 Abdominal muscles.

Diaphragm

Left psoas major

Right psoas major

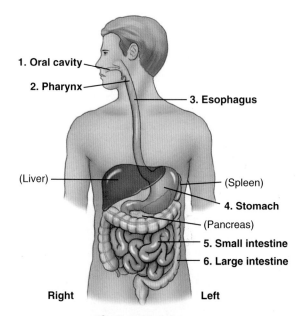

1. Oral cavity
2. Pharynx
3. Esophagus
(Liver)
(Spleen)
4. Stomach
(Pancreas)
5. Small intestine
6. Large intestine

Right   **Left**

Fig. 3.3 Digestive tract.

Stomach and Small and Large Intestines

The three digestive organs within the abdominal cavity are the **stomach** and **small** and **large intestines** (Fig. 3.3).

Stomach The stomach is the first organ of the digestive system that is located entirely within the abdominal cavity. The stomach is an expandable reservoir for swallowed food and fluids. The size and shape of the stomach vary depending on the volume of its contents and on the body habitus of the patient

Gastro is a common combining form denoting a relationship to the stomach (the Greek word *gaster* means "stomach"). The term *gastrointestinal (GI) tract* or *system* describes the entire digestive system, starting with the stomach and continuing through the small and large intestines.

Small Intestine The small intestine continues from the stomach as a long, tubelike convoluted structure about 15 to 18 feet (4.5 to 5.5 m) in length. The three parts of the small intestine, as labeled in descending order in Figs. 3.4 and 3.5, are as follows: duodenum *(doo″-o-de′-num)* (A); jejunum *(je-joo′-num)* (B); and ileum *(il′-eum)* (C).

Duodenum (A) The first portion of the small intestine, the duodenum, is the shortest, but widest, in diameter of the three segments. It is about 10 inches (25 cm) in length. When filled with contrast medium, the duodenum looks like the letter C. The proximal portion of the duodenum is the *duodenal bulb,* or *cap.* It has a characteristic shape that is usually well demonstrated on barium studies of the upper GI tract. Ducts from the liver, gallbladder, and pancreas drain into the duodenum to aid in digestive functions.

Jejunum and ileum (B and C) The remainder of the small bowel lies in the central and lower abdomen. The first two-fifths, following the duodenum, are the **jejunum,** and the distal three-fifths are the **ileum.** The orifice (valve) between the distal ileum and the cecum portion of the large intestine is the **ileocecal valve.**

Radiographic Images of Stomach and Small Intestine Air seldomly fills the entire stomach or small intestine on an abdominal image of a healthy, ambulatory adult. Fig. 3.5 demonstrates the stomach, small intestine, and proximal large intestine filled with radiopaque barium sulfate . Note the duodenal bulb and the long, convoluted loops of the three labeled parts of the small intestine located in the mid-abdomen and lower abdomen.

Large Intestine The sixth and last organ of digestion is the large intestine, which begins in the right lower quadrant at the junction of the small intestine and the **ileocecal valve.** The portion of the large intestine below the ileocecal valve is a saclike portion named the **cecum.** The **appendix (vermiform appendix)** is attached to the posteromedial aspect of the cecum (Fig. 3.6).

The vertical portion of the large bowel, above the cecum, the **ascending colon,** joins the **transverse colon** at the **right colic** (kol′-ik, referring to colon) **flexure.** The transverse colon joins the **descending colon** at the **left colic flexure.** Alternative secondary names for the two colic flexures are **hepatic** *(right)* and **splenic** *(left)* **flexures,** based on their proximity to the liver and spleen, respectively.

The descending colon continues as the S-shaped **sigmoid colon** in the lower left abdomen. The **rectum** is the final 6 inches (15 cm) of the large intestine. The rectum ends at the **anus,** the sphincter muscle at the terminal opening of the large intestine.

As seen in body habitus illustrations, the shape and location of the large intestine varies greatly, with the transverse colon located high in the abdomen of wide hypersthenic body types and low in the abdomen of slender hyposthenic and asthenic body types (see also Chapter 13).

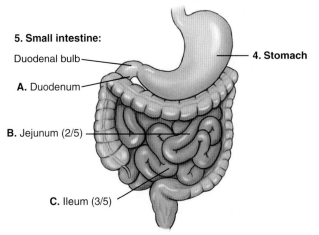

5. Small intestine:
Duodenal bulb
A. Duodenum
B. Jejunum (2/5)
C. Ileum (3/5)
4. Stomach

Fig. 3.4 Stomach and small intestine.

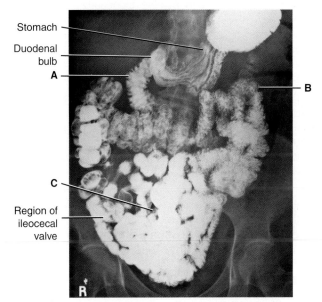

Stomach
Duodenal bulb
A
B
C
Region of ileocecal valve
R

Fig. 3.5 Stomach and small intestine radiograph.

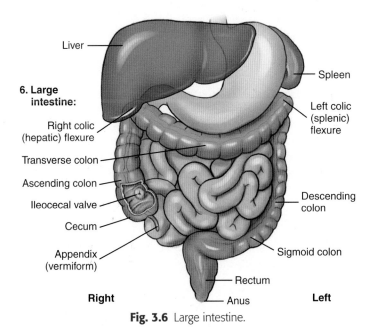

Liver
Spleen
6. Large intestine:
Right colic (hepatic) flexure
Left colic (splenic) flexure
Transverse colon
Ascending colon
Ileocecal valve
Cecum
Appendix (vermiform)
Descending colon
Sigmoid colon
Rectum
Right
Anus
Left

Fig. 3.6 Large intestine.

SPLEEN

The spleen is the part of the **lymphatic system** that, along with the heart and blood vessels, is part of the circulatory system. It is an important abdominal organ that occupies a space posterior and to the left of the stomach in the **left upper quadrant,** as shown in Fig. 3.7.

The spleen may be visualized faintly on abdominal images, particularly if the organ is enlarged. The spleen is a fragile organ and is sometimes lacerated during trauma to the lower left posterior rib cage.

ACCESSORY DIGESTIVE ORGANS

Three accessory organs of digestion, also located in the abdominal cavity, are the (1) pancreas, (2) liver, and (3) gallbladder. Accessory organs of digestion are outside the digestive tract but aid in digestion via the materials they secrete into the digestive tract.

Pancreas

The pancreas, which is not visualized on an abdominal image, is an elongated gland that is located **posterior to the stomach** and near the posterior abdominal wall, between the duodenum and the spleen. The average length is about 6 inches (12.5 cm). The head of the pancreas is nestled in the C-loop of the duodenum, and the body and tail of the pancreas extend toward the upper left quadrant of the abdomen. This relationship of the duodenum and the head of the pancreas sometimes is referred to as "the romance of the abdomen."

The pancreas is part of the **endocrine** (internal) secretion system and the **exocrine** (external) secretion system. The endocrine portion of the pancreas produces essential hormones, such as insulin, which aids in controlling the blood sugar level of the body. As part of its exocrine functions, the pancreas produces large amounts (1½ quarts [1500 mL] daily) of digestive juices that move to the duodenum, through a main pancreatic duct, as needed for digestion.

Liver

The liver is the largest solid organ in the body, occupying the majority of the **right upper quadrant** of the abdomen. The liver has numerous functions, one of which is the production of bile that assists in the emulsification (breakdown) of fats.

Gallbladder

The gallbladder is a pear-shaped sac located posterior and inferior to the liver. If bile produced in the liver is not necessary at the current time for fat emulsification, it is stored and concentrated for future use in the gallbladder. The gallbladder contracts and releases the stored bile when stimulated by an appropriate hormone (cholecystokinin). In most cases, the gallbladder cannot be visualized without the use of contrast media. This is because the gallbladder and the biliary ducts are similar in tissue density and subject contrast to the surrounding abdominal soft tissues. The anatomy of the gallbladder and biliary ducts is described in greater detail in Chapter 12.

Cholelithiasis Cholelithiasis is the presence of one or more calculi (gallstones) in the gallbladder.[1] Gallstones are composed of either cholesterol or a pigment made of bile salts, phosphate, and carbonate. Cholesterol-based gallstones are more commonly found in populations within the United States (80%), whereas the pigment-based stones are more commonly found in populations within Asia. These variances are most generally associated with diet.

Only about 20% of all gallstones contain enough calcium to allow visualization on an abdominal image. The majority of gallstones are radiolucent (not visible radiographically).[2] Alternative imaging modalities, such as diagnostic ultrasound, are better able to detect the presence and location of radiolucent gallstones.

CT SECTIONAL IMAGES

Computed tomography (CT) images through various levels of the abdomen are used to demonstrate anatomic relationships of the

digestive organs and their accessory organs, in addition to the spleen.

Fig. 3.8 demonstrates an axial view of the upper abdomen at the level of T10 or T11 (tenth or eleventh thoracic vertebra) just below the diaphragm. Note the proportionately large size of the liver at this level in the right upper quadrant of the abdomen and the cross-sectional view through the stomach to the patient's left of the liver. The spleen is visualized posterior to the stomach in the left upper quadrant of the abdomen.

Fig. 3.9 is an axial image inferior to Fig. 3.8 through the mid-abdomen at the approximate level of L2 (second lumbar vertebra). The abdominal aorta and inferior vena cava lie anterior to the

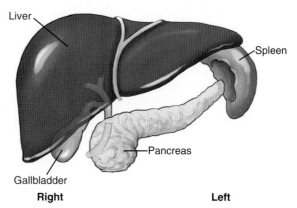

Fig. 3.7 Spleen and accessory organs of digestion—pancreas, liver, and gallbladder.

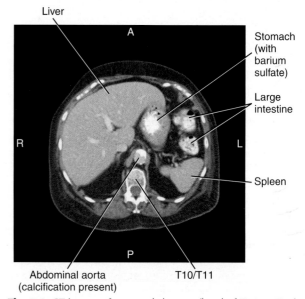

Fig. 3.8 CT image of upper abdomen (level of T10 or T11).

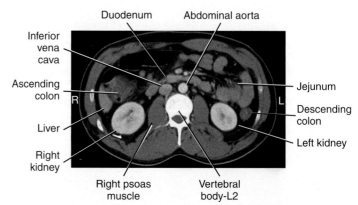

Fig. 3.9 CT image of abdomen demonstrating liver, gallbladder, pancreas, and **major vessels (aorta and inferior vena cava).**

vertebral body. The kidneys are seen lateral to the psoas muscles. The dark air-filled portion of the transverse colon is on top (anteriorly), indicating that the patient was lying in a supine position for this CT scan.

Urinary System

The urinary system is another important abdominal system. Although this system is introduced in this chapter, it is discussed in detail in Chapter 14.

The urinary system comprises the following (Fig. 3.10):
- Two kidneys
- Two ureters (u-re′-tersor yoo-ret′-ers)[3]
- One urinary bladder
- One urethra (u-re′-thrah or yoo-re′-thra)[4]

Each **kidney** drains via its own **ureter** to the single **urinary bladder.** The bladder, which is situated superior and posterior to the symphysis pubis, stores urine. Under voluntary control, the stored urine passes to the exterior environment via the **urethra.** The two **suprarenal** (adrenal) **glands** of the endocrine system are located at the superomedial portion of each kidney. The bean-shaped kidneys are located on either side of the lumbar vertebral column. The right kidney is typically situated a little more inferior than the left kidney because of the presence of the liver on the right.

Waste materials and excess water are eliminated from the blood by the kidneys and are transported through the ureters to the urinary bladder.

EXCRETORY OR INTRAVENOUS UROGRAM

The kidneys are usually faintly demonstrated on an abdominal image because of a fatty capsule that surrounds each kidney. The contrast medium examination shown in Fig. 3.11 is an **excretory** or **intravenous urogram** (IVU), which is an examination of the urinary system performed with intravenous contrast medium. During this examination, the hollow organs of this system are visualized with the use of the contrast medium that has been filtered from the blood flow by the kidneys. The organs as labeled are the **left kidney** (A), the **left proximal ureter** (B), the **left distal ureter** (C) before emptying into the urinary bladder (D), and the **right kidney** (E).

NOTE: The term **intravenous pyelogram (IVP)** often was previously used for this examination. However, this is *not* an accurate term for this examination. The terms *excretory urogram* (EU) and *intravenous urogram* (IVU) are both current and correct terms.

SECTIONAL IMAGE

The sectional CT image (Fig. 3.12) may appear confusing at first because of the numerous small, odd-shaped structures that are demonstrated. However, as you study the relationships between these structures and imagine a thin "slice" view through the level of about L2–L3 of the drawings (see Fig. 3.10) and on the previous page (see Fig. 3.7), you may use the image to identify the anatomic positions and relationships of the structures previously discussed. The structures labeled in Fig. 3.12 are:

A. Inferior lobe of liver
B. Ascending colon
C. Right kidney
D. Right ureter
E. Right psoas major
F. L2–L3 vertebra
G. Left kidney
H. Left ureter
I. Descending colon
J. Loops of small intestines (jejunum)

Two major blood vessels of the abdomen are also seen, labeled K and L. K is the large abdominal aorta, and L is the inferior vena cava.

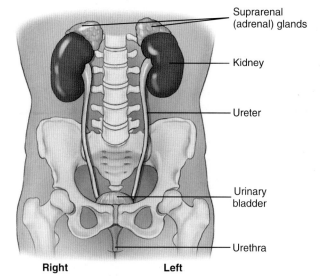

Fig. 3.10 Urinary system.

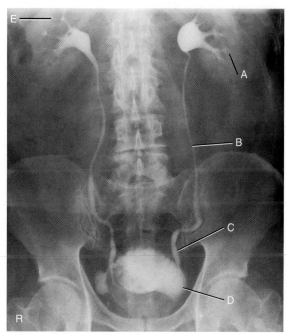

Fig. 3.11 Intravenous urogram (IVU). **A,** Left kidney. **B,** Left midureter. **C,** Left distal ureter. **D,** Bladder. **E,** Right kidney.

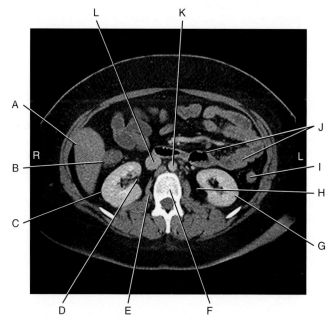

Fig. 3.12 CT image of abdomen, level of mid-kidneys, and proximal ureters. See text for label identifications.

Abdominal Cavity

Four important terms that describe the anatomy of the abdominal cavity appear on the drawings to the right and are described subsequently. These four terms are:

1. **Peritoneum** *(per"-i-to-ne'-um)*
2. **Mesentery** *(mes'-en-ter'-e)*
3. **Omentum** *(o-men'-tum)*
4. **Mesocolon** *(mez'-o-ko'-lon)*

PERITONEUM

Most of the abdominal structures and organs, in addition to the wall of the abdominal cavity in which they are contained, are covered to varying degrees by a large serous, double-walled, saclike membrane called the **peritoneum.** The total surface area of the peritoneum is approximately equal to the total surface area of the skin that covers the entire body.

A greatly simplified cross-section of the abdominal cavity is shown in Fig. 3.13. Two types of peritoneum exist: parietal and visceral. The two-layered peritoneum that adheres to the abdominal cavity wall is the **parietal peritoneum,** whereas the portion that covers an organ is the **visceral peritoneum.** The space or cavity between the parietal and visceral portions of the peritoneum is the **peritoneal cavity.** This space is only a potential cavity because normally it is filled with various organs, such as the loops of bowel. This cavity also contains some serous lubricating-type fluid, which allows organs to move against each other without friction. An abnormal accumulation of this serous fluid is a condition called **ascites** (see Clinical Indications section later in the chapter).

A layer of visceral peritoneum only **partially** covers certain organs that are more closely attached to the posterior abdominal wall (see Fig. 3.13). At this level, the ascending and descending colon, the aorta, and the inferior vena cava are only partially covered; therefore, this lining would *not* be considered mesentery, and these structures and organs are called **retroperitoneal,** as described in the next section.

MESENTERY

The peritoneum forms large folds that bind the abdominal organs to each other and to the walls of the abdomen. Blood and lymph vessels, and the nerves that supply these abdominal organs, are contained within these folds of peritoneum. One of these double folds that hold the small intestine in place is known as **mesentery.** Mesentery is the **double fold of peritoneum** that extends anteriorly from the posterior abdominal wall to completely envelop a loop of **small bowel. Mesentery** is the specific term for a double fold of peritoneum that loosely connects the small intestine to the posterior abdominal wall (Fig. 3.14).

OMENTUM

The term **omentum** refers to a specific type of double-fold peritoneum that extends from the **stomach** to another organ (see Fig. 3.14). The **lesser omentum** extends superiorly from the lesser curvature of the stomach to portions of the liver. The **greater omentum** connects the transverse colon to the greater curvature of the stomach inferiorly. The greater omentum drapes over the small bowel, then folds back on itself to form an apron along the anterior abdominal wall.

If one dissected the abdomen through the mid-anterior wall, the first structure encountered beneath the parietal peritoneum would be the greater omentum. Varying amounts of fat are deposited in the greater omentum, which serves as a layer of insulation between the abdominal cavity and the exterior. This is sometimes called the "fatty apron" because of its location and the amount of fat contained therein (Fig. 3.15).

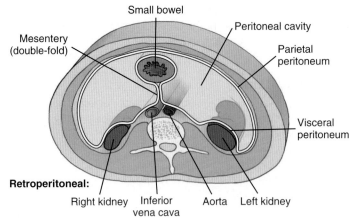

Fig. 3.13 Cross-section—abdominal cavity (demonstrates peritoneum, mesentery, and retroperitoneal structures).

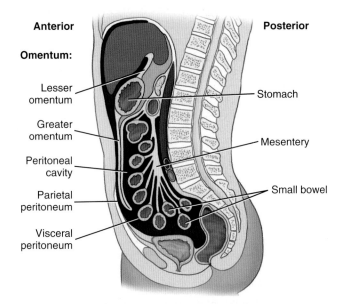

Fig. 3.14 Midsagittal section—abdominal cavity (demonstrates peritoneum, mesentery, and omentum).

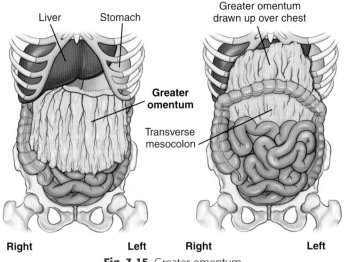

Fig. 3.15 Greater omentum.

MESOCOLON

The peritoneum that attaches the **colon** to the posterior abdominal wall is the **mesocolon**. The prefix *meso-* is used to refer to mesentery-type folds from which other abdominal organs are suspended. Four forms of mesocolon exist, each named according to the portion of the colon to which it is attached: ascending, transverse, descending, and sigmoid or pelvic. The **transverse mesocolon** is shown in Fig. 3.15 as the visceral peritoneum that loosely connects the transverse colon to the posterior abdominal wall.

GREATER SAC AND LESSER SAC

The illustration in Fig. 3.16 shows the two parts of the peritoneal cavity. The major portion of the peritoneal cavity is the **greater sac** and is commonly referred to as simply the **peritoneal cavity**. A smaller portion of the upper posterior peritoneal cavity located posterior to the stomach is the **lesser sac**. This sac has a special name, the **omentum bursa**.

This drawing shows the **mesentery** connecting one loop of **small intestine** (ileum) to the posterior abdominal wall. A full drawing of a normal abdomen would have many loops of small bowel connected to the posterior wall by mesentery.

RETROPERITONEAL AND INFRAPERITONEAL ORGANS

The organs shown in Fig. 3.17 are considered either **retroperitoneal** (*retro*, meaning "backward" or "behind") or **infraperitoneal** (*infra*, meaning "under" or "beneath") in relation to the peritoneal cavity (Table 3.1).

Retroperitoneal Organs

Structures closely attached to the posterior abdominal wall that are retroperitoneal are the kidneys and ureters, adrenal glands, pancreas, C-loop of duodenum (aspect adjacent to head of pancreas), ascending and descending colon, upper rectum, abdominal aorta, and inferior vena cava.

These retroperitoneal structures are less mobile, within the abdomen, than other intraperitoneal organs. For example, Fig. 3.16 shows that the **stomach, small intestine,** and **transverse colon** are only loosely attached to the abdominal wall by long loops of different types of peritoneum; these structures change, or vary greatly, in their position within the abdomen compared with retroperitoneal or infraperitoneal structures.

Infraperitoneal Organs

Located under or beneath the peritoneum, in the true pelvis, are the lower rectum, urinary bladder, and reproductive organs.

INTRAPERITONEAL ORGANS

Organs within the abdominal cavity that are partially or completely covered by some type of visceral peritoneum, but are not retroperitoneal or infraperitoneal, may be called **intraperitoneal** (*intra*, meaning "within"). These organs, which have been removed from the drawing in Fig. 3.17, include the **liver, gallbladder, spleen, stomach, jejunum, ileum, cecum,** and **transverse** and **sigmoid colon.**

MALE VERSUS FEMALE PERITONEAL ENCLOSURES

One significant difference exists between male and female peritoneal enclosures. The lower aspect of the peritoneum is a **closed sac in the male** but **not in the female.** In males, the lower peritoneal sac lies above the urinary bladder, totally separating the reproductive organs from the organs within the peritoneal cavity. In females, the uterus, uterine (fallopian) tubes, and ovaries pass directly into the peritoneal cavity (see Fig. 3.16).

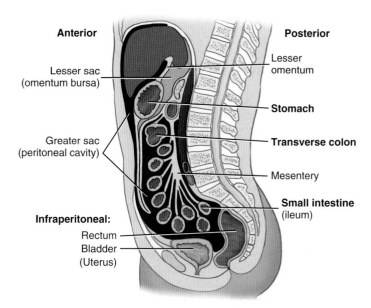

Fig. 3.16 Sagittal section—abdominal cavity (demonstrates greater and lesser sacs, transverse mesocolon, and infraperitoneal structures).

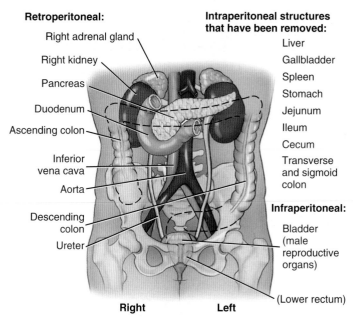

Fig. 3.17 Retroperitoneal and infraperitoneal organs.

TABLE 3.1 **SUMMARY OF ABDOMINAL ORGANS IN RELATION TO THE PERITONEAL CAVITY**		
INTRAPERITONEAL ORGANS	**RETROPERITONEAL ORGANS**	**INFRAPERITONEAL (PELVIC) ORGANS**
Liver	Kidneys	Lower rectum
Gallbladder	Ureters	Urinary bladder
Spleen	Adrenal glands	Reproductive organs
Stomach	Pancreas	Male—closed sac
Jejunum	C-loop of duodenum	Female—open sac
Ileum	Ascending and	(female uterus, tubes,
Cecum	descending colon	and ovaries, extending
Transverse colon	Upper rectum	into the peritoneal
Sigmoid colon	Major abdominal blood	cavity)
	vessels (aorta and	
	inferior vena cava)	

Quadrants and Regions

To facilitate description of the locations of various organs or other structures within the abdominopelvic cavity, the abdomen may be divided into **four quadrants** or **nine regions.**

FOUR ABDOMINAL QUADRANTS

If two imaginary perpendicular planes (at right angles) were passed through the abdomen at the umbilicus (or navel), they would divide the abdomen into four quadrants (Figs. 3.18 and 3.19). One plane would be transverse through the abdomen at the **level of the umbilicus,** which on most people is at the level of the **intervertebral disk between L4 and L5** (fourth and fifth lumbar vertebrae), which is at about the level of the iliac crests on a female.

The vertical plane would coincide with the **midsagittal plane,** or midline, of the abdomen and would pass through both the umbilicus and the symphysis pubis. These two planes would divide the abdominopelvic cavity into four quadrants: **right upper quadrant** (RUQ), **left upper quadrant** (LUQ), **right lower quadrant** (RLQ), and **left lower quadrant** (LLQ).

NOTE: The four-quadrant system is used most frequently in imaging for localizing a particular organ or for describing the location of abdominal pain or other symptoms (Table 3.2).

TABLE 3.2 **ANATOMY SUMMARY CHART: FOUR-QUADRANT ABDOMEN**[a]			
RUQ	**LUQ**	**RLQ**	**LLQ**
Liver	Spleen	Ascending colon	Descending colon
Gallbladder	Stomach	Appendix	Sigmoid colon
Right colic	Left colic	(vermiform)	2/3 of jejunum
(hepatic)	(splenic)	Cecum	
flexure	flexure	2/3 of ileum	
Duodenum	Tail of pancreas	Ileocecal valve	
(C-loop)	Left kidney		
Head of	Left suprarenal		
pancreas	gland		
Right kidney			
Right suprarenal			
gland			

[a]Quadrant locations of structures and organs (primary location on average adult).

NINE ABDOMINAL REGIONS

The abdominopelvic cavity also can be divided into nine regions through the use of two horizontal or transverse planes and two vertical planes. The two transverse/horizontal planes are the **transpyloric plane** and the **transtubercular plane.** The two vertical planes are the **right** and **left lateral planes** (Fig. 3.20).

The transpyloric plane is at the level of the lower border of L1 (first lumbar vertebra), and the transtubercular plane is at the level of L5. The right and left lateral planes are parallel to the midsagittal plane and are located midway between it and each anterior superior iliac spine (ASIS).

Names of Regions

The names of these nine regions are given in the following list. Technologists should be familiar with the locations and names of these nine regions. However, in general, locating most structures and organs within the four-quadrant system is sufficient for imaging purposes because of variables that affect specific locations of organs, such as body habitus, body position, and age (see organ outlines in Fig. 3.20 for general locations of organs within these nine regions).

1. Right hypochondriac
2. Epigastric
3. Left hypochondriac
4. Right lateral (lumbar)
5. Umbilical
6. Left lateral (lumbar)
7. Right inguinal (iliac)
8. Pubic (hypogastric)
9. Left inguinal (iliac)

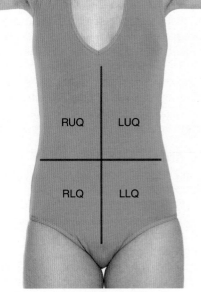

Fig. 3.18 Four abdominal quadrants.

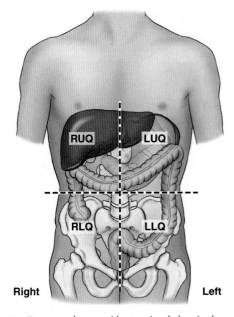

Fig. 3.19 Four quadrants with certain abdominal structures.

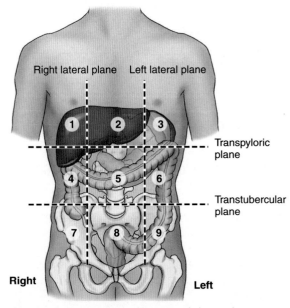

Fig. 3.20 Nine regions with certain abdominal structures.

TOPOGRAPHIC LANDMARKS

Abdominal borders and organs within the abdomen are not visible from the exterior, and because these soft tissue organs cannot be palpated directly, certain bony landmarks are used for this purpose.

NOTE: Palpation must be performed gently because the patient may have painful or sensitive areas within the abdomen and pelvis. Also, ensure the patient is informed of the purpose of palpation before beginning.

SEVEN LANDMARKS OF THE ABDOMEN

The following seven palpable landmarks are important in positioning the abdomen or locating organs within the abdomen (Figs. 3.21 and 3.22). You should practice finding these bony landmarks on yourself before attempting to locate them on another person or on a patient for the first time.

Positioning for abdominal radiographs in AP or posteroanterior (PA) projections requires quick and accurate localization of these landmarks on all patient body types.

1. **Xiphoid process (level of T9–T10):** The tip of the xiphoid process is the most inferior process of the sternum. This landmark can be palpated best by first gently pressing on the soft abdomen below the distal sternum, then moving upward carefully against the firm, distal margin of the xiphoid process. This landmark approximates the superior anterior portion of the diaphragm, which is also the **superior margin of the abdomen.** However, this is not a primary landmark for positioning the abdomen because of variation in body types and the importance of including all of the lower abdomen on images of the abdomen.
2. **Inferior costal (rib) margin (level of L2–L3):** This landmark is used to locate upper abdominal organs, such as the gallbladder and stomach.
3. **Iliac crest (level of L4–L5 vertebral interspace):** The crest of the ilium is the uppermost portion of the curved border of the ilium. The iliac crest can be palpated easily by pressing inward and downward along the mid-lateral margin of the abdomen. The uppermost, or most superior, portion of this crest is the **most commonly used abdominal landmark** and corresponds approximately to the level of the **mid-abdominopelvic region,** which is also at or just slightly below the level of the umbilicus on most people.

NOTE: Ensuring the entire upper abdomen, including the diaphragm, is included on the radiographic image may require centering about 2 inches (5 cm) above the level of the crest for most patients, which subsequently may cause some of the important lower abdomen not to be included in the image. Therefore, a second projection centered lower would be required to include this lower region.

4. **Anterior superior iliac spine:** The ASIS can be found by locating the iliac crest, then palpating anteriorly and inferiorly until a prominent projection or "bump" is felt (more prominent on females). This landmark is commonly used for positioning of pelvic and vertebral structures but can also serve as a secondary landmark for general abdominal positioning (Fig. 3.23).
5. **Greater trochanter:** This landmark is more easily palpated on thin patients. Gentle but very firm palpation is required to feel the movement of the trochanter with one hand, while rotating the leg internally and externally at the knee area with the other hand. This is not as precise a landmark as the other bony landmarks of the pelvis, but the prominence of the greater trochanter is at about the same level as the superior border of the symphysis. With practice, the greater trochanter can be used as a secondary landmark for abdominal positioning.

6. **Symphysis pubis:** The symphysis pubis is the anterior junction (joint) of the two pelvic bones. The most superior anterior portion of the pubis can be palpated when the patient is in a supine position. This landmark corresponds to the **inferior margin of the abdomen.** However, palpation of this area may be embarrassing to some patients and palpating the greater trochanter may be a better option.
7. **Ischial tuberosity:** This landmark can be used to determine the lower margin on a PA abdomen with the patient in a **prone position.** These two bony prominences, which can be palpated most easily on thin patients, bear most of the weight of the trunk when one is seated. The lower margins of the ischial tuberosities are about 0.4 to 1.5 inches (1 to 4 cm) below or distal to the symphysis pubis. This landmark may be used for positioning a PA projection of the colon when the rectal area is to be included on the IR. However, this may be uncomfortable and embarrassing for the patient, and other landmarks can and should be used when possible.

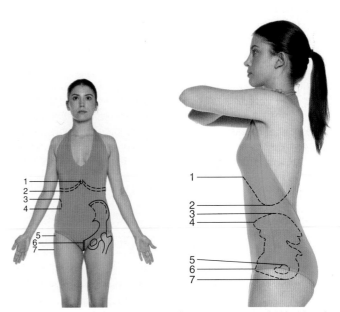

Fig. 3.21 Topographic landmarks. **Fig. 3.22** Topographic landmarks.

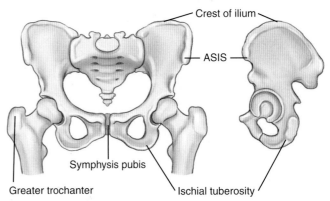

Fig. 3.23 Topographic landmarks of pelvis.

RADIOGRAPHIC POSITIONING

Patient Preparation

Patient preparation for abdominal imaging includes removal of all clothing and any radiopaque items that may be in the area to be imaged. The patient should wear a hospital gown with the opening and ties in the back (if this type of gown is used). Shoes and socks may remain on the feet. Generally, no patient instructions are required before the examination unless contrast media studies are also scheduled.

General Positioning Considerations

Make patients as comfortable as possible on the radiographic table. A pillow under the head and support under the knees enhance comfort for a supine abdomen. Place clean linen on the table and cover patients to keep them warm and to protect their modesty.

Breathing Instructions

A key factor in quality abdominal imaging is the prevention of motion. Motion may result from **voluntary** movement, such as breathing, or from **involuntary** movement, such as peristaltic action of the bowel. The difference between these two types of motion is illustrated in Chapter 1. However, to prevent any potential motion in abdominal radiography, the **shortest exposure time possible** should be used.

A second method to prevent voluntary motion is by providing **careful breathing instructions** to the patient. Most abdominal radiographs are taken on expiration; the patient is instructed to "take in a deep breath—let it all out and hold it—do not breathe." Before making the exposure, ensure the patient is following instructions and sufficient time has been allowed for all breathing movements to cease.

Abdominal images are exposed on **expiration,** with the diaphragm in a superior position for better visualization of abdominal structures.

Image Markers

Correctly placed R and L markers corresponding to the appropriate side of the patient and "up side" indicator markers, such as short arrows, for erect and decubitus projections should be visible without superimposing abdominal structures. The marker(s) must be placed on the IR before exposure. It is not acceptable practice to indicate the side of the body postexposure.

Radiation Protection

Good radiation protection practices are especially important in abdominal imaging because of the proximity of the radiation-sensitive gonadal organs.

REPEAT EXPOSURES

Careful positioning and selection of correct exposure factors are means to reduce unnecessary exposure from repeat examinations. Providing clear breathing instructions also assists in eliminating repeat exposures that often result from motion caused by breathing during the exposure.

CLOSE COLLIMATION

For abdominal radiographs of small patients, some side collimation to skin borders is possible; ensure it does not exclude any pertinent abdominal anatomy.

Collimation on the top and bottom for adults should be adjusted directly to the margins of the IR, allowing for divergence of the x-ray beam.

NOTE: Vertical collimation (up/down) may result in collimating off essential anatomy on average-sized adults when using a typical 14 × 17-inch (35 × 43-cm) field size.

GONADAL SHIELDING

For abdominal images, gonadal shields should be used for male patients, with the upper edge of the shield carefully placed at the pubic symphysis (Fig. 3.24). For female patients, gonadal shields should be used only when such shields do not obscure essential anatomy in the lower abdominopelvic region (Fig. 3.25). Generally, the decision to shield female gonads on abdominal radiographs should be made by a physician to determine whether essential anatomy would be obscured. The top of an ovarian shield should be at or slightly above the level of ASIS, and the lower border should be at the symphysis pubis.

PREGNANCY PROTECTION

See Chapter 1, regarding safeguards for potential early pregnancies with abdominal or pelvic projections.

Exposure Factors

The principal exposure factors for abdominal images are as follows:
- Medium kVp of 70 to 85
- Short exposure time
- Adequate mAs based on part thickness

Correctly exposed abdominal images on an average-sized patient should faintly demonstrate the lateral borders of the psoas muscles, lower liver margin, kidney outlines, and the transverse processes of the lumbar vertebrae. The kVp should be set at a level that will allow for appropriate penetrability to visualize various abdominal structures, including possible small semiopaque stones in the gallbladder or kidneys.

NOTE: Placing the patient in a prone position (rather than supine) can reduce part thickness by compressing the abdominal region; this will allow for lower mAs settings.

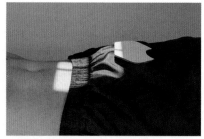

Fig. 3.24 Gonadal shielding—male.

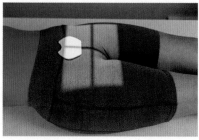

Fig. 3.25 Gonadal shielding—female (use only if shielding does not obscure essential anatomy).

Special Patient Considerations

PEDIATRIC APPLICATIONS

Motion prevention is of utmost importance in pediatric patients, and short exposure times are essential. Children younger than 13 years of age require a reduction in kVp and mAs based on measured part thickness. Confirmed technique factors for children of various sizes and ages for the equipment that is being used should always be available to minimize repeat exposures. Grids may not be necessary for pediatric abdominal radiographic procedures (if measured thickness is less than 10 cm).

GERIATRIC APPLICATIONS

Older patients often require extra care and patience in explaining what is expected of them. Careful breathing instructions are essential, as is assistance in helping patients move into the required position. Extra radiolucent padding under the back and buttocks for thin patients and blankets to keep patients warm add greatly to their comfort on supine abdomen radiographic procedures.

BARIATRIC PATIENT CONSIDERATIONS

Positioning of the bariatric patient for abdomen projections is similar to that for the sthenic patient. The challenge is often in palpation for bony landmarks, such as the iliac crest and symphysis pubis, on the morbidly obese patient. The technologist may need to move folds of adipose tissue and skin to locate these landmarks, which may be embarrassing for the patient. It may be more feasible to use the xiphoid process (T9–T10) or the lower costal margin (L2–L3) to determine the upper margin of the IR. The ASIS may be easier to palpate to determine the lower abdomen margin. Some technologists may use the umbilicus ("belly button") as an alternative to the iliac crest. However, due to extension of the abdomen, skin folds, and possible past surgeries, this often proves to be an inaccurate landmark.

It is critical to image the entire abdomen to the skin margins because the large intestine often extends the width of the abdomen. This is accomplished by taking two exposures of the abdomen with a landscape alignment to capture any abnormal anatomy, gas patterns, or pathology. The first projection would image the upper abdomen (top of IR at the level of the xiphoid process), whereas the second projection would slightly overlap about 1 to 2 inches (3 to 5 cm) to visualize all abdominal anatomy. The bottom of the second IR should be placed at the level of the symphysis pubis to image the lower abdominopelvic structures (Figs. 3.26 and 3.27). This alteration in the routine protocol would be recommended for the supine abdomen (KUB) and erect abdomen studies.

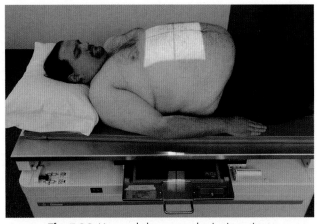

Fig. 3.26 Upper abdomen on bariatric patient.

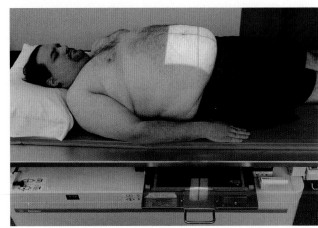

Fig. 3.27 Lower abdomen on bariatric patient.

Digital Imaging Considerations

The guidelines that should be followed with digital imaging of the abdomen as described in this chapter are summarized as follows:

1. **Four-sided collimation:** Collimation to the body part being imaged and **accurate centering** are most important in digital imaging of the abdomen.
2. **Exposure factors:** It is important that the ALARA principle (as low as reasonably achievable) be followed in regard to patient exposure to radiation and that the **lowest exposure factors required to obtain a diagnostic image** be used. This includes the highest kVp and the lowest mAs that result in desirable image quality.
3. **Post-processing evaluation of exposure indicator:** The exposure indicator on the final processed image must be checked to verify that the exposure factors used were in the correct range to ensure optimal quality with the least amount of radiation to the patient. The technologist should assess these after each image.

Alternative Modalities

CT AND MRI

CT and magnetic resonance imaging (MRI) are very useful in the evaluation and early diagnosis of small neoplasms involving abdominal organs, such as the liver and pancreas. With the use of intravenous, iodinated contrast media, CT imaging can discriminate between a simple cyst and a solid neoplasm.

Both CT and MRI also provide valuable information in assessing the extent to which neoplasms have spread to surrounding tissues or organs. For example, MRI may be used to demonstrate blood vessels within neoplasms and to assess their relationship and involvement with surrounding organs without the need for contrast media injection.

MRI is also used to visualize the biliary and pancreatic ducts. Endoscopic retrograde cholangiopancreatography (ERCP), a fluoroscopic procedure in which a contrast medium is injected endoscopically, is used to visualize the biliary and pancreatic ducts as well (described in Chapter 19).

SONOGRAPHY

Ultrasound has become the method of choice when imaging the **gallbladder** for detection of gallstones (in the gallbladder or bile ducts). Ultrasound is of limited use in the evaluation of the hollow viscus of the GI tract for bowel obstruction or perforation, but along with CT, it is very useful in detecting and evaluating lesions or inflammation of soft tissue organs such as the liver or pancreas. Ultrasound is widely used, along with CT, for demonstrating abscesses, cysts, or tumors involving the kidneys, ureters, or bladder.

Ultrasound with graded compression, in combination with clinical evaluation, can be used successfully to diagnose **acute appendicitis**; this is the recommended approach for pediatric patients. However, CT is considered the ideal imaging modality to demonstrate an abscess or thickened wall surrounding the inflamed appendix. CT, with the use of intravenous contrast media, can demonstrate the location, extent, and degree of involvement of the surrounding tissues.[5]

NUCLEAR MEDICINE

Nuclear medicine is useful as a noninvasive means of evaluating GI motility and reflux as related to possible bowel obstruction. It is also useful for evaluation of suspected lower GI bleeding.

With the injection of specific radionuclides, nuclear medicine imaging can be used to examine the entire liver, the major bile ducts and gallbladder.

Clinical Indications

An **AP supine image** of the abdomen **(KUB)** is generally taken before contrast medium is introduced into the various abdominal organ systems for evaluation and diagnosis of diseases and conditions involving these systems (Table 3.3). Clinical indications and terms specifically related to each of these systems are provided in Chapters 12 and 13.

The **acute abdomen series,** as described in this chapter, is performed most commonly to evaluate and diagnose conditions or diseases related to **bowel obstruction or perforation.** This evaluation requires visualization of air-fluid levels and possible intraperitoneal "free" air with the use of a horizontal beam and erect or decubitus body positions. Following are terms and pathologic diseases or conditions that are related to the acute abdominal series examination.

Ascites *(ah-si´-tez)* is an abnormal accumulation of fluid in the peritoneal cavity of the abdomen. It is usually caused by long-standing (chronic) conditions such as cirrhosis of the liver or by metastatic disease to the peritoneal cavity.

Pneumoperitoneum refers to free air or gas in the peritoneal cavity. This is a serious condition for which surgery is required when it is caused by perforation of a gas-containing viscus, such as a gastric or duodenal ulcer. It also can be caused by trauma that penetrates the abdominal wall. Small amounts of residual air may be evident radiographically 2 to 3 weeks after abdominal surgery. Air is best demonstrated with a horizontal beam, erect abdomen, or chest image, with which even a small amount of free air can be seen as it rises to the highest position under the diaphragm.

Dynamic (with power or force) or **mechanical bowel obstruction** is the complete or nearly complete blockage of the flow of intestinal contents. Causes include the following:

- **Fibrous adhesions:** The most common cause of mechanically based obstruction, in which a fibrous band of tissue interrelates with the intestine, creating a blockage.
- **Crohn's** *(krons)* **disease:** Also known as **regional enteritis,** a chronic inflammation of the intestinal wall that results in bowel obstruction in at least half of affected patients. The cause is unknown. Crohn's disease is most common in young adults and is characterized by loops of small intestine joined by fistulas or connected openings with adjacent loops of intestine. The two most common sites of intestinal involvement in **Crohn's disease** are the terminal ileum and proximal colon.[5]
- **Intussusception:** The telescoping of a section of bowel into another loop, which creates an obstruction. Intussusception is most common in the distal small intestine region (terminal

TABLE 3.3 SUMMARY OF CLINICAL INDICATIONS

CONDITION OR DISEASE	MOST COMMON RADIOGRAPHIC EXAMINATION	POSSIBLE RADIOGRAPHIC APPEARANCE	EXPOSURE FACTOR ADJUSTMENT[a]
Ascites	Acute abdomen series	General abdominal haziness	Increase, depending on severity (+ or + +)
Pneumoperitoneum (air in peritoneal cavity)	Acute abdomen series—erect chest or abdomen	Thin, crest-shaped radiolucency under dome of right hemidiaphragm on erect	Decrease (−)
Dynamic (Mechanical Bowel) Obstruction			
Fibrous adhesions	Acute abdomen series	Distended loops of air-filled small intestine	Decrease, depending on severity of distention (− or − −)
Crohn's disease	Acute abdomen series	Distended loops of air-filled small intestine (cobblestone appearance)	Decrease, depending on severity of distention (− or − −)
Intussusception (most common in children)	Acute abdomen series	Air-filled "coiled spring" appearance	Decrease (−)
Volvulus (most common in sigmoid colon)	Acute abdomen series	Large amounts of air in sigmoid with tapered narrowing at site of volvulus (beak sign)	Slight decrease (−)
Ileus (nonmechanical obstruction), adynamic or paralytic	Acute abdomen series	Large amounts of air in entire dilated small and large intestine with air-fluid levels visualized	Decrease, depending on severity of distention (− or − −)
Ulcerative Colitis Severe case may lead to toxic megacolon and bowel perforation	AP abdomen	Deep air-filled mucosal protrusions of colon wall, usually in rectosigmoid region	Decrease (−)
	Acute abdomen series for possible free air (barium enema contraindicated)	Dilated loop of colon	Decrease (−)

[a]Automatic exposure control (AEC) systems are designed to optimize mAs. Digital radiographic systems will correct exposure brightness automatically for patient size variances and for these pathologic conditions through processing algorithms. If they are calibrated correctly and are used as intended, manual adjustments generally are not needed when AEC systems are used. However, these exposure adjustments may be needed for more extreme cases, or for repeats, even with AEC.

ileum), and it is more common in children than in adults. This condition requires treatment within 48 hours to prevent necrosis (tissue death).
- **Volvulus:** The twisting of a loop of intestine, which creates an obstruction. Volvulus may require surgery for correction.

Ileus (nonmechanical bowel obstruction) is categorized as *adynamic* (without power or force) ileus and most frequently is caused by peritonitis, or *paralytic* (paralysis) ileus, which is caused by a lack of intestinal motility. Paralytic ileus occurs frequently in postoperative patients, usually 24 to 72 hours after abdominal surgery. In contrast to mechanical obstruction, it rarely leads to perforation, and the radiographic appearance is characterized by a large amount of air and fluid, with air-fluid levels visible in a significantly dilated small and large intestine and no visible distinct point of obstruction (in contrast to a mechanical obstruction).

Ulcerative colitis is a chronic disease involving inflammation of the colon that occurs primarily in young adults and most frequently involves the rectosigmoid region. In some cases, it becomes a very severe acute process, causing serious complications, such as toxic megacolon (extreme dilation of a segment of colon) with potential perforation into the peritoneal cavity. **Barium enema is strongly contraindicated** with symptoms of toxic megacolon.

Routine and Special Projections

Routine, alternate, and special projections of the abdomen are demonstrated and described on the following pages.

AP PROJECTION: SUPINE POSITION—ABDOMEN

KUB

Clinical Indications
- Pathology of the abdomen, including bowel obstruction, neoplasms, calcifications, ascites, and scout image for contrast media studies of abdomen

> **Abdomen**
> ROUTINE
> - AP supine (KUB)

Technical Factors
- Minimum SID—40 inches (100 cm)
- IR size—14 × 17 inches (35 × 43 cm), portrait
- Grid
- kVp range—70–85

Shielding Shield radiosensitive tissues outside region of interest.

Patient Position
- Supine with midsagittal plane centered to midline of table or IR
- Arms placed at patient's sides, away from body
- Legs bent with support under knees (to lessen lordotic lumbar curvature)

Part Position
- Center of IR to **level of iliac crests,** with bottom margin at symphysis pubis (Fig. 3.28) (see NOTES)
- **No rotation** of pelvis or shoulders (check that both ASIS are the same distance from the tabletop)

CR
- CR perpendicular to and directed to **center of IR** (to level of iliac crest)

Recommended Collimation 14 × 17 inches (35 × 43 cm), field of view or collimate on four sides to anatomy of interest

Respiration Make the exposure at end of expiration (allow about 1 second delay after expiration to allow involuntary motion of bowel to cease).

NOTES: A tall hyposthenic or asthenic patient may require **two images placed portrait** (Fig. 3.30)—one centered lower to include the symphysis pubis (bottom margin of first IR at symphysis) and the second centered higher to include the upper abdomen and diaphragm (top margin of second IR at xiphoid).

A broad hypersthenic patient may require two 14 × 17-inch (35 × 43-cm) IRs placed landscape, one centered lower to include the symphysis pubis and the second for the upper abdomen, with a minimum of 1 to 2 inches (3 to 5 cm) overlap (Fig. 3.29).

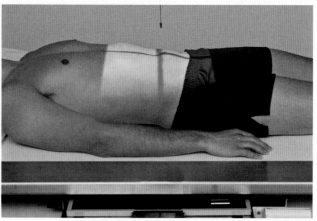

Fig. 3.28 AP abdomen (KUB).

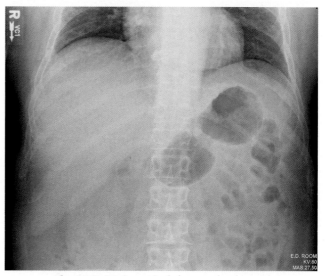

Fig. 3.29 AP (upper) abdomen—landscape.

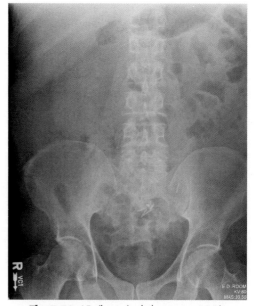

Fig. 3.30 AP (lower) abdomen—portrait.

Evaluation Criteria

Anatomy Demonstrated: • Outline of liver, spleen, kidneys, psoas muscles, and air-filled stomach and bowel segments and the arch of the symphysis pubis for the urinary bladder region (Fig. 3.31 and 3.32).

Position: • No rotation; iliac wings, obturator foramina (if visible), and ischial spines have symmetric appearance, and outer lower rib margins are the same distance from spine (elongation of iliac wing indicates rotation in that direction). Bilateral structure should also be on the same plane (if not the patient is tilted on the table) • Collimation to area of interest. • See preceding NOTES regarding the possibility of two images per projection.

Exposure: • No motion; ribs and all gas bubble margins appear sharp. • Sufficient exposure factors (kVp and mAs) to visualize psoas muscle outlines, lumbar transverse processes, and ribs. • Margins of liver and kidneys should be visible on smaller to average-sized patients.

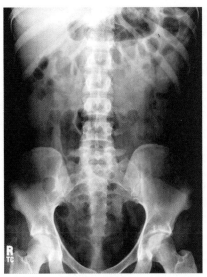

Fig. 3.31 AP abdomen (KUB).

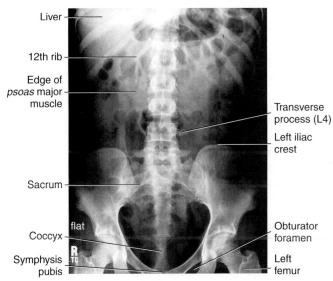

Fig. 3.32 AP abdomen.

PA PROJECTION—PRONE POSITION: ABDOMEN

Clinical Indications

- Pathology of abdomen, including bowel obstruction, neoplasms, calcifications, ascites, and scout image for contrast medium studies of abdomen

Abdomen
SPECIAL
• PA prone
• Lateral decubitus (AP)
• AP erect
• Dorsal decubitus (lateral)
• Lateral

NOTE: This projection is **less desirable** than AP if the kidneys are of primary interest because of the **increased object–image receptor distance (OID)**. However, this projection is helpful to lower exposure due to tissue compression as it leads to reduced part thickness.

Technical Factors

- Minimum SID—40 inches (100 cm)
- IR size—14 × 17 inches (35 × 43 cm), portrait
- Grid
- kVp range—70–85

Shielding Shield radiosensitive tissues outside region of interest

Patient Position

- Prone with midsagittal plane of body centered to midline of table or IR (Fig. 3.33)
- Legs extended with support under ankles
- Arms up beside head; clean pillow provided

Part Position

- **No rotation** of pelvis or shoulders and thorax
- Center of IR to **iliac crest**

CR

- CR perpendicular to and directed to **center of IR** (to level of iliac crest)

Recommended Collimation 14 × 17 inches (35 × 43 cm), field of view or collimate on four sides to anatomy of interest

Respiration Make exposure at end of **expiration.**

NOTE: Tall, asthenic patients may require two images placed portrait; broad, hypersthenic and bariatric patients may require two images placed landscape.

Evaluation Criteria

Anatomy Demonstrated: • Outline of liver, spleen, kidneys, psoas muscles, and air-filled stomach and bowel segments and the arch of the symphysis pubis for the urinary bladder region (Figs. 3.34 and 3.35).

Position: • No rotation; iliac wings appear symmetric, and sacroiliac joints and outer lower rib margins (if visible) should be the same distance from spine. • Collimation to area of interest. • See *Notes* regarding the possibility of two images.

Exposure: • No motion; ribs and all gas bubble margins appear sharp. • Exposure (mAs) and long-scale contrast (kVp) are sufficient to visualize psoas muscle outlines, lumbar transverse processes, and ribs. • Margins of liver and kidneys should be visible on smaller to average-sized patients.

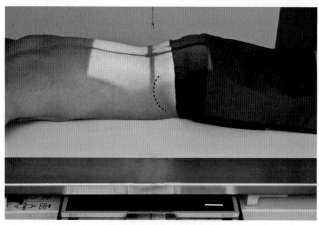

Fig. 3.33 PA abdomen.

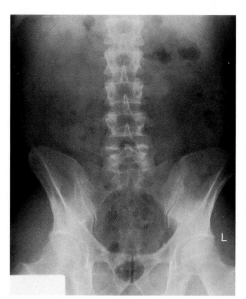

Fig. 3.34 PA abdomen.

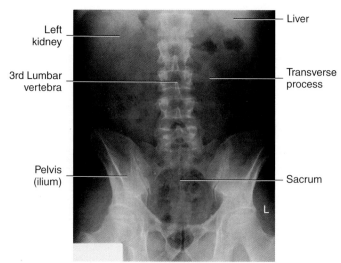

Fig. 3.35 PA abdomen.

Left kidney

Liver

3rd Lumbar vertebra

Transverse process

Pelvis (ilium)

Sacrum

LATERAL DECUBITUS POSITION (AP PROJECTION)—ABDOMEN

Clinical Indications
- Abdominal masses, air-fluid levels, and possible accumulations of intraperitoneal air are demonstrated.
- Small amounts of free intraperitoneal air are best demonstrated with chest technique on erect PA chest.

Important: Patient should be on his or her side a **minimum of 5 minutes** before exposure (to allow air to rise or abnormal fluids to accumulate); **10 to 20 minutes is preferred,** if possible, for best visualization of potentially small amounts of intraperitoneal air

Left lateral decubitus position best visualizes free intraperitoneal air in the area of the liver in the right upper abdomen away from the gastric bubble

Abdomen
SPECIAL
• PA prone
• Lateral decubitus (AP)
• AP erect
• Dorsal decubitus (lateral)
• Lateral

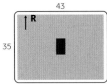

Technical Factors
- Minimum SID—40 inches (100 cm)
- IR size—14 × 17 inches (35 × 43 cm), landscape
- Grid
- kVp range—70–85

Marker: Place arrow or other appropriate marker to indicate "up" side.

Shielding Shield radiosensitive tissues outside region of interest.

Patient Position
- Lateral recumbent on radiolucent pad, firmly against table or vertical grid device (with wheels on cart locked so as not to move away from table)
- Patient on firm surface, such as a cardiac or back board, positioned under the sheet to prevent sagging and anatomy cutoff (Fig. 3.36)
- Knees partially flexed, one on top of the other, to stabilize patient
- Arms up near head; clean pillow provided

Part Position
- Adjust patient and cart/table so that center of IR and CR are approximately **2 inches (5 cm) above level of iliac crests** (to include diaphragm). Upper margin of IR is approximately at level of axilla.
- Ensure **no rotation** of pelvis or shoulders.

- Adjust height of IR to center midsagittal plane of patient to center of IR, but ensure that **upside of abdomen is clearly included on the IR.**

CR
- CR **horizontal,** directed to **center of IR,** at about 2 inches (5 cm) above level of iliac crest; use of a horizontal beam to demonstrate air-fluid levels and free intraperitoneal air

Recommended Collimation
- 14 × 17 inches (35 × 43 cm), field of view or collimate on four sides to anatomy of interest
- Must include elevated side of the abdomen

Respiration Make exposure at end of **expiration.**

Evaluation Criteria
Anatomy Demonstrated: • Air-filled stomach and loops of bowel and air-fluid levels where present. • Should include bilateral diaphragm (Figs. 3.37 and 3.38).

Position: • No rotation; iliac wings appear symmetric, and outer rib margins are the same distance from spine. • No tilt: Spine should be straight (unless scoliosis is present), aligned to center of IR. • Collimation to area of interest.

Exposure: • No motion; ribs and all gas bubble margins sharp. • Exposure sufficient to visualize spine and ribs and soft tissue but not to overexpose possible intraperitoneal air in upper abdomen.

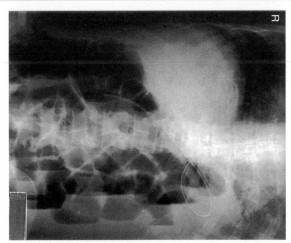

Fig. 3.37 Left lateral decubitus (AP). (Modified from McQuillen Martensen K: *Radiographic image analysis,* ed 4, St Louis, 2015, Saunders.)

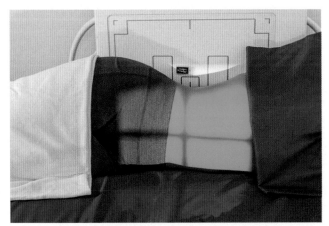

Fig. 3.36 Left lateral decubitus position (AP).

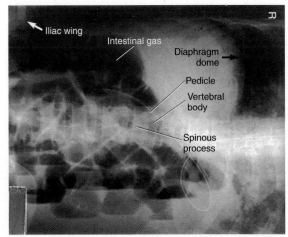

Fig. 3.38 Left lateral decubitus (AP). (From McQuillen Martensen K: *Radiographic image analysis,* ed 4, St Louis, 2015, Saunders.)

AP PROJECTION: ERECT POSITION—ABDOMEN

Clinical Indications
- Abnormal masses, air-fluid levels, and accumulations of intraperitoneal air under diaphragm

  Perform erect abdominal image first if the patient comes to the department ambulatory or in a wheelchair in an erect position.

Abdomen
SPECIAL
• PA prone
• Lateral decubitus (AP)
• AP erect
• Dorsal decubitus (lateral)
• Lateral

Technical Factors
- Minimum SID—40 inches (100 cm)
- IR size—14 × 17 inches (35 × 43 cm), portrait
- Grid
- kVp range—70–85

  Marker: Include erect marker on IR.

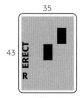

Shielding
- Shield radiosensitive tissues outside region of interest.
- Use gonadal shields on male patients. An adjustable freestanding mobile shield can be used.

Patient Position
- Upright, legs slightly spread apart, back against table or grid device (see NOTE regarding weak or unsteady patients)
- Arms at sides away from body
- Midsagittal plane of body centered to midline of table or erect bucky

Part Position
- Do not rotate pelvis or shoulders.
- Adjust height of IR so that the center is approximately **2 inches (5 cm) above iliac crest** (to include diaphragm), which for the average patient places the **top of the IR approximately at the level of the axilla** (Fig. 3.39).

CR
- CR perpendicular, to center of IR

Recommended Collimation
- 14 × 17 inches (35 × 43 cm), field of view or collimate on four sides to anatomy of interest
- Must include upper abdomen

Respiration Exposure should be made at end of expiration.

NOTE: Patient should be upright a minimum of **5 minutes**, but **10 to 20 minutes** is desirable, if possible, before exposure for visualizing small amounts of intraperitoneal air. If a patient is too weak to maintain an erect position, a lateral decubitus should be performed. For hypersthenic patients, two landscape IRs may be required to include the entire abdomen.

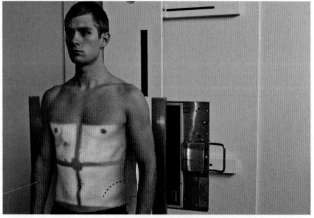

Fig. 3.39 Erect AP—to include diaphragm.

Evaluation Criteria
Anatomy Demonstrated: • Air-filled stomach and loops of bowel and air-fluid levels where present. • Should include **bilateral diaphragms** and as much of lower abdomen as possible. • Small free, intraperitoneal crescent-shaped air bubble if present seen under **right** hemidiaphragm, away from gas in stomach (Figs. 3.40 and 3.41).

Position: • No rotation; iliac wings appear symmetric, and outer rib margins are the same distance from spine. • No tilt: Spine should be straight (unless scoliosis is present), aligned with center of IR. • Collimation to area of interest.

Exposure: • No motion; ribs and all gas bubble margins appear sharp. • Exposure is sufficient to visualize spine and ribs and soft tissue but not to overexpose possible intraperitoneal air in upper abdomen. • Slightly less overall density (brightness) than supine abdomen is preferred.

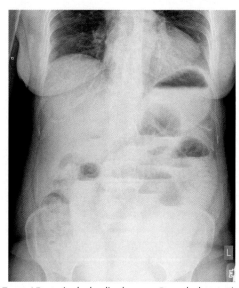

Fig. 3.40 Erect AP—to include diaphragm. Bowel obstruction is present (note air-fluid level).

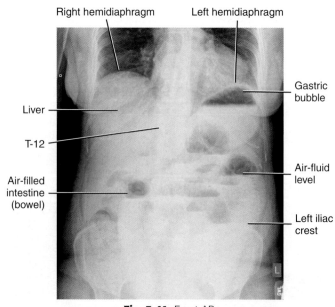

Fig. 3.41 Erect AP.

DORSAL DECUBITUS POSITION (RIGHT OR LEFT LATERAL)—ABDOMEN

Clinical Indications

- Abnormal masses, accumulations of gas, air-fluid levels, **aneurysms** (widening or dilation of the wall of an artery, vein, or the heart)
- **Calcification of aorta or other vessels**
- **Umbilical hernia**

Abdomen
SPECIAL
• PA prone
• Lateral decubitus (AP)
• AP erect
• Dorsal decubitus (lateral)
• Lateral

Technical Factors

- Minimum SID—40 inches (100 cm)
- IR size—14 × 17 inches (35 × 43 cm), landscape
- Grid
- kVp range—70–85

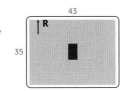

Shielding

- Shield radiosensitive tissues outside region of interest.
- Use gonadal shields on male patients.

Patient Position

- Supine on radiolucent pad, side against table or vertical grid device; secure cart so that it does not move away from table or grid device.
- Ensure that neither the patient nor the cart is tilted in relation to the IR.
- Pillow under head, arms up beside head; support under partially flexed knees may be more comfortable for the patient (Fig. 3.42).

Part Position ⊞

- Adjust patient and cart so that center of IR and CR is at level of iliac crest or 2 inches (5 cm) above iliac crest to include diaphragm.
- Ensure that **no rotation** of pelvis or shoulders exists (both ASIS should be the same distance from tabletop).
- Adjust height of IR to align midcoronal plane with centerline of IR.

CR

- CR **horizontal** to **center of IR** at iliac crest and/or 2 inches (5 cm) above iliac crest to include diaphragm

Recommended Collimation Collimate to upper and lower abdomen soft tissue borders. Close collimation is important because of increased scatter produced by exposure of tissue outside the area of interest

Respiration Exposure is made at end of **expiration.**

NOTE: This may be taken as a right or left lateral; appropriate R or L lateral marker should be used, indicating the side closest to IR.

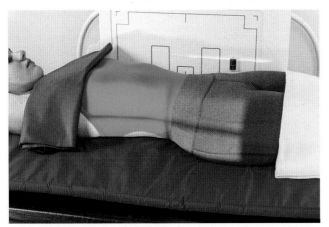

Fig. 3.42 Dorsal decubitus—right lateral position.

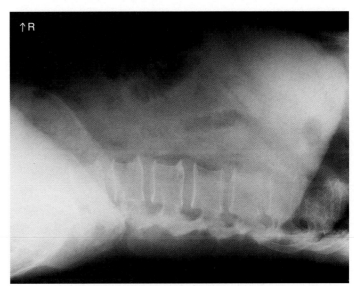

Fig. 3.43 Dorsal decubitus—right lateral position.

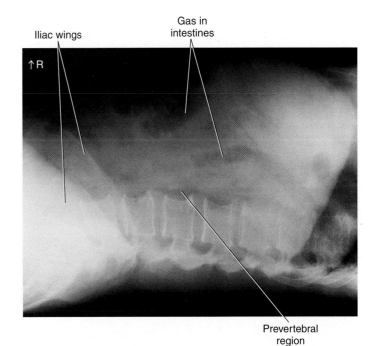

Iliac wings

Gas in intestines

Prevertebral region

Fig. 3.44 Dorsal decubitus—right lateral position.

LATERAL POSITION—ABDOMEN

Clinical Indications
- Abnormal soft tissue masses, umbilical hernia, prevertebral region for possible aneurysms of aorta or calcifications
- May be performed for localization of foreign bodies

Abdomen

SPECIAL
- PA prone
- Lateral decubitus (AP)
- AP erect
- Dorsal decubitus (lateral)
- Lateral

Technical Factors
- Minimum SID—40 inches (100 cm)
- IR size—14 × 17 inches (35 × 43 cm), portrait
- Grid
- kVp range—70–85

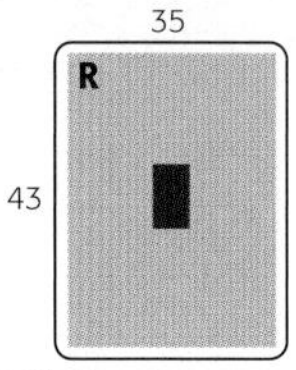

35

R

43

Shielding
- Shield radiosensitive tissues outside region of interest.
- Use gonadal shields on male patients.

Patient Position
- Patient in lateral recumbent position on right or left side, pillow for head
- Elbows flexed, arms up, knees and hips partially flexed, pillow between knees to maintain a lateral position (Fig. 3.45)
- Ensure patient is not tilted

Part Position
- Align midcoronal plane with CR and midline of table.
- Ensure that pelvis and thorax are **not rotated** but are in a true lateral position.

CR
- CR perpendicular to table, centered at level of the **iliac crest** to midcoronal plane
- IR centered to CR

Recommended Collimation Collimate closely to upper and lower IR borders and to anterior and posterior skin borders to minimize scatter.

Respiration Suspend breathing on **expiration.**

Evaluation Criteria
Anatomy Demonstrated: • Diaphragm and as much of lower abdomen as possible should be included. • Air-filled loops of bowel in abdomen with soft tissue detail should be visible in prevertebral and anterior abdomen regions (Figs. 3.46 and 3.47).
Position: • **No rotation** as evident by superimposition of posterior ribs and posterior borders of iliac wings and bilateral ASIS. • Collimation to area of interest.
Exposure: • No motion; rib and gas bubble margins appear sharp. • Lumbar vertebrae may appear about 50% underexposed with soft tissue detail visible in anterior abdomen and in prevertebral region of lower lumbar vertebra.

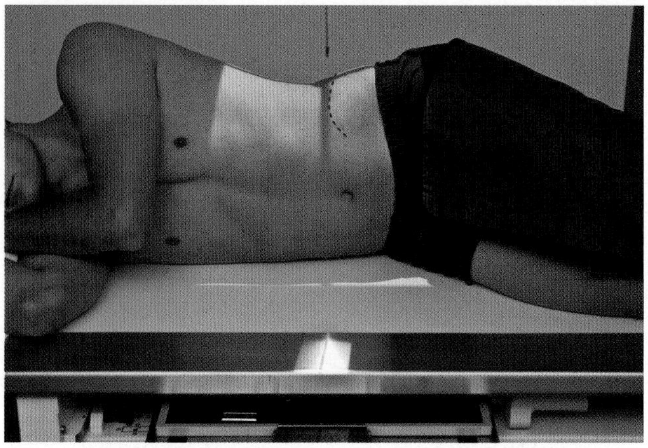

Fig. 3.45 Right lateral abdomen.

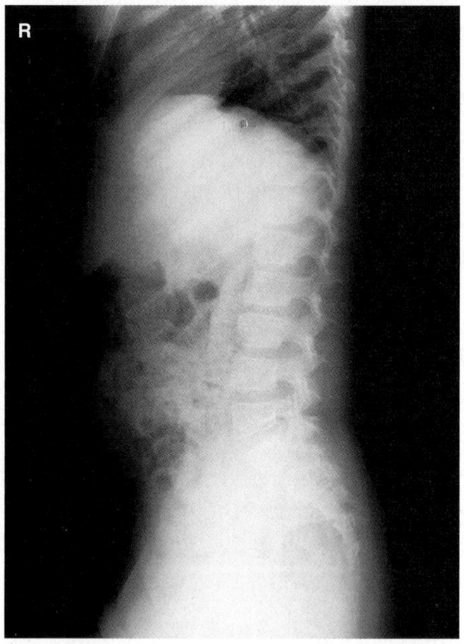

Fig. 3.46 Right lateral abdomen.

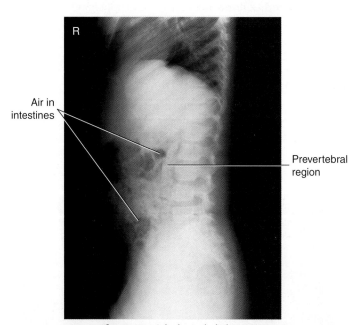

Air in intestines

Prevertebral region

Fig. 3.47 Right lateral abdomen.

ACUTE ABDOMINAL SERIES—ACUTE ABDOMEN

(1) AP SUPINE, (2) ERECT (OR LATERAL DECUBITUS) ABDOMEN, (3) PA CHEST

Departmental Routine The acute abdomen series typically consists of three projections: AP supine abdomen (Fig. 3.48), AP erect abdomen, and a PA chest projection. However, acute abdomen routines may vary, depending on the institution. Students and technologists should be aware of the routine for their departments.

> **Acute Abdomen**
> ROUTINE
> • AP supine
> • AP erect
> • PA chest
> SPECIAL
> • Left lateral decubitus (can be used in place of the AP erect abdomen projection for nonambulatory patients)

The PA chest is commonly included in the acute abdomen series because the erect chest allows free intraperitoneal air under the diaphragm to be visualized. The erect abdomen also visualizes free air, if the IR is centered high enough to include the diaphragm; however, the exposure technique for the chest best visualizes small amounts of this free air if present.

NOTE: Acute abdomen routines for pediatric patients generally include only an AP supine abdomen and one horizontal beam projection to demonstrate air-fluid levels. For patients younger than 2 or 3 years of age, a left lateral decubitus may be difficult to obtain, and an AP erect abdomen with an immobilization device such as a Pigg-O-Stat (Modern Way Immobilizers, Inc, Clifton, Tennessee) is preferred (see Chapter 16).

Specific Clinical Indications for Acute Abdominal Series
• **Ileus** (nonmechanical small bowel obstruction) or mechanical ileus (obstruction of bowel from hernia, adhesions)
• **Ascites** (abnormal fluid accumulation in abdomen)
• **Perforated hollow viscus** (e.g., bowel or stomach, evident by free intraperitoneal air)
• **Intra-abdominal mass** (neoplasms—benign or malignant)
• **Postoperative** (abdominal surgery)
Perform erect images first if patient comes to the department in an erect position.

Positional Guidelines Review positional guidelines as described on preceding pages for AP supine, AP erect, and PA chest.

Patient and Part Positioning
Most department routines for the erect abdomen include centering high to demonstrate possible free intraperitoneal air under the diaphragm, even if a PA chest is included in the series.

Breathing Instructions Chest projections exposed on full inspiration; abdomen exposed on expiration.

CR CR to level of iliac crest on supine and approximately 2 inches (5 cm) above level of crest to include diaphragm on erect or decubitus radiographs

NOTES: Left lateral decubitus replaces erect position if the patient is too ill to stand.

Horizontal beam is necessary for visualization of air-fluid levels.

Erect PA chest (Fig. 3.49) or AP erect abdomen (Fig. 3.50) best visualizes free air under diaphragm.

For left lateral decubitus, patient should be on the right side for a minimum of 5 minutes before exposure (10 to 20 minutes preferred) to demonstrate potential small amounts of intraperitoneal air (Fig. 3.51).

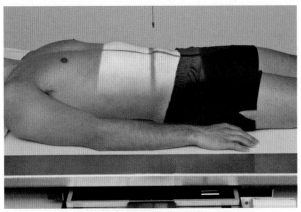

Fig. 3.48 AP supine.

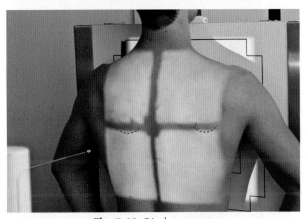

Fig. 3.49 PA chest erect.

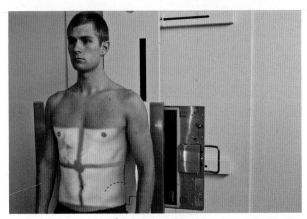

Fig. 3.50 AP erect.

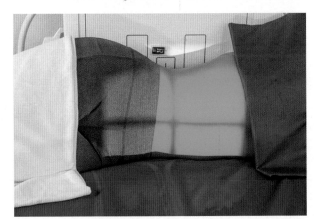

Fig. 3.51 Left lateral decubitus (special projection, if patient cannot stand for AP erect abdomen).

RADIOGRAPHS FOR CRITIQUE

This section consists of an ideal projection (Image A) along with one or more projections that may demonstrate positioning and/or technical errors. Critique Figures C3.52 through C3.54. Compare Image A to the other projections and identify the errors. While examining each image, consider the following questions:

1. Is all essential anatomy demonstrated on the image?

2. What positioning errors are present that compromise image quality?
3. Are technical factors optimal?
4. Is there evidence of collimation and pre-exposure anatomical side markers visible on the image?
5. Do these errors require a repeat exposure?

Feedback for each set of images is located on the faculty Evolve site.

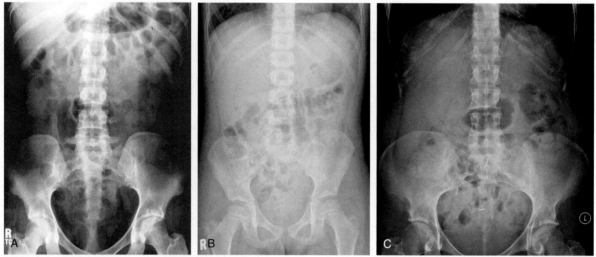

Fig. C3.52 AP supine abdomen—KUB. (Image **C** courtesy of Dr. Jeremy Jones, Radiopaedia.org, rID: 34067.)

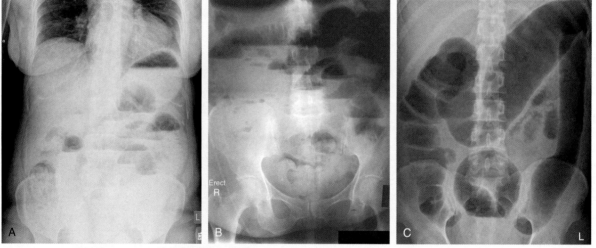

Fig. C3.53 Erect abdomen. (Image **C** courtesy of Abdominal X-ray Interpretation. Available at https://geekymedics.com/abdominal-x-ray-interpretation/.)

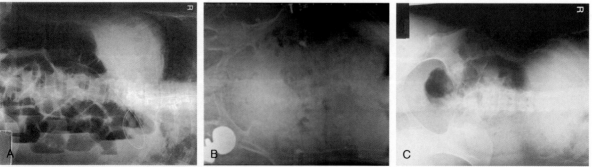

Fig. C3.54 Left lateral decubitus. (Image **A** modified from McQuillen Martensen K: *Radiographic image analysis*, ed 4, St Louis, 2015, Saunders; **B** copyright Nicholas Joseph Jr. [Radiograph #95; http://www.ceessentials.net/article24.html].)

CHAPTER 4

Upper Limb

CONTRIBUTIONS BY **Janelle M. Black,** B.S.(DMIT), R.T.(R)(ARRT)

CONTRIBUTORS TO PAST EDITIONS   Nancy Johnson, MEd, RT(R)(CV)(CT)(QM)(ARRT), FASRT, Kathy M. Martensen, BS, RT(R), Donna Davis, MEd, RT(R)(CV), Linda S. Lingar, MEd, RT(R)(M)

CONTENTS

Upper Limb

The bones of the upper limb can be divided into four main groups: (1) **hand and wrist,** (2) **forearm,** (3) **arm** (humerus), and (4) **shoulder girdle** (Fig. 4.1). The first two groups are discussed in this chapter. The important wrist and elbow joints are included; the shoulder joint and proximal humerus are discussed in Chapter 5.

The shape and structure of each of the bones and articulations, or joints, of the upper limb must be thoroughly understood by technologists so that each part can be identified and demonstrated on radiographs.

HAND AND WRIST

The 27 bones in each hand and wrist are divided into the following three groups (Fig. 4.2):

Phalanges (fingers and thumb)	14
Metacarpals (palm)	5
Carpals (wrist)	8
Total	27

The most distal bones of the hand are the **phalanges** *(fa-lan'-jez),* which constitute the digits (fingers and thumb). The second group of bones is the **metacarpals** *(met″-ah-kar'-palz);* these bones make up the palm of each hand. The third group of bones, the **carpals** *(kar'-palz),* consists of the bones of the wrist.

Phalanges: Fingers and Thumb (Digits)

Each finger and thumb is called a *digit,* and each digit consists of two or three separate small bones called *phalanges* (singular, **phalanx** *[fa'-lanks]*). The digits are numbered, starting with the thumb as 1 and ending with the little finger as 5.

Each of the four fingers (digits 2, 3, 4, and 5) is composed of three phalanges—**proximal, middle,** and **distal.** The thumb, or first digit, has two phalanges—**proximal** and **distal.**

Each phalanx consists of three parts: a distal rounded **head,** a **body** (shaft), and an expanded **base,** similar to that of the metacarpals.

Metacarpals (Palm)

The second group of bones of the hand, which make up the palm, consists of the five **metacarpals.** These bones are numbered the same way as the digits are, with the first metacarpal being on the thumb, or lateral, side when the hand is in the anatomic position.

Each metacarpal is composed of three parts, similar to the phalanges. Distally, the rounded portion is the **head.** The **body** (shaft) is the long curved portion; the anterior part is concave in shape, and the posterior, or dorsal, portion is convex. The **base** is the expanded proximal end, which articulates with associated carpals.

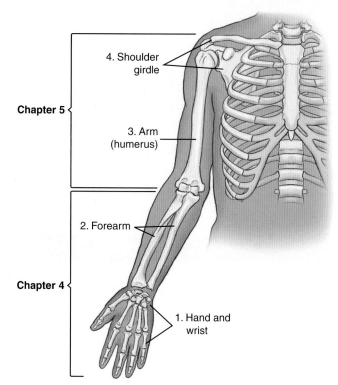

Fig. 4.1 Right upper limb (anterior view).

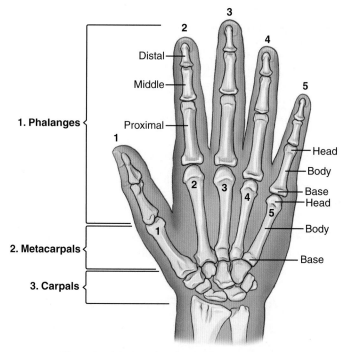

Fig. 4.2 Right hand and wrist (posterior view).

JOINTS OF THE HAND

The joints, or articulations, between the individual bones of the upper limb are important in radiology because small chip fractures may occur near the joint spaces. Therefore, accurate identification of all joints of the phalanges and metacarpals of the hand is required (Fig. 4.3).

Thumb (First Digit)

The thumb has only two phalanges, so the joint between them is called the **interphalangeal (IP) joint.** The joint between the first metacarpal and the proximal phalanx of the thumb is called the **first metacarpophalangeal (MCP) joint.** The name of this joint consists of the names of the two bones that make up this joint. The proximal bone is named first, followed by the distal bone.

For radiographic purposes, the first metacarpal is considered part of the thumb and must be included in its entirety in a radiograph of the thumb—**from the distal phalanx to the base of the first metacarpal.** This inclusion is not the case with the fingers, which for positioning purposes include only the three phalanges—distal, middle, and proximal.

Fingers (Second through Fifth Digits)

Each of the second through fifth digits has three phalanges, and they have three joints each. Starting from the most distal portion of each digit, the joints are the **distal interphalangeal (DIP) joint,** followed by the **proximal interphalangeal (PIP) joint,** and, most proximally, the **MCP joint.**

MPJ and CMC Joints

The metacarpals articulate with the phalanges at their distal ends and are called **metacarpophalangeal (MCP) joints.** At the proximal end, the metacarpals articulate with the respective carpals and are called **carpometacarpal (CMC) joints.** The five metacarpals articulate with specific carpals as follows:
- First metacarpal with trapezium
- Second metacarpal with trapezoid
- Third metacarpal with capitate
- Fourth and fifth metacarpal with hamate

REVIEW EXERCISE WITH RADIOGRAPHS

In identifying the joints and phalanges of the hand, the specific digit and hand must be included in the descriptions. A PA radiograph of the hand (Fig. 4.4) shows the phalanges and metacarpals and the joints described previously. A good review exercise is to identify each part labeled A through R on Fig. 4.4 (cover up the answers listed next). Then check your answers against the following list:

A. First carpometacarpal joint of right hand
B. First metacarpal of right hand
C. First metacarpophalangeal joint of right hand
D. Proximal phalanx of first digit (or thumb) of right hand
E. Interphalangeal joint of first digit (or thumb) of right hand
F. Distal phalanx of first digit (or thumb) of right hand
G. Second metacarpophalangeal joint of right hand
H. Proximal phalanx of second digit of right hand
I. Proximal interphalangeal joint of second digit of right hand
J. Middle phalanx of second digit of right hand
K. Distal interphalangeal joint of second digit of right hand
L. Distal phalanx of second digit of right hand
M. Middle phalanx of fourth digit of right hand
N. Distal interphalangeal joint of fifth digit of right hand
O. Proximal phalanx of third digit of right hand
P. Fifth metacarpophalangeal joint of right hand
Q. Fourth metacarpal of right hand
R. Fifth carpometacarpal joint of right hand

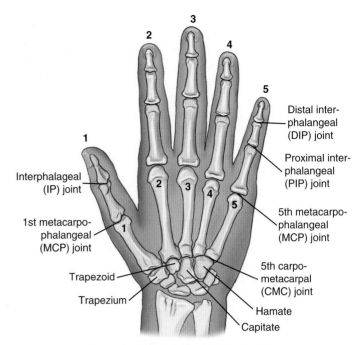

Fig. 4.3 Joints of right hand and wrist.

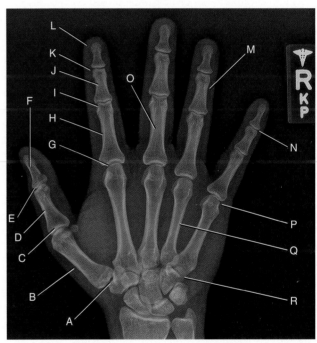

Fig. 4.4 PA radiograph of right hand.

CARPALS (WRIST)

The third group of bones of the hand and wrist are the **carpals,** the bones of the wrist. Learning the names of the eight carpals is easiest when they are divided into two rows of four each (Fig. 4.5).

Proximal Row

Beginning on the lateral, or thumb, side is the **scaphoid** *(skaf'-oyd),* sometimes referred to as the *navicular.* One of the tarsal bones of the foot also is sometimes called the *navicular* or *scaphoid.* However, the correct term for the tarsal bone of the **foot** is the **navicular,** and the correct term for the carpal bone of the **wrist** is the **scaphoid.**

The scaphoid, a boat-shaped bone, is the largest bone in the proximal row and **articulates with the radius proximally.** Its location and articulation with the forearm make it important radiographically because it is the **most frequently fractured carpal bone.**

The **lunate** (moon shaped) is the second carpal in the proximal row; it **articulates with the radius.** It is distinguished by the deep concavity on its distal surface, where it articulates with the capitate of the distal row of carpals (best seen on anterior view; Fig. 4.6).

The **third** carpal is the **triquetrum** *(tri-kwe'-trum),* which has three articular surfaces and is distinguished by its pyramidal shape and anterior articulation with the small pisiform.

The **pisiform** *(pi'-si-form)* (pea shaped), the smallest of the carpal bones, is located anterior to the triquetrum and is most evident in the carpal canal or tangential projection (Fig. 4.7).

Distal Row

The second, more distal row of four carpals articulates with the five metacarpal bones. Starting again on the lateral, or thumb, side is the **trapezium** *(trah-pe'-ze-um),* a four-sided, irregularly shaped bone that is located medial and distal to the scaphoid and proximal to the first metacarpal. The wedge-shaped **trapezoid** *(trap'-e-zoyd),* also four sided, is the smallest bone in the distal row. This bone is followed by the largest of the carpal bones, the **capitate** *(kap'-i-tate)* (capitate means "large bone"). It is identified by its large rounded head that fits proximally into a concavity formed by the scaphoid and lunate bones.

The last carpal in the distal row on the medial aspect is the **hamate** *(ham'-ate),* which is easily distinguished by the hooklike process called the **hamulus** *(ham'-u-lus),* or hamular process, which projects from its palmar surface (see Fig. 4.7).

Carpal Sulcus (Canal or Tangential Projection)

Fig. 4.7 is a drawing of the carpals as they would appear in a tangential projection down the wrist and arm from the palm or volar side of a hyperextended wrist. This view demonstrates the carpal sulcus formed by the concave anterior or palmar aspect of the carpals. The anteriorly located pisiform and the hamulus process of the hamate are visualized best on this view. This concave area or groove is called the *carpal sulcus (carpal tunnel* or *canal),* through which major nerves and tendons pass.

The term *hamate* means hooked, which describes the shape of the hamate in the illustration. The trapezium and its relationships to the thumb and trapezoid are well demonstrated.

Summary Chart of Carpal Terminology

The terms listed in Table 4.1 are used throughout this text. The names of these eight carpals may be remembered more easily with the use of a mnemonic (in which a sentence or phrase is formed by using the first letter of each carpal). Two mnemonic samples are provided in Table 4.1.

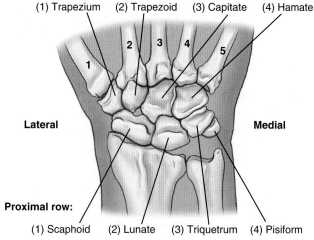

Distal row:
(1) Trapezium   (2) Trapezoid   (3) Capitate   (4) Hamate

Lateral   Medial

Proximal row:
(1) Scaphoid   (2) Lunate   (3) Triquetrum   (4) Pisiform

Fig. 4.5 Right carpals (dorsal or posterior view).

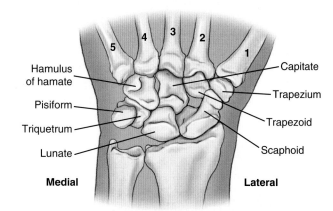

Hamulus of hamate — Capitate
Pisiform — Trapezium
Triquetrum — Trapezoid
Lunate — Scaphoid

Medial   **Lateral**

Fig. 4.6 Right carpals (palmar or anterior view).

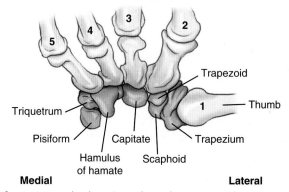

Trapezoid
Triquetrum — Thumb
Pisiform — Capitate — Trapezium
Hamulus of hamate   Scaphoid

Medial   **Lateral**

Fig. 4.7 Carpal sulcus (carpal canal or tangential projection).

TABLE 4.1 MNEMONIC FOR THE CARPALS

MNEMONIC			CARPAL
Send		Steve	Scaphoid
Letter		Left	Lunate
To		The	Triquetrum
Peter	Or	Party	Pisiform
To		To	Trapezium
Tell 'em (to)		Take	Trapezoid
Come		Carol	Capitate
Home		Home	Hamate

REVIEW EXERCISE WITH RADIOGRAPHS

Five projections for the wrist are shown in Figs. 4.8 through 4.12. A good review exercise is to identify each carpal bone as labeled (first cover the answers that follow). Check your answers against the following list.

In the lateral position (see Fig. 4.12), the trapezium (E) and the scaphoid (A) are located more anteriorly. Also, the ulnar deviation projection (see Fig. 4.10) best demonstrates the scaphoid without the foreshortening and overlapping seen on the posteroanterior (PA) (see Fig. 4.8).

The radial deviation projection (see Fig. 4.9) best demonstrates the interspaces and the carpals on the ulnar (lateral) side of the wrist-hamate (H), triquetrum (C), pisiform (D), and lunate (B). The outline of the end-on view of the hamulus process of the hamate (h) also can be seen on this radial deviation radiograph. The hamulus process also is demonstrated well on the carpal canal projection in Fig. 4.11, as is the pisiform (D), which is projected anteriorly and is seen in its entirety. Answers are as follows:

A. Scaphoid
B. Lunate
C. Triquetrum
D. Pisiform
E. Trapezium
F. Trapezoid
G. Capitate
H. Hamate
h. Hamulus (hamular process of hamate)

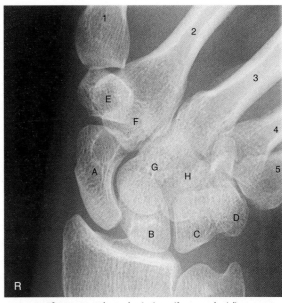
Fig. 4.10 Ulnar deviation (for scaphoid).

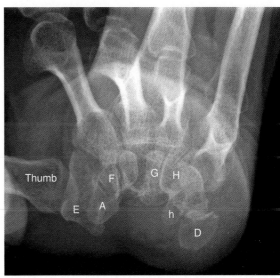
Fig. 4.11 Carpal canal. The scaphoid (A) is partially superimposed with the trapezium (E) and the trapezoid (F) on this projection.

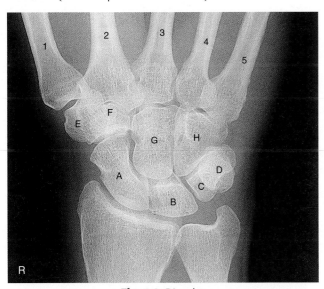
Fig. 4.8 PA wrist.

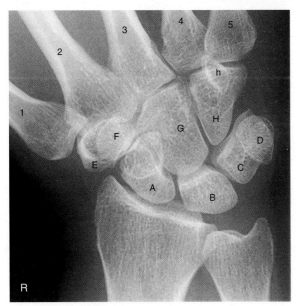
Fig. 4.9 Radial deviation.

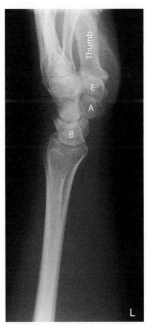
Fig. 4.12 Lateral wrist.

4

FOREARM—RADIUS AND ULNA

The second group of upper limb bones consists of the bones of the forearm—the radius on the lateral or thumb side and the ulna on the medial side (Fig. 4.13). The radius and ulna articulate with each other at the proximal radioulnar joint and at the distal radioulnar joint, as shown in Fig. 4.14. These two joints allow for the rotational movement of the wrist and hand, as described later in this chapter.

Radius and Ulna

Small conical projections, called **styloid processes,** are located at the extreme distal ends of both the radius and the ulna (see Fig. 4.14). The radial styloid process can be palpated on the thumb side of the wrist joint. The radial styloid process extends more distally than the ulnar styloid process.

The **ulnar notch** is a small depression on the medial aspect of the distal radius. The head of the ulna fits into the ulnar notch to form the distal radioulnar joint.

The **head of the ulna** is located near the wrist at the **distal** end of the ulna. When the hand is pronated, the ulnar head and the styloid process are easily felt and seen on the "little finger" side of the distal forearm.

The **head of the radius** is located at the **proximal** end of the radius near the elbow joint. The long midportion of both the radius and the ulna is called the **body** (shaft).

The radius, the shorter of the two bones of the forearm, is the only one of the two that is directly involved in the wrist joint. During the act of pronation, the radius is the bone that rotates around the more stationary ulna.

The proximal radius shows the round, disklike **head** and the **neck** of the radius as a tapered constricted area directly below the head. The rough oval process on the medial and anterior side of the radius, just distal to the neck, is the **radial tuberosity.**

Proximal Ulna The ulna, the longer of the two bones of the forearm, is primarily involved in the formation of the elbow joint. The two beaklike processes of the proximal ulna are called the **olecranon** and the **coronoid processes** (Figs. 4.14 and 4.15). The olecranon process can be palpated easily on the posterior aspect of the elbow joint.

The medial margin of the coronoid process opposite the radial notch *(lateral)* is commonly referred to as the **coronoid tubercle** (see Fig. 4.14 and anteroposterior [AP] elbow radiograph in Fig 4.19).

The large concave depression, or notch, that articulates with the distal humerus is the **trochlear** *(trok'-le-ar)* **notch** (semilunar notch). The small, shallow depression located on the lateral aspect of the proximal ulna is the **radial** *(ra'-de-al)* **notch.** The head of the radius articulates with the ulna at the radial notch, forming the proximal radioulnar joint. This joint, or articulation, is the proximal radioulnar joint that combines with the distal radioulnar joint to allow rotation of the forearm during pronation. During the act of pronation, the radius crosses over the ulna near the upper third of the forearm (see Fig. 4.25).

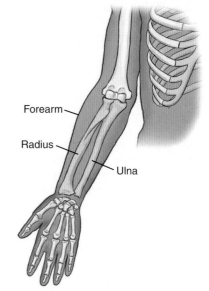

Fig. 4.13 Right upper limb (anterior view).

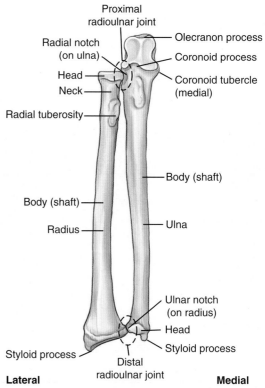

Fig. 4.14 Right radius and ulna (anterior view).

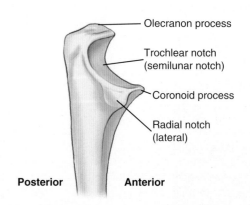

Fig. 4.15 Proximal ulna (lateral view).

DISTAL HUMERUS

Specific structures of the proximal humerus are discussed along with the shoulder girdle in Chapter 5. However, the anatomy of the midhumerus and distal humerus is included in this chapter as part of the elbow joint.

The **body** (shaft) of the humerus is the long center section, and the expanded distal end of the humerus is the **humeral condyle.** The articular portion of the humeral condyle is divided into two parts: the **trochlea** (troke'-le-ah) (medial condyle) and the **capitulum** (kah-pit'-u-lum) (lateral condyle).

The **trochlea** (meaning "pulley") is shaped like a pulley or spool; it has two rimlike outer margins and a smooth depressed center portion called the **trochlear sulcus,** or groove. This depression of the trochlea, which begins anteriorly and continues inferiorly and posteriorly, appears circular on a lateral end-on view; on a lateral elbow radiograph, it appears as a less dense (more radiolucent) area (see Figs. 4.17 and 4.20). The **trochlea** is located more medially and articulates with the **ulna.**

The **capitulum,** meaning "little head," is located on the lateral aspect and articulates with the head of the **radius.** (A memory aid is to associate the **cap**itulum ["cap"] with the "head" of the radius.) In earlier literature, the capitulum was called the **capitellum** (kap"-i-tel'-um).

The articular surface that makes up the rounded articular margin of the capitulum is just slightly smaller than that of the trochlea (Fig. 4.18). This structure becomes significant in the evaluation for a true lateral position of the elbow, as does the direct superimposition of the two **epicondyles** (ep"-e-kon'-dylz).

The **lateral epicondyle** is the small projection on the lateral aspect of the distal humerus above the capitulum. The **medial epicondyle** is larger and more prominent than the lateral epicondyle and is located on the medial edge of the distal humerus. In a true lateral position, the directly superimposed epicondyles (which are difficult to recognize) are seen as proximal to the circular appearance of the trochlear sulcus (see Fig. 4.17).

The distal humerus has specific **depressions** on both anterior and posterior surfaces. The two shallow **anterior depressions** are the **coronoid fossa** and the **radial fossa** (see Figs. 4.16 and 4.17. As the elbow is completely flexed, the coronoid process and the radial head are received by these respective fossae, as the names indicate.

The deep **posterior depression** of the distal humerus is the **olecranon fossa** (not specifically shown on these illustrations). The olecranon process of the ulna fits into this depression when the arm is fully extended. Soft tissue detail as depicted by specific fat pads located within the deep olecranon fossa is important in trauma diagnosis of the elbow joint.

The lateral view of the elbow (see Fig. 4.17) clearly shows specific parts of the proximal radius and ulna. The **head** and **neck** of the radius are well demonstrated, as are the **radial tuberosity** (partially seen on the proximal radius) and the large concave **trochlear (semilunar) notch.**

TRUE LATERAL ELBOW

Specific positions, such as an **accurate lateral** with **90° flexion,** along with possible associated visualization of fat pads, are essential for evaluation of joint pathology of the elbow.

A good criterion by which to evaluate a true lateral position of the elbow when it is flexed 90° is the appearance of the three concentric arcs, as labeled in Fig. 4.18. The first and smallest arc is the **trochlear sulcus.** The second, intermediate arc appears double lined as the outer ridges or rounded edges of the **capitulum and trochlea.**[1] (The smaller of the double-lined ridges is the capitulum; the larger is the medial ridge of the trochlea.) The **trochlear notch of the ulna** appears as a third arc of a true lateral elbow. If the elbow is rotated even slightly from a **true** lateral, the arcs do not appear symmetrically aligned in this way, and the elbow joint space is not as open.

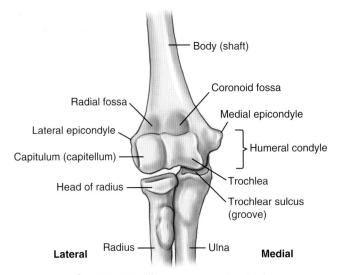
Fig. 4.16 Distal humerus (anterior view).

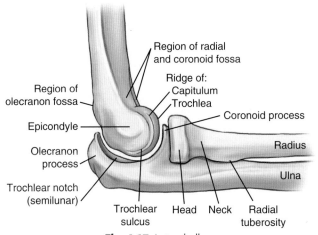
Fig. 4.17 Lateral elbow.

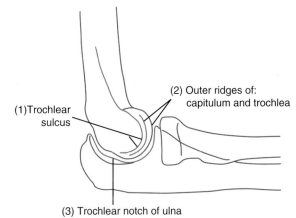
Fig. 4.18 True lateral elbow—three concentric arcs.

REVIEW EXERCISE WITH RADIOGRAPHS

The AP and lateral radiographs of the elbow provide a review of anatomy and demonstrate the three concentric arcs as evidence of a true lateral position (Figs. 4.19 and 4.20). Answers to the labels are as follows:

A. Medial epicondyle
B. Trochlea (medial aspect)
C. Coronoid tubercle
D. Radial head
E. Capitulum
F. Lateral epicondyle
G. Superimposed epicondyles of humerus
H. Olecranon process
I. Trochlear sulcus
J. Trochlear notch
K. Double outer ridges of capitulum and trochlea (capitulum being the smaller of the two areas and trochlea the larger)
L. Coronoid process of ulna
M. Radial head
N. Radial neck

CLASSIFICATION OF JOINTS

Table 4.2 provides a summary of hand, wrist, forearm, and elbow joints. Refer back to Chapter 1 for a general description of joints or articulations, along with the various classifications and movement types. These classifications are reviewed and described here more specifically for each joint of the hand, wrist, forearm, and elbow.

All joints of the upper limb as described in this chapter are classified as **synovial** and are freely movable, or **diarthrodial.** Only the movement types differ.

Hand and Wrist

Interphalangeal Joints Beginning distally with the phalanges, all IP joints are **ginglymus,** or hinge-type, joints with movement in two directions only—**flexion** and **extension** (Fig. 4.21). This movement occurs in one plane only, around the transverse axis. This includes the single IP joint of the thumb (first digit) and the distal and proximal IP joints of the fingers (second to fifth digits).

Metacarpophalangeal Joints The second to fifth MCP joints are ellipsoidal (condyloid)-type joints that allow movement in four directions—flexion, extension, abduction, and adduction. Circumduction movement, which also occurs at these joints, is conelike sequential movement in these four directions.

The first MCP joint (thumb) also is generally classified as an ellipsoidal (condyloid) joint, although it has very limited abduction and adduction movements because of the wider and less-rounded head of the first metacarpal (see Fig. 4.21).

Carpometacarpal Joints The first CMC joint of the thumb is a **saddle** (sellar)-type joint. This joint best demonstrates the shape and movement of a saddle joint, which allows a great range of movement, including flexion, extension, abduction, adduction, circumduction, opposition, and some degree of rotation.

The second through fifth CMC joints are **plane** (gliding)-type joints, which allow the least amount of movement of the synovial class joints. The joint surfaces are flat or slightly curved, with movement limited by a tight fibrous capsule.

Intercarpal Joints The intercarpal joints between the various carpals have only a **plane (gliding)** movement.

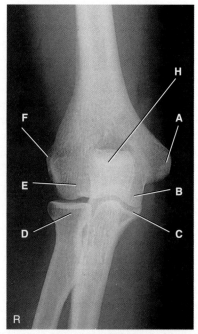

Fig. 4.19 AP elbow.

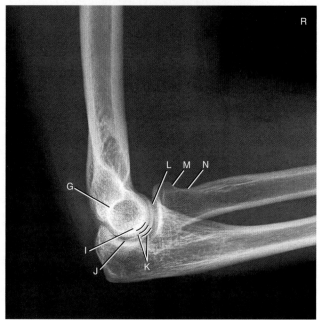

Fig. 4.20 Lateral elbow.

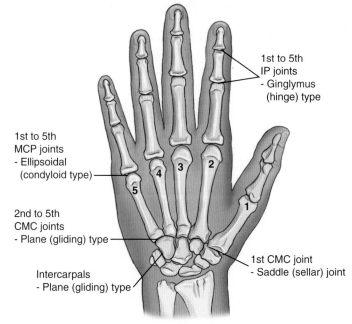

Fig. 4.21 Joints of left hand and wrist (posterior view).

Wrist Joint

The wrist joint is an **ellipsoidal** (condyloid)-type joint and is the most freely movable, or **diarthrodial**, of the **synovial classification**. Of the two bones of the forearm, only the radius articulates directly with two carpal bones—the **scaphoid** and the **lunate**. This wrist joint is called the **radiocarpal joint.**

The **triquetral** bone is also part of the wrist joint in that it is opposite the **articular disk.** The articular disk is part of the total wrist articulation, including a joint between the distal radius and ulna of the forearm—the **distal radioulnar joint.**

The articular surface of the distal radius along with the total articular disk forms a smooth, concave-shaped articulation with the three carpals to form the complete wrist joint.

The total wrist joint is enclosed by an articular synovial capsule that is strengthened by ligaments that allow movement in four directions, plus circumduction.

The synovial membrane lines the synovial capsule and the four wrist ligaments as they pass through the capsule, in addition to lining the distal end of the radius and the articular surfaces of adjoining carpal bones.

Wrist Ligaments

The wrist has numerous important ligaments that stabilize the wrist joint. Two of these are shown in the drawing in Fig. 4.22. The **ulnar collateral ligament** is attached to the styloid process of the ulna and fans out to attach to the triquetrum and the pisiform. The **radial collateral ligament** extends from the styloid process of the radius primarily to the lateral side of the scaphoid (scaphoid tubercle), but it also has attachments to the trapezium.

Five additional ligaments not shown in this drawing are crucial to the stability of the wrist joint and often are damaged during trauma. These five ligaments are commonly imaged with conventional arthrography or magnetic resonance imaging (MRI):

- Dorsal radiocarpal ligament
- Palmar radiocarpal ligament
- Triangular fibrocartilage complex (TFCC)
- Scapholunate ligament
- Lunotriquetral ligament

Elbow Joint

The elbow joint is also of the **synovial classification** and is freely movable, or **diarthrodial.** The elbow joint generally is considered a **ginglymus** (hinge)-type joint with flexion and extension movements between the humerus and the ulna and radius. However, the complete elbow joint includes three joints enclosed in one articular capsule. In addition to the hinge joints between the humerus and ulna and the humerus and radius, the **proximal radioulnar joint** (**pivot** or trochoidal type) is considered part of the elbow joint (Fig. 4.23).

The importance of accurate lateral positioning of the elbow for visualization of certain fat pads within the elbow joint is discussed later in this chapter.

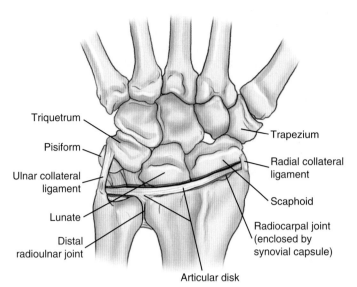

Fig. 4.22 Left wrist joint with articular disk (posterior view).

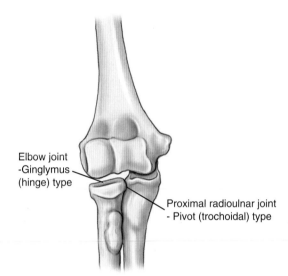

Fig. 4.23 Elbow joint.

TABLE 4.2 **SUMMARY OF HAND, WRIST, FOREARM, AND ELBOW JOINTS**	
Classification	
Synovial (articular capsule containing synovial fluid)	
Mobility Type	
Diarthrodial (freely movable)	
Movement Type	
1. Interphalangeal joints	**Ginglymus** (hinge)
2. Metacarpophalangeal joints	**Ellipsoidal** (condyloid)
3. Carpometacarpal joints	
First digit (thumb)	**Saddle** (sellar)
Second to fifth digits	**Plane** (gliding)
4. Intercarpal joints	**Plane** (gliding)
5. Wrist (radiocarpal) joint	**Ellipsoidal** (condyloid)
6. Proximal: radioulnar	**Pivot** (trochoidal) joint
7. Elbow joint	
Humeroulnar and humeroradial	**Ginglymus** (hinge)

WRIST JOINT MOVEMENT TERMINOLOGY

Certain terminology involving movements of the wrist joint may be confusing, but these terms must be understood by technologists because special projections of the wrist are described by these movements. These terms were described in Chapter 1 as turning or bending the hand and wrist from its natural position toward the side of the ulna for **ulnar deviation** and toward the radius for **radial deviation** (Fig. 4.24).

Ulnar Deviation

The ulnar deviation movement of the wrist "opens up" and best demonstrates the carpals on the opposite side (the radial or lateral side) of the wrist—the scaphoid, trapezium, and trapezoid. Because the scaphoid is the most frequently fractured carpal bone, this ulnar deviation projection is commonly known as a *special scaphoid projection.*

Radial Deviation

A less frequent PA wrist projection involves the radial deviation movement that opens and best demonstrates the carpals on the opposite, or ulnar, side of the wrist—the hamate, pisiform, triquetrum, and lunate.

FOREARM ROTATIONAL MOVEMENTS

The radioulnar joints of the forearm also involve some special rotational movements that must be understood for accurate imaging of the forearm. For example, the forearm generally should not be radiographed in a pronated position (a PA projection), which may appear to be the most natural position for the forearm and hand. The forearm routinely should be radiographed in an AP projection with the hand supinated, or palm up (anatomic position). The reason becomes clear in studying the "cross-over" position of the radius and ulna when the hand is pronated (Fig. 4.25). This cross-over results from the unique pivot-type rotational movements of the forearm that involve both the proximal and the distal radioulnar joints.

Summary To prevent superimposition of the radius and ulna that may result from these pivot-type rotational movements, the forearm is radiographed with the **hand supinated** for an **AP projection.**

ELBOW ROTATIONAL MOVEMENTS

The appearance of the proximal radius and ulna changes as the elbow and distal humerus are rotated or positioned obliquely either medially or laterally as shown on these radiographs. On the AP radiograph with no rotation, the proximal radius is superimposed only slightly by the ulna (Fig. 4.26).

The radius and ulna can be separated through lateral rotation (40-45 degrees) of the elbow, as shown in Fig. 4.27, whereas medial rotation (pronated hand) completely superimposes them, as can be seen in Fig. 4.28. This relationship is crucial in evaluation of AP projections of the elbow; **lateral rotation separates** and **medial rotation superimposes** the proximal radius and ulna.

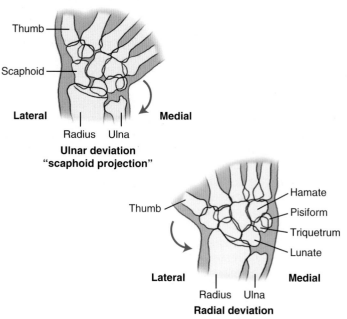

Fig. 4.24 Wrist movements.

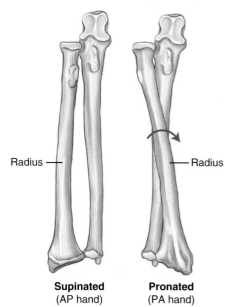

Fig. 4.25 Forearm rotational movements.

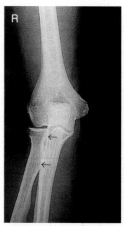

Fig. 4.26 AP, no rotation—radius and ulna partially superimposed.

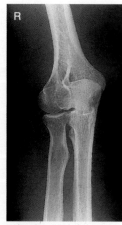

Fig. 4.27 AP, lateral rotation—separation of radius and ulna.

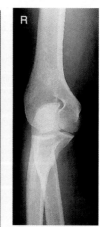

Fig. 4.28 AP, medial rotation—superimposed radius and ulna.

IMPORTANCE OF VISUALIZING FAT PADS

Radiographs of the upper and lower limbs are taken not only to evaluate for disease or trauma to bony structures but also to assess associated soft tissues, such as certain accumulations of fat called **fat pads, fat bands,** or **stripes.** In some cases, displacement of an adjoining fat pad or band may be the only indication of disease or significant injury or fracture within a joint region.

For diagnostic purposes, the most important fat pads or bands are those located around certain joints of the upper and lower limbs. These fat pads are extrasynovial (outside the synovial sac) but are located within the joint capsule. Therefore, any changes that occur within the capsule itself alter the normal position and shape of the fat pads. Most often, such changes result from fluid accumulation (effusion) within the joint, which indicates the presence of an injury involving the joint.

Radiolucent fat pads are seen as densities that are slightly more lucent than surrounding structures. Fat pads and their surrounding soft tissue are of only slightly different tissue density (brightness), making them difficult to visualize on radiographs. This visualization requires optimum exposure for visualization of these soft tissue structures.[2] (They generally are not visible on published radiographs without enhancement, as is shown on the illustrations on this page.)

Wrist Joint

The wrist joint includes two important fat stripes. First, a **scaphoid fat stripe** (A) is visualized on the PA (Fig. 4.29) and oblique (Fig. 4.30) projections. It is elongated and slightly convex in shape and is located between the radial collateral ligament and adjoining muscle tendons immediately lateral to the scaphoid. Absence or displacement of this fat stripe may be the only indicator of a fracture on the radial aspect of the wrist.

A second fat stripe is visualized on the lateral view of the wrist. This **pronator fat stripe** (B) is normally visualized approximately ¼ inch (1 cm) from the anterior surface of the radius (Fig. 4.31). Subtle fractures of the distal radius can be indicated by displacement or obliteration of the plane of this fat stripe.[2]

Elbow Joint

The three significant fat pads or stripes of the elbow are visualized only on the lateral projection. They are not seen on the AP because of their superimposition over bony structures. On the lateral projection, the **anterior fat pad** (Fig. 4.32C), which is formed by the superimposed coronoid and radial pads, is seen as a slightly radiolucent teardrop shape located just anterior to the distal humerus. Trauma or infection can cause the anterior fat pad to be elevated and more visible and distorted in shape. This is usually visible only on a true lateral elbow projection flexed 90°.

The **posterior fat pad** (see Fig. 4.32D) is located deep within the olecranon fossa and normally is **not visible** on a negative elbow examination. Visualization of this fat pad on a 90° flexed lateral elbow radiograph indicates that a change within the joint has caused its position to change, suggesting the presence of a joint pathologic process.

To ensure an accurate diagnosis, the elbow **must be flexed 90°** on the lateral view. If the elbow is extended beyond the 90° flexed position, the olecranon slides into the olecranon fossa, elevates the posterior fat pad, and causes it to appear. In this situation, the pad is visible whether the examination is negative or positive. Generally, visualization of the posterior fat pad is considered more reliable than visualization of the anterior fat pads.

The **supinator fat stripe** (see Fig. 4.32E) is a long, thin stripe just anterior to the proximal radius. It may indicate the diagnosis of radial head or neck fractures that are not obviously apparent.[2,3]

Summary For the anterior and posterior fat pads to be useful diagnostic indicators on the lateral elbow, the elbow must be (1) flexed 90° and (2) in a true lateral position; (3) optimum exposure techniques, including soft tissue detail for visualization of fat pads, must be used.

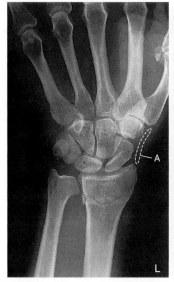
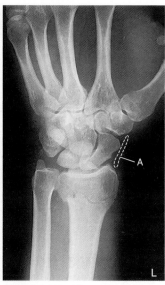

Fig. 4.29 PA wrist—**scaphoid fat stripe** (A).   **Fig. 4.30** PA oblique wrist—scaphoid fat stripe (A).

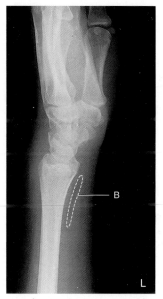

Fig. 4.31 Lateral wrist view—**pronator fat stripe (B).**

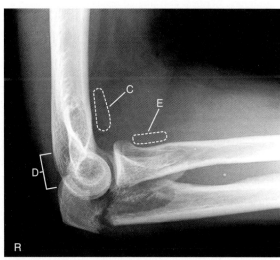

Fig. 4.32 Lateral elbow—fractured olecranon process (anterior and posterior fat pads), as follows: anterior fat pad (C); posterior fat pad (D), not visible; supinator fat stripe (E).

RADIOGRAPHIC POSITIONING

General Positioning Considerations

Radiographic examinations involving the upper limb on ambulatory patients generally are performed with the patient seated sideways at the end of the table, in a position that is neither strained nor uncomfortable. An extended tabletop may make this position more comfortable, especially if the patient is in a wheelchair. The patient's body should be moved away from the x-ray beam and the region of scatter radiation as much as possible. The height of the tabletop should be near shoulder height so that the arm can be fully supported (Fig. 4.33). The bucky tray should be moved to the opposite side of the radiographic table to reduce the amount of scatter radiation produced by the bucky device.

Lead Shielding

Shielding is important for examinations of the upper limb because of the proximity of the gonads to the divergent x-ray beam and scatter radiation, a risk for patients seated at the end of the table and for trauma patients taken on a stretcher. A lead, vinyl-covered shield should be draped over the patient's lap or gonadal area. Although the gonadal rule states that shielding should be provided to patients of reproductive age when the gonads lie within or close to the primary field, a good practice is to provide shielding for all patients.

Distance

A common minimum source to image receptor distance (SID) is 40 to 44 inches (100 to 110 cm). When radiographs are taken with the image receptor (IR) directly on the tabletop, to maintain a constant SID, the tube height must be increased compared with radiographs taken with the IR in the bucky tray. From the bucky tray to the tabletop, this difference is generally 3 to 4 inches (8 to 10 cm) for floating-type tabletops.

Special Patient Considerations

TRAUMA PATIENTS

Trauma patients can be radiographed on the table, or radiographs can be taken directly on the stretcher (Fig. 4.34). The patient should be moved to one side to provide the necessary space on the stretcher for the IR.

PEDIATRIC APPLICATIONS

Patient motion plays an important role in pediatric radiography. Immobilization is needed in many cases to assist children in maintaining the proper position. Sponges and tape are useful; however, sandbags should be used with caution because of their weight. Parents frequently are asked to assist with radiographic examination of their children. If parents are permitted in the radiography room during the exposure, proper shielding must be provided.

It is also important for the technologist to speak to the child in a soothing manner in language the child can readily understand to ensure maximal cooperation. (See Chapter 16 for more detailed explanations regarding upper limb radiography of young children.)

GERIATRIC APPLICATIONS

Providing **clear and complete instructions** is essential with elderly patients. Routine upper limb examinations may have to be altered to accommodate an older patient's physical condition. Geriatric patients may have greater difficulty in holding some of the strenuous positions required, so the technologist needs to ensure that adequate immobilization is used to prevent movement during the exposure. Radiographic exposure techniques may have to be reduced because of certain destructive pathologies commonly seen in elderly patients, such as osteoporosis.

Exposure Factors

The principal exposure factors for radiography of the upper limbs are as follows:

1. Lower to medium kVp (60 to 80—digital)
2. Short exposure time
3. Small focal spot
4. Adequate mAs for sufficient density (brightness)

Correctly exposed images of the upper limbs should reveal soft tissue margins for fat pad visualization and fine trabecular markings of all bones being radiographed.

Image Receptors

Grids are not generally used for the upper limb examinations unless the body part (e.g., the shoulder) measures greater than 10 cm.

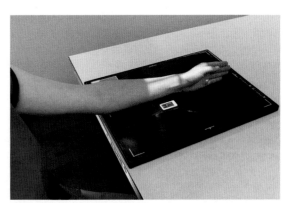

Fig. 4.33 Ambulatory patient—lateral wrist (lead shield across lap covering gonads).

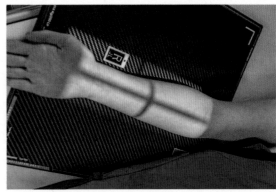

Fig. 4.34 Trauma patient—AP forearm.

TABLE 4.3 **CAST CONVERSION CHART**	
TYPE OF CAST	**INCREASE IN EXPOSURE**
Small to medium plaster cast	Increase 5 to 7 kVp
Large plaster cast	Increase 8 to 10 kVp
Fiberglass cast	Increase 3 to 4 kVp

Increased Exposure with Casts

An upper limb with a cast requires an increase in exposure (Table 4.3). This increase depends on the thickness and type of cast, as outlined in the table. These increases apply to analog imaging. Digital imaging does not require exposure adjustments in most cases.

Collimation, General Positioning, and Markers

The collimation rule should be followed: Collimation borders should be visible on all four sides if the IR is large enough to allow this without cutting off essential anatomy.

A general rule regarding IR size is to use the smallest possible receptor size for the specific part that is being imaged. Four-sided collimation is generally possible even with an IR of minimum size for most, if not all, radiographic examinations of the upper limb.

A general positioning rule that is especially applicable to the upper limbs is **always to place the long axis of the part being imaged parallel to the long axis of the portion of the IR being exposed.**

Side markers within the collimation borders must be demonstrated on each image.

Correct Centering

Accurate centering and alignment of the body part with the IR and the central ray (CR) are important for examinations of the upper limb to avoid shape and size distortion and to demonstrate narrow joint spaces clearly. The following three positioning principles should be remembered for upper limb examinations:

1. Part should be parallel to plane of IR.
2. CR should be 90° or perpendicular to part and IR, unless a specific CR angle is indicated.
3. CR should be directed to correct centering point.

Digital Imaging Considerations

Specific guidelines should be followed when upper limb images are acquired through digital imaging technology (computed radiography or digital radiography).

1. **Collimation:** In addition to the benefit of reducing radiation dose to the patient, collimation that is closely restricted to the part being examined is key in ensuring that the image processed by the computer is of optimal quality. Close collimation also allows the computer to provide accurate information regarding the exposure indicator.
2. **Accurate centering:** Because of the way the image plate reader scans the exposed imaging plate, it is important in digital imaging, as in all radiographic imaging, that the body part and the CR be accurately centered to the IR.

3. **Grid use with digital systems (computed radiography/digital radiography):** As already mentioned, grids generally are not used for body parts measuring 10 cm or less. However, with direct digital radiography, grids may be used if the grid is an integral part of the IR mechanism. In such cases, because it may be impractical and difficult to remove the grid, it may be left in place even for smaller body parts, such as for upper and lower limb examinations.

NOTE: Keep x-ray tube centered to grid to avoid cutoff.

4. **Evaluation of exposure indicator:** After the image has been processed and is ready for viewing, the image is critiqued for exposure accuracy. It must be checked for an acceptable exposure indicator to verify that the exposure factors used were in the correct range to ensure an optimal quality image with the least possible radiation dose to the patient.

EXPOSURE FACTORS

Digital imaging systems are known for their wide exposure latitude; they are able to process an acceptable image from a broad range of exposure factors (kVp and mAs). It is still important, however, that the ALARA principle (as low as reasonably achievable) be followed regarding exposure to the patient; the lowest exposure factors that produce an optimal image should be used. This principle includes using the highest possible kVp and the lowest mAs consistent with desirable image quality as viewed on a radiologist-type interpretation monitor. Insufficient mAs results in a noisy (grainy) image on an interpretation monitor, even though it may appear satisfactory on a workstation monitor. Optimal kVp will provide the proper penetration to demonstrate the bony cortex and bony trabecular markings.

Alternative Modalities and Procedures
ARTHROGRAPHY

Arthrography is commonly used to image tendinous, ligamentous, and capsular pathology associated with diarthrodial joints, such as the wrist, elbow, shoulder, and ankle. This procedure requires the use of a radiographic contrast medium injected into the joint capsule under sterile conditions (see Chapter 19).

CT AND MRI

Computed tomography (CT) and MRI often are used on upper limbs to evaluate soft tissue and skeletal involvement of lesions and soft tissue injuries. Sectional CT images are also excellent for determination of displacement and alignment relationships with certain fractures that may be difficult to visualize with conventional radiographs.

NUCLEAR MEDICINE

Nuclear medicine bone scans are useful for demonstrating osteomyelitis, metastatic bone lesions, stress fractures, and cellulitis. Nuclear medicine scans demonstrate the pathologic process within 24 hours of onset. Nuclear medicine is more sensitive than radiography because it assesses the **physiologic aspect** instead of the anatomic aspect.

4

Clinical Indications

Clinical indications that technologists should be most familiar with in relation to the upper limb include the following (not an inclusive list).

Bone metastases refers to transfer of disease or cancerous lesions from one organ or part that may not be directly connected. All malignant tumors have the ability to metastasize, or transfer malignant cells from one body part to another, through the bloodstream or lymphatic vessels or by direct extension. Metastases are the most common of malignant bone tumors.

Bursitis *(ber-sy-tis)* is inflammation of the bursae or fluid-filled sacs that enclose the joints; the process generally involves the formation of calcification in associated tendons,[4] which causes pain and limited joint movement.

Carpal *(kar'-pul)* **tunnel syndrome** is a common painful disorder of the wrist and hand that results from compression of the median nerve as it passes through the center of the wrist; it is most commonly found in middle-aged women.

Fracture *(frak'-chur)* is a break in the structure of bone caused by a force (direct or indirect).[4] Numerous types of fractures have been identified; these are named by the extent of fracture, direction of fracture lines, alignment of bone fragments, and integrity of overlying tissue (see Chapter 15 for additional trauma and fracture terminology). Some common examples are as follows:

- **Barton fracture:** Fracture and dislocation of the **posterior lip of the distal radius** involving the wrist joint.
- **Bennett fracture:** Fracture of the **base of the first metacarpal bone,** extending into the carpometacarpal joint, complicated by subluxation with some posterior displacement.
- **Boxer fracture:** Transverse fracture that extends through the **metacarpal neck;** most commonly seen in the **fifth metacarpal.**
- **Colles fracture:** Transverse fracture of the **distal radius** in which the distal fragment is **displaced posteriorly;** an associated ulnar styloid fracture is seen in 50% to 60% of cases.
- **Smith fracture:** Reverse of Colles fracture, or transverse fracture of the **distal radius** with the distal fragment displaced **anteriorly.**

Joint effusion refers to **accumulated fluid** (synovial or hemorrhagic) in the joint cavity. It is a sign of an underlying condition, such as fracture, dislocation, soft tissue damage, or inflammation.

Osteoarthritis *(os"-te-o-ar-thry'-tis)*, also known as **degenerative joint disease (DJD),** is a noninflammatory joint disease characterized by gradual deterioration of the articular cartilage with hypertrophic (enlarged or overgrown) bone formation. This is the most common type of arthritis and is considered a normal part of the aging process.

Osteomyelitis *(os"-te-o-my"-e-ly'-tis)* is a local or generalized **infection of bone or bone marrow** that may be caused by bacteria introduced by trauma or surgery. However, it is more commonly the result of an infection from a contiguous source, such as a diabetic foot ulcer.

Osteopetrosis *(os"-te-o-pe-tro'-sis)* is a hereditary disease marked by **abnormally dense bone.** It commonly occurs as a result of fracture of affected bone and may lead to obliteration of the marrow space. This condition is also known as *marble bone.*

Osteoporosis *(os"-te-o-po-ro'-sis)* refers to **reduction in the quantity of bone** or **atrophy** of skeletal tissue. It occurs in postmenopausal women and elderly men, resulting in bone trabeculae that are scanty and thin. Most fractures sustained by women older than 50 years are secondary to osteoporosis.

Paget disease (osteitis deformans) is a common chronic skeletal disease; it is characterized by bone destruction followed by a reparative process of overproduction of very dense yet soft bones that tend to fracture easily. It is most common in men older than age 40. The cause is unknown, but evidence suggests involvement of a viral infection. Paget disease can occur in any bone but most commonly affects the pelvis, femur, tibia, skull, vertebrae, and clavicle.[4]

Rheumatoid *(ru'-ma-toyd)* **arthritis** is a chronic systemic disease with inflammatory changes throughout the connective tissues; the earliest change is soft tissue swelling that is most prevalent around the ulnar styloid of the wrist. Early bone erosions typically occur first at the second and third MCP joints or the third PIP joint. Rheumatoid arthritis is three times more common in women than in men.

Skier's thumb is a sprain or tear of the **ulnar collateral ligament of the thumb** near the MCP joint of the hyperextended thumb. The sprain or tear may result from an injury such as falling on an outstretched arm and hand, which causes the thumb to be bent back toward the arm. (The PA stress projection of bilateral thumbs [Folio method] best demonstrates this condition.)

Tumors (neoplasms, bone neoplasia) are most often benign (noncancerous) but may be malignant (cancerous). CT and MRI are helpful in determining the type and exact location and size of the tumor. Specific types of tumors are listed on p. 139.

- Malignant bone tumors
  - **Multiple myeloma** is the most common **primary cancerous bone tumor.** Multiple myeloma generally affects persons between ages 40 and 70 years. As the name implies, these tumors occur in various parts of the body, arising from bone marrow or marrow plasma cells. Therefore, these are not truly exclusively bone tumors. They are highly malignant and usually are fatal within a few years. The typical radiographic appearance includes multiple "punched-out" osteolytic (loss of calcium in bone) lesions scattered throughout the affected bones.[4]
  - **Osteogenic sarcoma (osteosarcoma)** is the second most common type of **primary cancerous bone tumor** and generally affects persons aged 10 to 20 years but can occur at any age. It may develop in older persons with Paget disease.
  - **Ewing sarcoma** is a common primary **malignant bone tumor** in children and young adults that arises from bone marrow. Symptoms are similar to symptoms of osteomyelitis with low-grade fever and pain. Stratified new bone formation results in an "onion peel" appearance on radiographs. The prognosis is poor by the time Ewing sarcoma is evident on radiographs.
  - **Chondrosarcoma** is a slow-growing **malignant tumor of the cartilage.** The appearance is similar to that of other malignant tumors, but dense calcifications are often seen within the cartilaginous mass.
- Benign bone or cartilaginous tumors (chondromas)
  - **Enchondroma** is a slow-growing **benign cartilaginous tumor** most often found in small bones of the hands and feet of adolescents and young adults. Generally, enchondromas are well-defined, radiolucent-appearing tumors with a thin cortex that often lead to pathologic fracture with only minimal trauma.
  - **Osteochondroma** (exostosis) is the most common type of **benign bone tumor,** usually occurring in persons aged 10 to 20 years. Osteochondromas arise from the outer cortex with the tumor growing parallel to the bone, pointing away from the adjacent joint. These are most common at the knee but also occur on the pelvis and scapula of children or young adults.

Table 4.4 provides a summary of clinical indications.

Routine and Special Projections

Routine and special projections for the hand, wrist, forearm, elbow, and humerus are demonstrated and described on the following pages.

TABLE 4.4 SUMMARY OF CLINICAL INDICATIONS

CONDITION OR DISEASE	MOST COMMON RADIOGRAPHIC EXAMINATION	POSSIBLE RADIOGRAPHIC APPEARANCE	EXPOSURE FACTOR ADJUSTMENT[a]
Conditions not Requiring an Exposure Factor Adjustment			
Select optimal exposure factors			
Bursitis	AP and lateral joint	Fluid-filled joint space with possible calcification	
Carpal tunnel syndrome	PA and lateral wrist; Gaynor-Hart method Sonography	Possible calcification in carpal sulcus Enlargement of wrist ligaments and median nerve compression	
Fractures	AP and lateral of long bones; AP, lateral, and oblique if joint involved	Disruption in bony cortex with soft tissue swelling	
Joint effusion	AP and lateral joint	Fluid-filled joint cavity	
Osteoarthritis (DJD)	AP and lateral affected area	Narrowing of joint space with periosteal growths on joint margins	None or decrease (−) in severe cases
Osteomyelitis	AP and lateral affected bone; nuclear medicine bone scan	Soft tissue swelling and loss of fat pad detail visibility	Visualize soft tissue structures
"Skier's thumb" (ulnar collateral ligament injury)	PA bilateral stress projection thumbs (Folio method)	Widening of inner MCP joint space of thumb and increase in degrees of angle of MCP line	
Tumors (neoplasms)—malignant and benign	AP and lateral affected area	Appearance dependent on type and stage of tumor	
Conditions Requiring an Increased Exposure Factor Adjustment			
Osteopetrosis (marble bone)	AP and lateral long bone	Chalky white or opaque appearance with lack of distinction between the bony cortex and trabeculae	
Paget disease	AP and lateral affected area	Mixed areas of sclerotic and cortical thickening along with radiolucent lesions; "cotton wool" appearance	May require increase (+) in advanced stages
Conditions Requiring a Decreased Exposure Factor Adjustment			
Osteoporosis	AP and lateral affected area	Best visibility in distal extremities and joints as decrease in bone density (brightness); long bones demonstrating thin cortex	
Rheumatoid arthritis (RA)	AP and lateral hand/wrist. Brewerton method can detect early signs of RA in hands	Closed joint spaces with subluxation of MCP joints	Decrease (−)

AP, Anteroposterior; *DJD,* degenerative joint disease; *MCP,* metacarpophalangeal; *PA,* posteroanterior.
[a]Depends on stage or severity of disease or condition. Adjustments primarily apply to manual exposure factors.

4

PA PROJECTION—FINGERS

Clinical Indications
- Fractures and dislocations of the distal, middle, and proximal phalanges; distal metacarpal; and associated joints
- Pathologic processes, such as osteoporosis and osteoarthritis

Fingers
ROUTINE
• PA
• PA oblique
• Lateral

Technical Factors
- Minimum SID—40 inches (100 cm)
- IR size—8 × 10 inches (18 × 24 cm), portrait; smallest IR available and collimate to area of interest
- Nongrid
- kVp range—55 to 65

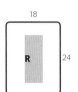

NOTE: A possible alternative routine involves a larger IR to include the entire hand for the PA projection of the finger for possible secondary trauma or pathology to other aspects of the hand and wrist. Then oblique and lateral projections of the affected finger only would be taken.

Shielding Shield radiosensitive tissues outside region of interest.

Patient Position Seat patient at end of table, with elbow flexed about 90° and with hand and forearm resting on the table (Fig. 4.35).

Part Position
- Pronate hand with fingers extended
- Center and align long axis of affected finger with long axis of IR
- Separate adjoining fingers from affected finger (Fig. 4.36)

CR
- CR perpendicular to IR, directed to **PIP joint**

Recommended Collimation Collimate on four sides to area of affected finger and distal aspect of metacarpal

---

Evaluation Criteria

Anatomy Demonstrated: • Distal, middle, and proximal phalanges; distal metacarpal; and associated joints.
Position: • Long axis of finger should be aligned with and parallel to side border of IR. • **No rotation** of fingers is evidenced by symmetric appearance of both sides or concavities of the shafts of the phalanges and distal metacarpals. • The amount of tissue on each side of the phalanges should appear equal. • Fingers should be separated with no overlapping of soft tissues. • Interphalangeal joints should appear open, indicating that hand was fully pronated and the correct CR position was used (Figs. 4.37 and 4.38). • CR and midpoint of collimation field should be to the **PIP joint.**
Exposure: • Optimal density (brightness) and contrast with **no motion** demonstrate soft tissue margins and clear, sharp bony trabecular markings.

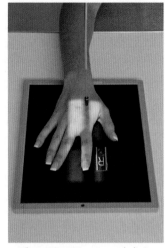

Fig. 4.35 PA—second digit.

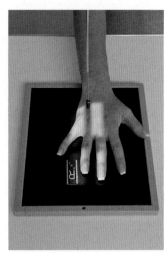

Fig. 4.36 PA—fourth digit.

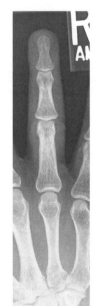

Fig. 4.37 PA—fourth digit.

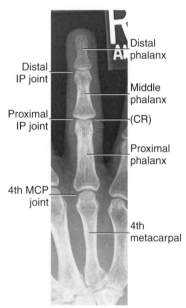

Distal phalanx

Distal IP joint

Middle phalanx

Proximal IP joint

(CR)

Proximal phalanx

4th MCP joint

4th metacarpal

Fig. 4.38 PA—fourth digit.

PA OBLIQUE PROJECTION—MEDIAL OR LATERAL ROTATION: FINGERS

Clinical Indications
- Fractures and dislocations of the distal, middle, and proximal phalanges; distal metacarpal; and associated joints
- Pathologies such as osteoporosis and osteoarthritis

Fingers
ROUTINE
• PA
• PA oblique
• Lateral

Technical Factors
- Minimum SID—40 inches (100 cm)
- IR size—8 × 10 inches (18 × 24 cm), portrait; smallest IR available and collimate to area of interest
- Nongrid
- kVp range—55 to 65
- Accessories—45° foam wedge block or step wedge

Shielding Shield radiosensitive tissues outside region of interest.

Patient Position Seat patient at end of table, with elbow flexed about 90° with hand and wrist resting on IR and fingers extended.

Part Position
- With fingers extended against 45° foam wedge block, place hand in a 45° lateral oblique (thumb side up) (Fig. 4.39).
- Position hand on image receptor so that the long axis of the finger is aligned with the long axis of the IR.
- Separate fingers and carefully place finger that is being examined against block, so it is supported in a 45° oblique and **parallel to IR.**

CR
- CR perpendicular to IR, directed to **PIP joint**

Recommended Collimation Collimate on four sides to affected finger and distal aspect of metacarpal.

Optional Medial Oblique Second digit also may be taken in a 45° medial oblique (thumb side down) with thumb and other fingers flexed to prevent superimposition (Fig. 4.40). This position places the part closer to the IR for improved definition but may be more painful for the patient. Lateral rotation of hand is recommended to demonstrate the third, fourth, and fifth digits (Figs. 4.41 and 4.42)

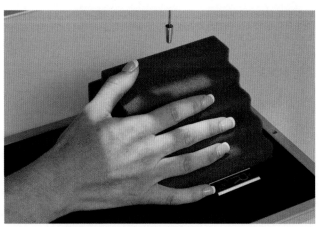

Fig. 4.39 Second digit (lateral rotation).

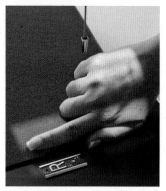

Fig. 4.40 Second digit (medial rotation).

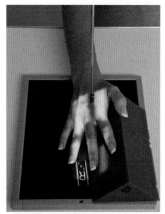

Fig. 4.41 Third digit (lateral rotation).

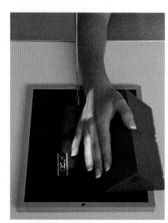

Fig. 4.42 Fifth digit (lateral rotation).

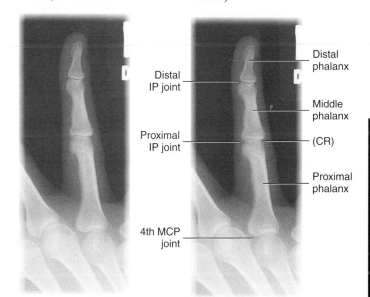

Fig. 4.43 Fourth digit (lateral rotation).

Fig. 4.44 Fourth digit.

Evaluation Criteria

Anatomy Demonstrated: • Oblique view of distal, middle, and proximal phalanges; distal metacarpal; and associated joints.

Position: • Long axis of finger should be aligned with side border of IR. • View of finger being examined should be 45° oblique. • No superimposition of adjacent fingers should occur. • IP and MCP joint spaces should be open, indicating correct CR location and that the phalanges are parallel to IR. • CR and center of collimation field should be to the **PIP joint** (Figs. 4.43 and 4.44).

Exposure: • Optimal density (brightness) and contrast with **no motion** demonstrate soft tissue margins and clear, sharp bony trabecular markings.

LATEROMEDIAL OR MEDIOLATERAL PROJECTIONS—FINGERS

Clinical Indications
- Fractures and dislocations of the distal, middle, and proximal phalanges; distal metacarpal; and associated joints
- Pathologic processes, such as osteoporosis and osteoarthritis

Fingers
ROUTINE
• PA
• PA oblique
• Lateral

Technical Factors
- Minimum SID—40 inches (100 cm)
- IR size—8 × 10 inches (18 × 24 cm), portrait; smallest IR available and collimate to area of interest
- Nongrid
- kVp range—55 to 65
- Accessories—sponge support block

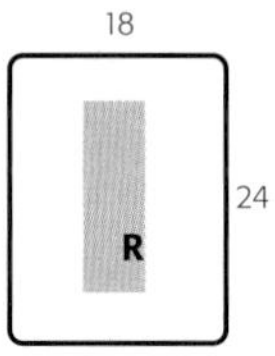

Shielding Shield radiosensitive tissues outside region of interest

Patient Position Seat patient at end of table, with elbow flexed about 90° with hand and wrist resting on IR and fingers extended.

Part Position
- Place hand in lateral position (thumb side up) with finger to be examined fully extended and centered to portion of IR being exposed (see NOTE for second digit lateral).
- Align and center finger to long axis of IR and to CR.
- Use sponge block or other radiolucent device to support finger and prevent motion. Flex unaffected fingers (Fig. 4.45).
- Ensure that long axis of finger is **parallel to IR** (Figs. 4.46 to 4.48).

CR
- CR perpendicular to IR, directed to **PIP joint**

Recommended Collimation Collimate on four sides to affected finger and distal aspect of metacarpal

NOTE: For second digit, a mediolateral is advised (Fig. 4.45) if the patient can assume this position. Place the second digit in contact with IR. (Definition is improved with less object–image receptor distance [OID].)

Evaluation Criteria
Anatomy Demonstrated: • Lateral views of distal, middle, and proximal phalanges; distal metacarpal; and associated joints are visible (Figs. 4.49 and 4.50).

Position: • Long axis of finger should be aligned with the side border of IR. • Finger should be in **true lateral position,** as indicated by the concave appearance of the anterior surface of the shaft of the phalanges. • Interphalangeal and metacarpophalangeal joint spaces should be open, indicating correct CR location and that the phalanges are parallel to the IR. • CR and center of collimation field should be to the **PIP joint.**

Exposure: • Optimal density (brightness) and contrast with **no motion** demonstrate soft tissue margins and clear, sharp bony trabecular markings.

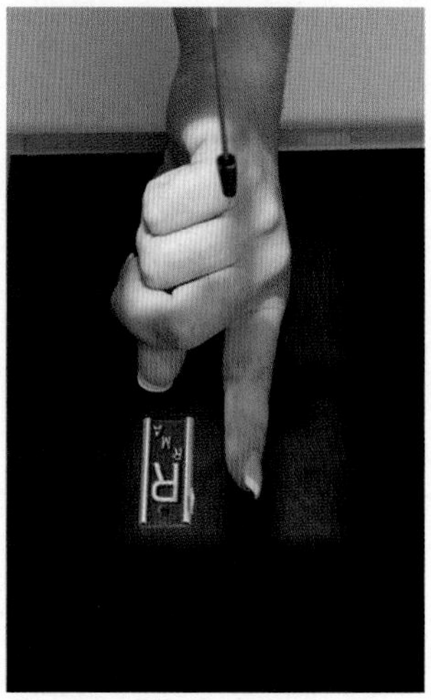

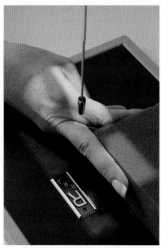
Fig. 4.45 Second digit (mediolateral).

Fig. 4.46 Third digit (lateromedial).

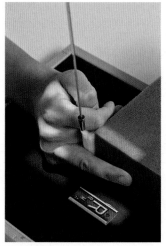
Fig. 4.47 Fourth digit (lateromedial).

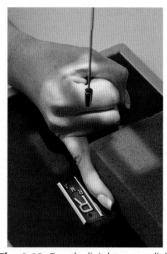
Fig. 4.48 Fourth digit lateromedial.

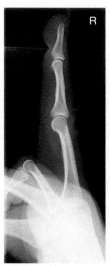
Fig. 4.49 Fourth digit.

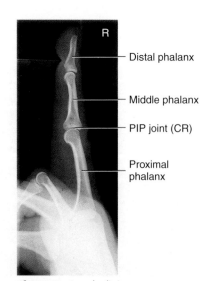
Fig. 4.50 Fourth digit.

Distal phalanx

Middle phalanx

PIP joint (CR)

Proximal phalanx

AP PROJECTION—THUMB

Clinical Indications

- Fractures and dislocations of the distal and proximal phalanges, distal metacarpal, and associated joints
- Pathologic processes, such as osteoporosis and osteoarthritis

See special AP modified Robert projection for Bennett fracture at base of first metacarpal.

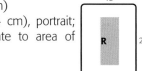

Thumb
ROUTINE
• AP
• PA oblique
• Lateral

Technical Factors

- Minimum SID—40 inches (100 cm)
- IR size—8 × 10 inches (18 × 24 cm), portrait; smallest IR available and collimate to area of interest
- Nongrid
- kVp range—55 to 65

Shielding Shield radiosensitive tissues outside region of interest.

Patient Position—AP Seat patient facing table, arms extended in front, with hand rotated internally to supinate thumb for AP projection (Fig. 4.51).

Part Position—AP

First, demonstrate this awkward position on yourself, so the patient can see how it is done and better understand what is expected.

- Internally rotate hand with fingers extended until posterior surface of thumb is in contact with IR. Immobilize other fingers with tape to isolate thumb if necessary (see Fig. 4.51).
- Align thumb with long axis of the IR.
- Center **first MCP joint** to CR and to center of IR.

Exception—PA (Only if Patient Cannot Position for Previous AP)

- Place hand in near-lateral position and rest thumb on sponge support block that is high enough so the thumb is not rotated but is in position for a **true PA projection** (Fig. 4.52)

NOTE: As a rule, the PA is *not* advisable because it results in loss of definition caused by increased OID.

CR

- CR perpendicular to IR, to **first MCP joint**

Recommended Collimation

Collimate on four sides to area of thumb, remembering that **thumb includes entire first metacarpal and trapezium**

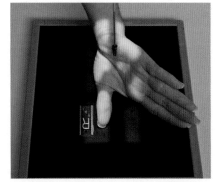

Fig. 4.51 AP thumb—CR to first MCP joint.

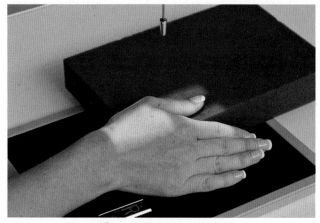

Fig. 4.52 PA (exception).

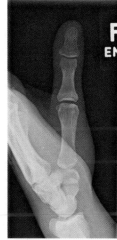 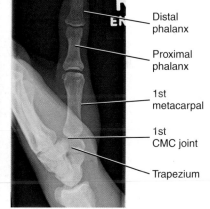

Distal phalanx

Proximal phalanx

1st metacarpal

1st CMC joint

Trapezium

Fig. 4.53 AP thumb. **Fig. 4.54** AP thumb.

Evaluation Criteria

Anatomy Demonstrated: • Distal and proximal phalanges, first metacarpal, trapezium, and associated joints are visible. • Interphalangeal and metacarpophalangeal joints should appear open (Figs. 4.53 and 4.54).

Position: • Long axis of thumb should be aligned with side border of IR. • **No rotation,** as evidenced by the concave sides of the phalanges and by equal amounts of soft tissue appearing on each side of the phalanges, should be present. Interphalangeal joint should appear open, indicating that thumb was fully extended and correct CR location was used. • CR and center of collimation field should be at the **first MCP joint.**

Exposure: • Optimal density (brightness) and contrast with **no motion** demonstrate soft tissue margins and clear, sharp bony trabecular markings.

4

PA OBLIQUE PROJECTION—MEDIAL ROTATION: THUMB

Clinical Indications
- Fractures and dislocations of the distal and proximal phalanges, distal metacarpal, and associated joints
- Pathologic processes, such as osteoporosis and osteoarthritis

Thumb
ROUTINE
• AP
• PA oblique
• Lateral

Technical Factors
- Minimum SID—40 inches (100 cm)
- IR size—8 × 10 inches (18 × 24 cm), portrait; smallest IR available and collimate to area of interest
- Nongrid
- kVp range—55 to 65

Shielding Shield radiosensitive tissues outside region of interest.

Patient Position Seat patient at end of table with hand resting on IR.

Part Position
- Abduct thumb slightly with palmar surface of hand in contact with IR (this action naturally places thumb in a 45° oblique position).
- Align long axis of thumb with long axis of IR.
- Center **first MCP joint** to CR and to center of IR (Fig. 4.55).

CR
- CR perpendicular to IR, directed to **first MCP joint**

Recommended Collimation Collimate on four sides to thumb, ensuring that all of first metacarpal and trapezium is included.

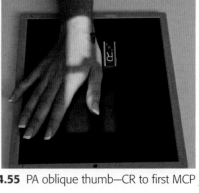

Fig. 4.55 PA oblique thumb—CR to first MCP joint.

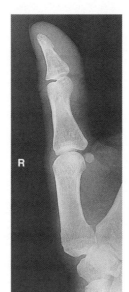

Fig. 4.56 PA oblique thumb.

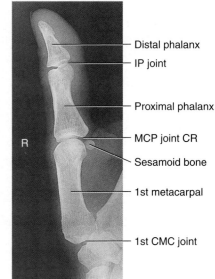

Fig. 4.57 PA oblique thumb.

- Distal phalanx
- IP joint
- Proximal phalanx
- MCP joint CR
- Sesamoid bone
- 1st metacarpal
- 1st CMC joint

Evaluation Criteria
Anatomy Demonstrated: • Distal and proximal phalanges, first metacarpal, trapezium, and associated joints are visualized in a 45° oblique position (Figs. 4.56 and 4.57).
Position: • Long axis of thumb should be aligned with side border of IR. • Interphalangeal and metacarpophalangeal joints should appear open if the phalanges are parallel to the IR and if the CR location is correct. • CR and center of collimation field should be at **first MCP joint.**
Exposure: • Optimal density (brightness) and contrast with **no motion** demonstrate soft tissue margins and clear, sharp bony trabecular markings.

4

LATERAL POSITION—THUMB

Clinical Indications
- Fractures and dislocations of the distal and proximal phalanges, distal metacarpal, and associated joints
- Pathologic processes, such as osteoporosis and osteoarthritis

Thumb
ROUTINE
• AP
• PA oblique
• Lateral

Technical Factors
- Minimum SID—40 inches (100 cm)
- IR size—8 × 10 inches (18 × 24 cm), portrait; smallest IR available and collimate to area of interest
- Nongrid
- kVp range—55 to 65

Shielding Shield radiosensitive tissues outside region of interest.

Patient Position Seat patient at end of table, with elbow flexed about 90° with hand resting on IR, palm down.

Part Position
- Start with hand pronated and thumb abducted, with fingers and hand slightly arched; then rotate hand slightly medial until thumb is in **true lateral position** (You may need to provide a sponge or other support under lateral portion of hand)
- Align long axis of thumb with long axis of the IR.
- Center **first MCP joint** to CR and to center of IR.
- Entire lateral aspect of thumb should be in direct contact with IR (Fig. 4.58)

CR
- CR perpendicular to IR, directed to **first MCP joint**

Recommended Collimation Collimate on four sides to thumb area (remember that first metacarpal and **trapezium** must be within the field of view).

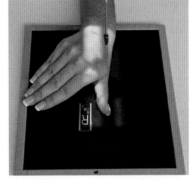

Fig. 4.58 Part position—lateral thumb; CR to first MCP joint.

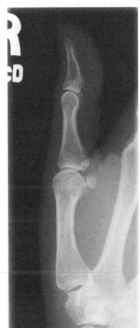

Fig. 4.59 Lateral thumb.

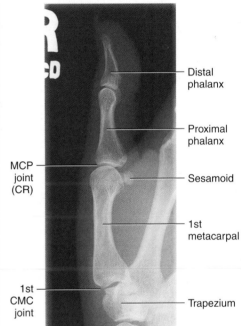

Distal phalanx

Proximal phalanx

MCP joint (CR)

Sesamoid

1st metacarpal

1st CMC joint

Trapezium

Fig. 4.60 Lateral thumb.

Evaluation Criteria
Anatomy Demonstrated: • Distal and proximal phalanges, first metacarpal, trapezium (superimposed), and associated joints are visualized in the lateral position (Figs. 4.59 and 4.60).
Position: • Long axis of thumb should be aligned with side border of IR. • Thumb should be in a true lateral position, evidenced by the concave-shaped anterior surface of the proximal phalanx and first metacarpal and relatively straight posterior surfaces. • Interphalangeal and metacarpophalangeal joints should appear open if the phalanges are parallel to the IR and if the CR location is correct. • CR and center of collimation field should be at the **first MCP joint.**
Exposure: • Optimal density (brightness) and contrast with **no motion** demonstrate soft tissue margins and clear, sharp bony trabecular markings.

4

AP AXIAL PROJECTION (MODIFIED ROBERT METHOD)[5]—THUMB

Clinical Indications
- Base of first metacarpal is demonstrated for ruling out **Bennett fracture.**
  This special projection demonstrates fractures, dislocations, or pathology of the base of the first metacarpal and trapezium

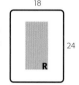

Thumb
SPECIAL
- AP axial, modified Robert method

Technical Factors
- Minimum SID—40 inches (100 cm)
- IR size—8 × 10 inches (18 × 24 cm), portrait; smallest IR available and collimate to area of interest
- Nongrid
- kVp range—55 to 65

Shielding Shield radiosensitive tissues outside region of interest.

Patient Position Seat patient parallel to end of table, with hand and arm fully extended.

Part Position
- Rotate arm internally until posterior aspect of thumb rests on IR.
- Place thumb in center of IR, parallel to side border of IR.
- Extend fingers.

CR
- CR directed **15° proximally** (toward wrist), entering at the **first CMC joint**
- Lewis modification—CR angle 10° to 15° proximal to MCP joint (see NOTE)

Recommended Collimation Collimate on four sides to area of thumb and first CMC joint.

NOTE: This projection was first described by M. Robert in 1936 to demonstrate the first CMC joint with the use of a **perpendicular** CR. The projection was later modified to include **15°** proximal CR angle to the first CMC joint.[6] The **Lewis modification** centers the CR to the first MCP joint with a **10° to 15°** proximal angle[7] (Fig. 4.61).

Evaluation Criteria
Anatomy Demonstrated: • An AP projection of the thumb and first CMC joint are visible without superimposition. • Base of first metacarpal and trapezium should be well visualized (Figs. 4.62 and 4.63).
Position: • Long axis of the thumb should be aligned with side border of IR. • **No rotation,** as evidenced by the symmetric appearance of both concave sides of the phalanges and by the equal amounts of soft tissue that appear on each side of the phalanges. • First CMC and MCP joints should appear open. • CR and center of collimation field should be at **first CMC joint.**
Exposure: • Optimal density (brightness) and contrast with **no motion** demonstrate soft tissue margins and clear, sharp bony trabecular markings.

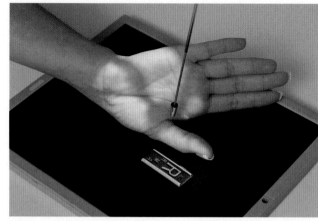

Fig. 4.61 AP axial projection—Lewis modification, CR 10° to15° to MCP joint.

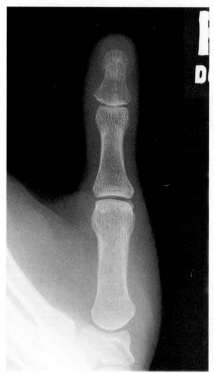

Fig. 4.62 AP axial projection—Lewis modification.

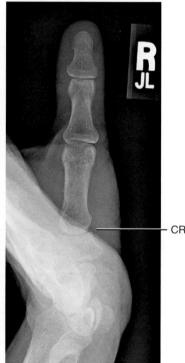

CR

Fig. 4.63 AP axial projection—modified Robert method.

PA STRESS THUMB PROJECTION

FOLIO METHOD[8]

Clinical Indications
- Sprain or tearing of ulnar collateral ligament of thumb at MCP joint as a result of acute hyperextension of thumb; also referred to as a "skier's thumb" injury

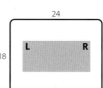

Thumb
SPECIAL
• AP axial, modified Robert method
• PA stress (Folio method)

Technical Factors
- Minimum SID—40 inches (100 cm)
- IR size—8 × 10 inches (18 × 24 cm), landscape; smallest IR available and collimate to area of interest
- Nongrid
- kVp range—55 to 65

Shielding Shield radiosensitive tissues outside region of interest.

Patient Position Seat patient at end of table with both hands extended and pronated on IR.

Part Position
- Position both hands side by side to center of IR, rotated laterally into ±45° oblique position, resulting in PA projection of both thumbs.
- Place supports as needed under both wrist and proximal thumb regions to prevent motion. Ensure that hands are rotated enough to place thumbs parallel to IR for **PA projection** of both thumbs.
- Place round spacer, such as a roll of medical tape, between proximal thumb regions; wrap rubber bands around distal thumbs (Fig. 4.64).
- Immediately before exposure, ask patient to pull thumbs apart firmly and hold.

NOTE: Explain procedure carefully to patient and observe patient while applying tension on rubber band without motion before initiating exposure. Work quickly because this can be painful for patient.

CR
- CR perpendicular to IR directed to midway between MCP joints

Recommended Collimation Collimate on four sides to include second metacarpals and entire thumbs, from CMC joints proximally to distal phalanges distally.

Evaluation Criteria

Anatomy Demonstrated: • Entire thumbs from first metacarpals to distal phalanges (Fig. 4.65). • Demonstrates metacarpophalangeal angles and joint spaces at MCP joints (Fig. 4.66).

Position: • No rotation of thumbs as evidenced by symmetric appearance of concavities of shafts of first metacarpals and phalanges. • Distal phalanges should appear to be pulled together, indicating that tension was applied. • MCP and IP joints should appear open, indicating that thumbs were parallel to IR and perpendicular to CR. • CR and center of collimation field should be **midway between the two MCP joints.**

Exposure: • Optimal density (brightness) and contrast with **no motion** demonstrates soft tissue margins and clear, sharp bony edges and trabecular markings.

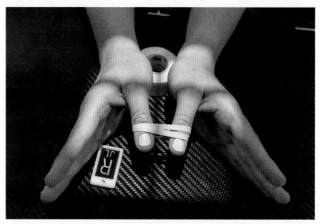

Fig. 4.64 PA stress projection of bilateral thumbs; CR perpendicular to midway between MCP joints, firm tension applied.

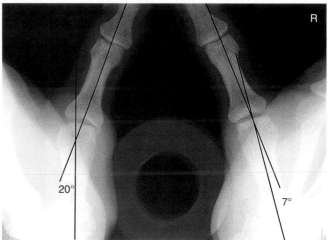

Fig. 4.65 PA stress projection of bilateral thumbs with tension applied. 20° MCP angle on left indicates sprain or torn ulnar collateral ligament. (From Frank ED, Long BW, Smith BJ. *Merrill's atlas of radiographic positions and radiologic procedures,* ed 11, St Louis, 2007, Mosby.)

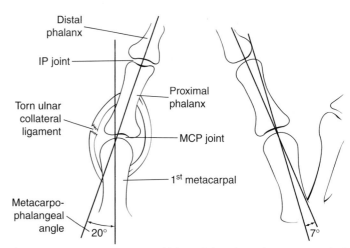

Fig. 4.66 PA stress projection of bilateral thumbs with tension applied (demonstrates torn ulnar collateral ligament on left).

PA PROJECTION—HAND

Clinical Indications
- Fractures, dislocations, or foreign bodies of the phalanges, metacarpals, and all joints of the hand
- Pathologic processes such as osteoporosis and osteoarthritis

Hand
ROUTINE
• **PA**
• PA oblique
• Lateral

Technical Factors
- Minimum SID—40 inches (100 cm)
- IR size—10 × 12 inches (24 × 30 cm), portrait; smallest IR available and collimate to area of interest
- Nongrid
- kVp range—55 to 65

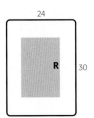

Shielding Shield radiosensitive tissues outside region of interest.

Patient Position Seat patient at end of table with hand and forearm extended.

Part Position
- Pronate hand with palmar surface in contact with IR; spread fingers slightly (Fig. 4.67)
- Align long axis of hand and forearm with long axis of IR.
- Center hand and wrist to IR

CR
- CR perpendicular to IR, directed to **third MCP joint**

Recommended Collimation Collimate on four sides to outer margins of hand and wrist.

NOTE: If examinations of both hands or wrists are requested, generally the body parts should be positioned and exposed separately for correct CR placement.

Evaluation Criteria
Anatomy Demonstrated: • PA projection of entire hand and wrist and about 1 inch (2.5 cm) of distal forearm are visible. • PA projection of hand demonstrates oblique view of the thumb.

Position: • Long axis of hand and wrist aligned with long axis of IR. • **No rotation** of hand, as evidenced by symmetric appearance of both sides or concavities of shafts of metacarpals and phalanges of digits 2 through 5 and the appearance of equal amounts of soft tissue on each side of phalanges 2 through 5. • Digits should be separated slightly with soft tissues not overlapping. • MCP and IP joints should appear open, indicating correct CR location and that hand was fully pronated (Figs. 4.68 and 4.69). • CR and center of collimation field should be to **third MCP joint.**

Exposure: • Optimal density (brightness) and contrast with **no motion** demonstrate soft tissue margins and clear, sharp bony trabecular markings.

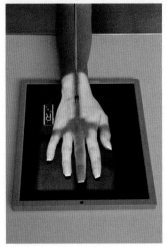

Fig. 4.67 PA hand, CR to third MCP joint.

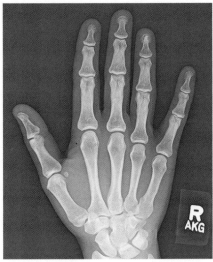

Fig. 4.68 PA hand.

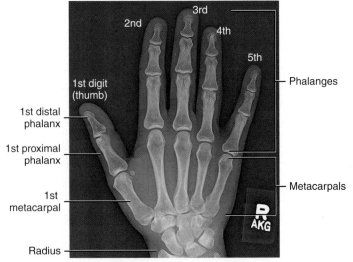

2nd 3rd 4th 5th

1st digit (thumb)

1st distal phalanx

1st proximal phalanx

1st metacarpal

Radius

Phalanges

Metacarpals

Fig. 4.69 PA of right hand.

PA OBLIQUE PROJECTION—HAND

Clinical Indications
- Fractures and dislocations of the phalanges, metacarpals, and all joints of the hand
- Pathologic processes, such as osteoporosis and osteoarthritis

Hand
ROUTINE
• PA
• PA oblique
• Lateral

Technical Factors
- Minimum SID—40 inches (100 cm)
- IR size—10 × 12 inches (24 × 30 cm), portrait; smallest IR available and collimate to area of interest
- Nongrid
- kVp range—55 to 65

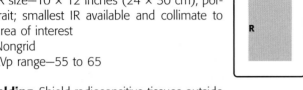

Shielding Shield radiosensitive tissues outside region of interest.

Patient Position Seat patient at end of table with hand and forearm extended.

Part Position ⊞
- Pronate hand on IR; center and align long axis of hand with long axis of IR.
- Rotate entire hand and wrist laterally 45° and support with radiolucent wedge or step block, as shown, so that all digits are separated and **parallel to IR** (see Exception).

CR
- CR perpendicular to IR, directed to **third MCP joint**

Recommended Collimation Collimate on four sides to hand and wrist.

Exception For a routine oblique hand, use a support block to place digits parallel to IR (Fig. 4.70). This block prevents foreshortening of phalanges and obscuring of interphalangeal joints. If the **metacarpals only** are of interest, the image can be taken with thumb and fingertips touching IR (Figs. 4.71 and 4.73).

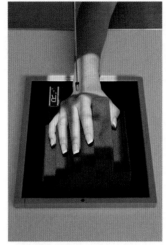 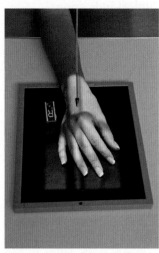

Fig. 4.70 Routine oblique hand (digits parallel).

Fig. 4.71 *Exception:* Oblique hand for metacarpals (digits not parallel)—not recommended for digits.

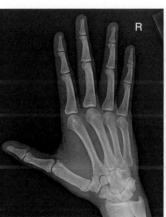 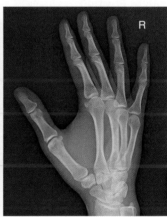

Fig. 4.72 PA oblique hand (digits parallel).

Fig. 4.73 PA oblique hand (digits not parallel)—joint spaces not open.

Evaluation Criteria
Anatomy Demonstrated: • Oblique projection of the entire hand and wrist and about 1 inch (2.5 cm) of distal forearm are visible.

Position: • Long axis of hand and wrist should be aligned with IR. • 45° oblique is evidenced by: midshafts of metacarpals should not overlap; some overlap of distal heads of third, fourth, and fifth metacarpals but no overlap of distal second and third metacarpals should occur; excessive overlap of metacarpals indicates over-rotation, and too much separation indicates under-rotation. • MCP and IP joints are open without foreshortening of midphalanges or distal phalanges, indicating that fingers are parallel to IR (Figs. 4.72 and 4.74). • CR and center of collimation field should be at **third MCP joint.**

Exposure: • Optimal density (brightness) and contrast with **no motion** demonstrate soft tissue margins and clear, sharp bony trabecular markings.

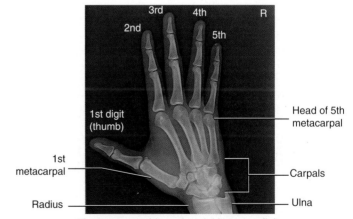

Fig. 4.74 PA oblique hand (digits parallel).

"FAN" LATERAL–LATEROMEDIAL PROJECTION: HAND

Clinical Indications
- Fractures and dislocations of the phalanges, anterior/posterior displaced fractures, and dislocations of the metacarpals
- Pathologic processes, such as osteoporosis and osteoarthritis especially in the phalanges

Hand
ROUTINE
• PA
• PA oblique
• Lateral

Technical Factors
- Minimum SID—40 inches (100 cm)
- IR size—10 × 12 inches (24 × 30 cm), portrait; smallest IR available and collimate to area of interest
- Nongrid
- kVp range—55 to 65
- Accessories—45° foam step support

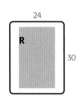

Compensation Filter A filter may be used to ensure optimum exposure of phalanges and metacarpals because of differences in part thickness.

Shielding Shield radiosensitive tissues outside region of interest.

Patient Position Seat patient at end of table with hand and forearm extended.

Part Position
- Align long axis of hand with long axis of IR.
- Rotate hand and wrist into lateral position with thumb side up.
- Spread fingers and thumb into a "fan" position, and support each digit on radiolucent block as shown. Ensure that all digits, including the thumb, are separated and **parallel to IR** and that the metacarpals are *not* rotated but remain in a true lateral position (Fig. 4.75)

CR
- CR perpendicular to IR, directed to **second MCP joint**

Recommended Collimation Collimate on four sides to outer margins of hand and wrist.

NOTE: The "fan" lateral position is the preferred lateral for the hand if phalanges are the area of interest. (See next page for alternative projections.)

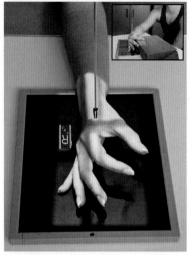

Fig. 4.75 Patient position—fan lateral hand (digits kept separated and parallel to IR); CR to second MCP joint.

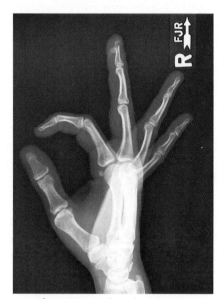

Fig. 4.76 Fan lateral projection.

Evaluation Criteria
Anatomy Demonstrated: • Entire hand and wrist and about 1 inch (2.5 cm) of distal forearm are visible (Figs. 4.76 and 4.77).
Position: • Long axis of hand and wrist should be aligned with long axis of IR. • Fingers should appear equally separated, with phalanges in the lateral position and joint spaces open, indicating that fingers were parallel to IR. • Thumb should appear in slightly oblique position completely free of superimposition, with joint spaces open. • Hand and wrist should be in a true lateral position, as evidenced by: distal radius and ulna are superimposed; metacarpals are superimposed. • CR and center of collimation field should be at **second MCP joint.**
Exposure: • Optimal density (brightness) and contrast with **no motion** demonstrate soft tissue margins and clear, sharp bony trabecular markings. • Outlines of individual metacarpals demonstrated are superimposed. • Midphalanges and distal phalanges of thumb and fingers should appear sharp but may be slightly overexposed.

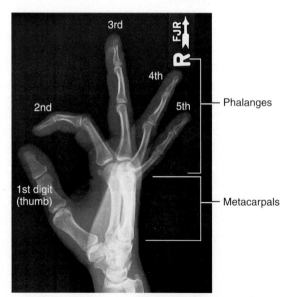

Fig. 4.77 Fan lateral projection of right hand.

LATERAL IN EXTENSION AND FLEXION–LATEROMEDIAL PROJECTIONS: HAND

ALTERNATIVES TO FAN LATERAL

Clinical Indications
- The lateral in either extension or flexion is an alternative to the fan lateral for localization of foreign bodies of the hand and fingers; it also demonstrates anterior or posterior displaced fractures of the metacarpals.

Hand
ALTERNATE
• Extension lateral
• Flexion lateral

The lateral in a natural flexed position may be less painful for the patient.

Technical Factors
- Minimum SID—40 inches (100 cm)
- IR size—10 × 12 inches (24 × 30 cm), portrait; smallest IR available and collimate to area of interest
- Nongrid
- kVp range—55 to 65

Shielding Shield radiosensitive tissues outside region of interest.

Patient Position Seat patient at end of table with hand and forearm extended.

Part Position
Rotate hand and wrist, with thumb side up, into **true lateral position,** with second to fifth MCP joints centered to IR and CR.
- **Lateral in extension:** Extend fingers and thumb, and support against a radiolucent support block. Ensure that all fingers and metacarpals are superimposed directly for true lateral position (Fig. 4.78)
- **Lateral in flexion:** Flex fingers into a natural flexed position, with thumb lightly touching the first finger; maintain true lateral position (Fig. 4.79)

CR
- CR perpendicular to IR, directed to the **second to fifth MCP joints**

Recommended Collimation Collimate to outer margins of hand and wrist.

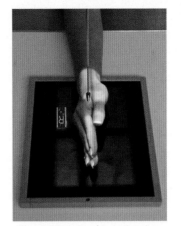
Fig. 4.78 Lateral in extension.

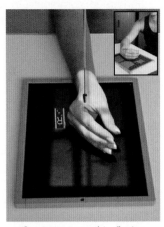
Fig. 4.79 Lateral in flexion.

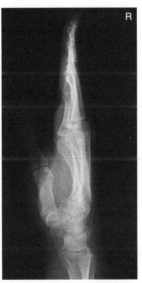
Fig. 4.80 Lateral in extension.

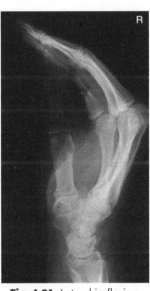
Fig. 4.81 Lateral in flexion.

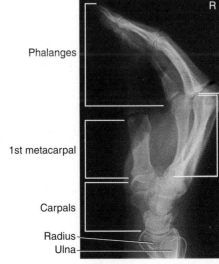
Fig. 4.82 Lateral in flexion.

Evaluation Criteria
Anatomy Demonstrated: • Entire hand and wrist and about 1 inch (2.5 cm) of distal forearm are visible. • Thumb should appear in slightly oblique position and free of superimposition with joint spaces open.
Position: • Long axis of the hand and wrist is aligned with long axis of the IR. • Hand and wrist should be in **true lateral position,** as evidenced by: distal radius and ulna are superimposed; metacarpals and phalanges are superimposed. • **Lateral in extension:** The phalanges and metacarpals should be superimposed and extended (Fig. 4.80). • **Lateral in flexion:** The phalanges and metacarpals should be superimposed with hand in natural flexed position (Figs. 4.81 and 4.82). • CR and center of collimation field should be at **second to fifth MCP joints.**
Exposure: • Optimal density (brightness) and contrast with **no motion** demonstrate soft tissue margins and clear, sharp bony trabecular markings. • Margins of individual metacarpals and phalanges are visible but mostly superimposed.

AP AXIAL PROJECTION—HAND

BREWERTON METHOD[9,10]

Clinical Indications

- Performed commonly to evaluate for early evidence of rheumatoid arthritis at the second through fifth metacarpophalangeal (MCP) joints. Evident by slight erosion of the head of the metacarpal.
- May demonstrate fractures of the base of the fourth and fifth metacarpal.

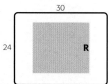

Hand
SPECIAL
- AP Axial

Technical Factors

- Minimum SID—40 inches (100 cm)
- IR size—10 × 12 inches (24 × 30 cm) portrait or 14 × 17 inches (35 × 43 cm) for bilateral study, landscape; smallest IR available and collimate to area of interest
- Nongrid
- kVp range—55 to 65

Shielding Shield radiosensitive tissues outside region of interest.

Patient Position Stand patient at end of table with hand supinated and flexed.

Part Position

- Supinate hand and place at the center of the IR.
- From this position, keeping fingers in contact with the IR, flex the hand to create a 65° angle between the dorsum of hand and IR (Fig. 4.83).
- Extend fingers and ensure they are relaxed, slightly separated and parallel to IR.
- Abduct thumb to avoid superimposition.

CR

- Angle CR 15° proximally, toward ulna, directed to the **third MCP joint.**

Recommended Collimation Collimate on four sides to outer margins of hand and wrist.

Evaluation Criteria

Anatomy Demonstrated: • Entire hand from the carpal area to the tips of digits are visible (Figs. 4.84 and 4.85).

Position: • Second through fifth MCP joints open and visible with no superimposition of the palmer soft tissue; thumb should be free of superimposition with second through fifth digits. Midshafts of second through fifth metacarpals and phalanges should not overlap • CR and center of collimation field should be **at the third MCP joint.**

Exposure: • Optimal density (brightness) and contrast with **no motion** are demonstrated by clear, sharp bony trabecular markings and joint space margins of MCP joints.

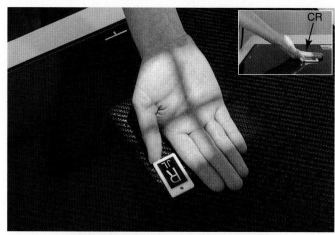

Fig. 4.83 AP axial—Brewerton method.

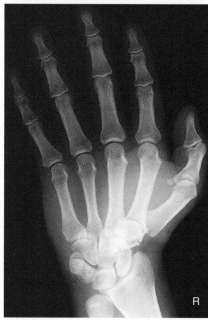

Fig. 4.84 AP axial. (From Wilson DJ et al. *Musculoskeletal imaging,* ed 2, Philadelphia, 2015, Elsevier.)

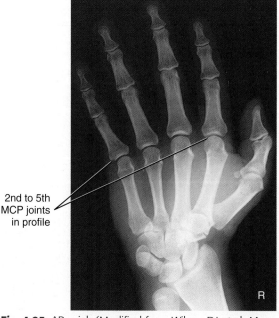

2nd to 5th MCP joints in profile

Fig. 4.85 AP axial. (Modified from Wilson DJ et al. *Musculoskeletal imaging,* ed 2, Philadelphia, 2015, Elsevier.)

Clinical Indications

- Fractures of distal radius or ulna, isolated fractures of radial or ulnar styloid processes, and fractures of individual carpal bones
- Pathologic processes, such as osteomyelitis and arthritis

Wrist
ROUTINE
- PA
- PA oblique
- Lateral

Technical Factors

- Minimum SID—40 inches (100 cm)
- IR size—8 × 10 inches (18 × 24 cm), portrait; smallest IR available and collimate to area of interest
- Nongrid
- kVp range—55 to 65

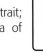

Shielding Shield radiosensitive tissues outside region of interest.

Patient Position Seat patient at end of table with hand and forearm extended. Drop shoulder so that shoulder, elbow, and wrist are on same horizontal plane.

Part Position

- Align and center long axis of hand and wrist to IR, with carpal area centered to CR.
- With hand pronated, arch hand slightly to **place wrist and carpal area in close contact with IR** (Fig. 4.86).

CR

- CR perpendicular to IR, directed to **midcarpal area**

Recommended Collimation Collimate to wrist on all four sides; include distal radius and ulna and midmetacarpal area.

Alternative AP An AP wrist may be taken, with hand slightly arched to place **wrist and carpals in close contact with IR,** to demonstrate intercarpal spaces and wrist joint better and to place the intercarpal spaces more parallel to the divergent rays (Fig. 4.87). This wrist projection is good for visualizing the carpals if the patient can assume this position easily.

Evaluation Criteria

Anatomy Demonstrated: • Midmetacarpals and proximal metacarpals; carpals; distal radius, ulna, and associated joints; and pertinent soft tissues of the wrist joint, such as fat pads and fat stripes, are visible. • All the intercarpal spaces do not appear open because of irregular shapes that result in overlapping (Figs. 4.88 and 4.89).

Position: • Long axis of the hand, wrist, and forearm is aligned with IR. • True PA is evidenced by: equal concavity shapes are on each side of the shafts of the proximal metacarpals; near-equal distances exist among the proximal metacarpals; separation of the distal radius and ulna is present except for possible minimal superimposition at the distal radioulnar joint. • CR and center of collimation field should be to the **midcarpal area.**

Exposure: • Optimal density (brightness) and contrast with **no motion** should visualize soft tissue, such as pertinent fat pads, and sharp, bony margins of the carpals and clear trabecular markings.

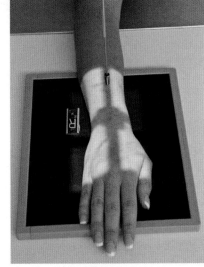

Fig. 4.86 PA wrist.

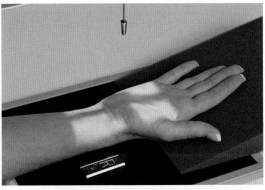

Fig. 4.87 Alternative AP wrist.

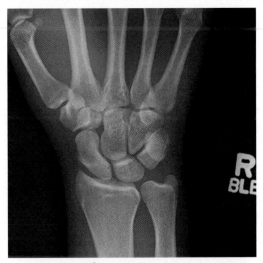

Fig. 4.88 PA wrist.

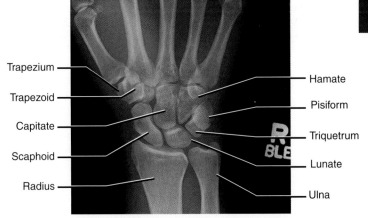

Trapezium
Trapezoid
Capitate
Scaphoid
Radius

Hamate
Pisiform
Triquetrum
Lunate
Ulna

Fig. 4.89 PA of right wrist.

4

PA OBLIQUE PROJECTION—LATERAL ROTATION: WRIST

Clinical Indications
- Fractures of distal radius or ulna, isolated fractures of radial or ulnar styloid processes, and fractures of individual carpal bones
- Pathologic processes, such as osteomyelitis and arthritis

Wrist
ROUTINE
• PA
• PA oblique
• Lateral

Technical Factors
- Minimum SID—40 inches (100 cm)
- IR size—8 × 10 inches (18 × 24 cm), portrait; smallest IR available and collimate to area of interest
- Nongrid
- kVp range—60 to 70

Shielding Shield radiosensitive tissues outside region of interest.

Patient Position Seat patient at end of table with hand and forearm extended. Drop shoulder so that shoulder, elbow, and wrist are on same horizontal plane.

Part Position
- Align and center hand and wrist to IR.
- From pronated position, rotate wrist and hand laterally 45°.
- For stability, place a 45° support under thumb side of hand to support hand and wrist in a 45° oblique position (Fig. 4.90) or partially flex fingers to arch hand so that fingertips rest lightly on IR without support (Fig. 4.91).

CR
- CR perpendicular to IR, directed to **midcarpal area**

Recommended Collimation Collimate to wrist on four sides; include distal radius and ulna and midmetacarpal area.

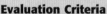

Evaluation Criteria
Anatomy Demonstrated: • Distal radius, ulna, carpals, and at least to midmetacarpal area are visible. • Trapezium and scaphoid should be well visualized, with only slight superimposition of other carpals on their medial aspects (Figs. 4.92 and 4.93).
Position: • Long axis of the hand, wrist, and forearm should be aligned with IR. • True 45° oblique of the wrist is evidenced by: ulnar head partially superimposed by distal radius; proximal third through fifth metacarpals (metacarpal bases) should appear mostly superimposed. • CR and center of collimation field should be to **midcarpal area.**
Exposure: • Optimal density (brightness) and contrast with **no motion** demonstrate carpals and their overlapping borders; soft tissue margins; and clear, sharp bony trabecular markings.

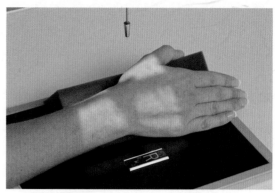

Fig. 4.90 PA oblique wrist (with 45° support).

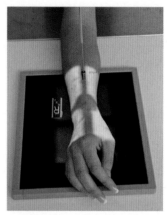

Fig. 4.91 PA oblique wrist without support.

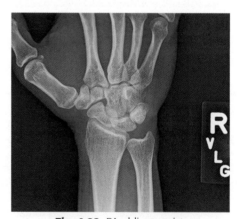

Fig. 4.92 PA oblique wrist.

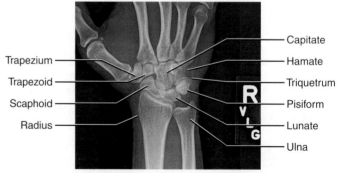

Trapezium — Capitate
Trapezoid — Hamate
Scaphoid — Triquetrum
Radius — Pisiform
— Lunate
— Ulna

Fig. 4.93 PA oblique of right wrist.

LATEROMEDIAL PROJECTION—WRIST

Clinical Indications

- Fractures or dislocations of the distal radius or ulna, specifically anteroposterior fragment displacements for **Barton**, **Colles**, or **Smith fractures**
- Osteoarthritis also may be demonstrated primarily in the trapezium and first CMC joint

ROUTINE
- PA
- PA oblique
- Lateral

Technical Factors

- Minimum SID—40 inches (100 cm)
- IR size—8 × 10 inches (18 × 24 cm), portrait; smallest IR available and collimate to area of interest
- Nongrid
- kVp range—60 to 70

Shielding Shield radiosensitive tissues outside region of interest.

Patient Position Seat patient at end of table, with arm and forearm resting on the table. Place wrist and hand on IR in thumb-up lateral position. Shoulder, elbow, and wrist should be on same horizontal plane.

Part Position

- Align and center hand and wrist to long axis of IR.
- Adjust hand and wrist into a **true lateral** position, with fingers comfortably extended (Fig. 4.94); if support is needed to prevent motion, use a radiolucent support block and sandbag, and place block against extended hand and fingers (Fig. 4.95).

CR

- CR perpendicular to IR, directed to **midcarpal area**

Recommended Collimation Collimate on four sides, including distal radius and ulna and metacarpal area.

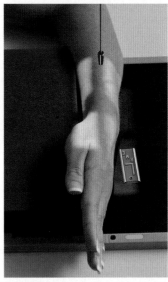

Fig. 4.94 Part position—lateral wrist

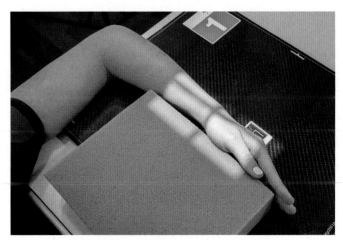

Fig. 4.95 Patient position—lateral wrist with support.

Evaluation Criteria

Anatomy Demonstrated: • Distal radius and ulna, carpals, and at least the midmetacarpal area are visible.
Position: • Long axis of the hand, wrist, and forearm should be aligned with long axis of IR. • **True lateral** position is evidenced by: ulnar head should be superimposed over distal radius; proximal second through fifth metacarpals all should appear aligned and superimposed (Figs. 4.96 and 4.97). • CR and center of collimation field should be to **midcarpal region**.
Exposure: • Optimal density (brightness) and contrast with **no motion** demonstrate clear, sharp bony 'trabecular markings and soft tissue, such as margins of pertinent fat pads of the wrist and borders of the distal ulna, seen through the superimposed radius.

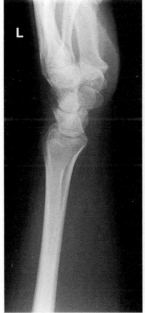

Fig. 4.96 Lateral projection of left wrist.

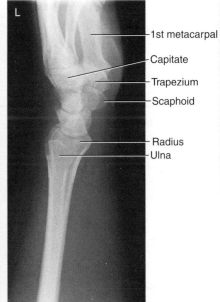

- 1st metacarpal
- Capitate
- Trapezium
- Scaphoid
- Radius
- Ulna

Fig. 4.97 Lateral wrist.

PA AND PA AXIAL SCAPHOID—WITH ULNAR DEVIATION: WRIST

WARNING: If patient has possible wrist trauma, do *not* attempt this position before a routine wrist series has been completed and evaluated to rule out possible fracture of distal forearm or wrist or both.

Clinical Indications
- Possible fractures of the **scaphoid** Nondisplaced fractures may require additional projections or CT scan of the wrist

Wrist
SPECIAL
• Scaphoid projections: CR angle with ulnar deviation

Technical Factors
- Minimum SID—40 inches (100 cm)
- IR size—8 × 10 inches (18 × 24 cm), portrait; smallest IR available and collimate to area of interest
- Nongrid
- kVp range—55 to 65

Shielding Shield radiosensitive tissues outside region of interest.

Patient Position Seat patient at end of table, with wrist and hand on IR, palm down, and shoulder, elbow, and wrist on same horizontal plane.

Part Position ⊞
- Position wrist as for a PA projection—palm down and hand and wrist aligned with center of long axis of IR, with scaphoid centered to CR.
- Without moving forearm, gently evert hand (move toward ulnar side) as far as patient can tolerate without lifting or rotating distal forearm (Fig. 4.98).

NOTE: See terminology in Chapter 1 for explanation of ulnar deviation versus radial deviation.

CR
- Angle CR **10° to 15° proximally,** along long axis of forearm and toward elbow (CR angle should be perpendicular to long axis of scaphoid).
- Center CR to **scaphoid** (Locate scaphoid at a point ¾ inch (2 cm) distal and medial to radial styloid process).

Recommended Collimation Collimate on four sides to carpal region.

NOTE: Obscure fractures of scaphoid may require several projections taken with different CR angles. Rafert and Long[11] described a four-projection series with the CR angled proximally 0°, 10°, 20°, and 30°.

Evaluation Criteria
Anatomy Demonstrated: • Distal radius and ulna, carpals, and proximal metacarpals are visible. • Scaphoid should be demonstrated clearly without foreshortening, with adjacent carpal interspaces open (evidence of CR angle) (Figs. 4.99 and 4.100).
Position: • Long axis of wrist and forearm should be aligned with side border of IR. • Ulnar deviation should be evident by the angle of the long axis of the metacarpals to that of the radius and ulna. • **No rotation** of wrist is evidenced by appearance of distal radius and ulna, with minimal superimposition of distal radioulnar joint (Fig. 4.101). • CR and center of collimation field should be to the **scaphoid.**
Exposure: • Optimal density (brightness) and contrast with **no motion** visualize the scaphoid borders and clear, sharp bony trabecular markings.

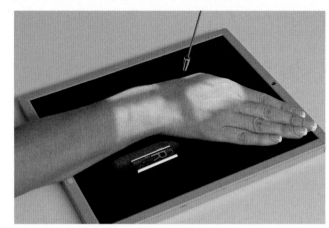

Fig. 4.98 PA axial wrist (scaphoid)—ulnar deviation with 15° CR angle.

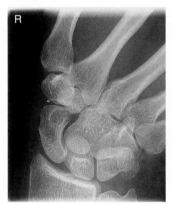
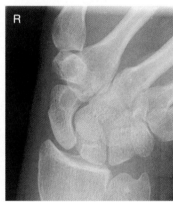

Fig. 4.99 15° CR angle.   **Fig. 4.100** 25° CR angle.

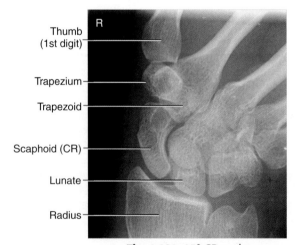

Thumb (1st digit)
Trapezium
Trapezoid
Scaphoid (CR)
Lunate
Radius

Fig. 4.101 15° CR angle.

PA SCAPHOID–HAND ELEVATED AND ULNAR DEVIATION: WRIST

MODIFIED STECHER METHOD[12]

WARNING: If patient has possible wrist trauma, do *not* attempt this position before a routine wrist series has been completed and evaluated to rule out possible fracture of distal forearm or wrist or both.

Clinical Indications
- Possible fractures of the **scaphoid**
  This is an alternative projection to the CR angle ulnar deviation method demonstrated on the preceding page.

Wrist
ALTERNATE
• Scaphoid projections: CR angle with ulnar deviation
• Scaphoid projections: Hand elevated and ulnar deviation, modified Stecher method

Technical Factors
- Minimum SID—40 inches (100 cm)
- IR size—8 × 10 inches (18 × 24 cm), portrait; smallest IR available and collimate to area of interest
- Nongrid
- kVp range—55 to 65

Shielding Shield radiosensitive tissues outside region of interest.

Patient Position Seat patient at end of table with hand and forearm extended. Drop shoulder so that shoulder, elbow, and wrist are on same horizontal plane.

Part Position
- Place hand and wrist palm down on IR with hand elevated on 20° angle sponge (Fig. 4.102).
- Ensure that wrist is in direct contact with IR.
- Gently evert or turn hand outward (toward ulnar side) unless contraindicated because of severe injury (Fig. 4.103).

Alternative Method Have patient clench the fist with ulnar deviation to obtain a similar position of the scaphoid.

CR
- Center CR **perpendicular to IR** and directed to **scaphoid** (locate scaphoid at a point ¾ inch [2 cm] distal and medial to radial styloid process).

Recommended Collimation Collimate on four sides to carpal region.

NOTE: Stecher[12] indicated that elevation of the hand 20° rather than angling of CR places the scaphoid parallel to the IR. Stecher also suggested that clenching of the fist is an alternative to elevation of the hand or angling of the CR. Bridgman[13] recommended ulnar deviation in addition to hand elevation, for less scaphoid superimposition.

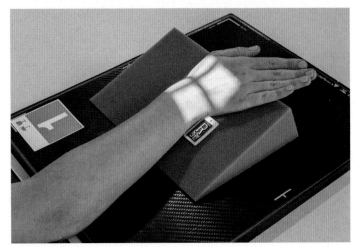

Fig. 4.102 PA wrist for scaphoid as follows: hand elevated 20°; ulnar deviation, if possible; no CR angle.

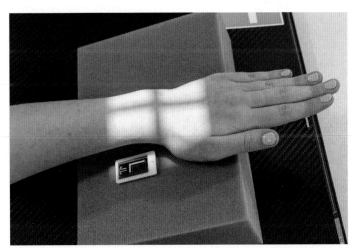

Fig. 4.103 Severe pain as follows: hand elevated 20°; **no** ulnar deviation; no CR angle.

Evaluation Criteria
Anatomy Demonstrated: • Distal radius and ulna, carpals, and proximal metacarpals are visible. • Carpals are visible, with adjacent interspaces more open on the lateral (radial) side of the wrist. • Scaphoid is shown, without foreshortening or superimposition of adjoining carpals (Figs. 4.104 and 4.105).
Position: • Long axis of wrist and forearm should be aligned with side border of IR. • Ulnar deviation is evidenced by only minimal, if any, superimposition of distal scaphoid. • **No rotation** of wrist is evidenced by the appearance of distal radius and ulna with no or only minimal superimposition of distal radioulnar joint. • CR and center of collimation field should be to **scaphoid**.
Exposure: • Optimal density (brightness) and contrast with **no motion** visualize the scaphoid borders and clear, sharp bony trabecular markings.

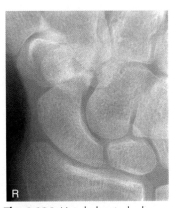

Fig. 4.104 Hand elevated, ulnar deviation, and no CR angle.

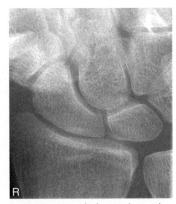

Fig. 4.105 Hand elevated, no ulnar deviation or CR angle.

PA PROJECTION—RADIAL DEVIATION: WRIST

WARNING: If patient has possible wrist trauma, do *not* attempt this position before a routine wrist series has been completed and evaluated to rule out possible fracture of distal forearm or wrist or both.

Clinical Indications
- Possible fractures of the carpal bones on the ulnar side of the wrist, especially the lunate, triquetrum, pisiform, and hamate

Wrist
SPECIAL
• Scaphoid projections: CR angle with ulnar deviation, or alternate modified Stecher method
• Radial deviation

Technical Factors
- Minimum SID—40 inches (100 cm)
- IR size—8 × 10 inches (18 × 24 cm), portrait; smallest IR available and collimate to area of interest
- Nongrid
- kVp range—55 to 65

Shielding Shield radiosensitive tissues outside region of interest.

Patient Position Seat patient at end of table with hand and forearm extended. Drop shoulder so that shoulder, elbow, and wrist are on same horizontal plane.

Part Position
- Position wrist as for PA projection—palm down with wrist and hand aligned with center of long axis of IR.
- Without moving forearm, gently invert the hand (move medially toward thumb side) as far as patient can tolerate without lifting or rotating distal forearm (Fig. 4.106).

CR
- CR perpendicular to IR, directed to midcarpal area

Recommended Collimation Collimate on four sides to carpal region.

Evaluation Criteria
Anatomy Demonstrated: • Distal radius and ulna, carpals, and proximal metacarpals are visible. • Carpals are visible, with adjacent interspaces more open on the medial (ulnar) side of the wrist (Figs. 4.107 and 4.108).
Position: • Long axis of the forearm is aligned with the side border of IR • Extreme radial deviation is evidenced by the angle of the long axis of the metacarpals to that of the radius and ulna and the space between the triquetrum/pisiform and the styloid process of the ulna. • **No rotation** of the wrist is evidenced by the appearance of the distal radius and ulna. • CR and center of the collimation field should be to the **midcarpal area.**
Exposure: • Optimal density (brightness) and contrast with **no motion** visualize the carpal borders and clear, sharp bony trabecular markings.

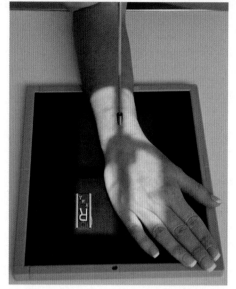

Fig. 4.106 PA wrist—radial deviation.

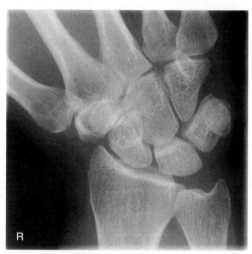

Fig. 4.107 Radial deviation.

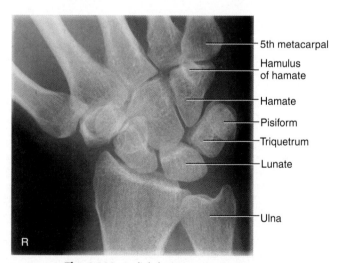

- 5th metacarpal
- Hamulus of hamate
- Hamate
- Pisiform
- Triquetrum
- Lunate
- Ulna

Fig. 4.108 Radial deviation.

CARPAL CANAL (TUNNEL)—TANGENTIAL, INFEROSUPERIOR PROJECTION: WRIST

GAYNOR-HART METHOD

WARNING: If patient has possible wrist trauma, do *not* attempt this position before a routine wrist series has been completed and evaluated to rule out possible fracture of distal forearm or wrist or both.

Clinical Indications

- Rule out abnormal calcification and bony changes in the carpal sulcus that may impinge on the **median nerve,** as with **carpal tunnel syndrome**
- Possible fractures of the hamulus process of the hamate, pisiform, and trapezium

> **Wrist**
> SPECIAL
> - Scaphoid projections: CR angle with ulnar deviation, or alternate modified Stecher method
> - Radial deviation
> - Carpal canal

Technical Factors

- Minimum SID—40 inches (100 cm)
- IR size—8 × 10 inches (18 × 24 cm), portrait; smallest IR available and collimate to area of interest
- Nongrid
- kVp range—55 to 65

Shielding Shield radiosensitive tissues outside region of interest.

Patient Position Seat patient at end of table, with wrist and hand on IR and palm down (pronated).

Part Position

- Align hand and wrist with long axis of the IR.
- Ask patient to hyperextend wrist (dorsiflex) as far as possible by the use of a piece of tape or band, gently but firmly hyperextending the wrist until the long axis of the metacarpals and the fingers are as near vertical (90° to forearm) as possible (without lifting the wrist and forearm from the IR).
- Rotate entire hand and wrist about **10° internally** (toward radial side) to prevent superimposition of pisiform and hamate (Fig. 4.109).

CR

- Angle CR **25° to 30° proximally, to the long axis of the hand** (the total CR angle in relationship to the IR must be increased if patient cannot hyperextend wrist as far as indicated).
- Direct CR to a point about 1 inch (2 to 3 cm) distal to the base of third metacarpal (center of palm of hand).

Recommended Collimation Collimate on four sides to area of interest.

Alternative Imaging Sonography for carpal tunnel: High-resolution ultrasonography allows for noninvasive imaging of the carpal tunnel and related anatomy. Fig. 4.110 demonstrates the "bowing" of the flexor retinaculum (arrows) with the "flattening" of the median nerve below it, indicating compression.[14]

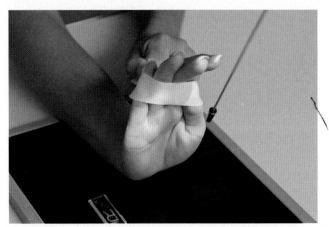

Fig. 4.109 Tangential projection. CR 25° to 30° to long axis of hand.

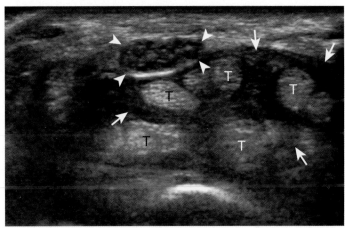

Fig. 4.110 Carpal tunnel syndrome: tenosynovitis. Ultrasound image in short axis. (From Jacobson J. *Fundamentals of musculoskeletal ultrasound,* ed 2, Philadelphia, 2013, Elsevier.)

Evaluation Criteria

Anatomy Demonstrated: • The carpals are demonstrated in a tunnel-like, arched arrangement (Figs. 4.111 and 4.112).

Position: • The pisiform and the hamulus process should be separated and visible in profile without superimposition. • The rounded palmar aspects of the capitate and the scaphoid should be visualized in profile, in addition to the aspect of the trapezium that articulates with the first metacarpal. • CR and center of collimation field should be to **midpoint of the carpal canal.**

Exposure: • Optimal density (brightness) and contrast should visualize soft tissues and possible calcifications in carpal canal region, and outlines of superimposed carpals should be visible without overexposure of these carpals in profile. • Trabecular markings and bony margins should appear clear and sharp, indicating **no motion.**

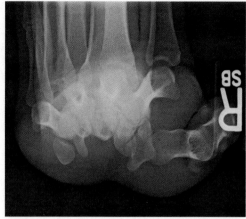

Fig. 4.111 Tangential (Gaynor-Hart method) projection.

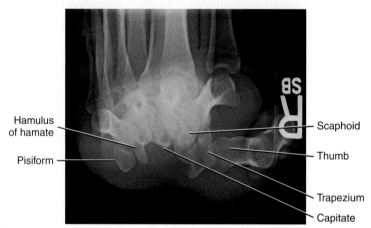

Hamulus of hamate

Pisiform

Scaphoid

Thumb

Trapezium

Capitate

Fig. 4.112 Tangential projection of right wrist.

4

CARPAL BRIDGE—TANGENTIAL PROJECTION: WRIST

WARNING: If patient has possible wrist trauma, do *not* attempt this position before a routine wrist series has been completed and evaluated to rule out possible fracture of distal forearm or wrist or both.

Clinical Indications
- Calcification or other pathology of the dorsal (posterior) aspect of the carpal bones

> **Wrist**
> SPECIAL
> - Scaphoid projections: CR angle with ulnar deviation, alternate modified Stecher method
> - Radial deviation
> - Carpal canal
> - Carpal bridge

Technical Factors
- Minimum SID—40 inches (100 cm)
- IR size—8 × 10 inches (18 × 24 cm), portrait; smallest IR available and collimate to area of interest
- Nongrid
- kVp range—55 to 65

Shielding Shield radiosensitive tissues outside region of interest.

Patient Position Have patient stand or sit at end of the table and then lean over and place dorsal surface of hand, **palm upward,** on IR.

Part Position
- Center dorsal aspect of carpals to IR.
- Gently flex wrist as far as patient can tolerate, or until the hand and forearm form as near a 90° (right) angle as possible (Fig. 4.113).

CR
- Angle CR 45°distally, to the long axis of the forearm.
- Direct CR to a midpoint of the distal forearm about 1½ inches (4 cm) proximal to wrist joint.

Recommended Collimation Collimate all four sides of carpal region.

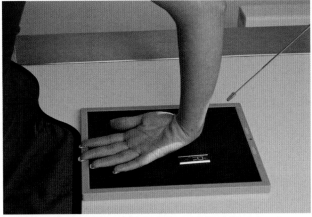
Fig. 4.113 Carpal bridge—tangential projection; CR 45° to forearm.

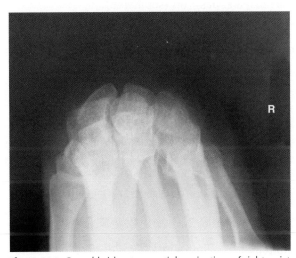
Fig. 4.114 Carpal bridge tangential projection of right wrist.

> **Evaluation Criteria**
> **Anatomy Demonstrated:** • Tangential view of the dorsal aspect of the scaphoid, lunate, and triquetrum is visible. • Outline of the capitate and trapezium superimposed is visible (Figs. 4.114 and 4.115).
> **Position:** • Dorsal aspect of the carpal bones should be visualized clear of superimposition and centered to IR. • CR and center of collimation field should be to the area of the **dorsal carpal bones.**
> **Exposure:** • Optimal density (brightness) and contrast with **no motion** should demonstrate the dorsal aspect of carpal bones, with sharp borders and clear, sharp bony trabecular markings. • Outlines of proximal metacarpals should be visualized through superimposed structures without overexposure of the dorsal aspects of carpals seen in profile.

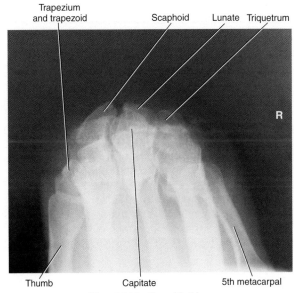
Trapezium and trapezoid   Scaphoid   Lunate   Triquetrum
Thumb   Capitate   5th metacarpal
Fig. 4.115 Carpal bridge.

AP PROJECTION—FOREARM

Clinical Indications
- Fractures and dislocations of the radius or ulna
- Pathologic processes such as osteomyelitis or arthritis

Forearm
ROUTINE
• AP
• Lateral

Technical Factors
- Minimum SID—40 inches (100 cm)
- IR size 14 × 17 inches (35 × 43 cm), portrait or smallest IR available and collimate to area of interest
- Nongrid
- kVp range—65 to 75

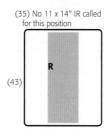

(35) No 11 x 14" IR called for this position

(43)

R

Shielding Shield radiosensitive tissues outside region of interest.

Patient Position Seat patient at end of table, with hand and arm fully extended and **palm up (supinated).**

Part Position
- Drop shoulder to place entire upper limb on same horizontal plane.
- Align and center forearm to long axis of IR, ensuring that both wrist and elbow joints are included (use as large an IR as necessary).
- Instruct patient to lean laterally as necessary to place entire wrist, forearm, and elbow in as near a true frontal position as possible (Fig. 4.116). Palpate the medial and lateral epicondyles to ensure they are the same distance from IR.

CR
- CR perpendicular to IR, directed to **mid-forearm**

Recommended Collimation Collimate lateral borders to actual forearm area with minimal collimation at both ends to avoid excluding anatomy at either joint. Considering divergence of the x-ray beam, ensure that a **minimum** of 1 to 1½ inches (3 to 4 cm) distal to wrist and elbow joints is included on IR.

Evaluation Criteria
Anatomy Demonstrated: • AP projection of the entire radius and ulna is shown, with a minimum of proximal row carpals and distal humerus and pertinent soft tissues, such as fat pads and stripes of the wrist and elbow joints (Fig. 4.117).
Position: • Long axis of forearm should be aligned with long axis of IR. • **No rotation** is evidenced by humeral epicondyles visualized in profile, with radial head, neck, and tuberosity slightly superimposed by the ulna. • Wrist and elbow joint spaces are only partially open because of beam divergence. • CR and center of collimation field should be to the **approximate midpoint of the radius and ulna.**
Exposure: • Optimal density (brightness) and contrast with **no motion** should visualize soft tissue and sharp, cortical margins and clear, bony trabecular markings.

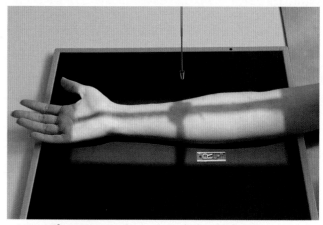
Fig. 4.116 AP forearm (including both joints).

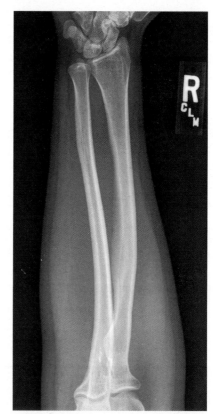
Fig. 4.117 AP forearm (both joints).

4

LATEROMEDIAL PROJECTION—FOREARM

Clinical Indications

- Fractures and dislocations of the radius or ulna
- Pathologic processes, such as osteomyelitis or arthritis

Forearm
ROUTINE
• AP
• Lateral

Technical Factors

- Minimum SID—40 inches (100 cm)
- IR size—14 × 17 inches (35 × 43 cm), portrait; smallest IR available and collimate to area of interest
- Nongrid
- kVp range—65 to 75
- To make best use of the anode heel effect, place elbow at cathode end of x-ray beam

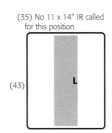

(35) No 11 x 14" IR called for this position

(43)   L

Shielding Shield radiosensitive tissues outside region of interest.

Patient Position Seat patient at end of table, with elbow flexed 90°.

Part Position

- Drop shoulder to place entire upper limb on same horizontal plane.
- Align and center forearm to long axis of IR; ensure that both wrist and elbow joints are included on IR (Fig. 4.118).
- Rotate hand and wrist into **true lateral position,** and support hand to prevent motion, if needed (ensure that distal radius and ulna are superimposed directly).
- For heavy muscular forearms, place support under hand and wrist as needed to place radius and ulna parallel to IR.

CR

- CR perpendicular to IR, directed to **mid-forearm**

Recommended Collimation Collimate both lateral borders to the actual forearm area. Also, collimate at both ends to avoid excluding anatomy at either joint. Considering divergence of the x-ray beam, ensure that a **minimum** of 1 to 1½ inches (3 to 4 cm) distal to wrist and elbow joints is included on IR.

Evaluation Criteria

Anatomy Demonstrated: • Lateral projection of entire radius and ulna, proximal row of carpal bones, elbow, and distal end of the humerus are visible, in addition to pertinent soft tissue, such as fat pads and stripes of the wrist and elbow joints (Fig. 4.119).
Position: • Long axis of forearm should be aligned with long axis of IR. • Elbow should be flexed 90°. • **No rotation** as evidenced by head of ulna being superimposed over the radius, and humeral epicondyles should be superimposed. • Radial head should superimpose coronoid process, with radial tuberosity demonstrated. • CR and center of collimation field should be to **midpoint of the radius and ulna.**
Exposure: • Optimal density (brightness) and contrast with **no motion** should visualize sharp cortical margins and clear, sharp bony trabecular markings and fat pads and stripes of the wrist and elbow joints.

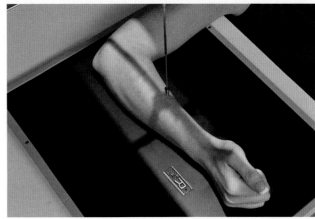

Fig. 4.118 Lateral forearm (including both joints).

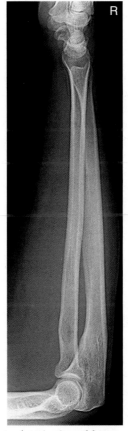

Fig. 4.119 Lateral projection of forearm (both joints).

4

AP PROJECTION—ELBOW

ELBOW FULLY EXTENDED

Clinical Indications
- Fractures and dislocations of the elbow
- Pathologic processes, such as osteomyelitis and arthritis

Elbow
ROUTINE
• AP
• Alternate AP—partial flexion
• Alternate AP—acute flexion
• Oblique
• Lateral (external)
• Medial (internal)
• Lateral

Technical Factors
- Minimum SID—40 inches (100 cm)
- IR size—10 × 12 inches (24 × 30 cm), portrait; smallest IR available and collimate to area of interest
- Nongrid
- kVp range—65 to 75

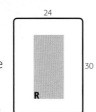

Shielding Shield radiosensitive tissues outside region of interest.

Patient Position Seat patient at end of table, with elbow fully extended, if possible (See following page if patient cannot fully extend elbow).

Part Position
- Extend elbow, supinate hand, and align arm and forearm with long axis of IR (Fig. 4.120).
- Center elbow joint to center of IR.
- Ask patient to lean laterally as necessary for **true AP projection.** Palpate humeral epicondyles to ensure that the interepicondylar plane is parallel to the IR. (The interepicondylar plane is an imaginary plane between the medial and lateral epicondyles of the distal humerus. This plane is useful for elbow and humerus positioning.)
- Support hand as needed to prevent motion.

CR
- CR perpendicular to IR, directed to **mid-elbow joint,** which is approximately ¾ inch (2 cm) distal to midpoint of a line between epicondyles

Recommended Collimation Collimate on four sides to area of interest.

Evaluation Criteria
Anatomy Demonstrated: • Distal humerus, elbow joint space, and proximal radius and ulna are visible (Figs. 4.121 and 4.122).
Position: • Long axis of arm should be aligned with long axis of IR. • **No rotation** is evidenced by the appearance of bilateral epicondyles seen in profile and radial head, neck, and tubercles separated or only slightly superimposed by ulna. • Olecranon process should be seated in the olecranon fossa with fully extended arm • Elbow joint space appears open with fully extended arm and proper CR centering. • CR and center of collimation field should be to the **mid-elbow joint.**
Exposure: • Optimal density (brightness) and contrast with **no motion** should visualize soft tissue detail; sharp, bony cortical margins; and clear, bony trabecular markings.

Fig. 4.120 AP elbow (fully extended).

Fig. 4.121 AP (extended).

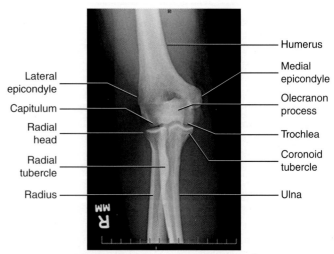

Fig. 4.122 AP right elbow (extended).

AP PROJECTION—ALTERNATE PARTIAL FLEXION: ELBOW

WHEN ELBOW CANNOT BE FULLY EXTENDED

Clinical Indications
- Fractures and dislocations of the elbow
- Pathologic processes, such as osteomyelitis and arthritis

Technical Factors
- Minimum SID—40 inches (100 cm)
- IR size—10 × 12 inches (24 × 30 cm), portrait; smallest IR available and collimate to area of interest
- Nongrid
- kVp range—65 to 75

Shielding Shield radiosensitive tissues outside region of interest.

Patient Position Seat patient at end of table, with elbow partially flexed.

Part Position
- Obtain **two** AP projections—one with **forearm parallel** to IR and one with **humerus parallel** to IR (Figs. 4.123 and 4.124).
- Place support under wrist and forearm for projection with humerus parallel to IR, if needed, to prevent motion.

CR
- CR **perpendicular** to IR, directed to **mid-elbow joint,** which is approximately ¾ inch (2 cm) distal to midpoint of a line between epicondyles

Recommended Collimation Collimate on four sides to area of interest.

NOTE: If patient cannot partially extend elbow as shown (see Fig. 4.123) and elbow remains **flexed near 90°,** take the two AP projections as described, but **angle CR 10° to 15°** into elbow joint, or if flexed **more than 90°,** use the **acute flexion projection** (see p. 166).

Elbow
ROUTINE
• AP
• Alternate AP—partial flexion
• Alternate AP—acute flexion
• Oblique
• Lateral (external)
• Medial (internal)
• Lateral

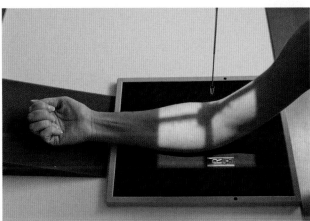

Fig. 4.123 AP elbow (partially flexed); humerus parallel to IR.

Fig. 4.124 AP elbow (partially flexed); forearm parallel to IR.

Evaluation Criteria
Anatomy Demonstrated: • Distal humerus is best visualized on "humerus parallel" projection, and proximal radius and ulna are best visualized on "forearm parallel" projection (Figs. 4.125 and 4.126).

NOTE: Structures in elbow joint region are partially obscured and slightly distorted, depending on amount of elbow flexion possible.

Position: • Long axis of arm should be aligned with side border of IR. • **No rotation** is evidenced by the epicondyles seen in profile and radial head and neck separated or only slightly superimposed over ulna on forearm parallel projection. • CR and center of collimation field should be to the **mid-elbow joint.**

Exposure: • Optimal density (brightness) and contrast with **no motion** should visualize soft tissue detail; sharp, bony cortical margins; and clear, bony trabecular markings. • Distal humerus, including epicondyles, should be demonstrated with sufficient density on "humerus parallel" projection. • On "forearm parallel" projection, proximal radius and ulna should be well visualized with density to allow visualization of both soft tissue and bony detail.

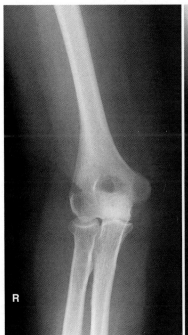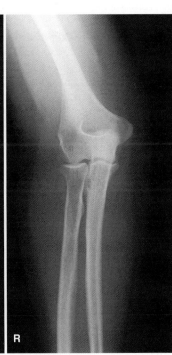

Fig. 4.125 Humerus parallel. **Fig. 4.126** Forearm parallel.

ACUTE FLEXION PROJECTIONS—ELBOW

AP PROJECTIONS OF ELBOW IN ACUTE FLEXION

Clinical Indications
- Fractures and moderate dislocations of the elbow in acute flexion when the elbow cannot be extended to any degree

NOTE: To visualize both the distal humerus and the proximal radius and ulna, **two** projections are required—one with **CR perpendicular to the humerus** and one with CR angled so that it is **perpendicular to the forearm.**

Elbow
ROUTINE
• AP
• Alternate AP—partial flexion
• Alternate AP—acute flexion
• Oblique
• Lateral (external)
• Medial (internal)
• Lateral

Technical Factors
- Minimum SID—40 inches (100 cm)
- IR size—10 × 12 inches (24 × 30 cm), portrait; smallest IR available and collimate to area of interest
- Nongrid
- kVp range—70 to 80

Shielding Shield radiosensitive tissues outside region of interest.

Patient Position Seat patient at end of table, with acutely flexed arm resting on IR.

Part Position ⊞
- Align and center humerus to long axis of IR, with forearm acutely flexed and fingertips resting on shoulder.
- Adjust IR to center of elbow joint region.
- Palpate humeral epicondyles and ensure interepicondylar plane is parallel to IR for **no rotation**

CR
- **Distal humerus:** CR perpendicular to IR and humerus, directed to a point midway between epicondyles (Fig. 4.127)
- **Proximal forearm:** CR perpendicular to forearm (angling CR as needed), directed to a point approximately 2 inches (5 cm) proximal or superior to olecranon process (Fig. 4.128)

Recommended Collimation Collimate on four sides to area of interest.

Evaluation Criteria
- Four-sided collimation borders should be visible with CR and center of collimation field midway between epicondyles.

Distal Humerus: • Forearm and humerus should be directly superimposed. • Medial and lateral epicondyles and parts of trochlea, capitulum, and olecranon process all should be seen in profile. • Optimal exposure should visualize distal humerus and olecranon process through superimposed structures. • Soft tissue detail is not readily visible on either projection (Figs. 4.129 and 4.131).

Proximal Forearm: • Proximal ulna and radius, including outline of radial head and neck, should be visible through superimposed distal humerus. • Optimal exposure visualizes outlines of proximal ulna and radius superimposed over humerus (Figs. 4.130 and 4.132).

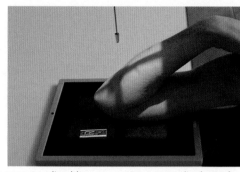

Fig. 4.127 For distal humerus—CR perpendicular to **humerus.**

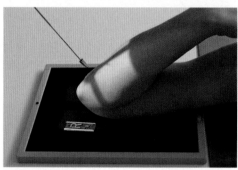

Fig. 4.128 For proximal forearm—CR perpendicular to **forearm.**

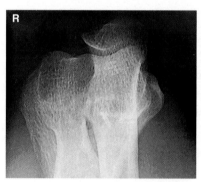

Fig. 4.129 Distal humerus.

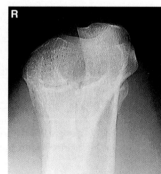

Fig. 4.130 Proximal forearm.

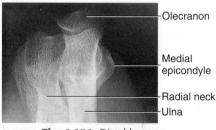

Olecranon

Medial epicondyle

Radial neck
Ulna

Fig. 4.131 Distal humerus.

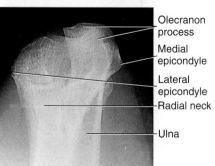

Olecranon process

Medial epicondyle

Lateral epicondyle

Radial neck

Ulna

Fig. 4.132 Proximal forearm.

AP OBLIQUE PROJECTION—LATERAL (EXTERNAL) ROTATION: ELBOW

Clinical Indications
- Fractures and dislocations of the elbow, primarily the radial head and neck
- Certain pathologic processes, such as osteomyelitis and arthritis

Lateral (External Rotation) Oblique Best visualizes radial head and neck of the radius and capitulum of humerus

Elbow
ROUTINE
• AP
• Alternate AP—partial flexion
• Alternate AP—acute flexion
• Oblique
• Lateral (external)
• Medial (internal)
• Lateral

Technical Factors
- Minimum SID—40 inches (100 cm)
- IR size—10 × 12 inches (24 × 30 cm), portrait; smallest IR available and collimate to area of interest
- Nongrid
- kVp range —65 to 75

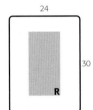

Shielding Shield radiosensitive tissues outside region of interest.

Patient Position Seat patient at end of table, with arm fully extended and shoulder and elbow on same horizontal plane (lowering shoulder as needed).

Part Position
- Align arm and forearm with long axis of IR (Fig. 4.133).
- Center elbow joint to CR and to IR.
- Supinate hand and **rotate laterally** the entire arm so that the distal humerus and the anterior surface of the elbow joint are approximately 45° to IR. (Patient must lean laterally for sufficient lateral rotation.) Place interepicondylar plane approximately 45° to the IR (Fig. 4.134).

CR
- CR perpendicular to IR, directed to **mid-elbow joint** (a point approximately ¾ inch [2 cm] distal to midpoint of line between the epicondyles as viewed from the x-ray tube)

Recommended Collimation Collimate on four sides to area of interest.

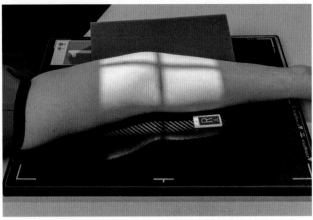

Fig. 4.133 45° lateral (external) oblique.

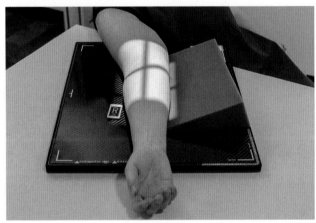

Fig. 4.134 End view, showing 45° external rotation.

4

Evaluation Criteria
Anatomy Demonstrated: • Oblique projection of distal humerus and proximal radius and ulna is visible (Figs. 4.135 and 4.136).
Position: • Long axis of arm should be aligned with side border of IR. • Correct 45° lateral oblique should visualize **radial head, neck,** and **tuberosity,** free of superimposition by ulna. • Lateral epicondyle and capitulum should appear elongated and in profile. • CR and center of collimation field should be to **mid-elbow joint.**
Exposure: • Optimal density (brightness) and contrast with **no motion** should visualize soft tissue detail; sharp, bony cortical margins; and clear, bony trabecular markings.

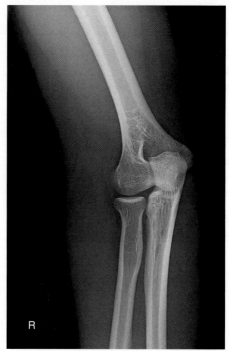

Fig. 4.135 Lateral oblique of right elbow—external rotation.

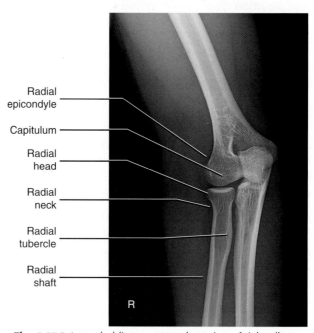

Radial epicondyle
Capitulum
Radial head
Radial neck
Radial tubercle
Radial shaft

Fig. 4.136 Lateral oblique—external rotation of right elbow.

AP OBLIQUE PROJECTION—MEDIAL (INTERNAL) ROTATION: ELBOW

Clinical Indications
- Fractures and dislocations of the elbow, primarily the coronoid process
- Certain pathologic processes, such as osteoporosis and arthritis

Medial (Internal Rotation) Oblique Best visualizes **coronoid process** of ulna and **trochlea** in profile.

Elbow
ROUTINE
• AP
• Alternate AP—partial flexion
• Alternate AP—acute flexion
• Oblique
• Lateral (external)
• Medial (internal)
• Lateral

Technical Factors
- Minimum SID—40 inches (100 cm)
- IR size—10 × 12 inches (24 × 30 cm), portrait; smallest IR available and collimate to area of interest
- Nongrid
- kVp range—65 to 75

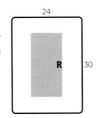

Shielding Shield radiosensitive tissues outside region of interest.

Patient Position Seat patient at end of table, with arm fully extended and shoulder and elbow on same horizontal plane.

Part Position
- Align arm and forearm with long axis of IR. Center elbow joint to CR and to IR.
- Pronate hand into a natural palm-down position and rotate arm as needed until distal humerus and anterior surface of elbow are rotated **45°** (place interepicondylar plane approximately 45° to the IR) (Figs. 4.137 and 4.138).

CR
- CR perpendicular to IR, directed to **mid-elbow joint** (approximately ¾ inch [2 cm] distal to midpoint of line between epicondyles as viewed from x-ray tube)

Recommended Collimation Collimate on four sides to area of interest.

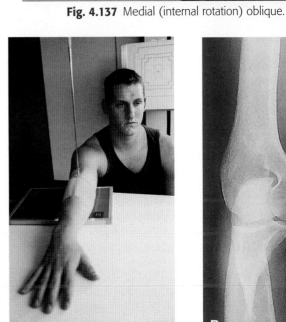

Fig. 4.137 Medial (internal rotation) oblique.

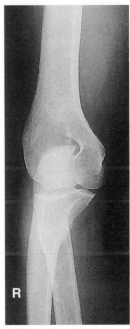

Fig. 4.138 End view, showing 45° medial oblique.

Fig. 4.139 Medial (internal rotation) oblique.

Evaluation Criteria
Anatomy Demonstrated: • Oblique view of distal humerus and proximal radius and ulna is visible (Figs. 4.139 and 4.140).
Position: • Long axis of arm should be aligned with side border of IR. • Correct 45° medial oblique should visualize coronoid process of the ulna in profile. • Radial head and neck should be superimposed and centered over the proximal ulna. • Medial epicondyle and trochlea should appear elongated and in partial profile. • Olecranon process should appear seated in olecranon fossa and trochlear notch partially open and visualized with arm fully extended. • CR and center of collimation field should be at **mid-elbow joint.**
Exposure: • Optimal density (brightness) and contrast with **no motion** should visualize soft tissue detail; bony cortical margins; and clear, bony trabecular markings.

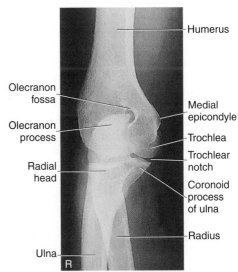

Fig. 4.140 Medial oblique of right elbow.

LATEROMEDIAL PROJECTION—ELBOW

Clinical Indications
- Fractures and dislocations of the elbow
- Certain bony pathologic processes, such as osteomyelitis and arthritis
- Elevated or displaced fat pads of the elbow joint may be visualized

Elbow
ROUTINE
• AP
• Alternate AP—partial flexion
• Alternate AP—acute flexion
• Oblique
• Lateral (external)
• Medial (internal)
• Lateral

Technical Factors
- Minimum SID—40 inches (100 cm)
- IR size—10 × 12 inches (24 × 30 cm), portrait; smallest IR available and collimate to area of interest
- Nongrid
- kVp range—65 to 75

Shielding Shield radiosensitive tissues outside region of interest.

Patient Position Seat patient at end of table, with elbow flexed 90° (see NOTE).

Part Position
- Align long axis of forearm with long axis of IR.
- Center elbow joint to CR and to center of IR.
- Drop shoulder so that humerus and forearm are on same horizontal plane.
- Rotate hand and wrist into true lateral position, thumb side up. Place interepicondylar plane perpendicular to the IR (Fig. 4.141).
- Place support under hand and wrist to elevate hand and distal forearm as needed for heavy muscular forearm so that forearm is parallel to IR for true lateral elbow.

CR
- CR perpendicular to IR, directed to **mid-elbow joint** (a point approximately 1½ inches [4 cm] medial to easily palpated posterior surface of olecranon process)

Recommended Collimation Collimate on four sides to area of interest.

NOTE: Diagnosis of certain important joint pathologic processes (e.g., possible visualization of the posterior fat pad) depends on 90° flexion of the elbow joint.[3]

EXCEPTION: Certain soft tissue diagnoses may require less flexion (30° to 35°), but these views should be taken only when specifically indicated.

Evaluation Criteria
Anatomy Demonstrated: • Lateral projection of distal humerus and proximal forearm, olecranon process, and soft tissues and fat pads of the elbow joint are visible (Figs. 4.142 and 4.143).
Position: • Long axis of the forearm should be aligned with long axis of IR, with the elbow joint flexed 90°. • About one-half of radial head should be superimposed by the coronoid process, and olecranon process should be visualized in profile. • True lateral view is indicated by three concentric arcs of the trochlear sulcus, double ridges of the capitulum and trochlea, and the trochlear notch of the ulna. In addition, superimposition of the humeral epicondyles occurs. • CR and center of collimation field should be **midpoint of the elbow joint.**
Exposure: • **No motion** and optimal density (brightness) and contrast should visualize sharp cortical margins and clear trabecular markings as well as soft tissue margins of the anterior and posterior fat pads.

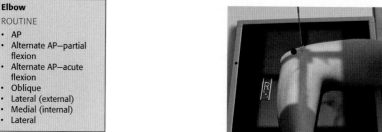

Fig. 4.141 Lateral—elbow flexed 90° (forearm parallel to IR).

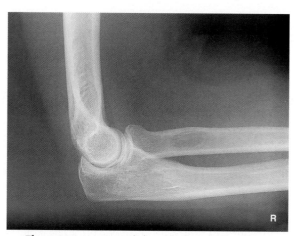

Fig. 4.142 Lateromedial projection of right elbow.

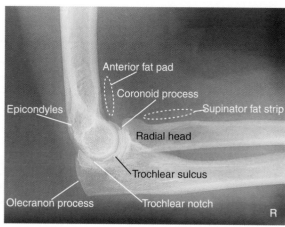

Fig. 4.143 Lateromedial projection of right elbow.

TRAUMA AXIAL LATEROMEDIAL AND MEDIOLATERAL PROJECTIONS: ELBOW

COYLE METHOD[15]

These are special projections taken for pathologic processes or trauma to the area of the radial head or the coronoid process of ulna. These are effective projections when the patient cannot extend the elbow fully for medial or lateral oblique projections of the elbow.

Clinical Indications
- Fractures and dislocations of the elbow, particularly the radial head (part position 1) and coronoid process (part position 2 for coronoid process)

Elbow
SPECIAL
- Trauma axial laterals (Coyle method)

Technical Factors
- Minimum SID—40 inches (100 cm)
- IR size—10 × 12 inches (24 × 30 cm), portrait; smallest IR available and collimate to area of interest
- Nongrid
- kVp range—70 to 80

30 R

24

Shielding Shield radiosensitive tissues outside region of interest.

Patient Position Seat patient at the end of the table for the erect position or supine on the table for horizontal beam imaging.

Part Position 1: Radial Head–Axial Lateromedial Projection
- Elbow flexed 90° if possible; **hand pronated**
- CR directed at **45° angle toward shoulder,** centered to radial head, mid-elbow joint (Figs. 4.144 and 4.146)

Part Position 2: Coronoid Process–Axial Mediolateral Projection
- Elbow flexed **only 80°** from extended position (because >80° may obscure coronoid process) and hand pronated
- CR angled **45° from shoulder,** into mid-elbow joint (Figs. 4.145 and 4.147)

Recommended Collimation Collimate on four sides to area of interest.

NOTE: Increase exposure factors by 4 to 6 kVp from lateral elbow because of angled CR. These projections are effective with or without a splint.

Evaluation Criteria
Radial Head: • Joint space between radial head and capitulum should be open and clear. • Radial head, neck, and tuberosity should be in profile and free of superimposition except for a small part of the coronoid process. • Distal humerus and epicondyles appear distorted because of 45° angle (Figs. 4.148 and 4.150).
Coronoid Process: • Anterior portion of the coronoid appears elongated but in profile. • Joint space between coronoid process and trochlea should be open and clear. • Radial head and neck should be superimposed by ulna. • Optimal exposure factors should visualize clearly the coronoid process in profile. Bony margins of superimposed radial head and neck should be visualized faintly through proximal ulna (Figs. 4.149 and 4.151).

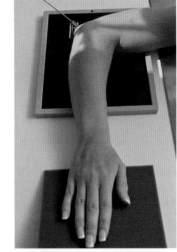
Fig. 4.144 Erect for **radial head**—flexed **90°**.

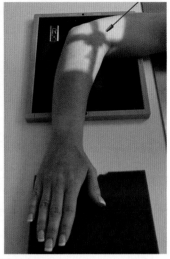
Fig. 4.145 Erect for **coronoid process**—flexed **80°**.

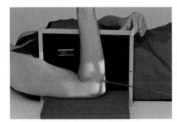
Fig. 4.146 Supine, angled 45° for radial head—flexed **90°**.

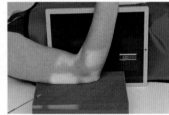
Fig. 4.147 Supine, angled 45° for coronoid process—flexed **80°**.

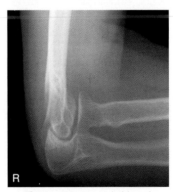
Fig. 4.148 For radial head.

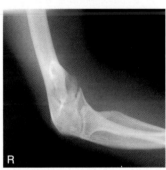
Fig. 4.149 For coronoid process.

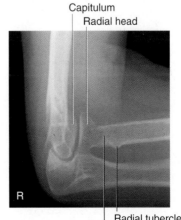
Capitulum
Radial head

Radial tubercle
Radial neck
Fig. 4.150 Axial lateromedial projection for radial head.

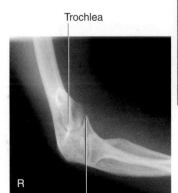
Trochlea

Coronoid process
Fig. 4.151 Axial mediolateral projection for coronoid process.

4

RADIAL HEAD—LATEROMEDIAL PROJECTIONS: ELBOW

Clinical Indications
- Occult fractures of the radial head or neck

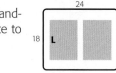

Elbow

SPECIAL
- Trauma axial laterals (Coyle method)
- Radial head laterals

Technical Factors
- Minimum SID—40 inches (100 cm)
- IR size—8 × 10 inches (18 × 24 cm), land-scape; smallest IR available and collimate to area of interest
- Nongrid
- kVp range—65 to 75

Shielding
Shield radiosensitive tissues outside region of interest.

Patient Position
Seat patient at end of table, with arm **flexed 90°** and resting on IR with humerus, forearm, and hand on same horizontal plane. Place support under hand and wrist if needed.

Part Position
- Center radial head area to center of IR, positioned so that distal humerus and proximal forearm are placed "square" with, or parallel with, the borders of IR.
- Center radial head region to CR.
- Take **four projections,** the only difference among the four being rotation of the hand and wrist from (1) maximum external rotation to (4) maximum internal rotation; different parts of the radial head projected clear of the coronoid process are demonstrated. Near-complete rotation of the radial head occurs in these four projections, as follows:
  1. Supinate hand (palm up) and externally rotate as far as patient can tolerate (Fig. 4.152).
  2. Place hand in true lateral position (thumb up) (Fig. 4.154).
  3. Pronate hand (palm down) (Fig. 4.156).
  4. Internally rotate hand (thumb down) as far as patient can tolerate (Fig. 4.158).

CR
- CR perpendicular to IR, directed to **radial head** (approximately 1 inch [2 to 3 cm] distal to lateral epicondyle)

Recommended Collimation
- Collimate on four sides to area of interest (including at least 3 to 4 inches [10 cm] of proximal forearm and distal portion of humerus).

Evaluation Criteria
- Elbow should be flexed 90° in true lateral position, as evidenced by direct superimposition of epicondyles. • Radial head and neck should be partially superimposed by ulna but completely visualized in profile in various projections. • **Radial tuberosity** should be visualized in various positions and degrees of profile as follows (see small arrows): (1) Fig. 4.153, slightly anterior; (2) Fig. 4.155, not in profile, superimposed over radial shaft; (3) Fig. 4.157, slightly posterior; (4) Fig. 4.159, seen posteriorly, adjacent to ulna when hand and wrist are at maximum internal rotation. • Optimal exposure with **no motion** should clearly visualize sharp, bony margins and clear trabecular markings of radial head and neck area.

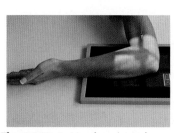

Fig. 4.152 1. Hand supinated (maximum external rotation).

Fig. 4.153 Hand supinated (maximum external rotation).

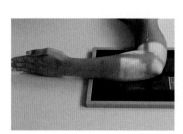
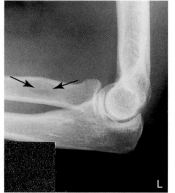

Fig. 4.154 2. Hand lateral.

Fig. 4.155 Hand lateral.

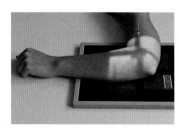
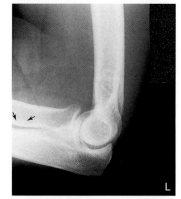

Fig. 4.156 3. Hand pronated.

Fig. 4.157 Hand pronated.

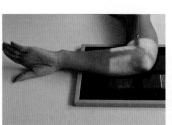
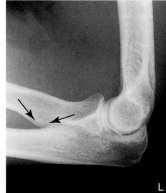

Fig. 4.158 4. Hand with maximum internal rotation.

Fig. 4.159 Hand with maximum internal rotation.

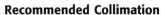

RADIOGRAPHS FOR CRITIQUE

This section consists of an ideal projection (Image A) along with one or more projections that may demonstrate positioning and/or technical errors. Critique Figures C4.160 through C4.165. Compare Image A to the other projections and identify the errors. While examining each image, consider the follow ing questions:

1. Is all essential anatomy demonstrated on the image?

2. What positioning errors are present that compromise image quality?
3. Are technical factors optimal?
4. Is there evidence of collimation and are pre-exposure anatomic side markers visible on the image?
5. Do these errors require a repeat exposure?
   Feedback for each set of images is located on the faculty Evolve site.

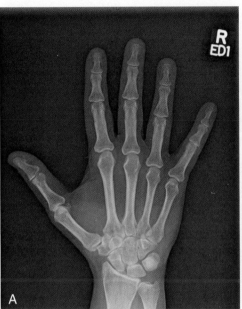 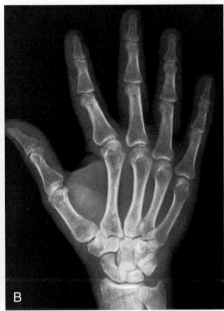 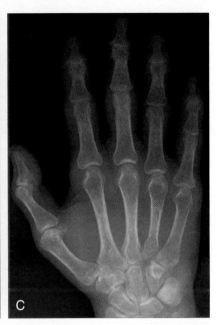

Fig. C4.160 PA hand.

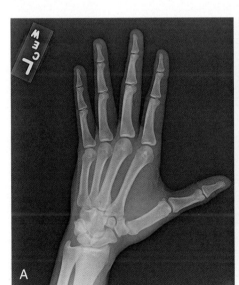 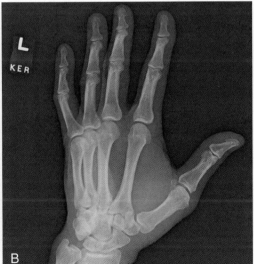 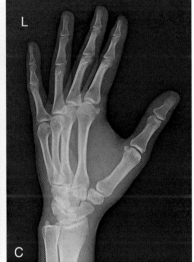

Fig. C4.161 PA oblique hand.

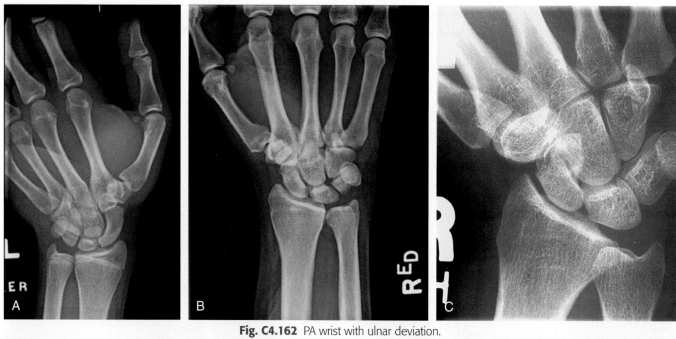

Fig. C4.162 PA wrist with ulnar deviation.

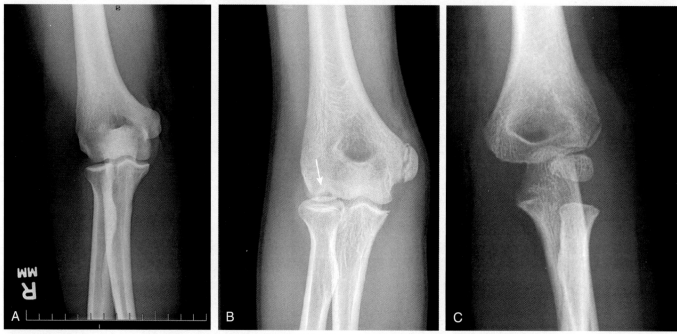

Fig. C4.163 AP elbow.

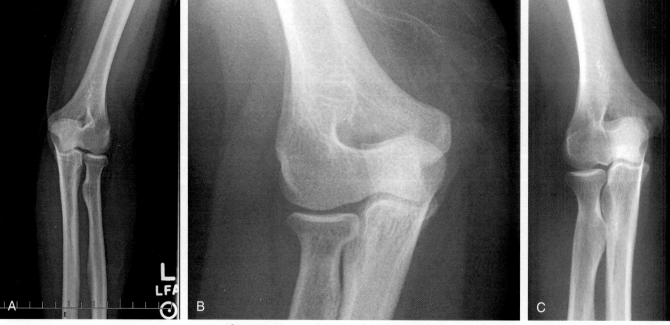

Fig. C4.164 Lateral (external) oblique elbow.

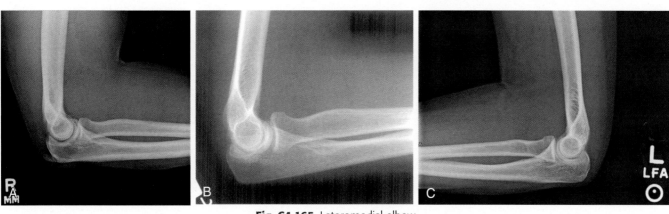

Fig. C4.165 Lateromedial elbow.

CHAPTER 5

Humerus and Shoulder Girdle

CONTRIBUTIONS BY **Christopher I. Wertz,** MSRS, RT(R)

CONTRIBUTORS TO PAST EDITIONS   John P. Lampignano, **MEd, RT(R)(CT)**, Dan L. Hobbs, MSRS, RT(R)(CT)(MR), Linda S. Lingar, MEd, RT(R)(M), Donna Davis, MEd, RT(R)(CV)

CONTENTS

RADIOGRAPHIC ANATOMY

Upper Limb (Extremity)

The hand, wrist, forearm, and elbow of the upper limb were described in Chapter 4. This chapter describes the humerus and the shoulder girdle, which includes the clavicle and scapula (Fig. 5.1).

HUMERUS

The **humerus** is the largest and longest bone of the upper limb. Its length on an adult equals approximately one-fifth of body height. The humerus articulates with the **scapula** (shoulder blade) at the shoulder joint. The anatomy of the distal humerus and of the elbow joint was described in Chapter 4.

Proximal Humerus

The proximal humerus is the part of the upper arm that articulates with the scapula, making up the shoulder joint. The most proximal part is the rounded **head** of the humerus. The slightly constricted area directly below and lateral to the head is the **anatomic neck,** which appears as a line of demarcation between the rounded head and the adjoining greater and lesser tubercles.

The process directly below the anatomic neck on the anterior surface is the **lesser tubercle** *(tu'-ber-k'l).* The larger lateral process is the **greater tubercle,** to which the pectoralis major and supraspinatus muscles attach. The deep groove between these two tubercles is the **intertubercular** *(in"-ter-tu-ber'-ku-lar)* sulcus (bicipital groove). The tapered area below the head and tubercles is the **surgical neck,** and distal to the surgical neck is the long **body** (shaft) of the humerus.

The surgical neck is so named because it is the site of frequent fractures requiring surgery. Fractures at the thick anatomic neck are rarer.

The **deltoid tuberosity** is the roughened raised triangular elevation along the anterolateral surface of the body (shaft) to which the deltoid muscle is attached.

Anatomy of Proximal Humerus on Radiograph

Fig. 5.2 shows a neutral rotation (natural position of the arm without internal or external rotation). This places the humerus in an oblique position midway between an anteroposterior (AP) (external rotation) and a lateral (internal rotation). Fig. 5.3 is an AP radiograph of the shoulder taken with **external rotation,** which places the humerus in a **true AP** or frontal position.

Some anatomic parts are more difficult to visualize on radiographs than on drawings. However, a good understanding of the location of various parts and the relationship between them helps in this identification. The following parts are shown in Fig. 5.3:

A. Head of humerus
B. Greater tubercle
C. Intertubercular sulcus
D. Lesser tubercle
E. Anatomic neck
F. Surgical neck
G. Body

The relative location of the greater and lesser tubercles is significant in determining a true frontal view or a true AP projection of the proximal humerus. The **lesser tubercle is located anteriorly and the greater tubercle is located laterally** in a true AP projection.

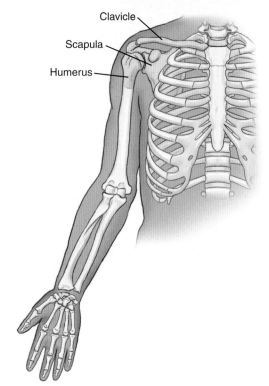

Fig 5.1 Shoulder girdle.

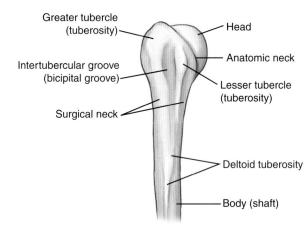

Fig 5.2 Frontal view of proximal humerus—neutral rotation (oblique position).

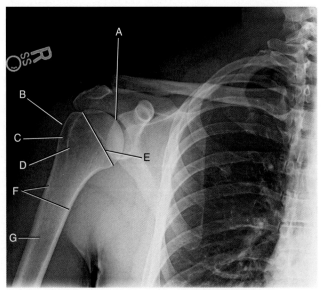

Fig 5.3 AP shoulder—external rotation.

SHOULDER GIRDLE

The shoulder girdle consists of two bones: the **clavicle** and the **scapula** (Fig. 5.4). The function of the clavicle and scapula is to connect each upper limb to the trunk or axial skeleton. Anteriorly, the shoulder girdle connects to the trunk at the upper sternum; however, posteriorly, the connection to the trunk is incomplete because the scapula is connected to the trunk by muscles only.

Each shoulder girdle and each upper limb connect at the shoulder joint between the scapula and the humerus. Each clavicle is located over the upper anterior rib cage. Each scapula is situated over the upper posterior rib cage.

The upper margin of the scapula is at the level of the **second posterior rib**, and the lower margin is at the level of the **seventh posterior rib** (T7). The lower margin of the scapula corresponds to T7, also used as a landmark for location of the central ray (CR) for chest positioning (see Chapter 2).

Clavicle

The **clavicle** (collarbone) is a long bone with a double curvature that has three main parts: two ends and a long central portion. The lateral or **acromial** *(ah-kro´-me-al)* extremity (end) of the clavicle articulates with the acromion of the scapula. This joint or articulation is called the **acromioclavicular** *(ah-kro´´-me-o-klah-vik´-u-lar)* joint and generally can be readily palpated.

The medial or **sternal extremity** (end) articulates with the manubrium, which is the upper part of the sternum. This articulation is called the **sternoclavicular** *(ster´´-no-klah-vik´-u-lar)* joint. This joint also is easily palpated, and the combination of the sternoclavicular joints on either side of the manubrium helps to form an important positioning landmark called the **jugular** *(jug´-u-lar)* **notch.**

The **body** (shaft) of the clavicle is the elongated portion between the two extremities. The acromial end of the clavicle is flattened and has a downward curvature at its attachment with the acromion. The sternal end is more triangular in shape, broader, and is directed downward to articulate with the sternum.

In general, the size and shape of the clavicle differ between males and females. The **female clavicle** is usually **shorter** and **less curved** than the male clavicle. The male clavicle tends to be thicker and more curved, usually being most curved in heavily muscled men.

Radiograph of the Clavicle The AP radiograph of the clavicle in Fig. 5.5 reveals the two joints and the three parts of the clavicle:
A. Sternoclavicular joint
B. Sternal extremity
C. Body
D. Acromial extremity
E. Acromioclavicular joint

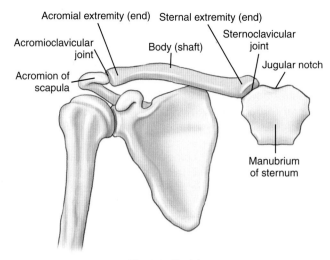

Fig 5.4 Clavicle.

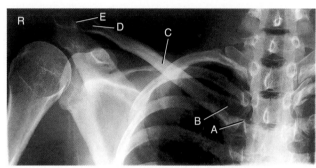

Fig 5.5 Radiograph of AP clavicle.

Scapula

The **scapula** (shoulder blade), which forms the posterior part of the shoulder girdle, is a flat triangular bone with three borders, three angles, and two surfaces. The three borders are the **medial (vertebral) border,** which is the long edge or border near the vertebrae; the **superior border,** or the uppermost margin of the scapula; and the **lateral (axillary) border,** or the border nearest the axilla *(ak-sil'-ah)* (Fig. 5.6). *Axilla* is the medical term for the armpit.

Anterior View The three corners of the triangular scapula are called *angles* (Fig. 5.7). The **lateral angle,** sometimes called the *head of the scapula,* is the thickest part and ends laterally in a shallow depression called the *glenoid cavity* (fossa).

The humeral head articulates with the glenoid cavity of the scapula to form the **scapulohumeral** *(skap"-u-lo-hu'-mer-al)* **joint,** also known as the *glenohumeral joint,* or *shoulder joint.*

The constricted area between the head and the body of the scapula is the **neck.** The **superior** and **inferior angles** refer to the upper and lower ends of the medial or vertebral border. The **body** (blade) of the scapula is arched for greater strength. The thin, flat, lower part of the body sometimes is referred to as the *wing* or *ala* of the scapula, although these are not preferred anatomic terms.

The anterior surface of the scapula is termed the **costal** *(kos'-tal)* **surface** because of its proximity to the ribs (*costa* literally means "rib"). The middle area of the costal surface presents a large concavity or depression, known as the **subscapular fossa.**

The **acromion** is a long, curved process that extends laterally over the head of the humerus. The **coracoid process** is a thick, beaklike process that projects anteriorly beneath the clavicle. The **suprascapular notch** is a notch on the superior border that is partially formed by the base of the coracoid process.

Posterior View Fig. 5.8 shows a prominent structure on the dorsal, or posterior, surface of the scapula, called the **spine.** The elevated spine of the scapula starts at the vertebral border as a smooth triangular area and continues laterally to end at the **acromion.** The acromion overhangs the shoulder joint posteriorly.

The posterior border or ridge of the spine is thickened and is termed the **crest** of the spine. The spine separates the posterior surface into an **infraspinous** *(in"-frah-spi'-nus)* **fossa** and a **supraspinous fossa.** Both fossae serve as surfaces of attachment for shoulder muscles. The names of these muscles are associated with their respective fossae.

Lateral View The lateral view of the scapula demonstrates relative positions of the various parts of the scapula (Fig. 5.9). The thin scapula looks like the letter Y in this position. The upper parts of the Y are the acromion and the coracoid process. The **acromion** is the expanded distal end of the spine that extends superiorly and posteriorly to the glenoid cavity (fossa). The **coracoid process** is located more anteriorly in relationship to the glenoid cavity or shoulder joint.

The lower portion of the Y is the body of the scapula. The posterior surface or back portion of the thin body portion of the scapula is the **dorsal surface.** The **spine** extends from the dorsal surface at its upper margin. The anterior surface of the body is the **ventral (costal) surface.** The **lateral (axillary) border** is a thicker edge or border that extends from the **glenoid cavity** to the **inferior angle** (see Fig. 5.9)

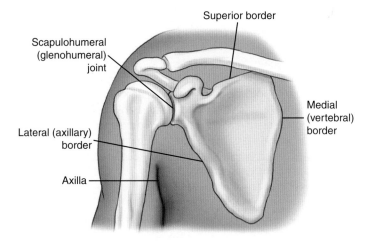

Fig 5.6 Scapula—three borders and scapulohumeral (glenohumeral) joint.

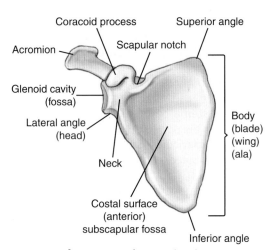

Fig 5.7 Scapula—anterior view.

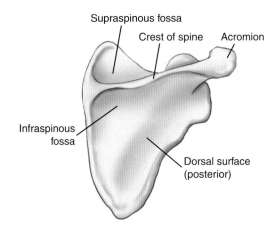

Fig 5.8 Scapula—posterior view.

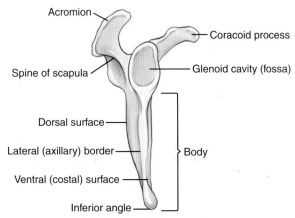

Fig 5.9 Scapula—lateral view.

REVIEW EXERCISE WITH RADIOGRAPHS

AP Projection

Fig. 5.10 is an AP projection of the scapula taken with the arm abducted so as not to superimpose the scapula. Knowing the shapes and relationships of anatomic parts should help one to identify each of the following parts:

A. Acromion
B. Neck of scapula (approximately 1 inch [2.5 cm] below the coracoid process)
C. Suprascapular notch
D. Superior angle
E. Medial (vertebral) border
F. Inferior angle
G. Lateral (axillary) border
H. Glenoid cavity (fossa) or scapulohumeral joint

Lateral Projection

In Fig. 5.11 the posteroanterior (PA) oblique–scapular Y lateral projection of the scapula was taken with the patient in an anterior oblique position and with the upper body rotated until the scapula is separated from the rib cage in a true end-on or lateral projection. This lateral view of the scapula presents a Y shape, wherein the acromion and the coracoid process make up the upper legs of the Y, and the body makes up the long lower leg. The scapular Y position gets its name from this Y shape, resulting from a true lateral view of the scapula.

The labeled parts as seen on this view are as follows:

A. Acromion
B. Coracoid process
C. Inferior angle
D. Spine of scapula
E. Body of scapula

Proximal Humerus and Scapula

Inferosuperior Axial Projection This projection (as shown in Fig. 5.12) results in a lateral view of the head and neck of the humerus. It also demonstrates the relationship of the humerus to the glenoid cavity, which makes up the scapulohumeral (glenohumeral) joint.

The anatomy of the scapula may appear confusing in this position, but understanding the relationships between the various parts facilitates identification.

Part A of Fig. 5.13 is the tip of the **coracoid process,** which is located anterior to the shoulder joint and would be seen superiorly with the patient lying on her back (see Fig. 5.12).

Part B is the **glenoid cavity,** which is the articulating surface of the **lateral angle** or **head** of the scapula.

Part C is the **spine** of the scapula, which is located posteriorly with the patient lying on her back (see Fig. 5.12).

Part D is the **acromion,** which is the extended portion of the spine that is superimposed over the humerus in this position.

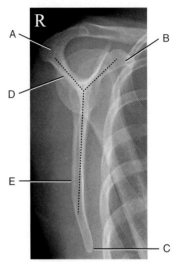

Fig 5.11 PA oblique (scapular Y position). (Courtesy Joss Wertz, DO.)

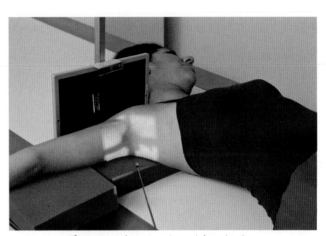

Fig 5.12 Inferosuperior axial projection.

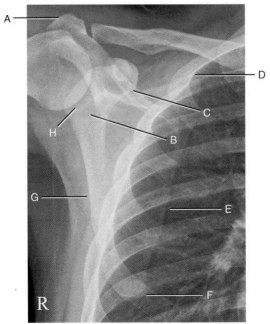

Fig 5.10 AP scapula projection. (Courtesy Joss Wertz, DO.)

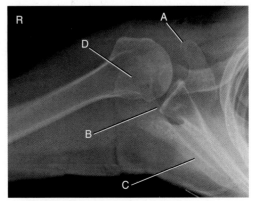

Fig 5.13 Inferosuperior axial projection.

CLASSIFICATION OF JOINTS

Three joints or articulations are involved in the shoulder girdle: **sternoclavicular joint, acromioclavicular joint,** and **scapulo-humeral joint** (glenohumeral or shoulder joint) (Fig. 5.14).

Classification

The three shoulder girdle joints (articulations) classified as **synovial joints** are characterized by a fibrous capsule that contains synovial fluid.

Mobility Type

The mobility type of all three of these joints is freely movable, or **diarthrodial.** All synovial joints are by nature of their structure freely movable. The only difference between these three joints is their movement type.

Movement Type

The **scapulohumeral** (glenohumeral) or shoulder joint involves articulation between the head of the humerus and the glenoid cavity of the scapula. The movement type is a **ball-and-socket (spheroidal) joint,** which allows great freedom of movement. These movements include **flexion, extension, abduction, adduction, circumduction,** and **medial** (internal) and **lateral** (external) **rotation.**

The glenoid cavity is very shallow, allowing the greatest freedom in mobility of any joint in the human body but at some expense to its strength and stability. Strong ligaments, tendons, and muscles surround the joint, providing stability. However, stretching of the muscles and tendons can cause separation or dislocation of the humeral head from the glenoid cavity. Dislocations at the shoulder joint occur more frequently than at any other joint in the body, creating the need for frequent radiographic examinations of the shoulder to evaluate for structural damage. The shoulder girdle also includes two joints involving both ends of the clavicle, called the *sternoclavicular* and *acromioclavicular joints.*

The **sternoclavicular joint** is a **double plane,** or **gliding, joint** because the sternal end of the clavicle articulates with the manubrium or upper portion of the sternum and the cartilage of the first rib. A limited amount of gliding motion occurs in nearly every direction.

The **acromioclavicular joint** is also a small synovial joint of the **plane, or gliding, movementtype** between the acromial end of the clavicle and the medial aspect of the acromion of the scapula. Two types of movement occur at this joint. The primary movement is a gliding action between the end of the clavicle and the acromion. Some secondary rotary movement also occurs as the scapula moves forward and backward with the clavicle. This movement allows the scapula to adjust its position as it remains in close contact with the posterior chest wall. However, the rotary type of movement is limited, and this joint generally is referred to as a plane, or gliding-type, joint. Table 5.1 presents a summary of the shoulder girdle joints.

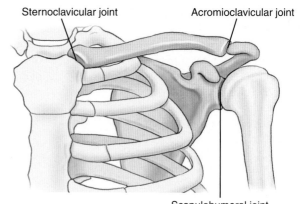

Fig 5.14 Joints of shoulder girdle.

TABLE 5.1 SUMMARY OF SHOULDER GIRDLE JOINTS

Classification
Synovial (articular capsule containing synovial fluid)
Mobility Type
Diarthrodial (freely movable)

Movement Types	
1. Scapulohumeral (glenohumeral) joint	**Ball and socket** or **spheroidal**
2. Sternoclavicular joint	**Plane** or **gliding**
3. Acromioclavicular joint	**Plane** or **gliding**

RADIOGRAPHIC POSITIONING

Proximal Humerus Rotation

RADIOGRAPHS OF THE PROXIMAL HUMERUS

Rotational views of the proximal humerus or shoulder girdle are commonly taken on nontrauma patients when gross fractures or dislocations of the humerus have been ruled out. These AP rotational projections delineate well the scapulohumeral joint (shoulder joint), revealing possible calcium deposits or other pathology. Note specifically the location and shapes of the **greater tubercle** (A) and the **lesser tubercle** (B) on these external, internal, and neutral rotation radiographs (Figs. 5.16, 5.18, and 5.20).

By studying the position and relationships of the greater and lesser tubercles on a radiograph of the shoulder, you can determine the rotational position of the arm. This understanding enables you to know which rotational view is necessary for visualization of specific parts of the proximal humerus.

External Rotation

The external rotation position represents a true **AP projection** of the humerus in the anatomic position, as determined by the epicondyles of the distal humerus. Positioning requires supination of the hand and external rotation of the elbow so that the interepicondylar line is **parallel to the image receptor (IR)** (Fig. 5.15).

NOTE: You can check this on yourself by dropping your arm at your side and externally rotating your hand and arm while palpating the epicondyles of your distal humerus.

On the external rotation radiograph (see Fig. 5.16), the **greater tubercle** (A), which is located anteriorly in a neutral position, is now seen **laterally in profile.** The **lesser tubercle** (B) now is located **anteriorly,** just medial to the greater tubercle.

Internal Rotation

For the internal rotation position, the hand and arm are rotated internally until the epicondyles of the distal humerus are **perpendicular to the IR**, placing the humerus in a **true lateral position.** The hand must be pronated and the elbow adjusted to place the epicondyles **perpendicular to the IR** (Fig. 5.17).

The AP projection of the shoulder taken in the internal rotation position (see Fig. 5.18) is a lateral position of the proximal humerus in which the **greater tubercle** (A) now is rotated around to the anterior and medial aspect of the proximal humerus. The **lesser tubercle** (B) is seen in profile medially.

Neutral Rotation

Neutral rotation is appropriate for a trauma patient when rotation of the part is unacceptable. The epicondyles of the distal humerus appear at an **approximate 45° angle to the IR** (Fig. 5.19). A 45° oblique position of the humerus results when the **palm of the hand is facing inward** toward the thigh. The neutral position is approximately midway between the external and internal positions and places the greater tubercle anteriorly but still lateral to the lesser tubercle, as can be seen on the radiograph in Fig. 5.20.

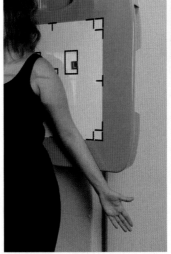
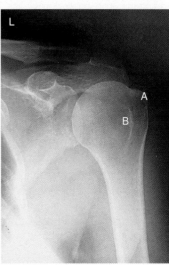

Fig. 5.15 External rotation (AP projection of humerus).

Fig. 5.16 External rotation (AP projection of humerus).

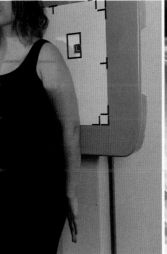
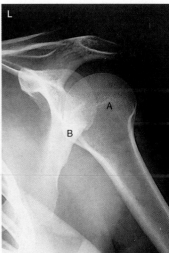

Fig. 5.17 Internal rotation (lateral projection of humerus).

Fig. 5.18 Internal rotation (lateral projection of humerus).

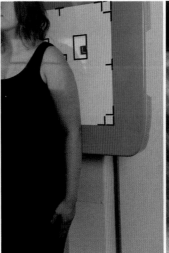
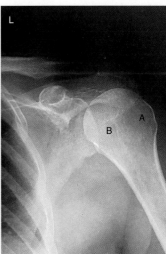

Fig. 5.19 Neutral rotation (oblique projection of humerus).

Fig. 5.20 Neutral rotation (oblique projection of humerus).

Positioning and Exposure Considerations

General positioning considerations for the humerus and shoulder girdle (clavicle and scapula) are similar to those for other upper and lower limb procedures.

Technical Considerations

Depending on part thickness, the humerus can be exposed with or without a grid. Grids generally are used when the humerus projection is performed erect with the use of a Bucky. However, adult shoulders generally measure 10 to 15 cm, and the use of a grid is required. Other technical considerations are listed subsequently. Children and thin, asthenic adults may measure less than 10 cm, requiring exposure factor adjustments without the use of grids. Acromioclavicular (AC) joints generally also measure less than 10 cm and require less kVp (70 to 75) without grids. However, this practice can vary, depending on department protocol, and grids are often used for AC joints to reduce scatter radiation. But the use of a grid results in added dose to the patient caused by the required increase in exposure factors.

AVERAGE ADULT HUMERUS AND SHOULDER

1. Medium kVp, 70 to 85, with grid for shoulder thickness >10 cm (<10 cm, 70 to 75 kVp without grid)
2. Higher milliampere (mA) with short exposure times
3. Small focal spot
4. Center cell for automatic exposure control (AEC) if used for the shoulder (manual techniques may be recommended with certain projections, such as humerus and AC joints)
5. Adequate mAs for sufficient density (brightness) (for visualization of soft tissues, bone margins, and trabecular markings of all bones)
6. 40- to 44-inch (100- to 110-cm) source–image receptor distance (SID) except for AC joints, which may use a 72-inch (180-cm) SID for less beam divergence. This is highly effective in demonstrating comparative studies of the AC joints with both joints in a single exposure.
7. Compensating filter: The use of a boomerang filter for AP projections of the shoulder and scapula permits both soft tissues and bony anatomy to be demonstrated clearly. It is especially effective in demonstrating the acromion and AC joint region while allowing for optimal visualization of the denser shoulder joint region (Figs. 5.21 and 5.22).

Radiation Protection

GONADAL SHIELDING

Generally, gonadal shielding is important for upper limb radiography because of the proximity of parts of the upper limb, such as the hands or wrists, to the gonads when radiography is performed with the patient in a supine position. The relationship of the divergent x-ray beam to the pelvic region when a patient is in an erect seated position also necessitates gonadal protection. Protecting radiosensitive regions of the body whenever possible for procedures is good practice and reassures the patient.

SHIELDING OF THYROID, LUNGS, AND BREASTS

Radiography of the shoulder region may deliver potentially significant doses to the thyroid, lung regions, and to the breasts, all of which are radiosensitive organs. **Close collimation** to the area of interest is important, as is providing **contact shields** over portions of the lungs, breast, and thyroid regions that do not obscure the area of interest.

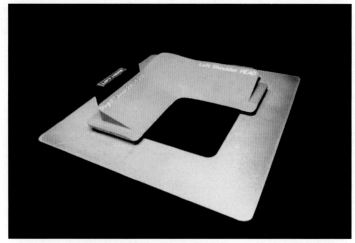

Fig 5.21 Boomerang filter. (Ferlic, Inc.)

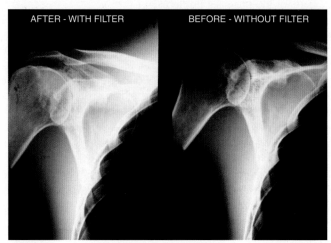

AFTER - WITH FILTER   BEFORE - WITHOUT FILTER

Fig 5.22 AP projection of shoulder with and without use of boomerang filter. (Ferlic, Inc)

Special Patient Considerations

PEDIATRIC APPLICATIONS

The routines used for radiographic examinations of the humerus and shoulder girdle generally do not vary significantly from adult to pediatric patients, although it is essential that exposure technique be decreased to compensate for the decrease in tissue quantity and density (brightness). **Patient motion** plays an important role in pediatric radiography. Immobilization often is necessary to assist the child in maintaining the proper position. Sponges and tape are very useful, but caution is necessary when sandbags are used because of the weight of the sandbags.

Parents frequently are asked to assist with the radiographic examination of their child. If parents are permitted in the radiography room during the exposure, proper shielding must be provided. To ensure maximum cooperation, the technologist should speak to the child in a soothing manner and should use words that the child can easily understand.

GERIATRIC APPLICATIONS

It is essential to provide clear and complete instructions to an older patient. Routine humerus and shoulder girdle examinations may have to be altered to accommodate the physical condition of an older patient. Reduction in radiographic technique may be necessary as a result of destructive pathologies commonly seen in geriatric patients.

BARIATRIC PATIENT CONSIDERATIONS

With bariatric patients, alternative palpation points (the jugular notch and AC joint) should be used for shoulder projections instead of the coracoid process. If you choose to use the AC joint to identify the shoulder joint, go 2 inches (5 cm) inferior to the AC joint and ½ inch (1.25 cm) medial to locate the scapulohumeral joint.

Use a boomerang compensating filter for AP projections of the shoulder and scapula because of the increased shoulder thickness. This permits greater visibility of both soft tissue and bony anatomy. Perform positions erect when possible for patient comfort and to reduce object–image receptor distance (OID) and part distortion as a result of curved shoulders. Collimation is critical to reduce scatter reaching the image receptor. The proximal humerus should be performed with a grid. Although it will add to the patient dose, it will reduce scatter radiation and increase image contrast and visibility of the anatomy.

Digital Imaging Considerations

Specific guidelines should be followed when digital imaging systems are used for imaging the humerus and shoulder girdle. These guidelines were described in greater detail in Chapter 4 for the upper limb and are summarized here:

1. **Collimation:** Close collimation is important for ensuring that the final image after processing is of optimal quality.
2. **Accurate centering:** Because of the way the digital image plate reader scans the exposed imaging plate, it is important that the body part and the CR be accurately centered to the IR.
3. **Exposure factors:** With regard to patient exposure, the ALARA principle (as low as reasonably achievable) must be followed: the lowest exposure factors required to obtain a diagnostic image should be used. This involves using the highest kVp and the lowest mAs that result in a final image of diagnostic quality.
4. **Post-processing evaluation of exposure indicator:** After the image has been processed and is ready for viewing, the technologist must assess the exposure indicator to verify that the exposure factors used met ALARA standards and produced a quality image.

Alternative Modalities and Procedures

ARTHROGRAPHY

Arthrography sometimes is used to image soft tissue pathologies such as rotator cuff tears associated with the shoulder girdle. This procedure, which is described in greater detail in Chapter 19, requires the use of a radiographic contrast medium injected into the joint capsule under fluoroscopy and sterile conditions.

COMPUTED TOMOGRAPHY (CT) AND MAGNETIC RESONANCE IMAGING (MRI)

CT and MRI often are used on the shoulder to evaluate soft tissue and skeletal involvement of lesions and soft tissue injuries. Sectional CT images also are excellent for determining the extent of fracture. MRI, with or without the use of a contrast agent, is useful in the diagnosis of rotator cuff injuries. CT arthrography, as described in Chapter 18, can be performed instead of or in conjunction with conventional arthrography.

NUCLEAR MEDICINE (NM)

Nuclear medicine bone scans are useful in demonstrating osteomyelitis, metastatic bone lesions, and cellulitis. Nuclear medicine scans demonstrate pathology within 24 hours of onset. Nuclear medicine is more sensitive than radiography because it assesses the physiologic aspect instead of the anatomic aspect.

SONOGRAPHY

Ultrasound is useful for musculoskeletal imaging of joints such as the shoulder to evaluate soft tissues within the joint for possible rotator cuff tears; bursa injuries; or disruption and damage to nerves, tendons, or ligaments. These studies can be used as an adjunct to more expensive MRI studies. Ultrasound also allows for dynamic evaluation during joint movement.

Clinical Indications

Clinical indications involving the shoulder girdle with which all technologists should be familiar include the following conditions.

AC joint separation refers to trauma to the upper shoulder region resulting in a partial or complete tear of the AC or coracoclavicular (CC) ligament or both ligaments. AC joint injuries represent nearly half of all athletic shoulder injuries, often resulting from a fall onto the tip of the shoulder with the arm in adduction. Currently there are six classifications of AC joint separation, ranging from a sprain to a complete separation of the distal clavicle from acromion as a result of ligament tears.[1]

Acromioclavicular dislocation refers to an injury in which the distal clavicle usually is displaced superiorly. This injury most commonly is caused by a fall and is more common in children than adults.[2]

Bankart lesion is an injury of the anteroinferior aspect of the glenoid labrum. This type of injury often is caused by anterior dislocation of the proximal humerus. Repeated dislocation may result in a small avulsion fracture in the anteroinferior region of the glenoid rim.

Bursitis *(ber-sy'-tis)* is an inflammation of the bursae, or fluid-filled sacs enclosing the joints. The shoulder is the most common joint to develop bursitis, with repetitive motion being the most common cause. However, trauma, rheumatoid arthritis, and infection can also produce bursitis.[3] It generally involves the formation of calcification in associated tendons, causing pain and limitation of joint movement.

Hill-Sachs defect is a compression fracture of the articular surface of the posterolateral aspect of the humeral head that often is associated with an anterior dislocation of the humeral head.

Idiopathic chronic adhesive capsulitis (frozen shoulder) is a disability of the shoulder joint that is caused by chronic inflammation in and around the joint. It is characterized by pain and limitation of motion. (*Idiopathic* means of unknown cause.)

Impingement syndrome is impingement of the greater tuberosity and soft tissues on the coracoacromial ligamentous and osseous arch, generally during abduction of the arm.[4]

Osteoarthritis, also called **degenerative joint disease (DJD),** is a noninflammatory joint disease characterized by gradual deterioration of the articular cartilage with hypertrophic bone formation. DJD is the most common type of arthritis and is considered part of the normal aging process. It generally occurs in persons older than 50 years, chronically bariatric persons, and athletes.

Osteoporosis (*os″-te-o-po-ro′-sis*) and resultant fractures are to the result of a reduction in the quantity of bone or atrophy of skeletal tissue. Osteoporosis occurs in postmenopausal women and elderly men, resulting in bony trabeculae that are scanty and thin. Most fractures sustained by women older than 50 years are related to osteoporosis.

Rheumatoid (*ru′-ma-toyd*) **arthritis (RA)** is a chronic systemic disease characterized by inflammatory changes that occur throughout the connective tissues of the body. The inflammation begins in synovial membranes and can later involve the articular cartilage and bony cortex. RA occurs more frequently in women than men. Radiographic evidence of RA includes loss of joint space, destruction cortical bone and bony deformity.[1]

Rotator cuff pathology is an acute or a chronic traumatic injury to one or more of the rotator cuff muscles: teres minor, supraspinatus, infraspinatus, and subscapularis. Rotator cuff injuries limit the range of motion of the shoulder. The most common injury of the rotator cuff is impingement of the supraspinatus tendon as it passes beneath the acromion, caused by a subacromial bone spur. Repeated irritation associated with the bone spur can lead to a partial or complete tear of the supraspinatus tendon, as evident on MRI and sonographic examination of the shoulder (Figs. 5.23 and 5.24).

Shoulder dislocation is traumatic removal of the humeral head from the glenoid cavity. Of shoulder dislocations, 95% are anterior, in which the humeral head is projected anterior to the glenoid cavity.

Tendonitis (*ten″-de-ni′-tis*) is an inflammatory condition of the tendon that usually results from a strain.

Table 5.2 presents a summary of clinical indications.

Routine, Alternate, and Special Projections

Routine, alternate, and special projections of the humerus, shoulder, clavicle, AC joints, and scapula are demonstrated and described on the following pages.

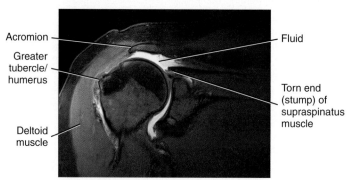

Fig 5.23 MRI showing full-thickness tear of supraspinatus tendon.

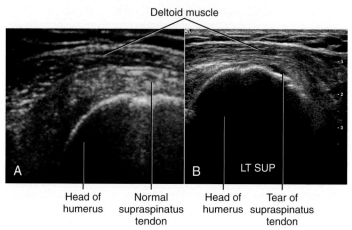

Fig 5.24 Ultrasound scans of normal supraspinatus tendon (A) and tear of supraspinatus tendon (B).

TABLE 5.2 **SUMMARY OF CLINICAL INDICATIONS**			
CONDITION OR DISEASE	**MOST COMMON RADIOGRAPHIC EXAMINATION**	**POSSIBLE RADIOGRAPHIC APPEARANCE**	**EXPOSURE FACTOR ADJUSTMENT[a]**
AC dislocation	Unilateral or bilateral, erect AC joints	Widening of AC joint space	None
AC joint separation	Unilateral or bilateral, erect AC joints (with and without weights) or Zanca method	Asymmetric widening of AC joint compared with contralateral (opposite) side[13]	None
Bankart lesion	AP internal rotation, PA oblique (scapular Y), and AP oblique (Grashey)	Possible small avulsion fracture of anteroinferior aspect of glenoid rim	None
Bursitis	AP and lateral shoulder	Fluid-filled joint space with possible calcification	None
Hill-Sachs defect	AP internal rotation and transaxillary with exaggerated external rotation	Compression fracture and possible anterior dislocation of humeral head	None
Idiopathic chronic adhesive capsulitis (frozen shoulder)	AP rotation shoulder and PA oblique (Scapular Y-Neer method) projection shoulder	Possible calcification or other joint space abnormalities	None
Impingement syndrome	Apical AP axial shoulder PA oblique (scapular Y), Neer method	Possible bone spurs near acromiohumeral space	None
Osteoarthritis	AP and lateral shoulder	Narrowing of joint space	Decrease (−)
Osteoporosis (resultant fractures)	AP and lateral shoulder	Thin bony cortex	Decrease (−)
Rheumatoid arthritis (RA)	AP and lateral shoulder	Loss of joint space, bony erosion, bony deformity	Decrease (−)
Rotator cuff injury	MRI or sonography	Partial or complete tear in musculature	Not applicable
Shoulder dislocation	PA oblique (scapular Y), transthoracic lateral, or Garth method	Separation between humeral head and glenoid cavity	None
Tendonitis	Neer method, MRI, or sonography	Calcified tendons	None

[a]Depends on stage or severity of disease or condition. Exposure adjustments apply primarily to the use of manual exposure factors.

AP PROJECTION: HUMERUS

WARNING: Do not attempt to rotate the arm if a fracture or dislocation is suspected.

Clinical Indications
- Fracture and dislocation of the humerus
- Pathologic processes, including osteoporosis

Humerus
ROUTINE
• AP
• Rotational lateral

Technical Factors
- Minimum SID—40 inches (100 cm)
- IR size—portrait (large enough to include entire humerus)
- 14 × 17 inches (35 × 43 cm) may be needed to place cassette diagonally to include both joints
- For pediatric patient, 10 × 12 inches (24 × 30 cm)
- Grid (nongrid for humerus <10 cm thickness)
- kVp range: 70–85

Shielding Shield radiosensitive tissues outside region of interest.

Patient Position Position patient erect or supine. Adjust the height of the cassette so that shoulder and elbow joints are equidistant from ends of IR (Figs. 5.25 and 5.26).

Part Position
- Rotate body toward affected side as needed to bring shoulder and proximal humerus into contact with cassette.
- Align humerus with long axis of IR, unless diagonal placement is needed to include both shoulder and elbow joints.
- Extend hand and forearm as far as patient can tolerate.
- Abduct arm slightly and gently supinate hand so that **epicondyles of elbow are parallel and equidistant** from IR.

CR
- CR perpendicular to IR, directed to **midpoint of humerus**

Recommended Collimation Collimate on sides to soft tissue borders of humerus and shoulder. (Lower margin of collimation field should include the elbow joint and approximately 1 inch (2.5 cm) minimum of proximal forearm.)

Respiration Suspend respiration during exposure.

Evaluation Criteria
Anatomy Demonstrated: • AP projection shows the entire humerus, including the shoulder and elbow joints (Figs. 5.27 and 5.28).
Position: • Long axis of humerus should be aligned with long axis of IR. • **True AP** projection is evidenced at proximal humerus by the following: greater tubercle is seen in profile laterally; humeral head is partially seen in profile medially, with minimal superimposition of the glenoid cavity. • Distal humerus: lateral and medial epicondyles both are visualized in profile. • Collimation to area of interest.
Exposure: • Optimal density (brightness) and contrast with **no motion** visualize sharp cortical margins and clear, bony trabecular markings at both proximal and distal portions of the humerus.

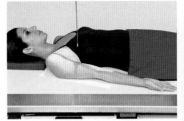

Fig 5.25 AP supine.

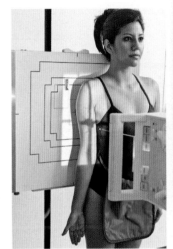

Fig 5.26 AP—erect.

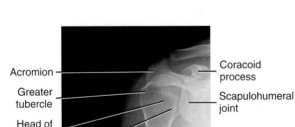

Fig 5.27 AP humerus projection.

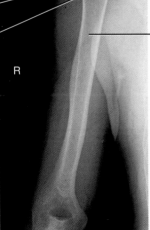

Acromion
Greater tubercle
Head of humerus
Lesser tubercle
Coracoid process
Scapulohumeral joint
Proximal humerus

Fig 5.28 AP humerus projection.

5

ROTATIONAL LATERAL–LATEROMEDIAL OR MEDIOLATERAL PROJECTIONS: HUMERUS

WARNING: Do not attempt to rotate the arm if a fracture or dislocation is suspected (see Trauma Horizontal Beam Lateral, p. 189).

Clinical Indications
- Fracture and dislocation of the humerus
- Pathologic processes including osteoporosis

Humerus
ROUTINE
• AP
• Rotational lateral

Technical Factors
- Minimum SID—40 inches (100 cm)
- IR size—portrait (large enough to include entire humerus)
- 14 × 17 inches (35 × 43 cm)
- For pediatric patient, 10 × 12 inches (24 × 30 cm)
- Grid (nongrid for humerus <10 cm thickness)
- kVp range: 70–85

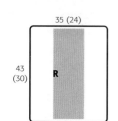

Shielding Shield radiosensitive tissues outside region of interest.

Patient and Part Position
- Position patient erect or supine as for lateromedial or mediolateral projection.
- **Lateromedial:** Position patient erect with back to IR and elbow partially flexed, with body rotated toward affected side as needed to bring humerus and shoulder in contact with cassette. **Internally rotate arm** as needed for lateral position; **epicondyles are perpendicular** to IR (Figs. 5.29 and 5.30).
- **Mediolateral:** Face patient toward IR (Fig. 5.31) and oblique as needed (20° to 30° from PA) to allow close contact of humerus with IR; flex elbow 90° as shown.
- Adjust image receptor height so that shoulders and elbow joints are equidistant from ends of it.

CR
- CR perpendicular to IR, centered to **midpoint of humerus**

Recommended Collimation Collimate on four sides to soft tissue border of humerus, ensuring that all of shoulder and elbow joints are included (Fig. 5.32).

Respiration Suspend respiration during exposure.

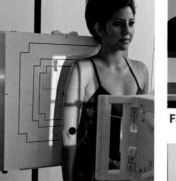

Fig 5.29 Erect lateral-lateromedial projection, back to IR.

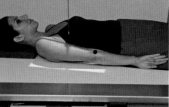

Fig 5.30 Supine lateral projection.

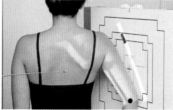

Fig 5.31 Erect lateral-mediolateral projection, facing IR.

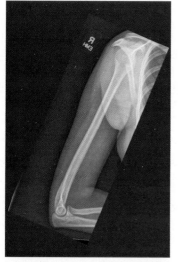

Fig 5.32 Erect mediolateral humerus projection. (Courtesy Joss Wertz, DO.)

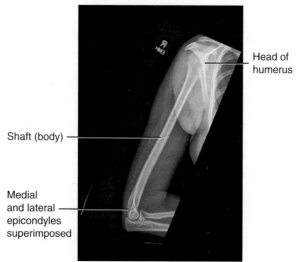

Head of humerus

Shaft (body)

Medial and lateral epicondyles superimposed

Fig 5.33 Mediolateral projection. (Courtesy Joss Wertz, DO.)

Evaluation Criteria
Anatomy Demonstrated: • Lateral projection of the entire humerus, including elbow and shoulder joints, is visible (see Fig. 5.32 and also Fig. 5.33).
Position: • True lateral projection is evidenced by the following: epicondyles are directly superimposed; lesser tubercle is shown in profile medially, partially superimposed by lower portion of glenoid cavity. • Collimation to area of interest.
Exposure: • Optimal density (brightness) and contrast with **no motion** visualize clear, sharp bony trabecular markings of entire humerus.

TRAUMA HORIZONTAL BEAM LATERAL—LATEROMEDIAL PROJECTION: MID-TO-DISTAL HUMERUS

DISTAL HUMERUS

WARNING: Do not attempt to rotate the arm if a fracture or dislocation is suspected.

This projection is used in conjunction with the Transthoracic Lateral, p. 14.

Clinical Indications

- Fractures and dislocations of the mid-humerus and distal humerus
- Pathologic processes, including osteoporosis

Humerus
ROUTINE
• AP
• Rotational lateral
SPECIAL (TRAUMA)
• Horizontal beam lateral
• Transthoracic lateral

Technical Factors

- Minimum SID—40 inches (100 cm)
- IR size—14 × 17 inches (35 × 43 cm); for smaller patient, 10 × 12 inches (24 × 30 cm) landscape
- Nongrid
- kVp range: 70–85

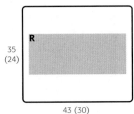

35 (24)

R

43 (30)

Shielding Shield radiosensitive tissues outside region of interest.

Patient and Part Position

- With patient recumbent, perform image as a horizontal beam lateral, placing support under the arm (Fig. 5.34).
- Flex elbow if possible, but do not attempt to rotate arm; projection should be 90° from AP.
- Gently place image receptor between arm and thorax (top of IR to axilla).

CR

- CR perpendicular to midpoint of distal two-thirds of humerus

Recommended Collimation Collimate to soft tissue margins. Include distal humerus and midhumerus, elbow joint, and proximal forearm.

Respiration Suspend respiration during exposure. (This step is important in preventing movement of the image receptor during the exposure.)

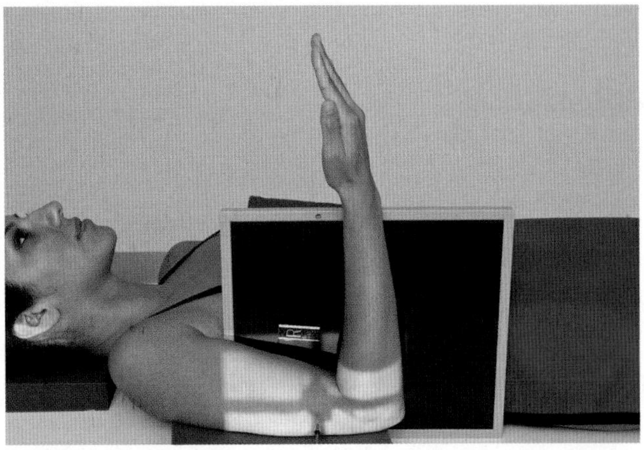

Fig 5.34 Horizontal beam lateral (midhumerus and distal humerus).

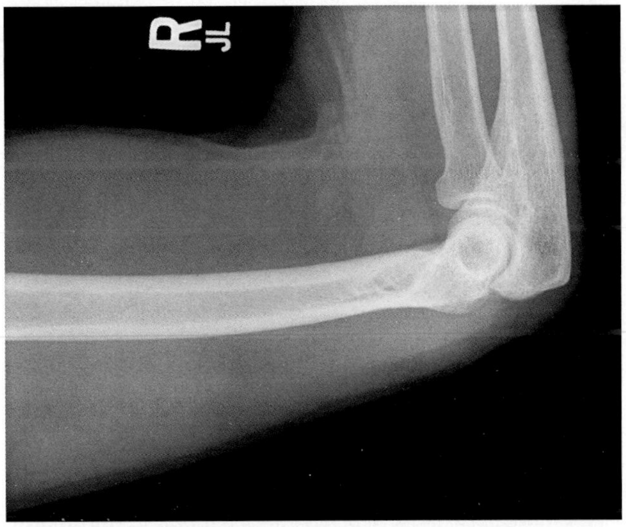

Fig 5.35 Lateromedial projection of mid-to-distal humerus.

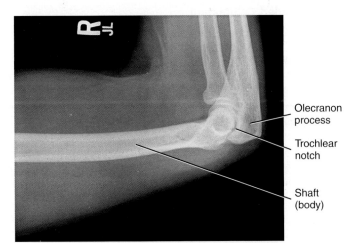

Olecranon process

Trochlear notch

Shaft (body)

Fig 5.36 Lateromedial projection of mid-to-distal humerus.

TRANSTHORACIC LATERAL PROJECTION: HUMERUS (TRAUMA)

Clinical Indications
- Fractures of the diaphysis of the humerus (In addition to a transthoracic lateral projection (Fig. 5.37), an AP projection with neutral rotation (Fig. 5.38) is required.)

Humerus (Nontrauma)
ROUTINE
• AP
• Rotational lateral
• Horizontal beam lateral
SPECIAL (TRAUMA)
• Horizontal beam lateral
• Transthoracic lateral

Technical Factors
- Minimum SID—40 inches (100 cm)
- IR size—14 × 17 inches (35 × 43 cm), portrait
- Grid, vertical, CR to centerline
- kVp range: 75–90
- **If orthostatic (breathing) lateral technique performed**—minimum of 3 seconds exposure time (4 to 5 seconds is desirable)

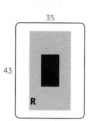

Shielding
Shield radiosensitive tissues outside region of interest.

Patient Position
Place patient in an erect or a supine position. (The erect position, which may be more comfortable for the patient, is preferred.) Place patient in lateral position with side of interest closest to IR (Fig. 5.37). With patient supine, place portable grid lines **horizontally** and **center CR to centerline** to prevent grid cutoff (Fig. 5.37, *inset*).

Part Position
- Place affected arm at patient's side in **neutral rotation; drop** shoulder if possible.
- Raise opposite arm and place hand over top of head; elevate shoulder as much as possible to prevent superimposition of affected shoulder.
- Center mid-diaphysis of affected humerus and center of IR to CR as projected through thorax.
- Ensure that thorax is in a true lateral position or has slight anterior rotation of unaffected shoulder to minimize superimposition of humerus by thoracic vertebrae.

CR
- CR perpendicular to IR, directed through thorax to **mid-diaphysis** (see NOTE)

Recommended Collimation
Collimate on four sides to area of interest.

Respiration
Orthostatic (breathing) technique is **preferred** if patient can cooperate. Patient should be asked to breathe gently in short, shallow breaths without moving affected arm or shoulder.

Evaluation Criteria (Transthoracic Lateral)
Anatomy Demonstrated: • Lateral view of entire humerus and glenohumeral joint should be visualized through the thorax without superimposition of the opposite humerus.
Position: • Outline of the shaft of the humerus should be clearly visualized anterior to the thoracic vertebrae. • Relationship of the humeral head and the glenoid cavity should be demonstrated. • Collimation to area of interest.
Exposure: • Optimal density (brightness) and contrast demonstrate entire outline of the humerus (Fig. 5.39).
• Overlying ribs and lung markings should appear blurred because of breathing technique, but bony outlines of the humerus should appear sharp, indicating **no motion** of the arm during the exposure.

(This allows best visualization of humerus by blurring out ribs and lung structures.)

NOTE: If patient is in too much pain to drop injured shoulder and elevate uninjured arm and shoulder high enough to prevent superimposition of shoulders, **angle CR 10° to 15° cephalad.**

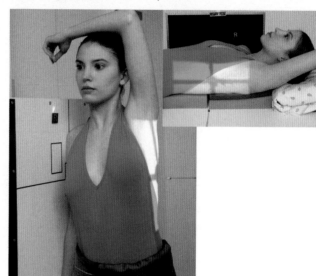

Fig 5.37 Erect and recumbent transthoracic lateral projecton of humerus.

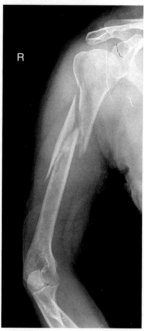

Fig 5.38 Fracture of proximal humerus, neutral rotation. This is a required projection for a trauma humerus in addition to a transthoracic lateral projection.

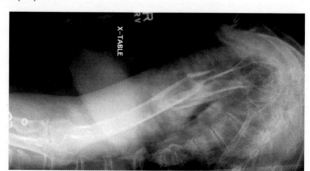

Fig 5.39 Recumbent transthoracic lateral projection of humerus.

AP PROJECTION—EXTERNAL ROTATION: SHOULDER (NONTRAUMA)

AP PROXIMAL HUMERUS

WARNING: Do *not* attempt to rotate the arm if a fracture or dislocation is suspected (see preceding trauma routine).

Clinical Indications
- Fractures or dislocations of proximal humerus and shoulder girdle
- Calcium deposits in muscles, tendons, or bursal structures
- Degenerative conditions, including osteoporosis and osteoarthritis

Shoulder (Nontrauma)
ROUTINE
- AP external rotation (AP)
- AP internal rotation (lateral)

Technical Factors
- Minimum SID—40 inches (100 cm)
- IR size—10 × 12 inches (24 × 30 cm), landscape (or portrait to demonstrate proximal aspect of humerus)
- Grid
- kVp range: 70–85

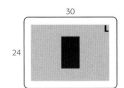

Shielding Shield radiosensitive tissues outside region of interest.

Patient Position Perform radiograph with patient in an erect or a supine position. (The erect position is usually less painful for patient, if condition allows.) Rotate body slightly toward affected side if necessary to place shoulder in contact with IR or tabletop (Fig. 5.40).

Part Position
- Position patient to center scapulohumeral joint to center of IR.
- Abduct extended arm slightly; **externally rotate arm** (supinate hand) until epicondyles of distal humerus are **parallel** to IR.

CR
- CR perpendicular to IR, directed to 1 inch (2.5 cm) inferior to coracoid process (see NOTE)

Recommended Collimation Collimate on four sides, with lateral and upper borders adjusted to soft tissue margins.

Respiration Suspend respiration during exposure.

NOTE: The coracoid process may be difficult to palpate directly on most patients, but it can be approximated; it is approximately 2 inches (5 cm) inferior to the lateral portion of the more readily palpated AC joint.

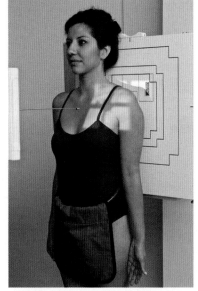

Fig 5.40 External rotation—AP.

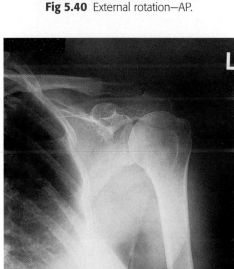

Fig 5.41 External rotation—AP.

Evaluation Criteria
Anatomy Demonstrated: • AP projection of proximal humerus and lateral two-thirds of clavicle and upper scapula, including relationship of the humeral head to the glenoid cavity (Figs. 5.41 and 5.42).
Position: • Full external rotation is evidenced by **greater tubercle visualized in full profile** on the lateral aspect of the proximal humerus. • Lesser tubercle is superimposed over humeral head. • Collimation to area of interest.
Exposure: • Optimal density (brightness) and contrast with **no motion** demonstrate clear, sharp bony trabecular markings with soft tissue detail visible for possible calcium deposits.

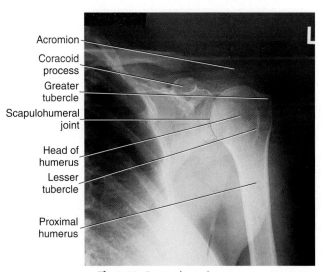

Acromion
Coracoid process
Greater tubercle
Scapulohumeral joint
Head of humerus
Lesser tubercle
Proximal humerus

Fig 5.42 External rotation.

AP PROJECTION—INTERNAL ROTATION: SHOULDER (NONTRAUMA)

LATERAL PROXIMAL HUMERUS

WARNING: Do *not* attempt to rotate the arm if a fracture or dislocation is suspected (see trauma projections, p. 200–203).

Clinical Indications
- Fractures or dislocations of proximal humerus and shoulder girdle
- Calcium deposits in muscles, tendons, or bursal structures
- Degenerative conditions, including osteoporosis and osteoarthritis

> **Shoulder (Nontrauma)**
> ROUTINE
> - AP external rotation (AP)
> - AP internal rotation (lateral)

Technical Factors
- Minimum SID—40 inches (100 cm)
- IR size—10 × 12 inches (24 × 30 cm), landscape (or portrait to demonstrate proximal aspect of humerus)
- Grid
- kVp range: 70–85

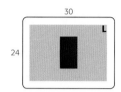

Shielding Shield radiosensitive tissues outside region of interest.

Patient Position Perform radiograph with patient in an erect or supine position. (The erect position is usually less painful for patient, if condition allows.) Rotate body slightly toward affected side, if necessary, to place shoulder in contact with IR or tabletop (Fig. 5.43).

Part Position
- Position patient to center scapulohumeral joint to center of IR.
- Abduct extended arm slightly; **internally rotate arm** (pronate hand) until epicondyles of distal humerus are **perpendicular to IR.**

CR
- CR perpendicular to IR, directed to **1 inch (2.5 cm) inferior to coracoid process** (see NOTE on p. 15)

Recommended Collimation Collimate on four sides, with lateral and upper borders adjusted to soft tissue margins.

Respiration Suspend respiration during exposure.

Evaluation Criteria
Anatomy Demonstrated: • Lateral view of proximal humerus and lateral two-thirds of clavicle and upper scapula are shown, including the relationship of the humeral head to the glenoid cavity (Figs. 5.44 and 5.45).
Position: • Full internal rotation position is evidenced by **lesser tubercle visualized in full profile** on the medial aspect of the humeral head. • An outline of the greater tubercle should be visualized superimposed over the humeral head. • Collimation to area of interest.
Exposure: • Optimal density (brightness) and contrast with **no motion** demonstrate clear, sharp bony trabecular markings with soft tissue detail visible for possible calcium deposits.

Fig 5.43 Internal rotation—lateral.

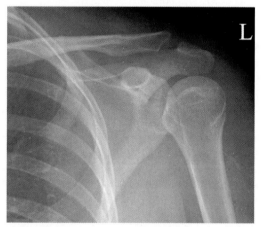

Fig 5.44 Internal rotation—lateral. (Courtesy Joss Wertz, DO.)

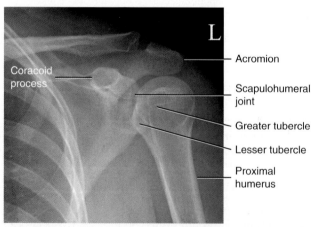

Coracoid process

Acromion

Scapulohumeral joint

Greater tubercle

Lesser tubercle

Proximal humerus

Fig 5.45 Internal rotation—lateral. (Courtesy Joss Wertz, DO.)

INFEROSUPERIOR AXIAL PROJECTION: SHOULDER (NONTRAUMA)

LAWRENCE METHOD[5]

WARNING: Do *not* attempt to rotate the arm or force abduction if a fracture or dislocation is suspected.

Clinical Indications
- Degenerative conditions, including osteoporosis and osteoarthritis
- Hill-Sachs defect with exaggerated rotation of affected limb

> **Shoulder (Nontrauma)**
> SPECIAL
> - Inferosuperior axial (Lawrence method)

Technical Factors
- Minimum SID—40 inches (100 cm).
- IR size—8 × 10 inches (18 × 24 cm) or 10 × 12 inches (24 × 30 cm), landscape
- Grid (CR to centerline of grid, landscape to prevent grid cutoff caused by CR angle); can be performed nongrid for smaller shoulder
- kVp range: 70–85

Shielding Shield radiosensitive tissues outside region of interest.

Patient Position Position patient supine with shoulder raised approximately 2 inches (5 cm) from tabletop by placing support under arm and shoulder to place body part near center of IR (Fig. 5.46).

Part Position
- Move patient toward the front edge of tabletop and place a cart or other arm support against front edge of table to support abducted arm.
- Rotate head toward opposite side, place vertical cassette on table as close to neck as possible, and support with sandbags.
- Abduct arm 90° from body if possible; keep in **external rotation**, palm up, with support under arm and hand.

CR
- Direct CR **medially 25° to 30°**, centered **horizontally to axilla and humeral head.** If abduction of arm is less than 90°, the CR medial angle also should be decreased to 15° to 20°. The greater the arm abduction, the greater the CR angle.

Recommended Collimation Collimate closely on four sides.

Respiration Suspend respiration during exposure.

An **alternative position** is exaggerated **external** rotation[4] (Fig. 5.47). Anterior dislocation of the humeral head may result in a compression fracture of the articular surface of the humeral head, called the *Hills-Sachs defect.* This pathology is best demonstrated by exaggerated external rotation, wherein the thumb is pointed down and posteriorly approximately 45°.

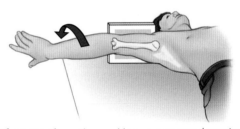

Fig 5.47 Alternative position—exaggerated rotation.

Evaluation Criteria
Anatomy Demonstrated: • Lateral view of proximal humerus in relationship to scapulohumeral cavity • Coracoid process of scapula and lesser tubercle of humerus are seen in profile. • The spine of the scapula is seen on edge below the scapulohumeral joint (Figs. 5.48 and 5.49).
Position: • Arm is seen to be abducted approximately 90° from the body. • Superior and inferior borders of the glenoid cavity should be directly superimposed, indicating correct CR angle. • Collimation to area of interest.
Exposure: • Optimal density (brightness) and contrast with **no motion** demonstrate clear, sharp bony trabecular markings. • Bony margins of the acromion and distal clavicle are visible through the humeral head.

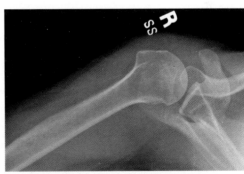

Fig 5.48 Inferosuperior axial projection.

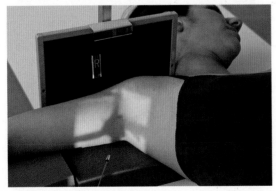

Fig 5.46 Inferosuperior axial (Lawrence method) projection.

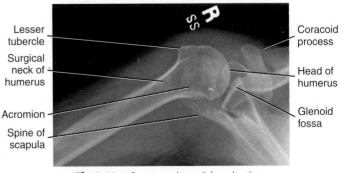

Lesser tubercle
Surgical neck of humerus
Acromion
Spine of scapula
Coracoid process
Head of humerus
Glenoid fossa

Fig 5.49 Inferosuperior axial projection.

PA AXIAL TRANSAXILLARY PROJECTION: SHOULDER (NONTRAUMA)

MODIFIED BERNAGEAU METHOD

WARNING: Do *not* attempt to rotate, force extension, or abduct the arm if a fracture or dislocation is suspected.

Clinical Indications
- Fractures or dislocations of the proximal humerus
- Bursitis, shoulder impingement, osteoporosis, osteoarthritis, and tendonitis

> **Shoulder (Nontrauma)**
> SPECIAL
> • PA transaxillary (modified Bernageau method)

Technical Factors
- Minimum SID—40 inches (100 cm).
- IR size—8 × 10 inches (18 × 24 cm) or 10 × 12 inches (24 × 30 cm), portrait
- Grid (CR to centerline of grid) or nongrid for smaller shoulders
- kVp range: 70–85

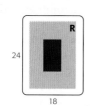

Shielding
Shield radiosensitive tissues outside region of interest.

Patient Position
Take radiograph with the patient in an erect (Fig. 5.50) or a recumbent position. The patient is positioned 70° from PA, rotating toward the affected side.[6]

Part Position
- The arm is raised superiorly to 160° to 180° flexion.[6]
- The head is turned away from the affected arm.

CR
- CR is directed 30° caudally and centered at the level of the scapular spine to pass through the scapulohumeral joint.[6]

Recommended Collimation
Collimate closely on four sides.

Respiration
Suspend respiration during exposure.

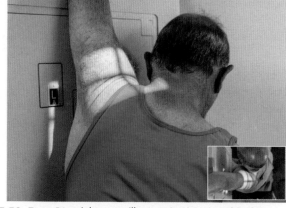

Fig 5.50 Erect PA axial transaxillary projection (modified Bernageau).

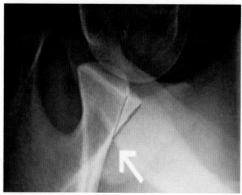

Fig 5.51 PA axial transaxillary projection (modified Bernageau). (From Pansard E et al. Reliability and validity assessment of a glenoid bone loss measurement using the Bernageau profile view in chronic anterior shoulder instability *Journal of Shoulder and Elbow Surgery* 22(9):1193–1198.)

Evaluation Criteria
Anatomy Demonstrated: • Lateral view of proximal humerus in relationship to scapulohumeral (glenohumeral) articulation is visualized. • Coracoid process of scapula is seen on end (Figs. 5.51 and 5.52).
Position: • Arm is seen to be raised superiorly above the body. • Collimation to area of interest.
Exposure: • Optimal density (brightness) and contrast with **no motion** demonstrate clear, sharp bony trabecular markings and pertinent soft tissue anatomy. • Bony margins of the acromion and coracoid process are visible through the humeral head.

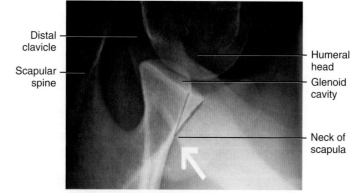

Distal clavicle — Scapular spine — Humeral head — Glenoid cavity — Neck of scapula

Fig 5.52 PA axial transaxillary projection. (modified Bernageau). (From Pansard E et.al. Reliability and validity assessment of a glenoid bone loss measurement using the Bernageau profile view in chronic anterior shoulder instability *Journal of Shoulder and Elbow Surgery* 22(9):1193–1198.)

INFEROSUPERIOR AXIAL PROJECTION: SHOULDER (NONTRAUMA)

CLEMENTS MODIFICATION[7]

WARNING: Do *not* attempt to rotate the arm or force abduction if a fracture or dislocation is suspected.

Clinical Indications
- Degenerative conditions, including osteoporosis and osteoarthritis
- Hill-Sachs defect with exaggerated rotation of affected limb

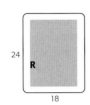

Shoulder (Nontrauma)
SPECIAL
- Inferosuperior axial (Clements modification)

Technical Factors
- Minimum SID—40 inches (100 cm)
- IR size—8 × 10 inches (18 × 24 cm) or 10 × 12 inches (24 × 30 cm), portrait
- Nongrid (can use grid if CR is perpendicular to it)
- kVp range: 70–85

24 R 18

Shielding Shield radiosensitive tissues outside region of interest.

Patient Position Place patient in the lateral recumbent position with the affected arm up.

Part Position
- Abduct arm 90° from body if possible (Fig. 5.53A).

CR
- Direct horizontal CR perpendicular to IR.
- If patient cannot abduct the arm 90°, angle the tube 5° to 15° toward the axilla (Fig. 5.53B).

Recommended Collimation Collimate closely on four sides.

Respiration Suspend respiration during exposure.

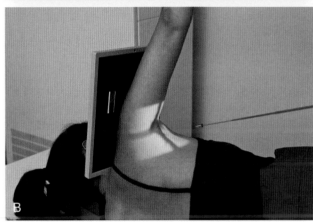

Fig 5.53 A, Inferosuperior axial projection. B, Alternative projection, 5° to 15° medial angle.

Evaluation Criteria
Anatomy Demonstrated: • Lateral view of proximal humerus in relationship to scapulohumeral cavity is shown.
Position: • Arm is abducted approximately 90° from the body. • Relationship of the humeral head and glenoid cavity should be evident (Fig. 5.54). • Collimation to area of interest.
Exposure: • Optimal density (brightness) and contrast with **no motion** demonstrate clear, sharp bony trabecular markings and pertinent soft tissue anatomy. • Bony margins of the acromion and distal clavicle are visible through the humeral head.

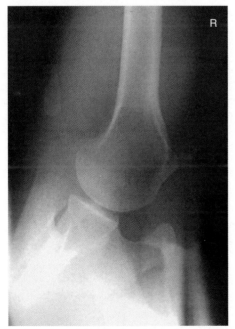

Fig 5.54 Inferosuperior axial projection (Clements modification). (From Frank ED, Long BW, Smith BJ: *Merrill's atlas of radiographic positioning and procedures,* ed 11, St Louis, 2007, Mosby.)

5

AP OBLIQUE PROJECTION—GLENOID CAVITY: SHOULDER (NONTRAUMA)

GRASHEY METHOD

Clinical Indications

- Fractures or dislocations of proximal humerus
- Fractures of glenoid labrum or brim
- Bankart lesion, erosion of glenoid rim, the integrity of the scapulohumeral joint, and other degenerative conditions

Shoulder (Nontrauma)
SPECIAL
• AP oblique projection (Grashey method)
• Apical AP axial projection

Technical Factors

- Minimum SID—40 inches (100 cm).
- IR size—8 × 10 inches (18 × 24 cm) or 10 × 12 inches (24 × 30 cm), landscape
- Grid
- kVp range: 70–85

Shielding Shield radiosensitive tissues outside region of interest.

Patient Position Perform radiograph with patient in an erect or a supine position. (The erect position is usually less painful for patient, if condition allows.)

Part Position

- Rotate body **35° to 45°** toward affected side (see NOTE) (Fig. 5.55). If the position is performed with the patient in the recumbent position, place supports under elevated shoulder and hip to maintain this position.
- Center mid-scapulohumeral joint to CR and to center of IR.
- Adjust image receptor so that top of IR is approximately 2 inches (5 cm) above shoulder and side of IR is approximately 2 inches (5 cm) from lateral border of humerus (Fig. 5.56).
- Abduct arm slightly with arm flexed and in neutral rotation.

Evaluation Criteria

Anatomy Demonstrated: • Glenoid cavity should be seen in profile without superimposition of humeral head (Figs. 5.57 and 5.58).
Position: • Scapulohumeral joint space should be open. • Anterior and posterior rims of glenoid cavity are superimposed. • Collimation to area of interest.
Exposure: • Optimal density (brightness) and contrast with **no motion** visualize soft tissue margins and clear, sharp bony trabecular markings. • Soft tissue detail of the joint space and axilla should be visualized.

CR

- CR perpendicular to IR, centered to scapulohumeral joint, which is approximately 2 inches (5 cm) inferior and 2 inches (5 cm) medial from the superolateral border of shoulder

Recommended Collimation Collimate so that upper and lateral borders of the field are to the soft tissue margins.

Respiration Suspend respiration during exposure.

NOTE: Degree of rotation varies, depending on how flat or round the patient's shoulders are or if position is performed recumbent rather than erect. Having a rounded or curved shoulder or using the recumbent position requires more rotation to place the body of the scapula parallel to the IR.

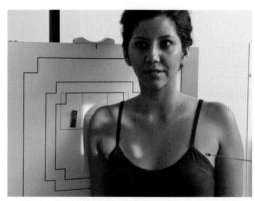
Fig 5.56 AP oblique projection—right posterior oblique (RPO) position.

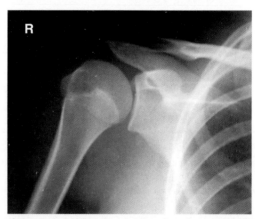
Fig 5.57 AP oblique projection (Grashey method).

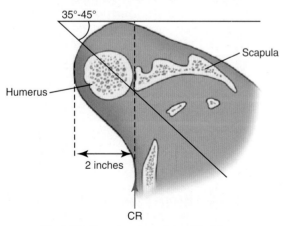
Fig 5.55 Superior view of the AP oblique.

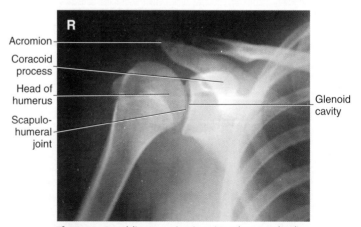
Fig 5.58 AP oblique projection (Grashey method).

APICAL AP AXIAL PROJECTION: SHOULDER[8]

Clinical Indications

- Demonstrate narrowing of acromio-humeral space and possible spurring of the anteroinferior aspect of acromion. Spurring may lead to injury to supraspinatus tendon partial or complete tears.
- May demonstrate signs of shoulder impingement syndrome

Shoulder (Nontrauma)
SPECIAL
• AP oblique projection (Grashey method)
• **Apical AP axial projection**

Technical Factors

- Minimum SID—40 inches (100 cm).
- IR size—8 × 10 inches (18 × 24 cm) or 10 × 12 inches (24 × 30 cm), landscape
- Grid
- kVp range: 70–85

Shielding Shield radiosensitive tissues outside region of interest.

Patient Position Perform radiograph with patient in an erect or a recumbent position. (The erect position is usually less painful for patient, if condition allows.)

Part Position

- Position patient into AP, erect position with no rotation.
- Extend and slightly abduct arm and hand is placed into neutral rotation.
- Adjust image receptor so that top of IR is approximately 1 inch (2.5 cm) above shoulder and side of IR is approximately 2 inches (5 cm) from lateral border of humerus (Fig. 5.59).

CR

- CR is angled 30° caudad and enters ½ inch (1.25 cm) above coracoid process.

Recommended Collimation Collimate so that upper and lateral borders of the field are to the soft tissue margins.

Respiration Suspend respiration during exposure.

Evaluation Criteria

Anatomy Demonstrated: • The anteroinferior aspect of the acromion process and acromiohumeral joint space is open (Figs. 5.60 and 5.61).
Position: • Proximal humerus is projected in neutral rotation position. • Acromiohumeral space is more open compared with routine AP shoulder projection. • Anteroinferior aspect of acromion is demonstrated.
Exposure: • Optimal density (brightness) and contrast with **no motion** visualize soft tissue margins and clear, sharp bony trabecular markings. • Soft tissue detail of the acromiohumeral space.

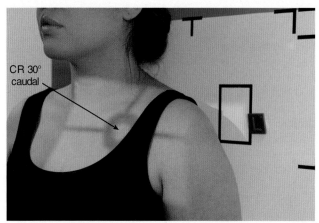

CR 30° caudal

Fig 5.59 Apical AP axial projection.

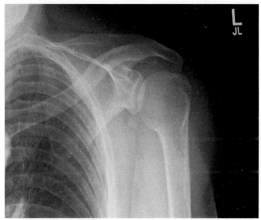

Fig 5.60 Apical AP axial.

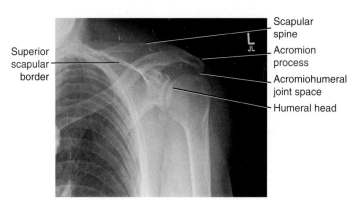

Superior scapular border

Scapular spine

Acromion process

Acromiohumeral joint space

Humeral head

Fig 5.61 Apical AP axial projection.

TANGENTIAL PROJECTION—INTERTUBERCULAR (BICIPITAL) SULCUS: SHOULDER (NONTRAUMA)

FISK MODIFICATION

Clinical Indications
- Pathologies of intertubercular sulcus (groove), including bony spurs of the humeral tubercles

Shoulder (Nontrauma)
SPECIAL
• Tangential projection (Fisk modification)

Technical Factors
- Minimum SID—40 inches (100 cm)
- IR size—8 × 10 inches (18 × 24 cm) or 10 × 12 inches (24 × 30 cm), landscape
- Nongrid
- kVp range: 70–80

Shielding Shield radiosensitive tissues outside region of interest.

Patient and Part Position

Erect (Fisk Modification)
- Patient standing, leaning over end of table with elbow flexed and posterior surface of forearm resting on table, hand supinated holding image receptor, head turned away from affected side (lead shield placed between back of IR and forearm reduces backscatter to IR) (Fig. 5.62)
- Patient leaning forward slightly to place humerus **10° to 15° from vertical**

Supine
- Patient supine, arm at side, hand supinated
- Vertical image receptor placed on table against top of shoulder and against neck (head turned away from affected side) (Fig. 5.63)
- CR **10° to 15° posterior from horizontal,** directed to groove at midanterior margin of humeral head

CR
- CR perpendicular to IR, directed to groove area at midanterior margin of humeral head (groove can be located by careful palpation)

Recommended Collimation Collimate closely on four sides to area of anterior humeral head.

Respiration Suspend respiration during exposure.

Evaluation Criteria
Anatomy Demonstrated: • Anterior margin of the humeral head is seen in profile. • Humeral tubercles and the intertubercular sulcus are seen in profile (Figs. 5.64 and 5.65).
Position: • Correct CR angle of 10° to 15° to the long axis of the humerus demonstrates the intertubercular sulcus and the tubercles in profile without superimposition of the acromion process. • Collimation to area of interest.
Exposure: • Optimal density (brightness) and contrast with **no motion** visualize sharp borders and sharp bony trabecular markings and demonstrate the complete intertubercular sulcus seen through soft tissue without excessive density.

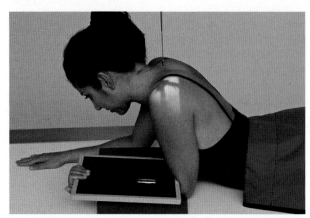
Fig 5.62 Erect superoinferior tangential projection.

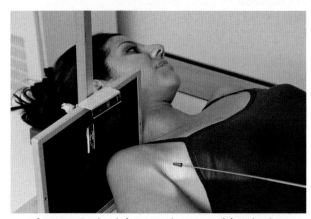
Fig 5.63 Supine inferosuperior tangential projection.

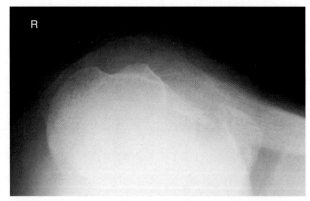
Fig 5.64 Erect tangential projection for intertubercular sulcus.

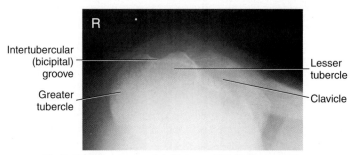
Fig 5.65 Erect tangential (Fisk modification) projection.

AP PROJECTION—NEUTRAL ROTATION: SHOULDER (TRAUMA)

WARNING: Do *not* attempt to rotate the arm if a fracture or dislocation is suspected; perform in neutral rotation, which generally places humerus in an oblique position.

Clinical Indications
- Fractures or dislocations of proximal humerus and shoulder girdle
- Calcium deposits in muscles, tendons, or bursal structures may be evident, along with degenerative diseases

Shoulder (Trauma)
ROUTINE
- AP (neutral rotation)
- Transthoracic lateral *or*
- PA oblique (scapular Y lateral)

Technical Factors
- Minimum SID—40 inches (100 cm)
- IR size—10 × 12 inches (24 × 30 cm), landscape (or portrait to show more of humerus if injury includes proximal half of humerus)
- Grid
- kVp range: 70–85

Shielding Shield radiosensitive tissues outside region of interest.

Patient Position Perform radiograph with patient in erect or supine position. (The erect position is usually less painful for patient, if condition allows.) Rotate body slightly toward affected side if necessary to place shoulder in contact with IR or tabletop (Figs. 5.66 and 5.67).

Part Position ⊡
- Position patient to center scapulohumeral joint to IR.
- Place patient's arm at side in "as is" neutral rotation. (Epicondyles generally are approximately 45° to plane of IR.)

CR
- CR **perpendicular** to IR, directed to **mid-scapulohumeral joint,** which is approximately ¾ inch (2 cm) inferior and slightly lateral to coracoid process (see NOTE, p. 191).

Recommended Collimation Collimate on four sides, with lateral and upper borders adjusted to soft tissue margins.

Respiration Suspend respiration during exposure.

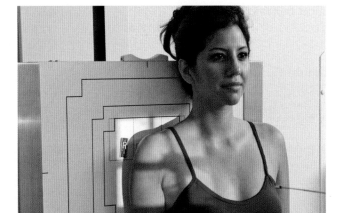
Fig 5.66 AP erect—neutral rotation.

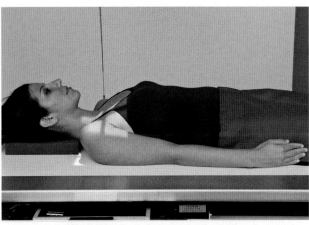
Fig 5.67 AP supine—neutral rotation.

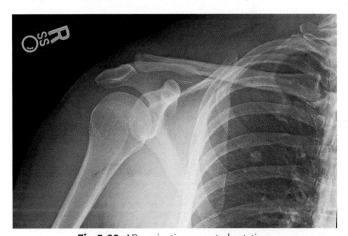
Fig 5.68 AP projection—neutral rotation.

Evaluation Criteria
Anatomy Demonstrated: • The proximal one-third of the humerus and upper scapula and the lateral two-thirds of the clavicle are shown, including the relationship of the humeral head to the glenoid cavity.
Position: • With neutral rotation, both the greater and the lesser tubercles most often are superimposed by the humeral head (Figs. 5.68 and 5.69). • Collimation to area of interest.
Exposure: • Optimal density (brightness) and contrast with **no motion** visualize sharp bony trabecular markings and pertinent soft tissue anatomy. • The outline of the medial aspect of the humeral head is visible through the glenoid cavity, and soft tissue detail should be visible to demonstrate possible calcium deposits.

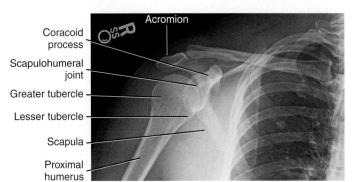

Acromion
Coracoid process
Scapulohumeral joint
Greater tubercle
Lesser tubercle
Scapula
Proximal humerus

Fig 5.69 AP projection—neutral rotation.

TRANSTHORACIC LATERAL PROJECTION: PROXIMAL HUMERUS (TRAUMA)

LAWRENCE METHOD

Clinical Indications
- Fractures or dislocations of proximal humerus

Shoulder (Trauma)
ROUTINE
• AP (neutral rotation)
• Transthoracic lateral *or*
• PA oblique (scapular Y lateral)

Technical Factors
- Minimum SID—40 inches (100 cm)
- IR size—10 × 12 inches (24 × 30 cm), portrait
- Grid, vertical, CR to centerline
- kVp range: 70–80
- Minimum of 3 seconds exposure time with orthostatic (breathing) technique (4 or 5 seconds is desirable). This technique will blur the surrounding pulmonary structures while keeping the proximal humerus in a relatively stationary position.

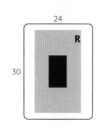

Shielding Shield radiosensitive tissues outside region of interest.

Patient Position Perform radiograph with patient in erect or supine position. (The erect position is preferred and may be more comfortable for patient.) Place patient in lateral position with side of interest against IR. With patient supine, place grid lines **vertically** and **center CR to centerline** to prevent grid cutoff (Figs. 5.70 and 5.71).

Part Position
- Place affected arm at patient's side in **neutral rotation**; drop shoulder if possible.
- Raise opposite arm and place hand over top of head; elevate shoulder as much as possible to prevent superimposition of affected shoulder.
- Center surgical neck and center of IR to CR as projected through thorax.
- Ensure that thorax is in a true lateral position or has slight anterior rotation of unaffected shoulder to minimize superimposition of humerus by thoracic vertebrae.

CR
- CR perpendicular to IR, directed through thorax to level of affected **surgical neck** (see NOTE)

Recommended Collimation Collimate on four sides to area of interest.

Respiration Expose on full inspiration. **Orthostatic (breathing) technique is preferred** if patient can cooperate. Patient should be asked to breathe gently short, shallow breaths without moving affected arm or shoulder. (This best visualizes proximal humerus by blurring out ribs and lung structures.)

NOTE: If patient is in too much pain to drop injured shoulder and elevate uninjured arm and shoulder fully to prevent superimposition of shoulders, **angle CR 10° to 15° cephalad.**

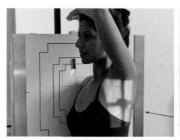

Fig 5.70 Erect transthoracic lateral projection (R lateral). **Fig 5.71** Supine transthoracic lateral projection (R lateral).

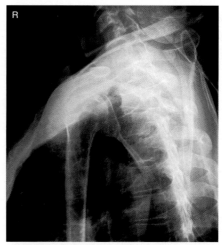

Fig 5.72 Erect transthoracic lateral.

Evaluation Criteria
Anatomy Demonstrated: • Lateral view of proximal half of the humerus and scapulohumeral joint should be visualized through the thorax without superimposition of the opposite shoulder (Figs. 5.72 and 5.73).
Position: • Outline of the shaft of the proximal humerus should be clearly visualized anterior to the thoracic vertebrae. • Relationship of the humeral head and the glenoid cavity should be demonstrated. • Collimation to area of interest.
Exposure: • Optimal density (brightness) and contrast demonstrate entire outline of the humeral head and the proximal half of the humerus. • Overlying ribs and lung markings should appear blurred because of breathing technique, but bony outlines of the humerus should appear sharp, indicating **no motion** of the arm during the exposure.

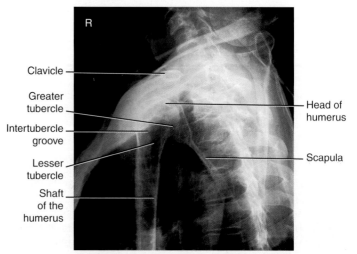

Clavicle

Greater tubercle

Intertubercle groove

Lesser tubercle

Shaft of the humerus

Head of humerus

Scapula

Fig 5.73 Erect transthoracic lateral.

PA OBLIQUE PROJECTION—SCAPULAR Y LATERAL: SHOULDER (TRAUMA)

WARNING: Do *not* attempt to rotate the arm if a fracture or dislocation is suspected.

Clinical Indications

- Fractures or dislocations of proximal humerus and scapula
- Humeral head is demonstrated inferior to coracoid process with anterior dislocations; for less common posterior dislocations, humeral head is demonstrated inferior to acromion process

Shoulder (Trauma)
ROUTINE
• AP (neutral rotation)
• Transthoracic lateral *or*
• PA oblique (scapular Y lateral)

Technical Factors

- Minimum SID—40 inches (100 cm).
- IR size—10 × 12 inches (24 × 30 cm), portrait
- Grid, vertical, CR to centerline
- kVp range: 70–85

Shielding Shield radiosensitive tissues outside region of interest.

Patient Position Perform radiograph with patient in erect or recumbent position. (The erect position is usually more comfortable for the patient.)

Part Position

- Rotate into an anterior oblique position as for a lateral scapula with patient facing IR. **Palpate the superior angle of the scapula and AC joint articulation.** Rotate the patient until an imaginary line between those two points is perpendicular to IR. Because of differences among patients, the amount of body obliquity may range from 45° to 60° (Fig. 5.74). Center scapulohumeral joint to CR and to center of IR.
- Abduct arm slightly if possible so as not to superimpose proximal humerus over ribs; do *not* attempt to rotate arm.

CR

- CR perpendicular to IR, directed to **scapulohumeral joint** (2 inches [5 cm] below AC joint) (see NOTE)

Recommended Collimation Collimate on four sides to area of interest.

Respiration Suspend respiration during exposure.

NOTE: If necessary, because of the patient's condition, this PA oblique (scapular Y lateral) may be taken recumbent in the opposite AP oblique position with injured shoulder elevated (see Lateral Scapula, Recumbent).

Evaluation Criteria

Anatomy Demonstrated: • True lateral view of the scapula, proximal humerus, and scapulohumeral joint.
Position: • The thin body of the scapula should be seen on end without rib superimposition (Fig. 5.75). • The acromion and coracoid processes should appear as nearly symmetric upper limbs of the Y. • The humeral head should appear superimposed over the base of the Y if the humerus is not dislocated (Fig. 5.76). Fig. 5.77 shows an anterior dislocation of the proximal humerus. • Collimation to area of interest.
Exposure: • Optimal density (brightness) and contrast with no motion visualize sharp bony borders and the outline of the body of the scapula through the proximal humerus.

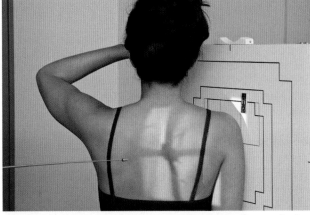

Fig 5.74 PA oblique (scapular Y lateral) with CR perpendicular.

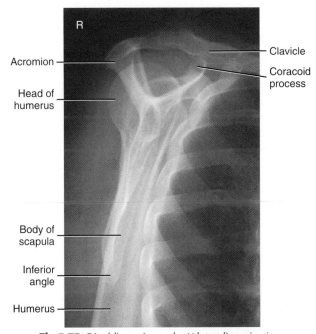

Fig 5.75 PA oblique (scapular Y lateral) projection.

Clavicle
Coracoid process
Acromion
Head of humerus
Body of scapula
Inferior angle
Humerus

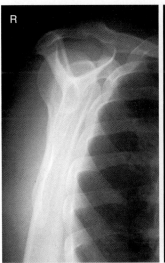
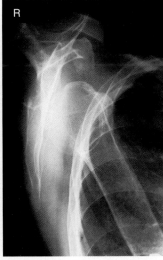

Fig 5.76 PA oblique (scapular Y lateral) with no dislocation.   **Fig 5.77** PA oblique (scapular Y lateral) with anterior dislocation.

TANGENTIAL PROJECTION—SUPRASPINATUS OUTLET: SHOULDER (TRAUMA)

NEER METHOD[9]

WARNING: Do *not* attempt to rotate the arm if a fracture or dislocation is suspected.

Clinical Indications
- Fractures or dislocations of proximal humerus and scapula
- Specifically demonstrates **coracoacromial arch** for **supraspinatus outlet** region for possible **shoulder impingement**[10]

Shoulder (Trauma)
SPECIAL
• Supraspinatus outlet (Neer method)

Technical Factors
- Minimum SID—40 inches (100 cm)
- IR size—10 × 12 inches (24 × 30 cm), portrait
- Grid, vertical, CR to centerline
- kVp range: 70–85
- AEC not recommended

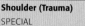

Shielding Shield radiosensitive tissues outside region of interest.

Patient Position Take radiograph with patient in erect or recumbent position. (The erect position is usually more comfortable for patient.)

Part Position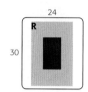
- With patient facing IR, rotate into anterior oblique position as for a lateral scapula.
- **Palpate superior angle of scapula and AC joint articulation.** Rotate patient until an imaginary line between those two points is perpendicular to IR. Because of differences among patients, the amount of body obliquity may range from 45° to 60°. Center scapulohumeral joint to CR and to center of IR (Fig. 5.78).
- Abduct arm slightly so as not to superimpose proximal humerus over ribs; do not attempt to rotate arm.

CR
- Requires **10° to 15° CR caudal angle,** centered posteriorly to pass through superior margin of humeral head, which is located approximately 1 inch (2.5 cm) superior to medial aspect of scapular spine.[11]

Recommended Collimation Collimate on four sides to area of interest.

Respiration Suspend respiration during exposure.

Evaluation Criteria
Anatomy Demonstrated: • Proximal humerus is superimposed over thin body of the scapula, which should be seen on end without rib superimposition.
Position: • Acromion and coracoid processes should appear as nearly symmetric upper limbs of the Y. • The humeral head should appear superimposed and centered to the glenoid fossa just below the supraspinatus outlet region. • The supraspinatus outlet region appears open, free of superimposition by the humeral head (see arrow in Fig. 5.79). • Collimation to area of interest.
Exposure: • Optimal density (brightness) and contrast demonstrate the Y appearance of the upper lateral scapula superimposed by the humeral head with outline of the body of the scapula visible through the humerus. • Bony margins appear clear and sharp, indicating **no motion.**

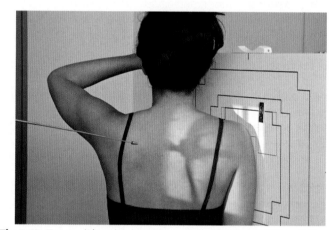

Fig 5.78 Tangential projection—Neer method with CR 10° to 15° caudal angle.

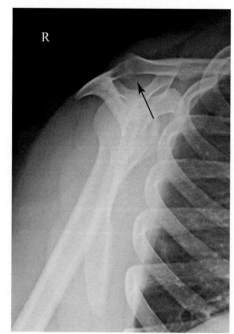

Fig 5.79 Tangential projection—Neer method. (Courtesy Joss Wertz, DO.)

AP APICAL OBLIQUE AXIAL PROJECTION: SHOULDER (TRAUMA)

GARTH METHOD

Clinical Indications
- Optimal trauma projection for possible scapulohumeral dislocations (especially posterior dislocations) (Figs. 5.80 and 5.81)
- Glenoid process fractures, Hill-Sachs lesions, and soft tissue calcifications[12,13]

Shoulder (Trauma)
SPECIAL
- Supraspinatus outlet (Neer method)
- AP apical oblique axial (Garth method)

Technical Factors
- Minimum SID—40 inches (100 cm)
- IR size—10 × 12 inches (24 × 30 cm), portrait
- Grid
- kVp range: 70–85

24
R
30

Shielding Shield radiosensitive tissues outside region of interest.

Patient Position Perform radiograph with patient in erect or supine position. (The erect position is usually less painful, if patient's condition allows.) Rotate body 45° toward affected side (posterior surface of affected shoulder against IR) (Fig. 5.82).

Part Position
- Center scapulohumeral joint to CR and mid-IR.
- Adjust IR so that 45° CR projects scapulohumeral joint to the center of IR.
- Flex elbow and place arm across chest, or with trauma, place arm at side as is.

CR
- CR 45° caudad, centered to scapulohumeral joint. Hint: CR enters just inferior to coracoid process.

Recommended Collimation Collimate closely to area of interest.

Respiration Suspend respiration during exposure.

Evaluation Criteria
Anatomy Demonstrated: • Humeral head, glenoid cavity, and neck and head of the scapula are well demonstrated free of superimposition.
Position: • The coracoid process is projected over part of the humeral head, which appears elongated. • Acromion and AC joint are projected superior to the humeral head (Figs. 5.83 and 5.84). • Collimation to area of interest.
Exposure: • Optimal density (brightness) and contrast with **no motion** demonstrate clear, sharp bony trabecular markings and soft tissue detail for possible calcifications.

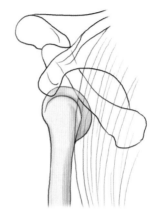
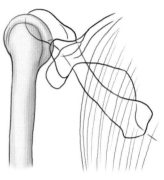

Fig 5.81 Posterior dislocation, humerus projected superiorly.

Fig 5.80 Appearance of humerus when a dislocation has occurred. Anterior dislocation (most common), humerus projected inferiorly.

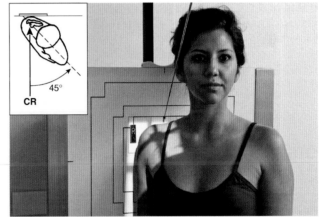

Fig 5.82 Erect apical oblique axial projection—45° posterior oblique, CR 45° caudad.

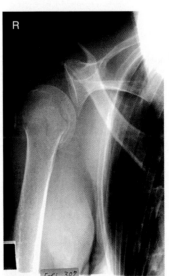
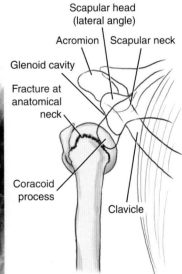

Scapular head (lateral angle)
Acromion | Scapular neck
Glenoid cavity
Fracture at anatomical neck
Scapular neck
Coracoid process
Clavicle

Fig 5.83 AP apical oblique projection. (Note impacted fracture of humeral head but no major scapulohumeral dislocation.)

Fig 5.84 AP apical oblique projection (Garth method). (Note impacted fracture of humeral head but no major scapulohumeral dislocation.)

AP AND AP AXIAL PROJECTIONS: CLAVICLE

Clinical Indications
- Fractures or dislocations of clavicle
- Departmental routines commonly include both AP and AP axial projections

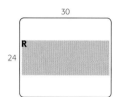

Clavicle
ROUTINE
- AP and AP axial

Technical Factors
- Minimum SID—40 inches (100 cm)
- IR size—10 × 12 inches (24 × 30 cm), landscape
- Grid
- kVp range: 70–85
- AEC not recommended

Shielding Shield radiosensitive tissues outside region of interest.

Patient Position Perform radiograph with patient in erect or supine position with arms at sides, chin raised, and looking straight ahead. Posterior shoulder should be in contact with IR or tabletop, without rotation of body (Fig. 5.85).

Part Position
- Center clavicle and IR to CR. (Clavicle can be readily palpated with medial aspect at jugular notch and lateral portion at AC joint above shoulder.)

CR
AP
- CR perpendicular to midclavicle

AP Axial
- CR 15° to 30° cephalad to midclavicle (Fig. 5.86) (see NOTE)

Evaluation Criteria

AP 0°	AP AXIAL
Anatomy Demonstrated:	**Anatomy Demonstrated:**
• Entire clavicle visualized, including both AC and sternoclavicular joints and acromion.	• Entire clavicle visualized, including both AC and sternoclavicular joints and acromion.
Position:	**Position:**
• Clavicle is demonstrated without any foreshortening.	• Correct angulation of CR projects most of the clavicle above the scapula and second and third ribs.
• The midclavicle is superimposed on the superior scapular angle (Fig. 5.87A).	• Only the medial portion of the clavicle is superimposed by the first and second ribs (Fig. 5.87B).
• Collimation borders should be visible.	
Exposure:	**Exposure:**
• Midclavicle, sternal, and acromial extremities demonstrate clear, sharp bony trabecular markings and soft tissue detail.	• Optimal exposure demonstrates the distal clavicle and AC joint without excessive density (brightness). • Bony margins and trabecular markings should appear sharp, indicating no motion, and medial clavicle and sternoclavicular joint should be visualized through the thorax.

Recommended Collimation Collimate to area of clavicle. (Ensure that both AC and sternoclavicular joints are included.)

Respiration Suspend respiration at end of inhalation (helps to elevate clavicles).

Alternative PA Radiograph also may be taken as PA projection or PA axial with 15° to 30° caudal angle.

NOTE: Thin (asthenic) patients require 25° to 30° CR angle; patients with thick shoulders and chest (hypersthenic) require 15° to 20° CR angle.

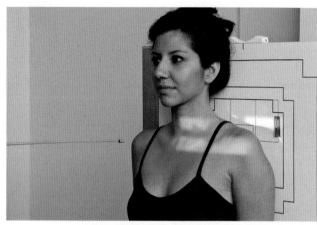

Fig 5.85 AP clavicle—CR 0°.

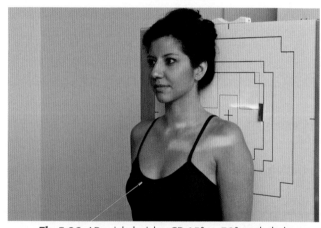

Fig 5.86 AP axial clavicle—CR 15° to 30° cephalad.

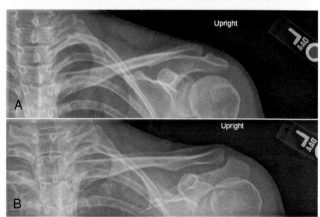

Fig 5.87 A, AP—CR 0°. B, AP axial clavicle—25°. (Courtesy Joss Wertz, DO.)

AP PROJECTION (PEARSON METHOD): AC JOINTS

BILATERAL WITH AND WITHOUT WEIGHTS

WARNING: Shoulder or clavicle projections should be completed first to rule out fracture, or this radiograph may be taken without weights first and checked before it is taken with weights.

Clinical Indications

- Possible AC joint separation: AC joint studies may be taken unilateral if comparative study is not requested or bilateral study for comparison of both joints is requested.
- Widening of one joint space compared with the other view with weights usually indicates AC joint separation

AC Joints
ROUTINE
• AP bilateral with weights *and*
• AP bilateral without weights
• Unilateral study (if requested) with and without weights

Technical Factors

- Minimum SID—40 inches (100 cm) or **72 inches (180 cm)** to include both joints on the same study for broad-shouldered adult.
- IR size—14 × 17 inches (35 × 43 cm), landscape; or two 10 × 12 inch (24 × 30 cm) landscapes for unilateral exposures
- For broad-shouldered patients, **two 8 × 10 inch (18 × 24 cm) IRs, landscape,** placed side by side and exposed simultaneously to include both AC joints on a single exposure
- "With weight" and "without weight" markers
- Grid or nongrid (depending on size of shoulder)
- kVp range: 70–75 nongrid; 80–85 with grid on larger patients
- AEC not recommended

Shielding Secure gonadal shield around waist.

Patient Position Perform radiograph with patient in erect position, posterior shoulders against cassette with equal weight on both feet; arms at side; no rotation of shoulders or pelvis; and looking straight ahead (may be taken seated if patient's condition requires). **Two sets** of bilateral AC joints are taken in the same position, one **without weights** and one **stress view with weights** (Figs. 5.88 and 5.89).

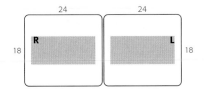

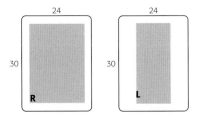

Part Position

- Position patient to direct CR to midway between AC joints.
- Center midline of IR to CR (top of IR should be approximately 2 inches [5 cm] above shoulders).

CR

- CR perpendicular to **midpoint between AC joints,** 1 inch (2.5 cm) above jugular notch
- Unilateral study: CR center 1 inch (2.5 cm) below affected AC joint (see NOTE)

Recommended Collimation Collimate with a long, narrow light field to area of interest; upper light border should be to upper shoulder soft tissue margins.

Respiration Suspend respiration during exposure.

Weights After the first exposure is made without weights and the cassette has been changed, for large adult patients, strap 8- to 10-lb **minimum** weights to each wrist and, with shoulders relaxed, **gently** allow weights to hang from wrists while pulling down on each arm and shoulder. The same amount of weight must be used on each wrist. Less weight (5 to 8 lb per limb) may be used for smaller or asthenic patients, and more weight may be used for larger or hypersthenic patients. (Check department protocol for the amount of applied weight.)

NOTE: Patients should *not* be asked to hold onto the weights with their hands; the **weights should be attached to the wrists so that the hands, arms, and shoulders are relaxed** and possible AC joint separation can be determined. Holding onto weights may result in false-negative radiographs because they tend to pull on the weights, resulting in contraction rather than relaxation of the shoulder muscles.

Alternative AP Axial Projection (Alexander Method) This method requires a 15° cephalic angle centered at the level of the affected AC joint. It projects the AC joint superior to the acromion, providing optimal visualization. This projection may be performed for suspected AC joint subluxation or dislocation.

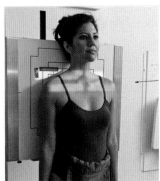

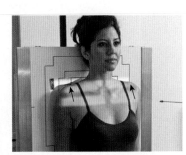

Fig 5.89 AC joints marked by arrows.

Fig 5.88 Stress view with weights (weights tied to wrists). Female, 8 to 10 lb minimum per limb.

Alternative AP Axial Projection (Zanca Method) This method uses a 10° to 15° cephalic angle centered at the level of the affected AC joint. It projects the AC joint superior to the acromion, providing optimal visualization (Fig. 5.90). The Zanca method also uses 50% less kilovoltage than a standard glenohumeral exposure to better visualize the soft tissue and joint detail of the AC joint.[14] This projection may be performed for suspected AC joint subluxation or dislocation and for soft tissue pathologies (Figs. 5.91 and 5.92).

Alternative Supine Position If the patient's condition requires, the radiograph may be taken supine. Tie both ends of a long strip of gauze to the patient's wrists and place the strip around the patient's feet with the knees partially flexed. Then, **slowly** and **gently** straighten the legs and pull down on the shoulders. Alternatively an assistant (with proper protective shielding) can **gently** pull down on the arms and shoulders (Fig. 5.93).

WARNING: This method should be used only by experienced and qualified personnel to prevent additional injury.

Evaluation Criteria
Anatomy Demonstrated: • Both AC joints, entire clavicles, and SC joints are demonstrated.
Position: • Both AC joints are on the same horizontal plane. • **No rotation** occurred, as is evidenced by the symmetric appearance of the sternoclavicular (SC) joints on each side of the vertebral column.
Exposure and Markers: • Optimal density (brightness) and contrast clearly demonstrate AC joints and soft tissues. Bony margins and trabecular markings appear sharp indicating **no motion.** • **Right and left markers** and markers indicating **with** and **without weights** should be visible without superimposing essential anatomy (Fig. 5.94).

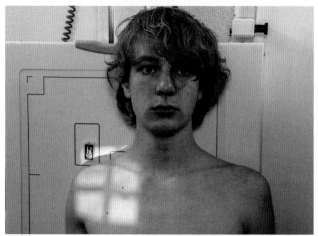

Fig 5.90 AP axial projection (Zanca method) for acromioclavicular joint.

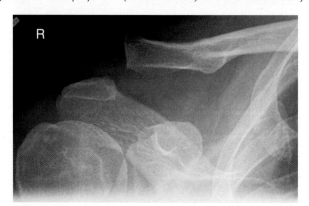

Fig 5.91 AC joints—Zanca method. (From Cvetanovich GL et al. Biological solutions to anatomical acromioclavicular joint reconstruction. *Operative Techniques in Sports Medicine* 23(1):52–59.)

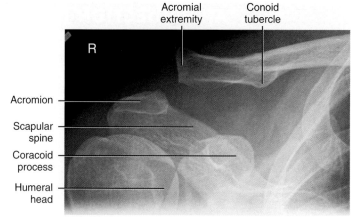

Fig 5.92 AC joints—Zanca method. (From Cvetanovich GL et al. Biological solutions to anatomical acromioclavicular joint reconstruction. *Operative Techniques in Sports Medicine* 23(1):52–59.)

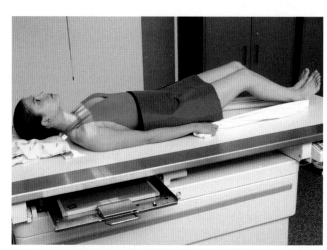

Fig 5.93 Alternative supine position.

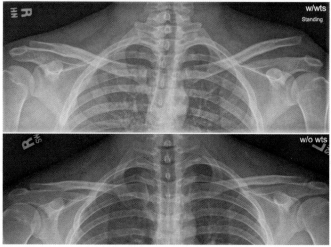

Fig 5.94 AP acromioclavicular joints with and without weights. (Courtesy Joss Wertz, DO.)

AP PROJECTION: SCAPULA

Clinical Indications
- Fractures and other pathology of scapula

Scapula
ROUTINE
• AP
• Lateral

Technical Factors
- Minimum SID—40 inches (100 cm)
- IR size—10 × 12 inches (24 × 30 cm), portrait
- Grid
- kVp range: 70–85
- Minimum of 3 seconds exposure time with optional breathing technique (4 to 5 seconds is desirable)
- Manual exposure factors (AEC is not recommended)

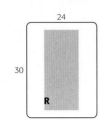

Shielding Shield radiosensitive tissues outside region of interest.

Patient Position Perform radiograph with patient in erect or supine position. (The erect position may be more comfortable for the patient.) Posterior surface of shoulder is in direct contact with tabletop or IR without rotation of thorax. (Rotation toward affected side would place the scapula into a truer posterior position, but this also would result in greater superimposition of the rib cage.)

Part Position ⊞
- Position patient so that midscapular area is centered to CR.
- Adjust cassette to center to CR. Top of IR should be approximately 2 inches (5 cm) above shoulder, and lateral border of IR should be approximately 2 inches (5 cm) from lateral margin of rib cage.
- Gently **abduct arm 90°** and supinate hand. (Abduction moves scapula laterally to clear more of the thoracic structures (Figs. 5.95 and 5.96).

CR
- CR perpendicular to midscapula, 2 inches (5 cm) inferior to coracoid process, or to level of axilla, and approximately 2 inches (5 cm) medial from lateral border of patient

Recommended Collimation Closely collimate on four sides to area of scapula.

Respiration Orthostatic (breathing) technique is preferred if patient can cooperate. Ask patient to breathe gently without moving affected shoulder or arm. Or suspend respiration if orthostatic technique is not preferred.

Evaluation Criteria
Anatomy Demonstrated: • Lateral portion of the scapula is free of superimposition. • Medial portion of the scapula is seen through the thoracic structures (Figs. 5.97 and 5.98).
Position: • Affected arm seen to be abducted 90° and hand supinated, as evidenced by the lateral border of the scapula free of superimposition. • Collimation to area of interest.
Exposure: • Optimal density (brightness) and contrast with **no motion** demonstrate clear, sharp bony trabecular markings of the lateral portion of the scapula. • Ribs and lung structures appear blurred with proper breathing technique.

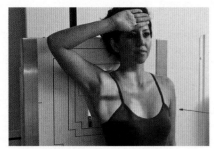

Fig 5.95 AP scapula erect.

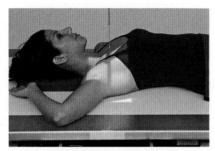

Fig 5.96 AP supine.

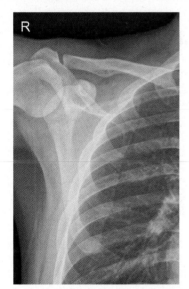

Fig 5.97 AP scapula. (Courtesy Joss Wertz, DO.)

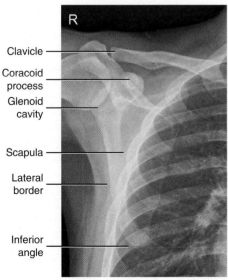

Fig 5.98 AP scapula. (Courtesy Joss Wertz, DO.)

Clavicle
Coracoid process
Glenoid cavity
Scapula
Lateral border
Inferior angle

LATERAL POSITION: SCAPULA—PATIENT ERECT

See Patient Recumbent, p. 209.

Clinical Indications
- Horizontal fractures of the scapula; arm placement should be determined by scapular area of interest

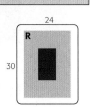

Scapula
ROUTINE
• AP
• Lateral
• Erect
• Recumbent

Technical Factors
- Minimum SID—40 inches (100 cm).
- IR size—10 × 12 inches (24 × 30 cm), portrait
- Grid
- kVp range: 70–85
- Manual exposure factors (AEC is not recommended)

Shielding Secure gonadal shield around waist.

Patient Position Perform radiograph with patient in erect or recumbent position. (Erect position is preferred if patient's condition allows.) Face patient toward IR in anterior oblique position.

Part Position
- Have patient reach across front of chest and grasp opposite shoulder to demonstrate **body** of scapula (Figs. 5.99 and 5.100).
  or
- Have patient drop affected arm, flex elbow, and place arm behind lower back with arm partially abducted, or just let arm hang down at patient's side. This best demonstrates **acromion and coracoid processes** (Figs. 5.101 and 5.102).
- **Palpate superior angle of the scapula** and **AC joint articulation.** Rotate the patient until an imaginary line between the two points is perpendicular to IR; this results in a lateral position of the body of the scapula. The position of the humerus (down at side or up across anterior chest) has an effect on the amount of body rotation required. Less rotation is required with arm up across anterior chest. (The flat posterior surface of body of scapula should be perpendicular to IR.)
- Align patient to center midvertebral border to CR and to IR.

CR
- CR to midvertebral border of scapula

Recommended Collimation Closely collimate to area of scapula.

Respiration Suspend respiration during exposure.

Evaluation Criteria
Anatomy Demonstrated and Position: • Entire scapula should be visualized in a lateral position, as evidenced by direct superimposition of vertebral and lateral borders. • True lateral is shown by direct superimposition of vertebral and lateral borders. • Body of scapula should be in profile, free of superimposition by ribs. • As much as possible, the humerus should not superimpose area of interest of the scapula. • Collimation to area of interest.
Exposure: • Optimal exposure with **no motion** demonstrates sharp bony borders and trabecular markings without excessive density (brightness) in area of inferior angle. • Bony borders of both acromion and coracoid processes should be seen through the head of the humerus.

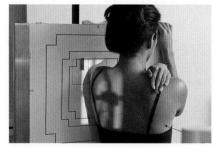

Fig 5.99 Lateral for body of scapula (approximately 45° LAO).

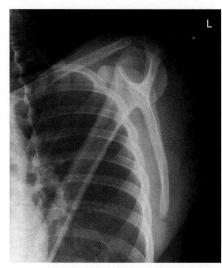

Fig 5.100 Lateral for body of scapula (approximately 45° LAO).

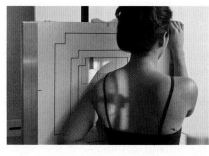

Fig 5.101 Lateral for acromion or coracoid process (approximately 60° LAO).

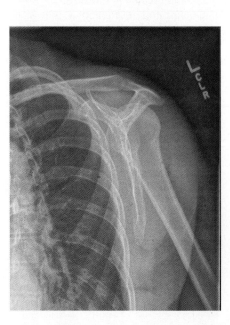

Fig 5.102 Lateral for acromion or coracoid process (approximately 60° LAO). (Courtesy Joss Wertz, DO.)

LATERAL POSITION: SCAPULA–PATIENT RECUMBENT

See Patient Erect, p. 208.

Scapula
ROUTINE
• AP
• Lateral

Clinical Indications
• Fractures of the scapula

NOTE: This position results in a magnified image because of increased OID.

Technical Factors
• Minimum SID–40 inches (100 cm).
• IR size–10 × 12 inches (24 × 30 cm), portrait
• Grid
• kVp range: 70–85
• Manual exposure factors (AEC is not recommended)

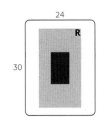

Shielding Shield radiosensitive tissues outside region of interest.

Patient Position Perform radiograph with patient in a supine position, and place affected arm across chest. Palpate AC joint articulation and superior border of the scapula and rotate patient until an imaginary line between these two points is perpendicular to the IR; this elevates the affected shoulder until body of scapula is in a true lateral position. Flex knee of affected side to help patient maintain this oblique body position.

Part Position
• Align patient on tabletop so that center of the midlateral (axillary) border of scapula is centered to CR and IR. (Fig. 5.103)
• Palpate borders of scapula by grasping medial and lateral borders of body of scapula with fingers and thumb (Fig. 5.103, *inset*). Carefully adjust body rotation as needed to bring the plane of the scapular body **perpendicular to the IR.**)

CR
• CR to midscapula lateral border

Recommended Collimation Closely collimate to area of scapula.

Respiration Suspend respiration during exposure.

Evaluation Criteria
Anatomy Demonstrated: • Entire scapula should be visualized in a lateral position.
Position: • True lateral is shown by direct superimposition of vertebral and lateral borders (Fig. 5.104). • Body of scapula should be seen in profile, free of superimposition by ribs. • As much as possible, the humerus should not superimpose area of interest of the scapula. • Collimation to area of interest.
Exposure: • Optimal exposure with **no motion** demonstrates sharp bony borders and trabecular markings. • Entire scapula should be visualized without excessive density in area of inferior angle. • Bony borders of both acromion and coracoid processes should be seen through the head of the humerus.

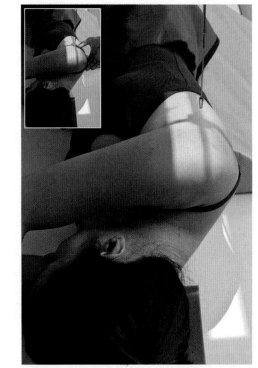

Fig 5.103 Recumbent lateral scapula position. Inset shows palpating the borders of the scapula.

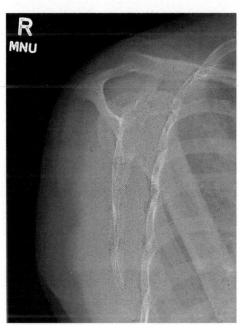

Fig 5.104 Erect lateral scapula. (Courtesy Joss Wertz, DO.)

5

RADIOGRAPHS FOR CRITIQUE

This section consists of an ideal projection (Image A) along with one or more projections that may demonstrate positioning and/or technical errors. Critique Figures C5.105 through C5.107. Compare Image A to the other projections and identify the errors. While examining each image, consider the following questions:

1. Is all essential anatomy demonstrated on the image?
2. What positioning errors are present that compromise image quality?

3. Are technical factors optimal?
4. Is there evidence of collimation, and are pre-exposure anatomic side markers visible on the image?
5. Do these errors require a repeat exposure?
   Feedback for each set of images is located on the faculty Evolve site.

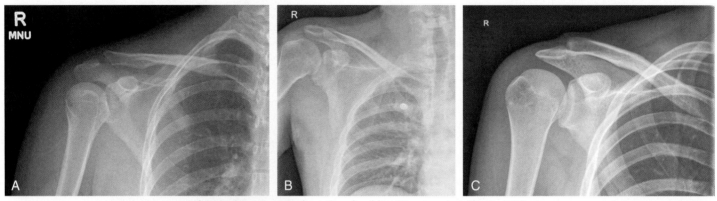

Fig C5.105 AP Internal rotation shoulder. (Courtesy Joss Wertz, DO.)

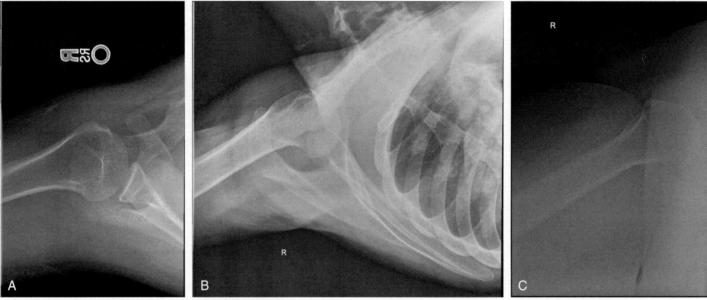

Fig C5.106 Inferiosuperior axillary shoulder. (Courtesy Joss Wertz, DO.)

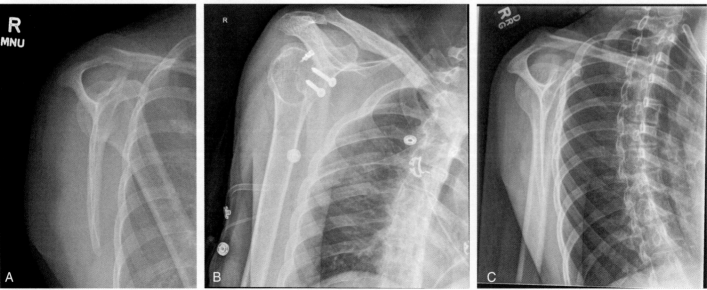

Fig C5.107 Scapular Y. (Courtesy Joss Wertz, DO.)

CHAPTER 6

Lower Limb

CONTRIBUTIONS BY **Christopher I. Wertz,** MSRS, RT(R)

CONTRIBUTORS TO PAST EDITIONS Dan L. Hobbs, MSRS, RT(R)(CT)(MR), Beth L. Vealé, BSRS, MEd, PhD, RT(R)(QM), Jeannean Hall-Rollins, MRC, BS, RT(R)(CV)

CONTENTS

6

Distal Lower Limb

The bones of the distal lower limb are divided into the foot, lower leg, and distal femur (Fig. 6.1). The ankle and knee joints are also discussed in this chapter. The proximal femur and the hip are included in Chapter 7, along with the pelvic girdle.

FOOT

The bones of the foot are fundamentally similar to the bones of the hand and wrist, which are described in Chapter 4.

The 26 bones of one foot (Fig. 6.2) are divided into three groups as follows:

1. Phalanges (toes or digits)	14
2. Metatarsals (instep)	5
3. Tarsals	7
Total	26

Phalanges—Toes (Digits)

The most distal bones of the foot are the **phalanges,** which make up the toes, or digits. The five digits of each foot are numbered 1 through 5, starting on the medial or big-toe side of the foot. The large toe, or first digit, has only two phalanges, similar to the thumb: the **proximal phalanx** and the **distal phalanx.** Each of the second, third, fourth, and fifth digits has a **middle phalanx,** in addition to a proximal phalanx and a distal phalanx. Because the first digit has two phalanges and digits 2 through 5 have three phalanges apiece, **14 phalanges** are found in each foot.

Similarities to the hand are obvious because there are also 14 phalanges in each hand. However, two noticeable differences exist: the phalanges of the foot are smaller, and their movements are more limited than those of the phalanges of the hand.

When any of the bones or joints of the foot are described, the specific digit and foot should also be identified. For example, referring to the "distal phalanx of the first digit of the right foot" would leave no doubt as to which bone is being described.

The distal phalanges of the second through fifth toes are very small and may be difficult to identify as separate bones on a radiograph.

Metatarsals

The five bones of the instep are the **metatarsal** bones. These are numbered along with the digits, with number 1 on the medial side and number 5 on the lateral side.

Each of the metatarsals consists of three parts. The small, rounded distal part of each metatarsal is the **head.** The centrally located, long, slender portion is termed the **body** (shaft). The expanded, proximal end of each metatarsal is the **base.**

The **base of the fifth metatarsal** is expanded laterally into a prominent rough **tuberosity,** which provides for the attachment of a tendon. The proximal portion of the fifth metatarsal, including this tuberosity, is readily visible on radiographs and is a **common trauma site** for the foot; this area must be well visualized on radiographs.

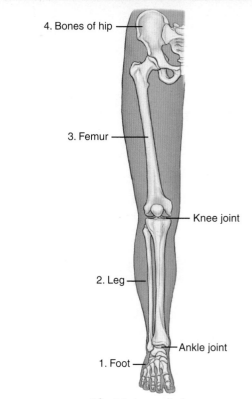

4. Bones of hip

3. Femur

Knee joint

2. Leg

Ankle joint

1. Foot

Fig 6.1 Lower limb.

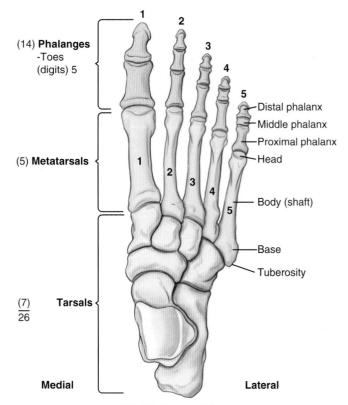

(14) **Phalanges** -Toes (digits) 5

Distal phalanx
Middle phalanx
Proximal phalanx
Head

(5) **Metatarsals**

Body (shaft)

Base
Tuberosity

(7)/26 **Tarsals**

Medial   Lateral

Fig 6.2 Bones of foot.

Joints of Phalanges (Digits) and Metatarsals

Joints of Digits The joints or articulations of the digits of the foot are important to identify because fractures may involve the joint surfaces. Each joint of the foot has a name derived from the two bones on either side of that joint. Between the proximal and distal phalanges of the first digit is the **interphalangeal (IP) joint.**

Because digits 2 through 5 each comprise three bones, these digits also have two joints each. Between the middle and distal phalanges is the **distal interphalangeal (DIP) joint.** Between the proximal and middle phalanges is the **proximal interphalangeal (PIP) joint.**

Joints of Metatarsals Each of the joints at the head of the metatarsal is a **metatarsophalangeal (MTP) joint,** and each of the joints at the base of the metatarsal is a **tarsometatarsal (TMT) joint.** The base of the third metatarsal or the third tarsometatarsal joint is important because this is the centering point or the central ray (CR) location for anteroposterior (AP) and oblique foot projections.

When joints of the foot are described, the name of the joint should be stated first, followed by the digit or metatarsal, and finally the foot. For example, an injury or fracture may be described as near the DIP joint of the fifth digit of the left foot.

Sesamoid Bones Several small, detached bones, called **sesamoid** bones, often are found in the feet and hands. These extra bones, which are embedded in certain tendons, are often present near various joints. In the upper limbs, sesamoid bones are quite small and most often are found on the palmar surface near the metacarpophalangeal joints or occasionally at the interphalangeal joint of the thumb.

In the **lower limbs,** sesamoid bones tend to be larger and more significant radiographically. The largest sesamoid bone in the body is the *patella,* or *kneecap,* as described later in this chapter. The sesamoid bones illustrated in Figs. 6.3 and 6.4 are almost always present on the posterior or **plantar surface at the head of the first metatarsal** near the first MTP joint. Specifically, the sesamoid bone on the medial side of the lower limb is termed the **tibial** sesamoid and the lateral is the **fibular** sesamoid bone. Sesamoid bones also may be found near other joints of the foot. Sesamoid bones are important radiographically because fracturing these small bones is possible. Because of their plantar location, such fractures can be quite painful and may cause discomfort when weight is placed on that foot. Special tangential projections may be necessary to demonstrate a fracture of a sesamoid bone, as shown later in this chapter (p. 231).

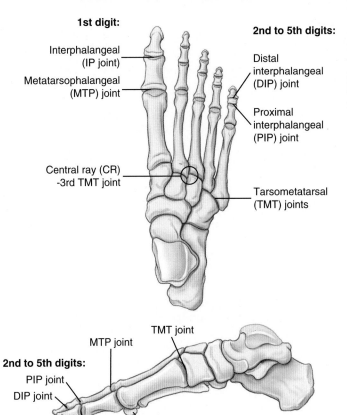

Fig 6.3 Joints of right foot.

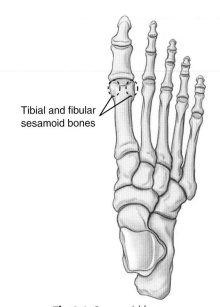

Fig 6.4 Sesamoid bones.

6

Tarsals

The seven large bones of the proximal foot are called *tarsal bones* (Fig. 6.5). The names of the tarsals can be remembered with the aid of a mnemonic: **C**ome **t**o **C**olorado (the) **n**ext **3** **C**hristmases.

(1) **C**ome	Calcaneus (os calcis)
(2) **T**o	Talus (astragalus)
(3) **C**olorado	Cuboid
(4) **N**ext	Navicular (scaphoid)
(5, 6, 7) **3** **C**hristmases	First, second, and third **c**uneiforms

The calcaneus, talus, and navicular bones are sometimes known by alternative names: the *os calcis, astragalus,* and *scaphoid.* However, correct usage dictates that the tarsal bone of the foot should be called the *navicular,* and the carpal bone of the wrist, which has a similar shape, should be called the *scaphoid.* (The carpal bone more often has been called the *navicular* rather than the preferred *scaphoid.*)

Similarities to the upper limb are less obvious with the tarsals in that there are only **seven tarsal bones,** compared with **eight carpal bones** in the wrist. Also, the tarsals are larger and less mobile because they provide a basis of support for the body in an erect position, compared with the more mobile carpals of the hand and wrist.

The seven tarsal bones sometimes are referred to as the *ankle bones,* although only one of the tarsals, the talus, is directly involved in the ankle joint. Each of these tarsals is described individually, along with a list of the bones with which they articulate.

Calcaneus The largest and strongest bone of the foot is the *calcaneus (kal-kay′-ne-us).* The posterior portion is often called the *heel bone.* The most posterior-inferior part of the calcaneus contains a process called the tuberosity. The tuberosity can be a common site for bone spurs, which are sharp outgrowths of bone that can be painful on weight bearing.

Certain large tendons, the largest of which is the Achilles tendon, are attached to this rough and striated process, which at its widest point includes two small, rounded processes. The largest of these is labeled the lateral process. The medial process is smaller and less pronounced.

Another ridge of bone that varies in size and shape and is visualized laterally on an axial projection is the peroneal trochlea *(per″-o-ne′-al trok′-le-ah).* Sometimes, in general, this is also called the *trochlear process.* On the medial proximal aspect is a larger, more prominent bony process called the *sustentaculum (sus″-ten-tak′-u-lum) tali,* which literally means a support for the talus.

Articulations The calcaneus articulates with **two** bones: anteriorly with the **cuboid** and superiorly with the **talus.** The superior articulation with the talus forms the important **subtalar** (talocalcaneal) joint. Three specific articular facets appear at this joint with the talus through which the weight of the body is transmitted to the ground in an erect position: the larger **posterior articular facet** and the smaller **anterior** and **middle articular facets.** The middle articular facet is the superior portion of the prominent sustentaculum tali, which provides medial support for this important weight-bearing joint.

The deep depression between the posterior and middle articular facets is called the **calcaneal sulcus** (Fig. 6.6). This depression, combined with a similar groove or depression of the talus, forms an opening for certain ligaments to pass through. This opening in the middle of the subtalar joint is the **sinus tarsi,** or tarsal sinus (Fig. 6.7).

Talus The talus, the second largest tarsal bone, is located between the lower leg and the calcaneus. The weight of the body is transmitted by this bone through the important ankle and talocalcaneal joints.

Articulations The talus articulates with **four** bones: superiorly with the **tibia** and **fibula,** inferiorly with the **calcaneus,** and anteriorly with the **navicular.**

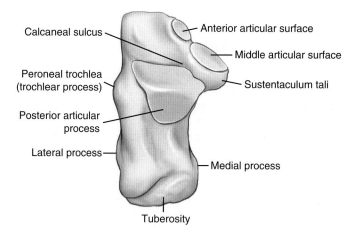

Fig 6.6 Right calcaneus (superior or proximal surface).

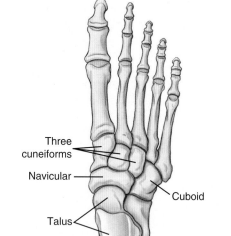

Fig 6.5 Tarsals (7).

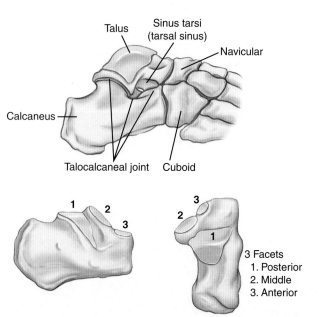

Fig 6.7 Calcaneus and talus (with ankle and subtalar joints).

Navicular

The navicular is a flattened, oval bone located on the medial side of the foot between the talus and the three cuneiforms.

Articulations The **navicular** articulates with **five** bones: posteriorly with the talus, laterally with the cuboid, and anteriorly with the three cuneiforms (Fig. 6.8).

Cuneiforms The three cuneiforms (meaning "wedge shaped") are located on the medial and mid aspects of the foot between the first three metatarsals distally and the navicular proximally. The largest cuneiform, which articulates with the first metatarsal, is the **medial** (first) cuneiform. The **intermediate** (second) cuneiform, which articulates with the second metatarsal, is the smallest of the cuneiforms. The **lateral** (third) cuneiform articulates with the third metatarsal distally and with the cuboid laterally. All three cuneiforms articulate with the navicular proximally.

Articulations The **medial cuneiform** articulates with **four** bones: the navicular proximally, the first and second metatarsals distally, and the intermediate cuneiform laterally.

The **intermediate cuneiform** also articulates with **four** bones: the navicular proximally, the second metatarsal distally, and the medial and lateral cuneiforms on each side.

The **lateral cuneiform** articulates with **six** bones: the navicular proximally; the second, third, and fourth metatarsals distally; the intermediate cuneiform medially; and the cuboid laterally.

Cuboid The cuboid is located on the lateral aspect of the foot, distal to the calcaneus and proximal to the fourth and fifth metatarsals.

Articulations The **cuboid** articulates with **five** bones: the calcaneus proximally, the lateral cuneiform and navicular medially, and the fourth and fifth metatarsals distally.

Arches of Foot

Longitudinal Arch The bones of the foot are arranged in **longitudinal** and **transverse arches,** providing a strong, shock-absorbing support for the weight of the body. The springy, longitudinal arch comprises a medial and a lateral component, with most of the arch located on the medial and mid aspects of the foot.

Transverse Arch The transverse arch is located primarily along the plantar surface of the distal tarsals and the tarsometatarsal joints. The transverse arch is primarily made up of the wedge-shaped cuneiforms, especially the smaller second and third cuneiforms, in combination with the larger first cuneiform and the cuboid (Fig. 6.9).

Box 6.1 presents a summary of the tarsals and articulating bones.

BOX 6.1 **SUMMARY OF TARSALS AND ARTICULATING BONES**	
CALCANEUS (2)[A]	**INTERMEDIATE CUNEIFORM (4)**
1. Cuboid	1. Navicular
2. Talus	2. Second metatarsal
TALUS (4)	3. Medial and lateral cuneiforms
1. Tibia and fibula	**LATERAL CUNEIFORM (6)**
2. Calcaneus	1. Navicular
3. Navicular	2. Second, third, and fourth metatarsals
NAVICULAR (5)	3. Intermediate cuneiform
1. Talus	4. Cuboid
2. Cuboid	
3. Three cuneiforms	**CUBOID (5)**
MEDIAL CUNEIFORM (4)	1. Calcaneus
	2. Lateral cuneiform
1. Navicular	3. Navicular
2. First and second metatarsals	4. Fourth and fifth metatarsals
3. Intermediate cuneiform	

[a] Numbers in parentheses indicate total number of bones with which each of these tarsals articulates.

Fig 6.8 Navicular, cuneiforms (3), and cuboid.

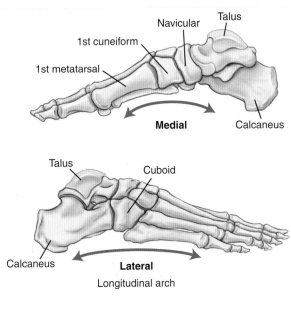

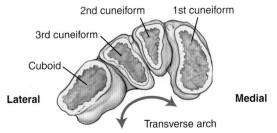

Fig 6.9 Arches and tarsal relationships.

ANKLE JOINT

Frontal View

The **ankle joint** is formed by three bones: the two long bones of the lower leg, the **tibia** and **fibula**, and one tarsal bone, the **talus.** The expanded distal end of the slender fibula, which extends well down alongside the talus, is called the **lateral malleolus.**

The distal end of the larger and stronger tibia has a broad articular surface for articulation with the similarly shaped broad upper surface of the talus. The medial elongated process of the tibia that extends down alongside the medial talus is called the **medial malleolus.**

The inferior portions of the tibia and fibula form a deep "socket," or three-sided opening, called a **mortise,** into which the superior talus fits. However, the entire three-part joint space of the ankle mortise is **not seen** on a true frontal view (AP projection) because of overlapping of portions of the distal fibula and tibia by the talus. This overlapping is caused by the more posterior position of the distal fibula, as is shown on these drawings. A 15° internally rotated AP oblique projection, called the **mortise position,**[1] is performed (see Fig. 6.15) to demonstrate the mortise of the joint, which should have an even space over the entire talar surface.

The **anterior tubercle** is an expanded process at the distal anterior and lateral tibia that has been shown to articulate with the superolateral talus, while partially overlapping the fibula anteriorly (Figs. 6.10 and 6.11).

The **distal tibial joint surface** that forms the roof of the ankle mortise joint is called the **tibial plafond** (ceiling). Certain types of fractures of the ankle in children and youth involve the distal tibial epiphysis and the tibial plafond.

Lateral View

The ankle joint, seen in a true lateral position in Fig. 6.11, demonstrates that the **distal fibula is located about ⅜ inch (1 cm) posterior in relation to the distal tibia.** This relationship becomes important in evaluation for a **true lateral** radiograph of the lower leg, ankle, or foot. A common mistake in positioning a lateral ankle is to rotate the ankle slightly so that the medial and lateral malleoli are directly superimposed; however, this results in a partially oblique ankle, as these drawings illustrate. A true lateral requires the **lateral malleolus** to be **about (⅜) inch (1 cm) posterior** to the medial malleolus. The lateral malleolus extends **about ⅜ inch (1 cm) more distal** than its counterpart, the medial malleolus (best seen on frontal view, Fig. 6.10).

Axial View

An axial view of the inferior margin of the distal tibia and fibula is shown in Fig. 6.12; this visualizes an "end-on" view of the ankle joint looking from the bottom up, demonstrating the concave inferior surface of the tibia (tibial plafond). Also demonstrated are the relative positions of the **lateral** and **medial malleoli** of the fibula and tibia. The smaller **fibula** is shown to be **more posterior.** A horizontal plane drawn through the midportions of the two malleoli would be approximately **15° to 20°** from the coronal plane (the true side-to-side plane of the body). This positioning line is termed the **intermalleolar plane.** The lower leg and ankle must be rotated 15° to 20° to bring the intermalleolar plane parallel to the coronal plane. This relationship of the distal tibia and fibula becomes important in positioning for various views of the ankle joint or ankle mortise, as described in the positioning sections of this chapter.

Joint Structure

The ankle joint is a **synovial joint** of the saddle (**sellar**) **type** with flexion and extension (dorsiflexion and plantar flexion) movements only. This joint requires strong collateral ligaments that extend from the medial and lateral malleoli to the calcaneus and talus. Lateral stress can result in a "sprained" ankle with stretched or torn collateral ligaments and torn muscle tendons leading to an increase in parts of the mortise joint space. AP stress views of the ankle can be performed to evaluate the stability of the mortise joint space.

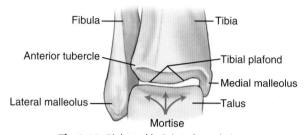

Fig 6.10 Right ankle joint—frontal view.

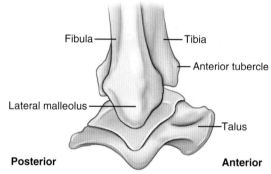

Fig 6.11 Right ankle joint—true lateral view.

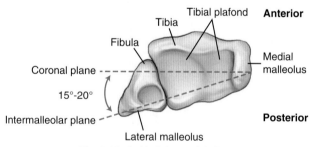

Fig 6.12 Ankle joint—axial view.

REVIEW EXERCISE WITH RADIOGRAPHS

Three common projections of the foot and ankle are shown with labels for an anatomy review of the bones and joints. A good review exercise is to cover up the answers that are listed here and identify all the labeled parts before checking the answers.

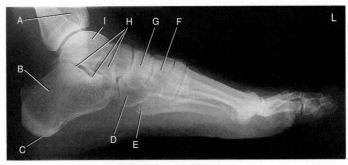

Fig 6.13 Lateral left foot.

Lateral Left Foot (Fig. 6.13)
A. Tibia
B. Calcaneus
C. Tuberosity of calcaneus
D. Cuboid
E. Fifth metatarsal tuberosity
F. Superimposed cuneiforms
G. Navicular
H. Subtalar joint
I. Talus

Oblique Right Foot (Fig. 6.14)
A. Interphalangeal joint of first digit of right foot
B. Proximal phalanx of first digit of right foot
C. Metatarsophalangeal joint of first digit of right foot
D. Head of first metatarsal
E. Body of first metatarsal
F. Base of first metatarsal
G. Second or intermediate cuneiform (partially superimposed over first or medial cuneiform)
H. Navicular
I. Talus
J. Tuberosity of calcaneus
K. Third or lateral cuneiform
L. Cuboid
M. Tuberosity of the base of the fifth metatarsal
N. Fifth metatarsophalangeal joint of right foot
O. Proximal phalanx of fifth digit of right foot

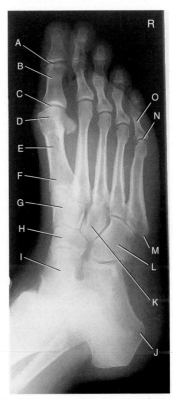

Fig 6.14 AP medial oblique right foot.

AP Mortise View Right Ankle (Fig. 6.15)
A. Fibula
B. Lateral malleolus
C. "Open" mortise joint of ankle
D. Talus
E. Medial malleolus
F. Tibial epiphyseal plate (epiphyseal fusion site)

Lateral Right Ankle (Fig. 6.16)
A. Fibula
B. Calcaneus
C. Cuboid
D. Tuberosity at base of fifth metatarsal
E. Navicular
F. Talus
G. Sinus tarsi
H. Anterior tubercle
I. Tibia

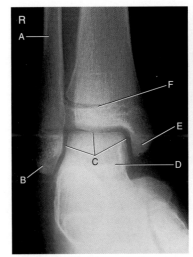

Fig 6.15 AP right ankle (mortise view—15° medial oblique).

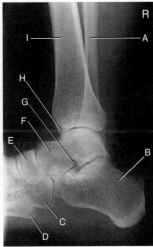

Fig 6.16 Lateral right ankle.

LOWER LEG—TIBIA AND FIBULA

The second group of bones of the lower limb to be studied in this chapter consists of the two bones of the lower leg: the **tibia** and **fibula** (Fig. 6.17).

Tibia

The tibia, as one of the larger bones of the body, is the weight-bearing bone of the lower leg. The tibia can be felt easily through the skin in the anteromedial part of the lower leg. It is made up of three parts: the central **body** (shaft) and **two extremities.**

Proximal Extremity The **medial** and **lateral condyles** are the two large processes that make up the medial and lateral aspects of the proximal tibia.

The **intercondylar eminence** (also known as the **tibial spine**) includes two small pointed prominences, called the **medial** and **lateral intercondylar tubercles,** which are located on the superior surface of the tibial head between the two condyles.

The upper articular surface of the condyles includes two smooth concave **articular facets,** commonly called the **tibial plateau,** which articulate with the femur. As can be seen on the lateral view, the **articular facets making up the tibial plateau slope posteriorly from 10° to 20°** in relation to the long axis of the tibia[2] (Fig. 6.18). This is an important anatomic consideration because when an AP knee is positioned, the CR must be angled as needed in relation to the image receptor (IR) and the tabletop to be parallel to the tibial plateau. This CR angle is essential in demonstrating an "open" joint space on an AP knee projection.

The **tibial tuberosity** on the proximal extremity of the tibia is a rough-textured prominence located on the midanterior surface of the tibia just distal to the condyles. This tuberosity is the distal attachment of the patellar tendon, which connects to the large muscle of the anterior thigh. Sometimes in young persons the tibial tuberosity separates from the body of the tibia, a condition known as *Osgood-Schlatter disease* (see Clinical Indications, p. 226).

Body The **body** (shaft) is the long portion of the tibia between the two extremities. Along the anterior surface of the body, extending from the tibial tuberosity to the medial malleolus, is a sharp ridge called the **anterior crest** or **border.** This sharp anterior crest is just under the skin surface and often is referred to as the *shin* or *shin bone.*

Distal Extremity The distal extremity of the tibia is smaller than the proximal extremity and ends in a short pyramid-shaped process called the **medial malleolus,** which is easily palpated on the medial aspect of the ankle.

The lateral aspect of the distal extremity of the tibia forms a flattened, triangular **fibular notch** for articulation with the distal fibula.

Fibula

The smaller fibula is located **laterally** and **posteriorly** to the larger tibia. The fibula articulates with the tibia proximally and the tibia and talus distally. The proximal extremity of the fibula is expanded into a **head,** which articulates with the lateral aspect of the posteroinferior surface of the lateral condyle of the tibia. The extreme proximal aspect of the head is pointed and is known as the **apex** of the head of the fibula. The tapered area just below the head is the **neck** of the fibula.

The **body** (shaft) is the long, slender portion of the fibula between the two extremities. The enlarged distal end of the fibula can be felt as a distinct "bump" on the lateral aspect of the ankle joint and, as described earlier, is called the **lateral malleolus.**

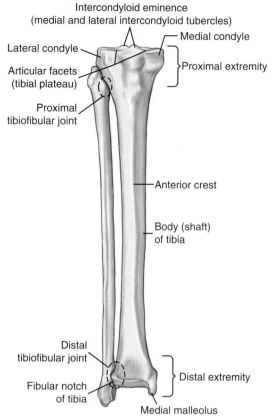

Fig 6.17 Tibia—anterior view.

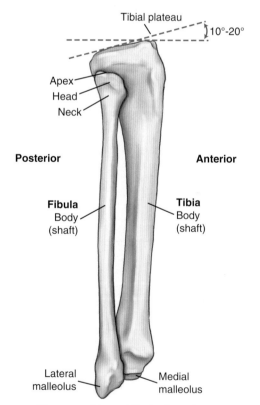

Fig 6.18 Tibia and fibula—lateral view.

Midfemur and Distal Femur–Anterior View Similar to all long bones, the body or shaft of the femur is the slender, elongated portion of the bone. The distal femur viewed anteriorly demonstrates the position of the patella or kneecap (Fig. 6.19). The **patella**, which is the largest sesamoid bone in the body, is located anteriorly to the distal femur. The most distal part of the patella is **superior** or **proximal** to the actual knee joint by approximately ½ inch (1.25 cm) in this position with the lower leg fully extended. This relationship becomes important in positioning for the knee joint.

The **patellar surface** is the smooth, shallow, triangular depression at the distal portion of the anterior femur that extends up under the lower part of the patella, as seen in Fig. 6.19. This depression sometimes is referred to as the **intercondylar sulcus**. (*Sulcus* means a groove or depression.) Some literature also refers to this depression as the **trochlear groove**. (*Trochlea* means pulley or pulley-shaped structure in reference to the medial and lateral condyles.) All three of these terms should be recognized as referring to this smooth, shallow depression.

The patella itself most often is superior to the patellar surface with the leg fully extended. However, as the leg is flexed, the patella, which is attached to large muscle tendons, moves distally or downward over the patellar surface. This is best shown on the lateral knee drawing (see Fig. 6.21).

Midfemur and Distal Femur–Posterior View The posterior view of the distal femur best demonstrates the two large, rounded condyles that are separated distally and posteriorly by the deep **intercondylar fossa** or notch, above which is the popliteal surface (see Fig. 6.20; also Fig. 6.21).

The rounded distal portions of the **medial** and **lateral condyles** contain smooth articular surfaces for articulation with the tibia. The **medial condyle extends lower or more distally** than the lateral condyle when the femoral shaft is vertical, as in Fig. 6.20. This explains why the **CR must be angled 5° to 7° cephalad for a lateral knee** to cause the two condyles to be directly superimposed when the femur is parallel to the IR. The explanation for this is apparent in Fig. 6.19, which demonstrates that in an erect anatomic position, wherein the distal femoral condyles are parallel to the floor at the knee joint, the femoral shaft is at an angle of approximately 10° from vertical for an average adult. The range is 5° to 15°.[3] This angle would be greater on a person of short stature and a wider pelvis. The angle would be less on a person of tall stature with a narrow pelvis. In general, this angle is greater on a woman than on a man.

A distinguishing difference between the medial and lateral condyles is the presence of the **adductor tubercle,** a slightly raised area that receives the tendon of an adductor muscle. This tubercle is present on the **posterolateral aspect of the medial condyle**. It is best seen on a slightly rotated lateral view of the distal femur and knee. The presence of this adductor tubercle on the medial condyle is important in critiquing a lateral knee for rotation. It allows the viewer to determine whether the knee is under-rotated or over-rotated to correct a positioning error when the knee is not in a true lateral position (see the radiograph in Fig. 6.33).

The **medial** and **lateral epicondyles,** which can be palpated, are rough prominences for attachments of the medial and lateral collateral ligaments and are located on the outermost portions of the condyles. The medial epicondyle, along with the adductor tubercle, is the more prominent of the two.

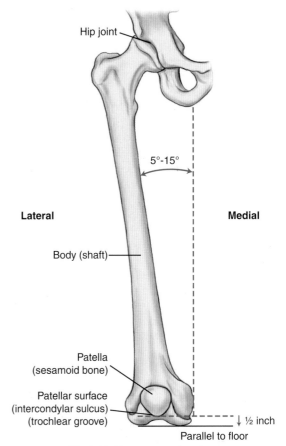

Fig 6.19 Femur–anterior view.

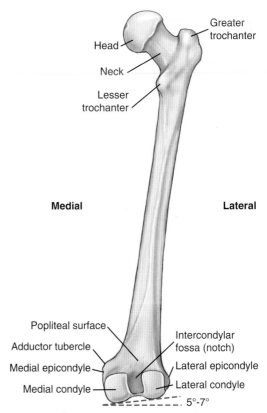

Fig 6.20 Femur–posterior view.

Distal Femur and Patella (Lateral View) The lateral view in Fig. 6.21 shows the relationship of the patella to the **patellar surface** of the distal femur. The patella, as a large sesamoid bone, is embedded in the tendon of the large quadriceps femoris muscle. As the lower leg is flexed, the patella moves downward and is drawn inward into the intercondylar groove or sulcus. A partial flexion of almost 45°, as shown in Fig. 6.21, demonstrates the patella being pulled only partially downward. With 90° flexion, the patella would move down farther over the distal portion of the femur. This movement and the relationship of the patella to the distal femur become important in positioning for the knee joint and for the tangential projection of the patellofemoral (femoropatellar) joint (articulation between patella and distal femur).

The posterior surface of the distal femur just proximal to the intercondylar fossa is called the **popliteal surface,** over which popliteal blood vessels and nerves pass.

Distal Femur and Patella (Axial View) The axial or end-on view of the distal femur demonstrates the relationship of the patella to the **patellar surface** (intercondylar sulcus or trochlear groove) of the distal femur. The patellofemoral joint space is visualized in this axial view (Fig. 6.22). Other parts of the distal femur are also well visualized.

The **intercondylar fossa** (notch) is shown to be very deep on the posterior aspect of the femur. The **epicondyles** are seen as rough prominences on the outermost tips of the large **medial** and **lateral condyles.**

PATELLA

The **patella** (kneecap) is a flat triangular bone approximately 2 inches (5 cm) in diameter (Fig. 6.23). The patella appears to be upside down because its pointed **apex** is located along the **inferior border,** and its **base** is the **superior** or **upper border.** The outer or **anterior surface** is convex and rough, and the inner or **posterior surface** is smooth and oval shaped for articulation with the femur. The patella serves to protect the anterior aspect of the knee joint and acts as a pivot to increase the leverage of the large quadriceps femoris muscle, the tendon of which attaches to the tibial tuberosity of the lower leg. The patella is loose and movable in its more superior position when the leg is extended and the quadriceps muscles are relaxed. However, as the leg is flexed and the muscles tighten, it moves distally and becomes locked into position. The patella articulates only with the femur, not with the tibia.

KNEE JOINT

The knee joint proper is a large complex joint that primarily involves the **femorotibial joint** between the two condyles of the **femur** and the corresponding condyles of the **tibia.** The **patellofemoral joint** is also part of the knee joint, wherein the patella articulates with the anterior surface of the distal femur.

Proximal Tibiofibular Joint and Major Knee Ligaments

The proximal fibula is not part of the knee joint because it does not articulate with any aspect of the femur, even though the **fibular (lateral) collateral ligament (LCL)** extends from the femur to the lateral proximal fibula, as shown in Fig. 6.24. However, the head of the fibula does articulate with the lateral condyle of the tibia, to which it is attached by this ligament.

Additional major knee ligaments shown on this posterior view are the tibial (medial) collateral ligament (MCL), located medially, and the major posterior and anterior cruciate *(kroo'-she-at)* ligaments (PCL and ACL), located within the knee joint capsule (Fig. 6.25). (The abbreviations ACL, PCL, LCL, and MCL are commonly used to refer to these four ligaments.[2]) The knee joint is highly dependent on these two important pairs of major ligaments for stability.

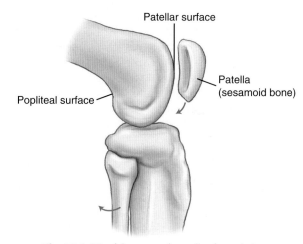

Fig 6.21 Distal femur and patella—lateral view.

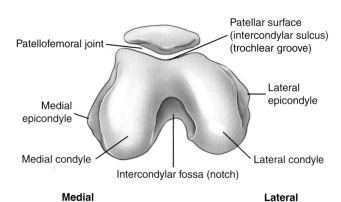

Medial   **Lateral**

Fig 6.22 Distal femur and patella—axial view.

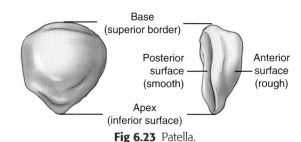

Fig 6.23 Patella.

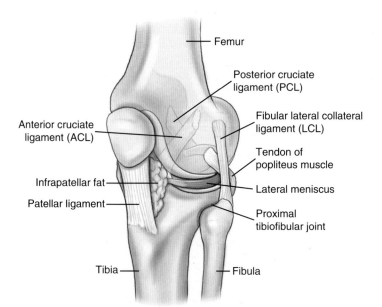

Fig 6.24 Knee joint and proximal tibiofibular joint—anterior oblique view.

The two **collateral ligaments** are strong bands at the sides of the knee that **prevent adduction and abduction** movements at the knee. The two **cruciate ligaments** are strong, rounded cords that cross each other as they attach to the respective anterior and posterior aspects of the intercondylar eminence of the tibia. They stabilize the knee joint by **preventing anterior or posterior movement** within the knee joint.

In addition to these two major pairs of ligaments, an anteriorly located **patellar ligament** and various minor ligaments help to maintain the integrity of the knee joint (Fig. 6.26). The patellar ligament is shown as part of the tendon of insertion of the large quadriceps femoris muscle, extending over the patella to the tibial tuberosity. The **infrapatellar fat pad,** posterior to this ligament, aids in protecting the anterior aspect of the knee joint.

Synovial Membrane and Cavity

The articular cavity of the knee joint is the largest joint space of the human body. The total knee joint is a synovial type enclosed in an **articular capsule, or bursa.** It is a complex, saclike structure filled with a lubricating-type synovial fluid. This is demonstrated in the arthrogram radiograph, wherein a combination of negative and positive contrast media has been injected into the articular capsule or bursa (Fig. 6.27).

The articular cavity or bursa of the knee joint extends upward under and superior to the patella, identified as the **suprapatellar bursa** (see Fig. 6.26). Distal to the patella, the **infrapatellar bursa** is separated by a large **infrapatellar fat pad,** which can be identified on radiographs. The spaces posterior and distal to the femur also can be seen and are filled with negative contrast media on the lateral arthrogram radiograph.

Menisci (Articular Disks)

The **medial** and **lateral menisci** *(me-nis'-ci)* are crescent-shaped fibrocartilage disks between the articular facets of the tibia (tibial plateau) and the femoral condyles (Fig. 6.28). They are thicker at their external margins, tapering to a very thin center portion. They act as shock absorbers to reduce some of the direct impact and stress that occur at the knee joint. The synovial membrane and the menisci produce synovial fluid, which lubricates the articulating ends of the femur and tibia that are covered with a tough, slick hyaline membrane.

Knee Trauma

The knee has great potential for traumatic injury, especially in activities such as skiing or snowboarding or in contact sports such as football or basketball. A tear of the tibial MCL frequently is associated with a tear of the ACL and a tear of the medial meniscus. Patients with these injuries typically come to the imaging department for magnetic resonance imaging (MRI) to visualize these soft tissue structures or for knee arthrography.

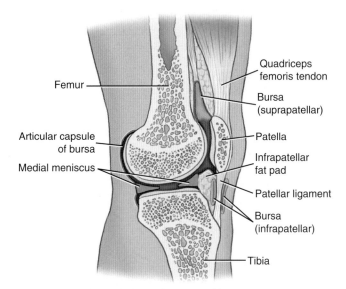

Fig 6.26 Sagittal section of knee joint.

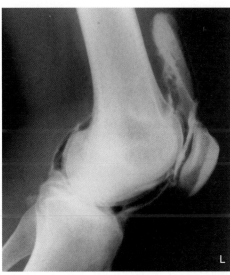

Fig 6.27 Lateral knee arthrogram radiograph (demonstrates articular capsule or bursa as outlined by a combination of negative and positive contrast media).

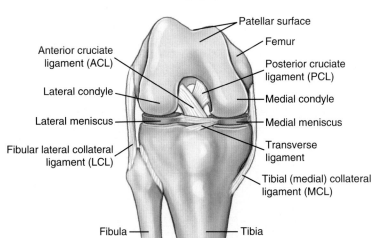

Fig 6.25 Right knee joint (flexed)—anterior view.

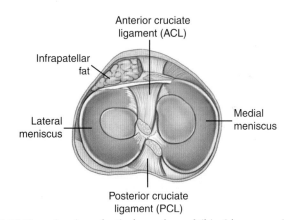

Fig 6.28 Superior view of articular surface of tibia (shows menisci and cruciate ligament attachments).

REVIEW EXERCISE WITH RADIOGRAPHS

Common projections of the lower leg, knee, and patella are shown with labels for an anatomy review.

AP Lower Leg (Fig. 6.29)

A. Medial condyle of the tibia
B. Body or shaft of tibia
C. Medial malleolus
D. Lateral malleolus
E. Body or shaft of fibula
F. Neck of fibula
G. Head of fibula
H. Apex (styloid process) of head of fibula
I. Lateral condyle of tibia
J. Intercondylar eminence (tibial spine)

Lateral Lower Leg (Fig. 6.30)

A. Intercondylar eminence (tibial spine)
B. Tibial tuberosity
C. Body or shaft of tibia
D. Body or shaft of fibula
E. Medial malleolus
F. Lateral malleolus

AP Knee (Fig. 6.31)

A. Medial and lateral intercondylar tubercles; extensions of intercondylar eminence (tibial spine)
B. Lateral epicondyle of femur
C. Lateral condyle of femur
D. Lateral condyle of tibia
E. Articular facets of tibia (tibial plateau)
F. Medial condyle of tibia
G. Medial condyle of femur
H. Medial epicondyle of femur
I. Patella (seen through femur)

Lateral Knee (Fig. 6.32)

A. Base of patella
B. Apex of patella
C. Tibial tuberosity
D. Neck of fibula
E. Head of fibula
F. Apex (styloid process) of head of fibula
G. Superimposed medial and lateral condyles
H. Patellar surface (intercondylar sulcus or trochlear groove)

Rotated Lateral Knee (*Fig. 6.33*) Projection demonstrates some rotation.

I. Adductor tubercle
J. Lateral condyle
K. Medial condyle

Tangential Projection (Patellofemoral Joint) (Fig. 6.34)

A. Patella
B. Patellofemoral (femoropatellar) joint
C. Lateral condyle
D. Patellar surface (intercondylar sulcus, trochlear groove)
E. Medial condyle

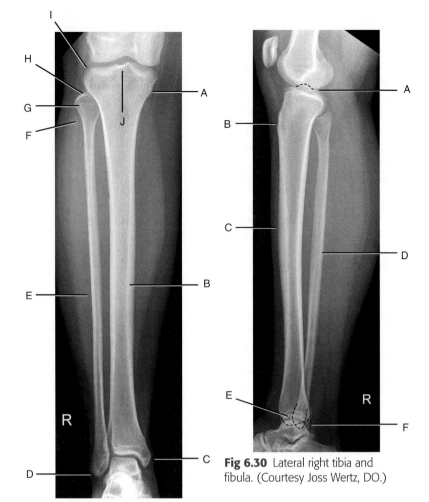

Fig 6.29 AP right tibia and fibula. (Courtesy Joss Wertz, DO.)

Fig 6.30 Lateral right tibia and fibula. (Courtesy Joss Wertz, DO.)

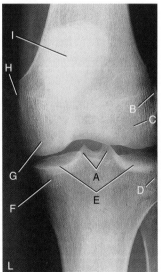

Fig 6.31 AP left knee.

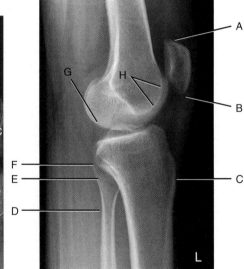

Fig 6.32 Lateral left knee—true lateral. (Courtesy Joss Wertz, DO.)

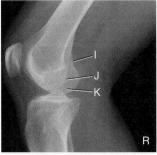

Fig 6.33 Rotated lateral knee (medial condyle more posterior).

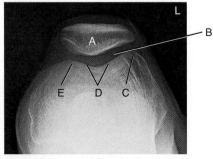

Fig 6.34 Tangential projection (patellofemoral joint). (Courtesy Joss Wertz, DO.)

CLASSIFICATION OF JOINTS

The joints or articulations of the lower limb (Fig. 6.35) all (with one exception) are classified as **synovial joints** and are characterized by a fibrous-type capsule that contains synovial fluid. They also are (with one exception) **diarthrodial,** or freely movable.

The single exception to the synovial joint is the **distal tibiofibular joint,** which is classified as a **fibrous joint** with fibrous interconnections between the surfaces of the tibia and fibula. It is of the **syndesmosis type** and is only slightly movable, or **amphiarthrodial.** However, the most distal part of this joint is smooth and is lined with a synovial membrane that is continuous with the ankle joint.

Box 6.2 summarizes the foot, ankle, lower leg, and knee joints.

SURFACES AND PROJECTIONS OF THE FOOT
Surfaces

The surfaces of the foot are sometimes confusing because the top or anterior surface of the foot is called the **dorsum.** *Dorsal* usually refers to the posterior part of the body. *Dorsum,* in this case, comes from the term **dorsum pedis,** which refers to the upper surface, or the surface opposite the sole of the foot.

The sole of the foot is the **posterior** surface or **plantar surface.** These terms are used to describe common projections of the foot.

Projections

The **AP projection** of the foot is the same as a **dorsoplantar (DP) projection.** The less common **posteroanterior (PA) projection** can also be called a **plantodorsal (PD) projection** (Fig. 6.36). Technologists should be familiar with each of these projection terms and should know which projection they represent.

MOTIONS OF THE FOOT AND ANKLE

Other potentially confusing terms involving the ankle and intertarsal joints are **dorsiflexion, plantar flexion, inversion,** and **eversion** (Fig. 6.37). To decrease the angle (flex) between the dorsum pedis and the anterior part of the lower leg is to **dorsiflex** at the ankle joint. Extending the ankle joint or pointing the foot and toe downward with respect to the normal position is called *plantar flexion.*

Inversion, or **varus,** is an inward turning or bending of the ankle and subtalar (talocalcaneal) joints, and **eversion,** or **valgus,** is an outward turning or bending. The lower leg does not rotate during inversion or eversion. Most sprained ankles result from an accidental forced inversion or eversion.

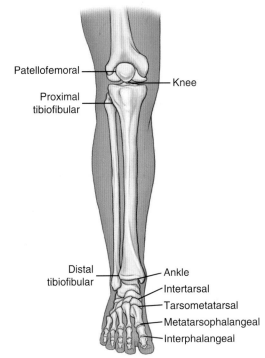

Fig 6.35 Joints of lower limb.

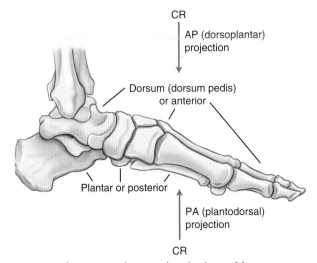

Fig 6.36 Surfaces and projections of foot.

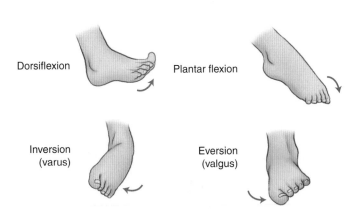

Fig 6.37 Motions of foot and ankle.

BOX 6.2 **SUMMARY OF FOOT, ANKLE, LOWER LEG, AND KNEE JOINTS**	
ALL JOINTS OF LOWER LIMB EXCEPT DISTAL TIBIOFIBULAR	
Classification: Synovial (articular capsule containing synovial fluid)	
Mobility Type: Diarthrodial (freely movable)	
Movement Types	
1. Interphalangeal joints	**Ginglymus (hinge):** Flexion and extension movements
2. Metatarsophalangeal joints	**Modified ellipsoidal (condyloid):** Flexion, extension, abduction, and adduction (circumduction similar to metacarpophalangeal joints of hand is generally not possible)
3. Tarsometatarsal joints	**Plane (gliding):** Limited gliding movement
4. Intertarsal joints	**Plane (gliding):** Subtalar in combination with some other intertarsal joints provides for gliding and rotation; results in inversion and eversion of foot
5. Ankle joint	**Saddle (sellar):** Alignment between talus and lateral and medial malleolus creates a saddle type of joint. Dorsiflexion and plantar flexion only (side-to-side movements occur only with stretched or torn ligaments)
6. Knee joints Femorotibial	**Bicondylar:** Flexion and extension and some gliding and rotational movements when knee is partially flexed
Patellofemoral	**Saddle (sellar):** Considered a saddle type because of its shape and relationship of patella to anterior, distal femur
7. Proximal tibiofibular joint	**Plane (gliding):** Limited gliding movement between lateral condyle and head of fibula
DISTAL TIBIOFIBULAR	
Classification: Fibrous	
Mobility Type: Amphiarthrodial (slightly movable) of syndesmosis type	

RADIOGRAPHIC POSITIONING

Positioning Considerations

Radiographic examinations involving the lower limb below the knee generally are done on a tabletop, as shown in Fig. 6.38. Patients with severe trauma or patients who are difficult to move can be radiographed directly on the cart.

DISTANCE

A common minimum source–image receptor distance (SID) is 40 inches (100 cm). When you are radiographing with IRs directly on the tabletop, to maintain a constant SID, increase the tube height compared with radiographs taken with the IR in the bucky tray. This difference is generally 3 to 4 inches (8 to 10 cm) for floating-type tabletops. The same minimum 40-inch (100-cm) SID should be used when you are radiographing directly on the cart, unless exposure factors are adjusted to compensate for a change in SID.

SHIELDING

Shielding of radiation-sensitive regions is important for examinations of the lower limb because of these regions' proximity to the divergent x-ray beam and scatter radiation. Red bone marrow in the hips and gonadal tissues are two of the key radiation-sensitive regions. A lead vinyl-covered shield should be draped over the patient's gonadal area. Although the gonadal rule states that this should be done on patients of reproductive age, when the gonads lie within or close to the primary field, providing gonadal shielding for all patients is good practice.

COLLIMATION

The collimation rule should be followed: collimation borders should be visible on all four sides if the IR is large enough to allow this without cutting off essential anatomy. A general rule concerning IR size is to use the smallest IR size possible for the specific part that is being radiographed. However, four-sided collimation is generally possible, even with a minimum-sized IR, for most if not all radiographic examinations of the lower limb.

With film-screen radiography and sometimes with CR, two or more projections may be taken on one IR for some examinations, such as for the toes, foot, ankle, or lower leg. Close collimation of the part that is being radiographed is required, and lead masking should be used to cover the parts of the IR not in the collimation field.

With **digital imaging,** multiple exposures on the same imaging plate are not suggested; however, when this is done, lead masking should be used to protect aspects of the IR not within the collimation field. The reason for this is to prevent unwanted exposure from scatter radiation from reaching the hypersensitive IR plate.

Four-sided collimation permits checking of radiographs for accuracy of centering and positioning by placing a large imaginary X from the four corners of the collimation field. The center point of the X indicates the CR location.

GENERAL POSITIONING

A general positioning rule that is especially applicable to both the upper and the lower limbs is **always to place the long axis of the part that is being radiographed parallel to the long axis of the IR.** If more than one projection is taken on the same IR, the part should be parallel to the long axis of the part of the IR being used. Also, **all body parts should be oriented in the same direction** when two or more projections are taken on the same IR.

An exception to this rule is the lower leg of an adult. This limb generally can be placed diagonally to include both the knee and the ankle joints.

CORRECT CENTERING

Accurate centering and alignment of the body part to the IR and correct CR location are especially important for examinations of the upper and lower limbs, in which shape and size distortion must be avoided and the narrow joint spaces clearly demonstrated. In general, the part being radiographed should be parallel to the plane of the IR, and the CR should be 90° or perpendicular and should be directed to the correct centering point, as indicated on each positioning page. (Exceptions to the 90° or perpendicular CR do occur, as indicated in the following pages.)

Multiple Exposures Per Imaging Plate

Placing multiple images on the same digital imaging plate (IP) is not commonly performed. Most experts would recommend that one exposure be placed centered to the IP for computed radiography and digital radiography imaging systems. But if multiple images are placed on the same IP, careful collimation and lead masking must be used to prevent pre-exposure or fogging of other images.

EXPOSURE FACTORS

The principal exposure factors for radiographs of the lower limbs are as follows:
1. Low-to-medium kVp (50–85)
2. Short exposure time
3. Small focal spot
4. Adequate milliamperes (mAs) for sufficient density (brightness)

Correctly exposed radiographs of the lower limbs generally should visualize both soft tissue margins and fine bony trabecular markings of the bones being radiographed.

IMAGE RECEPTORS

For examinations distal to the knee, IRs without grids are generally used. High resolution IRs may be used for extremities to obtain better detail.

Grids

A general rule is that grids should be used with body parts that measure more than 10 cm. (Some references suggest a grid for body parts greater than 13 cm.) This rule places the average knee (measuring 9 to 13 cm) at a size for which either a nongrid or a grid technique may be used, depending on patient size and departmental preferences. This text recommends a nongrid technique on smaller patients with knees measuring 10 cm or less and a grid for larger patients with knees measuring more than 10 cm, especially on the AP knee. Anything proximal to the knee, such as the midfemur or distal femur, requires the use of a grid. When grids are used, you may choose either the moving bucky or a fine-lined portable grid.

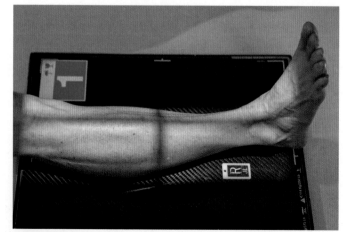

Fig 6.38 Tabletop mediolateral projection of lower limb demonstrating *(A)* correct CR location and *(B)* collimation.

Special Patient Considerations

PEDIATRIC APPLICATIONS

Pediatric patients should be addressed in language they are able to understand. Parents are often helpful in positioning younger children in nontrauma situations. If parents are allowed to stay in the room, they must be provided appropriate shielding, and females must be asked their current pregnancy status according to facility policy. Immobilization is needed in many cases to assist in holding the limb in the proper position. Sponges and tape are useful, but sandbags should be used with caution because of their weight. Accurate part measurement is critical in setting technical factors.

Generally, exposure factors must be decreased because of reduced tissue quantity and density (brightness). Shorter exposure times, along with the highest mA possible, help to eliminate motion on the radiograph.

GERIATRIC APPLICATIONS

Older patients must be handled carefully when they are being moved, and radiography of the lower limbs is no exception. Look for telltale signs of hip fracture (i.e., foot in extreme external rotation position). Routine positioning maneuvers may have to be adjusted to accommodate potential pathology and lack of joint flexibility. Positioning aids and supports should be used to enhance patient comfort and assist in immobilizing the limb in the correct position.

Exposure factors may require adjustment because of underlying pathologic conditions such as osteoarthritis or osteoporosis. Shorter exposure time and higher mA are desirable for reducing the possibility of imaging involuntary or voluntary motion.

BARIATRIC PATIENT CONSIDERATIONS

Properly dressing patients for radiographic examinations is important to maintain radiographic quality. It is especially important in digital imaging and with bariatric patients. The increased sensitivity of digital imaging can cause clothing and other artifacts to appear on the image. Also, tight-fitting clothing on bariatric patients can interfere with radiographic quality. For example, increased compression due to improper clothing and added soft tissue can make it difficult to visualize fad pad signs indicative of fractures.

When imaging bariatric patients, proper alignment of the central ray with the body part remains the same. The increase in soft tissue does not change the position of the osseous anatomy. Increases in soft tissue may warrant changes in exposure factors. These changes may include an increase in kVp to improve penetration through additionally thick tissue. mA and time may also be increased, but sparingly to avoid excessive skin exposure. Care should also be taken to decrease scatter radiation to the IR due to the increased amount of tissue. The use of a grid for anatomic structures over 10 cm can be used to eliminate the demonstration of scatter.

Although most factors remain the same when imaging bariatric patients, there are factors to be considered. The largest consideration involves imaging of the knee. An increased cephalad CR angle may be required to visualize an open joint space when a patient has a greater thickness of the lower torso. Also, bariatric patients may require modifications to conventional imaging positions for the ease and comfort of the patient. For example, tissue may interfere with performing a tangential view of the patella using the Merchant method, requiring the use of the inferosuperior projection. Bariatric patients may also have difficulty internally rotating for a medial oblique knee, requiring instead the CR and IR to be adjusted to compensate.

PLACEMENT OF MARKERS AND PATIENT IDENTIFICATION INFORMATION

At the top of each of the following positioning pages is a small rectangular diagram that shows the correct IR size and placement (portrait or landscape). When film-screen technology is used, a suggested corner placement for the patient identification blocker is shown for each IR. However, this is only a suggested location because the location of the blocker changes with each manufacturer. The important consideration is **always to place it in the location that is least likely to superimpose anatomy of interest** for that projection. This concern is eliminated when computed radiography or digital radiography applications are used. The size and location of multiple projections on one IR are also shown.

When final radiographs are evaluated, as part of the evaluation criteria, right (R) and left (L) markers should always be visible on the lateral margin of the collimation field **on at least one projection on each IR** without superimposing any anatomy of interest. If film-screen systems are used, the patient identification information should always be checked to see whether it is legible and to ensure that it is not superimposing essential anatomy.

INCREASED EXPOSURE WITH CAST

A lower limb with a cast requires an increase in exposure. The thickness of the cast and the body part and the type of cast affect the increase in exposure required. See Table 6.1 for a recommended conversion guide for casts.

Digital Imaging Considerations

Following is a summary of guidelines that should be followed when digital imaging technology (computed radiography or digital radiography) is used for the lower limbs:

1. **Four-sided collimation:** Collimate to the area of interest with a minimum of two collimation parallel borders clearly demonstrated in the image. Four-sided collimation is always preferred if the study permits it.
2. **Accurate centering:** It is important that the body part and the central ray be centered to the IR.
3. **Grid use with cassette-less systems:** Anatomy thickness and kVp range are deciding factors if a grid is to be used. With these systems, it may be impractical and difficult to remove the grid, so the grid is commonly left in place even for smaller body parts measuring 10 cm or less (i.e., some upper and lower limb examinations). If the grid is left in place, ensure that the CR is centered to the grid.
4. **Exposure factors:** Patient exposure should follow the ALARA (as low as reasonably achievable) principle, and the lowest exposure factors required to obtain a diagnostic image should be used. This includes the highest kVp and the lowest mAs that would result in desirable image quality. The kVp may need to be higher than that used for analog (film-screen) imaging for larger body parts, with 50 kVp as the general minimum used on any procedure (exception is mammography).
5. **Post-processing evaluation of exposure indicator:** The exposure indicator value on the final processed image must be checked to verify that the exposure factors used were in the correct range to ensure optimal quality with the least radiation to the patient. If the index is outside of the acceptable range, the technologist must adjust the kVp or mAs or both accordingly for any repeat exposures.

TABLE 6.1 CAST CONVERSION CHART	
TYPE OF CAST	**INCREASE IN EXPOSURE**
Small to medium plaster cast	Increase 5 to 7 kVp
Large plaster cast	Increase 8 to 10 kVp
Fiberglass cast	Increase 3 to 4 kVp

Alternative Modalities and Procedures

ARTHROGRAPHY

Arthrography sometimes is used to image large diarthrodial joints such as the knee. This procedure requires the use of a contrast medium injected into the joint capsule under sterile conditions. Disease or traumatic damage to the menisci, ligaments, and articular cartilage may be evaluated with arthrography (see Chapter 19).

COMPUTED TOMOGRAPHY (CT)

CT often is used on the lower limbs to evaluate soft tissue involvement of lesions. The cross-sectional images are also excellent for determining the extent of fractures and for evaluating bone mineralization.

MAGNETIC RESONANCE IMAGING (MRI)

MRI may be used to image the lower limbs when soft tissue injuries are suspected. The knee is the most often evaluated portion of the lower limb, and MRI is invaluable in detecting ligament damage or meniscal tears of the joint capsule. MRI also may be used to evaluate lesions in the skeletal system.

BONE DENSITOMETRY

Bone densitometry may be used to evaluate loss of bone in geriatric patients or in patients with a lytic (bone-destroying) type of bone disease (see Chapter 20 for more information on bone density measurement procedures).

NUCLEAR MEDICINE (NM)

NM uses radioisotopes injected into the bloodstream. These isotopes are absorbed in great concentration in areas where pathologic conditions exist. Nuclear medicine bone scans are particularly useful in showing osteomyelitis and metastatic bone lesions.

Clinical Indications

Radiographers should be familiar with common pathologic indications that relate to the lower limb, as follows:

Bone cysts are benign, neoplastic bone lesions filled with clear fluid that most often occur near the knee joint in children and adolescents. Generally, these are not detected on radiographs until a pathologic fracture occurs. When bone cysts are detected on radiographs, they appear as lucent areas with a thin cortex and sharp boundaries.

Chondromalacia patellae (commonly known as *runner's knee*) involves a softening of the cartilage under the patella, which results in erosion of this cartilage, causing pain and tenderness in this area. Cyclists and runners are vulnerable to this condition.

Chondrosarcomas are malignant tumors of the cartilage that usually occur in the pelvis and long bones of men older than 45 years.

Enchondroma is a slow-growing **benign cartilaginous tumor** that most often is found in small bones of the hands and feet in adolescents and young adults. Generally, these are well-defined, radiolucent-appearing tumors with a thin cortex, and they often lead to pathologic fracture with only minimal trauma.

Ewing sarcoma is a common **primary malignant bone tumor** that arises from bone marrow in children and young adults. Symptoms are similar to those of osteomyelitis, with low-grade fever and pain. Bone has stratified new bone formation, resulting in an "onion peel" look on radiographs. Ewing sarcoma generally occurs in the diaphysis of long bones. The prognosis is poor by the time it is evident on radiographs.

Exostosis (osteochondroma) is a benign, neoplastic bone lesion that is caused by consolidated overproduction of bone at a joint (usually the knee). The tumor grows parallel to the bone and away from the adjacent joint. Tumor growth stops as soon as the epiphyseal plates close. Pain is an associated symptom if the tumor is large enough to irritate surrounding soft tissues.

Fractures are breaks in the structure of bone caused by a force (direct or indirect). The types of fracture are named according to the extent of fracture, direction of fracture lines, alignment of bone fragments, and integrity of overlying skin (see Chapter 15 for fracture types and descriptions).

Gout is a form of arthritis that may be hereditary in which uric acid appears in excessive quantities in the blood and may be deposited in the joints and other tissues; common initial attacks occur in the **first MTP joint** of the foot. Later attacks may occur in other joints, such as the first metacarpophalangeal (MCP) joint of the hand, but generally these are not evident radiographically until more advanced conditions develop. Most cases occur in men, and first attacks rarely occur before the age of 30.

Joint effusions occur as accumulated fluid (synovial or hemorrhagic) in the joint cavity. These are signs of an underlying condition (e.g., fracture, dislocation, soft tissue damage).

The **Lisfranc ligament** is a large band that spans the articulation of the medial cuneiform and the first and second metatarsal base. Because no transverse ligament exists between the first and second metatarsal bases, this region of the foot is prone to stress injury caused by motor vehicle crashes, twisting falls, and falls from high places. Athletes often may acquire a Lisfranc injury that is due to high stress placed on the midfoot. **Lisfranc joint injuries** range from sprains to fracture-dislocations of the bases of the first and second metatarsals. A moderate sprain of the Lisfranc ligament is characterized by an abnormal separation between the first and second metatarsals. A small avulsion fracture may indicate a more severe injury. Lisfranc joint injuries may be missed if weight-bearing AP and lateral foot projections are not performed.

Multiple myeloma is the most common type of **primary cancerous bone tumor.** Generally, these tumors affect persons 40 to 70 years old. As the name implies, they occur in various parts of the body. Because this tumor arises from bone marrow or marrow plasma cells, it is not a truly exclusive bony tumor. Multiple myelomas are highly malignant and usually are fatal within a few years. The typical radiographic appearance consists of multiple "punched-out" osteolytic (loss of calcium in bone) lesions scattered throughout the affected bones.

Osgood-Schlatter disease, which involves inflammation of the bone and cartilage of the anterior proximal tibia, is most common in boys 10 to 15 years old. The cause is believed to be an injury that occurs when the large patellar tendon detaches part of the **tibial tuberosity** to which it is attached. Severe cases may require immobilization by plaster cast.

Osteoarthritis, also called **degenerative joint disease (DJD),** is a noninflammatory joint disease that is characterized by gradual deterioration of the articular cartilage with hypertrophic (enlargement or overgrown) bone formation. This is the most common type of arthritis and is considered part of the normal aging process.

Osteoclastomas (giant cell tumors) are benign lesions that typically occur in the long bones of young adults; they usually occur in the proximal tibia or distal femur after epiphyseal closure. These tumors appear on radiographs as large "bubbles" separated by thin strips of bone.

Osteogenic sarcomas (osteosarcomas) are **highly malignant primary bone tumors** that occur from childhood to young adulthood (peak age, 20 years). The neoplasm usually is seen in long bones and may cause gross destruction of bone.

Osteoid osteomas are **benign bone lesions** that usually occur in teenagers or young adults. Symptoms include localized pain that typically worsens at night but is relieved by over-the-counter anti-inflammatory or pain medications. The tibia and the femur are the most likely locations of these lesions.

Osteomalacia (rickets) literally means "bone softening." This disease is caused by lack of bone mineralization secondary to a deficiency of calcium, phosphorus, or vitamin D in the diet or an inability to absorb these minerals. Because of the softness of the bones, bowing defects in weight-bearing parts often result. This disease is known as *rickets* in children and commonly results in bowing of the tibia.

Paget disease (osteitis deformans) is one of the most common diseases of the skeleton. It is most common in midlife and is twice as common in men as in women. It is a non-neoplastic bone disease that disrupts new bone growth, resulting in over-production of very dense yet soft bone. Bone destruction creates lytic or lucent areas; this is followed by reconstruction of bone, by which sclerotic or dense areas are created. The result is a very characteristic radiographic appearance that sometimes is described as cotton wool. Lesions typically occur in the skull, pelvis, femurs, tibias, vertebrae, clavicles, and ribs. Long bones generally bow or fracture because of softening of the bone; the associated joint may develop arthritic changes. The **pelvis** is the most common initial site of this disease.

Reiter syndrome affects the sacroiliac joints and lower limbs of young men; the radiographic hallmark is a specific area of bony erosion at the Achilles tendon insertion on the **posterosuperior margin of the calcaneus.** Involvement is usually bilateral, and arthritis, ure-thritis, and conjunctivitis are characteristic of this syndrome. Reiter syndrome is caused by a previous infection of the gastrointestinal tract, such as salmonella, or by a sexually transmitted infection. See Table 6.2 for a summary of clinical indications.

Routine, Alternate, and Special Projections

Routine, alternate, and special projections for the toes, foot, ankle, lower leg, and knee are demonstrated and described on the following pages.

TABLE 6.2 SUMMARY OF CLINICAL INDICATIONS

CONDITION OR DISEASE	MOST COMMON RADIOGRAPHIC EXAMINATION	POSSIBLE RADIOGRAPHIC APPEARANCE	EXPOSURE FACTOR ADJUSTMENT[a]
Bone cyst	AP and lateral of affected limb	Well-circumscribed lucency	None
Chondromalacia patellae	AP and lateral knee, tangential (axial) of patellofemoral joint	Pathology of patellofemoral joint space, possible misalignment of patella	None
Chondrosarcoma	AP and lateral of affected limb, CT, MRI	Bone destruction with calcifications in cartilaginous tumor	None
Enchondroma (benign cartilaginous tumor)	AP and lateral of affected limb	Well-defined radiolucent tumor with thin cortex (often results in pathologic fracture with minimal trauma)	None
Ewing sarcoma (malignant bone tumor)	AP and lateral of affected limb, CT, MRI	Ill-defined area of bone destruction with surrounding "onion peel" (layers of periosteal reaction)	None
Exostosis (osteochondroma)	AP and lateral of affected limb	Projection of bone with cartilaginous cap; grows parallel to shaft and away from nearest joint	None
Gout (a form of arthritis)	AP (oblique) and lateral of affected part (most common initially in MTP joint of foot)	Uric acid deposits in joint space; destruction of joint space	None
Lisfranc joint injury	Weight-bearing AP and lateral and 30° medial oblique projections, CT, MRI	Abnormal separation or avulsion fracture between base of first and second metatarsals and cuneiforms	Slight increase in exposure factors to penetrate tarsal region of foot
Multiple myeloma (most common primary cancerous bone tumor)	AP and lateral of affected part	Multiple "punched-out" osteolytic lesions throughout affected bone	None
Osgood-Schlatter disease	AP and lateral of knee	Fragmentation or detachment of tibial tuberosity by patellar tendon	None
Osteoarthritis (degenerative joint disease)	AP, oblique, and lateral of affected part	Narrowed, irregular joint spaces with sclerotic articular surfaces and spurs	Advanced stage may require slight decrease (−)
Osteoclastoma (giant cell tumor)	AP and lateral of affected part	Large radiolucent lesions with thin strips of bone between	None
Osteogenic sarcoma (primary bone tumor)	AP and lateral of affected part, CT, MRI	Extensively destructive lesion with irregular periosteal reaction; classic appearance is sunburst pattern that is diffuse periosteal reaction	None
Osteoid osteoma (benign bone lesions)	AP and lateral of affected part	Small, round-to-oval density with lucent center	None
Osteomalacia (rickets)	AP and lateral of affected limb	Decreased bone density, bowing deformity in weight-bearing limbs	Loss of bone matrix requires decrease (−)
Paget disease (osteitis deformans)	AP and lateral of affected parts	Mixed areas of sclerotic and cortical thickening and lytic or radiolucent lesions; cotton wool appearance	Extensive sclerotic areas may require increase (+)
Reiter syndrome	AP and lateral of affected part	Asymmetric erosion of joint spaces; calcaneus erosion, usually bilateral	None

[a]Dependent on stage or severity of disease or condition.

6

AP PROJECTION: TOES

Clinical Indications

- Fractures or dislocations of the phalanges of the digits in question
- Pathologies such as osteoarthritis and gouty arthritis (gout), especially in the first digit

Toes
ROUTINE
• AP
• Oblique
• Lateral

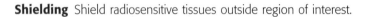

Technical Factors

- Minimum SID—40 inches (100 cm)
- IR size—8 × 10 inches (18 × 24 cm), landscape
- Nongrid
- kVp range: 50–65

NOTE: Some departmental routines include centering and collimation for AP toes to include all the toes and distal metatarsals. Most routines involve centering to the toe of interest with closer collimation to include only one digit on each side of injury.

Shielding Shield radiosensitive tissues outside region of interest.

Patient Position Place patient supine or seated on table; knee should be flexed with plantar surface of foot resting on IR.

Part Position ⊞

- Center and align long axis of digit to CR and long axis of portion of IR being exposed.
- Ensure that MTP joint of digit in question is centered to CR.

CR

- Angle CR **10° to 15° toward calcaneus** (CR perpendicular to phalanges) (Fig. 6.39).
- If a **15° wedge** is placed under the foot for parallel part-film alignment, the CR is **perpendicular** to the IR (Fig. 6.40).
- Center CR to **MTP joint** in question.

Recommended Collimation Collimate on four sides to area of interest. On side margins, include a minimum of at least part of one digit on each side of the digit in question.

Computed Radiography or Digital Radiography Close collimation is important over unexposed portions of IR to prevent fogging from scatter radiation.

Evaluation Criteria

Anatomy Demonstrated: • Digits of interest and a minimum of the distal half of metatarsals should be included (Figs. 6.41 and 6.42).
Position: • Individual digits should be separated with no overlapping of soft tissues. • Long axis of foot is aligned to long axis of portion of IR being exposed. • **No rotation** is present if shafts of the phalanges and distal metatarsals appear equally concave on both sides. • Rotation appears as one side being more concave than the other. • Side with increased concavity has been rolled away from IR.[4] • IP and MTP joint spaces are open. Incorrect CR angulation or insufficient elevation of forefoot may distort or close joint spaces.[4] • Collimation to **area of interest**.
Exposure: • **No motion** as evidenced by sharply defined cortical margins of the bone and detailed bony trabeculae.
• Optimal contrast and density (brightness) allow visualization of bony cortical margins and trabeculae and soft tissue structures.

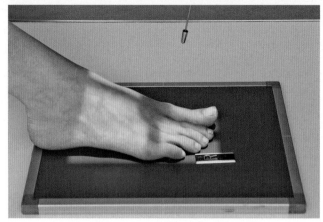

Fig 6.39 Second digit (CR, 10° to 15°).

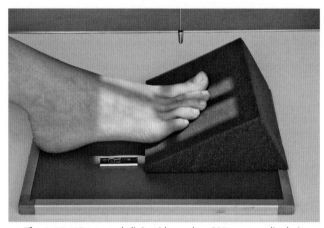

Fig 6.40 AP second digit with wedge (CR perpendicular).

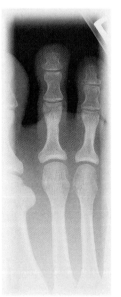

Fig 6.41 AP second digit.

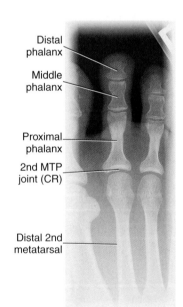

Distal phalanx
Middle phalanx
Proximal phalanx
2nd MTP joint (CR)
Distal 2nd metatarsal

Fig 6.42 AP second digit.

AP OBLIQUE PROJECTION—MEDIAL OR LATERAL ROTATION: TOES

Clinical Indications
- Fractures or dislocations of the phalanges of the digits in question
- Pathologies such as osteoarthritis and gouty arthritis (gout), especially in the first digit

Toes
ROUTINE
- AP
- Oblique
- Lateral

Technical Factors
- Minimum SID—40 inches (100 cm).
- IR size—8 × 10 inches (18 × 24 cm), landscape
- Nongrid
- kVp range: 50–60

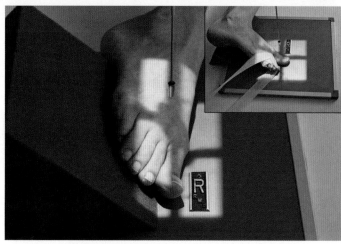
Fig 6.43 Medial oblique rotation—first digit.

Shielding Shield radiosensitive tissues outside region of interest.

Patient Position Place patient supine or seated on table; knee should be flexed with plantar surface of foot resting on IR.

Part Position
- Center and align long axis of digit to CR and long axis of portion of IR being exposed.
- Ensure that MTP joint of digit in question is centered to CR.
- Rotate the leg and foot 30° to 45° medially for the first, second, and third digits (Fig. 6.43) and laterally for the fourth and fifth digits (Fig. 6.44). (See oblique foot projections for degree of obliquity.)
- Use 45° radiolucent support under elevated portion of foot to prevent motion.

CR
- CR **perpendicular** to IR, directed to MTP joint in question

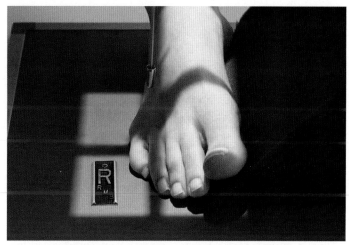
Fig 6.44 Lateral oblique rotation—fourth digit.

Recommended Collimation Collimate on four sides to include phalanges and a minimum of distal half of metatarsals. On side margins, include a minimum of one digit on each side of digit in question.

Computed Radiography or Digital Radiography Close collimation is important over unexposed portions of IR to prevent fogging from scatter radiation.

Evaluation Criteria
Anatomy Demonstrated: • Digits in question and distal half of metatarsals should be included without overlap (superimposition) (Figs. 6.45 and 6.46).
Position: • Long axis of foot is aligned to long axis of portion of IR being exposed. • Correct obliquity should be evident by increased concavity on one side of shafts and by overlapping of soft tissues of digits. • Heads of metatarsals should appear directly side by side with no (or only minimal) overlapping.[4] • Collimation to **area of interest.**
Exposure: • No motion as evidenced by sharply defined cortical margins of bone and detailed bony trabeculae. • Optimal contrast and density (brightness) allow visualization of bony cortical margins and trabeculae and soft tissue structures.

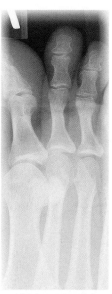
Fig 6.45 Medial oblique—second digit.

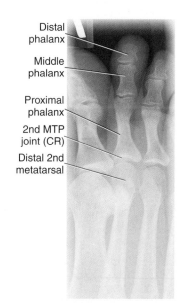

Distal phalanx
Middle phalanx
Proximal phalanx
2nd MTP joint (CR)
Distal 2nd metatarsal

Fig 6.46 Medial oblique—second digit.

6

LATERAL—MEDIOLATERAL OR LATEROMEDIAL PROJECTIONS: TOES

Clinical Indications

- Fractures or dislocations of the phalanges of the digits in question
- Pathologies such as osteoarthritis and gouty arthritis (gout), especially in the first digit

Toes
ROUTINE
- AP
- Oblique
- Lateral

Technical Factors

- Minimum SID—40 inches (100 cm).
- IR size—8 × 10 inches (18 × 24 cm), landscape
- Nongrid
- kVp range: 50–60

Shielding Shield radiosensitive tissues outside region of interest.

Patient and Part Position

- Rotate affected leg and foot medially (lateromedial) for first, second, and third digits (Figs. 6.47 and 6.48) and laterally (mediolateral) for fourth and fifth digits (Fig. 6.49).
- Adjust IR to center and align long axis of toe in question to CR and to long axis of portion of IR being exposed.
- Ensure that interphalangeal joint or proximal interphalangeal joint in question is centered to CR.
- Use tape, gauze, or tongue blade to flex and separate unaffected toes to prevent superimposition.

CR

- CR perpendicular to IR
- CR directed to interphalangeal joint for first digit and to proximal interphalangeal joint for second to fifth digits

Recommended Collimation Collimate closely on four sides to affected digit.

Computed Radiography or Digital Radiography Close collimation is important over unexposed portions of IR to prevent fogging from scatter radiation.

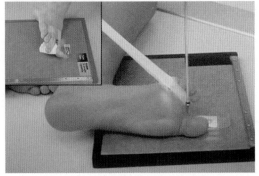

Fig 6.47 Lateromedial—first digit.

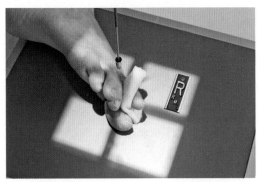

Fig 6.48 Lateromedial—second digit.

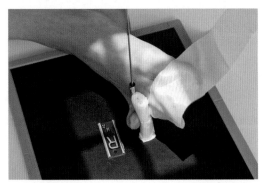

Fig 6.49 Mediolateral—fourth digit.

Evaluation Criteria

Anatomy Demonstrated: • Phalanges of digit in question should be seen in lateral position free of superimposition by other digits, if possible (Figs. 6.50 and 6.51). • (When total separation of toes is impossible, especially third to fifth digits, the distal phalanx at least should be separated, and the proximal phalanx should be visualized through superimposed structures.)

Position: • Long axis of digit is aligned to long axis of portion of IR being used. • True lateral of digit demonstrates increased concavity on anterior surface of the distal phalanx and posterior surface of the proximal phalanx. • Opposing surface of each phalanx appears straighter.[4] • Collimation to area of interest.

Exposure: • No motion as evidenced by sharply defined cortical margins of bone and detailed bony trabeculae. • Optimal contrast and density (brightness) allow visualization of bony cortical margins and trabeculae and soft tissue structures.

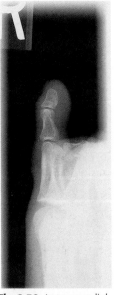

Fig 6.50 Lateromedial—second digit.

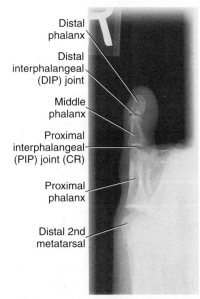

Distal phalanx
Distal interphalangeal (DIP) joint
Middle phalanx
Proximal interphalangeal (PIP) joint (CR)
Proximal phalanx
Distal 2nd metatarsal

Fig 6.51 Lateromedial—second digit.

TANGENTIAL PROJECTION: TOES—SESAMOIDS

Clinical Indications
- This projection provides a profile image of the sesamoid bones at the first MTP joint for evaluation of extent of injury

NOTE: A lateral of the first digit in dorsiflexion also may be taken to visualize these sesamoids.

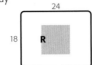

Toes
SPECIAL
- Sesamoids (tangential)

Technical Factors
- Minimum SID—40 inches (100 cm)
- IR size—8 × 10 inches (18 × 24 cm), landscape
- Nongrid
- kVp range: 50–60

Shielding Shield radiosensitive tissues outside region of interest.

Patient Position Place patient prone; provide a pillow for patient's head and a small sponge or folded towel under lower leg for comfort.

Part Position
- Dorsiflex the foot so that the plantar surface of the foot forms a **15° to 20° angle** from vertical (Figs. 6.52 and 6.53).
- Dorsiflex the first digit (great toe) and rest on IR to maintain position.
- Ensure that long axis of foot is not rotated; place sandbags or other support on both sides of foot to prevent movement.

NOTE: This is an uncomfortable and often painful position; do not keep patient in this position longer than necessary.

CR
- CR **perpendicular** to IR, directed tangentially to posterior aspect of **first MTP joint** (depending on amount of dorsiflexion of foot, may need to angle CR slightly for a true tangential projection)

Recommended Collimation Collimate closely to area of interest. Include at least the first, second, and third distal metatarsals for possible sesamoids but with CR at first MTP joint.

Evaluation Criteria
Anatomy Demonstrated: • Sesamoids should be seen in profile free of superimposition. • A minimum of the first three distal metatarsals should be included in collimation field for possible sesamoids, with the center of the four-sided collimation field (CR) at the posterior portion of the first MTP joint (Figs. 6.54 and 6.55).
Position: • Borders of posterior margins of first to third distal metatarsals are seen in profile, indicating correct dorsiflexion of foot. • Centering and CR angulation are correct if the sesamoids are free of any bony superimposition and open space is demonstrated between sesamoids and first metatarsal.
Exposure: • No motion as evidenced by sharp bony cortical margins and detailed trabeculae. • Optimal contrast and density (brightness) allow visualization of bony cortical margins and trabeculae and soft tissue structures without sesamoids appearing overexposed.

Alternative Projection If the patient cannot tolerate the previously described prone position, this radiograph may be performed in a reverse projection with the patient supine and the use of a long strip of gauze for the patient to hold the toes as shown. The CR would be directed tangential to the posterior aspect of the first MTP joint. Use support to prevent motion. However, this is not a desirable projection because of the increased object–image receptor distance (OID) with accompanying magnification and loss of definition.

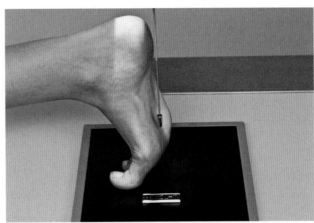

Fig 6.52 Tangential projection—patient prone.

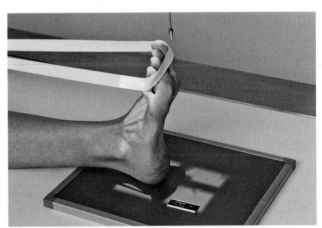

Fig 6.53 Alternative projection—patient supine.

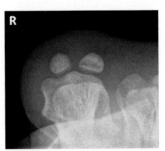

Fig 6.54 Tangential projection. (Courtesy Joss Wertz, DO.)

Tibial and fibular sesamoids   Distal 1st metatarsal

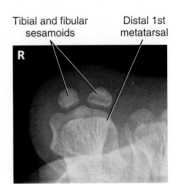

Fig 6.55 Tangential projection. (Courtesy Joss Wertz, DO.)

AP PROJECTION: FOOT

DORSOPLANTAR PROJECTION

Clinical Indications
- Location and extent of fractures and fragment alignments, joint space abnormalities, soft tissue effusions
- Location of opaque foreign bodies

Foot
ROUTINE
• AP
• Oblique
• Lateral

Technical Factors
- Minimum SID—40 inches (100 cm)
- IR size—10 × 12 inches (24 × 30 cm), portrait
- Nongrid
- kVp range: 55–65

Shielding Shield radiosensitive tissues outside region of interest.

Patient Position Place patient supine; provide a pillow for patient's head; flex knee and place plantar surface (sole) of affected foot flat on IR.

Part Position
- Extend (plantar flex) foot but maintain plantar surface resting flat and firmly on IR (Fig. 6.56).
- Align and center long axis of foot to CR and to long axis of portion of IR being exposed. (Use sandbags if necessary to prevent IR from slipping on tabletop.)
- If immobilization is needed, flex opposite knee also and rest against affected knee for support.

CR
- Angle CR **10° posteriorly** (toward heel) with CR perpendicular to metatarsals (see **NOTE**).
- Direct CR to base of third metatarsal.

Recommended Collimation Collimate to outer margins of foot on four sides.

Evaluation Criteria
Anatomy Demonstrated: • Entire foot should be demonstrated, including all phalanges and metatarsals and navicular, cuneiforms, and cuboids (Figs. 6.57 and 6.58).
Position: • Long axis of foot should be aligned to long axis of portion of IR being exposed. • **No rotation** as evidenced by nearly equal distance between second through fifth metatarsals. • Bases of first and second metatarsals generally are separated, but bases of second to fifth metatarsals appear to overlap. • Intertarsal joint space between first and second cuneiforms should be demonstrated. • Collimation to **area of interest.**
Exposure: • Optimal density (brightness) and contrast with **no motion** should visualize sharp borders and trabecular markings of distal phalanges and tarsals distal to talus. • Higher kVp technique used for more uniform densities between phalanges and tarsals. • Sesamoid bones (if present) should be seen through head of first metatarsal.

Computed Radiography or Digital Radiography Close collimation is important over unexposed portions of IR to prevent fogging from scatter radiation.

NOTE: A high arch requires a greater angle (15°) and a low arch nearer 5° to be perpendicular to the metatarsals. For a foreign body, CR should be perpendicular to IR with no CR angle.

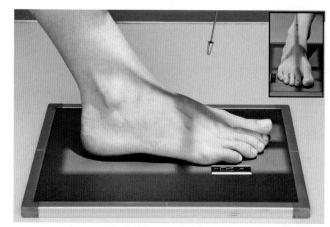

Fig 6.56 AP foot—CR 10°.

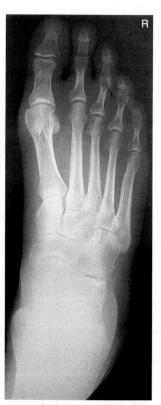

Fig 6.57 AP foot.

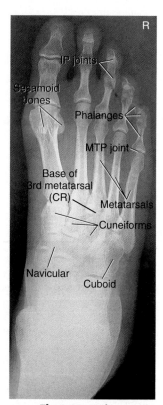

IP joints

Sesamoid bones

Phalanges

MTP joint

Base of 3rd metatarsal (CR)

Metatarsals

Cuneiforms

Navicular

Cuboid

Fig 6.58 AP foot.

AP OBLIQUE PROJECTION—MEDIAL ROTATION: FOOT

Clinical Indications

- Location and extent of fractures and fragment alignments, joint space abnormalities, soft tissue effusions
- Location of opaque foreign bodies

Foot
ROUTINE
• AP
• Oblique
• Lateral

Technical Factors

- Minimum SID—40 inches (100 cm)
- IR size—10 × 12 inches (24 × 30 cm), portrait
- Nongrid
- kVp range: 60–70

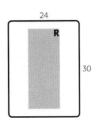

Shielding Shield radiosensitive tissues outside region of interest.

Patient Position Place patient supine or sitting; flex knee, with plantar surface of foot on table; turn body slightly away from side in question.

Part Position

- Align and center long axis of foot to CR and to long axis of portion of IR being exposed.
- Rotate foot **medially** to place **plantar surface 30° to 40° to plane of IR** (see NOTE). The general plane of the dorsum of the foot should be parallel to IR and perpendicular to CR (Fig. 6.59).
- Use 45° radiolucent support block to prevent motion. Use sandbags if necessary to prevent IR from slipping on tabletop.

CR

- CR perpendicular to IR, directed to base of third metatarsal

Recommended Collimation Collimate to outer margins of skin on four sides.

NOTE: Some references suggest only a 30° oblique routinely. This text recommends greater obliquity, 40°, to demonstrate tarsals and proximal metatarsals best relatively free of superimposition for the foot with an average transverse arch.

Evaluation Criteria (Medial Oblique)

Anatomy Demonstrated: • Entire foot should be demonstrated from distal phalanges to posterior calcaneus and proximal talus (Figs. 6.61 and 6.62).

Position: • Long axis of foot should be aligned to long axis of IR. • Correct obliquity is demonstrated when third through fifth metatarsals are free of superimposition. • First and second metatarsals also should be free of superimposition except for base area. • Tuberosity at base of fifth metatarsal is seen in profile and is well visualized. • Joint spaces around cuboid and the sinus tarsi are open and well demonstrated when foot is positioned obliquely correctly. • Collimation to area of interest.

Exposure: • Optimal density (brightness) and contrast with no motion should visualize sharp borders and trabecular markings of phalanges, metatarsals, and tarsals.

Optional Lateral Oblique (Fig. 6.60)

- Rotate the foot laterally 30° (less obliquity is required because of the natural arch of the foot).
- A lateral oblique best demonstrates the space between first and second metatarsals and between first and second cuneiforms. The navicular also is well visualized on the lateral oblique.

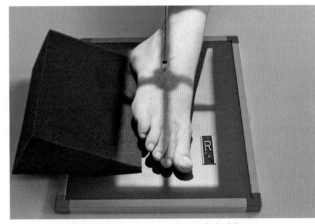

Fig 6.59 30° to 40° AP medial oblique.

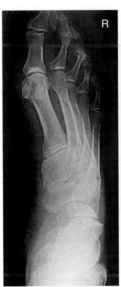
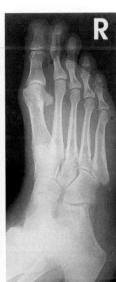
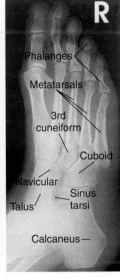

Fig 6.60 30° AP lateral oblique.

Fig 6.61 40° AP medial oblique.

Fig 6.62 40° medial oblique.

6

LATERAL—MEDIOLATERAL OR LATEROMEDIAL PROJECTIONS: FOOT

Clinical Indications
- Location and degree of anterior or posterior displacement of fracture fragments, joint abnormalities, and soft tissue effusions
- Location of opaque foreign bodies

Foot
ROUTINE
• AP
• Oblique
• Lateral

Technical Factors
- Minimum SID—40 inches (100 cm)
- IR size—8 × 10 inches (18 × 24 cm), for smaller foot, or 10 × 12 inches (24 × 30 cm) for larger foot, portrait
- Nongrid
- kVp range: 60–70

24 (30)

18 (24)

R

Shielding Shield radiosensitive tissues outside region of interest.

Patient Position Place patient in lateral recumbent position; provide pillow for patient's head.

Part Position (Mediolateral Projection)
- Flex knee of affected limb about 45°; place opposite leg **behind** the injured limb to prevent over-rotation of affected leg.
- Carefully dorsiflex foot if possible to assist in positioning for a true lateral foot and ankle (Fig. 6.63).
- Place support under leg and knee as needed so that **plantar surface is perpendicular to IR.** Do not **over-rotate** foot.
- Align long axis of foot to long axis of IR (unless diagonal placement is needed to include entire foot).
- Center mid area of base of metatarsals to CR.

CR
- CR **perpendicular** to IR, directed to **medial cuneiform** (at level of base of third metatarsal)

Recommended Collimation Collimate to the outer skin margins of the foot to include approximately 1 inch (2.5 cm) proximal to ankle joint.

Digital Imaging Systems Close collimation is important over unexposed portions of IR to prevent fogging from scatter radiation. Close collimation and lead masking are important over unused portions of IP to prevent fogging from scatter radiation to the hypersensitive IP or IR.

Evaluation Criteria
Anatomy Demonstrated: • Entire foot should be demonstrated, with a minimum of 1 inch (2.5 cm) of distal tibia-fibula. • Heads of metatarsals are superimposed with the tuberosity of the fifth metatarsal seen in profile (Figs. 6.65 and 6.66).
Position: • Long axis of the foot should be aligned to the long axis of IR. • True lateral position is achieved when tibiotalar joint is open, distal fibula is superimposed by the posterior tibia, and distal metatarsals are superimposed. • Collimation to **area of interest.**
Exposure: • Optimal density (brightness) and contrast should visualize borders of superimposed tarsals and metatarsals. • **No motion;** cortical margins and trabecular markings of calcaneus and nonsuperimposed portions of other tarsals should appear sharply defined.

Alternative Lateromedial Projection A lateromedial projection may be taken as an alternative lateral. This position can be more uncomfortable or painful for the patient, but it may be easier to achieve a true lateral (Fig. 6.64).

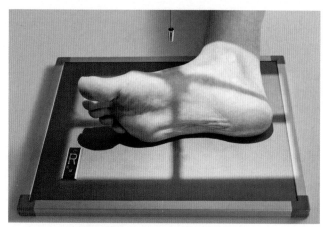
Fig 6.63 Mediolateral projection.

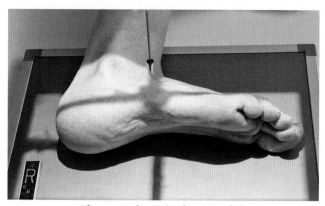
Fig 6.64 Alternative lateromedial.

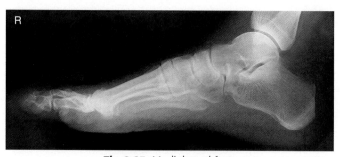
Fig 6.65 Mediolateral foot.

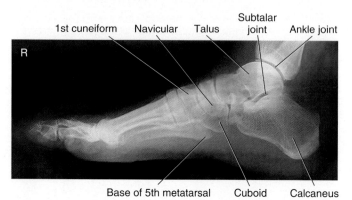

1st cuneiform   Navicular   Talus   Subtalar joint   Ankle joint

Base of 5th metatarsal   Cuboid   Calcaneus
Fig 6.66 Mediolateral foot.

AP WEIGHT-BEARING PROJECTIONS: FOOT

Clinical Indications
- Demonstrate the bones of the feet to show the condition of the longitudinal arches under the full weight of the body
- May demonstrate injury to structural ligaments of the foot such as a Lisfranc joint injury

Foot
SPECIAL
• AP and lateral (weight-bearing)

NOTE: Bilateral projections of both feet often are taken for comparison. Some AP routines include separate projections of each foot taken with CR centered to individual foot.

43

35

R   L

AP both feet

Technical Factors
- Minimum SID—40 inches (100 cm)
- IR size—10 × 12 inches (24 × 30 cm), 14 × 17 inches (35 × 43 cm) for bilateral study, landscape
- Nongrid
- kVp range: 60–70

Shielding Shield radiosensitive tissues outside region of interest.

Patient Position
AP
- Place patient erect, with full weight evenly distributed on *both* feet.
- Feet should be directed straight ahead, parallel to each other (Fig. 6.67).

CR
- Angle CR 15° posteriorly to midpoint between feet at level of base of metatarsals.

Recommended Collimation Collimate to outer skin margins of the feet.

Evaluation Criteria
Anatomy Demonstrated: • For **AP,** projection shows bilateral feet from soft tissue surrounding phalanges to distal portion of talus (Fig. 6.68).
Position: • For **AP,** proper angulation is demonstrated by open tarsometatarsal joint spaces and visualization of joint between first and second cuneiforms. • Metatarsal bases should be at center of the collimated field (CR) with four-sided collimation, including the soft tissue surrounding the feet.
Exposure: • Optimal density (brightness) and contrast should visualize soft tissue and bony borders of superimposed tarsals and metatarsals. • Adequate penetration of midfoot region. • Bony trabecular markings should be sharp.

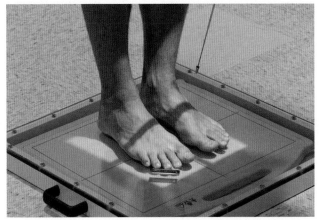

Fig 6.67 AP—bilateral feet (projection taken on digital IR).

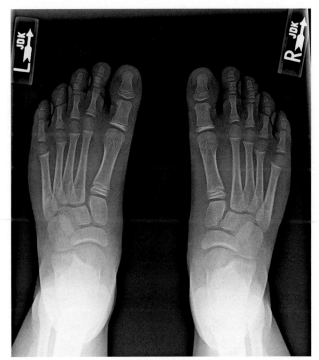

Fig 6.68 AP weight-bearing—bilateral feet. (Courtesy Joss Wertz, DO.)

6

LATERAL WEIGHT-BEARING PROJECTIONS: FOOT

Clinical Indications
- Demonstrate the bones of the feet to show the condition of the longitudinal arches under the full weight of the body
- May demonstrate injury to structural ligaments of the foot such as a Lisfranc joint injury

> **Foot**
> SPECIAL
> - AP and lateral (weight-bearing)

NOTE: Bilateral projections of both feet often are taken for comparison. Some AP routines include separate projections of each foot taken with CR centered to individual foot.

Technical Factors
- Minimum SID—40 inches (100 cm)
- IR size—10 × 12 inches (24 × 30 cm), 14 × 17 inches (35 × 43 cm) for bilateral study, landscape
- Nongrid
- kVp range: 60–70

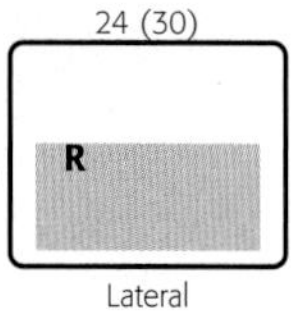

24 (30)

18 (24) R

Lateral

Shielding Shield radiosensitive tissues outside region of interest.

Patient Position
- Have patient stand erect, with weight placed on affected foot (Fig. 6.69).
- Have patient stand on wood blocks placed on a step stool or the foot rest attached to the table. You also may use a special wooden box with a slot for the IR. (It has to be high enough from the floor to get the x-ray tube down into a horizontal beam position.)
- Provide some support for patient to hold onto for security.

Part Position
- Align long axis of foot to long axis of IR.
- Change IR and turn patient for lateral of other foot for comparison after first lateral has been taken.

CR
- Direct CR horizontally to level of base of third metatarsal.

Recommended Collimation Collimate to margins of feet.

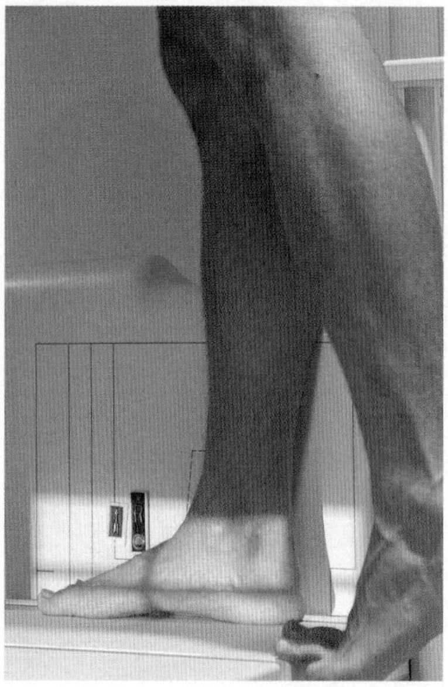

Fig 6.69 Lateral weight-bearing—right foot (projection taken on digital IR).

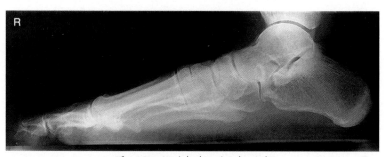

Fig 6.70 Weight-bearing lateral.

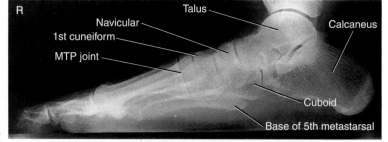

Talus
Navicular
1st cuneiform
MTP joint
Calcaneus
Cuboid
Base of 5th metastarsal

Fig 6.71 Weight-bearing lateral.

Evaluation Criteria
Anatomy Demonstrated: • For lateral, entire foot should be demonstrated, along with a minimum of 1 inch (2.5 cm) of distal tibia-fibula. • Distal fibula should be seen superimposed over posterior half of the tibia, and plantar surfaces of heads of metatarsals should be superimposed if no rotation is present. • The longitudinal arch of the foot must be demonstrated in its entirety (Figs. 6.70 and 6.71).
Position: • For lateral, center of collimated field (CR) should be to level of base of third metatarsal. • Four-sided collimation should include all surrounding soft tissue from the phalanges to the calcaneus and from the dorsum to the plantar surface of the foot with approximately 1 inch (2.5 cm) of the distal tibia-fibula demonstrated.
Exposure: • Optimal density (brightness) and contrast should visualize borders of superimposed tarsals and metatarsals. • **No motion;** cortical margins and trabecular markings of calcaneus and nonsuperimposed portions of other tarsals should appear sharply defined.

PLANTODORSAL (AXIAL) PROJECTION: CALCANEUS

Clinical Indications
- Pathologies or fractures with medial or lateral displacement

Calcaneus
ROUTINE
• Plantodorsal (axial)
• Lateral

Technical Factors
- Minimum SID—40 inches (100 cm)
- IR size—8 × 10 inches (18 × 24 cm), portrait
- Nongrid
- kVp range: 65–75 (increase by 8 to 10 kVp over other foot projections)

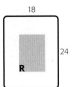

Shielding Shield radiosensitive tissues outside region of interest.

Patient Position Place patient supine or seated on table with leg fully extended.

Part Position
- Center and align ankle joint to CR and to portion of IR being exposed.
- Dorsiflex foot so that plantar surface is near perpendicular to IR (Fig. 6.72).

CR
- Direct CR to **base of third metatarsal** to emerge at a level just distal to lateral malleolus.
- Angle CR **40° cephalad from long axis of foot** (which also would be 40° from vertical *if* long axis of foot is perpendicular to IR). (See NOTE.)

Recommended Collimation Collimate closely to region of calcaneus.

Digital Imaging Systems Close collimation is important over unexposed portions of IR to prevent fogging from scatter radiation.

NOTE: CR angulation must be increased if long axis of plantar surface of foot is not perpendicular to IR.

Evaluation Criteria
Anatomy Demonstrated: • Entire calcaneus should be visualized from tuberosity posteriorly to talocalcaneal joint anteriorly (Figs. 6.73 and 6.74).
Position: • No rotation; a portion of the sustentaculum tali should appear in profile medially. • With the foot in proper 90° flexion, correct alignment and angulation of CR are evidenced by open talocalcaneal joint space, no distortion of the calcaneal tuberosity, and adequate elongation of the calcaneus. • Collimation to **area of interest.**
Exposure: • Optimal density (brightness) and contrast with no motion demonstrate sharp bony margins and trabecular markings and at least faintly visualize talocalcaneal joint without overexposing distal tuberosity area.

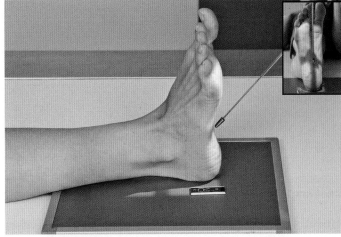

Fig 6.72 Plantodorsal (axial) projection of calcaneus.

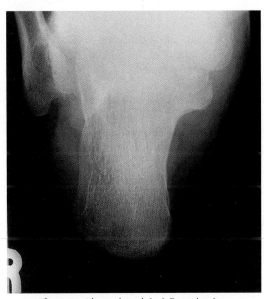

Fig 6.73 Plantodorsal (axial) projection.

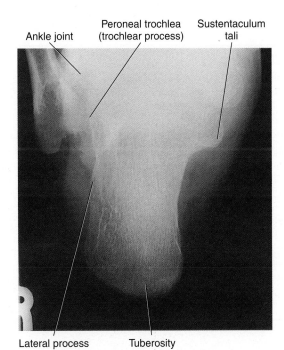

Ankle joint   Peroneal trochlea (trochlear process)   Sustentaculum tali

Lateral process   Tuberosity
Fig 6.74 Plantodorsal (axial) projection.

6

LATERAL—MEDIOLATERAL PROJECTION: CALCANEUS

Clinical Indications
- Bony lesions involving calcaneus, talus, and talocalcaneal joint
- Demonstrate extent and alignment of fractures

Calcaneus
ROUTINE
• Plantar dorsal
• Lateral

Technical Factors
- Minimum SID—40 inches (100 cm)
- IR size—8 × 10 inches (18 × 24 cm), portrait
- Nongrid
- kVp range: 60–75

Shielding Shield radiosensitive tissues outside region of interest.

Patient Position Place patient in lateral recumbent position, affected side down. Provide a pillow for patient's head. Flex knee of affected limb about 45°; place opposite leg behind injured limb.

Part Position ⊡
- Center calcaneus to CR and to unmasked portion of IR, with long axis of foot parallel to plane of IR (Fig. 6.75).
- Place support under knee and leg as needed to place plantar surface perpendicular to IR.
- Position ankle and foot for a **true lateral,** which places the lateral malleolus approximately 1 cm posterior to the medial malleolus.
- Dorsiflex foot so that plantar surface is at right angle to leg.

CR
- CR perpendicular to IR, directed to a point 1 inch (2.5 cm) inferior to medial malleolus

Recommended Collimation Collimate to outer skin margins to include ankle joint proximally and entire calcaneus.

Digital Imaging Systems Close collimation is important over unexposed portions of IR to prevent fogging from scatter radiation.

Evaluation Criteria
Anatomy Demonstrated: • Calcaneus is demonstrated in profile with talus and distal tibia-fibula demonstrated superiorly and navicular and open joint space of the calcaneus and cuboid demonstrated distally (Figs. 6.76 and 6.77).
Position: • **No rotation** as evidenced by superimposed superior portions of the talus, open talocalcaneal joint, and lateral malleolus superimposed over posterior half of the tibia and talus. • Tarsal sinus and calcaneocuboid joint space should appear open. • Four-sided collimation should include ankle joint proximally and talonavicular joint and base of fifth metatarsal anteriorly.
Exposure: • Optimal exposure visualizes some soft tissue and more dense portions of calcaneus and talus. • Outline of the distal fibula should be faintly visible through the talus. • Trabecular markings appear clear and sharp, indicating **no motion.**

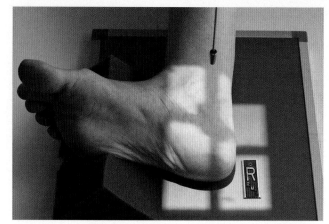

Fig 6.75 Mediolateral calcaneus.

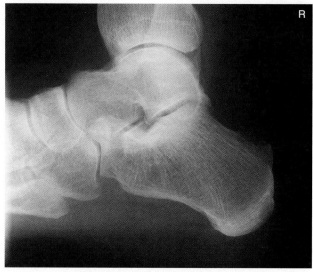

Fig 6.76 Mediolateral calcaneus.

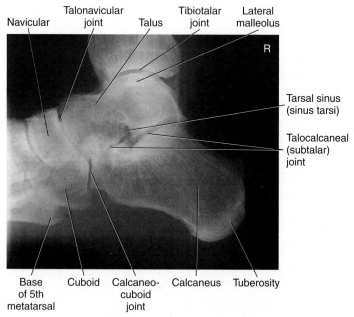

Fig 6.77 Mediolateral calcaneus.

AP PROJECTION: ANKLE

Clinical Indications

- Bony lesions or diseases involving the ankle joint, distal tibia and fibula, proximal talus, and proximal fifth metatarsal
  The lateral portion of the ankle joint space should not appear open on this projection—see AP Mortise Projection.

Ankle
ROUTINE
• **AP**
• AP mortise (15°)
• Lateral
SPECIAL
• Oblique (45°)
• AP stress

Technical Factors

- Minimum SID—40 inches (100 cm)
- IR size—10 × 12 inches (24 × 30 cm), portrait
- Nongrid
- kVp range: 60–75

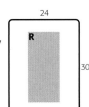

Shielding
Shield radiosensitive tissues outside region of interest.

Patient Position
Place patient in the supine position; place pillow under patient's head; legs should be fully extended.

Part Position

- Center and align ankle joint to CR and to long axis of portion of IR being exposed (Fig. 6.78).
- Do not force dorsiflexion of the foot; allow it to remain in its natural position (see NOTE 1).
- Adjust the **foot and ankle** for a **true AP projection.** Ensure that the entire lower leg is not rotated. The intermalleolar line should not be parallel to IR (see NOTE 2).

CR

- CR perpendicular to IR, directed to a point midway between malleoli

Recommended Collimation
Collimate to lateral skin margins; include proximal one-half of metatarsals and distal tibia-fibula.

Digital Imaging Systems
Close collimation is important over unexposed portions of IR to prevent fogging from scatter radiation.

NOTE 1: Forced dorsiflexion of the foot can be painful and may cause additional injury.

NOTE 2: The malleoli are *not* the same distance from the IR in the anatomic position with a true AP projection. (The lateral malleolus is approximately 15° more posterior.) The lateral portion of the mortise joint should *not* appear open. If this portion of the ankle joint does appear open on a true AP, it may suggest spread of the ankle mortise from ruptured ligaments.[1]

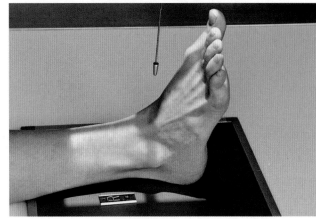

Fig 6.78 AP ankle.

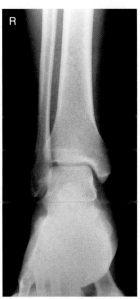

Fig 6.79 AP ankle. (Courtesy E. Frank, RT[R], FASRT.)

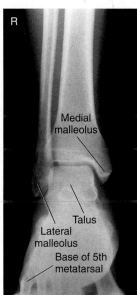

Fig 6.80 AP ankle. (Courtesy E. Frank, RT[R], FASRT.)

Labels in Fig 6.80: Medial malleolus · Talus · Lateral malleolus · Base of 5th metatarsal

Evaluation Criteria

Anatomy Demonstrated: • Distal one-third of tibia-fibula, lateral and medial malleoli, and talus and proximal half of metatarsals should be demonstrated (Figs. 6.79 and 6.80).

Position: • Long axis of the leg should be aligned to collimation field and to IR. • **No rotation** if the medial mortise joint is open and the lateral mortise is closed. • Some superimposition of the distal fibula by the distal tibia and talus exists. • Four-sided collimation should include the distal one-third of the lower leg to the proximal half of the metatarsals. • All surrounding soft tissue also should be included.

Exposure: • Optimal exposure with **no motion** demonstrates clear bony margins and trabecular markings. • Talus must be penetrated enough to demonstrate the cortical margins and trabeculae of the bone. • Soft tissue structures also must be visible.

6

AP MORTISE PROJECTION—15° TO 20° MEDIAL ROTATION: ANKLE

Clinical Indications

- Evaluation of pathology involving the entire ankle mortise[1] and the proximal fifth metatarsal, a common fracture site. This is a common projection taken during open reduction surgery of the ankle (see NOTE).

Ankle
ROUTINE
- **AP**
- **AP mortise (15°)**
- **Lateral**
SPECIAL
- Oblique (45°)
- AP stress

Technical Factors

- Minimum SID—40 inches (100 cm)
- IR size—10 × 12 inches (24 × 30 cm), portrait
- Nongrid
- kVp range: 60–75

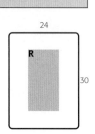

Shielding Shield radiosensitive tissues outside region of interest.

Patient Position Place patient in the supine position; place pillow under patient's head; legs should be fully extended.

Part Position

- Center and align ankle joint to CR and to long axis of portion of IR being exposed (Fig. 6.81).
- Do not dorsiflex foot; allow foot to remain in natural extended (plantar flexed) position (allows for visualization of base of fifth metatarsal, a common fracture site).[4]
- Internally rotate entire leg and foot approximately 15° to 20° until intermalleolar line is parallel to IR.
- Place support against foot if needed to prevent motion.

CR

- CR perpendicular to IR, directed midway between malleoli

Recommended Collimation Collimate to lateral skin margins, including proximal metatarsals and distal tibia-fibula.

Digital Imaging Systems Close collimation is important over unexposed portions of IR to prevent fogging from scatter radiation.

NOTE: This position should *not* be a substitute for either the AP projection or the oblique ankle position but rather should be a separate projection of the ankle that is taken routinely when potential trauma or sprains of the ankle joint are involved.[1]

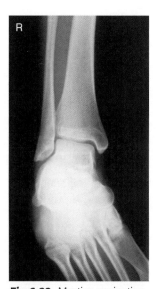

Fig 6.81 Mortise projection, demonstrating 15° to 20° medial rotation of lower leg and foot.

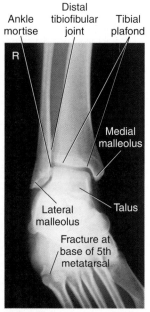

Fig 6.82 Mortise projection.   **Fig 6.83** Mortise projection.

Evaluation Criteria

Anatomy Demonstrated: • Distal one-third of tibia and fibula, tibial plafond involving the epiphysis if present, lateral and medial malleoli, talus, and proximal half of the metatarsals should be demonstrated. • Entire ankle mortise should be open and well visualized (3- to 4-mm space over entire talar surface is normal; an extra 2 mm of widening is abnormal)[2] (Figs. 6.82 and 6.83).

Position: • Proper obliquity for the mortise joint is evidenced by demonstration of open lateral and medial mortise joints with malleoli demonstrated in profile. • Only minimal superimposition should exist at distal tibiofibular joint. • Collimation to **area of interest.**

Exposure: • **No motion** as demonstrated by sharp bony outlines and trabecular markings. • Optimal exposure should demonstrate soft tissue structures and sufficient density (brightness) for talus and distal tibia and fibula.

AP OBLIQUE PROJECTION—45° MEDIAL ROTATION: ANKLE

Clinical Indications
- Pathologies including possible fractures involving distal tibiofibular joint
- Fractures of distal fibula and lateral malleolus and base of the fifth metatarsal

Ankle
ROUTINE
• AP
• AP mortise (15°)
• Lateral
SPECIAL
• Oblique (45°)
• AP stress

Technical Factors
- Minimum SID—40 inches (100 cm)
- IR size—10 × 12 inches (24 × 30 cm), portrait
- Nongrid
- kVp range: 60–75

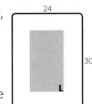

Shielding Shield radiosensitive tissues outside region of interest.

Patient Position
Place patient in the supine position; place pillow under patient's head; legs should be fully extended (small sandbag or other support under knee increases comfort of patient).

Part Position
- Center and align ankle joint to CR and to long axis of portion of IR being exposed (Fig. 6.84).
- If patient's condition allows, dorsiflex the foot if needed so that the plantar surface is at least 80° to 85° from IR (10° to 15° from vertical). (See NOTE 1.)
- **Rotate leg and foot** medially 45°.

CR
- CR perpendicular to IR, directed to a point midway between malleoli

Recommended Collimation
Collimate to include distal tibia and fibula to midmetatarsal area (see NOTE 2).

Digital Imaging Systems Close collimation is important over unexposed portions of IR to prevent fogging from scatter radiation.

NOTE 1: If the foot is extended or plantar flexed more than 10° or 15° from vertical, the calcaneus is superimposed over the lateral malleolus on this 45° oblique, obscuring an important area of interest.

NOTE 2: The base of the fifth metatarsal (a common fracture site) may be demonstrated in this projection and should be included in the collimation field. If fracture of the fifth metatarsal is suspected, a foot series should be ordered by physician.

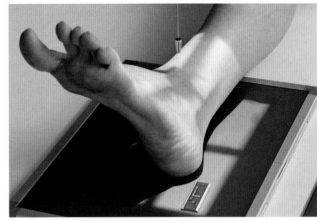

Fig 6.84 45° AP medial oblique.

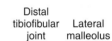

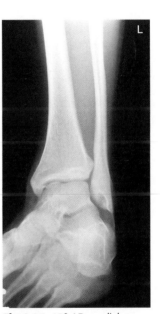

Fig 6.85 45° AP medial oblique. (Courtesy E. Frank, RT[R], FASRT.)

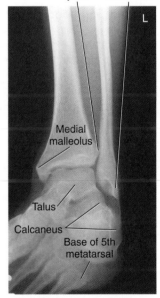

Fig 6.86 45° AP medial oblique. (Courtesy E. Frank, RT[R], FASRT.)

Evaluation Criteria

Anatomy Demonstrated: • Distal one-third of lower leg, malleoli, talus, and proximal half of metatarsals should be seen (Figs. 6.85 and 6.86).

Position: • A 45° medial oblique demonstrates distal tibiofibular joint open, with no or only minimal overlap on the average person. • Lateral malleolus and talus joint should show no or only slight superimposition, but medial malleolus and talus are partially superimposed. • Ankle joint should be in center of four-sided collimated field with distal one-third of lower leg to proximal half of metatarsals and surrounding soft tissues included.

Exposure: • Bony cortical margins and trabecular patterns should be sharply defined on image if no motion is present. • The talus should be sufficiently penetrated to demonstrate trabeculae; soft tissue structures also must be evident.

LATERAL–MEDIOLATERAL (OR LATEROMEDIAL) PROJECTION: ANKLE

Clinical Indications
- Projection is useful in the evaluation of fractures, dislocations, and joint effusions associated with other joint pathologies

Ankle
ROUTINE
• AP
• AP mortise (15°)
• Lateral
SPECIAL
• Oblique (45°)
• AP stress

Technical Factors
- Minimum SID—40 inches (100 cm)
- IR size—10 × 12 inches (24 × 30 cm), portrait
- Nongrid
- kVp range: 60–75

Shielding Shield radiosensitive tissues outside region of interest.

Patient Position Place patient in the lateral recumbent position, affected side down; provide a pillow for patient's head; flex knee of affected limb approximately 45°; place opposite leg behind injured limb to prevent over-rotation.

Part Position (Mediolateral Projection)
- Center and align ankle joint to CR and to long axis of portion of IR being exposed (Fig. 6.87).
- Place support under knee as needed to place leg and foot in **true lateral position.**
- Dorsiflex foot so that plantar surface is at a right angle to leg or as far as patient can tolerate; do *not* force. (This helps maintain a true lateral position.)

CR
- CR perpendicular to IR, directed to medial malleolus

Recommended Collimation Collimate to include distal tibia and fibula to midmetatarsal area.

Digital Imaging Systems Close collimation is important over unexposed portions of IR to prevent fogging from scatter radiation.

Alternative Lateromedial Projection This lateral may be performed rather than the more common mediolateral projection (Fig. 6.88). (This position is more uncomfortable for the patient but may make it easier to achieve a true lateral position.)

Evaluation Criteria
Anatomy Demonstrated: • Distal one-third of tibia and fibula with the distal fibula superimposed by the distal tibia, talus, and calcaneus appear in lateral profile. • Tuberosity of fifth metatarsal, navicular, and cuboid also are visualized (Figs. 6.89 and 6.90).
Position: • **No rotation** is evidenced by distal fibula being superimposed over the posterior half of tibia. • Tibiotalar joint is open with uniform joint space. • Collimation field should include distal one-third of lower leg, calcaneus, tuberosity of fifth metatarsal, and surrounding soft tissue structures. • Collimation to **area of interest.**
Exposure: • **No motion,** as evidenced by sharp bony margins and trabecular patterns. • Lateral malleolus should be seen through the distal tibia and talus, and soft tissue must be demonstrated for evaluation of joint effusion.

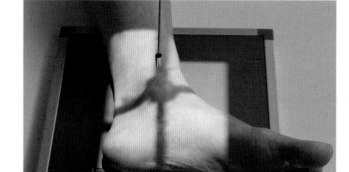
Fig 6.87 Mediolateral ankle.

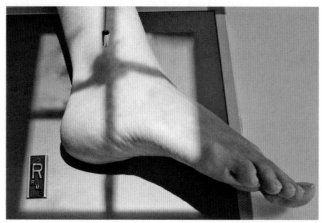
Fig 6.88 Alternative lateromedial ankle.

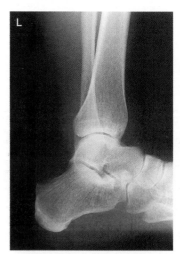
Fig 6.89 Mediolateral ankle.

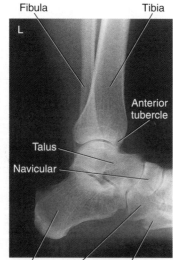
Fibula   Tibia

Anterior tubercle

Talus

Navicular

Calcaneus   Cuboid   Base of 5th metatarsal
Fig 6.90 Mediolateral ankle.

AP STRESS PROJECTIONS: ANKLE

INVERSION AND EVERSION POSITIONS

WARNING: Proceed with utmost care with injured patient.

Clinical Indications
- Pathology involving ankle joint separation secondary to ligament tear or rupture

Ankle
SPECIAL
• Oblique (45°)
• AP stress

Technical Factors
- Minimum SID—40 inches (100 cm)
- IR size—10 × 12 inches (24 × 30 cm), portrait
- Nongrid
- kVp range: 60–75

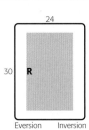

Eversion   Inversion

Shielding Shield radiosensitive tissues outside region of interest. Supply lead gloves and a lead apron for the individual who is applying stress if stress positions are handheld during exposures.

Patient Position Place patient in supine position; place pillow under patient's head; leg should be fully extended, with support under knee.

Part Position
- Center and align ankle joint to CR and to long axis of portion of IR being exposed.
- Dorsiflex the foot as near the right angle to the lower leg as possible.
- Stress is applied with leg and ankle in position for a **true AP** with no rotation, wherein the entire plantar surface is turned medially for inversion and laterally for eversion (Figs. 6.91 and 6.92) (see NOTE).

CR
- CR perpendicular to IR, directed to a point midway between malleoli

Recommended Collimation Collimate to lateral skin margins, including proximal metatarsals and distal tibia-fibula.

Digital Imaging Systems Close collimation is important over unexposed portions of IR to prevent fogging from scatter radiation.

NOTE: A physician or another health professional must be present to hold the foot and ankle in these stress views (or to strap into position with weights), or patient must hold this position with long gauze looped around ball of foot. If this is too painful for the patient, a local anesthetic may be injected by the physician.

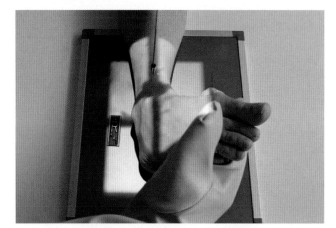

Fig 6.91 AP ankle—inversion stress.

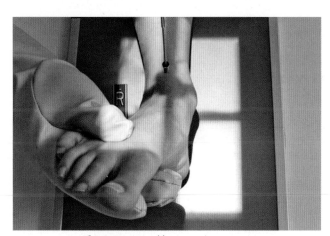

Fig 6.92 AP ankle—eversion stress.

Evaluation Criteria
Anatomy Demonstrated and Position: • Ankle joint for evaluation of joint separation and ligament tear or rupture is shown. • Appearance of joint space may vary greatly depending on the severity of ligament damage. • Collimation to **area of interest** (Figs. 6.93 and 6.94).
Exposure: • **No motion**, as evidenced by sharp bony margins and trabecular patterns. • Optimal exposure should visualize soft tissue, lateral and medial malleoli, talus, and distal tibia and fibula.

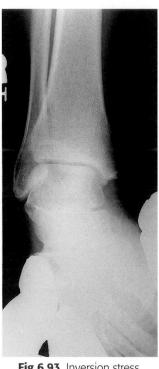

Fig 6.93 Inversion stress.

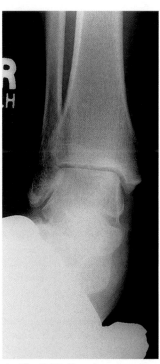

Fig 6.94 Eversion stress.

AP PROJECTION: LOWER LEG (TIBIA AND FIBULA)

Clinical Indications
- Pathologies involving fractures, foreign bodies, or lesions of the bone

Lower Leg
• AP
• Lateral

Technical Factors
- Minimum SID—40 inches (100 cm); may increase to 44 to 48 inches (110 to 120 cm) to reduce divergence of x-ray beam and to include more of body part
- IR size—14 × 17 inches (35 × 43 cm), portrait (or diagonal, which requires 44-inch [110-cm] minimum SID)
- Nongrid (unless lower leg measures >10 cm)
- kVp range: 70–80
- To make best use of anode heel effect, place knee at cathode end of x-ray beam

Shielding Shield radiosensitive tissues outside region of interest.

Patient Position Place patient in the supine position; provide a pillow for patient's head; entire leg should be fully extended.

Part Position
- Adjust pelvis, knee, and leg into true AP with no rotation (Fig. 6.95).
- Place sandbag against foot if needed for stabilization, and dorsiflex foot to 90° to lower leg if possible.
- Ensure that both ankle and knee joints are 1 to 2 inches (2.5 to 5 cm) from ends of IR (so that divergent rays do not project either joint off IR).
- If limb is too long, place the lower leg diagonally (corner to corner) on one 14 × 17 inch (35 × 43 cm) IR to ensure that both joints are included. (Also, if needed, a second smaller IR may be taken of the joint farthest from the injury site.)

CR
- CR perpendicular to IR, directed to midpoint of lower leg

Recommended Collimation Collimate on both sides to skin margins, with full collimation at ends of IR borders to include maximum knee and ankle joints.

Evaluation Criteria
Anatomy Demonstrated: • Entire tibia and fibula must include ankle and knee joints on this projection (or two if needed). • The exception is an alternative routine on follow-up examinations (Figs. 6.96 and 6.97).
Position: • No rotation as evidenced by demonstration of femoral and tibial condyles in profile with intercondylar eminence centered within intercondylar fossa. • Some overlap of the fibula and tibia is visible at both proximal and distal ends. • Collimation to **area of interest.**
Exposure: • Correct use of anode heel effect results in an image with nearer equal density at both ends of IR. • **No motion** is present, as evidenced by sharp cortical margins and trabecular patterns. • Contrast and density (brightness) should be optimum to visualize soft tissue and bony trabecular markings at both ends of tibia.

Alternative Follow-Up Examination Routine The routine for follow-up examinations of long bones in some departments is to include only the joint that is nearest the site of injury and to place this joint a minimum of 2 inches (5 cm) from the end of the IR for better demonstration of the joint. **However, for initial examinations, it is important, especially when the injury site is in the distal leg, to include the proximal tibiofibular joint area** because it is common to have a second fracture at this site. For very large patients, a second AP projection of the knee and proximal lower leg may be needed on a smaller IR.

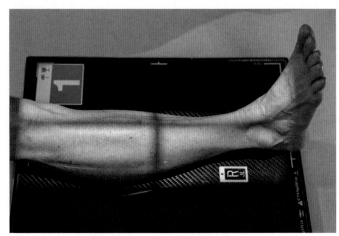

Fig 6.95 AP lower leg—include both joints.

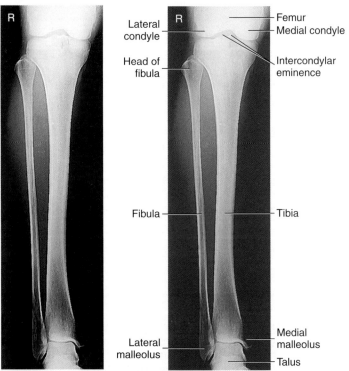

Fig 6.96 AP lower leg—both joints. (Courtesy J. Sanderson, RT.)

Fig 6.97 AP lower leg—both joints. (Courtesy J. Sanderson, RT.)

Lateral condyle
Head of fibula
Femur
Medial condyle
Intercondylar eminence
Fibula
Tibia
Lateral malleolus
Medial malleolus
Talus

LATERAL—MEDIOLATERAL PROJECTION: LOWER LEG (TIBIA AND FIBULA)

Clinical Indications
- Localization of lesions and foreign bodies and determination of extent
- Alignment of fractures demonstrated

Lower Leg
• AP
• Lateral

Technical Factors
- Minimum SID—40 inches (100 cm); may increase to 44 to 48 inches (110 to 120 cm) to reduce divergence of x-ray beam and to include more of body part
- IR size—14 × 17 inches (35 × 43 cm), portrait (or diagonal, which requires 44-inch [110-cm] minimum SID)
- Nongrid (unless lower leg measures >10 cm)
- kVp range: 65–80
- To make best use of anode heel effect, place knee at cathode end of x-ray beam

35

43

Diagonal placement

Shielding Shield all radiosensitive tissues outside region of interest.

Patient Position Place patient in the lateral recumbent position, injured side down; the opposite leg may be placed behind the affected leg and supported with a pillow or sandbags.

Part Position
- Ensure that leg is in true lateral position (plane of patella should be perpendicular to IR) (Fig. 6.98).
- Ensure that both ankle and knee joints are 1 to 2 inches (2.5 to 5 cm) from ends of IR so that divergent rays do not project either joint off IR.
- If limb is too long, place the lower leg diagonally (corner to corner) on one 14 × 17 inch (35 × 43 cm) IR to ensure that both joints are included (Fig. 6.98, *inset*). (Also, if needed, a second, smaller IR may be taken of the joint furthest from the injury site.)

CR
- CR perpendicular to IR, directed to midpoint of lower leg

Evaluation Criteria
Anatomy Demonstrated: • Entire tibia and fibula must include ankle and knee joints on this projection (or two if needed). • Exception is alternative routine on follow-up examinations (Fig. 6.99).
Position: • True lateral of tibia and fibula **without rotation** demonstrates tibial tuberosity in profile, a portion of the proximal head of the fibula superimposed by the tibia, and outlines of the distal fibula seen through posterior half of the tibia. • Posterior borders of femoral condyles should appear superimposed. • Collimation to **area of interest.**
Exposure: • **No motion** is present, as evidenced by sharp cortical margins and trabecular patterns. • Correct use of the anode heel effect results in near-equal density at both ends of the image. • Contrast and density (brightness) should be optimum to visualize soft tissue and bony trabecular markings.

Recommended Collimation Collimate on both sides to skin margins, with full collimation at ends to include maximum knee and ankle joints.

Alternative Follow-Up Examination Routine The routine for follow-up examinations of long bones in some departments is to include only the one joint nearest the site of injury and to place this joint a minimum of 2 inches (5 cm) from the end of the IR for better demonstration of the joint. However, for initial examinations, it is especially important when the injury site is in the distal lower leg to include the proximal tibiofibular joint area because it is common to have a second fracture at this site.

Horizontal Beam (Cross-Table) Lateral If patient cannot be turned, this image can be taken cross-table with IR placed on edge between lower legs. Place a support under injured leg to center the lower leg to IR, and direct horizontal beam from lateral side of patient.

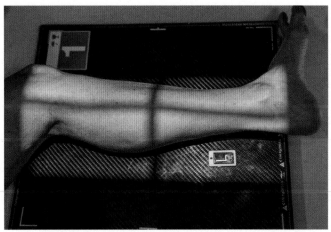

Fig 6.98 Mediolateral lower leg—include both joints.

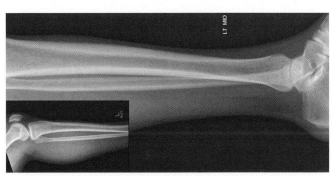

Fig 6.99 Mediolateral lower leg projection. Inset shows proximal lower leg to show both joints are included.

6

AP PROJECTION: KNEE

Clinical Indications
- Fractures, lesions, or bony changes related to degenerative joint disease involving the distal femur, proximal tibia and fibula, patella, and knee joint

Knee
ROUTINE
• AP
• Oblique (medial and lateral)
• Lateral

Technical Factors
- Minimum SID—40 inches (100 cm)
- IR size—10 × 12 inches (24 × 30 cm), portrait
- Grid or bucky, >10 cm
- Nongrid, tabletop, <10 cm
- kVp range: 65–80

Shielding Shield radiosensitive tissues outside region of interest.

Patient Position Place patient in supine position with no rotation of pelvis; provide pillow for patient's head; leg should be fully extended.

Part Position
- Align and center leg and knee to CR and to midline of table or IR (Fig. 6.100).
- Rotate leg internally 3° to 5° for true AP knee (or until **interepicondylar line is parallel** to plane of IR).
- Place sandbags by foot and ankle to stabilize if needed.

CR
- Align CR **parallel to articular facets (tibial plateau);** for average-sized patient, CR is perpendicular to IR (see NOTE).
- Direct CR to a point ½ inch (1.25 cm) distal to apex of patella.

Recommended Collimation Collimate on both sides to skin margins at ends to IR borders.

NOTE: A suggested guideline for determining that CR is parallel to articular facets (tibial plateau) for open joint space is to measure distance from anterior superior iliac spines (ASIS) to tabletop to determine CR angle as follows[5]:
- <19 cm: **5° caudad** (thin thighs and buttocks)
- 19 to 24 cm: **0° angle** (average thighs and buttocks)
- >24 cm: **5° cephalad** (thick thighs and buttocks)

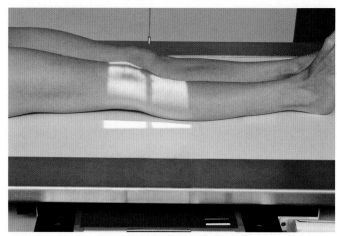

Fig 6.100 AP knee—CR perpendicular to IR (average patient—19 to 24 cm).

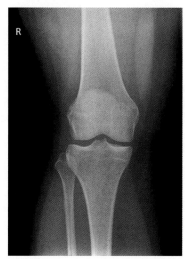

Fig 6.101 AP knee—0° CR. (Courtesy Joss Wertz, DO.)

Evaluation Criteria
Anatomy Demonstrated: • Distal femur and proximal tibia and fibula are shown. • Femorotibial joint space should be open, with the articular facets of the tibia seen on end with only minimal surface area visualized (Figs. 6.101 and 6.102).
Position: • No rotation, as evidenced by symmetric appearance of femoral and tibial condyles and the joint space. • The approximate medial half of the fibular head should be superimposed by tibia. • The intercondylar eminence is seen in the center of intercondylar fossa. • Center of collimation field (CR) should be to the midknee joint space.
Exposure: • Optimal exposure visualizes the outline of the patella through the distal femur, and the fibular head and neck do not appear overexposed. • **No motion** should occur; trabecular markings of all bones should be visible and appear sharp. • Soft tissue detail should be visible.

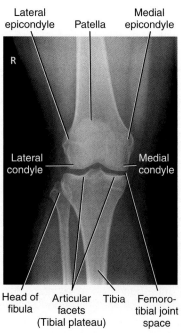

Fig 6.102 AP knee—0° CR. (Courtesy Joss Wertz, DO.)

AP OBLIQUE PROJECTION—MEDIAL (INTERNAL) ROTATION: KNEE

Clinical Indications
- Pathology involving the proximal tibio-fibular and femorotibial (knee) joint articulations
- Fractures, lesions, and bony changes related to degenerative joint disease, especially on the anterior and medial or posterior and lateral portions of knee

Knee
ROUTINE
• AP
• Oblique (medial and lateral)
• Lateral

NOTE: A common departmental routine is to include *both* medial and lateral rotation oblique projections for the knee. If only one oblique is routine, it is most commonly the medial rotation oblique.

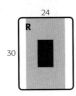

Technical Factors
- Minimum SID—40 inches (100 cm)
- IR size—10 × 12 inches (24 × 30 cm), portrait
- Grid or bucky, >10 cm
- Nongrid, tabletop, <10 cm
- kVp range: 65–80

Shielding Shield radiosensitive tissues outside region of interest.

Patient Position Place patient in semisupine position with entire body and leg rotated partially away from side of interest; place support under elevated hip; provide a pillow for patient's head.

Part Position
- Align and center leg and knee to CR and to midline of table or IR.
- Rotate entire leg **internally 45°**. (Interepicondylar line should be 45° to plane of IR.) (Fig. 6.103)
- If needed, stabilize foot and ankle in this position with sandbags.

CR
- Angle CR 0° on average patient (see AP Knee, p. 246).
- Direct CR to midpoint of knee at a level ½ inch (1.25 cm) distal to apex of patella.

Recommended Collimation Collimate on both sides to skin margins, with full collimation at ends to IR borders to include maximum femur and tibia-fibula.

NOTE: The terms *medial (internal) oblique* and *lateral (external) oblique positions* refer to the direction of rotation of the anterior or patellar surface of the knee. This is true for descriptions of AP or PA oblique projections.

Evaluation Criteria
Anatomy Demonstrated: • Distal femur and proximal tibia and fibula with the patella superimposing the medial femoral condyle are shown. • **Lateral condyles** of the femur and tibia are well demonstrated, and the medial and lateral knee joint spaces appear unequal (Figs. 6.104 and 6.105).
Position: • The proper amount of part obliquity demonstrates the proximal tibiofibular articulation open with the lateral condyles of the femur and tibia seen in profile. • The head and neck of the fibula are visualized without superimposition, and approximately half of the patella should be seen free of superimposition by the femur. The center of the collimated field is to the **femorotibial (knee) joint space**.
Exposure: • Optimal exposure with **no motion** should visualize soft tissue in the knee joint area, and trabecular markings of all bones should appear clear and sharp. • Head and neck area of fibula should not appear overexposed.

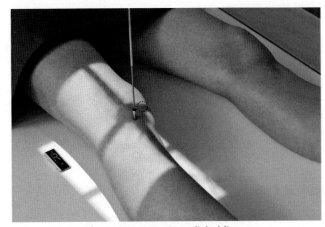

Fig 6.103 AP 45° medial oblique.

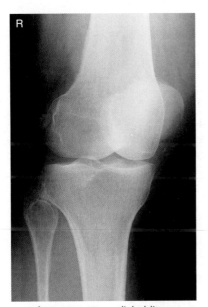

Fig 6.104 AP medial oblique.

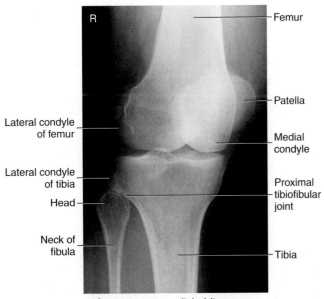

Femur

Patella

Medial condyle

Proximal tibiofibular joint

Tibia

Lateral condyle of femur

Lateral condyle of tibia

Head

Neck of fibula

Fig 6.105 AP medial oblique.

AP OBLIQUE PROJECTION—LATERAL (EXTERNAL) ROTATION: KNEE

Clinical Indications
- Pathology involving femorotibial (knee) articulation
- Fractures, lesions, and bony changes related to degenerative joint disease, especially on anterior and lateral or posterior and medial aspects of knee

Knee
ROUTINE
• AP
• Oblique (medial and lateral)
• Lateral

NOTE: A common departmental routine is to include *both* medial and lateral rotation oblique projections of the knee. If only one oblique is routine, it is most commonly the medial (internal) rotation oblique.

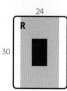

Technical Factors
- Minimum SID—40 inches (100 cm)
- IR size—10 × 12 inches (24 × 30 cm), portrait/grid or bucky, >10 cm
- Nongrid, tabletop, <10 cm
- kVp range: 65–80

Shielding Shield radiosensitive tissues outside region of interest.

Patient Position Place patient in semisupine position, with entire body and leg rotated partially away from side of interest; place support under elevated hip; give pillow for head.

Part Position
- Align and center leg and knee to CR and to midline of table or IR.
- Rotate entire leg **externally 45°** (interepicondylar line should be **45°** to plane of IR) (Fig. 6.106).
- If needed, stabilize foot and ankle in this position with sandbags.

CR
- Angle CR **0°** on average patient (see AP Knee Projection, p. 246).
- Direct CR to midpoint of knee at a level ½ inch (1.25 cm) distal to apex of patella.

Recommended Collimation Collimate on both sides to skin margins, with full collimation at ends to IR borders to include maximum femur and tibia-fibula.

NOTE: The terms *medial (internal) oblique* and *lateral (external) oblique positions* refer to the direction of rotation of the anterior or patellar surface of the knee. This is true for descriptions of either AP or PA oblique projections.

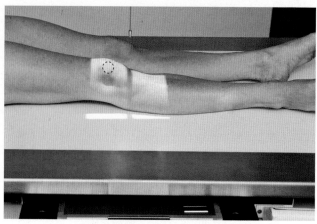

Fig 6.106 AP lateral oblique.

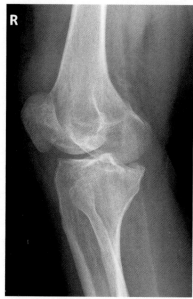

Fig 6.107 AP lateral oblique. (Courtesy Joss Wertz, DO.)

Evaluation Criteria
Anatomy Demonstrated: • Distal femur and proximal tibia and fibula, with the patella superimposing the lateral femoral condyle, are shown. • Medial condyles of the femur and tibia are demonstrated in profile (Figs. 6.107 and 6.108).
Position: • The proper amount of part obliquity demonstrates the proximal fibula superimposed by the proximal tibia, the medial condyles of the femur, and the tibia seen in profile. • Approximately half of patella should be seen free of superimposition by the femur. • Femorotibial (knee) joint space is the center of the collimated field.
Exposure: • Optimal exposure should visualize soft tissue in knee joint area, and trabecular markings of all bones should appear clear and sharp, indicating **no motion.** • Technique should be sufficient to demonstrate the head and neck area of the fibula through the superimposed tibia.

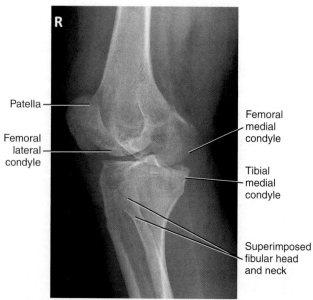

Patella

Femoral lateral condyle

Femoral medial condyle

Tibial medial condyle

Superimposed fibular head and neck

Fig 6.108 AP lateral oblique. (Courtesy Joss Wertz, DO.)

LATERAL—MEDIOLATERAL PROJECTION: KNEE

Clinical Indications
- Fractures, lesions, and joint space abnormalities

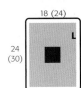

Knee
ROUTINE
- AP
- Oblique
- Lateral

Technical Factors
- Minimum SID—40 inches (100 cm)
- IR size—8 × 10 inches (18 × 24 cm) or 10 × 12 inches (24 × 30 cm), portrait
- Grid or bucky, >10 cm
- Nongrid, tabletop, <10 cm
- kVp range: 65–80

18 (24)

24 (30)

L

Shielding Shield radiosensitive tissues outside region of interest.

Patient Position This position may be taken in the lateral recumbent position or as a horizontal beam lateral.

Lateral Recumbent Position This projection is designed for patients who are able to flex the knee 20° to 30°. Take radiograph with patient in lateral recumbent position, affected side down; provide pillow for patient's head; provide support for knee of opposite limb placed behind knee being examined to prevent over-rotation (Fig. 6.109).

Horizontal Beam Projection This lateromedial beam projection is ideal for a patient who is unable to flex the knee because of pain or trauma. With the patient in the prone position, use a horizontal beam with IR placed beside knee. Place support under knee to avoid obscuring posterior soft tissue structures (see Fig. 6.109, inset).

Part Position
- Adjust rotation of body and leg until knee is in **true lateral** position (femoral epicondyles directly superimposed and plane of patella perpendicular to plane of IR).
- Flex knee **20° to 30°** for lateral recumbent projection (see NOTE 1).
- Align and center leg and knee to CR and to midline of table or IR.

CR
- Angle CR **5° to 7° cephalad** for lateral recumbent projection (see NOTES 2 and 3).
- Direct CR to a point **1 inch (2.5 cm) distal** to medial epicondyle.

Recommended Collimation Collimate on both sides to skin margins, with full collimation at ends to IR borders to include maximum femur, tibia, and fibula.

NOTE 1: Additional flexion tightens muscles and tendons that may obscure important diagnostic information in the joint space. The patella is drawn into the intercondylar sulcus, also obscuring soft tissue detail from effusion or fat pad displacement. Additional flexion may result in fragment separation of patellar fractures, if present.

NOTE 2: Angle CR 7° to 10° on a short patient with a wide pelvis and about 5° on a tall, male patient with a narrow pelvis for lateral recumbent projection.

NOTE 3: If the ankle and lower leg can be elevated to the same plane as the long axis of the femur, a perpendicular CR can be used.

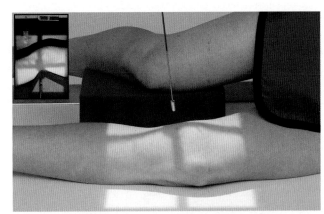

Fig 6.109 Mediolateral knee. *Inset,* Lateromedial—horizontal beam.

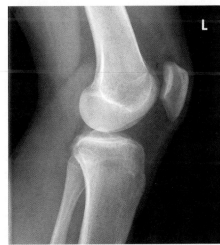

Fig 6.110 Mediolateral knee. (Courtesy Joss Wertz, DO.)

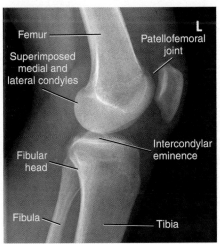

Femur
Patellofemoral joint
Superimposed medial and lateral condyles
Intercondylar eminence
Fibular head
Fibula
Tibia
L

Fig 6.111 Mediolateral knee. (Courtesy Joss Wertz, DO.)

AP WEIGHT-BEARING BILATERAL KNEE PROJECTION: KNEE

Clinical Indications

- Femorotibial joint spaces of the knees demonstrated for possible cartilage degeneration or other knee joint pathologies
- Bilateral knees included on same exposure for comparison

Knee
SPECIAL
• AP bilateral weight-bearing

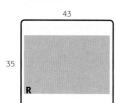

NOTE: This projection most commonly is taken AP but may be taken PA with a cephalic CR angle rather than caudal as with an AP. (This may be easier for patients who are unable to straighten their knee joints fully, such as patients with arthritic conditions or with certain neuromuscular disorders involving the lower limbs.)

Technical Factors

- Minimum SID—40 inches (100 cm)
- IR size—14 × 17 inches (35 × 43 cm), landscape
- Grid
- kVp range: 70–80

Shielding Shield radiosensitive tissues outside region of interest.

Patient and Part Position

- Position patient erect and standing on attached step or on step stool to place patient high enough for horizontal beam x-ray tube.
- Position feet straight ahead with weight evenly distributed on both feet; provide support handles for patient stability.
- Align and center bilateral legs and knees to CR and to midline of table and IR; IR height is adjusted to CR (Fig. 6.112).

CR

- CR perpendicular to IR (average-sized patient), or 5° to 10° caudad on thin patient, directed to midpoint between knee joints at a level ½ inch (1.25 cm) below apex of patellae.

Recommended Collimation Collimate to bilateral knee joint region, including some distal femurs and proximal tibia for alignment purposes.

Evaluation Criteria
Anatomy Demonstrated: • Distal femur, proximal tibia, and fibula and femorotibial joint spaces are demonstrated bilaterally (Fig. 6.113).
Position: • **No rotation** of both knees is evident by symmetric appearance of femoral and tibial condyles. • Approximately one-half of proximal fibula is superimposed by tibia. • Collimation field should be centered to knee joint spaces and should include sufficient femur and tibia to determine long axes of these long bones for alignment.
Exposure: • Optimal exposure should visualize faint outlines of patellae through femora. • Soft tissue should be visible, and trabecular markings of all bones should appear clear and sharp, indicating **no motion.**

Alternative PA If requested, an alternative PA may be performed with patient facing the table or IR holder, knees flexed at approximately 20°, feet straight ahead, and thighs against tabletop or IR holder. Direct CR **10° caudad** (parallel to tibial plateaus) to **level of knee joints** for PA projection.

NOTE: CR angle should be parallel to articular facets (tibial plateau) for best visualization of open knee joint spaces. See AP Knee Projection, p. 246, for correct CR angle.

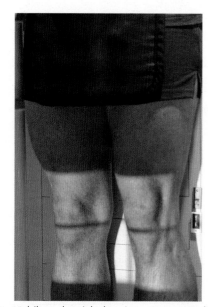

Fig 6.112 AP bilateral weight-bearing—CR perpendicular to IR.

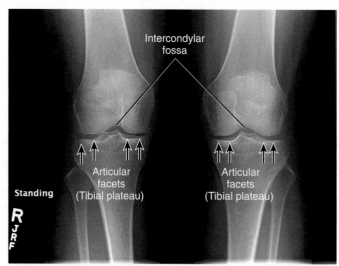

Fig 6.113 AP bilateral weight-bearing—CR 10° caudad. (Courtesy Joss Wertz, DO.)

PA AXIAL WEIGHT-BEARING BILATERAL KNEE PROJECTION: KNEE

ROSENBERG METHOD

Clinical Indications

- Femorotibial joint spaces of the knees demonstrated for possible cartilage degeneration or other knee joint pathologies
- Knee joint spaces and intercondylar fossa demonstrated
- Bilateral knees included on same exposure for comparison

Knee
SPECIAL
- AP bilateral weight-bearing
- PA axial bilateral weight-bearing

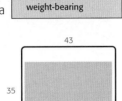

Technical Factors

- Minimum SID—40 inches (100 cm)
- IR size—14 × 17 inches (35 × 43 cm), landscape
- Grid
- kVp range: 70–80

Shielding Shield radiosensitive tissues outside region of interest.

Patient and Part Position

- Position patient erect, standing on attached step of x-ray table or on step stool if the upright bucky is used so that patient is placed high enough for 10° caudad angle.
- Position feet straight ahead with weight evenly distributed on both feet and knees flexed to 45°; have patient use bucky device for support, with patella touching the upright bucky (Fig. 6.114).
- Align and center bilateral legs and knees to CR and to midline of upright bucky and IR; IR height is adjusted to CR.

CR

- CR angled 10° caudad and centered directly to midpoint between knee joints at level ½ inch (1.25 cm) below apex of patellae when a bilateral study is performed (Fig. 6.115); alternatively, CR centered directly to midpoint of knee joint at level ½ inch (1.25 cm) below apex of patella when a unilateral study is performed.

Recommended Collimation Collimate to bilateral knee joint region, including some distal femurs and proximal tibia for alignment purposes.

Alternative Unilateral Projection If requested, this examination may be performed unilaterally with patient facing the upright bucky or IR holder, knees flexed to 45°, and feet straight ahead. The patient should put full weight on the affected extremity. This requires the patient to balance with minimal pressure placed on the contralateral side. Direct CR **10° caudad** (parallel to tibial plateau) to **level of knee joint** for this PA unilateral projection.

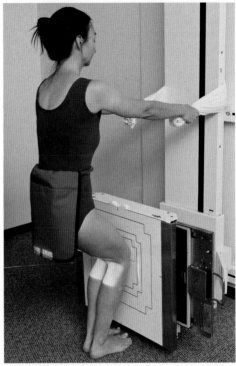

Fig 6.114 Rosenberg method. Position for standing 45° PA flexion weight-bearing for bilateral knees.

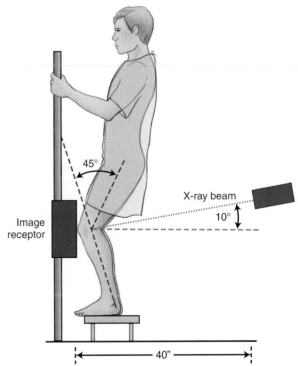

Fig 6.115 Rosenberg method—bilateral PA axial projection with 10° caudad.

Evaluation Criteria
Anatomy Demonstrated: • Distal femur, proximal tibia and fibula, femorotibial joint spaces, and intercondylar fossa are demonstrated bilaterally or unilaterally (Figs. 6.116 and 6.117).
Position: • **No rotation** of both knees is evident in symmetric appearance of femoral and tibial condyles. • Intercondylar fossa should be open. • Knee joint spaces should appear open if CR angle was correct and tibia was flexed 45°.
Exposure: • Optimal exposure should visualize intercondylar fossa and proximal tibia with open joint space • Trabecular markings of all bones should appear clear and sharp, indicating **no motion.**

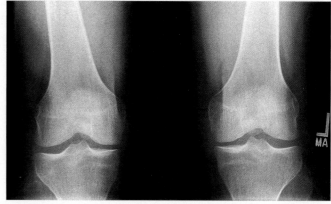

Fig 6.116 Normal bilateral knee radiograph performed using the Rosenberg method. Both medial and lateral compartments show no significant narrowing.

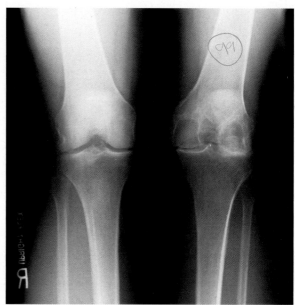

Fig 6.117 Abnormal bilateral knee radiograph performed using the Rosenberg method. Note the obliterated lateral compartment of the left knee with associated joint space narrowing medially. (Reprinted with permission from Hobbs, DL: Osteoarthritis and the Rosenberg method, *Radiol Technol* 77:181, 2006.)

PA AND AP AXIAL PROJECTIONS ("TUNNEL VIEWS"): INTERCONDYLAR FOSSA

CAMP COVENTRY METHOD, HOLMBLAD METHOD (AND VARIATIONS), AND BÉCLERE METHOD

Clinical Indications

- Intercondylar fossa, femoral condyles, tibial plateaus, and intercondylar eminence demonstrated
- Evidence of bony or cartilaginous pathology, osteochondral defects, or narrowing of joint space

Knee—Intercondylar Fossa Projections
ROUTINE
• PA axial

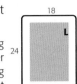

NOTE: Several methods are described for demonstrating these structures. The prone position (Fig. 6.118) is an easier position for the patient to assume. The Holmblad kneeling method provides another option with a slightly different projection of these structures (Fig. 6.119). The disadvantage is that this position is sometimes uncomfortable for the patient. As a result of the advent of x-ray tables that can be raised and lowered, several Holmblad variations can be used to alleviate the pain of kneeling on both knees. These methods do not require a complete kneeling position, but they do require a cooperative ambulatory patient.

Technical Factors

- Minimum SID—40 inches (100 cm)
- IR size—8 × 10 inches (18 × 24 cm), or 14 × 17 inches (35 × 43 cm) for bilateral studies, portrait
- Grid
- kVp range: 70–80

Shielding Place lead shield over gonadal area. Secure around waist in kneeling position and extend shield down to midfemur level.

Patient Position

1. Place patient prone; provide a pillow for patient's head (Camp Coventry method).
2. Have patient kneel on x-ray table (Holmblad method).
3. Have patient partially standing, straddling x-ray table with one leg (Holmblad variation, requires elevation of examination table).
4. Have patient partially standing with affected leg on a stool or chair (Holmblad variation).

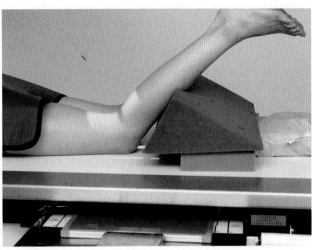

Fig 6.118 Camp Coventry method—prone position (40° to 50° flexion). (Position credited to Rosenberg TD, Paulos LE, Parker RD, et al: The 45° posteroanterior flexion weight-bearing radiograph of the knee, *J Bone Joint Surg Am* 70:1479, 1988.)

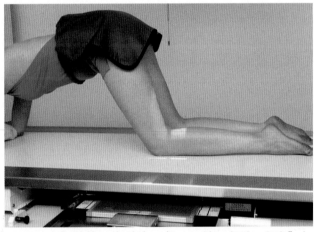

Fig 6.119 Holmblad method—kneeling position (60° to 70° flexion).

Evaluation Criteria

Anatomy Demonstrated: • Intercondylar fossa, articular facets (tibial plateaus), and knee joint space are demonstrated clearly (Figs. 6.120 and 6.121).
Position: • Intercondylar fossa should appear in profile, open without superimposition by patella. • **No rotation** is evidenced by symmetric appearance of distal posterior femoral condyles and superimposition of approximately half of fibular head by tibia. • Articular facets and intercondylar eminence of tibia should be well visualized without superimposition.
Exposure: • Optimal exposure should visualize soft tissue in knee joint space and an outline of the patella through the femur. • Trabecular markings of femoral condyles and proximal tibia should appear clear and sharp, with no motion.

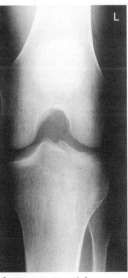

Fig 6.120 PA axial projection.

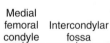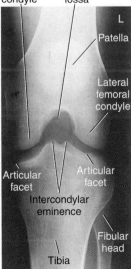

Medial femoral condyle — Intercondylar fossa

Patella

Lateral femoral condyle

Articular facet — Articular facet

Intercondylar eminence

Fibular head

Tibia

Fig 6.121 PA axial projection.

Part Position ⬦

1. **Prone (Camp Coventry method)** (see Fig. 6.118)
   - Flex knee **40° to 50°**; place support under ankle.
   - Center IR to knee joint, considering projection of CR angle.
2. **Kneeling (Holmblad method)** (see Fig. 6.119)
   - With patient kneeling on "all fours," place IR under affected knee and center IR to popliteal crease.
   - Ask patient to support body weight primarily on opposite knee.
   - Place padded support under ankle and leg of affected limb to reduce pressure on injured knee.
   - Ask patient to **lean forward slowly 20° to 30°** and to hold that position (results in **60° to 70°** knee flexion).
3. **Partially standing, straddling table (Holmblad variation)**
   - Lower examination table to a comfortable height for the patient, which is usually at the height of the knee joint.
   - Ask patient to support body weight primarily on unaffected knee.
   - Place affected knee over the bucky or IR.
   - Ask patient to **lean forward slowly 20° to 30°** and to hold that position (results in **60° to 70°** knee flexion).
4. **Partially standing, affected leg on stool or chair (Holmblad variation)** (Figs. 6.122 and 6.123)
   - Adjust stool height to a comfortable height for the patient, which is usually at the height of the knee joint.
   - Ask patient to support body weight primarily on the unaffected knee. **Provide a step stool for support.**
   - Place the affected knee on the IR, while resting on the stool or chair.
   - Ask patient to **lean forward slowly 20° to 30°** and to hold that position (results in **60° to 70°** knee flexion).

CR

1. **Prone:** Direct CR perpendicular to lower leg (40° to 50° caudad to match degree of flexion).
2. **Kneeling:** Direct CR perpendicular to IR and lower leg.
   - Direct CR to midpopliteal crease.

Recommended Collimation Collimate on four sides to knee joint area.

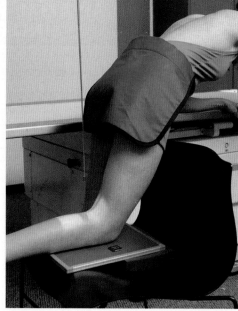

Fig 6.122 Holmblad variation—partially standing by examination table knee position (60° to 70° flexion).

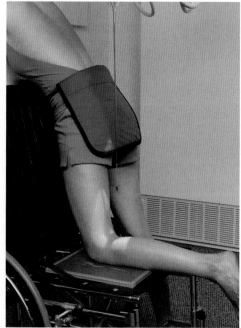

Fig 6.123 Holmblad variation—wheelchair version (60° to 70° flexion).

AP AXIAL PROJECTION: KNEE—INTERCONDYLAR FOSSA

BÉCLERE METHOD

Clinical Indications
- Intercondylar fossa, femoral condyles, tibial plateaus, and intercondylar eminence demonstrated to look for evidence of bony or cartilaginous pathology
- Osteochondral defects, or narrowing of the joint space

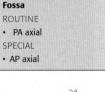

Knee—Intercondylar Fossa
ROUTINE
- PA axial
SPECIAL
- AP axial

NOTE: This is a reversal of the PA axial projection for patients who cannot assume the prone position. However, this is **not** a preferred projection because of distortion from the CR angle and increased part-IR distance. This projection also increases exposure for the gonadal region.

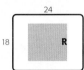

Technical Factors
- Minimum SID—40 inches (100 cm)
- IR size—8 × 10 inches (18 × 24 cm), landscape
- Grid
- kVp range: 65–80

Shielding Place lead shield over pelvic area, extending to midfemur.

Patient Position Place patient in supine position. Provide support under partially flexed knee with entire leg in anatomic position with no rotation.

Part Position
- Flex knee **40° to 45°,** and position support under IR as needed to place IR firmly against posterior thigh and lower leg, as shown in Figs. 6.124 and 6.125.
- Adjust IR as needed to center IR to midknee joint area.

CR
- Direct CR **perpendicular to lower leg** (approximately 40° to 45° cephalad).
- Direct CR to a point ½ inch (1.25 cm) distal to apex of patella.

Recommended Collimation Collimate on four sides to knee joint area.

Evaluation Criteria
Anatomy Demonstrated: • Intercondylar fossa, femoral condyles, tibial plateaus, and intercondylar eminence.
Position: • Center of four-sided collimation field should be to midknee joint area. • Intercondylar fossa should appear in profile, open without superimposition by patella. • Intercondylar eminence and tibial plateau and distal condyles of femur should be clearly visualized. • **No rotation** is evidenced by symmetric appearance of distal posterior femoral condyles and superimposition of approximately half of fibular head by tibia (Fig. 6.126).
Exposure: • Optimal exposure should visualize soft tissue in knee joint space and outline of patella through femur. • Trabecular markings of femoral condyles and proximal tibia should appear clear and sharp, with no motion.

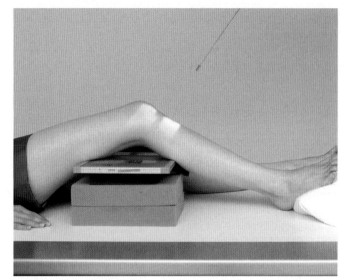

Fig 6.124 AP axial—(40° flexion, CR perpendicular to lower leg approximately 40°cephalad).

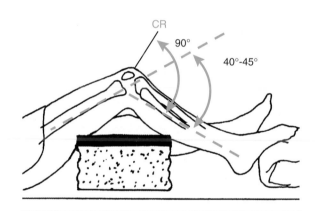

Fig 6.125 8 × 10 inches (18 × 24 cm) IR.

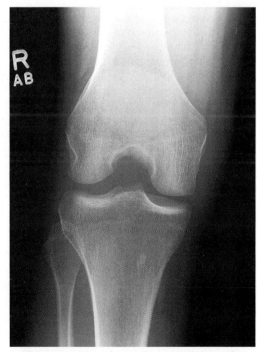

Fig 6.126 AP axial—40° flexion and CR angle.

PA PROJECTION: PATELLA AND PATELLOFEMORAL JOINT

Clinical Indications
- Evaluation of patellar fractures before knee joint is flexed for other projections

Patella
• PA
• Lateral
• Tangential

Technical Factors
- Minimum SID—40 inches (100 cm)
- IR size—8 × 10 inches (18 × 24 cm), portrait
- Grid
- Nongrid for knee thickness <10 cm
- kVp range: 70–80 (increase 4 to 6 kVp from PA knee)

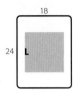

Shielding Shield radiosensitive tissues outside region of interest.

Patient Position Place patient in prone position, legs extended; provide a pillow for patient's head; place support under ankle and lower leg, with smaller support under femur above knee to prevent direct pressure on patella.

Part Position
- Align and center long axis of leg and knee to midline of table or IR (Fig. 6.127).
- **True PA:** Align interepicondylar line parallel to plane of IR. (This usually requires about **5° internal rotation of anterior knee.**)

CR
- CR is **perpendicular** to IR.
- Direct CR to **midpatella area** (which is usually at approximately the midpopliteal crease).

Recommended Collimation Collimate closely on four sides to include just the area of the patella and knee joint.

NOTE: With potential fracture of the patella, extra care should be taken **not to flex knee** and **provide support under thigh** (femur) so as not to put direct pressure on patellar area.

The projection also may be taken as an AP projection positioned similar to an AP knee if patient cannot assume a prone position.

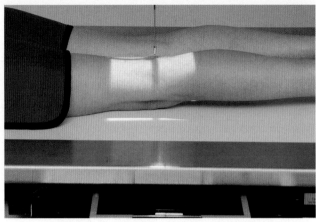

Fig 6.127 PA patella—CR 0° to midpatella.

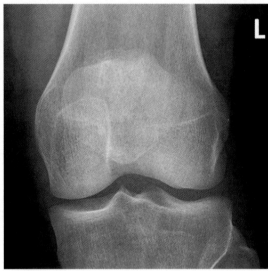

Fig 6.128 PA patella. (Courtesy Joss Wertz, DO.)

Evaluation Criteria
Anatomy Demonstrated: • Knee joint and patella are shown, with optimal recorded detail of patella because of decreased OID if taken as PA projection (Fig. 6.128).
Position: • **No rotation** is present, as evidenced by symmetric appearance of condyles. • Patella is centered to femur with correct slight internal rotation of anterior knee. • Patella is in center of collimated field.
Exposure: • Optimal exposure **without motion** visualizes soft tissue in joint area and clearly visualizes sharp bony trabecular markings and outline of patella as seen through distal femur.

LATERAL—MEDIOLATERAL PROJECTION: PATELLA

Clinical Indications
- Evaluation of patellar fractures in conjunction with the PA
- Abnormalities of patellofemoral and femorotibial joints

Patella
• PA
• Lateral
• Tangential

Technical Factors
- Minimum SID—40 inches (100 cm)
- IR size—8 × 10 inches (18 × 24 cm), portrait
- Grid
- Nongrid for knee thickness <10 cm
- kVp range: 70–80

Shielding Shield radiosensitive tissues outside region of interest.

Patient Position Place patient in lateral recumbent position, affected side down; provide a pillow for patient's head; provide support for knee of opposite limb placed behind affected knee.

Part Position
- Adjust rotation of body and leg until knee is in **true lateral** position (femoral epicondyles directly superimposed and plane of patella perpendicular to plane of IR).
- Flex knee **only 5° or 10°.** (Additional flexion may separate fracture fragments if present.)
- Align and center long axis of patella to CR and to centerline of table or IR (Fig. 6.129).

CR
- CR is **perpendicular** to IR.
- Direct CR to mid-patellofemoral joint.

Recommended Collimation Collimate closely on four sides to include just the area of the patella and knee joint.

NOTE: This also can be taken as a **horizontal beam lateral** with no knee flexion on a patient with severe trauma, as described in Chapter 15.

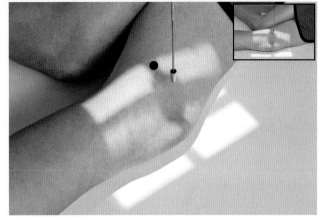
Fig 6.129 Lateral patella.

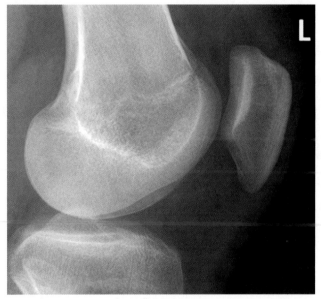
Fig 6.130 Lateral patella. (Courtesy Joss Wertz, DO.)

Evaluation Criteria
Anatomy Demonstrated: • Profile images of patella, patellofemoral joint, and femorotibial joint are demonstrated (Fig. 6.130).
Position: • True lateral: Anterior and posterior borders of medial and lateral femoral condyles should be directly superimposed, and patellofemoral joint space should appear open. • Centering and angulation are correct if patella is in center of the film and collimated field with joint spaces open.
Exposure: • Optimal exposure visualizes soft tissue detail and patella well without overexposure. • Trabecular markings of patella and other bones should appear clear and sharp.

TANGENTIAL–AXIAL OR SUNRISE/SKYLINE PROJECTION: PATELLA

MERCHANT BILATERAL METHOD

Clinical Indications
- Subluxation of patella and other abnormalities of the patella and patellofemoral joint

> **Patella**
> • Tangential

Technical Factors
- SID—48 to 72 inches (120 to 180 cm) (increased SID reduces magnification)
- IR size—10 × 12 inches (24 × 30 cm), or 14 × 17 inches (35 × 43 cm) for bilateral studies of the knees; landscape
- Nongrid (grid is not required because of air gap caused by increased OID)
- kVp range: 70–80
- Some type of leg support and cassette holder should be used

Shielding Shield radiosensitive tissues outside region of interest.

Patient Position Place patient in the supine position with knees flexed 40° over the end of the table, resting on a leg support. Patient must be comfortable and relaxed for quadriceps muscles to be relaxed (see NOTE).

Part Position
- Place support under knees to raise distal femurs as needed so that they are parallel to tabletop.
- Place knees and feet together and secure lower legs together to prevent rotation and to allow patient to be totally relaxed.
- Place IR on edge against legs approximately 12 inches (30 cm) below the knees, **perpendicular** to x-ray beam (Figs. 6.131 and 6.132).

CR
- Angle CR caudad, **30° from horizontal plane** (CR 30° to femur). Adjust CR angle if needed for true tangential projection of patellofemoral joint spaces.
- Direct CR to a point midway between patellae.

Recommended Collimation Collimate **tightly** on all sides to patellae.

NOTE: Patient comfort and total relaxation are essential. The quadriceps femoris muscles must be relaxed to prevent subluxation of the patellae, wherein they are pulled into the intercondylar sulcus or groove, which may result in false readings.[6]

Evaluation Criteria
Anatomy Demonstrated: • Intercondylar sulcus (trochlear groove) and patella of each distal femur should be visualized in profile with patellofemoral joint space open (Figs. 6.133 and 6.134).
Position: • No rotation of knee is present, as evidenced by symmetric appearance of patella, anterior femoral condyles, and intercondylar sulcus. • Correct CR angle and centering are evidenced by open patellofemoral joint spaces.
Exposure: • Optimal exposure should clearly visualize soft tissue and joint space margins and trabecular markings of patellae. • Femoral condyles appear underexposed with only anterior margins clearly defined.

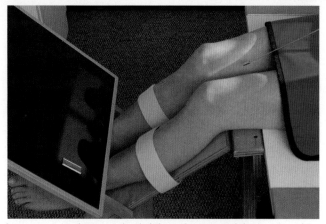

Fig 6.131 Merchant method—bilateral tangential, knees flexed 40°.

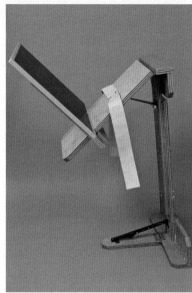

Fig 6.132 Adjustable-type leg support and IR holder. (Courtesy St. Joseph's Hospital and Medical Center, Phoenix, AZ.)

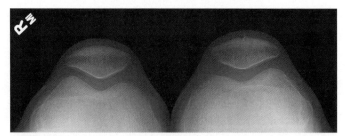

Fig 6.133 Merchant method—bilateral tangential. (Courtesy Joss Wertz, DO.)

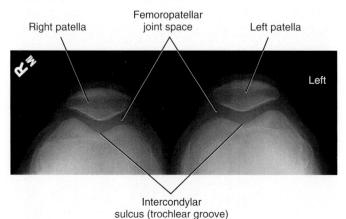

Right patella   Femoropatellar joint space   Left patella

Left

Intercondylar sulcus (trochlear groove)

Fig 6.134 Merchant method—bilateral tangential. (Courtesy Joss Wertz, DO.)

TANGENTIAL—AXIAL OR SUNRISE/SKYLINE PROJECTIONS: PATELLA

INFEROSUPERIOR AND HUGHSTON METHODS

Summary Three additional methods for tangential projections of the patellae and patellofemoral joints are described. Advantages and disadvantages of each are noted. **Both sides** generally are taken for comparison.

Patella
• Tangential

35   43

L   R

Technical Factors
- SID—40 to 48 inches (100 to 120 cm)
- IR size—14 × 17 inches (35 × 43 cm), landscape, for bilateral studies of the knees, or unilateral study 8 × 10 inches (18 × 24 cm), portrait
- Nongrid
- kVp range: 70–80

Inferosuperior Projection
- Place patient in supine position, legs together, with sufficient-sized support placed under knees for 40° to 45° knee flexion (legs relaxed).
- Ensure no leg rotation.
- Place IR on edge, resting on midthighs, tilted to be perpendicular to CR. Use sandbags and tape as shown, or use other methods to stabilize IR in this position. It is *not* recommended that patient be asked to sit up to hold IR in place because this may place patient's head and neck region in path of x-ray beam (Fig. 6.135).

CR
- Direct CR inferosuperiorly, at 10° to 15° angle from lower legs to be **tangential to patellofemoral joint**. Palpate borders of patella to determine specific CR angle required to pass through infrapatellar joint space.

NOTE 1: Major advantages of this method are that it does not require special equipment and a relatively comfortable position is required for the patient. Relaxation of the quadriceps muscle can be achieved with 40° to 45° knee flexion if properly sized support is placed under knees. The chief disadvantage is a potential problem with holding or supporting the IR in this position if the patient cannot cooperate fully.

Hughston Method[7]
This projection may be done bilaterally on one IR. Place patient in prone position, with IR placed under knee; slowly flex knee between 50° to 60° from full extension of lower leg (see NOTE 3); have patient hold foot with gauze, or rest foot on supporting device **(not on collimator)** (Fig. 6.136).

CR
- Angle CR 45° cephalad (CR tangential to patellofemoral joint).

NOTE 2: This is a relatively comfortable position for the patient, and relaxation of the quadriceps can be achieved. The major disadvantage is that this method requires the prone position, which is difficult for some patients. Additionally, image distortion is caused by awkward part alignment and difficulties encountered in angling the tube, which usually are caused by large collimators.

NOTE 3: Some authors suggest reduced flexion of only 20° to prevent the patella from being drawn into the patellofemoral groove, which may prevent detection of subtle abnormalities in alignment.[8]

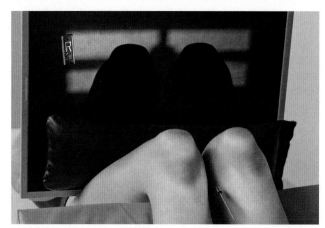

Fig 6.135 Inferosuperior projection—40° to 45° flexion of knees.

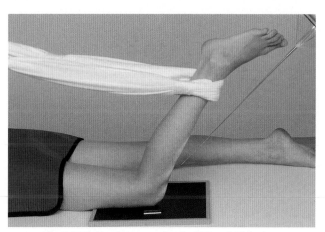

Fig 6.136 Hughston method—50° to 60° flexion.

TANGENTIAL—AXIAL OR SUNRISE/SKYLINE PROJECTIONS: PATELLA

SETTEGAST METHOD

WARNING: This acute flexion of the knee should not be attempted until fracture of the patella has been ruled out by other projections.

- Place patient in prone position, with IR under knee; slowly flex knee to a **minimum of 90°;** have patient hold onto gauze or tape to maintain position (Fig. 6.137). An alternative seated variation is possible but with the risk of increased exposure to hands and thorax. Close collimation is required (Fig. 6.138).

CR

- Direct CR tangential to **patellofemoral joint space** (15° to 20° from lower leg).
- Minimum SID is 40 inches (100 cm).

NOTE 4: The major disadvantage of this method is that acute knee flexion tightens the quadriceps and draws the patella into the intercondylar sulcus, reducing the diagnostic value of this projection.[9]

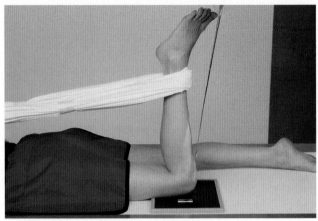

Fig 6.137 Settegast prone method—90° flexion of knee.

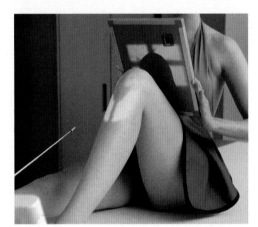

Fig 6.138 Settegast seated variation—90° flexion of knee.

SUPEROINFERIOR SITTING TANGENTIAL METHOD: PATELLA

HOBBS MODIFICATION

This method may be done bilaterally on one IR.

WARNING: This acute flexion of the knee should not be attempted until fracture of the patella has been ruled out by other projections.

- Place patient seated in a chair, with IR placed under knees resting on a step stool or support to help reduce OID; knees should be flexed with feet placed slightly underneath the chair (Fig. 6.139).

CR
- Align CR to be perpendicular to IR (tangential to patellofemoral joint).
- Direct CR to mid-patellofemoral joint.
- Minimum SID is 48 to 50 inches (120 to 125 cm) to reduce magnification because of increased OID.[10]

NOTE: The major advantage of this position is that the patient can be examined while sitting in a chair. This position also requires little manipulation of the x-ray tube. The major disadvantage is that it requires acute flexion of the knees.[10]

Evaluation Criteria
Anatomy Demonstrated: • Intercondylar sulcus (trochlear groove) and patella of each distal femur should be visualized in profile with patellofemoral joint space open. No superimposition of the patellae or tibial tuberosities[11] (Figs. 6.140 and 6.141).
Position: • No rotation of knee is present, as evidenced by symmetric appearance of patella, anterior femoral condyles, and intercondylar sulcus. • Correct CR angle and centering are evidenced by open patellofemoral joint space.
Exposure: • Optimal exposure should clearly visualize soft tissue and joint space margins and trabecular markings of patellae. • Femoral condyles appear underexposed with only anterior margins clearly defined.

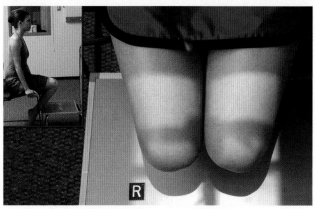
Fig 6.139 Hobbs modification.

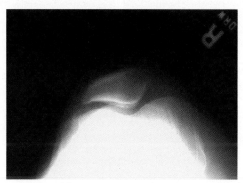
Fig 6.140 Hobbs modification—superoinferior sitting tangential method.

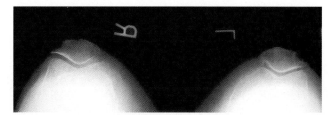
Fig 6.141 Superoinferior sitting tangential method.

RADIOGRAPHS FOR CRITIQUE

This section consists of an ideal projection (Image A) along with one or more projections that may demonstrate positioning and/or technical errors. Critique Figures C6.142 through C6.147. Compare Image A to the other projections and identify the errors. While examining each image, consider the following questions:

1. Is all essential anatomy demonstrated on the image?

2. What positioning errors are present that compromise image quality?
3. Are technical factors optimal?
4. Is there evidence of collimation and pre-exposure anatomic side markers visible on the image?
5. Do these errors require a repeat exposure?
   Feedback for each set of images is located on the faculty Evolve site.

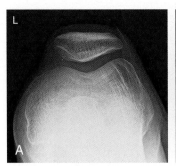
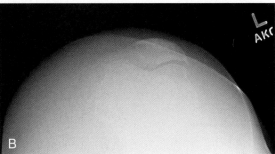
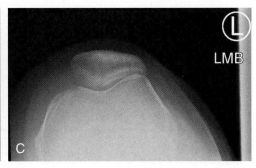

Fig C6.142 Bilateral tangential patella.

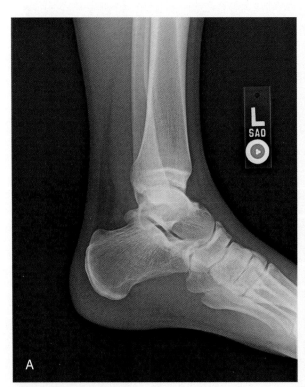
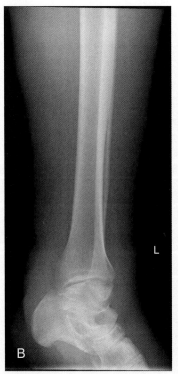
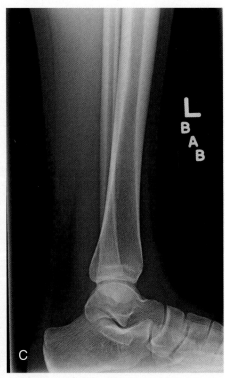

Fig C6.143 Lateral ankle.

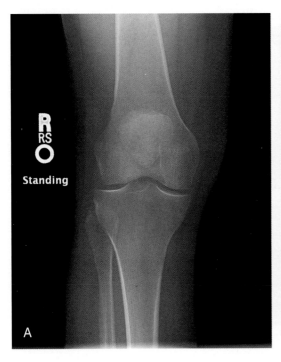
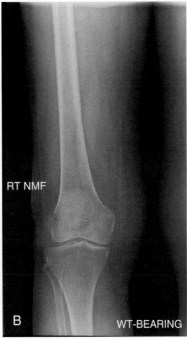
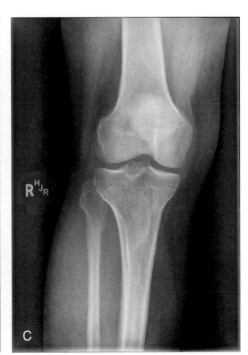

Fig C6.144 AP knee.

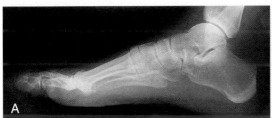
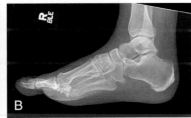
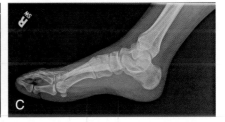

Fig C6.145 Lateral foot. (Courtesy Joss Wertz, DO.)

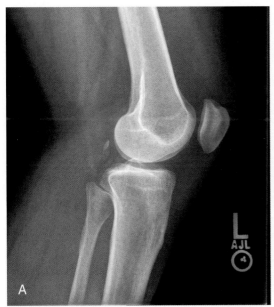
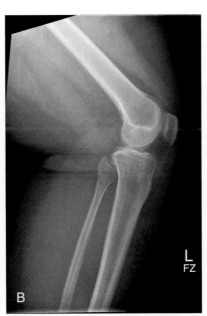
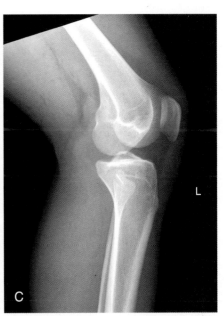

Fig C6.146 Mediolateral knee. (Courtesy Joss Wertz, DO.)

6

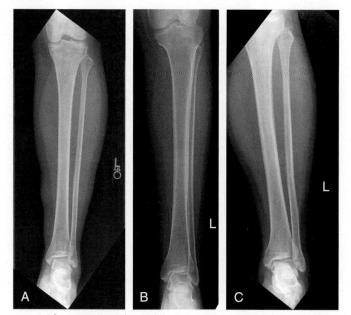

Fig C6.147 AP lower leg. (Courtesy Joss Wertz, DO.)

Femur and Pelvic Girdle

CONTRIBUTIONS BY **Beth L. Vealé,** PhD, RT(R)(QM)
CONTRIBUTOR TO PAST EDITIONS   Jeannean Hall-Rollins, MRC, BS, RT(R)(CV)

CONTENTS

Lower Limb (Extremity)

In Chapter 6, three groups of bones of the lower limb—the foot, lower leg, and distal femur—were described, along with the associated knee and ankle joints (Fig. 7.1).

The lower limb bones discussed in this chapter are the **proximal femur** and the **pelvic girdle.** The joints involving these two groups of bones, also included in this chapter, are the important **hip joint** and the **sacroiliac** and **symphysis pubis** joints of the pelvic girdle.

FEMUR

The **femur** is the longest and strongest bone in the body. The entire weight of the body is transferred through this bone and the associated joints at each end. Therefore, these joints are a frequent source of pathology when trauma occurs. The anatomy of the mid- to distal femur was discussed in Chapter 6.

Proximal Femur

The proximal femur consists of four essential parts, the head (1), neck (2), and greater (3) and lesser trochanters (4) *(tro-kan'-ters).*

The **head** of the femur is rounded and smooth for articulation with the hip bones. It contains a depression, or pit, near its center called the *fovea capitis (fo'-ve-ah cap'-i-tis),* wherein a major ligament called the *ligament of the head of the femur,* or the *ligament capitis femoris,* is attached to the head of the femur.

The **neck** of the femur is a strong pyramidal process of bone that connects the head with the body or shaft in the region of the trochanters.

The **greater trochanter** is a large prominence located **superiorly** and **laterally** to the femoral shaft and is palpable as a bony landmark. The **lesser trochanter** is a smaller, blunt, conical eminence that projects **medially** and **posteriorly** from the junction of the neck and shaft of the femur. The trochanters are joined posteriorly by a thick ridge called the **intertrochanteric** *(in"-ter-tro"-kan-ter'-ik)* **crest.** The **body** or **shaft** of the femur is long and almost cylindrical (Fig. 7.2).

Angles of the Proximal Femur The angle of the neck to the shaft on an average adult is approximately **125°,** with a variance of ±15°, depending on the width of the pelvis and the length of the lower limbs. For example, in a long-legged person with a narrow pelvis, the femur would be nearer vertical, which then would change the angle of the neck to about 140°. This angle would be less (110° to 115°) for a shorter person with a wider pelvis.

On an average adult in the anatomic position, the longitudinal plane of the femur is approximately **10° from vertical,** as shown on the left in Fig. 7.3. This vertical angle is nearer 15° on someone with a wide pelvis and shorter limbs and only about 5° on a long-legged person. This angle affects positioning and the central ray (CR) angles for a lateral knee, as described in Figs. 6.19 and 6.20.

Another angle of the neck and head of the femur that is important in radiography is the **15° to 20° anterior angle** of the head and neck in relation to the body of the femur (see right drawing of Fig. 7.3). The head projects somewhat anteriorly or forward as a result of this angle. This angle becomes important in radiographic positioning; the femur and lower leg must be rotated **15° to 20° internally** to place the femoral neck parallel to the image receptor (IR) for a true anteroposterior (AP) projection of the proximal femur.

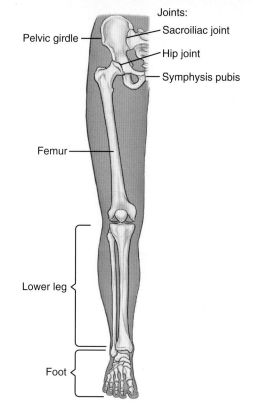

Fig. 7.1 Lower limb.

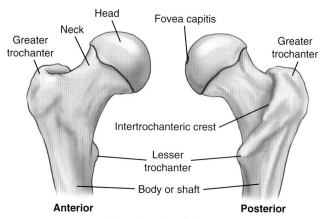

Fig. 7.2 Proximal femur.

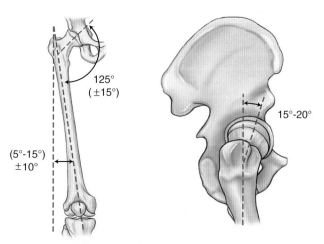

Fig. 7.3 Angles of proximal femur.

PELVIS

The complete **pelvis** (meaning a *basin*) serves as the base of the trunk and forms the connection between the vertebral column and lower limbs. The pelvis consists of four bones—two **hip bones** (also called **innominate bones**), one **sacrum** *(sa'-krum)*, and one **coccyx** *(kok'-siks)* (Fig. 7.4). The sacrum articulates superiorly with the fifth lumbar vertebra to form the lumbosacral joint (also called the L5–S1 joint). The right and left hip (iliac) bones articulate posteriorly with the sacrum to form the sacroiliac joints.[1]

NOTE: The sacrum and the coccyx also are considered parts of the distal vertebral column and in this textbook are discussed in Chapter 9, along with the lumbar spine.

HIP BONE

Each hip bone is composed of three divisions: (1) **ilium** *(il'-e-um)*, (2) **ischium** *(is'-ke-um)*, and (3) **pubis** *(pu'-bis)*. In a child, these three divisions are separate bones, but they fuse into one bone during the middle teens. The fusion occurs in the area of the **acetabulum** *(as''-e-tab'-u-lum)*. The acetabulum is a deep, cup-shaped cavity that accepts the head of the femur to form the hip joint (Fig. 7.5).

The ilium, the largest of the three divisions, is located superior to the acetabulum. The ischium is inferior and posterior to the acetabulum, whereas the pubis is inferior and anterior to the acetabulum. Each of these three parts is described in detail in the following sections.

Ilium

Each **ilium** is composed of a **body** and an **ala,** or wing (Fig. 7.6). The body of the ilium is the more inferior portion near the acetabulum and includes the superior two-fifths of the acetabulum. The ala, or wing portion, is the thin and flared superior part of the ilium.

The **crest** of the ilium is the superior margin of the ala; it extends from the **anterior superior iliac spine** (ASIS) to the **posterior superior iliac spine** (PSIS). In radiographic positioning, the uppermost peak of the crest often is referred to as the **iliac crest,** but it actually extends between the ASIS and the PSIS.

Below the ASIS is a less prominent projection referred to as the **anterior inferior iliac spine.** Similarly, inferior to the PSIS is the **posterior inferior iliac spine.**

Positioning Landmarks The two important positioning landmarks of these borders and projections are the **iliac crest** and the **ASIS.**

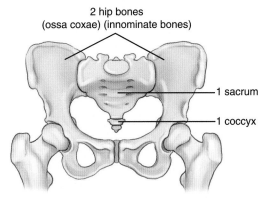

Fig. 7.4 Pelvis—four bones: two hip bones, sacrum, and coccyx.

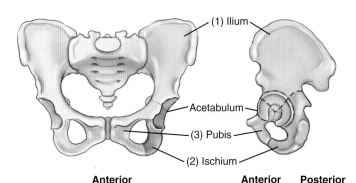

Fig. 7.5 Hip bone—three parts.

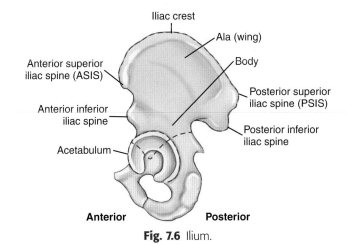

Fig. 7.6 Ilium.

Ischium

The **ischium** is that part of the hip bone that lies inferior and posterior to the acetabulum. Each ischium is divided into a **body** and a **ramus** (Fig. 7.7). The superior portion of the body of the ischium makes up the posteroinferior two-fifths of the acetabulum. The lower portion of the body of the ischium (formerly called the *superior ramus*) projects caudally and medially from the acetabulum, ending at the **ischial tuberosity.** Projecting anteriorly from the ischial tuberosity is the **ramus** of the ischium.

The rounded roughened area near the junction of the lower body and the inferior rami is a landmark called the **tuberosity** of the ischium, or the **ischial** *(is'-ke-al)* **tuberosity.**

Posterior to the acetabulum is a bony projection termed the ***ischial spine.*** A small part of the ischial spine also is visible on a frontal view of the pelvis, as shown in Fig. 7.8. (It is also seen in the anatomy review radiograph; see Fig. 7.16.)

Directly superior to the ischial spine is a deep notch termed the ***greater sciatic notch.*** Inferior to the ischial spine is a smaller notch termed the ***lesser sciatic notch.***

Positioning Landmarks The ischial tuberosities bear most of the weight of the body when an individual sits. They can be palpated through the soft tissues of each buttock in a prone position. However, because of discomfort and possible embarrassment to the patient, this landmark is not used as commonly as the previously described ASIS and crest of the ilium.

Pubis

The last of the three divisions of one hip bone is the **pubis,** or **pubic bone.** The **body** of the pubis is anterior and inferior to the acetabulum and includes the anteroinferior one-fifth of the acetabulum.

Extending anteriorly and medially from the body of each pubis is a **superior ramus.** The two superior rami meet in the midline to form an amphiarthrodial joint, the **symphysis pubis** *(sim'-fi-sis pu'-bis),* which also is correctly called the **pubic symphysis.** Each **inferior ramus** passes down and posterior from the symphysis pubis to join the ramus of the respective ischium.

The **obturator foramen** *(ob'-tu-ra"-tor fo-ra'-men)* is a large opening formed by the ramus and body of each ischium and by the pubis. The obturator foramen is the largest foramen in the human skeletal system.

Positioning Landmark The crests of the ilium and ASIS are important positioning landmarks. The superior margin of the symphysis pubis is a possible landmark for pelvis and hip positioning and for positioning of the abdomen, because it defines the inferior margin of the abdomen. However, if other associated landmarks are available, the symphysis pubis generally is not used as a palpated landmark because of patient modesty and potential embarrassment.

SUMMARY OF TOPOGRAPHIC LANDMARKS

Important positioning landmarks of the pelvis are reviewed in Fig. 7.9. The most superior aspects of the **iliac crest** and the **ASIS** are easily palpated. The ASIS is one of the more frequently used positioning landmarks of the pelvis. It also is commonly used to check for rotation of the pelvis and/or lower abdomen by determination of whether the distance between the ASIS and the tabletop is equal on both sides.

The **greater trochanter** of the femur can be located by firm palpation of the soft tissues of the upper thigh. Note that the prominence of the greater trochanter is at about the same level as the superior border of the **symphysis pubis,** whereas the **ischial tuberosity** is 1½ to 2 inches (4 to 5 cm) below the symphysis pubis. These distances vary between a male and a female pelvis because of general differences in shape, as described later in this chapter.

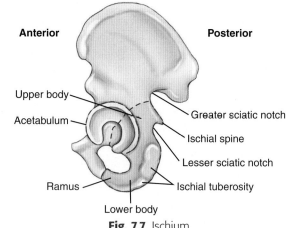

Fig. 7.7 Ischium.

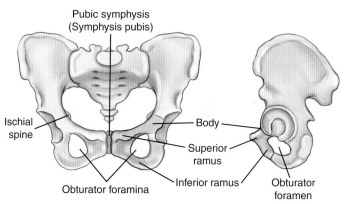

Fig. 7.8 Pubis (pubic bone).

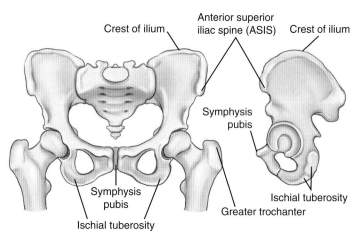

Fig. 7.9 Bony topographic landmarks of the pelvis.

TRUE AND FALSE PELVIS

A plane through the **brim** of the pelvis divides the pelvic area into two cavities. The pelvic brim is defined by the superior portion of the symphysis pubis anteriorly and by the superior, prominent part of the sacrum posteriorly. The general area above or superior to the oblique plane through the pelvic brim is termed the *greater,* or *false, pelvis.* The flared portion of the pelvis, which is formed primarily by the alae, or wings, of the ilia, forms the lateral and posterior limits of the false pelvis, whereas the abdominal muscles of the anterior wall define the anterior limits. The lower abdominal organs rest on the floor of the greater pelvis, as does the fetus within a pregnant uterus.

The area inferior to a plane through the pelvic brim is termed the *lesser,* or *true, pelvis.* The true pelvis is a cavity that is completely surrounded by bony structures. The size and shape of the true pelvis are of greatest importance during the birth process because the **true pelvis forms the actual birth canal** (Fig. 7.10).

True Pelvis

The oblique plane defined by the brim of the pelvis is termed the *inlet,* or *superior aperture,* of the true pelvis. The **outlet,** or *inferior aperture,* of the true pelvis is defined by the two ischial tuberosities and the tip of the coccyx (Fig. 7.11). The three sides of the triangularly shaped outlet are formed by a line between the ischial tuberosities and a line between each ischial tuberosity and the coccyx. The area between the inlet and outlet of the true pelvis is termed the *cavity* of the true pelvis. During the birth process, the baby must travel through the inlet, cavity, and outlet of the true pelvis.

Birth Canal

During a routine delivery, the baby's head first travels through the pelvic inlet, then to the midcavity, and finally through the outlet before it exits in a forward direction, as shown in Fig. 7.12.

Because of sensitivity of the fetus to radiation, radiographs of the pelvis generally are **not** taken during pregnancy. If the dimensions of the birth canal of the pelvis are in question, certain ultrasound procedures can be done to evaluate for potential problems during the birth process.

Pelvic Ring The pelvic ring is a term applied in orthopedics describing the sturdy, ringlike structure formed by the union of the ilium, ischium, and pubic bones, along with the sacrum and coccyx. This term is often used in described specific fractures that can disrupt the alignment of these bones.[2]

Male Versus Female Pelvis Differences[3]

There are four common shapes of the human pelvic inlet:
- Gynecoid: round
- Platypelloid: wider right to left than anterior to posterior
- Android: heart shaped
- Anthropoid: wider anterior to posterior than right to left

The general shape of the female pelvis is different enough from that of the male pelvis to enable discrimination of one from the other on pelvis radiographic images. In general, the **female pelvis** is wider, with the ilia more flared and more shallow from front to back (gynecoid or platypelloid). The **male pelvis** is narrower, deeper (anthropoid), or less flared with a heart-shaped pelvic inlet (android). In overall appearance on a frontal view, the female pelvis is wider with a round pelvic inlet. Therefore, the first difference between the male pelvis and female pelvis is the difference in the **overall general shape** of the entire pelvis, along with the shape differences of the pelvic inlet (Fig. 7.13).

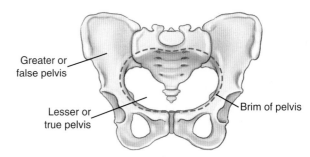
Fig. 7.10 Pelvic cavities.

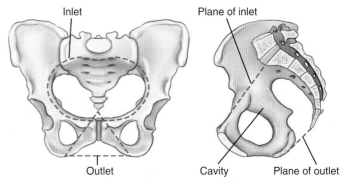
Fig. 7.11 Lesser or true pelvis.

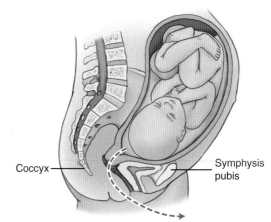
Fig. 7.12 Birth canal—sagittal sectional view.

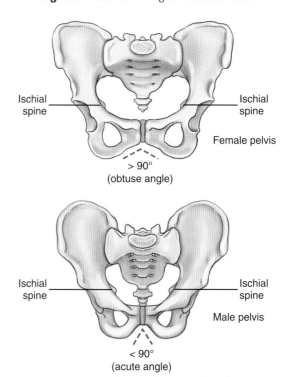
Fig. 7.13 Pelvis—male versus female.

A second major difference is the **angle of the pubic arch,** formed by the inferior rami of the pubis just inferior to the symphysis pubis. In the female, this angle is between 80° and 85°, whereas in the male, the pubic arch usually forms an acute angle between 50° and 60°.

A third difference is that the ischial spines generally do not project as far medially toward the pelvic cavity in the female as they do in males. They are more visible along the lateral margins of the pelvic cavity in the male than in the female in the AP pelvis projection.

NOTE: The general shape of the pelvis does vary considerably from one individual to another, so the pelvis of a slender female may resemble a male pelvis. In general, however, the differences are usually obvious enough that the gender of the patient can be determined from a radiographic image of the pelvis.

See Table 7.1 for a summary of male and female pelvic characteristics.

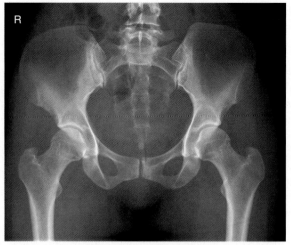

Fig. 7.14 Female pelvis.

TABLE 7.1 **SUMMARY OF MALE AND FEMALE PELVIC CHARACTERISTICS**		
	MALE	**FEMALE**
General shape (shape of pelvic inlet)	Narrower, deeper, less flared. Pelvic inlet is more oval or heart shaped (anthropoid or android)	Wider, more shallow, more flared. Pelvic inlet rounder (gynecoid or platypelloid)
Angle of pubic arch	Narrower angle (50° to 60°)	Wider angle (80° to 85°)
Ischial spines	More protrusion into pelvic inlet (or cavity)	Less protrusion into pelvic inlet

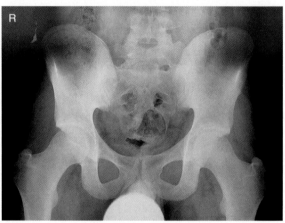

Fig. 7.15 Male pelvis.

Male Versus Female Pelvis Radiographs

Figs. 7.14 and 7.15 are pelvic radiographs of a female subject and a male subject, respectively. Note the three differences between the typical female pelvis and typical male pelvis.

1. In overall shape, the male pelvis appears narrower and deeper and has a less-flared appearance of the ilia. The shape of the inlet on the male pelvis is not as large or as rounded as that of the female pelvis.
2. The pubic arch of the male pelvis has a smaller angle compared to the greater angle on the female pelvis. This angle is commonly one of the more noticeable differences.
3. Radiographic presence of the ischial spines along the lateral margins of the pelvic cavity is less pronounced with the female pelvis.

REVIEW EXERCISE WITH RADIOGRAPHS

Key pelvic anatomy is labeled on the AP pelvis radiograph of Fig. 7.16. A good review exercise is to cover up the answers (listed below) while identifying the labeled parts.

A. Iliac crest
B. ASIS (anterior end of crest)
C. Body of left ischium
D. Ischial tuberosity
E. Symphysis pubis (pubic symphysis)
F. Inferior ramus of right pubis
G. Superior ramus of right pubis
H. Right ischial spine
I. Acetabulum of right hip
J. Neck of right femur
K. Greater trochanter of right femur
L. Head of right femur
M. Ala, or wing, of right ilium

Lateral Hip

Fig. 7.17 presents a lateral radiograph of the proximal femur and hip, taken with an axiolateral projection (Danelius-Miller method), as demonstrated by the positioning in Fig. 7.18. Answers to the labeled parts are as follows:

A. Acetabulum
B. Femoral head
C. Femoral neck
D. Shaft or body
E. Area of lesser trochanter
F. Area of greater trochanter
G. Ischial tuberosity

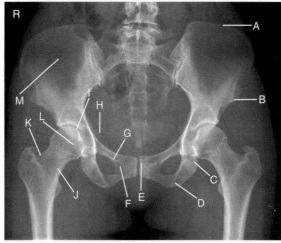

Fig. 7.16 AP Pelvis.

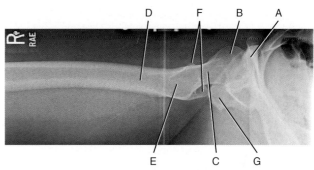

Fig. 7.17 Axiolateral projection.

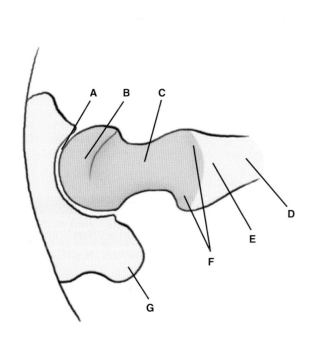

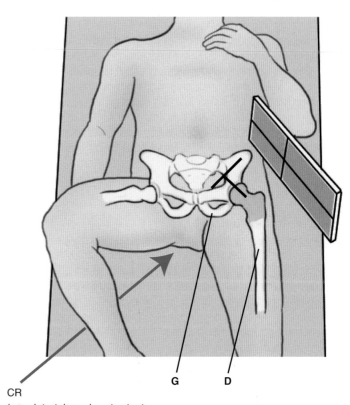

Fig. 7.18 Proximal femur and hip—lateral (axiolateral projection).

CLASSIFICATION OF JOINTS (FIG. 7.19)

The number of joints or articulations of the proximal femora and pelvis is limited, with the hip joint being the most obvious. These joints of the pelvis, in the following list, again are described according to their **classification, mobility type,** and **movement type.**

   Sacroiliac joints: joints between the sacrum and each ilium

   Symphysis pubis: structure between the right and left pubic bones

   Union of acetabulum: temporary growth joint of each acetabulum that solidifies in the midteen years

   Hip joints: joints between the head of the femur and the acetabulum of the pelvis

Sacroiliac Joints (Fig. 7.20)

The sacroiliac joints are wide flat joints located on each side obliquely between the sacrum and each ilium. These joints are situated at an unusual oblique angle, requiring special positioning to visualize the joint spaces radiographically.

The sacroiliac joint is classified as a **synovial joint** in that it is enclosed in a fibrous articular capsule that contains synovial fluid. The bones are joined by firm sacroiliac ligaments. Generally, synovial joints by their nature are considered freely movable, or diarthrodial, joints. However, the sacroiliac joint is a special type of synovial joint that permits little movement. Due to its unique structure and movement, it's type of movement is **irregular gliding**. The reason for this classification is that the joint surfaces are very irregularly shaped and the interconnecting bones are snugly fitted because they serve a weight-bearing function. This shape restricts movement, and the cavity of the joint or the joint space may be reduced in size or even nonexistent in older persons, especially in males. Positioning of the sacroiliac joints is described in Chapter 9.

Symphysis Pubis

The symphysis pubis is the articulation of the right and left pubic bones located in the midline of the anterior pelvis. The most superior anterior aspect of this joint is palpable and is an important positioning landmark, as described earlier.

The symphysis pubis is classified as a **cartilaginous joint** of the **symphysis subtype** in that only limited movement is possible **(amphiarthrodial).** The two articular surfaces are separated by a fibrocartilaginous disk and are held together by certain ligaments. This interpubic disk of fibrocartilage is a relatively thick pad (thicker in females than males) that is capable of being compressed or partially displaced, thereby allowing limited movement of these bones, as in the case of pelvic trauma or during the childbirth process in females.

Union of Acetabulum

The three divisions of each hip bone are separate bones in a child but come together in the acetabulum by fusing during the middle teens to become completely indistinguishable in an adult. Therefore, this structure is classified as a **cartilaginous-type** joint of the **synchondrosis subtype,** which is **immovable,** or **synarthrodial,** in an adult. This joint is considered a temporary type of growth joint that is similar to the joints between the epiphyses and diaphyses of long bones in growing children.

Hip Joint

The hip joint is classified as a **synovial type,** which is characterized by a large fibrous capsule that contains synovial fluid. It is a **freely movable,** or **diarthrodial,** joint and is the truest example of a **ball and socket** (spheroidal) movement type. See Table 7.2 for a summary of the pelvic joints.

The head of the femur forms more than half a sphere as it fits into the relatively deep, cup-shaped acetabulum. This connection makes the hip joint inherently strong as it supports the weight of the body while still permitting a high degree of mobility. The articular capsule surrounding this joint is strong and dense, with the thickest part being superior, as would be expected because it is in line with the weight-bearing function of the hip joints. A series of strong bands of ligaments surround the articular capsule and joint in general, making this joint very strong and stable.

Movements of the hip joint include **flexion** and **extension, abduction** and **adduction, medial** (internal) and **lateral** (external) **rotation,** and **circumduction.**

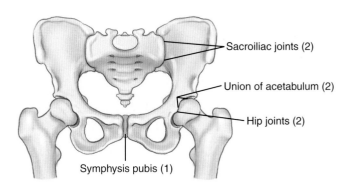

Fig. 7.19 Joints of pelvis.

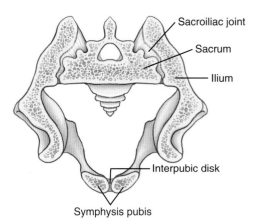

Fig. 7.20 Coronal view of a transverse section showing sacroiliac and symphysis pubis joints.

TABLE 7.2 SUMMARY OF PELVIC JOINTS			
JOINTS	**CLASSIFICATION**	**MOBILITY TYPE**	**MOVEMENT TYPE**
Sacroiliac joint	Synovial	Limited movement	Irregular gliding
Symphysis pubis	Cartilaginous	Amphiarthrodial	Limited
Union of acetabulum	Cartilaginous	Synarthrodial (for adults)	Nonmovable
Hip joint	Synovial	Diarthrodial	Ball and socket (spheroidal)

RADIOGRAPHIC POSITIONING

Positioning Considerations

LOCATING THE FEMORAL HEAD AND NECK

A long-standing traditional method used to locate the femoral head and neck is first to determine the midpoint of a line between the ASIS and the symphysis pubis. The **neck** is approximately 2½ inches (6 to 7 cm), and the **head** 1½ inches (4 cm) distal and at right angles to the midpoint of this line (Figs. 7.21 and 7.22).

The **greater trochanters** are shown to be located on the same horizontal line as the symphysis pubis. However, the greater trochanters are difficult to palpate accurately on large or bariatric patients, and palpation of the symphysis pubis can be embarrassing for the patient. Therefore, a second method is suggested for locating the femoral head or neck that uses only the **ASIS**, which is easily palpated on all types of patients. The level of the symphysis pubis is between 3 and 4 inches (8 to 10 cm) inferior to the level of the ASIS. Therefore, the femoral neck can be readily located as being **1 to 2 inches (3 to 5 cm) medial and 3 to 4 inches (8 to 10 cm) distal to the ASIS.** This level also places it on the same horizontal plane as the symphysis pubis and the greater trochanters.

As was previously demonstrated, significant differences exist between the male pelvis and the female pelvis, but with some practice and allowances for male and female differences, both of these methods work well for locating the femoral head or neck for hip positioning.

APPEARANCE OF PROXIMAL FEMUR IN ANATOMIC POSITION

As was described earlier in this chapter under anatomy of the proximal femur, the head and neck of the femur project approximately 15° to 20° anteriorly or forward with respect to the rest of the femur and the lower leg. Thus, when the leg is in the true anatomic position, as for a true AP leg, the proximal femur actually is rotated posteriorly 15° to 20° (Fig. 7.23). Therefore, the femoral neck appears shortened and the **lesser trochanter is visible** when the leg and ankle are truly AP, as in a true anatomic position.

INTERNAL ROTATION OF LEG

By **internally rotating the entire lower limb,** the proximal femur and hip joint are positioned in a **true AP** projection. The neck of the femur is now parallel to the imaging surface and will not appear foreshortened.

The **lesser trochanter** is key in determining the correct leg and foot position (on a radiographic image). If the entire leg is rotated internally a full 15° to 20° (Fig. 7.24A), the outline of the lesser trochanter generally is not visible at all or is only slightly visible on some patients, when it is obscured by the shaft of the femur. If the leg is straight AP, or when it is externally rotated, the lesser trochanter is visible (see page 274).

EVIDENCE OF HIP FRACTURE

The femoral neck is a common fracture site for an older patient who has fallen. The typical physical sign for such a fracture is the **external rotation** of the involved foot, where the lesser trochanter is clearly visualized in profile, as can be seen on the left hip depicted in Fig. 7.32 and the drawing on the right (Fig. 7.24B). This radiographic sign is demonstrated on the following page (see Figs. 7.31 and 7.32).

WARNING: If evidence of a hip fracture is present (external foot rotation), a pelvis radiograph should be taken "as is" **without** attempting to rotate the leg internally, as would be necessary for a true AP hip projection.

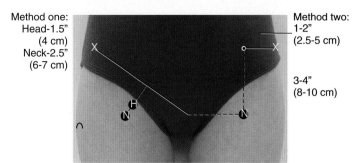

Method one:
Head-1.5" (4 cm)
Neck-2.5" (6-7 cm)

Method two:
1-2" (2.5-5 cm)

3-4" (8-10 cm)

Fig. 7.21 Femoral head *(H)* or neck *(N)* localization.

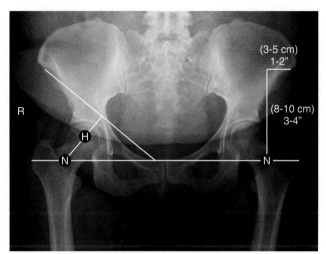

(3-5 cm) 1-2"

(8-10 cm) 3-4"

Fig. 7.22 Female pelvis, head *(H)*, and neck *(N)* locations.

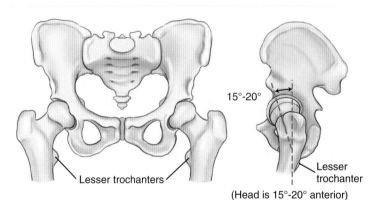

15°-20°

Lesser trochanters

Lesser trochanter

(Head is 15°-20° anterior)

Fig. 7.23 Anatomic position (true AP of knee, leg, and ankle—but not of hip).

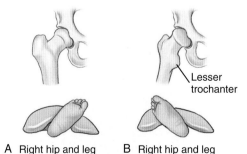

Lesser trochanter

A Right hip and leg   B Right hip and leg

Fig. 7.24 A, Internal rotation (true AP of hip). B, External rotation (typical hip fracture position).

SUMMARY: EFFECT OF LOWER LIMB ROTATION

The photographs and associated pelvis radiographs on this page demonstrate the effects of lower limb rotation on the appearance of the proximal femora.

1. **Anatomic position** (Figs. 7.25 and 7.26)
   - Long axes of feet vertical
   - Femoral necks partially foreshortened
   - Lesser trochanters **partially visible**
2. **15° to 20° medial rotation** (desired position to visualize pelvis and hips; Figs. 7.27 and 7.28)
   - Long axes of feet and lower limbs rotated internally 15° to 20°
   - Femoral heads and necks in profile
   - True AP projection of proximal femora
   - Lesser trochanters **not visible** or only slightly visible on some patients
3. **External rotation** (Figs. 7.29 and 7.30)
   - Long axes of feet and lower limbs equally rotated laterally in a normal relaxed position
   - Femoral necks greatly foreshortened
   - Lesser trochanters visible in profile internally
4. Typical rotation with hip fracture (Figs. 7.31 and 7.32)
   - Long axis of left foot externally rotated (on side of hip fracture)
   - Unaffected right foot and limb in neutral position
   - Lesser trochanter on externally rotated (left) limb more visible; neck area foreshortened

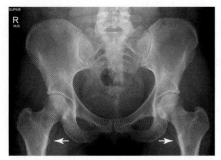

Fig. 7.28 2. 15° to 20° medial rotation.

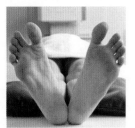

Fig. 7.29 External rotation.

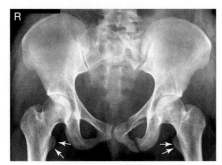

Fig. 7.30 3. External rotation.

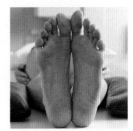

Fig. 7.25 Anatomic position.

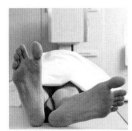

Fig. 7.31 Typical rotation with hip fracture.

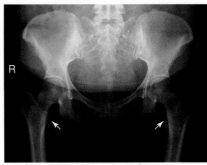

Fig. 7.26 1. Anatomic position without correction of lower limbs.

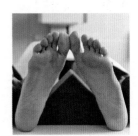

Fig. 7.27 15° to 20° medial rotation.

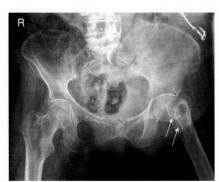

Fig. 7.32 4. Typical rotation with hip fracture.

SHIELDING GUIDELINES

Accurate gonadal shielding for pelvis and hip examinations is especially critical because of the proximity of radiation-sensitive gonads to the primary x-ray beam.

Male Shielding

Shielding is easier for males in that small contact shields, such as those shown in Fig. 7.33, can be used on **all males.** These shields are placed over the area of the testes without covering the essential anatomy of the pelvis or hips. However, care must be taken with pelvic radiographs that the top of the shield is placed at the **inferior margin of the symphysis pubis** to cover the testes adequately without obscuring the pubic and ischial areas of the pelvis.

Female Shielding

Ovarian contact shields for females require more critical placement to shield the area of the ovaries without covering essential pelvic or hip anatomy. Vinyl-covered lead material cut into various shapes and sizes can be used for this purpose for an AP pelvis or bilateral hip radiograph, as shown in Fig. 7.34. For a unilateral hip or proximal femur, larger contact shields can be used to cover the general pelvic area without covering the specific hip that is being examined, as shown in Fig. 7.35. Accurate location of the femoral head and neck makes this type of gonadal shielding possible.

Gonadal shielding may not be possible for females on certain AP pelvic projections in which the entire pelvis, including the sacrum and coccyx, must be demonstrated. Also, gonadal shielding may not be possible on lateral inferosuperior hip projections for males and females because shielding may obscure essential anatomy. However, **gonadal shielding should be used whenever possible for both males and females,** along with **close collimation** for all hip and pelvic projections. General pelvic trauma requiring visualization of the entire pelvis may prohibit ovarian shielding for females.

Exposure Factors and Patient Dose

To reduce total radiation dose to the patient, a higher kVp range of 80 to 90 may be used for hip and pelvic examinations. This higher kVp technique, with lower mAs, results in a lower radiation dose to the patient. Higher kVp, however, decreases subject contrast and may not be advisable, especially for older patients, who may have some loss of bone mass or density caused by osteoporosis; thus, they may require even lower kVp than average. Overexposure with high kVp on osteoporotic patients will decrease the visibility of the bony detail when using both analog and digital imaging systems.

Special Patient Considerations
PEDIATRIC APPLICATIONS

Pelvic and hip radiographic examinations are not performed often on children, except on newborns with developmental dysplasia of the hip (DDH). Correct shielding is especially important for infants and children because of the repeat radiographic examinations that are frequently required during the growth of the child. If holding the legs of an infant is required, an individual other than radiology personnel should do this while wearing a lead apron and lead gloves.

The degree and type of immobilization required for older children are dependent on the ability and willingness of the child to cooperate during the procedure. A mummy wrap (see Chapter 16) helps prevent the upper limbs from interfering with the anatomy of interest on a challenging patient. At the very least, tape or sandbags may be required to immobilize the legs at the proper degree of internal rotation.

GERIATRIC APPLICATIONS

Geriatric patients are prone to hip fractures resulting from falls and an increased incidence of osteoporosis. As noted earlier, the position of the patient's foot and leg must be observed in trauma cases. **It is critical that the injured limb not be moved if the leg is externally rotated.** An AP projection of both hips for comparison should be taken first, without movement of the affected limb, to check for fractures. This step may be followed by an inferosuperior (Danelius-Miller method) projection of the affected hip.

In nontrauma situations, most geriatric patients require (and appreciate) some immobilization to assist them in holding their feet and legs inverted for the AP pelvis and to support the limb for the lateral projection.

Patients who have undergone hip replacement surgery should **not** be placed in the frog-leg position for any postsurgical procedures. An inferosuperior lateral is indicated in addition to the AP projection.

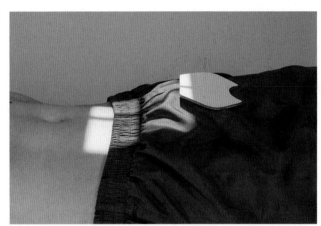

Fig. 7.33 Male gonadal shielding for hips and pelvis.

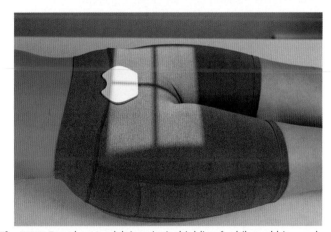

Fig. 7.34 Female gonadal (ovarian) shielding for bilateral hips and proximal femora.

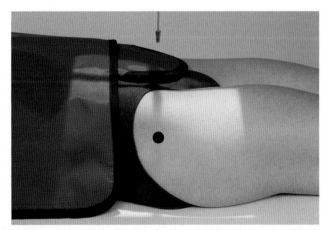

Fig. 7.35 General abdominal and pelvic shielding for proximal femur to include hip.

BARIATRIC PATIENT CONSIDERATIONS

Bariatric patients may present positioning challenges when imaging the pelvis, hips, and upper femurs. Increased adipose tissue adds subject density and may require an increase in technical factors. These changes may include an increase in kVp to improve penetration through additionally thick tissue. mA and time may also be increased, but sparingly to avoid excessive patient dose. The use of a grid for anatomic structures over 10 cm can be used to eliminate the demonstration of scatter.

Frequently used positioning landmarks may be difficult to palpate. Bony anatomy does not change unless major pathology, such as multiple fractures, has displaced the bones. Although the soft tissue may make it appear that the bones are larger or are farther apart, generally this is not the case. If common landmarks cannot be found, ask the patient to point out the ASIS, iliac crest, or the symphysis pubis on themselves. Additionally, bariatric patients may have difficulty holding oblique or lateral positions; the use of positioning sponges or other devices is recommended to ensure the patient's comfort and safety.

Digital Imaging Considerations

The following text provides a summary of the guidelines that should be followed with digital imaging of the procedures described in this chapter.

1. **Close collimation:** Collimating to the body part being imaged and **accurate centering** are most important when imaging the hip and pelvis.
2. **Exposure factors:** It is important that the ALARA principle (exposure to patient as low as reasonably achievable) be followed and the **lowest exposure factors required to obtain a diagnostic image be used.** This includes the highest kVp and lowest mAs that will result in desirable image quality.
3. **Post-processing evaluation of exposure indicator:** The exposure indicator on the final processed image must be checked to verify the exposure factors used were in the correct range **to ensure an optimum quality image with the least radiation dose to the patient.**
4. **Compensating filters:** The use of a compensating filter for axiolateral projections of the hip will allow better penetration of the femoral head while preventing overexposure of the femoral neck and shaft region.

Alternative Modalities

COMPUTED TOMOGRAPHY (CT)

CT is useful for evaluating soft tissue involvement of lesions or determining the extent of fractures. CT also is helpful for studying the relationship of the femoral head to the acetabulum before hip surgery or for performing a postreduction study of a developmental hip dislocation.

In general, CT is useful to add to the anatomic or pathologic information already obtained by conventional radiography. For children, the CT examination is useful for examining the relationship of the femoral head to the acetabulum after surgical reduction of a developmental hip dislocation.

Fractures of the pelvic ring missed on conventional radiographic projections, especially those involving the ischial and pubic rami, often are demonstrated during CT scanning.

MAGNETIC RESONANCE IMAGING (MRI)

Similar to CT, MRI can be useful for imaging the lower limb or pelvis when soft tissue injuries or possible abnormalities related to joints are suspected. In general, depending on clinical history, MRI may be used when additional information not obtained from conventional radiographs is needed.

SONOGRAPHY (ULTRASOUND)

Ultrasound is useful for evaluating newborns for hip dislocation and for assessing joint stability during movement of the lower limbs. This method usually is selected during the first 4 to 6 months of infancy to reduce ionizing radiation exposure.

NUCLEAR MEDICINE (NM)

NM scans can be useful in providing **early evidence** of certain bony pathologic processes, such as occult fractures, bone infections, metastatic carcinoma, or other metastatic or primary malignancies. NM is more sensitive and generally provides earlier evidence than other modalities because it assesses the physiologic aspect rather than the anatomic aspect of these conditions.

Clinical Indications

Clinical indications involving the pelvis and hips with which technologists should be familiar include the following (not necessarily an inclusive list):

Ankylosing spondylitis: The first effect demonstrated is fusion of the sacroiliac joints. The disease causes extensive calcification of the anterior longitudinal ligament of the spinal column. It is progressive, working up the vertebral column and creating a radiographic characteristic known as bamboo spine. Males are most often affected.

Avulsion fractures of the pelvis: These fractures cause extreme pain and are difficult to diagnose if not imaged properly. Fractures occur in adolescent athletes who experience sudden, forceful, or unbalanced contraction of the tendinous and muscular attachments, such as might occur while running hurdles. The force of the tendons and muscles sliding over the tuberosities, ASIS, anterior inferior iliac spine (AIIS), superior corner of the symphysis pubis, and iliac crest may cause avulsion fractures.[4]

Chondrosarcoma: A malignant tumor of the cartilage, it usually occurs in the pelvis and long bones of men older than 45 years. A chondrosarcoma may be completely removed surgically if it does not respond to radiation or chemotherapy.

Developmental dysplasia of the hip (DDH) (older term is *congenital dislocation of the hip* [CDH]): These hip dislocations are caused by conditions present at birth and may require frequent hip radiographs (see Chapter 16).

Legg-Calvé-Perthes disease: The most common type of aseptic or ischemic necrosis. Lesions typically involve only one hip (head and neck of femur). The disease occurs predominantly in 5- to 10-year-old boys, and a limp is usually the first clinical sign. Radiographs demonstrate a flattened femoral head that later can appear fragmented.

Metastatic carcinoma: The malignancy spreads to the bone via the circulatory system or lymphatic system, or by direct invasion. Metastatic tumors of the bone are much more common than primary malignancies. Bones that contain red bone marrow are the more common metastatic sites (spine, skull, ribs, pelvis, and femora).

Osteoarthritis: This condition is known as a *degenerative joint disease (DJD),* with degeneration of joint cartilage and adjacent bone causing pain and stiffness. It is the most common type of arthritis and may be considered a normal part of the aging process. It is common in weight-bearing joints such as the hips, and first evidence is seen on radiographic images of joints such as the hip before symptoms develop, in many persons by age 40. As the condition worsens, joints become less mobile, and new growths of cartilage and bone are seen as osteophytes (bony outgrowths).

Pelvic ring fractures: Because of the closed ring structure of the pelvis, a severe blow or trauma to one side of the pelvis may result in a fracture opposite from the site of primary trauma, thus requiring clear radiographic visualization of the entire pelvis. This type of trauma is referred to as a **contrecoup injury.**

Proximal femur (hip) fractures: These fractures are most common in older adult or geriatric patients with osteoporosis or avascular necrosis. Both osteoporosis (loss of bone mass from metabolic or other factors) and avascular (loss of blood circulation) necrosis (cell death) frequently lead to weakening or collapse of weight-bearing joints such as the hip joint; fractures occur with only minimal trauma.

Slipped capital femoral epiphysis (SCFE): This condition usually occurs in 10- to 16-year-olds during rapid growth, when even minor trauma can precipitate its development. The epiphysis appears shorter and the epiphyseal plate wider, with smaller margins.

Routine and Special Projections

Certain routine and special projections or positions for the proximal femora and pelvis are demonstrated and described on the following pages as suggested standard and special departmental procedures.

AP PROJECTION: FEMUR—MID AND DISTAL

NOTE: If the site of interest is in the area of the proximal femur, a unilateral hip routine or pelvis is recommended, as described in this chapter.

Femur—Mid and Distal
ROUTINE
• AP
• Lateral

Clinical Indications
• Mid- and distal femur, including knee joint, for detection and evaluation of fractures and/or bone lesions

Technical Factors
• Minimum SID—40 inches (100 cm)
• IR size—14 × 17 inches (35 × 43 cm), portrait
• Grid
• kVp range—75–85

Shielding Shield radiosensitive tissues outside the region of interest. Ensure that shielding does not obscure any aspect of the femur.

Patient Position Place patient in the supine position, with femur centered to midline of table; give pillow for head. (This projection also may be done on a stretcher with a portable grid placed under the femur.)

Part Position
• Align femur to CR and to midline of table or IR.
• Rotate leg internally approximately 5° for a true AP, as for an AP knee. (For proximal femur, 15° to 20° internal leg rotation is required, as for an AP hip.)
• Ensure that knee joint is included on IR, considering the divergence of the x-ray beam (Fig. 7.36). (Lower IR margin should be approximately 2 inches [5 cm] below knee joint.)

CR
• CR is **perpendicular** to femur and IR.
• Direct CR to **midpoint of IR.**

Recommended Collimation Collimate closely on both sides to femur with end collimation to film borders.

Including both Joints Common departmental routines include both joints on all initial femur exams. For a large adult, a second smaller IR then should be used for an AP of the knee or hip, ensuring that both hip and knee joints are included. If the hip is included, the leg should be rotated 15° to 20° internally to place the femoral neck in profile.

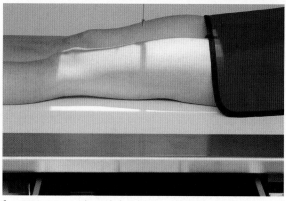
Fig. 7.36 AP—mid- and distal femur (head at cathode end).

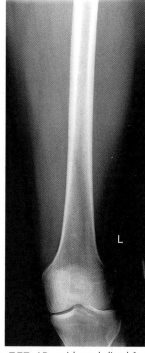
Fig. 7.37 AP—mid- and distal femur.

Evaluation Criteria
Anatomy Demonstrated: • Distal two-thirds of distal femur, including knee joint, is shown. • Knee joint space will not appear fully open because of divergent x-ray beam (Fig. 7.37). **Position:** • **No rotation** is evidenced; femoral and tibial condyles should appear symmetric in size and shape with the outline of patella slightly toward medial side of femur. • The approximate medial half of fibular head should be superimposed by tibia. Femur should be centered to collimation field and aligned with long axis of IR with knee joint space a minimum of 1 inch (2.5 cm) from distal IR margin. • Collimation to **area of interest.** **Exposure:** • Optimal exposure with correct use of anode heel effect or use of compensating filter will result in near uniform density (brightness) of entire femur. • **No motion** should occur; fine trabecular markings should be clear and sharp throughout length of femur.

LATERAL—MEDIOLATERAL OR LATEROMEDIAL PROJECTIONS: FEMUR—MID AND DISTAL

NOTE: For possible trauma, if the site of interest is in the area of the proximal femur, a unilateral trauma hip routine is recommended. For non-trauma, lateral of proximal femur (see p. 290).

Femur—Mid and Distal
ROUTINE
• AP
• Lateral

Clinical Indications
• Mid- and distal femur, including knee joint, for detection and evaluation of fractures and/or bone lesions

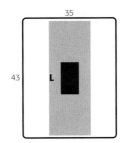

Technical Factors
• Minimum SID—40 inches (100 cm)
• IR size—14 × 17 inches (35 × 43 cm), portrait
• Grid
• kVp range—75–85

Shielding Shield radiosensitive tissues outside region of interest. Ensure shielding does not obscure any aspect of femur.

Patient Position Place patient in the lateral recumbent position, or supine for trauma patient.

Part Position
Lateral Recumbent (Fig. 7.38)
WARNING: Do not attempt this position if patient has severe trauma.

• Flex knee approximately 45° with patient on affected side, and align femur to midline of table or IR.
• Place unaffected leg behind affected leg to prevent over-rotation.
• Adjust IR to include knee joint (lower IR margin should be approximately 2 inches [5 cm] below knee joint). A second IR to include the proximal femur and hip generally will be required on an adult (see p. 290).

Trauma Lateromedial Projection (Fig. 7.39)
• Place support under affected leg and knee and support foot and ankle in true AP position.
• Place IR on edge against medial aspect of thigh to include knee, with horizontal x-ray beam directed from lateral side.

CR
• CR **perpendicular** to femur and directed to **midpoint of IR**

Recommended Collimation Collimate closely on both sides to femur with end collimation to IR borders.

Evaluation Criteria
Anatomy Demonstrated: • Distal two-thirds of distal femur, including the knee joint, is shown. • Knee joint will not appear open, and distal margins of the femoral condyles will not be superimposed because of divergent x-ray beam (Fig. 7.40).
Position, True Lateral: • Anterior and posterior margins of medial and lateral femoral condyles should be superimposed and aligned with open patellofemoral joint space. • Femur should be centered to collimation field with knee joint space a minimum of 1 inch (2.5 cm) from distal IR margin. • Collimation to **area of interest.**
Exposure: • Optimal exposure with correct use of anode heel effect or use of compensating filter will result in near-uniform density (brightness) of entire femur. • **No motion** is present; fine trabecular markings should be clear and sharp throughout length of femur.

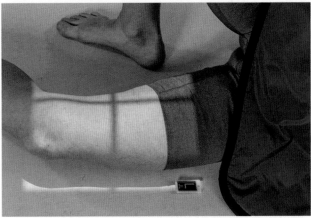

Fig. 7.38 Mediolateral mid- and distal femur.

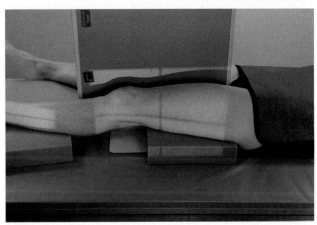

Fig. 7.39 Trauma lateromedial (horizontal beam) projection. Note: When a grid cassette is used, care must be taken to prevent grid cutoff.

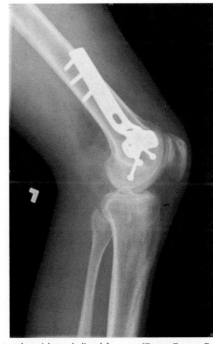

Fig. 7.40 Lateral—mid- and distal femur. (From Fagan R, Furey AJ. Use of large osteochondral allografts in reconstruction of traumatic uncontained distal femoral defects. *Journal of Orthopaedics* 11(1): 43–47, 2014.)

LATERAL–MEDIOLATERAL PROJECTION: FEMUR–MID AND PROXIMAL

WARNING: Do not attempt this position for patients with possible fracture of the hip or proximal femur. Refer to trauma lateral hip routine in this chapter.

Clinical Indications
- Mid- and proximal femur, including lateral hip, for detection and evaluation of fractures and bone lesions

Femur—Mid and Proximal
ROUTINE
• AP
• Lateral

Technical Factors
- Minimum SID—40 inches (100 cm)
- IR size—14 × 17 inches (35 × 43 cm), portrait
- Grid
- kVp range—75–85

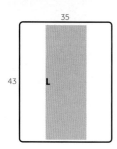

Shielding Shield radiosensitive tissues outside region of interest. Ensure shielding does not obscure any aspect of femur.

Patient Position Place patient in the lateral recumbent position, with affected side down; provide pillow for head.

Part Position
- Flex affected knee 45° and align femur to midline of table. (Remember the proximal and midportions of the femur are nearer to the anterior aspect of the thigh.)
- Extend and support unaffected leg behind affected knee and have patient roll back (posteriorly) 15° to prevent superimposition of proximal femur and hip joint (Fig. 7.41).
- Adjust IR to include hip joint, considering the divergence of the x-ray beam. (Palpate ASIS and place upper IR margin at the level of this landmark.)

CR
- CR **perpendicular** to femur
- CR directed to **midpoint of IR**

Recommended Collimation Collimate closely on both sides of femur with end collimation to IR borders.

NOTE: Alternate routine to include both joints: Common departmental routines include both joints on all initial femur examinations. On a large adult, this requires a second smaller IR (10 x 12 inches [24 x 30 cm]) of the hip or knee joint.

Evaluation Criteria
Anatomy Demonstrated: • Proximal one-half to two-thirds of the proximal femur, including the hip joint, is shown. • Proximal femur and hip joint should not be superimposed by opposite limb (Figs. 7.42 and 7.43).
Position, True Lateral: • Superimposition of the greater and lesser trochanters by the femur exists, with only a small part of the trochanters visible on medial side. • Most of the greater trochanter should be superimposed by the neck of the femur. Femur should be centered to collimation field with hip joint a minimum of 1 inch (2.5 cm) from proximal IR margin. • Collimation to **area of interest.**
Exposure: • Optimal exposure with correct use of anode heel effect or use of compensating filter will result in near-uniform density (brightness) of entire femur. • **No motion** is present; fine trabecular markings should be clear and sharp throughout length of femur.

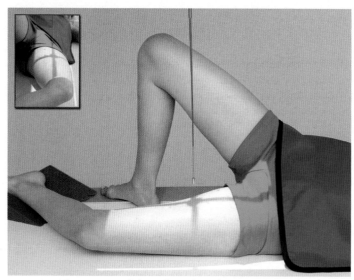

Fig. 7.41 Mediolateral—mid- and proximal femur.

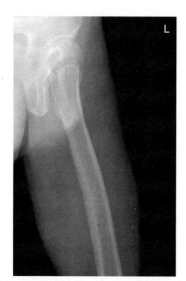

Fig. 7.42 Mediolateral—mid- and proximal femur.

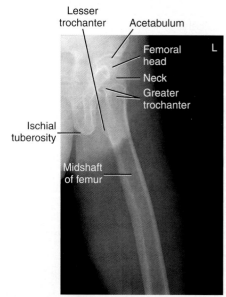

Fig. 7.43 Mediolateral—mid- and proximal femur.

AP PELVIS PROJECTION (BILATERAL HIPS): PELVIS

WARNING: Do not attempt to rotate legs internally if a hip fracture or dislocation is suspected. Perform position with minimal movement of affected leg.

Clinical Indications
- Fractures, joint dislocations, degenerative disease, and bone lesions

Pelvis
ROUTINE
• AP

Technical Factors
- Minimum SID—40 inches (100 cm)
- IR size—14 × 17 inches (35 × 43 cm), landscape
- Grid
- kVp range—80–90

Shielding Shield radiosensitive tissues outside the region of interest. Shield gonads on all male patients. Ovarian shielding on females, however, generally is not possible without obscuring essential pelvis anatomy (unless interest is in area of hips only).

Patient Position With patient supine, place arms at sides or across upper chest; provide pillow for head and support under knees; may be done erect with correction of lower limbs to rotate proximal femora into anatomic position and if **no fracture is suspected.** Position can also be performed erect.

Part Position ⊞
- Align midsagittal plane of patient to centerline of table and CR.
- Ensure that pelvis is **not rotated;** distance from tabletop to each ASIS should be equal.
- Separate legs and feet, then **internally rotate** long axes of feet and entire lower limb **15° to 20°** (see WARNING). Technologist may have to place sandbag between heels and tape top of feet together or use additional sandbags against feet to retain this position (Fig. 7.44, insert). Erect positioned similar to recumbent version (Fig. 7.44)

CR
- CR is perpendicular to IR, directed midway between level of ASIS and the symphysis pubis. This is approximately 2 inches (5 cm) inferior to level of ASIS (see NOTE).
- Center CR to IR.

Recommended Collimation Collimate on four sides to anatomy of interest.

Evaluation Criteria
Anatomy Demonstrated: • Pelvic girdle, L5, sacrum and coccyx, femoral heads and neck, and greater trochanters are visible (Figs. 7.45 and 7.46).
Position: • Lesser trochanters should not be visible at all; for many patients, only the tips are visible. Greater trochanters should appear equal in size and shape. • **No rotation** is evidenced by symmetric appearance of the iliac alae, or wings, the ischial spines, and the two obturator foramina. A foreshortened or closed obturator foramen indicates rotation in that direction. (A closed or narrowed right obturator foramen compared with the left indicates rotation toward the right.) • The right and left ischial spines (if visible) should appear equal in size. Correct centering evidenced by demonstration of entire pelvis and superior femora without foreshortening in collimated field. • Collimation to **area of interest.**
Exposure: • Optimal exposure visualizes L5 and sacrum area and margins of the femoral heads and acetabula, as seen through overlying pelvic structures, without overexposing the ischium and pubic bones. • Trabecular markings of proximal femora and pelvic structures appear sharp, indicating **no motion.**

Respiration Suspend respiration during exposure.

NOTE: If performed as part of a hip routine, centering should be 2 inches (5 cm) lower to level of midfemoral heads or necks to include more of proximal femora.

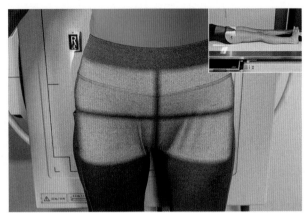
Fig. 7.44 Patient and part position—AP pelvis.

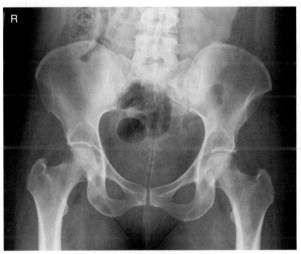
Fig. 7.45 AP pelvis.

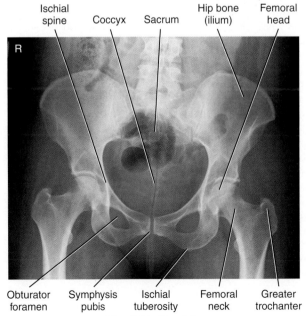

Ischial spine   Coccyx   Sacrum   Hip bone (ilium)   Femoral head

Obturator foramen   Symphysis pubis   Ischial tuberosity   Femoral neck   Greater trochanter
Fig. 7.46 AP pelvis.

7

AP BILATERAL FROG-LEG PROJECTION: PELVIS

MODIFIED CLEAVES METHOD

WARNING: Do not attempt this position on a patient with destructive hip disease or with potential hip fracture or dislocation.

Clinical Indications
- Demonstration of a nontrauma hip
- Developmental dysplasia of hip (DDH), also known as congenital hip dislocation (CHD)

Pelvis
ROUTINE
- AP
- AP bilateral frog-leg (modified Cleaves method)

Technical Factors
- Minimum SID—40 inches (100 cm)
- IR size—14 × 17 inches (35 × 43 cm), landscape
- Grid
- kVp range—80–90

No center AEC cell with shield in place.

Shielding Shield radiosensitive tissues outside the region of interest. Shield gonads for both males and females without obscuring essential anatomy (see NOTE 1).

Patient Position With patient supine, provide pillow for head and place arms across chest.

Part Position
- Align patient to midline of table and/or IR and to CR.
- Ensure pelvis is **not rotated** (equal distance of ASIS to tabletop).
- Center IR to CR, at level of femoral heads, with top of IR approximately at level of iliac crest.
- Flex both knees approximately 90°, as demonstrated.
- Place the plantar surfaces of feet together and **abduct both femora 40° to 45° from vertical** (see NOTE 2). Ensure that **both femora are abducted the same amount** and that pelvis is **not rotated** (Fig. 7.47).
- Place supports under each leg for stabilization if needed.

CR
- CR is **perpendicular** to IR, directed to a point **3 inches (7.5 cm) below level of ASIS** (1 inch [2.5 cm] above symphysis pubis).

Recommended Collimation Collimate on four sides to anatomy of interest.

Respiration Suspend respiration during exposure.

NOTE 1: This projection frequently is performed for periodic follow-up examinations on younger patients. Correct placement of gonadal shielding is important for male and female patients, ensuring that hip joints are not obscured (Fig. 7.48).

NOTE 2: Less abduction of femora of only 20° to 30° from vertical plane provides for the least foreshortening of femoral head and neck region, but this placement foreshortens the entire proximal femora, which may not be desirable.

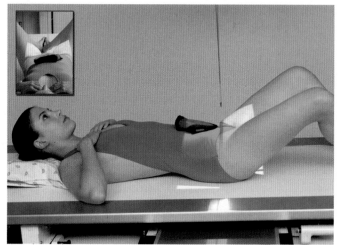

Fig. 7.47 Bilateral frog-leg—femora abducted 40° to 45°.

Evaluation Criteria
Anatomy Demonstrated: • Femoral heads and necks, acetabulum, and trochanteric areas are visible on one radiograph (see Fig. 7.48).
Position: • No rotation, as evidenced by symmetric appearance of the pelvic bones, especially the ala of the ilium, two obturator foramina, and ischial spines, if visible. • The femoral heads and necks and greater and lesser trochanters should appear symmetric if both thighs were abducted equally. • The lesser trochanters should appear equal in size, as projected beyond the lower or medial margin of the femora. • Most of the area of the greater trochanters appears superimposed over the femoral necks, which appear foreshortened (see NOTE 2). • Collimation to **area of interest.**
Exposure: • Optimal exposure visualizes the margins of the femoral head and the acetabulum through overlying pelvic structures, without overexposing the proximal femora. • Trabecular markings appear sharp, indicating **no motion.**

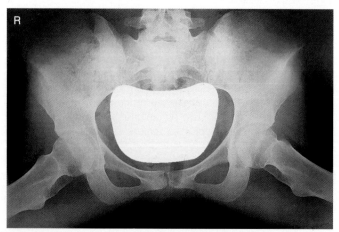

Fig. 7.48 Bilateral frog-leg (ovarian shield in place). (Courtesy Kathy Martensen, BS, RT[R].)

AP AXIAL OUTLET PROJECTION[5]
(FOR ANTERIOR-INFERIOR PELVIC BONES): PELVIS

TAYLOR METHOD

Clinical Indications
- Bilateral view of the bilateral pubis and ischium to allow assessment of pelvic trauma for fractures and displacement

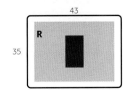

Pelvis
SPECIAL
- AP axial outlet projection

Technical Factors
- Minimum SID—40 inches (100 cm)
- IR size—14 × 17 inches (35 × 43 cm), landscape
- Grid
- kVp range—80–90

Shielding Shield radiosensitive tissues outside region of interest.

Patient Position With patient supine, provide pillow for head. With patient's legs extended, place support under knees for comfort (Fig. 7.49).

Part Position
- Align midsagittal plane to CR and to midline of table and/or IR.
- Ensure **no rotation** of pelvis (ASIS-to-tabletop distance equal on both sides).
- Center IR to projected CR.

CR
- Angle CR **cephalad 20° to 35° for males** and **30° to 45° for females.** (These different angles are caused by differences in the shape of male and female pelvises. See section *Male Versus Female Pelvis Differences* on pg. 270.)
- Direct CR to a midline point 1 to 2 inches (2.5 to 5 cm) distal to the superior border of the symphysis pubis or greater trochanters.

Recommended Collimation Collimate on four sides to anatomy of interest.

Respiration Suspend respiration during exposure.

Evaluation Criteria
Anatomy Demonstrated: • Superior and inferior rami of pubis and body and ramus of ischium are demonstrated well, with minimal foreshortening or superimposition (Figs. 7.50 and 7.51).
Position: • No rotation: Obturator foramina and bilateral ischia are equal in size and shape. Correct CR angle evidenced by demonstration of the anterior/inferior pelvic bones, with minimal foreshortening. Midpoint of symphysis joint should be at center of collimated field. • Collimation to area of interest.
Exposure: • Body and superior rami of pubis are well demonstrated without overexposure of ischial rami. • Bony margins and trabecular markings of pubic and ischial bones appear sharp, indicating **no motion.**

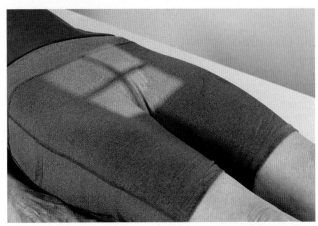

Fig. 7.49 AP axial outlet projection—CR 40° cephalad.

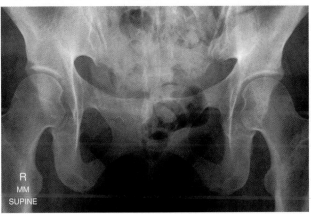

Fig. 7.50 AP axial outlet projection. (Courtesy Joss Wertz, DO.)

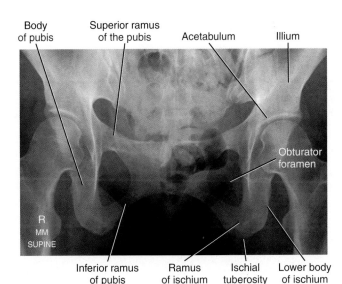

Fig. 7.51 AP axial outlet projection. (Courtesy Joss Wertz, DO.)

AP AXIAL INLET PROJECTION[5]: PELVIS

Clinical Indications
- Assessment of pelvic trauma for posterior displacement or inward or outward rotation of the anterior pelvis

Pelvis
SPECIAL
- AP axial outlet projection
- AP axial inlet projection

Technical Factors
- Minimum SID—40 inches (100 cm)
- IR size—14 × 17 inches (35 × 43 cm), landscape
- Grid
- kVp range—80–90

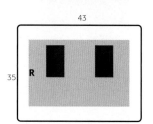

Shielding Shield radiosensitive tissues outside region of interest. Gonadal shielding is possible for males if care is taken not to obscure essential pelvic anatomy.

Patient Position
With patient supine, provide pillow for head. With patient's legs extended, place support under knees for comfort (Fig. 7.52).

Part Position
- Align midsagittal plane to CR and to midline of table and/or IR.
- Ensure **no rotation** of pelvis (ASIS-to-tabletop distance equal on both sides).
- Center IR to projected CR.

CR
- Angle CR **caudad 40°** (near perpendicular to plane of inlet).
- Direct CR to a midline point at level of ASIS.

Recommended Collimation Collimate closely on four sides to area of interest.

Respiration Suspend respiration during exposure.

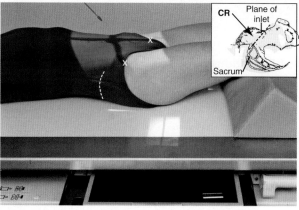

Fig. 7.52 AP axial inlet projection—CR 40° caudad (CR perpendicular to pelvic inlet).

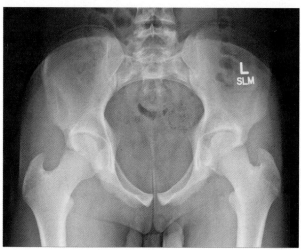

Fig. 7.53 AP axial inlet projection.

Evaluation Criteria
Anatomy Demonstrated: • Axial projection that demonstrates the pelvic ring or inlet (superior aperture) in its entirety (Figs. 7.53 and 7.54)
Position: • No rotation: Ischial spines are fully demonstrated and equal in size and shape. Proper centering and angulation are evidenced by demonstration of the superimposed anterior and posterior portions of the pelvic ring. • Center of pelvic inlet should be at center of collimated field. • Collimation to area of interest.
Exposure: • Optimal exposure demonstrates the superimposed anterior and posterior portions of the pelvic ring. Lateral aspects of ala generally are overexposed. • Bony margins and trabecular markings of pubic and ischial bones appear sharp, indicating **no motion.**

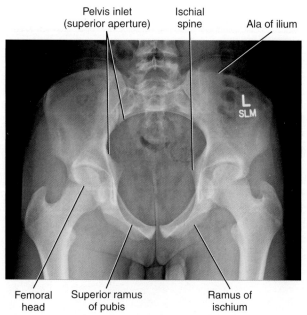

Pelvis inlet (superior aperture) | Ischial spine | Ala of ilium

Femoral head | Superior ramus of pubis | Ramus of ischium

Fig. 7.54 AP axial inlet projection.

POSTERIOR OBLIQUE PROJECTION: PELVIS—ACETABULUM

JUDET METHOD

Clinical Indications
- Acetabular fracture
- Pelvic ring fractures

  Right and **left oblique projections** generally are taken for comparison, with both centered for upside or both for downside acetabulum. Possible pelvic ring fractures due to a contrecoup injury, the entire pelvis must be included. In this case, centering should be adjusted to include both hips.

| **Pelvis** |
| SPECIAL |
| • AP axial outlet |
| • AP axial inlet |
| • Posterior oblique acetabulum (Judet method) |
| • Posterior axial oblique acetabulum (Teufel method) |

Technical Factors
- Minimum SID—40 inches (100 cm)
- IR size—10 × 12 inches (24 × 30 cm), portrait, or 14 × 17 (35 × 43 cm), landscape, if both hips must be seen on each projection
- Grid
- kVp range—80–90

Shielding Shield radiosensitive tissues outside region of interest.

Patient Position—Posterior Oblique Positions
- With patient semisupine, provide pillow for head and position for **affected side up or down,** depending on anatomy to be demonstrated.

Part Position
- Place patient in **45° posterior oblique,** with both pelvis and thorax 45° from tabletop. Support with wedge sponge.
- Align femoral head and acetabulum of interest to midline of tabletop and/or IR.
- Center IR longitudinally to CR at level of femoral head.

CR

Acetabulum
- Affected side **down:** direct CR perpendicular and centered to **2 inches** (5 cm) **distal and 2 inches** (5 cm) **medial to downside ASIS** (Fig. 7.55, insert).
- Affected side **up:** direct perpendicular and centered to **2 inches** (5 cm) **directly distal to upside ASIS** (Fig. 7.56, insert).

Pelvic Ring
- Direct CR perpendicular and centered to 2 inches (5 cm) inferior from level of ASIS and 2 inches (5 cm) medial to upside ASIS. (Figs. 7.55 and 7.56)

Recommended Collimation
- 10 × 12 inches (24 × 30 cm) or 14 × 17 inches (35 × 43 cm), depending on size of IR selected and field of view; or, collimate on four sides to anatomy of interest

Respiration Suspend respiration for the exposure.

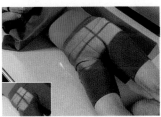 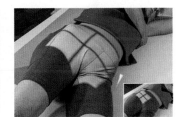

Fig. 7.55 RPO—centered for right (downside) acetabulum.

Fig. 7.56 LPO—centered for right (upside) acetabulum.

Evaluation Criteria

Anatomy Demonstrated:

Acetabulum: • When centered to the **downside** acetabulum, the **anterior rim** of the acetabulum and the **posterior (ilioischial) column** are demonstrated. The **iliac wing** also is well visualized (Figs. 7.57 and 7.58). • When centered to the **upside** acetabulum, the **posterior rim** of the acetabulum and the **anterior (iliopubic) column** are demonstrated. The **obturator foramen** also is visualized (Figs. 7.59 and 7.60).

Pelvic Ring: • Projections will demonstrate the ilioischial and iliopubic columns, along with other aspect of pelvic ring (Figs. 7.61 and 7.62).

Position: • Proper degree of obliquity is evidenced by an open and uniform hip joint space at the rim of acetabulum femoral head. • The obturator foramen should be open, if rotated correctly, for the upside oblique, and should appear closed on downside oblique. Acetabulum (or pelvis) should be centered to IR and to collimation field. • Collimation to **area of interest.**

Exposure: • Optimal exposure should clearly demonstrate bony margins and trabecular markings of the acetabulum and femoral head regions; such markings should appear sharp, indicating **no motion.**

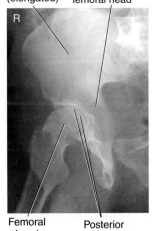

Area of anterior rim of acetabulum, partially superimposed by femoral head

Iliac wing (elongated)

Femoral head

Posterior ilioischial column

Fig. 7.57 RPO—downside (anterior rim and posterior [ilioischial] column).

Fig. 7.58 RPO—downside acetabulum.

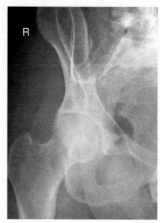

Fig. 7.59 LPO—upside (posterior rim and anterior [iliopubic] column.)

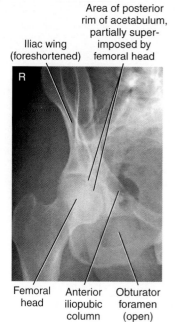

Iliac wing (foreshortened)

Area of posterior rim of acetabulum, partially super-imposed by femoral head

Femoral head

Anterior iliopubic column

Obturator foramen (open)

Fig. 7.60 LPO—upside acetabulum.

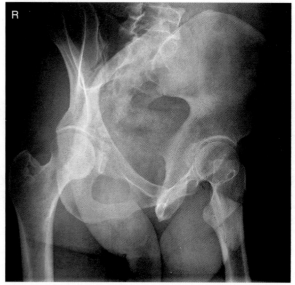

Fig. 7.61 LPO—full bilateral Judet method. (Case courtesy Dr Luke Danaher, Radiopaedia.org, rID: 39777.)

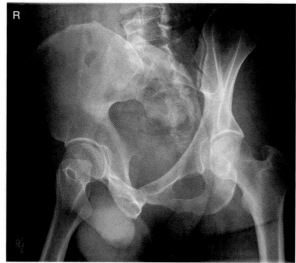

Fig. 7.62 RPO—Full bilateral Judet method. (Case courtesy Dr Luke Danaher, Radiopaedia.org, rID: 39777.)

PA AXIAL OBLIQUE PROJECTION: ACETABULUM

TEUFEL METHOD

Clinical Indications
- Acetabular fracture, especially the super-oposterior wall of the acetabulum

Right or left posterior **oblique** is taken to demonstrate the side of interest, centered to the downside acetabulum to demonstrate the hip joint and acetabulum in the center of the image, with the femoral head in profile. The concave area of the fovea capitis should be demonstrated, along with the superoposterior wall of the acetabulum.

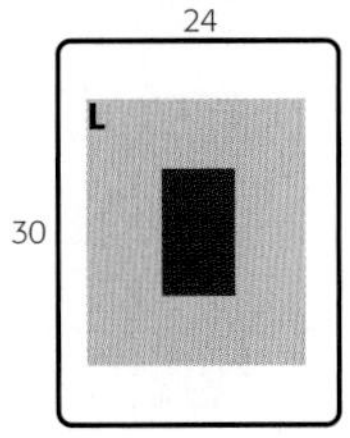

Technical Factors
- Minimum SID—40 inches (100 cm)
- IR size—10 × 12 inches (24 × 30 cm), portrait
- Grid
- kVp range—75–85

Shielding Shield radiosensitive tissues outside region of interest.

Patient Position—Axial Oblique Positions
- With patient semiprone, provide pillow for head and position for **affected side down.** Position can be performed erect

Part Position ⊞
- Place patient in **anterior oblique,** with both pelvis and thorax **35° to 40°** from tabletop or wall bucky. Support with wedge sponge (Fig. 7.63).
- Align femoral head and acetabulum of interest to midline of tabletop and/or IR.
- Center IR longitudinally to CR at level of femoral head.

CR
- When anatomy of interest is **downside,** direct CR perpendicular and centered to **1 inch** (2.5 cm) **superior to the level of the greater trochanter, approximately 2 inches** (5 cm) lateral to the midsagittal plane.
- Angle CR **12° cephalad.**

Recommended Collimation Collimate on four sides to anatomy of interest.

Respiration Suspend respiration for the exposure.

Pelvis
SPECIAL
- Acetabulum and femoral head, including the fovea capitis
- Posterior axial oblique acetabulum (Teufel method)

24
L
30

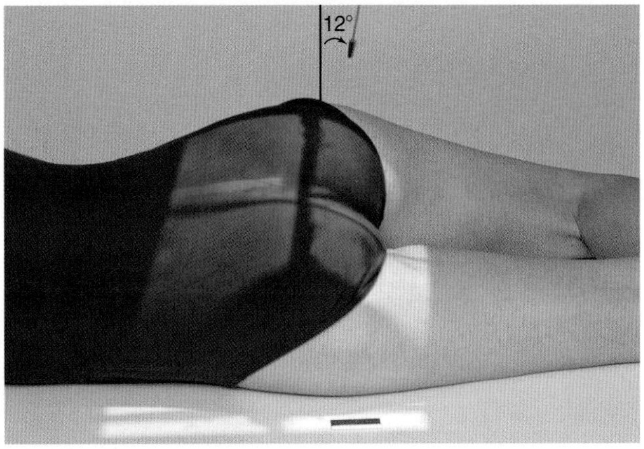

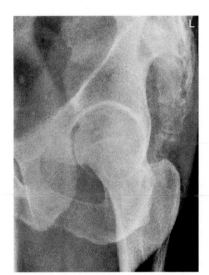

Fig. 7.63 PA axial oblique (Teufel) projection—12° cephalad angle.

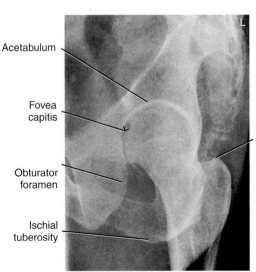

Fig. 7.64 PA axial oblique (Teufel) projection.

Evaluation Criteria
Anatomy Demonstrated: • Centered to the **downside** acetabulum, the **superoposterior wall** of the acetabulum is demonstrated (Figs. 7.64 and 7.65).
Position: • Proper degree of obliquity is evidenced by visualization of the concave area of the fovea capitis with the femoral head in profile. • The obturator foramen should be open, if rotated correctly. Acetabulum should be centered to IR and to collimation field. • Collimation to **area of interest.**
Exposure: • Optimal exposure should clearly demonstrate bony margins and trabecular markings of the acetabulum and femoral head regions; such markings should appear sharp, indicating **no motion.**

Acetabulum

Fovea capitis

Greater trochanter

Obturator foramen

Ischial tuberosity

Fig. 7.65 PA axial oblique projection.

AP UNILATERAL HIP PROJECTION: HIP AND PROXIMAL FEMUR

WARNING: Do not attempt to rotate legs if fracture is suspected. An AP pelvis projection to include both hips for comparison should be completed before an AP unilateral hip is performed for possible hip or pelvis trauma.

Clinical Indications
- Postoperative or follow-up examination to demonstrate the acetabulum, femoral head, neck, and greater trochanter
- Evaluation of condition and placement of any existing orthopedic appliance

> **Hip and Proximal Femur**
> ROUTINE
> - AP unilateral hip
> - Axiolateral (trauma hip) (inferosuperior)

Technical Factors
- Minimum SID—40 inches (100 cm)
- IR size—10 × 12 inches (24 × 30 cm), portrait
- Grid
- kVp range—80–85

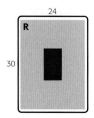

Shielding Shield radiosensitive tissues outside region of interest.

Patient Position With patient supine, place arms at sides or across superior chest.

Part Position
- Locate **femoral neck** and align to CR and to midline of table and/or IR.
- Ensure **no rotation** of pelvis (equal distance from ASISs to table).
- Rotate affected leg **internally 15° to 20°** (see WARNING).

CR
- CR is perpendicular to the femoral neck (see p. 273 for femoral head and neck localization methods). Femoral neck can also be located about 1 to 2 inches (2.5 to 5 cm) medial and 3 to 4 inches (8 to 10 cm) distal to ASIS (Fig. 7.66).

Recommended Collimation Collimate on four sides to anatomy of interest.

Respiration Suspend respiration during exposure.

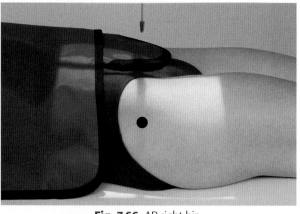
Fig. 7.66 AP right hip.

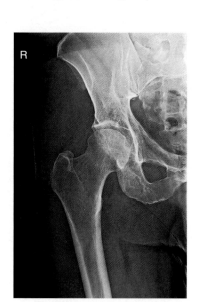
Fig. 7.67 AP hip.

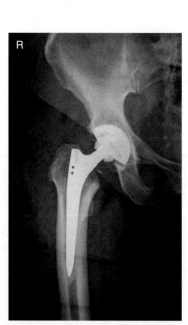
Fig. 7.68 AP hip. (Copyright Getty Images/DieterMeyrl.)

DANELIUS-MILLER METHOD

WARNING: Do not attempt to rotate leg internally on initial trauma examination.

NOTE: This is a common projection for trauma, surgery, and postsurgery patients, in addition to patients who cannot move or rotate the affected leg for frog-leg lateral.

Hip and Proximal Femur
ROUTINE
• AP unilateral hip
• Axiolateral (trauma) (inferosuperior)

Clinical Indications
- Lateral view for fracture or dislocation assessment in trauma hip situations when affected leg cannot be moved

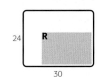

Technical Factors
- Minimum SID—40 inches (100 cm)
- IR size—10 × 12 inches (24 × 30 cm), landscape (**portrait to long axis of femur**)
- Grid (grid perpendicular to the CR to prevent grid cutoff)
- kVp range—80–95

Shielding Shield radiosensitive tissues outside region of interest. Gonadal shielding, if used, must be carefully placed to not obscure any anatomy of the affected hip. Close collimation is important for reducing patient dose and improving image quality.

Patient Position May be done on stretcher or bedside if patient cannot be moved (see Chapter 15). Patient is supine, with pillow provided for head; elevate pelvis 1 to 2 inches (2.5 to 5 cm) if possible by placing supports under pelvis (more important for thin patients and for patients on a soft pad or in a bed).

Part Position (Figs. 7.69 and 7.70)
- Flex and elevate unaffected leg so that thigh is near vertical position and outside collimation field. Support in this position. (**Do NOT** place leg on collimator or x-ray tube due to risk of burns or electrical shock.)
- Check to ensure **no rotation** of pelvis (equal ASIS-table distance).
- Use hip localization method to identify location and alignment of femoral neck.
- Place IR in the crease above iliac crest and adjust so that it is **parallel to femoral neck** and **perpendicular to CR** (see Fig. 7.18). Use cassette holder if available, or use sandbags to hold image receptor/grid in place.
- Internally rotate affected leg 15° to 20° **unless contraindicated** by possible fracture or other pathologic process (see warning above).

CR CR is **perpendicular** to femoral neck and to IR.

Recommended Collimation Collimate on four sides to anatomy of interest.

Respiration Suspend respiration during exposure.

NOTE: Demonstrating the most proximal portion of the femoral head and acetabulum on a patient with thick thighs may be challenging.

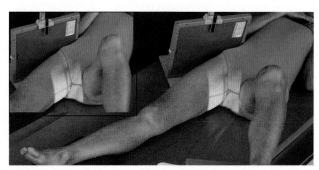

Fig. 7.69 Axiolateral hip. *Inset,* CR perpendicular and centered to femoral neck.

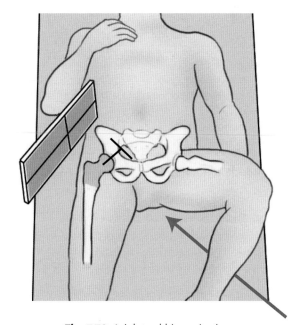

Fig. 7.70 Axiolateral hip projection.

Evaluation Criteria
Anatomy Demonstrated: • Entire femoral head and neck, trochanter, and acetabulum should be visualized along with any orthopedic prosthetic device in its entirety (Fig. 7.71).
Position: • Only a small part, if any, of lesser trochanter is visualized with inversion of affected leg. • Only the most distal part of femoral neck should be superimposed by greater trochanter. • Soft tissue from raised unaffected leg is not superimposed over affected hip if leg is raised sufficiently and CR is placed correctly. No grid lines are visible (grid lines indicate incorrect tube/IR alignment). • Collimation to **area of interest.**
Exposure: • Optimal exposure visualizes outline of entire femoral head and acetabulum without overexposing neck and proximal femoral shaft.

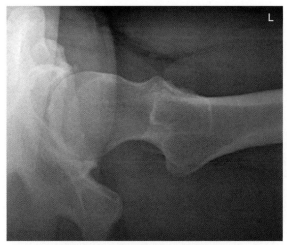

Fig. 7.71 Axiolateral hip projection.

UNILATERAL FROG-LEG PROJECTION—MEDIOLATERAL: HIP AND PROXIMAL FEMUR

MODIFIED CLEAVES METHOD

WARNING: Do not attempt this position on patient with destructive hip disease or potential hip fracture or dislocation. This could result in significant displacement of fracture fragments (see lateral trauma projections).

Clinical Indications
- Lateral view to assess hip joint and proximal femur for **nontraumatic hip** situations

> **Hip and Proximal Femur**
> SPECIAL—NONTRAUMA
> • Unilateral frog-leg

Technical Factors
- Minimum SID—40 inches (100 cm)
- IR size—10 × 12 inches (24 × 30 cm), portrait
- Grid
- kVp range—80–85

Shielding Shield radiosensitive tissues outside region of interest.

Patient Position With patient erect or supine, position affected hip area to be aligned to CR and midline of table and/or IR.

Part Position (Fig. 7.72)
- Flex knee and hip on affected side, as shown, with sole of foot against inside of opposite leg, near knee if possible.
- Abduct femur **45° from vertical** for general proximal femur region (see NOTE 1).
- Center affected femoral neck to CR and midline of IR and tabletop. Apply hip localization methods to determine location of femoral neck.
- CR is **perpendicular** to IR (see NOTE 2), directed to **midfemoral neck** (center of IR).

Recommended Collimation Collimate on four sides to anatomy of interest.

Respiration Suspend respiration during exposure.

NOTE 1: The optimum femur abduction for demonstration of the femoral neck with minimal distortion is **20° to 30°** from vertical on most patients. This results in significant foreshortening of the proximal femur region, which may be objectionable.

NOTE 2: A modification of this position is the Lauenstein-Hickey method, with the patient starting in a similar position, then rotating onto the affected side until the femur is in contact with the tabletop and parallel to the IR. This position foreshortens the neck region, but may demonstrate the head and acetabulum well if affected leg can be abducted sufficiently, as shown in Fig. 7.72, inset).

Evaluation Criteria
Anatomy Demonstrated: • Lateral views of acetabulum and femoral head and neck, trochanteric area, and proximal one-third of femur are visible.
Position: • Proper abduction (45°) of femur is demonstrated by femoral neck seen in profile, superimposed by greater trochanter (Fig. 7.73). Less abduction (20-30°) will prevent superimposition of greater trochanter on the femoral neck (Fig. 7.74). Proper centering is evidenced by femoral neck at center of collimated field. • Collimation to **area of interest.**
Exposure: • Optimal exposure visualizes the margins of the femoral head and the acetabulum through overlying pelvic structures without overexposing other parts of the proximal femur. • Trabecular markings and bony margins of proximal femur and pelvis should appear sharp, indicating **no motion.**

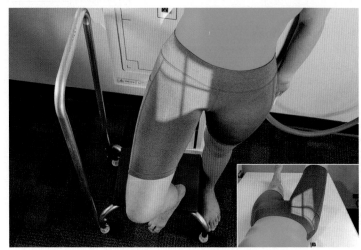

Fig. 7.72 45° abduction. Head and acetabulum are well demonstrated. *Inset,* 90° abduction. Unilateral frog-leg position (femoral neck parallel to IR). Femoral neck is foreshortened.

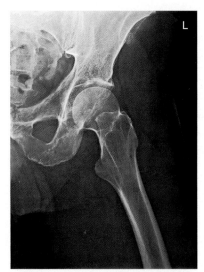

Fig. 7.73 For femoral neck—45° abduction.

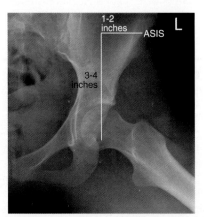

Fig. 7.74 Unilateral frog-leg, 20° to 30° abduction. (From McQuillen Martensen K. *Radiographic image analysis,* ed 4, St. Louis, 2015, Saunders Elsevier.)

MODIFIED AXIOLATERAL PROJECTION—POSSIBLE TRAUMA: HIP AND PROXIMAL FEMUR

CLEMENTS-NAKAYAMA METHOD[6]

Clinical Indications
- Lateral oblique view is useful for assessment of possible **hip fracture** or with **arthroplasty** (surgery for hip prosthesis) when the patient has limited movement in both lower limbs and the inferosuperior projection cannot be obtained

> **Hip and Proximal Femur**
> SPECIAL—NONTRAUMA
> - Unilateral frog-leg
> SPECIAL—TRAUMA
> - Modified axiolateral (Clements-Nakayama method)

Technical Factors
- Minimum SID—40 inches (100 cm)
- IR size—10 × 12 inches (24 × 30 cm), landscape (LW to long axis of femur)
- Grid (IR on edge with 15° tilt; grid lines parallel to CR angle.)
- kVp range—80–90

Shielding Shield radiosensitive tissues outside region of interest without obscuring essential anatomy.

Patient Position With patient supine, position affected side near edge of table with both legs fully extended. Provide pillow for head and place arms across superior chest.

Part Position
- Maintain leg in neutral (anatomic) position (15° posterior CR angle compensates for internal leg rotation).
- Rest IR on extended bucky tray, which places the bottom edge of the IR approximately 2 inches (5 cm) below the level of the tabletop (Fig. 7.75).
- Tilt IR about 15° from vertical and adjust alignment of IR to ensure that face of IR is **perpendicular** to CR to prevent grid cutoff (Fig. 7.75, inset).
- Center centerline of IR to projected CR.

CR Angle CR mediolaterally as needed so that it is perpendicular to and centered to femoral neck. It should be angled posteriorly 15° to 20° from horizontal.

Recommended Collimation Collimate on four sides to anatomy of interest.

Respiration Suspend respiration during exposure.

> ### Evaluation Criteria
> **Anatomy Demonstrated:** • Lateral oblique views of acetabulum, femoral head and neck, and trochanteric area are visible (Figs. 7.76 and 7.77).
> **Position:** • Femoral head and neck should be seen in profile, with only minimal superimposition by greater trochanter. • Lesser trochanter is seen projecting posterior to femoral shaft. (With leg in neutral or anatomic position, the amount of lesser trochanter seen is minimal, and with increased external rotation of leg, this amount decreases.) Femoral neck and trochanters should be centered to the image. • Collimation to **area of interest.**
> **Exposure:** • Optimal exposure visualizes femoral head and neck without overexposing proximal femoral shaft. • No excessive grid lines are visible on radiograph. • Bony margins and trabecular markings should be visible and sharp, indicating **no motion.**

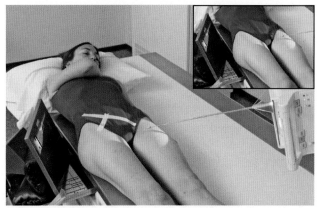

Fig. 7.75 Modified axiolateral—CR 15° tilt from horizontal perpendicular to femoral neck.

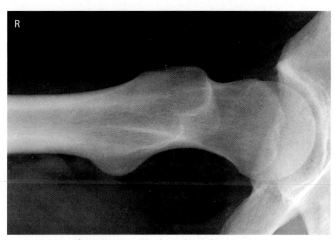

Fig. 7.76 Modified axiolateral projection.

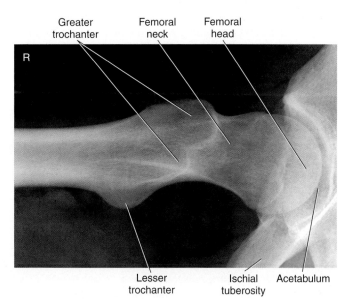

Greater trochanter   Femoral neck   Femoral head

Lesser trochanter   Ischial tuberosity   Acetabulum

Fig. 7.77 Modified axiolateral projection.

RADIOGRAPHS FOR CRITIQUE

This section consists of an ideal projection (Image A) along with one or more projections that may demonstrate positioning and/or technical errors. Critique Figs. C7.78 through C7.81 Compare Image A to the other projections and identify the errors. While examining each image, consider the following questions:

1. Is all essential anatomy demonstrated on the image?
2. What positioning errors are present that compromise image quality?

3. Are technical factors optimal?
4. Is there evidence of collimation and are pre-exposure anatomic side markers visible on the image?
5. Do these errors require a repeat exposure?

Feedback for each set of images is located on the faculty Evolve site.

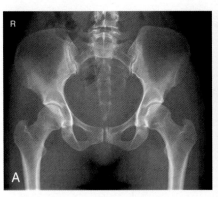
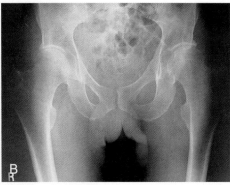
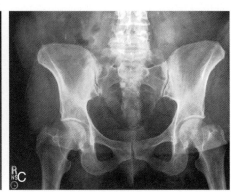

Fig. C7.78 AP pelvis projection.

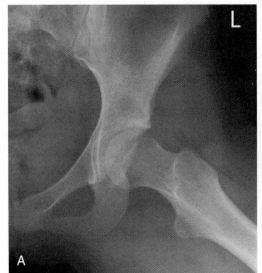
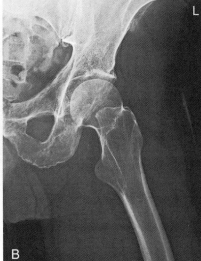
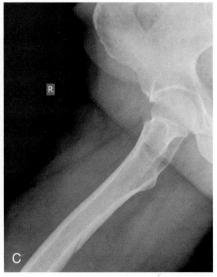

Fig. C7.79 **Unilateral modified Cleaves method.** (**A** from McQuillen Martensen K. *Radiographic image analysis*, ed 4, St. Louis, 2015, Saunders Elsevier; **C** from Dachs R et al. Double pathology, sarcoidosis associated with multiple myeloma: a case report. *Journal of Bone Oncology* 3(2):61–65.)

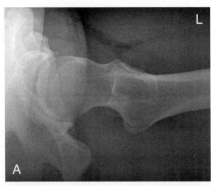
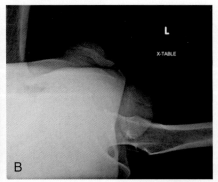
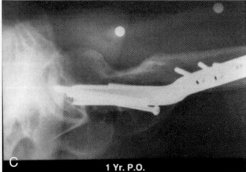

Fig. C7.80 **Axiolateral (Danelius-Miller) projection.** (**A** from Berry DJ. *Surgery of the hip,* ed 2, Philadelphia, 2020, Elsevier; **B** from Magee DJ. *Orthopedic physical assessment,* ed 6, Philadelphia, 2014, Saunders; **C** from Berry DJ. *Surgery of the hip,* Philadelphia, 2013, Saunders.)

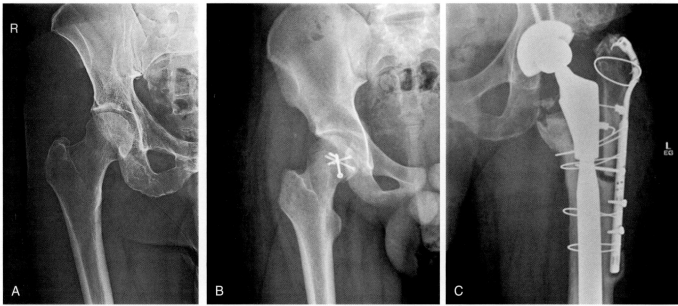

Fig. C7.81 **Unilateral AP hip projection.** (**B** from Ying LJ. A case of pathological fracture caused by vitamin D insufficiency in a young athlete and a review of the literature. *Journal of Clinical Orthopaedics and Trauma* 10(6):1111–1115 **C** From Berry DJ. *Surgery of the hip,* ed 2, Philadelphia, 2020, Elsevier.)

CHAPTER 8

Cervical and Thoracic Spine

CONTRIBUTIONS BY **Patti Ward,** PHD, RT(R)

CONTRIBUTORS TO PAST EDITIONS Alex Backus, MS, RT(R), April Apple, RT(R), Donna L. Wright, EdD, RT(R)

CONTENTS

RADIOGRAPHIC ANATOMY

Vertebral Column

The vertebral *(ver'-te-bral)* column, commonly called the spine or spinal column, is a complex succession of many bones called **vertebrae** *(ver'-te-bre)* (singular is **vertebra** *[ver'-te-brah]*) (Fig. 8.1). It provides a flexible supporting column for the trunk and head and also transmits the weight of the trunk and upper body to the lower limbs. This column is located in the midsagittal plane, forming the posterior or dorsal aspect of the bony trunk of the body. As adjacent vertebrae are stacked vertically, openings in each vertebra line up to create a tubelike, vertical spinal canal.

Spinal Canal

The spinal canal, which follows the various curves of the spinal column, begins at the base of the skull and extends distally into the sacrum. This canal contains the spinal cord and is filled with cerebrospinal fluid.

Spinal Cord

The spinal cord, which is enclosed and protected by the spinal canal, begins below the **medulla oblongata** *(me-dul'-ah ob''-long-ga'-tah)* of the brain, which passes through the foramen magnum of the skull. The spinal cord continues through the **first cervical vertebra** all the way down to the **lower border of the first lumbar vertebra,** where it tapers off to a point called the **conus medullaris** *(ko'-nus med''-u-lar'-is).*

NOTE: In some persons, the conus medullaris may extend to as low as the body of L2. Therefore, to avoid striking the spinal cord, the most common site for a lumbar puncture into the spinal canal is at the level of L3–L4. (See myelogram procedure description on p. 310.)

Intervertebral Disks

Tough fibrocartilaginous disks separate typical adult vertebrae. These cushion-like disks are tightly bound to the vertebrae for spinal stability, but allow for flexibility and movement of the vertebral column.

SECTIONS OF VERTEBRAL COLUMN

The vertebral column is divided into **five sections.** Within each of these five sections the vertebrae have distinctive characteristics.

Detailed anatomy and positioning of the first two sections, the cervical and thoracic vertebrae, are covered in this chapter. The last three sections, the lumbar vertebrae, sacrum, and coccyx, are covered in Chapter 9.

Cervical Vertebrae

The first seven vertebrae are known as **cervical vertebrae.** Although slight variation may be noted in the height of each vertebra among individuals, the average person has **seven** cervical vertebrae.

Thoracic Vertebrae

The next **12** vertebrae are the **thoracic vertebrae,** and each of these connects to a pair of ribs. Because all vertebrae are posterior or dorsal in the body, the term *thoracic* is more correct for describing this region than the older term, *dorsal spine.*

Lumbar Vertebrae

The largest individual vertebrae are the **five lumbar vertebrae.** These vertebrae are the strongest in the vertebral column because the load of body weight increases toward the inferior end of the column. For this reason, the cartilaginous disks between the inferior lumbar vertebrae are common sites of injury and pathology.

Sacrum and Coccyx

The **sacrum** *(sa'-krum)* and **coccyx** *(kok'-siks)* develop as multiple separate bones and then fuse into two distinct bones. A newborn has **five** sacral *(sa'-kral)* segments and from **three** to **five** (average, four) coccygeal *(kok-sij'-e-al)* segments, for an average of **33** separate bones in the vertebral column of a young child. After fusion into a single sacrum and a single coccyx, the adult vertebral column is composed of an average of **26 separate bones.**

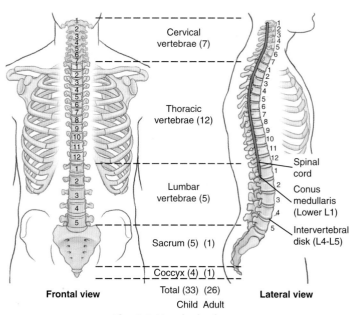

Fig. 8.1 Vertebral column.

Vertebral Column Curvatures

The vertebral column is composed of a series of anteroposterior (AP) curves (Fig. 8.2). The terms *concave* (a rounded inward or depressed surface like a cave) and *convex* (a rounded outward or elevated surface) are used to describe these curves. However, the curves are described as opposite, depending on whether one is describing them from an anterior perspective or a posterior perspective. For the purposes of this text, the curves are described as if the patient is being evaluated from the posterior perspective. The cervical and lumbar regions have concave curvatures and are described as **lordotic**. The thoracic and sacral regions have convex curvatures and are described as **kyphotic**.

Soon after birth, the **thoracic** and **sacral** (pelvic) curves begin to develop. These two convex curves are called **primary curves.** As children begin to raise their heads and sit up, the first **compensatory concave curve** forms in the cervical region. The second compensatory concave curve, the lumbar curvature, develops when children learn to walk. Both of the inferior curves, lumbar and sacral (pelvic), are usually more pronounced in women than in men.

These primary and compensatory curvatures are normal and serve an important function by increasing the strength of the vertebral column and helping maintain balance along a center line of gravity in the upright position.

Certain terms are commonly used to describe these curvatures when they become exaggerated or abnormal. These terms, *lordosis, kyphosis,* and *scoliosis,* are described as follows.

LORDOSIS

The term **lordosis** *(lor-do′-sis)* refers to an abnormal anterior concavity of the lumbar spine[1] (Fig. 8.3).

KYPHOSIS

Kyphosis *(ki-fo′-sis)* is an abnormal condition characterized by increased convexity of the thoracic spine curvature[1] (see Fig. 8.3).

SCOLIOSIS

If the spine is viewed from the posterior or anterior perspective (Fig. 8.4), the vertebral column usually is almost straight, with little lateral curvature. Occasionally, a slight lateral curvature occurs in the upper thoracic region of a healthy adult. This curvature usually is associated with the dominant extremity, so this curvature may be convex to the right in a right-handed person and convex to the left in a left-handed person.

An abnormal or **exaggerated lateral curvature of the spine** is called **scoliosis** *(sko″-le-o′-sis).*[1] Dextroscoliosis is an exaggerated curvature to the right, whereas levoscoliosis is an exaggerated curvature to the left. This is a more serious type of problem that occurs when a pronounced S-shaped lateral curvature exists. It may cause severe deformity of the entire thoracic and/or lumbar regions of the spine. The effect of scoliosis is more obvious if it occurs in the lower vertebral column, where it may create tilting of the pelvis with a resultant effect on the lower limbs, producing a limp or uneven walk. Table 8.1 presents a summary of spinal curvature terms.

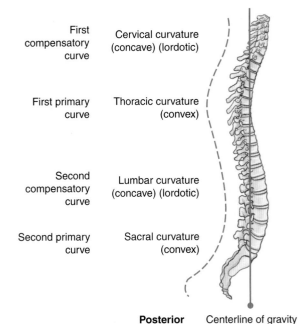

<table>
<tr><td>First compensatory curve</td><td>Cervical curvature (concave) (lordotic)</td></tr>
<tr><td>First primary curve</td><td>Thoracic curvature (convex)</td></tr>
<tr><td>Second compensatory curve</td><td>Lumbar curvature (concave) (lordotic)</td></tr>
<tr><td>Second primary curve</td><td>Sacral curvature (convex)</td></tr>
</table>

Posterior   Centerline of gravity   **Anterior**

Fig. 8.2 Normal adult curvature (side view).

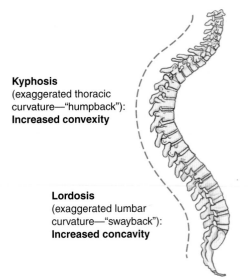

Kyphosis (exaggerated thoracic curvature—"humpback"): **Increased convexity**

Lordosis (exaggerated lumbar curvature—"swayback"): **Increased concavity**

Fig. 8.3 Lordosis-kyphosis.

TABLE 8.1	**SUMMARY OF SPINAL CURVATURE TERMS**
TERM	**DESCRIPTION**
Lordotic	Normal compensatory concave curvature of cervical and lumbar spine
	Or
	Abnormal exaggerated lumbar curvature with increased concavity (swayback)
Kyphotic	Normal primary (convex) curvature of thoracic and sacral region
Kyphosis	Abnormal exaggerated thoracic curvature with increased convexity
Scoliosis	Abnormal lateral curvature, dextroscoliosis (exaggerated curvature to the right) and levoscoliosis (exaggerated curvature to the left)

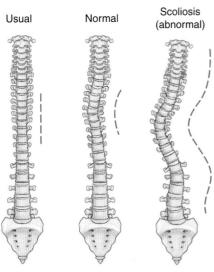

Usual   Normal   Scoliosis (abnormal)

Fig. 8.4 Scoliosis—lateral curvatures (anterior view).

Typical Vertebral Anatomy

Although the vertebrae in different regions vary in size and shape, all are similar in basic structure. A typical vertebra consists of two main parts, the **body** and the **vertebral arch.**

BODY

The body is the thick, weight-bearing anterior part of the vertebra. Its superior and inferior surfaces are flat and rough for attachment of the intervertebral disks.

VERTEBRAL ARCH

The second part of a typical vertebra consists of a ring or arch of bone that extends posteriorly from the vertebral body. The posterior surface of the body and arch form a circular opening, the **vertebral foramen,** which contains the spinal cord. When several vertebrae are stacked, as they are in the normal articulated vertebral column, the succession of vertebral foramina forms a tubelike opening, called the **vertebral (spinal) canal,** which encloses and protects the spinal cord (Fig. 8.5).

Superior Perspective

Fig. 8.6 illustrates the various parts of the vertebral arch. **Pedicles** *(ped'-i-kuls),* which extend posteriorly from either side of the vertebral body, form most of the sides of the vertebral arch.

The posterior part of the vertebral arch is formed by two somewhat flat layers of bone called **laminae** *(la-mə-nē).* Each **lamina** *(la-mə-nə)* extends posteriorly from each pedicle to unite in the midline.

Extending laterally from approximately the junction of each pedicle and lamina is a projection termed the ***transverse process.***

The **spinous process** extends posteriorly at the midline junction of the two laminae. The spinous processes, the most posterior extensions of the vertebrae, often can be palpated along the posterior surface of the neck and back.

Lateral Perspective

Fig. 8.7 illustrates a lateral orientation to the typical vertebra. The anterior vertebral body and posterior spinous process are readily identified. Extending posteriorly, directly from the vertebral body on each side, are the **pedicles,** which terminate in the area of the **transverse process.** Continuing posteriorly from the origin of the transverse process on each side are the two **laminae,** which end at the spinous process.

Additional obvious parts seen on this lateral view are the right and left superimposed **superior articular processes** and the lower pair of the right and left **inferior articular processes.** These processes allow for certain important joints that are unique and that must be visualized radiographically for each section of the vertebral column, as described on the following pages.

Summary

The typical vertebra consists of **two pedicles** and **two laminae** that form the vertebral arch and the vertebral foramen containing the spinal cord, **two transverse processes** extending laterally, **one spinous process** extending posteriorly, and the large anterior **body.** Each typical vertebra also has **four articular processes,** two superior and two inferior, which comprise the important joints of the vertebral column.

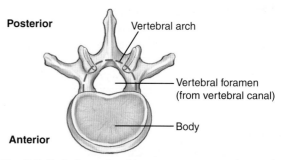

Fig. 8.5 Typical vertebra (demonstrates two main parts).

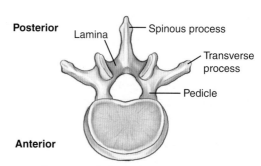

Fig. 8.6 Typical vertebra—superior view.

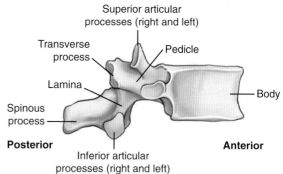

Fig. 8.7 Typical vertebra—lateral view.

JOINTS IN THE VERTEBRAL COLUMN

In addition to the **body** and the **vertebral arch**, the **joints** are a third important aspect of the vertebral column. The vertebral column would be rigidly immovable without the intervertebral disks and the zygapophyseal joints. Respiration could not occur without the spine, which serves as a pivot point for arch-like movement of the ribs.

Intervertebral Joints

The intervertebral joints are amphiarthrodial joints that are found between the vertebral bodies. The **intervertebral disks** located in these joints are tightly bound to adjacent vertebral bodies for spinal stability, but they also allow for flexibility and movement of the vertebral column.

Zygapophyseal Joints

The **four articular processes** described on the preceding page are seen projecting from the area of the junction of the pedicles and laminae (Fig. 8.8). The term *facet (fas'-et)* sometimes is used interchangeably with the term *zygapophyseal joint,* but the facet is actually only the articulating surface instead of the entire superior or inferior articular process. Zygapophyseal joints were once called by the older term *apophyseal joints.*

Costal Joints

Although not directly involved in the stability of the spinal column itself, a third type of joint is located along a portion of the vertebral column. In the thoracic region, the 12 ribs articulate with the transverse processes and vertebral bodies. These articulations of the ribs to the thoracic vertebrae, referred to as **costal joints,** are illustrated in later drawings of the thoracic vertebrae.

INTERVERTEBRAL FORAMINA

The fourth aspect of the vertebral column that is important radiographically involves the intervertebral foramina. Along the upper surface of each pedicle is a half-moon–shaped area termed the **superior vertebral notch,** and along the lower surface of each pedicle is another half-moon–shaped area called the **inferior vertebral notch** (see Fig. 8.8). When vertebrae are stacked, the superior and inferior vertebral notches line up. These two half-moon-shaped areas form a single opening, the **intervertebral foramen** (Fig. 8.9). Therefore, between every two vertebrae are **two** intervertebral foramina, **one on each side,** through which important spinal nerves and blood vessels pass.

The zygapophyseal joints and intervertebral foramina must be demonstrated radiographically by the appropriate projection in each of the three major portions of the vertebral column, as described and illustrated in later sections.

INTERVERTEBRAL DISK

The fifth and final aspect of the vertebral column that is important radiographically consists of the intervertebral disks. Typical adult vertebrae are separated by tough fibrocartilaginous disks between the bodies of every two vertebrae, except between the first and second cervical vertebrae. (The first cervical vertebra has no body.) These fibrocartilage disks provide a resilient cushion between vertebrae, helping to absorb shock during movement of the spine.

As labeled in Fig. 8.10, each disk consists of an outer fibrous portion termed the **annulus fibrosus** *(an'-u-lus)* and a soft, semi-gelatinous inner part termed the **nucleus pulposus** *(nu'-kle-us pul-po'-sus).* When this soft inner part protrudes through the outer fibrous layer, it presses on the spinal cord and causes severe pain and numbness that radiates into the upper or lower limbs. This condition, also known as a slipped disk, is termed the **herniated nucleus pulposus (HNP)** (see Clinical Indications, p. 311).

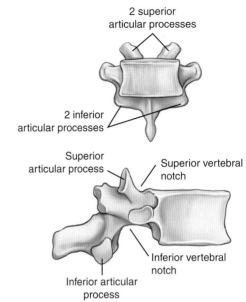

Fig. 8.8 Typical vertebra—articular processes (anterior and lateral views).

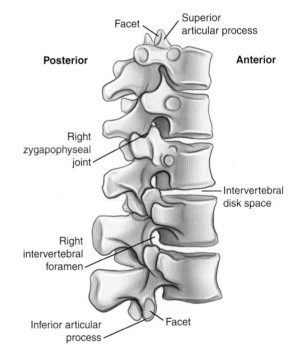

Fig. 8.9 Zygapophyseal joints and intervertebral foramina (lateral oblique view).

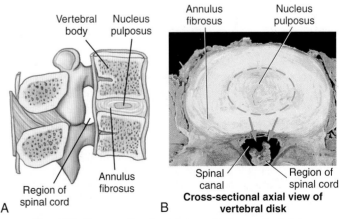

Fig. 8.10 Cross-sectional axial view of intervertebral disk.

Characteristics of Cervical Vertebrae

The cervical vertebrae show little resemblance to the lumbar or thoracic vertebrae, which are more typical in appearance. Although most of the parts that form typical vertebrae are present, various cervical vertebrae have unique characteristics such as **transverse foramina, bifid spinous process tips,** and **overlapping vertebral bodies.** Each cervical vertebra and vertebral body continues to get larger, progressing down to the seventh cervical vertebra.

C1 (the atlas) and C2 (the axis) are unusual and will be described separately. The third through sixth cervical vertebrae are typical cervical vertebrae. The last, or seventh, cervical vertebra, the **vertebra prominens,** has many features of thoracic vertebrae, including an extra long and more horizontal spinous process that can be palpated at the base of the neck. This palpable bony landmark is useful for radiographic positioning (Fig. 8.11).

Superior Perspective

Fig. 8.12 shows a typical cervical vertebra (C3 to C6) as viewed from above. The transverse processes are small and arise from both the pedicle and the body, rather than from the pedicle-lamina junction. The hole in each transverse process is called a **transverse foramen.** The vertebral artery and veins and certain nerves pass through these successive transverse foramina. Therefore, one unique characteristic of all cervical vertebrae is that each has **three foramina** that run vertically, the right and left transverse foramina and the single large vertebral foramen.

The **spinous processes** of C2 through C6 are fairly short and end in double-pointed or **bifid tips,** a second unique characteristic typical of cervical vertebrae.

Lateral Perspective

When viewed from the lateral perspective, typical (C3 to C6) cervical vertebral bodies are small and oblong in shape, with the anterior edge slightly more inferior, which causes slight overlapping of vertebral bodies (Fig. 8.13).

Located behind the transverse process at the junction of the pedicle and lamina are the cervical articular processes. Between the superior and inferior articular processes is a short column (pillar) of bone that is more supportive than the similar area in the rest of the spinal column. This column of bone is called the **articular pillar;** it sometimes is called the **lateral mass** when one is referring to C1.

CERVICAL ZYGAPOPHYSEAL JOINTS

The superior and inferior articular processes, located over and under the articular pillars, are directly lateral to the large vertebral foramen. The zygapophyseal joints of the second through seventh cervical vertebrae are located at **right angles,** or **90°,** to the midsagittal plane and thus are visualized only in a true lateral position (Fig. 8.14). However, in contrast to the other cervical zygapophyseal joints, those between C1 and C2 (atlantoaxial joints) are visualized only on an **AP open mouth projection** (see Fig. 8.18).

CERVICAL INTERVERTEBRAL FORAMINA

The intervertebral foramina can be identified by the pedicles, which form the superior and inferior boundaries of these foramina, as shown in Figs. 8.12 and 8.14. The intervertebral foramina are situated at a **45° angle** to the midsagittal plane, open anteriorly, as shown on the drawings. They also are directed at a **15° to 20° inferior angle** because of shape and overlapping of the cervical vertebrae. Therefore, to open and demonstrate the cervical intervertebral foramina radiographically, a 45° oblique position combined with a 15° to 20° cephalad angle of the x-ray beam would be required (see Figs. 8.31 and 8.33).

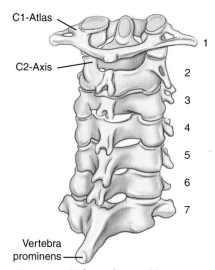

Fig. 8.11 Seven cervical vertebrae—oblique posterior view.

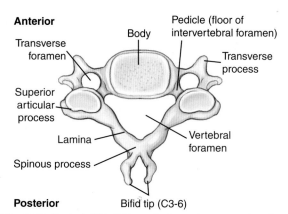

Fig. 8.12 Typical (C3–C6) cervical vertebra—superior view.

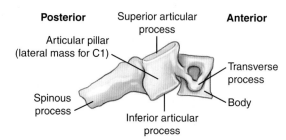

Fig. 8.13 Typical cervical vertebra—lateral view.

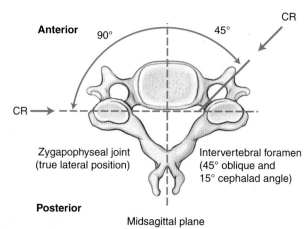

Fig. 8.14 Typical cervical vertebra—superior view: zygapophyseal joints, 90° (true lateral); intervertebral foramina, 45° oblique.

ATLAS (C1)

The first cervical vertebra, the **atlas,** a name derived from the Greek god who bore the world on his shoulders, least resembles a typical vertebra. Anteriorly, there is no body but simply a thick arch of bone called the **anterior arch,** which includes a small **anterior tubercle.**

The **odontoid process** or **dens** is part of the second cervical vertebra but a superior perspective of C1 shows its location and how it is held in place by the **transverse atlantal ligament** (Fig. 8.15). The positional relationship of C1 and C2 is illustrated in Fig. 8.17 and radiographically in Fig. 8.18.

Rather than the two laminae and a spinous process found in typical vertebrae, C1 has a **posterior arch** that generally bears a small **posterior tubercle** at the midline (see Fig. 8.15).

Each of the left and right C1 **superior articular processes** presents a large depressed surface called a **superior facet** for articulation with the respective left and right occipital condyles of the skull. These articulations, between C1 and the occipital condyles of the skull, are called **atlantooc-cipital joints**. The **transverse processes** of C1 are smaller but still contain the **transverse foramina** distinctive of all cervical vertebrae.

The **articular pillars,** the segments of bone between the superior and inferior articular processes, are called **lateral masses** for C1. Because the lateral masses of C1 support the weight of the head and assist in rotation of the head, these portions are the most bulky and solid parts of C1.

AXIS (C2)

The most distinctive feature of the second cervical vertebra, the **axis,** is the clinically important **odontoid process** or **dens,** the coni-cal process that projects up from the superior surface of the **body** (Fig. 8.16). Embryologically, the odontoid process is actually the body of C1, but it fuses to C2 during development. Therefore, it is considered part of C2 in mature skeletons.

Rotation of the head primarily occurs between C1 and C2, with the odontoid process acting as a pivot. The superior facets of the superior articular processes that articulate with the skull also assist in rotation of the head.

Severe stress as the possible result of a forced flexion-hyperextension, the so-called whiplash type of injury, may cause fracture of the dens. Any fracture of the vertebral column at this level could result in serious damage to the spinal cord as well.

The **inferior articular process** for articulation with C3 lies inferior to the **lamina** (Fig. 8.16). Below and lateral to the superior articular process is the transverse process, with its **transverse foramen.** The blunt **spinous process** with its bifid tip extends posteriorly.

RELATIONSHIP OF C1 AND C2

Radiographic demonstration of the relationship of C1 to C2 and the relationship of C1 to the base of the skull is clinically important because injury this high in the spinal canal can result in serious paralysis and death. Fig. 8.18 shows the radiographic image of an AP projection taken through an open mouth to demonstrate C1 and C2. The anterior arch of C1, which lies in front of the dens, is not clearly visible on this image because it is a fairly thin piece of bone compared with the larger denser dens.

Articulations between C2 and C1, the **atlantoaxial joints,** are normally **symmetric,** and so the **relationship of the odontoid process to C1 also must be perfectly symmetric.** Both injury and improper positioning can render these areas asymmetric. For example, **rotation of the skull** can alter the symmetry of these spaces and joints, thus imitating an injury. The median atlantoaxial joint is a pivot joint located between the odontoid process, anterior arch of C1, and the transverse atlantal ligament. There-fore, accurate positioning for this region is essential. The structures labeled on Fig. 8.17 correspond to the letters on Fig. 8.18 as follows:

A. Odontoid process (dens)
B. Left transverse process of C1
C. Left lateral mass of C1
D. Inferior articular surface of C1
E. Left atlantoaxial joint
F. Body of C2
G. Right superior articular surface of C2

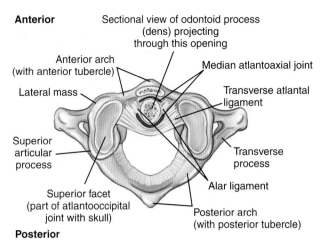

Fig. 8.15 Atlas (C1)—superior view.

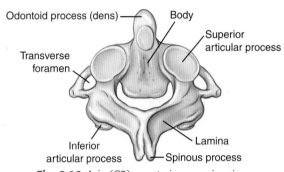

Fig. 8.16 Axis (C2)—posterior superior view.

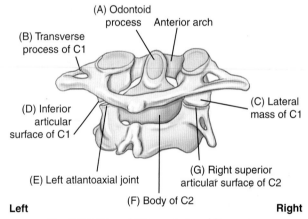

Fig. 8.17 C1 and C2—posterior oblique view.

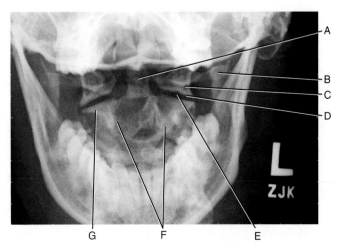

Fig. 8.18 AP open mouth radiograph.

Characteristics of Thoracic Vertebrae

An overview of the 12 thoracic vertebrae reveals marked progressive differences in the size and appearance of upper vertebrae compared with lower ones, as demonstrated in Fig. 8.19.

T5, T6, T7, and T8 are considered typical thoracic vertebrae. The upper four thoracic vertebrae are smaller and share features of the cervical vertebrae. The lower four thoracic vertebrae are larger and share characteristics of the lumbar vertebrae.

RIB ARTICULATIONS

A key distinguishing feature of all 12 thoracic vertebrae is their **facets for articulation with ribs.** Each thoracic vertebra is associated closely with one pair of ribs. Fig. 8.20 shows that the two lumbar vertebrae, L1 and L2, do not have facets for rib articulations.

Costovertebral Joints

Each thoracic vertebra has **a full facet** *(fas'-et)* or **two partial facets,** called **demifacets** *(dem'-e-fas'-ets),* on each side of the body. Each facet or combination of two demifacets accepts the head of a rib to form a **costovertebral joint** (Figs. 8.19 to 8.21).

.Vertebrae with two demifacets share articulations with the heads of ribs. For example, the head of the fourth rib straddles or articulates with demifacets on the vertebral bodies of both T3 and T4. The superior portion of the rib head articulates with the demifacet on the inferior margin of T3, and the inferior portion of the rib head articulates with the demifacet on the superior margin of T4.

Identifying ribs and the thoracic vertebrae is an important radiographic skill. T1 has a full facet and a demifacet on its inferior margin. T2 through T8 have demifacets on their upper and lower margins. T9 has only one demifacet on its upper margin. T10 through T12 have full facets. Knowing the facet arrangement makes it easy to predict the rib distribution. Rib 1 articulates with T1 only, rib 2 articulates with T1 and T2, and so forth. Ribs 11 and 12 articulate only with T11 and T12.

Costotransverse Joints

In addition to costovertebral joints, all of the **first 10 thoracic vertebrae** also have facets (one on each transverse process) that articulate with the tubercles of ribs 1 through 10. These articulations are termed **costotransverse joints.** Note in Figs. 8.19 and 8.20 that T11 and T12 do not show facets at the ends of the transverse process for rib articulations. Thus, as the first 10 pairs of ribs arch posteriorly from the upper 10 vertebral bodies, the tubercle of each rib articulates with one transverse process to form a costotransverse joint. **Ribs 11 and 12, however, articulate only at the costovertebral joints.**

The superior cross-sectional perspective of typical rib articulations (Fig. 8.21) shows that the articulations are closely spaced and are enclosed in synovial capsules. These **synovial joints** are **diarthrodial** and allow slight **gliding movements.** This anatomy is further demonstrated and described in Chapter 10.

Superior and Lateral Perspectives

Note the normal anatomic structures of a typical vertebra (vertebral body, pedicles, intervertebral foramina, superior and inferior articular processes, laminae, transverse processes, spinous processes). A unique characteristic of the thoracic region is that the long spinous process is projected so far inferiorly, as seen on a lateral view (Fig. 8.22). For example, on an AP radiographic projection of the thoracic spine, the spinous process of T4 will be superimposed on the body of T5.

Lateral Oblique Perspective

The **superior articular processes** (facing primarily posteriorly) and the **inferior articular processes** (facing more anteriorly) are shown to connect the successive thoracic vertebrae to form the **zygapophyseal (apophyseal) joints.**

On each side, between any thoracic vertebrae, are **intervertebral foramina,** which are defined on the superior and inferior margins by the pedicles (Fig. 8.23).

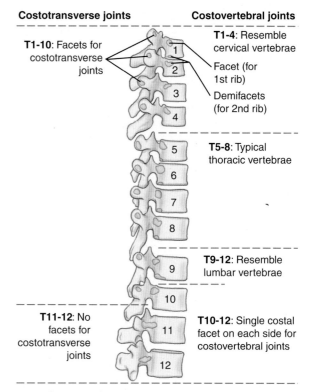

Fig. 8.19 Thoracic vertebrae (rib articulations).

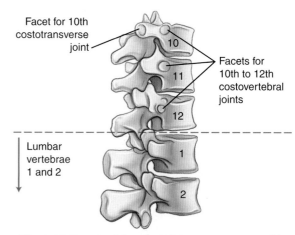

Fig. 8.20 T10–L2 (rib articulations on T10–T12 only).

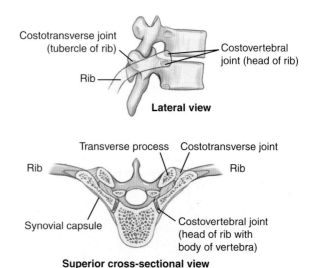

Fig. 8.21 Costovertebral and costotransverse joints—ribs 1 to 10.

THORACIC ZYGAPOPHYSEAL JOINTS

The structure and angles of the facets of the inferior and superior articular processes making up the zygapophyseal joints differ markedly from those of the cervical and lumbar vertebrae. In the thoracic vertebrae, the zygapophyseal joints form an angle of **70° to 75° from the midsagittal plane** (MSP). Therefore, for example, to open and demonstrate the thoracic zygapophyseal joints radiographically, a **70° to 75° oblique position** with a perpendicular central ray is required.

See Fig. 8.35 for a view of the thoracic portion of a skeleton in a left posterior oblique (LPO) position. Also see Fig. 8.37 for a radiographic image of the same LPO position. On both, one can easily see the right zygapophyseal joints.

THORACIC INTERVERTEBRAL FORAMINA

As demonstrated in Fig. 8.24, the openings of the intervertebral foramina on the thoracic vertebrae are located at right angles, or **90°, to the midsagittal plane.** This is best demonstrated again in Fig. 8.34, a photograph of the thoracic portion of a skeleton in a lateral position. See Fig. 8.36 for a radiographic image of the same lateral position. Both figures clearly show the left and right thoracic intervertebral foramina superimposed on each other.

UNIQUE C1–C2 JOINT CLASSIFICATIONS

Table 8.2 lists the **three** joints or articulations with two different movement types involved between the C1 and C2 vertebrae. The first two joints are the **right and left lateral atlantoaxial joints** between the inferior articular surface of C1 (atlas) and superior articular surface of C2 (axis). These are classified as **synovial** joints with **diarthrodial**, or freely movable, **plane** (or **gliding**) movements (see Figs. 8.17 and 8.18).

The third joint between C1 and C2 is the **medial atlantoaxial joint.** This articulation is located between the odontoid process of C2 and the anterior arch of C1 and is held in place by the transverse atlantal ligament, allowing a pivotal rotational movement between these two vertebrae. Therefore, this joint or articulation also is classified as a **synovial** joint that is freely movable, or **diarthrodial**, with a **pivot**, or **trochoid**, type of movement (see Figs. 8.15 and 8.17).

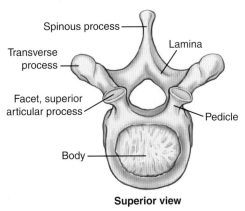

Fig. 8.22 Typical thoracic vertebrae.

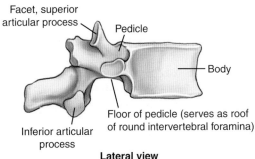

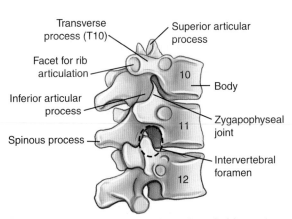

Fig. 8.23 Typical thoracic vertebrae—lateral oblique view.

TABLE 8.2 **SUMMARY OF VERTEBRAL JOINTS OF C AND T SPINES**			
JOINTS	**CLASSIFICATION**	**MOBILITY TYPE**	**MOVEMENT TYPE**
Skull–C1			
Atlanto-occipital	Synovial	Diarthrodial	Ellipsoid (condyloid)
C1–C2			
R and L lateral atlantoaxial (2)[a]	Synovial	Diarthrodial	Plane (gliding)
Median atlantoaxial (1)[b]	Synovial	Diarthrodial	Pivot (trochoid)
C2–T12			
Intervertebral	Cartilaginous (symphysis)	Amphiarthrodial (slightly movable)	N/A
Zygapophyseal	Synovial	Diarthrodial	Plane (gliding)
T1–T12			
Costovertebral	Synovial	Diarthrodial	Plane (gliding)
T1–T10			
Costotransverse	Synovial	Diarthrodial	Plane (gliding)

[a]Joint between odontoid process of C2 and anterior arch of C1.
[b]Joints between lateral masses of C1 and superior facets of C2.

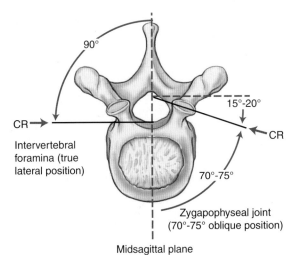

Fig. 8.24 Typical thoracic vertebrae: intervertebral foramina, 90° (true lateral); zygapophyseal joints, 70° to 75° (oblique).

Anatomy Review with Radiographic Images

AP CERVICAL SPINE IMAGE

Fig. 8.25 shows a conventional AP radiographic image of the cervical spine. Usually, the first two or three thoracic vertebrae, as well as C3 to C7, are seen well on this projection. Identifying specific cervical vertebrae is possible by starting with T1, which can be identified by the attachment of the first pair of ribs. Therefore, to localize T1, locate the most superior ribs and find the vertebra to which they appear to connect. After T1 is located, visible cervical vertebrae can be identified by starting at C7 and counting upward.

On Fig. 8.25:
- **A** is the first thoracic vertebra (T1); this can be determined by discovering that **B** is the first rib on the patient's right side
- **C** is the fourth cervical vertebra (count up from T1 and C7)
- **D** is the articular pillar or lateral mass region of C3
- **E** is the spinous process of C2 seen on end

NOTE: The white area at the top of the radiograph is created by the combined shadows of the base of the skull and mandible. These structures effectively obscure the first two cervical vertebrae on this type of radiograph.

LATERAL CERVICAL SPINE IMAGE

The single most important radiograph clinically for a cervical spine series is a well-positioned lateral, such as the one illustrated in Fig. 8.26. All seven cervical vertebrae and the alignment with T1 should be demonstrated on any lateral cervical spine radiograph. This is difficult in patients with thick, muscular, or wide shoulders and short necks. Additional projections may be necessary to supplement the routine lateral image. C1 and C7 have distinctive posterior structures that make it easier to identify them on radiographic images. The tubercle on the posterior arch of C1 resembles a spinous process and is easily identified. The spinous process of C7 is long and prominent, making it also easy to identify.

Fig. 8.26 shows that the lower anterior margins of the last four or five cervical vertebral bodies have a slightly lipped appearance. This characteristic, along with the general shape of the cervical vertebral bodies, requires that the central ray (CR) be angled approximately **15° to 20° cephalad** (toward the head) to open up these lower **intervertebral spaces** during an AP cervical spine projection:

A. Odontoid process (dens) extending up through the anterior arch of C1
B. Posterior arch of the atlas, C1
C. Body of C3
D. Zygapophyseal joint between C4 and C5 (best shown on a lateral projection for the cervical spine)
E. Body of C7
F. Spinous process of C7, vertebra prominens (a positioning landmark)

OBLIQUE (RPO) CERVICAL SPINE IMAGE

Fig. 8.27 illustrates how well the oblique position demonstrates the cervical **intervertebral foramina.** Spinal nerves to and from the cord are transmitted through these intervertebral foramina.
A. Posterior arch and tubercle of C1
B. Intervertebral foramen between C4 and C5 (count down from C1)
C. Pedicle of C6
D. Body of C7

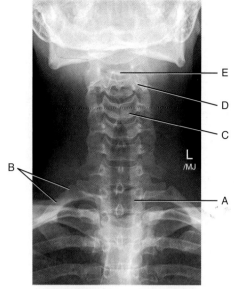

Fig. 8.25 AP cervical spine.

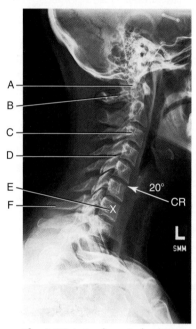

Fig. 8.26 Lateral cervical spine.

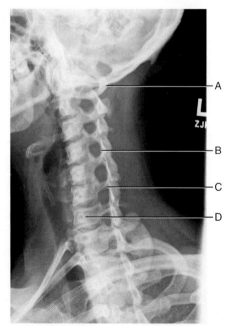

Fig. 8.27 Oblique cervical spine (RPO).

AP AND LATERAL THORACIC SPINE IMAGE

Individual thoracic vertebrae can best be identified on the AP projection through visual cues provided by the posterior rib articulations. The first rib has a distinctive sharp curvature and attaches to T1. The twelfth rib is very short and attaches to T12. After identifying T1 or T12, one can count superiorly or inferiorly to identify the other thoracic vertebrae.

AP Thoracic Spine Image (Fig. 8.28)
A. First posterior rib
B. Tenth posterior rib
C. Spinous process of T11, faintly seen on edge through body
D. Body of T12
E. Intervertebral disk space between T8 and T9
F. Body of T7 (center of T spine and of average chest)
G. Body of T1 (Remember, heads of first ribs articulate with upper portion of T1)

Lateral Thoracic Spine (Fig. 8.29)
A. Body of T3. (Count up from T12, assuming that the top edge of T12 is at the level of the costophrenic angle [posterior tip] of the diaphragm.
B. Body of T7
C. Intervertebral foramina between T11 and T12. (This is best demonstrated on a lateral image of the T spine.)
   Table 8.3 presents a summary of distinguishing features of the cervical and thoracic spine.

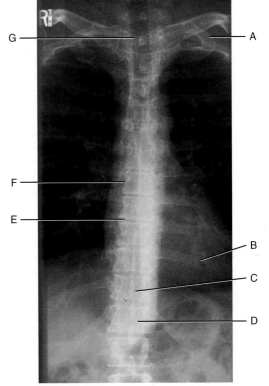

Fig. 8.28 AP thoracic spine.

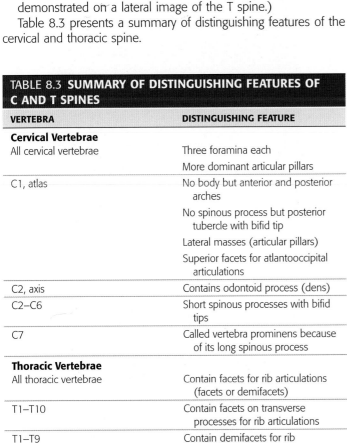

TABLE 8.3 SUMMARY OF DISTINGUISHING FEATURES OF C AND T SPINES

VERTEBRA	DISTINGUISHING FEATURE
Cervical Vertebrae	
All cervical vertebrae	Three foramina each
	More dominant articular pillars
C1, atlas	No body but anterior and posterior arches
	No spinous process but posterior tubercle with bifid tip
	Lateral masses (articular pillars)
	Superior facets for atlantooccipital articulations
C2, axis	Contains odontoid process (dens)
C2–C6	Short spinous processes with bifid tips
C7	Called vertebra prominens because of its long spinous process
Thoracic Vertebrae	
All thoracic vertebrae	Contain facets for rib articulations (facets or demifacets)
T1–T10	Contain facets on transverse processes for rib articulations
T1–T9	Contain demifacets for rib articulation
T10–T12	Contain single facet for rib articulation

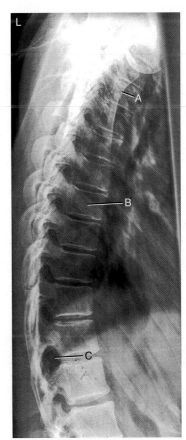

Fig. 8.29 Lateral thoracic spine.

Intervertebral Foramina Versus Zygapophyseal Joints

Two anatomic areas of the spine that generally need to be demonstrated by the proper radiographs are the **intervertebral foramina** and **zygapophyseal joints.** This is especially important for the cervical spine. The physician gains important information concerning the relationship of consecutive vertebrae by studying these two areas on the appropriate radiograph. To complicate matters, however, depending on the part of the spine to be radiographed (cervical, thoracic, or lumbar), a different body position is required to show each anatomic area best.

CERVICAL SPINE SKELETON

Two photographs of the cervical vertebrae (Figs. 8.30 and 8.31) are shown in position to visualize these areas on the cervical vertebrae. Fig. 8.30 is a cervical section of the vertebral column in a left lateral position, and Fig. 8.31 is a 45° LPO position. The **zygapophyseal joints** visualize well in the **lateral position** (see arrow).

On the right, the posterior oblique with a 45° rotation shows that the intervertebral foramina are clearly opened (see arrow). It is important to know that the **LPO** position opens up the foramina on the **right side** and a **15° to 20° CR cephalad angle** is needed. Therefore, on a **posterior oblique** cervical spine radiograph, the upside (side farthest from IR) is the side on which the intervertebral foramina are opened well. If this were taken in an **anterior** oblique position, with the foramina **closest** to the image receptor (IR), the downside would be open and a **15° to 20° caudad angle** would be required.

CERVICAL SPINE RADIOGRAPHS

The two radiographs of the cervical spine (Figs. 8.32 and 8.33) illustrate the same anatomy in the same two positions as shown on the skeleton above. The lateral position on the right best shows the **zygapophyseal joints.** The joint on each side is superimposed on the joint on the opposite side. It is important to remember that the zygapophyseal joints are located between the articular pillars of each vertebra.

The oblique cervical spine radiograph shows the circular **intervertebral foramina** opened. In each oblique radiograph, only one set of foramina are opened, whereas the ones on the opposite side are closed. Because this position is an **LPO,** the **right intervertebral foramina** or those on the **upside** are being shown.

Remember that the LPO will show the same anatomy as the right anterior oblique (RAO). Therefore, if the patient were placed in an **anterior** oblique position, the **downside** foramina to the IR would be shown. Thus, in either case, LPO or RAO, the right intervertebral foramina will be visualized.

Table 8.4 presents a summary of cervical spine joints and foramina.

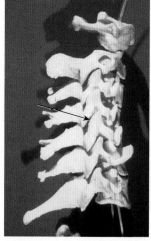

Fig. 8.30 Left lateral cervical spine—zygapophyseal joints.

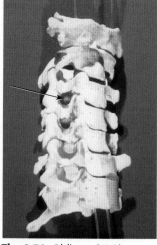

Fig. 8.31 Oblique (LPO) cervical spine—right intervertebral foramina (upside).

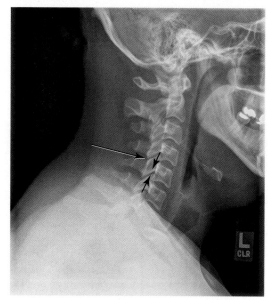

Fig. 8.32 Lateral (left) cervical spine—zygapophyseal joints demonstrated.

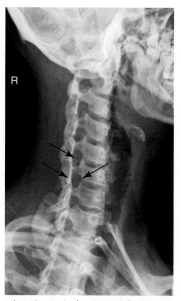

Fig. 8.33 Oblique (LPO) cervical spine—right intervertebral foramina (upside).

TABLE 8.4 SUMMARY OF CERVICAL SPINE JOINTS AND FORAMINA	
ZYGAPOPHYSEAL JOINTS—90° LATERAL	**INTERVERTEBRAL FORAMINA—45° OBLIQUE**
R or L lateral	**CR 15° to 20° Cephalad—Upside Visualized**
	LPO—right foramina
	RPO—left foramina
	CR 15° to 20° Caudad—Downside Visualized
	LAO—left foramina
	RAO—right foramina

THORACIC SPINE SKELETON

Two photographs of the thoracic vertebrae are shown in Figs. 8.34 and 8.35. The thoracic vertebrae on the left are in a lateral position; those on the right are in an oblique position. The **lateral position** of the thoracic spine best shows the **intervertebral foramina.** A **70° oblique** is necessary to open up the **zygapophyseal joints** on the thoracic spine.

The **posterior** oblique position on the right shows the zygapophyseal joint on the **upside.** Anterior oblique would demonstrate the **downside** joints.

THORACIC SPINE RADIOGRAPHS

Radiographs of the thoracic spine in the lateral position and in the 70° oblique position (Figs. 8.36 and 8.37) correspond to the position of the thoracic skeleton directly above. Observe that the round openings of the superimposed **intervertebral foramina** are best visualized on the **lateral** radiograph on the left (see arrow).

The **zygapophyseal joints** are best visualized on the **oblique** radiograph on the right. The oblique radiograph is in a 70° LPO position, which should best visualize the zygapophyseal joints on the **upside,** or those farthest away from the IR. The LPO position best shows the **right zygapophyseal** joints.

If the oblique was taken as **anterior** oblique, the opposite would be true and the **downside** joints would be demonstrated. A left anterior oblique would demonstrate the **left** zygapophyseal joints. Therefore, an LAO would show the same zygapophyseal joints as an RPO, as seen in Table 8.5.

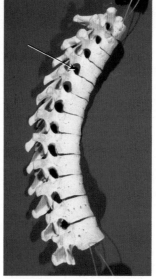

Fig. 8.34 Thoracic spine: left lateral, intervertebral foramina.

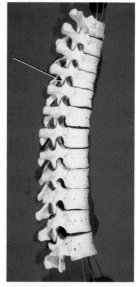

Fig. 8.35 Thoracic spine: oblique (LPO), upside zygapophyseal joints.

TABLE 8.5 SUMMARY OF THORACIC SPINE JOINTS AND FORAMINA

INTERVERTEBRAL FORAMINA—90° LATERAL	ZYGAPOPHYSEAL JOINTS—70° OBLIQUE
R or L lateral	Posterior oblique—upside
	LPO—right zygapophyseal
	RPO—left zygapophyseal
	Anterior oblique—downside
	LAO—left zygapophyseal
	RAO—right zygapophyseal

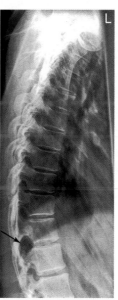

Fig. 8.36 Thoracic spine: left lateral, intervertebral foramina.

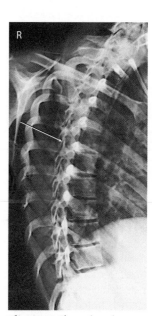

Fig. 8.37 Thoracic spine: oblique (LPO) right zygapophyseal joints.

8

RADIOGRAPHIC POSITIONING

Topographic Landmarks

Topographic landmarks are useful, palpable reference points for radiographic positioning that may be helpful when well-collimated radiographic images of specific vertebrae are required. Variations are seen among patients of different body habitus, but these landmarks show the anatomic relationships of an average patient.

CERVICAL LANDMARKS

Various anatomy correlates with levels of the cervical spine, as illustrated in Figs. 8.38 and 8.39. The **mastoid process (tip)** corresponds to the level of **C1.** Another way to localize the level of C1 is to go about 1 inch (2.5 cm) below the level of the external auditory meatus (EAM).

With the head in a neutral position, the angle of the mandible or **gonion,** is at the same level as **C3.** The most prominent part of the **thyroid cartilage,** or Adam's apple, is at the approximate level of C5. This thyroid cartilage landmark varies between the levels of **C4 and C6.**

The spinous process of the last cervical vertebra, **C7 vertebra prominens,** is at about the same level as the **body of T1.** It is more obvious with the patient's head tipped forward and should be used to help locate C7 and T1 rather than the top of the shoulders (too much variability exists in the position of shoulders because of relative fitness and posture). This is a useful landmark because of the importance of including all of C7 on a lateral cervical radiograph.

The shoulders should be depressed as much as possible for a lateral C spine radiograph; however, depending on the patient's body habitus, the shoulders may still occasionally superimpose the last cervical vertebra. Additional images may be necessary to demonstrate the alignment of C7 to T1 when the shoulders are too dense for adequate penetration on a routine lateral. In this case, the jugular notch or the vertebra prominens can be used as a landmark for centering.

STERNUM AND THORACIC SPINE LANDMARKS

Sternum anatomy correlates with levels of the thoracic spine, as illustrated in Figs. 8.40 and 8.41. The sternum is divided into three basic sections. The upper section is the **manubrium.** The easily palpated U-**shaped** dip in the superior margin is the **jugular** (suprasternal) **notch** (A). The jugular notch is at the level of T2 and T3. T1 is about 1.5 inches (4 cm) superior to the level of the jugular notch.

The first thoracic vertebra can be palpated posteriorly at the base of the neck for the prominent spinous process of C7, the **vertebra prominens.** Note that the long, sloping vertebra prominens extends downward, with its tip at the level of the body of T1.

The central portion of the sternum is called the **body.** The manubrium and the body connect at a slight, easily located angle termed the **sternal angle** (B), about 2 inches (5 cm) inferior to the manubrial notch. Posteriorly, this is the level of the junction of T4 and T5. Anteriorly, this is the level of the articulation of the second rib onto the sternum.

A frequently used landmark is the level of T7. Anteriorly, it is located about 3 to 4 inches (8 to 10 cm) inferior to the jugular notch or at the midpoint of the jugular notch and the xiphoid process. Posteriorly, this is about 7 to 8 inches (18 to 20 cm) below the vertebra prominens (C). This landmark indicates the approximate center of the 12 thoracic vertebrae because the inferior vertebrae are larger than the superior ones.

The most inferior end of the sternum is called the **xiphoid process, xiphoid tip,** or **ensiform process.** Locating the xiphoid process on a patient requires some pressure (D). The xiphoid tip is at the level of T9–T10.

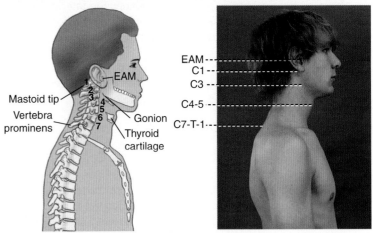

Fig. 8.38 Cervical spine landmarks. *EAM,* External auditory meatus.

Fig. 8.39 Cervical spine landmarks. *EAM,* External auditory meatus.

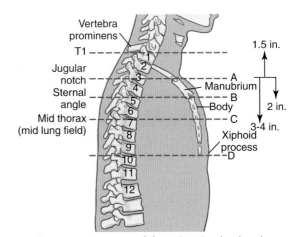

Fig. 8.40 Sternum and thoracic spine landmarks.

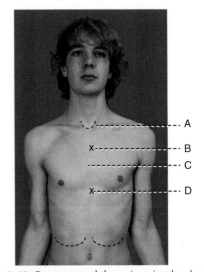

Fig. 8.41 Sternum and thoracic spine landmarks.

Positioning and Technical Considerations

ERECT VERSUS RECUMBENT

Radiographic examinations of the cervical spine generally are made with the patient erect to demonstrate alignment and ligament stability. An erect position also allows the natural curvature of the spine to be demonstrated, the shoulders to be depressed, and a 72-inch (180-cm) source–image receptor distance (SID) to be used for the lateral and oblique projections to improve image quality and reduce magnification.

The patient may be seated or standing in front of an upright bucky or a radiographic table. Some conditions, such as trauma, may require radiography of the cervical spine with the patient in a recumbent position.

Thoracic spines are radiographed in recumbent or erect positions, depending on the preference of the clinical facility. However, scoliosis examinations must be radiographed in the erect position (described in Chapter 9).

PATIENT RADIATION PROTECTION

Exposure to radiosensitive tissues such as the thyroid, parathyroid, breasts, testes, and ovaries can be minimized during radiography of the cervical and thoracic spine by **close collimation,** the use of **proper exposure factors,** and **minimization of repeats.** Theoretically, radiosensitive organs in the thoracic region (e.g., breast, thyroid) should be shielded from radiation, but because of the practicalities of maintaining the shields (e.g., erect positions, flexion-extension views), this is not a common practice when imaging the spinal column, especially for cervical spine projections. However, for radiation dose reduction measures, lead contact shielding over the gonads and other radiosensitive areas is a good practice when it is clinically practical. Also, the thyroid dose can be reduced significantly during cervical and thoracic spine oblique radiography by positioning the patient **in an anterior oblique rather than a posterior oblique** position (Figs. 8.42 and 8.43).

TECHNICAL AND IMAGE QUALITY FACTORS

For the purposes of this discussion, technical and image quality factors include the following: (1) exposure factors; (2) focal spot size; (3) compensating strategies; (4) SID; (5) scatter reduction; and (6) IR alignment.

During lateral and oblique cervical spinal radiography, the spinal column is unavoidably situated some distance from the IR (increased object–image receptor distance [OID]). Image geometry, therefore, results in reduced spatial resolution caused by magnification of spinal anatomy.

Exposure Factors

The kVp range for a cervical spine is 70 to 85 kVp and, for the thoracic spine, 75 to 90 kVp depending on the imaging system being used. Using higher kVp reduces patient dose, as long as lower mAs values are used.

The lateral thoracic spine image is usually obtained with the use of an orthostatic (breathing) technique to blur structures that overlie the thoracic vertebrae. This breathing technique involves the patient taking shallow breaths during the exposure and requires a minimum of a 3- or 4-second exposure time, with a low mA setting. The technologist must be sure the thorax, in general, is not moving during the exposure other than from the gentle breathing motion.

Focal Spot Size

Use of a small focal spot can improve spatial resolution. Orthostatic techniques require a long exposure time at low mA settings that have smaller focal spot sizes.

Compensating Strategies

The range of vertebral sizes and the different types of surrounding tissues in the thoracic region, in particular, present a radiographic challenge. For example, on an AP image, exposure factors could overexpose the superior end (smaller vertebral bodies surrounded by air-filled lungs) and underexpose the inferior end (larger vertebral bodies surrounded by dense abdominal tissues below the diaphragm).

The anode heel effect may be applied for AP thoracic spine projections by positioning the anode end of the tube (less intense portion of the field) over the thinner anatomic part (superior thoracic spine). However, the use of a compensating filter is generally a more effective method of equalizing density along an AP thoracic spine. See Chapter 1 for more information on compensating filters.

SID

Cervical spine radiographs should be imaged with a minimum of 40 inches (100 cm). An increased SID of 60 to 72 inches (150 to 180 cm) should be used for lateral, cervicothoracic ("swimmer's") and oblique projections to compensate for the increased OID.

Thoracic spine images usually are obtained at a minimum SID of 40 inches (100 cm).

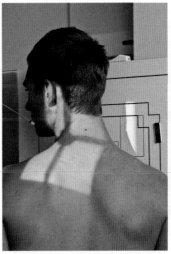 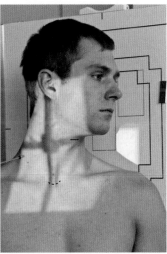

Fig. 8.42 Anterior cervical oblique: minimum 40-inch (100-cm) SID; small focal spot; anterior oblique, reduce thyroid doses.

Fig. 8.43 Posterior cervical oblique: 60-inch (150-cm) SID; small focal spot.

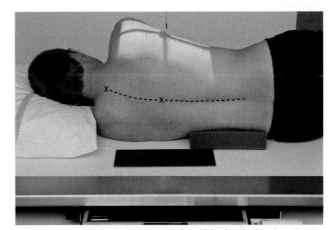

Fig. 8.44 Lateral thoracic spine: with lead blocker behind patient; vertebral column near parallel to tabletop.

Scatter Radiation

Use of higher kVp in thick or dense tissue results in increased production of scatter radiation, which degrades the radiographic image. The effects of scatter radiation can be minimized in three ways: (1) with close collimation; (2) with a lead blocker placed on the tabletop next to the patient during lateral radiography (Fig. 8.44); and (3) with grids. Collimation reduces the amount of scatter produced, and lead blockers and grids prevent scatter radiation from reaching the IR. Manufacturers have created post-processing software for digital systems that will eliminate the presentation of scatter radiation on the image; however, as a post-processing tool, this does not reduce or prevent scatter radiation from reaching the image as to the measures listed above.

Spine radiography requires a grid, with the exception of certain situations. When a patient's neck measures less than 10 cm, a grid is unnecessary. Placement of the IR far from the spine during lateral cervical radiography creates an air gap which also reduces the amount of scatter radiation that reaches the IR. This increased OID does however contribute to greater magnification of the image, which accounts for an above-mentioned increase in SID to compensate.

Part-IR Alignment

Correct part-IR alignment is important during spine radiography because the beam must pass through specific anatomic structures. For example, this may require placing a radiolucent sponge under the patient's waist to keep the spine near parallel to the IR during lateral thoracic positioning (see Fig. 8.44).

Optimal object-IR alignment is a challenge for lateral thoracic and lumbar spine radiography because of the wide range of body builds in male and female patients. This is illustrated in the positioning pages for those projections.

Special Patient Considerations
PEDIATRIC APPLICATIONS

Two primary concerns in pediatric radiography are **patient motion** and **patient radiation dose.** A clear explanation of the procedure is required to obtain maximal trust and cooperation from the patient and guardian.

Careful immobilization is important for achieving proper positioning and reducing patient motion. A **short exposure time** with optimal mA and kVp helps reduce the chance of motion. To reduce dose to the pediatric patient, use optimal kVp.

To ensure safety from falls or other physical injury, continuously watch and care for pediatric patients. Refer to Chapter 16 for detailed communication strategies, immobilization techniques, and explanations.

GERIATRIC APPLICATIONS

The physical effects associated with aging may cause the geriatric patient to require additional assistance, time, and patience if the required positions for spinal radiography are to be obtained. Patient care for the geriatric patient should include special attention in the areas of **communication, patient safety,** and **patient handling.** These patients may require extra time and assistance in achieving the required position.

Communication

Varying degrees of vision and hearing loss can reduce patient understanding and cooperation. To improve communication, do the following: (1) avoid background noise; (2) face the patient; (3) gain the patient's attention; and (4) use clear, simple instructions. Allow the patient to retain his or her hearing aids and eyeglasses, if possible, or wait until the last moment if it is necessary to remove them. Use touch to emphasize positioning instructions. For the patient with significant hearing loss, a lowered voice with increased volume improves the likelihood that the patient will hear you. To verify understanding, ask the patient to repeat instructions. Always treat the geriatric patient with dignity and respect.

Safety

The aging process can affect changes in balance and coordination that can bring about dizziness, vertigo, and an increased incidence of falling. Geriatric patients often fear falling. To ensure good patient safety, always assist the patient with the following: (1) to get onto and off the radiographic table; (2) to change position; and (3) to sit down. Reassurance and additional care from the technologist enable the patient to feel more secure and comfortable.

Patient Handling and Comfort

The geriatric patient experiences skin changes and a diminished ability to regulate temperature. As the skin ages, it becomes thinner, is more easily torn, and is more prone to bleeding and bruising. Use special care when holding or moving the patient. Avoid using adhesive tape and use special care when removing tape from skin. Use a radiolucent pad on the examination table to minimize skin damage and to provide comfort and added warmth. Extra blankets may be required to keep the patient warm. The patient with exaggerated kyphosis needs extra pillows under the head or may be more comfortable in the erect position for some procedures.

Technical Factors

Because of the high incidence of osteoporosis in geriatric patients, the kVp and/or mAs may require a decrease if manual exposure factors are being used. Older patients may have tremors or difficulty holding steady. Use of short exposure times (associated with the use of a high mA) is recommended to reduce the risk of motion.

BARIATRIC PATIENT CONSIDERATIONS

Bariatric patients may present some challenges when positioning for cervical and thoracic spine images. Additional tissue density from adipose tissue may require an increase in technical factors. An increase in kVp to improve penetration through additionally thick tissue may be necessary. mA and time may also be increased; however, a technologist must always use as low as reasonably achievable (ALARA) recommendations to avoid excessive radiation dose.

Measures must also be taken to reduce scatter radiation exposure to the IR because of the increased amount of tissue. The use of a grid for anatomic structures over 10 cm can be used to reduce the demonstration of scatter. Tight collimation to the anatomy of interest will also help to reduce the amount of scatter radiation reaching the IR. The location of the cervical and thoracic spine anatomy will be aligned similarly in the general population of patients. Use known external landmarks to aid in identifying the beginning and terminal ends of the cervical and thoracic spine regions. The swimmer's method of demonstrating the C7–T1 junction may be necessary for completion of both lateral cervical and thoracic spine views.

Digital Imaging Considerations

The following guidelines are important for digital imaging of the cervical and thoracic spines:

1. **Correct centering** to allow accurate processing by the image reader
2. **Close collimation, tabletop lead masking,** and **use of grids** to reduce scatter exposure to the highly sensitive image receptors
3. **Following the ALARA principle** in determining exposure factors, including the highest kVp and the lowest mAs that result in desirable image quality.
4. **Evaluation of exposure indicator** to help verify optimum image quality with the least radiation to the patient.

Alternative Modalities and Procedures
MYELOGRAPHY

Myelography is an alternative radiographic procedure that involves fluoroscopic and radiographic examination of the spinal canal for evaluation of lesions in the spinal canal, intervertebral disks, or nerve roots. Water-soluble iodinated contrast is injected into the subarachnoid space of the spinal canal at the level of L3–L4. If no obstruction exists, the contrast will flow freely with the cerebrospinal fluid throughout the spinal canal and around nerve roots. Lesions will appear as filling defects.

Magnetic resonance imaging (MRI) and computed tomography (CT) are other modalities of choice for evaluating spinal canal–related symptoms; however radiographic myelography is still being performed in many institutions and is described in greater detail in Chapter 19.

COMPUTED TOMOGRAPHY

CT scans are useful for evaluating spinal trauma such as fractures, subluxations, herniated disks, tumors, and pathologic conditions such as stenosis and arthritis.

MAGNETIC RESONANCE IMAGING

MRI of the cervical and thoracic spine is especially useful for demonstrating soft tissue (noncalcified) structures associated with the spine, such as the intervertebral disks, ligaments and the spinal cord itself. The MRI midsagittal image of a cervical spine in Fig. 8.45 clearly demonstrates not only bony structure but soft tissue as well. The vertebral canal which contains the spinal cord (Fig. 8.45, label B) is seen as a tubelike column that is directly posterior to the vertebral bodies. The spinal cord is seen to be a continuation of the medulla oblongata of the brain (Fig. 8.45, label A). A herniation of the disk between C6 and C7 is demonstrated by a slight posterior displacement, which causes mild spinal cord displacement.

NUCLEAR MEDICINE

NM studies involve the injection of pharmaceuticals tagged with tracer elements to demonstrate specific physiologic processes, including those that affect bone. For example, a technetium phosphate compound is injected and circulates with the blood. It will concentrate in areas of increased bone activity, creating a "hot spot" on the nuclear medicine scan image. (A hot spot is a region of nonsymmetrical uptake of the radioisotope.) Nuclear medicine scans can demonstrate several conditions related to the spine, such as bone tumors, healing fractures, metastases of cancer to the spine, osteomyelitis (bone infections), and additive or degenerative disease processes, such as Paget disease.

Clinical Indications

Clinical indications involving the cervical and thoracic spine that all technologists should be familiar with include the following (not necessarily an inclusive list).

Clay shoveler's fracture: This fracture, which results from hyperflexion of the neck, results in avulsion fractures on the spinous processes of C6 through T1. The fracture is best demonstrated on a lateral cervical spine radiograph.

Compression fracture: Frequently associated with osteoporosis, a compression fracture often involves collapse of a vertebral body, which results from flexion or axial loading most often in the thoracic or lumbar regions. It also can result from severe kyphosis caused by other diseases. The anterior edge collapses, changing the shape of the vertebral body into a wedge instead of a block. This induces kyphosis and may compromise respiratory and cardiac function; it also frequently results in injury to the spinal cord. Compression fractures are best demonstrated on a lateral projection of the affected region of the spine.

Facets – unilateral subluxation and bilateral locks: Zygapophyseal joints in the cervical region can be disrupted during trauma. If the patient's injury involves flexion, distraction, and rotation, only one zygapophyseal joint may be out of alignment, with a unilateral subluxation. Radiographically, the vertebral body will be rotated on its axis, creating a bowtie artifact on the lateral cervical spine image. If the patient's injury involves extreme flexion and distraction, both right and left zygapophyseal joints on the same level can be disrupted, creating bilateral locked facets. Radiographically, the vertebral body will appear to have jumped over the vertebral body immediately inferior to it. In either case, the spine is not stable because the spinal cord is distressed by this manipulation. Following the AP and lateral projections of the cervical spine, CT scanning of the spine generally is indicated.

Hangman's fracture: This fracture extends through the pedicles of C2, with or without subluxation of C2 on C3. This cervical fracture occurs when the neck is subjected to extreme hyperextension. The patient is not stable because the intact odontoid process is pressed posteriorly against the brainstem. A lateral projection of the cervical spine will demonstrate the anterior displacement of C2 characteristic of a hangman's fracture.

Herniated nucleus pulposus (HNP): If the soft inner part (nucleus pulposus) of an intervertebral disk protrudes through the fibrous cartilage outer layer (annulus) into the spinal canal, it may press on the spinal cord or spinal nerves, causing severe pain and possible numbness that radiate into the extremities. This condition sometimes is called a slipped disk. This is well demonstrated by MRI of the cervical spine region, as seen in Fig. 8.45. Although it can affect cervical vertebrae, HNP more frequently involves levels L4 through L5.

Jefferson fracture: This comminuted fracture (splintered or crushed at site of impact) occurs as a result of axial loading, such as that produced by landing on one's head or abruptly on one's feet. The anterior and posterior arches of C1 are fractured as the skull slams onto the ring. The AP open mouth projection and lateral cervical spine projections will demonstrate a Jefferson fracture.

Kyphosis: This condition is an abnormal or exaggerated convex curvature of the thoracic spine that results in stooped posture and reduced height. Kyphosis may be caused by compression fractures of the anterior edges of the vertebral bodies in osteoporotic patients, particularly postmenopausal women. It also may be caused by poor posture, rickets, or other diseases involving the spine (see Scheuermann disease). A lateral projection of the spine will best demonstrate the extent of kyphosis.

Odontoid fracture: This fracture involves the dens and can extend into the lateral masses or arches of C1. An AP open mouth projection will demonstrate any disruption of the arches of C1.

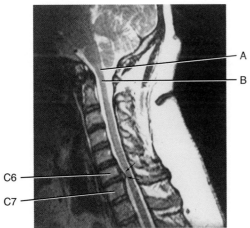

Fig. 8.45 MRI cervical spine (demonstrates herniated disk between C6 and C7).

Osteoarthritis This type of arthritis is characterized by degeneration of one or many joints. In the spine, changes may include bony sclerosis, degeneration of cartilage, and formation of osteophytes (bony outgrowths).

Osteoporosis: This condition is characterized by loss of bone mass. Bone loss increases with age, immobilization, long-term steroid therapy, and menopause. The condition predisposes individuals to vertebral and hip fractures. Bone densitometry is a relatively low-dose imaging modality for measuring the degree of osteoporosis, as described in Chapter 20.

Scheuermann disease: A relatively common disease of unknown origin that generally begins during adolescence, Scheuermann disease results in the abnormal spinal curvature of kyphosis and scoliosis. It is more common in males than females. Most cases are mild and continue for several years, after which symptoms disappear but some spinal curvature remains.

Scoliosis: Although many individuals normally have some slight lateral curvature of the thoracic spine, an **abnormal or exaggerated lateral curvature of the spine is called scoliosis.** Scoliosis is most common in children between the ages of 10 and 14 years and is more common in females. It may require the use of a back brace for a time, until the condition of vertebral stability improves. This deformity, if severe enough, may complicate cardiac and respiratory function. The effect of scoliosis is more obvious if it occurs in the lower vertebral column, where it may create tilting of the pelvis with a resultant effect on the lower limbs, producing a limp or uneven walk. Procedures for diagnosing and determining the degree of scoliosis are described in Chapter 9.

Spondylitis: This condition is inflammation of the vertebrae.

Spondylosis: The characteristic of this condition is neck stiffness due to age-related degeneration of intervertebral disks. The condition can contribute to arthritic changes that may affect the zygapophyseal joints and intervertebral foramen.

Teardrop burst fracture: The mechanism of injury is compression with hyperflexion in the cervical region. The vertebral body is comminuted, with triangular fragments avulsed from the antero-inferior border and fragments from the posterior vertebral body displaced into the spinal canal. Neurologic damage (usually quadriplegia) is a high probability. Based on the extent of the fracture and possible spinal cord involvement, CT scanning usually is indicated once a baseline lateral and AP projections of the cervical spine have been taken.

Transitional vertebra: A transitional vertebra is an incidental finding that occurs when the vertebra takes on a characteristic of the adjacent region of the spine. A transitional vertebra occurs most often in the lumbosacral region in which the vertebrae possess enlarged transverse processes. Another example of transitional vertebra involves the cervical and lumbar ribs. A cervical rib is a rudimentary rib that projects laterally from C7 but does not reach the sternum. A lumbar rib occurs as an outgrowth of bone extending from the transverse process(es) of L1.

See Table 8.6 for a summary of clinical indications.

Routine and Special Projections

Protocols and positioning routines vary among facilities, depending on administrative structure, liabilities, and other factors. Technologists should become familiar with the current standards of practice, protocols, and routine and special projections for any facility in which they are working.

Certain routine and special projections for the cervical and thoracic spine are demonstrated and described on the following pages.

TABLE 8.6 **SUMMARY OF CLINICAL INDICATIONS**

CONDITION OR DISEASE	MOST COMMON RADIOGRAPHIC EXAMINATION	POSSIBLE RADIOGRAPHIC APPEARANCE	EXPOSURE FACTOR ADJUSTMENT[a]
Fractures			
Clay shoveler's fracture	Lateral and AP cervical, CT	Avulsion fracture of the spinous process of any vertebra C6–T1; may see double spinous process sign on AP radiograph because of displacement of avulsed fractured segment	None
Compression fracture	Lateral and AP of affected spine, CT	Wedge-shaped vertebral body from lateral perspective; irregular spacing from AP perspective	None
Hangman's fracture	Lateral cervical, CT	Fracture of the anterior C2 arch, usually also with anterior subluxation of C2 on C3	None
Jefferson fracture	AP open mouth C1–C2 image, CT	Bilateral offset or spreading of the lateral masses of C1 relative to dens	None
Odontoid fracture	AP open mouth of C1–C2 and lateral horizontal beam , CT	Fracture line through base of dens, possibly extending into lateral masses or arches of C1	None
Teardrop burst fracture	Lateral cervical, CT	Comminuted vertebral body fragments avulsed from anteroinferior border and fragments from posterior vertebral body displaced into the spinal canal	None
Other Conditions			
Facets—unilateral subluxations and bilateral locks	Lateral cervical spine	Unilateral—bowtie deformity because vertebra is rotated on its axis; bilateral—jumped deformity because entire vertebra is located more anteriorly than it should be	None
Herniated nucleus pulposus (HNP)	AP and lateral of affected spine, CT, MRI	Possible narrowing in disk spacing between vertebrae and protrusion of disk into spinal canal on CT or MRI	None
Kyphosis	Lateral thoracic spine, scoliosis series, including erect PA-AP and lateral	Abnormal or exaggerated convex thoracic curvature	None
Scoliosis	Erect AP-PA spine, scoliosis series, including lateral bending	Abnormal or exaggerated lateral curvature of spine	None
Osteoarthritis	AP and lateral C and/or T spine	Degeneration of cartilage and formation of osteophytes (bony outgrowths)	None
Osteoporosis	DXA bone density examination of AP L spine and lateral hip	BMD	None or decreased (−) if severe
Scheuermann disease	Scoliosis series	Mild kyphosis and/or scoliosis, most commonly involvement of thoracic spine	None
Spondylitis, ankylosing spondylitis	Sacroiliac joints, spinal series, nuclear medicine bone scan	Calcification with ossification (formation of bony ridges between vertebrae), creating stiffness and lack of joint mobility	None
Spondylosis	AP, oblique, and lateral C spine, MRI	Decreased intervertebral joint space, foraminal stenosis, osteophytes,	None
Transitional vertebra	AP cervical and lumbar spine projections	Bony projections extended laterally from transverse processes	None

BMD, Bone mineral density; *DXA,* dual-energy x-ray absorptiometry.
[a]Depends on stage or severity of disease or condition.

AP OPEN MOUTH PROJECTION (C1 AND C2): CERVICAL SPINE

WARNING: For trauma patients, do not remove cervical collar and do not move the head or neck until authorized by a physician who has evaluated the horizontal beam lateral image or CT scan of the cervical spine.

Clinical Indications
- Pathology (particularly fractures) involving C1 and C2 and adjacent soft tissue structures
- Demonstrates odontoid and Jefferson fractures

Cervical Spine
ROUTINE
- AP open mouth (C1 and C2)
- AP axial
- Oblique
- Lateral

Technical Factors
- Minimum SID—40 inches (100 cm)
- IR size—8 × 10 inches (18 × 24 cm), portrait
- Grid
- kVp range: 70–85
- AEC not recommended because of small field

Shielding Shield radiosensitive tissues outside region of interest.

Patient Position—Supine or Erect Position Position patient in supine or erect position with arms by sides. Place head on table surface, providing immobilization if needed.

Part Position
- Align midsagittal plane to central ray (CR) and midline of table and/or IR.
- Adjust head so that, with mouth open, a line from **lower margin of upper incisors to the base of the skull** (mastoid tips) is **perpendicular** to table and/or IR, or angle the CR accordingly.
- Ensure that **no rotation** of the head (mandibular angles and mastoid tips equal distances from IR) or thorax exists.
- Ensure that **mouth is wide open** during exposure. Do this as the last step and work quickly, because it is difficult to maintain this position (Fig. 8.46).

CR
- CR perpendicular to IR
- Direct CR through center of open mouth.
- **Center IR to CR.**

Recommended Collimation Collimate tightly on four sides to anatomy of interest.

Respiration Suspend respiration.

NOTE: Make sure that when patient is instructed to open the mouth, only the lower jaw moves. Instruct the patient to keep the tongue in the lower jaw to prevent its shadow from superimposing the atlas and axis.

If the upper odontoid process cannot be demonstrated with correct positioning, perform Fuchs or Judd method (p. 321).

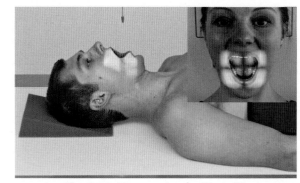

Fig. 8.46 AP open mouth—C1 to C2.

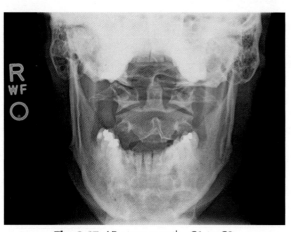

Fig. 8.47 AP open mouth—C1 to C2.

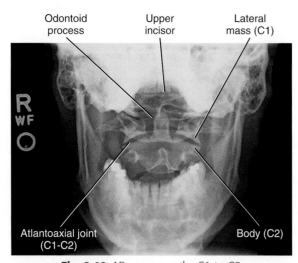

Odontoid process • Upper incisor • Lateral mass (C1) • Atlantoaxial joint (C1-C2) • Body (C2)

Fig. 8.48 AP open mouth—C1 to C2.

Evaluation Criteria
Anatomy Demonstrated: • Odontoid process (dens) and vertebral body of C2, lateral masses and transverse processes of C1, and atlantoaxial joints demonstrated through the open mouth (Figs. 8.47 and 8.48).
Position • Optimal flexion/extension of the neck, indicated by superimposition of the lower margin of the **upper incisors** on the **base of the skull**. Neither the teeth nor the skull base should superimpose the dens. • If the teeth are superimposed on the upper dens, reposition by slight hyperextension of the neck or angle the CR slightly cephalic. • If the base of the skull is superimposed on the upper dens, reposition by slight hyperflexion of the neck or angle the CR slightly caudal (the base of the skull and/or the upper incisors will be projected about 1 inch [2.5 cm] for every 5° of caudal angulation). • **No rotation** indicated by equal distances from lateral masses and/or transverse processes of C1 to condyles of mandible, and by center alignment of spinous process of C2. Rotation can imitate pathology by causing unequal spaces between lateral masses and dens. • Collimation to **area of interest.**
Exposure • Clear demonstration of soft tissue margins and of bony margins and trabecular markings of cervical vertebrae. • **No motion.**

AP AXIAL PROJECTION: CERVICAL SPINE

Clinical Indications
- Pathology involving the mid and lower cervical spine (C3 to C7)
- Demonstrates clay shoveler's fracture, compression fractures, HNP, and degenerative disease

> **Cervical Spine**
> ROUTINE
> - AP open mouth (C1 and C2)
> - AP axial
> - Oblique
> - Lateral

Technical Factors
- Minimum SID—40 inches (100 cm)
- IR size—8 × 10 inches (18 × 24 cm) or 10 × 12 inches (24 × 30 cm), portrait
- Grid
- kVp range: 70–85

Shielding Shield radiosensitive tissues outside region of interest.

Patient Position—Supine or Erect Position Position patient in the supine or erect position, with arms by sides.

Part Position
- Align midsagittal plane to CR and midline of table and/or IR.
- Adjust head so that a line from lower margin of upper incisors to the base of the skull (mastoid processes) is perpendicular to table and/or IR. Line from tip of mandible to base of skull should be **parallel to angled CR** (Fig. 8.49).
- Ensure no rotation of the head or thorax exists.

CR
- Angle CR 15° to 20° cephalad (see NOTE).
- Direct CR to enter at the level of the upper margin of thyroid cartilage to pass through C4.
- Center IR to CR.

Recommended Collimation Collimate on four sides to anatomy of interest.

Respiration Suspend respiration. Patient should not swallow during exposure.

NOTE: Cephalad angulation directs the beam between the overlapping cervical vertebral bodies to demonstrate the intervertebral disk spaces better. Angle the CR 15° when the patient is supine, or if there is less lordotic curvature. Angle the CR 20° when the patient is erect, or when more lordotic curvature is evident. The kyphotic (exaggerated curvature of the thoracic spine) patient will require an angle of more than 20°.

> **Evaluation Criteria**
> **Anatomy Demonstrated** • C3 to T2 vertebral bodies; space between pedicles and intervertebral disk spaces clearly seen (Figs. 8.50 and 8.51).
> **Position** • **No rotation** indicated by spinous processes and sternoclavicular joints (if visible) equidistant from the spinal column lateral borders. • The mandible and the base of the skull should superimpose the first two cervical vertebrae.
> • Collimation to **area of interest.**
> **Exposure** • Clear demonstration of soft tissue margins and of bony margins and trabecular markings of cervical vertebrae.
> • No motion.

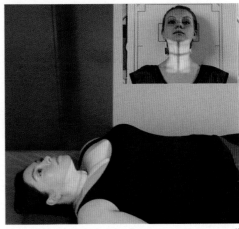

Fig. 8.49 AP axial, 15° cephalad angle. *Inset,* 20° CR, parallel to plane of intervertebral disk spaces, centered to C4.

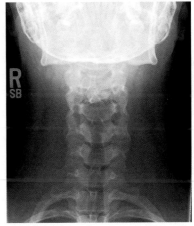

Fig. 8.50 AP axial, 15° cephalad angle.

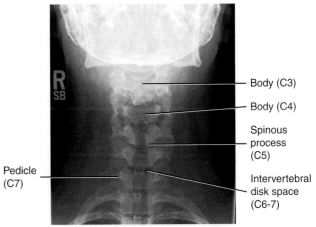

Body (C3)
Body (C4)
Spinous process (C5)
Pedicle (C7)
Intervertebral disk space (C6-7)

Fig. 8.51 AP axial, 15° cephalad angle.

ANTERIOR AND POSTERIOR OBLIQUE POSITIONS: CERVICAL SPINE

WARNING: For trauma patients, do not remove cervical collar and do not move head or neck until authorized by a physician who has evaluated the horizontal beam lateral image or CT scan of the cervical spine.

Clinical Indications
- Pathology involving the cervical spine and adjacent soft tissue structures, including stenosis involving the intervertebral foramen
- Both right and left oblique projections should be taken for comparison purposes. **Anterior oblique** positions—RAO, LAO—are preferred because of reduced thyroid doses.

Cervical Spine
ROUTINE
• AP open mouth (C1 and C2)
• AP axial
• Oblique
• Lateral

Technical Factors
- SID—40–72 inches (100–180 cm), longer SID recommended
- IR size—10 × 12 inches (24 × 30 cm), portrait
- Grid (optional because of air gap) but recommended when using higher kVp ranges
- kVp range: 70–85

Shielding Shield radiosensitive tissues outside region of interest.

Patient Position—Erect or Recumbent Position
The erect position preferred (sitting or standing), but recumbent is possible if the patient's condition requires.

Part Position
- Align midsagittal plane to CR and midline of table and/or IR.
- Place patient's arms at side; if patient is recumbent, place arms as needed to help maintain position.
- Rotate body and head into 45° oblique position. Use protractor or other angle gauge as needed to ensure 45° angle (see NOTE) (Figs. 8.52 and 8.53).
- Protract chin to prevent mandible from superimposing vertebrae. Elevate chin to place acanthiomeatal line (AML) parallel with floor (insert). Excessive skull and neck extension will superimpose base of skull over posterior arch of C1.

CR
Anterior Oblique (RAO, LAO)
- Direct CR 15° to 20° caudad to C4 (level of upper margin of thyroid cartilage).

Posterior Oblique (RPO, LPO)
- Direct CR 15° to 20° cephalad to C4.
- Center IR to CR.

Recommended Collimation Collimate on four sides to anatomy of interest.

Respiration
- Suspend respiration.

NOTE: Departmental option: The head may be turned toward IR to a near-lateral position. This results in some rotation of upper vertebrae but may help to prevent superimposition of mandible on upper vertebrae.

Evaluation Criteria
Anatomy Demonstrated • **Anterior:** Oblique (RAO and LAO): intervertebral foramina and pedicles on the side of the patient **closest to the IR** (right and left pedicles respectively). • **Posterior:** Oblique (RPO and LPO): intervertebral foramina and pedicles on the side of the patient **farthest from the IR** (left and right pedicles, respectively) (Figs. 8.54 and 8.55).
Position • Intervertebral disk spaces and intervertebral foramina of interest (C2 through C7) should be open and uniform in size and shape. The pedicles of interest should be demonstrated in full profile and the opposite, on-end pedicles should be aligned along the anterior cervical body. • On-end pedicles aligned at the midline of the cervical body and visualization of zygapophyseal joints indicate over-rotation. • Obscured intervertebral foramina and pedicles indicate under-rotation. • The mandibular rami should not superimpose the upper cervical vertebrae, and the base of the skull should not superimpose C1. • Collimation to **area of interest.**
Exposure • Clear demonstration of soft tissue margins and of bony margins and trabecular markings of cervical vertebrae. • **No motion.**

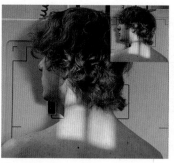

Fig. 8.52 Erect RAO position—CR 15°–20° caudad (less thyroid dose).

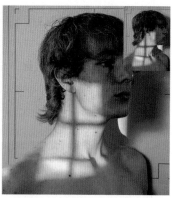

Fig. 8.53 Optional AP oblique, LPO—CR 15°–20° cephalad.

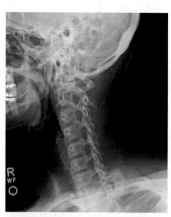

Fig. 8.54 Right posterior oblique.

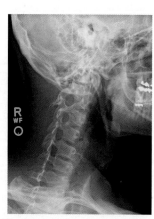

Fig. 8.55 Left posterior oblique.

LATERAL POSITION (ERECT): CERVICAL SPINE

Trauma patients: See lateral horizontal beam, p. 318.

Cervical Spine
ROUTINE
• AP open mouth (C1 and C2)
• AP axial
• Oblique
• Lateral

Clinical Indications

• Pathology involving the cervical spine and adjacent soft tissue structures, degenerative diseases including spondylosis and osteoarthritis

Technical Factors

• SID—60–72 inches (150 to 180 cm; see NOTE 1)
• IR size—10 × 12 inches (24 × 30 cm), portrait
• Grid (optional because of air gap) but required when using higher kVp ranges
• kVp range: 70–85

Shielding Shield radiosensitive tissues outside region of interest.

Patient Position—Lateral Position Position patient in the erect lateral position, either sitting or standing, with shoulder against vertical IR.

Part Position

• Align midcoronal plane to CR and midline of table and/or IR.
• Center IR to CR, which should place top of IR about 1 to 2 inches (2.5 to 5 cm) above the external auditory meatus (EAM) (Fig. 8.56).
• Depress shoulders (for equal weights to both arms [see NOTE 2]). Ask patient to **relax** and **drop shoulders down and forward as far as possible.** (Do this as the last step before exposure because this position is difficult to maintain.)
• Elevate chin to place AML parallel with floor. Protract chin (to prevent superimposition of the mandible on upper vertebrae).

CR

• CR perpendicular to IR.
• Direct CR horizontally to C4 (level of upper margin of thyroid cartilage).
• Center IR to CR.

Recommended Collimation Collimate on four sides to anatomy of interest.

Respiration Suspend respiration on **full expiration** (for maximum shoulder depression).

NOTE 1: Long (72 inches [180 cm]) SID compensates for increased OID and provides for greater spatial resolution.
NOTE 2: Adding weights (5–10 lb [2.3–4.5 kg]) with straps suspended from each wrist may help in pulling down shoulders.

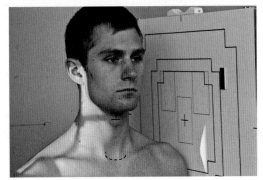

Fig. 8.56 Erect left lateral.

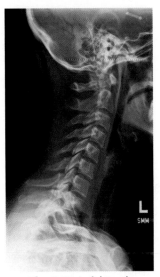

Fig. 8.57 Left lateral.

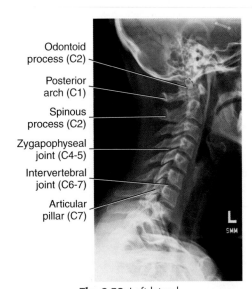

Odontoid process (C2)
Posterior arch (C1)
Spinous process (C2)
Zygapophyseal joint (C4-5)
Intervertebral joint (C6-7)
Articular pillar (C7)

Fig. 8.58 Left lateral.

Evaluation Criteria
Anatomy Demonstrated • Cervical vertebral bodies, intervertebral joint spaces, articular pillars, spinous processes, and zygapophyseal joints (Figs. 8.57 and 8.58).
Position • C1 through C7–T1 intervertebral joint spaces are clearly seen. If upper margin of T1 is not demonstrated, additional images such as the cervicothoracic lateral should be obtained. • The rami of the mandible do not superimpose C1 to C2. • The right and left articular pillars and zygapophyseal joints should be superimposed for each vertebra. • The bodies should be free of superimposition of the articular pillars and the spinous process seen in profile. • Collimation to **area of interest.**
Exposure • Clear demonstration of soft tissue margins, including margins of the trachea, and of bony margins and trabecular markings of cervical vertebrae. • **No motion.**

LATERAL, HORIZONTAL BEAM—TRAUMA: CERVICAL SPINE

WARNING: For trauma patients, do not remove cervical collar and do not move head or neck until authorized by a physician who has evaluated the horizontal beam lateral image or CT of the cervical spine. Many emergency departments routinely order CT to rule out fracture, subluxation, or other indications of cervical instability prior to performance of any radiographic procedures.

Clinical Indications
- Pathology involving the cervical spine, such as clay shoveler's fracture, compression fracture, hangman's fracture, odontoid fracture, teardrop burst fracture, and subluxation

Cervical Spine (Trauma Patient)
ROUTINE
- Lateral (horizontal beam)

Technical Factors
- SID—60–72 inches (150–180 cm) (see NOTE 1)
- IR size—10 × 12 inches (24 × 30 cm), portrait to the cervical spine
- IR with or without grid (see NOTE 2)
- kVp range: 70–85 with grid

Shielding Shield radiosensitive tissues outside region of interest.

Patient Position
Place patient in the supine position on stretcher or radiographic table.

Part Position
- Do **not** manipulate or move head or neck or remove cervical collar if present.
- Support IR vertically against shoulder, or place stretcher next to vertical grid device.
- Center IR to CR, which should place top of image receptor about 1 to 2 inches (2.5 to 5 cm) above EAM (Fig. 8.59).
- Depress shoulders (see NOTE 3).

CR
- CR perpendicular to IR.
- Direct CR horizontally to C4 (level of upper margin of thyroid cartilage).
- Center IR to CR.

Recommended Collimation Collimate on four sides to anatomy of interest.

Respiration Suspend respiration on **full expiration** (for maximum shoulder depression).

NOTE 1: Longer SID results in less magnification with increased image sharpness.
NOTE 2: Generally, a nongrid image receptor can be used for smaller or average-sized patients because of increased OID and the resultant air gap effect.
NOTE 3: Traction on arms will help depress shoulders but should be done only by a qualified assistant and/or with the consent or assistance of a physician. Protective apron must be worn and close collimation must be done to reduce any excessive exposure to assistant or physician.

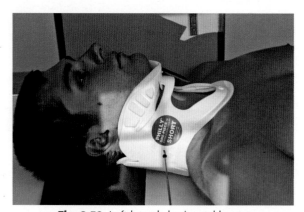
Fig. 8.59 Left lateral—horizontal beam.

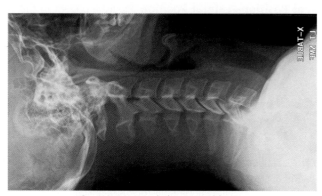
Fig. 8.60 Lateral—horizontal beam.

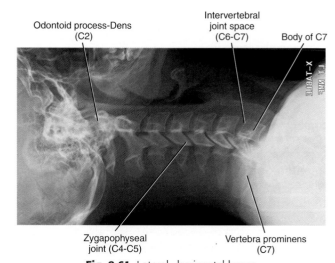

Odontoid process-Dens (C2)
Intervertebral joint space (C6-C7)
Body of C7
Zygapophyseal joint (C4-C5)
Vertebra prominens (C7)

Fig. 8.61 Lateral—horizontal beam.

Evaluation Criteria
Anatomy Demonstrated • Cervical vertebral bodies, intervertebral joint spaces, articular pillars, spinous processes, and zygapophyseal joints (Figs. 8.60 and 8.61).
Position • C1 through C7–T1 intervertebral joint spaces are clearly seen. • If the upper margin of T1 is not demonstrated, additional images, such as the cervicothoracic lateral, should be obtained. • The right and left articular pillars and zygapophyseal joints should be superimposed for each vertebra. • The bodies should be free of superimposition of the articular pillars and the spinous process seen in profile. • Collimation to **area of interest.**
Exposure • Clear demonstration of soft tissue margins and of bony margins and trabecular markings of cervical vertebrae. • **No motion.**

CERVICOTHORACIC (C5-T3) LATERAL POSITION: CERVICAL SPINE

SWIMMER'S

Clinical Indications
- Pathology involving the inferior cervical spine, superior thoracic spine, and adjacent soft tissue structures
- Various fractures (including compression fractures) and subluxation
- This is a good projection when C7 to T1 is not visualized on the lateral cervical spine, or when the upper thoracic vertebrae are of special interest on a lateral thoracic spine.

> Cervical Spine
> SPECIAL
> • Cervicothoracic lateral (Swimmer's)

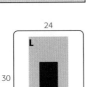

Technical Factors
- SID—60–72 inches (150–180 cm)
- IR size—10 × 12 inches (24 × 30 cm), portrait
- Grid
- Specially designed compensating filter useful for obtaining uniform brightness (see Chapter 1 for more information on compensating filters)
- kVp range: 75–95

Shielding Shield radiosensitive tissues outside region of interest.

Patient Position—Erect or Recumbent Position Place patient in preferred erect position (sitting or standing). The radiograph may be performed in the recumbent position if the patient's condition requires.

Part Position
- Align midcoronal plane to CR and midline of table and/or IR.
- Place patient's arm and shoulder closest to the IR up, flexing elbow and resting forearm on head for support.
- Position arm and shoulder furthest from the IR down and rotate slightly posterior, to place the remote humeral head posterior to vertebrae (Fig. 8.62).
- Ensure that no rotation of thorax and head exists.

CR
- CR perpendicular to IR (see NOTE).
- Direct CR to T1, which is approximately 1 inch (2.5 cm) above level of jugular notch anteriorly and at level of vertebra prominens posteriorly.
- Center IR to CR.

Recommended Collimation Collimate on four sides to anatomy of interest.

Respiration Suspend respiration on **full expiration**.

NOTE: A slight caudad angulation of 3° to 5° may be necessary to help separate the two shoulders farthest from the IR.

Optional Breathing Technique If patient can cooperate and remain immobilized, a low mA and 3- or 4-second exposure time can be used, with patient breathing short, even breaths during the exposure to blur out overlying lung structures.

Evaluation Criteria
Anatomy Demonstrated • Vertebral bodies and intervertebral disk spaces of C5 to T3 are shown. • The humeral head and arm farthest from the IR are magnified and appear inferior to T4 or T5 (if visible) (Figs. 8.63 and 8.64).
Position • Minimal vertebral rotation indicated by superimposition of cervical zygapophyseal joints and articular pillars, and posterior ribs. • The humeral heads should be separated vertically. • Collimation to area of interest.
Exposure • Clear demonstration of bony margins and trabecular markings of lower cervical and upper thoracic vertebrae. • **No motion.**

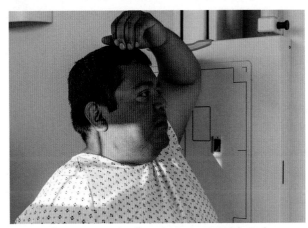

Fig. 8.62 Cervicothoracic (swimmer's) lateral.

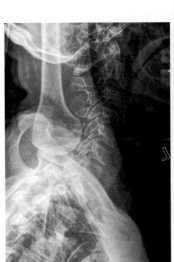

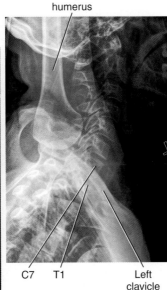

Fig. 8.63 Cervicothoracic (swimmer's) lateral.

Fig. 8.64 Cervicothoracic (swimmer's) lateral.

LATERAL POSITIONS—HYPERFLEXION AND HYPEREXTENSION: CERVICAL SPINE

WARNING: Never attempt these positions on a trauma patient until authorized by a physician who has evaluated the horizontal beam lateral image or CT scan of the cervical spine.

Clinical Indications
- Functional study to demonstrate antero-posterior vertebral mobility
- Frequently performed to rule out "whip-lash" type of injury or to follow up after spinal fusion surgery

Cervical Spine
SPECIAL
• Cervicothoracic lateral (Swimmer's)
• Lateral—hyperflexion and hyperextension

Technical Factors
- SID—60–72 inches (150–180 cm)
- IR size—10 × 12 inches (24 × 30 cm), portrait
- Grid or nongrid (with higher kVp ranges, grid should be used to minimize scatter radiation)
- kVp range: 70–85

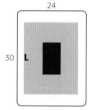

Shielding Shield radiosensitive tissues outside region of interest.

Patient Position—Erect Lateral Position Place patient in erect lateral position, either sitting or standing, with arms at sides.

Part Position
- Align midcoronal plane to CR and midline of table and/or IR.
- Ensure a **true lateral position,** with no rotation of pelvis, shoulders, or head.
- **Relax** and **depress shoulders** as far as possible (weights on each arm may be used).
- For **hyperflexion:** Depress chin until it touches the chest or as much as patient can tolerate (do not allow patient to move forward to ensure that entire cervical is included on IR) (Fig. 8.65).
- For **hyperextension:** Raise chin and tilt head back as much as possible (do not allow patient to move backward to ensure that entire cervical spine is included on IR) (Fig. 8.66).

CR
- CR perpendicular to IR.
- Direct CR horizontally to C4 (level of upper margin of thyroid cartilage).
- Center IR to CR.

Recommended Collimation Collimate on four sides to anatomy of interest.

Respiration Suspend respiration on **full expiration.**

NOTE: These are uncomfortable for patient; do not keep patient in these positions longer than necessary.

Evaluation Criteria
Anatomy Demonstrated • C1 through C7 should be included on IR, although C7 may not be completely visualized on some patients (Figs. 8.67 and 8.68).
Position • **No rotation** of head is indicated by superimposition of mandibular rami. • For **hyperflexion:** Spinous processes should be well separated. • For **hyperextension:** Spinous processes should be in close proximity.
Exposure • Clear demonstration of soft tissue margins, including margins of the trachea, and of bony margins and trabecular markings of cervical vertebrae. • **No motion.**

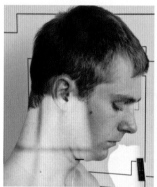
Fig. 8.65 Hyperflexion.

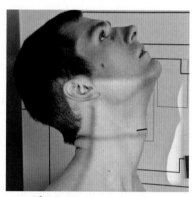
Fig. 8.66 Hyperextension.

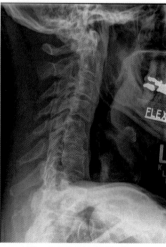
Fig. 8.67 Hyperflexion.

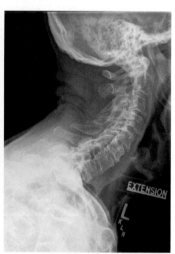
Fig. 8.68 Hyperextension.

AP OR PA PROJECTION FOR C1–C2 (ODONTOID PROCESS–DENS): CERVICAL SPINE

FUCHS METHOD (AP) OR JUDD METHOD (PA)

WARNING: For trauma patients, do not remove cervical collar and do not move head or neck until authorized by a physician who has evaluated the horizontal beam lateral image or CT scan of the cervical spine. The cervical spine must be cleared for fracture or subluxation prior to performing these projections.

One of these projections is useful for demonstrating the superior portion of the dens when this area is not well visualized on the AP open mouth cervical spine projection.

Cervical Spine
SPECIAL
• Cervicothoracic lateral (Swimmer's)
• Lateral—hyperflexion and hyperextension
• AP (Fuchs method)
• PA (Judd method)

Clinical Indications
• Pathology involving the dens and surrounding bony structures of the C1 ring

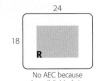

No AEC because of small field of view

Technical Factors
• Minimum SID—40 inches (100 cm)
• IR size—8 × 10 inches (18 × 24 cm), landscape
• Grid
• kVp range: 70–85

Shielding Shield radiosensitive tissues outside region of interest.

Patient and Part Position
Position patient supine (AP) or prone (PA) with midsagittal plane aligned to CR and midline of table and/or IR.

AP (Fuchs Method)
• Elevate chin as needed to bring mentomeatal line (MML) **near perpendicular to tabletop** (adjust CR angle as needed to be parallel to MML) (Fig. 8.69).
• Ensure that **no rotation** of head exists (angles of mandible equidistant to tabletop).
• CR is parallel to MML, directed to inferior tip of mandible.
• Center IR to CR.

PA (Judd Method)
• This is a reverse position to the supine position. Chin is resting on tabletop and is extended to bring MML near perpendicular to table (may adjust CR as needed to be parallel to MML) (Fig. 8.70).
• Ensure that **no rotation of head** exists.
• Ensure that CR is **parallel to MML,** through midoccipital bone, about 1 inch (2.5 cm) inferior to mastoid tips and angles of mandible.
• Center IR to CR.

Recommended Collimation Collimate tightly on four sides to anatomy of interest.

Respiration Suspend respiration.

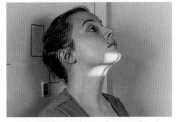
Fig. 8.69 AP—Fuchs method.

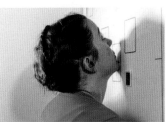
Fig. 8.70 PA—Judd method (less thyroid dose).

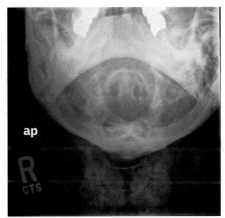
Fig. 8.71 AP projection.

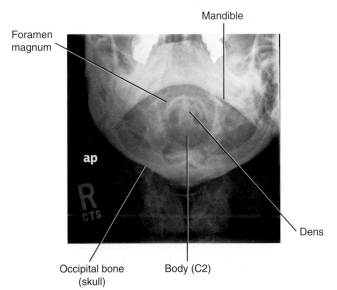
Fig. 8.72 AP projection for C1 to C2, odontoid process.

Evaluation Criteria
Anatomy Demonstrated • Odontoid process (dens) and other structures of C1 to C2 (Figs. 8.71 and 8.72).
Position • Dens should be centered within the foramen magnum. • **No rotation indicated** by the symmetric appearance of the mandible arched over the foramen magnum.

• **Correct extension** of head and neck indicated by the tip of the mandible clearing the superior portion of the dens and foramen magnum. • Collimation to **area of interest.**
Exposure • Clear demonstration of bony margins and trabecular markings of dens and other structures of C1 and C2 within foramen magnum • **No motion.**

AP "WAGGING JAW" PROJECTION: CERVICAL SPINE

OTTONELLO METHOD

WARNING: For trauma patients, do not remove cervical collar and do not move head or neck until authorized by a physician who has evaluated the horizontal beam lateral image or CT scan of the cervical spine.

Clinical Indications
- Pathology involving the odontoid process and surrounding bony structures of the C1 ring, as well as the entire cervical column

Cervical Spine
SPECIAL
- Cervicothoracic lateral (Swimmer's)
- Lateral—hyperflexion and hyperextension
- AP (Fuchs method), PA (Judd method)
- AP moving or "wagging jaw" (Ottonello method)

Technical Factors
- Minimum SID—40 inches (100 cm)
- IR size—8 × 10 inches (18 × 24 cm) or 10 × 12 inches (24 × 30 cm), portrait
- Grid
- Low mA and long (>2 seconds) exposure time
- kVp range: 70–85

18

24 R

No AEC because of long exposure

Shielding Shield radiosensitive tissues outside region of interest.

Patient Position—Supine Position Position patient in the supine position with arms at side and head on table surface, providing immobilization if needed.

Part Position
- Align midsagittal plane to CR and midline of table and/or IR.
- Adjust head so that a line drawn from lower margin of upper incisors to the base of the skull (mastoid tips) is perpendicular to table and/or IR (Figs. 8.73 and 8.74).
- Ensure **no rotation** of the head or thorax exists.
- Mandible must be in **continuous motion** during exposure.
- Ensure that only the mandible moves. The head must not move, and the teeth must not make contact.

CR
- CR perpendicular to IR.
- Direct CR to C4 (upper margin of thyroid cartilage).
- Center IR to CR.

Recommended Collimation Collimate on four sides to anatomy of interest.

Respiration Suspend respiration.

NOTE: Practice with patient before exposure to ensure that only the mandible is moving continuously, and that teeth do not make contact.

Evaluation Criteria
Anatomy Demonstrated: • C1 to C7 vertebral bodies with overlying blurred mandible (Figs. 8.75 and 8.76)
Position: • Accurate positioning indicated by demonstration of C1 and C2 without superimposition of maxillae or occipital bones. Optimal movement of mandible indicated by visualization of underlying cervical vertebrae. • Collimation to area of interest.
Exposure: • Clear demonstration of soft tissue margins and of bony margins and trabecular markings of cervical vertebrae. • Trabecular markings of upper vertebrae are somewhat masked by blurred mandible.

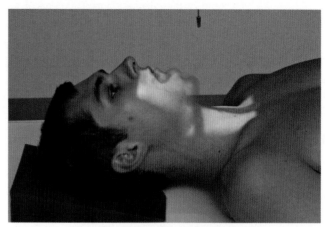

Fig. 8.73 Position for AP "wagging jaw."

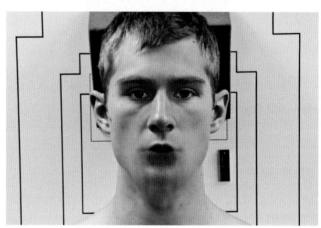

Fig. 8.74 AP "wagging jaw."

Odontoid process (dens)

Mandible (C2)

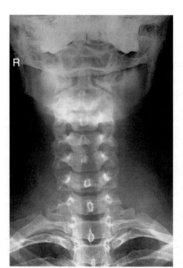

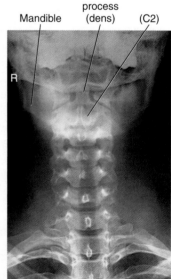

Fig. 8.75 AP radiograph of "wagging jaw" during exposure. (From Frank ED, Long BW, Smith BJ: *Merrill's atlas of radiographic positioning and procedures,* ed 11, St. Louis, 2007, Mosby.)

Fig. 8.76 AP "wagging jaw." (Modified from Frank ED, Long BW, Smith BJ: *Merrill's atlas of radiographic positioning and procedures,* ed 11, St. Louis, 2007, Mosby.)

AP AXIAL PROJECTION—VERTEBRAL ARCH (PILLARS): CERVICAL SPINE

WARNING: For trauma patients, do not remove cervical collar and do not move head or neck until authorized by a physician who has evaluated the horizontal beam lateral image or CT scan of the cervical spine.

Clinical Indications Pathology or trauma involving the posterior vertebral arch (particularly the pillars) of C4 to C7 and spinous processes of cervicothoracic vertebrae with whiplash-type injuries (see previous warning)

Cervical Spine
SPECIAL
• Cervicothoracic lateral (Swimmer's)
• Lateral—hyperflexion and hyperextension
• AP (Fuchs method), PA (Judd method)
• AP wagging jaw (Ottonello method)
• AP axial (pillars)

Technical Factors
- Minimum SID—40 inches (100 cm)
- IR size—10 × 12 inches (24 × 30 cm), portrait
- Grid
- kVp range: 70–85

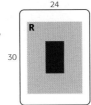

Shielding Shield radiosensitive tissues outside region of interest.

Patient Position—Supine Position Position patient in the supine position with arms at side.

Part Position
- Align midsagittal plane to CR and midline of table and/or IR.
- Hyperextend the neck if patient is able (see warning above) (Fig. 8.77).
- Ensure that **no rotation** of the head or thorax exists.

CR
- Angle CR 20° to 30° caudal.
- Direct CR to the lower margin of the thyroid cartilage and pass through C5 (see NOTE).
- Center IR to CR.

Recommended Collimation Collimate on four sides to anatomy of interest.

Respiration Suspend respiration. Ask patient to not swallow during the exposure.

NOTE: Sufficient hyperextension of neck and caudal CR angle is essential for demonstrating the posterior aspects of the mid and lower cervical vertebrae. The amount of the CR angle (20° to 30°) is determined by the amount of natural cervical lordotic curvature. Some support may have to be placed under the shoulders for sufficient hyperextension.

Evaluation Criteria
Anatomy Demonstrated • Posterior elements of mid and distal cervical and proximal thoracic vertebrae. • In particular, the articulations (zygapophyseal joints) between the lateral masses (or pillars) are open and well demonstrated, along with the laminae and spinous processes (Figs. 8.78 and 8.79).
Position • **No rotation** indicated by spinous processes equidistant from the lateral borders of the spinal column.
• The mandible and the base of the skull should be superimposed over the first two or three cervical vertebrae.
• Collimation to **area of interest.**
Exposure • Clear demonstration of soft tissue margins and of bony margins and trabecular markings of cervical vertebrae.

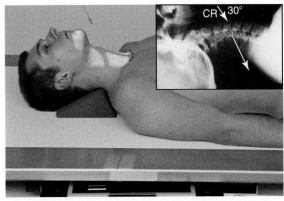

Fig. 8.77 AP axial (pillars), 20°–30° caudal angle. *Inset,* Demonstrates caudal CR angle parallel with zygapophyseal joint spaces.

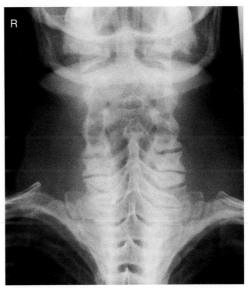

Fig. 8.78 AP axial (pillars). (Courtesy Teresa Easton-Porter.)

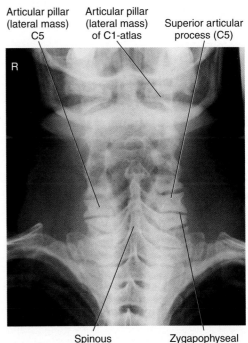

Articular pillar (lateral mass) C5   Articular pillar (lateral mass) of C1-atlas   Superior articular process (C5)

Spinous process (T1)   Zygapophyseal joint (C5-C6)

Fig. 8.79 AP axial (pillars).

AP PROJECTION: THORACIC SPINE

Clinical Indications
- Pathology involving the thoracic spine, such as compression fractures, subluxation, or kyphosis

Thoracic Spine
ROUTINE
• AP
• Lateral

Technical Factors
- Minimum SID—40 inches (100 cm)
- IR size—14 × 17 inches (35 × 43 cm), portrait
- Grid
- kVp range: 75–90
- Compensating filter useful in obtaining uniform brightness, density (thicker part of filter toward the upper vertebrae)

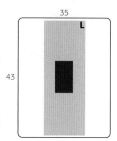

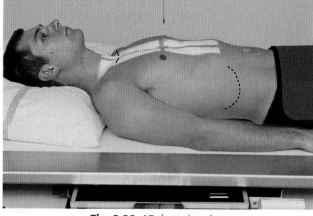

Fig. 8.80 AP thoracic spine.

Shielding Shield all radiosensitive tissues outside region of interest.

Patient Position—Recumbent and Erect Position
- Position patient supine (preferred) with arms at side and head on table or on a thin pillow. If patient cannot tolerate the supine position, place erect with arms at side and weight evenly distributed on both feet.
- The **anode heel effect** will create more uniform density throughout the thoracic spine. Place patient so the more intense aspect of the beam (cathode side) is over the thoracolumbar region of the spine.

Part Position
- Align midsagittal plane to CR and midline of table and/or IR (Fig. 8.80).
- **Flex knees and hips** to reduce thoracic curvature.
- Ensure that no rotation of thorax or pelvis exists.

CR
- CR perpendicular to IR.
- Direct CR to T7 (3 to 4 inches [8 to 10 cm] below jugular notch or 1 to 2 inches [2.5 to 5 cm] below sternal angle). Centering is similar to that used with AP chest.
- Center IR to CR.

Recommended Collimation Collimate on two sides of anatomy (four sides if possible).

Respiration Suspend respiration on **expiration**. Expiration reduces air volume in thorax for more uniform brightness and density.

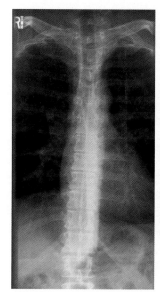

Fig. 8.81 AP thoracic spine. **Fig. 8.82** AP thoracic spine.

Left clavicle

First rib

Body (T8)

Posterior rib (T9)

Body (T12)

Evaluation Criteria
Anatomy Demonstrated • Thoracic vertebral bodies, intervertebral joint spaces, spinous and transverse processes, posterior ribs, and costovertebral articulations (Figs. 8.81 and 8.82).
Position • The spinal column from C7 to L1 centered to the midline of the IR. • **No rotation** indicated by sternoclavicular joints equidistant from the spine. • Collimation to **area of interest.**
Exposure • Clear demonstration of bony margins and trabecular markings of thoracic vertebrae. • **No motion.**

LATERAL POSITION: THORACIC SPINE

Clinical Indications
- Pathology involving the thoracic spine, such as compression fractures, subluxation, or kyphosis

NOTE: When upper thoracic vertebrae are of interest, perform the cervicothoracic (swimmer's) lateral position in addition to routine thoracic spine projections (see p. 319).

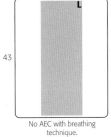

Thoracic Spine
ROUTINE
- AP
- Lateral

35
L

43

No AEC with breathing technique.

Technical Factors
- Minimum SID—40 inches (100 cm)
- IR size—14 × 17 inches (35 × 43 cm), portrait
- Grid
- kVp range: 80–95
- With orthostatic (breathing) technique, low mA and 2 to 3 seconds of exposure
- Lead mat placed on table behind patient to reduce scatter to IR (see NOTE 1)

Shielding Shield all radiosensitive tissues outside region of interest.

Patient Position—Lateral Recumbent or Erect Position Position patient in the lateral recumbent position, with head on pillow and knees flexed. For the erect position, place arms outstretched, with weight evenly distributed on both feet.

Part Position
- Align posterior half of thorax (between midcoronal plane and posterior aspect of thorax) to CR and midline of table and/or IR (Fig. 8.83).
- Raise patient's arms to right angles to body with elbows flexed.
- Support waist so entire spine is near parallel to table. Palpate spinous processes to determine alignment (see NOTE 2).
- Flex hips and knees, with support between the knees.
- Ensure that **no rotation** of shoulders or pelvis exists.

CR
- CR perpendicular to long axis of thoracic spine (see NOTE 2).
- Direct CR to T7 (3 to 4 inches [8 to 10 cm] below jugular notch or 7 to 8 inches [18 to 20 cm] below the vertebra prominens).
- Center IR to CR.

Recommended Collimation Collimate on two sides of anatomy (four sides if possible).

Respiration Use orthostatic breathing technique or suspend respiration. Suspended full inspiration can provide maximum uniform density of the vertebrae visualized above the diaphragm. A breathing technique is useful to blur unwanted rib and lung markings overlying thoracic vertebrae if the patient can cooperate. This breathing technique requires a minimum of 2 or 3 seconds of exposure time with a low mA setting.

NOTE 1: Significant amounts of secondary and scatter radiation are generated. Close collimation and placement of a lead mat posterior to the part are essential to maintaining image quality. This is particularly important with digital imaging.
NOTE 2: The optimal amount of support under the waist will cause the lower vertebrae to be the same distance from the tabletop as the upper vertebrae. A patient with wide hips will require substantially more support under the waist to prevent sag. A patient with broad shoulders may require a 10° to 15° cephalic CR angle if waist is not supported.

Evaluation Criteria
Anatomy Demonstrated • Thoracic vertebral bodies, intervertebral joint spaces, and intervertebral foramina. • T1 to T3 will not be well visualized. • Obtain a lateral image using a cervicothoracic (swimmer's) lateral if the upper thoracic vertebrae are of special interest (Figs. 8.84 and 8.85).
Position • Intervertebral disk spaces should be open. • **No rotation** indicated by superimposition of posterior aspects of vertebral bodies. • Because of greater OID on one side, the posterior ribs will not be directly superimposed, especially if a patient has a wide thorax. **No rotation** indicated by less than ½ inch (1.25 cm) of space between posterior ribs. • Collimation to **area of interest**.
Exposure • Clear demonstration of bony margins and trabecular markings of thoracic vertebrae. • **No motion**.

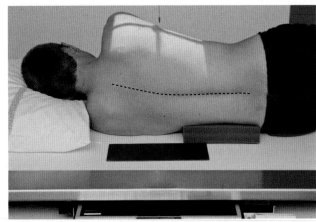

Fig. 8.83 Left lateral thoracic spine, with proper waist support.

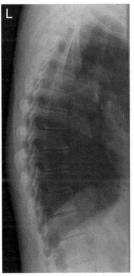

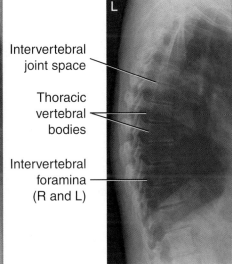

Intervertebral joint space

Thoracic vertebral bodies

Intervertebral foramina (R and L)

Fig. 8.84 Lateral thoracic with breathing technique.

Fig. 8.85 Lateral thoracic spine.

8

ANTERIOR OR POSTERIOR OBLIQUE POSITION: THORACIC SPINE

Clinical Indications
- Pathology involving the zygapophyseal joints of the thoracic spine
- Both right and left oblique projections are taken for comparison.

Thoracic Spine
SPECIAL
- Oblique

Technical Factors
- Minimum SID—40 inches (100 cm)
- IR size—14 × 17 inches (35 × 43 cm), portrait
- Grid
- kVp range: 80–95

Shielding Shield all radiosensitive tissues outside region of interest.

Patient Position—Oblique Anterior or Posterior Recumbent or Erect Positions
Initially position patient in the lateral recumbent position (preferred), with head on pillow and knees flexed. For the erect position, ensure equal distribution of weight on both feet.

Part Position
- Rotate the body 20° from true lateral to create a **70° oblique** from plane of table. Ensure equal rotation of shoulders and pelvis.
- Flex hips, knees, and arms for stability as needed.
- Align spinal column to CR and midline of table and/or IR.

Posterior Oblique Position (Recumbent)
- LPO or RPO: Place arm nearest table up and forward; arm nearest tube down and posterior (Fig. 8.86).

Anterior Oblique Position (Recumbent)
- LAO or RAO: Place arm nearest table down and posterior; arm nearest tube up and forward (Fig. 8.87).

Erect Anterior Oblique Position
- Distribute patient's weight equally on both feet.
- Rotate total body, shoulders, and pelvis 20° anterior from lateral.
- Flex elbow and place arm nearest IR on hip.
- Raise opposite arm and rest on top of head (Fig. 8.88).

CR
- CR perpendicular to IR.
- Direct CR to T7 (3 to 4 inches [8 to 10 cm] below jugular notch or 2 inches [5 cm] below sternal angle).
- Center IR to CR.

Recommended Collimation Collimate on two sides of anatomy (four sides if possible).

Respiration Suspend respiration on **full expiration**.

NOTE: Patient's thorax is 20° from lateral; some type of angle guide may be used to determine correct rotation (see Figs. 8.86 and 8.87).

Radiographs may be taken as posterior or anterior obliques. **Anterior obliques** are recommended because of significantly lower breast dose.

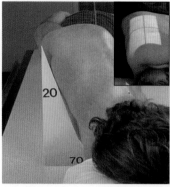 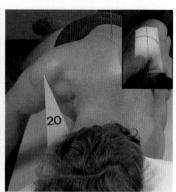

Fig. 8.86 Posterior oblique (RPO). **Fig. 8.87** Anterior oblique (LAO).

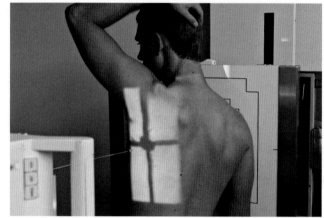

Fig. 8.88 Erect anterior oblique (RAO) thoracic spine.

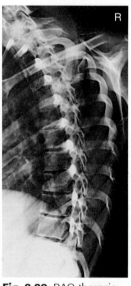 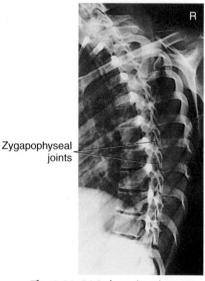

Zygapophyseal joints

Fig. 8.89 RAO thoracic spine. **Fig. 8.90** RAO thoracic spine.

Evaluation Criteria
Anatomy Demonstrated: • Zygapophyseal joints: Anterior oblique positions (RAO and LAO) demonstrate the downside zygapophyseal joints (Figs. 8.89 and 8.90), and posterior oblique positions (RPO and LPO) demonstrate the upside joints.

Position • The zygapophyseal joints of the side of interest should be open. However, the amount of kyphosis will determine how many zygapophyseal joints will be clearly seen.
Exposure • Clear demonstration of bony margins and trabecular markings of thoracic vertebrae.

RADIOGRAPHS FOR CRITIQUE

This section consists of an ideal projection (Image A) along with one or more projections that may demonstrate positioning and/or technical errors. Critique Figures C8.91 through C8.96. Compare Image A to the other projections and identify the errors. While examining each image, consider the following questions:

1. Is all essential anatomy demonstrated on the image?
2. What positioning errors are present that compromise image quality?
3. Are technical factors optimal?

4. Is there evidence of collimation and pre-exposure anatomic side markers visible on the image?
5. Do these errors require a repeat exposure? Feedback for each set of images is located on the faculty Evolve site.

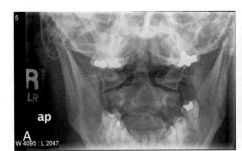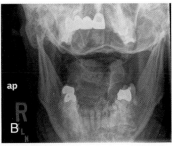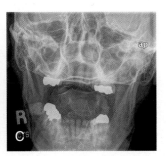

Fig. C8.91 AP open mouth (C1–C2).

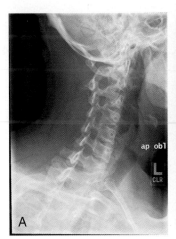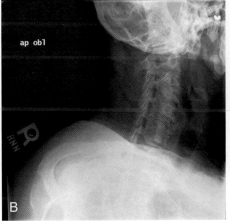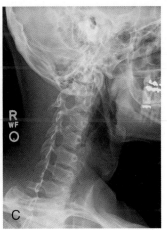

Fig. C8.92 Left posterior oblique (LPO).

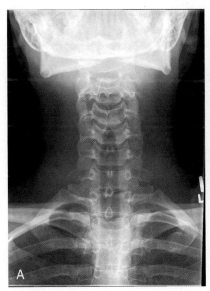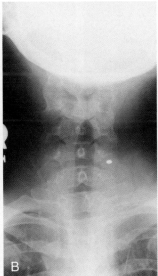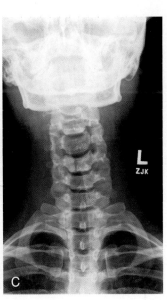

Fig. C8.93 AP axial C spine.

8

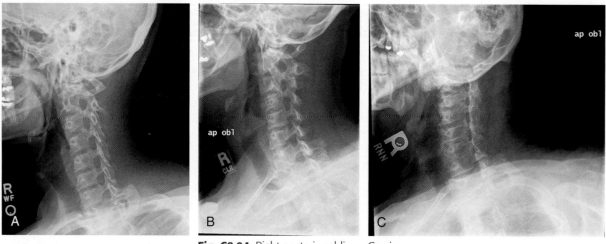

Fig. C8.94 Right posterior oblique C spine.

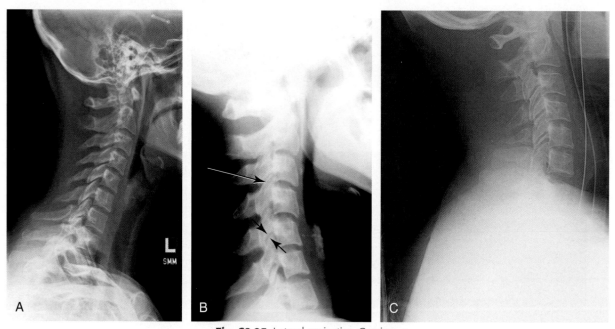

Fig. C8.95 Lateral projection C spine.

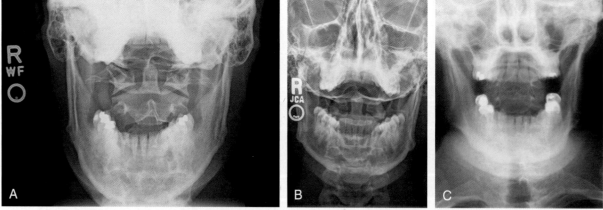

Fig. C8.96 AP open mouth (C1–C2).

CHAPTER 9

Lumbar Spine, Sacrum, and Coccyx

CONTRIBUTIONS BY **Patti Ward,** PHD, RT(R)

CONTRIBUTORS TO PAST EDITIONS Alex Backus, MS, RT(R), Cindy Murphy, BHSc, RT(R), ACR

CONTENTS

RADIOGRAPHIC ANATOMY

This chapter describes anatomy and positioning of the **lumbar, sacrum,** and **coccyx** sections of the vertebral column. Refer to Chapter 8 for more detailed information about vertebral anatomy.

Lumbar Vertebrae

The largest individual vertebrae are the **five lumbar vertebrae.** These vertebrae are the strongest in the vertebral column because the load of body weight increases toward the inferior end of the column. For this reason, the cartilaginous disks between the inferior lumbar vertebrae are common sites for injury and pathologic processes.

LATERAL AND SUPERIOR PERSPECTIVES

Patients typically have five lumbar vertebrae located just inferior to the 12 thoracic vertebrae. Fig. 9.1 illustrates the lateral perspective of a typical lumbar vertebra. Lumbar vertebral bodies are larger in comparison with thoracic and cervical vertebral bodies. The most inferior body, L5, is the largest. The **transverse processes** are small, whereas the posteriorly projecting **spinous process** is bulky and blunt. The palpable lower tip of each lumbar spinous process lies at the level of the intervertebral disk space inferior to each vertebral body.

Intervertebral Foramina

Fig. 9.2 shows the **intervertebral foramen** situated 90° relative to the midsagittal plane. Intervertebral foramina are spaces or openings between **pedicles** when two vertebrae are stacked on each other. Along the upper surface of each pedicle is a half-moon-shaped area called the *superior vertebral notch,* and along the lower surface of each pedicle is another half-moon-shaped area called the *inferior vertebral notch.* When vertebrae are stacked, the superior and inferior vertebral notches line up, and the two half-moon-shaped areas form a single opening, the **intervertebral foramina** (see Chapter 8, Figs. 8.8 and 8.9). Therefore, between every two vertebrae are two intervertebral foramina, one on each side, through which important spinal nerves and blood vessels pass. The intervertebral foramina in the lumbar region are demonstrated best on a lateral radiographic image.

Zygapophyseal Joints

Each typical vertebra has four articular processes that project from the area of the junction of the pedicles and laminae. The processes that project upward are called the *superior articular processes* and the processes that project downward are the *inferior articular processes.* The term *facet (fas-ət)* sometimes is used interchangeably with the term *zygapophyseal joint;* the facet is actually only the articulating surface instead of the entire superior or inferior articular process. Fig. 9.1 shows the relative positions of the superior and inferior lumbar articular processes from the lateral perspective.

The zygapophyseal joints form an angle open from **30° to 50°** to the midsagittal plane, as shown in Fig. 9.2. The upper or proximal lumbar vertebrae are nearer the 50° angle and the lower or distal lumbar vertebrae are nearer 30°. Radiographic demonstration of the zygapophyseal joints is achieved by rotating the patient's body an average of 45°.

The **laminae** form a bridge between the transverse processes, lateral masses, and spinous process (see Fig. 9.2). The portion of each lamina between the superior and inferior articular processes is the *pars interarticularis.* The pars interarticularis is demonstrated radiographically on the oblique lumbar image.

POSTERIOR AND ANTERIOR PERSPECTIVES

Fig. 9.3 demonstrates the general appearance of a lumbar vertebra as seen from the anterior and posterior perspectives. Anteroposterior (AP) or posteroanterior (PA) radiographic projections of the lumbar spine demonstrate the **spinous processes** superimposed on the vertebral bodies. The **transverse processes** are demonstrated protruding laterally beyond the edges of the vertebral body.

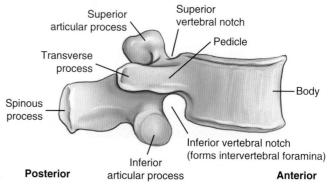

Fig. 9.1 Lumbar vertebra—lateral view.

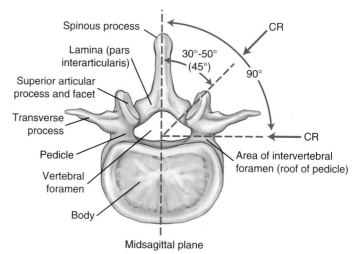

Fig. 9.2 Lumbar vertebra—superior view.

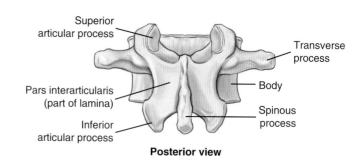

Posterior view

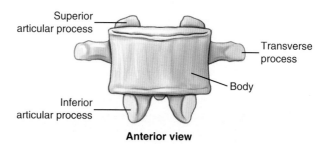

Anterior view

Fig. 9.3 Lumbar vertebra—posterior and anterior views.

Sacrum

The **sacrum** is inferior to the lumbar vertebrae.

ANTERIOR PERSPECTIVE

Fig. 9.4 illustrates the concave anterior surface of a sacrum. The bodies of the original five segments fuse into a single bone in the adult. The sacrum is shovel-shaped, with the apex pointed inferiorly and anteriorly. Four sets of **pelvic (anterior) sacral foramina** (similar to intervertebral foramina in more superior sections of the spine) transmit nerves and blood vessels.

The **alae,** or wings, of the sacrum are large masses of bone lateral to the first sacral segment. The two **superior articular processes** of the sacrum form zygapophyseal joints with the inferior articular processes of the fifth lumbar vertebrae.

LATERAL PERSPECTIVE

Fig. 9.5 clearly illustrates the dominant **convex** curve **(posterior perspective)** of the sacrum and forward projection of the coccyx. These curves determine how the central ray must be angled differently for AP radiographic projections of the sacrum or coccyx.

The anterior ridge of the body of the first sacral segment helps form the posterior wall of the inlet of the true pelvis and is termed the *promontory* of the sacrum; it is best demonstrated from a lateral perspective (see Fig. 9.5).

Posterior to the body of the first sacral segment is the opening to the **sacral canal,** which is a continuation of the vertebral canal and contains certain sacral nerves. The **median sacral crest** is formed by fused spinous processes of the sacral vertebrae.

Figs. 9.5 and 9.6 illustrate the relative roughness and irregularity of the posterior surface of the sacrum compared with the anterior or pelvic surface.

The sacrum articulates with the ilium of the pelvis at the **auricular surface** (marked A in Figs. 9.5 and 9.6) to form the sacroiliac joint. The auricular surface is so named because of its resemblance in shape to the auricle of the ear. Refer to Chapter 7 for more detailed information about the sacroiliac joints.

The **sacral horns** (cornua) (marked D in Figs. 9.5 and 9.6) are small tubercles that represent the inferior articular processes projecting inferiorly from each side of the fifth sacral segment. They project inferiorly and posteriorly to articulate with the corresponding **horns** (cornua) of the **coccyx.**

POSTERIOR SACRUM

Fig. 9.6 is a photograph of an actual sacrum, as seen from the posterior aspect. Clearly seen is the large, wedge-shaped **auricular surface** (A), which articulates with a similar surface on the ilium to form the **sacroiliac joint.** Each sacroiliac joint opens **obliquely at an angle of 30°.**

The **articulating facets of the superior articular processes** (B) also open to the rear and are shown on this photograph. There are eight **posterior sacral foramina** (C), four on each side, corresponding to the same number of anterior sacral foramina.

The **sacral horns** (cornua; D) are seen as small bony projections at the very inferoposterior aspect of the sacrum. Remnants of the enclosed sacral canal (E) also can be seen. (Deteriorating bone leaves the canal partially open on this bone specimen.)

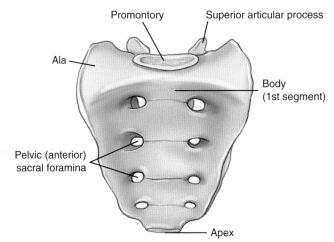

Fig. 9.4 Sacrum—anterior view.

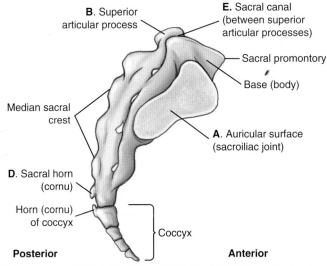

Fig. 9.5 Sacrum and coccyx—lateral view.

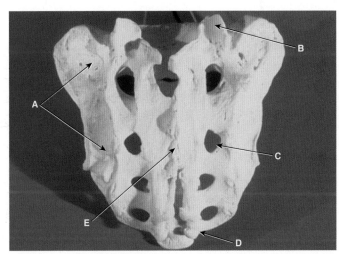

Fig. 9.6 Sacrum—posterior view.

Coccyx

ANTERIOR COCCYX

The most distal portion of the vertebral column is the **coccyx.** The anterior surface of the tailbone, or coccyx, is illustrated in Fig. 9.7. This portion of the vertebral column has greatly regressed in humans, so little resemblance to vertebrae remains. Three to five coccygeal segments (an average of four) have fused in the adult to form the single coccyx. The drawing in Fig. 9.7 demonstrates four formerly separate segments present in a child, now fused into a single bone as an adult. The photograph of a coccyx in Fig. 9.8 demonstrates five segments now mostly fused in the adult coccyx.

The most superior segment is the largest and broadest of the four sections and even has two lateral projections that are small *transverse processes.* The distal pointed tip of the coccyx is termed the *apex,* whereas the broader superior portion is termed the *base.*

Occasionally, the second segment does not fuse solidly with the larger first segment (see Fig. 9.8); however, the coccyx usually is one small, insignificant end of the vertebral column.

POSTERIOR COCCYX

The posterior aspect of an actual coccyx is pictured in Fig. 9.8 along with a common U.S. postage stamp to allow comparison of the two sizes. (Note that a portion of the transverse process is missing on the upper right aspect of this specimen.)

LATERAL SACRUM AND COCCYX RADIOGRAPH

The lateral sacrum on the radiograph in Fig. 9.9 is seen as a large solid bone as compared with the much smaller coccyx. The long axis of the sacrum is shown to be angled posteriorly, requiring a cephalad angle of the central ray (CR) on an AP projection. This angle is greater in an average woman as compared with an average man.

Ordinarily, the coccyx curves anteriorly, as can be seen and identified on this lateral radiograph, so that the apex points toward the symphysis pubis of the anterior pelvis. This forward curvature frequently is more pronounced in men and is less pronounced, with less curvature, in women. The coccyx projects into the birth canal in the woman and, if angled excessively forward, can impede the birth process.

The most common injury associated with the coccyx results from a direct blow to the lower vertebral column when a person is in a sitting position. This type of injury results from falling backward with a forceful sitting action. Also of note is that because of the shape of the female pelvis and the more vertical orientation of the coccyx, a female patient is more likely to experience a fracture of the coccyx than a male patient.

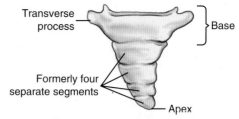

Fig. 9.7 Coccyx—anterior view.

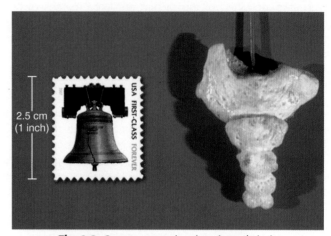

Fig. 9.8 Coccyx—posterior view (actual size).

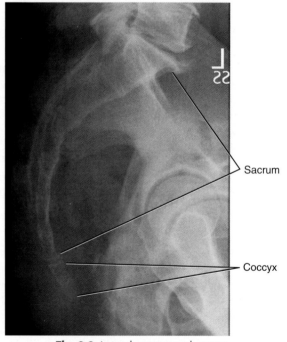

Fig. 9.9 Lateral sacrum and coccyx.

9

Anatomy Review
SUPEROINFERIOR PROJECTION
The radiograph in Fig. 9.10 demonstrates certain parts of an individual lumbar vertebra taken from a disarticulated skeleton; these parts are labeled as follows:

    A. Spinous process
    B. Lamina
    C. Pedicle
    D. Vertebral foramen
    E. Body
    F. Transverse process

LATERAL POSITION
Parts labeled A through F on the lateral view (Fig. 9.11) of a disarticulated lumbar vertebra are as follows:

    A. Body
    B. Inferior vertebral notch, or the floor of the pedicle making up the upper portion of the rounded intervertebral foramen
    C. Area of the articulating facet of the inferior articular process (actual articular facet not shown on this lateral view); makes up the zygapophyseal joints when vertebrae are stacked
    D. Spinous process
    E. Superior articular process
    F. Pedicle

Note that this lateral view would open and demonstrate the intervertebral foramina well (the larger round opening directly under B, the inferior vertebral notch). However, it would not demonstrate the zygapophyseal joints; this would require a 45° oblique view.

AP PROJECTION
Individual structures are more difficult to identify when the vertebrae are superimposed by the soft tissues of the abdomen, as demonstrated on the AP lumbar spine radiograph in Fig. 9.12. These structures, labeled A through F, are as follows:

    A. Right transverse process of L5
    B. Lower lateral portion of the body of L4
    C. Lower part of the spinous process of L4, as visualized on end
    D. Right inferior articular process of L3
    E. Left superior articular process of L4
    F. L1–L2 intervertebral disk space

The facets of the inferior and superior articular processes (D and E) create the zygapophyseal joint not visualized on this AP projection. However, the joint is demonstrated on a 45° oblique projection of lumbar vertebrae (see Fig. 9.16).

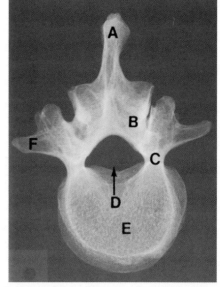

Fig. 9.10 Lumbar vertebra (superoinferior projection).

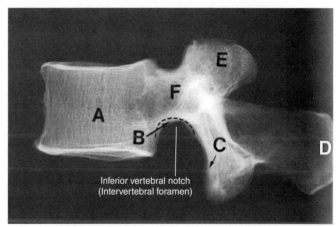

Inferior vertebral notch
(Intervertebral foramen)

Fig. 9.11 Lumbar vertebra (lateral projection).

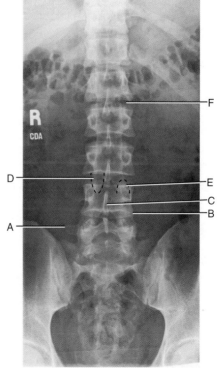

Fig. 9.12 Lumbar spine (AP projection).

LATERAL LUMBOSACRAL SPINE

A radiograph of the entire lumbosacral spine in the lateral position (Fig. 9.13) shows the following:
   A. Body of L1
   B. Body of L3
   C. Intervertebral disk space between L4 and L5
   D. Body of L5
   E. Superimposed intervertebral foramina between L1 and L2

AP LUMBOSACRAL SPINE

The AP projection of the entire lumbosacral spine, shown in Fig. 9.14, is labeled as follows:
   A. Last thoracic vertebra (T12)
   B. First lumbar vertebra (L1)
   C. Third lumbar vertebra (L3)
   D. Fifth lumbar vertebra (L5)

Oblique Lumbar Vertebrae

APPEARANCE OF "SCOTTIE DOG"

Any bone and its parts, when seen in an oblique position, are more difficult to recognize than the same bone seen in the conventional frontal or lateral view. A vertebra is no exception; however, imagination can help us in the case of the lumbar vertebrae. A good 45° oblique projects the various structures in such a way that a "Scottie dog" seems to appear. Fig. 9.15 shows the various components of the Scottie dog. The head and neck of the dog are probably the easiest features to recognize. The neck is one **pars interarticularis** (part of the lamina that primarily makes up the shoulder region of the dog). The **ear** of the dog is one **superior articular process,** whereas the **eye** is formed by one **pedicle.** One **transverse process** forms the **nose.** The **front legs** are formed by one **inferior articular process.**

OBLIQUE LUMBAR RADIOGRAPH

Fig. 9.16 shows the Scottie dog appearance that should be visible on oblique radiographs of the lumbar spine. The right posterior oblique (RPO) radiograph is labeled as follows:
   A. Nose of the Scottie dog, formed by one transverse process
   B. Eye, one pedicle seen on end
   C. Neck of the dog, which is the pars interarticularis
   D. Front leg of the dog, formed by one inferior articular process
   E. Pointed ear, one of the superior articular processes
   F. Zygapophyseal joint, formed by front leg of the Scottie above and ear of the Scottie below

Each of the five lumbar vertebrae should assume a similar Scottie dog appearance, with zygapophyseal joint spaces open on a correctly rotated lumbar radiograph.

Classification of Joints

Two types of classifications of joints, or articulations, involve the vertebral column.

ZYGAPOPHYSEAL JOINTS

The zygapophyseal joints between the superior and inferior articular processes are classified as **synovial** joints. These joints are lined with synovial membrane. They are **diarthrodial,** or freely movable, with a **plane (gliding) type** of movement.

INTERVERTEBRAL JOINTS

The intervertebral joints between the bodies of any two vertebrae contain intervertebral disks that are made up of fibrocartilage and are only slightly movable. These joints, which are tightly bound by cartilage, thus are classified as **cartilaginous joints.** They are **amphiarthrodial** (slightly movable) joints of the **symphysis subclass,** similar to the intervertebral joints of the cervical and thoracic spine, as described in the preceding chapter.

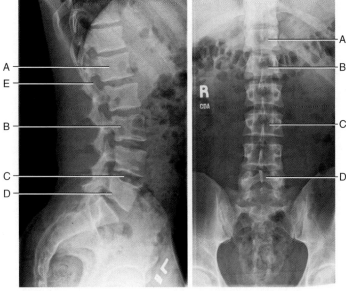

Fig. 9.13 Lumbosacral spine—lateral. **Fig. 9.14** Lumbosacral spine—AP.

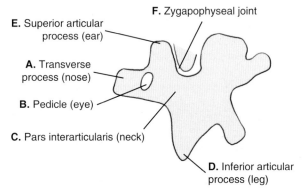

E. Superior articular process (ear)
F. Zygapophyseal joint
A. Transverse process (nose)
B. Pedicle (eye)
C. Pars interarticularis (neck)
D. Inferior articular process (leg)

Fig. 9.15 The "Scottie dog."

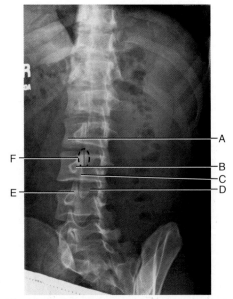

Fig. 9.16 Oblique lumbar spine (Scottie dog).

A great deal of motion is not evident between any two vertebrae, but the combined effects of all vertebrae in the column allow a considerable range of motion. Possible movements include flexion, extension, lateral flexion (bending), and rotation. Certain radiographic examinations of the spinal column involving hyperflexion and hyperextension and/or right- and left-bending routines can measure this range of motion.

Intervertebral Foramina Versus Zygapophyseal Joints

INTERVERTEBRAL FORAMINA—LATERAL LUMBAR SPINE
The intervertebral foramina for the lumbar spine are visualized on a true lateral projection, as demonstrated in Fig. 9.13.

ZYGAPOPHYSEAL JOINTS—OBLIQUE LUMBAR SPINE
Positioning for oblique projections of the lumbar spine requires a good understanding of the anatomy of the vertebrae and the zygapophyseal joints. It is important to know how much to rotate the patient and which joint is being demonstrated.

Posterior Oblique
As the drawing and photographs of the skeleton demonstrate, the **downside** joints are visualized on **posterior** oblique positions. The downside zygapophyseal joints are not visible on the skeleton because they are "under" the bodies of the vertebrae (Fig. 9.17), but as seen on the inferosuperior sectional drawing, the downside joints would be demonstrated on a posterior oblique (Fig. 9.18). The RPO radiograph in Fig. 9.19, clearly shows the ears and legs of the Scottie dogs, or the right zygapophyseal joints (arrow).

Anterior Oblique
The anterior oblique position may be more comfortable for the patient and may allow the natural lumbar curvature of the spine to coincide with the divergence of the x-ray beam.

As demonstrated, an **anterior** oblique visualizes the **upside** joints. Therefore, a right anterior oblique (RAO) visualizes the upside, or left, zygapophyseal joints (Figs. 9.20, 9.21, and 9.22).

The degree of rotation depends on which area of the lumbar spine is of specific interest. A 45° oblique is used for the general lumbar region, but if interest is specifically focused on **L1** or **L2**, the degree of rotation may be increased to **50°**. If interest is in the **L5–S1** area, rotation may be decreased to **30°** from an AP or PA projection. Some variance is seen among patients but in general, the upper lumbar region requires more degrees of rotation than the lower regions. The reason is that the upper lumbar vertebrae take on some shape characteristics of the thoracic vertebrae, which require 70° of rotation to demonstrate the zygapophyseal joints, as described in Chapter 8.

Table 9.1 lists lumbar (L) spine joint and foramina positioning, and Table 9.2 lists joint classifications of the L spine.

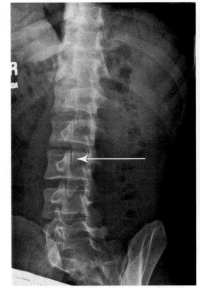
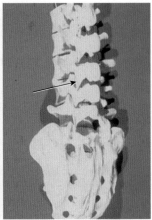

Fig. 9.20 Anterior oblique lumbar spine. RAO—upside, or left, joints.

Fig. 9.19 Posterior oblique lumbar spine. RPO—downside, or right, joints.

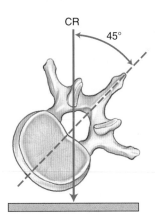

Fig. 9.21 Anterior oblique—upside joints.

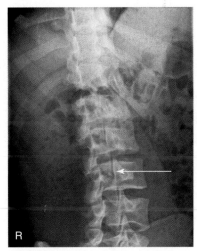

Fig. 9.22 Anterior oblique lumbar spine. RAO—upside, or left, joints.

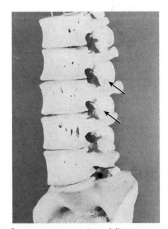

Fig. 9.17 Posterior oblique—downside joints.

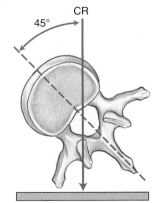

Fig. 9.18 Posterior oblique—downside joints.

TABLE 9.1 SUMMARY OF LUMBAR SPINE JOINT AND FORAMINA POSITIONING

INTERVERTEBRAL FORAMINA—90° LATERAL	ZYGAPOPHYSEAL JOINTS—45° OBLIQUE
R or L Lateral	Posterior oblique—downside
	RPO—Right joints
	LPO—Left joints
	Anterior oblique—upside
	RAO—Left joints
	LAO—right joints

TABLE 9.2 SUMMARY OF JOINT CLASSIFICATIONS OF LUMBAR SPINE

JOINTS	CLASSIFICATION	MOBILITY TYPE	MOVEMENT TYPE
Zygapophyseal joints	Synovial	Diarthrodial	Plane (gliding)
Intervertebral joints	Cartilaginous (symphysis)	Amphiarthrodial (slightly movable)	N/A

RADIOGRAPHIC POSITIONING

Topographic Landmarks

Correct positioning for the coccyx, sacrum, and lumbar spine requires a thorough understanding of specific topographic landmarks that can be easily palpated.

The most reliable landmarks for the spine are various palpable bony prominences that are consistent from one person to another. However, the landmarks presented refer to an average-sized, healthy, erect, typically developed male or female. These landmarks vary in subjects with anatomic and, especially, skeletal anomalies. The very young and the very old also have slightly different features from those of the average adult. Refer to the bariatric patient considerations in the following pages for tips to locate bony anatomy when palpation is inadequate.

LOWER SPINE LANDMARKS

The drawings on the right illustrate various landmarks relative to the lower vertebral column (Fig. 9.23).

A. This corresponds to the superior margin of the **symphysis pubis.** The **prominence** of the **greater trochanter** is at about the same level as the superior border of the symphysis pubis.

B. The **anterior superior iliac spine** (ASIS) is approximately the same level (B) as the **first or second sacral segment.**

C. This is the most superior portion of the **iliac crest** and is at approximately the same level as the junction of the **L4–L5 vertebrae.**

D. The lowest margin of the ribs or **lower costal margin** (D) is at the approximate level of **L2** to **L3.**

E. The **xiphoid tip** is approximately at the level of **T9–T10.**

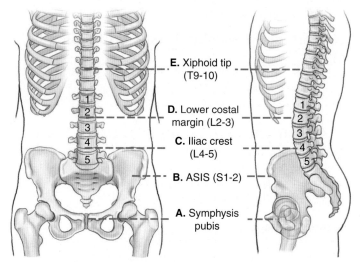

E. Xiphoid tip (T9-10)

D. Lower costal margin (L2-3)

C. Iliac crest (L4-5)

B. ASIS (S1-2)

A. Symphysis pubis

Fig. 9.23 Lower spine landmarks.

Positioning Considerations

PATIENT RADIATION PROTECTION

Use of gonadal shielding and close collimation is especially important in dose reduction because of the proximity of the lumbar spine, sacrum, and coccyx to the gonads. Gonadal shielding can and should **always be used on male patients** of reproductive age on coccyx, sacrum, or lumbar spine radiographs. The gonadal shield should be placed with the top edge of the shield at the lower margin of the symphysis pubis (Fig. 9.24).

If the area of interest includes the sacrum and/or coccyx, gonadal shielding for females may not be possible without obscuring essential anatomy.

Females of childbearing age always must be questioned regarding the possibility of pregnancy before any radiographic examination of the lower vertebral column is begun.

PATIENT POSITION

AP projections of the lumbar spine when the patient is recumbent are obtained with the **knees flexed.** Flexing the knees (Fig. 9.25) reduces the lumbar curvature (lordosis), bringing the back closer to the radiographic examination table and the lumbar vertebral column more parallel to the image receptor (IR). Also, **flexing the knees allows for greater patient comfort.**

The incorrect position is shown in Fig. 9.26, where the pelvis is tipped forward slightly when the lower limbs are extended, exaggerating the lumbar curvature.

PA Versus AP Projections

Even though the AP projection (with knees flexed) is a common part of the routine for the lumbar spine, the PA projection offers an advantage. The prone position places the lumbar spine with its natural lumbar curvature in such a way that the intervertebral disk spaces are almost parallel to the divergent x-ray beam. This position opens and provides better visualization of the margins of the intervertebral disk spaces. Another advantage of the PA projection in females is a lower ovarian dose, 25% to 30% less for a PA projection compared with an AP. However, a disadvantage of the PA projection is the increased object–image receptor distance (OID) of the lumbar vertebrae, which results in magnification unsharpness, especially for a patient with a large abdomen.

EXPOSURE FACTORS

Higher kVp and lower mAs reduces patient doses for all imaging systems. Typically, digital kVp ranges are higher than analog systems. Although higher kVp will produce more scatter radiation, close collimation, use of grids, and table masking for lateral projections will minimize its impact on image quality.

Lead Masking on Tabletop

See the section Digital Imaging Considerations later in the chapter, which details the importance of this practice along with close collimation, especially with digital imaging.

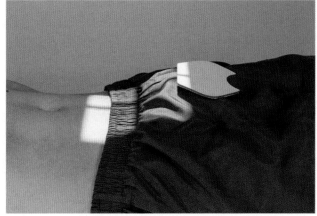

Fig. 9.24 Male gonadal shielding.

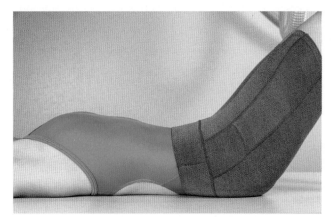

Fig. 9.25 Correct—knees and hips flexed (AP lumbar spine).

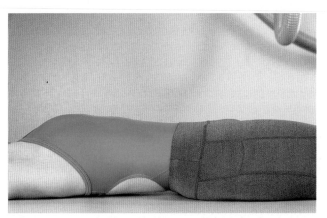

Fig. 9.26 Incorrect—lower limbs extended (AP lumbar spine).

SID

The minimum SID is typically 40 inches (100 cm), but an increased SID of 42, 44, or even 48 inches (105, 110, or 120 cm) may be used in some departments to reduce magnification. This depends on equipment specifications and on department protocol.

PART-IR ALIGNMENT

Correct part-IR alignment is important during radiography of the lower vertebral column to ensure that the beam passes through the intervertebral disk spaces. This alignment may require placement of a radiolucent sponge under the patient's waist while in the lateral position to ensure that the spine is parallel with the IR (Fig. 9.27). If a sponge is required, the appropriate size is determined by the patient's body habitus.

Special Patient Considerations

PEDIATRIC APPLICATIONS

Patient Motion and Safety

Two primary concerns in pediatric radiography are **patient motion** and **safety.** A clear explanation of this procedure is required if maximal trust and cooperation are to be obtained from the patient and guardian.

Careful immobilization is important for achieving proper positioning and reducing patient motion. A short exposure time helps reduce patient motion.

To secure their safety, pediatric patients should be continuously watched and cared for. See Chapter 16 for detailed communication strategies, immobilization techniques, and explanations.

Communication

Clear, simple instructions and communication are important, and distraction techniques such as toys or stuffed animals are effective in maintaining patient cooperation.

Immobilization

Pediatric patients (depending on age and condition) often are unable to maintain the required position. Use of immobilization devices to support the patient is recommended to reduce the need for the patient to be held, thus reducing radiation exposure. (Chapter 16 provides an in-depth description of these devices.) If the patient must be held by the guardian, the technologist must provide a lead apron and/or gloves and, if the guardian is female, it must be ensured that there is no possibility of pregnancy.

Technical Factors

Technical factors vary with patient size. Use of **short exposure times** (associated with the use of high mA) is recommended to reduce the risk of patient motion.

GERIATRIC APPLICATIONS

Communication and Comfort

Sensory loss (e.g., eyesight, hearing) associated with aging may result in the need for additional assistance, time, and patience in achieving the required positions for spinal radiography in the geriatric patient. Decreased position awareness may cause these patients to fear falling off the radiography table when they are imaged in the recumbent position. Reassurance and additional care from the technologist help the patient to feel secure and comfortable.

If the examination is performed with the patient in the recumbent position, a radiolucent mattress or pad placed on the examination table provides comfort. Extra blankets may be required to keep the patient warm. Patients with severe kyphosis may be more comfortable if positioned for images in the erect position.

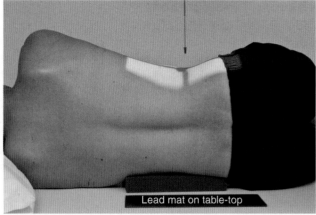

Fig. 9.27 Lateral lumbar spine with lead masking on tabletop.

Technical Factors

Because of the high incidence of osteoporosis in geriatric patients, the kVp or mAs may require a decrease.

Older patients may have tremors or difficulty holding steady. Use of short exposure times (associated with the use of higher mA) is recommended to reduce the risk of motion.

BARIATRIC PATIENT CONSIDERATIONS

Palpation of topographic landmarks can be difficult with the bariatric patient. The top of the gonadal shield must not be above the symphysis pubis. To locate the symphysis pubis, ask the patient to flex the knees and hips. The symphysis pubis is slightly superior to the level of the crease of the thigh. It may be necessary to lift the abdominal panniculus adiposus (fatty apron) to visualize the crease.[1]

Bariatric patients may present some challenges when positioning for lumbar spine, sacral, and coccygeal images. Additional density from adipose tissue and pannicular folds may require an increase in technical factors. An increase in kVp to improve penetration through additionally thick tissue may be necessary. mA and time may also be increased; however, a technologist must always follow recommendations based on the ALARA principle (exposure to the patient *as low as reasonably achievable*) to avoid excessive radiation exposure. Measures must also be taken to reduce scatter radiation exposure to the IR because of the increased amount of tissue. A grid can be used for anatomic structures over 10 cm to decrease the amount of scatter reaching the IR. Tight collimation to the anatomy of interest will also help to reduce the amount of scatter radiation reaching the IR. The location of the lumbar spine sacral and coccygeal anatomy will be aligned similarly in the general population of patients. Use known external landmarks and previously discussed tips for identifying the location of the anatomy of interest.

Digital Imaging Considerations

The following guidelines are important for digital imaging of the lumbar spine, sacrum, and coccyx:

1. **Correct centering** (this allows for accurate processing by the image reader): This is especially important for projections such as the L5–S1 joint, the sacrum, and/or the coccyx.
2. **Close collimation and tabletop lead masking:** This improves image quality by reducing scatter and secondary exposure to the highly sensitive digital image receptors.
3. **Adherence to the ALARA principle** in determining exposure factors: Increasing kVp for lumbar spine studies reduces patient dose.
4. **Post-processing evaluation of exposure indicator:** This becomes an important consideration with lumbar spine, sacrum, and coccyx projections to ensure **optimum image**

quality with the least radiation to the patient. (Remember, some of these projections may include primary exposure, in addition to secondary and scatter radiation to the reproductive organs.)

Alternative Modalities and Procedures
COMPUTED TOMOGRAPHY
Computed tomography (CT) is useful for evaluation of the vertebral column. A wide range of pathologic conditions is demonstrated on sectional images, including the presence and extent of fractures, disk disease, and neoplastic disease.

MAGNETIC RESONANCE IMAGING
Magnetic resonance imaging (MRI) is superior for the evaluation of soft tissue structures of the lumbar spine (i.e., the spinal cord and intervertebral disk spaces).

NUCLEAR MEDICINE TECHNOLOGY
Nuclear medicine (NM) provides a sensitive diagnostic procedure, the radionuclide bone scan, for detection of skeletal pathologic processes. A radiopharmaceutical-tagged tracer element is injected that concentrates in areas of increased bone activity, demonstrating a hot spot on the nuclear medicine image. Any abnormal area is then investigated further with radiography.

Commonly, patients who are at risk or are symptomatic for skeletal metastases undergo a bone scan; patients with multiple myeloma are an exception to this. The vertebral column is a common site of skeletal metastases. Inflammatory conditions, Paget disease, neoplastic processes, and osteomyelitis also may be demonstrated on the bone scan.

BONE DENSITOMETRY
Bone densitometry is the noninvasive measurement of bone mass (see Chapter 20). The lumbar spine is often assessed in a bone density study. Causes for loss of bone mass (osteoporosis) include long-term steroid use, hyperparathyroidism, estrogen deficiency, advancing age, and lifestyle factors (e.g., smoking, sedentary lifestyle, alcoholism). Bone densitometry is accurate to within 1%, and the radiation skin dose is very low. Conventional radiography does not detect loss of bone until bone mass has been reduced by at least 30%.

MYELOGRAPHY
Myelography requires injection of contrast medium into the subarachnoid space via a lumbar or cervical puncture to visualize the soft tissue structures of the spinal canal. Lesions of the spinal canal, nerve roots, and intervertebral disks are demonstrated. Post-injection CT imaging may be included.

The increase in availability of CT and MRI has greatly reduced the number of myelograms performed. In addition to the superior diagnostic quality of these modalities, avoidance of invasive puncture and contrast injection is beneficial for the patient.

Clinical Indications
Ankylosing spondylitis: This systemic illness of unknown origin involves the spine and larger joints. It predominantly affects men from ages 20 to 40 years and results in pain and stiffness that result from inflammation of the sacroiliac, intervertebral, and costovertebral joints, in addition to paraspinal calcification, with ossification and ankylosis (union of bones) of the spinal joints.

It may cause complete rigidity of the spine and thorax, which usually is seen first in the sacroiliac joints.

Fractures reflect lack of continuity of a structure:
- **Compression fractures** may be due to trauma, osteoporosis, or metastatic disease. The superior and inferior surfaces of the vertebral body are driven together, producing a wedge-shaped vertebra. For patients with osteoporosis or other vertebral pathologic processes, the force needed to cause this fracture type may be minor (e.g., lifting light objects). This type of fracture rarely causes a neurologic deficit.
- **Chance fractures** result from a hyperflexion force that causes fracture through the vertebral body and posterior elements (e.g., spinous process, pedicles, facets, transverse processes). Patients wearing lap-type seat belts are at risk because these belts act as a fulcrum during sudden deceleration.

Herniated nucleus pulposus (HNP), also commonly known as a *herniated lumbar disk* (slipped disk), is usually due to trauma or improper lifting. The soft inner part of the intervertebral disk (nucleus pulposus) protrudes through the fibrous outer layer, pressing on the spinal cord or nerves. It occurs most frequently at the L4–L5 levels, causing **sciatica** (an irritation of the sciatic nerve that passes down the posterior leg). Plain radiographs do not demonstrate this condition but can be used to rule out other pathologic processes, such as neoplasia and spondylolisthesis. Myelography once was indicated to visualize this pathologic process. CT and MRI are now the modalities of choice.

Lordosis describes the normal concave curvature of the lumbar spine and an abnormal or exaggerated concave lumbar curvature. This condition may result from pregnancy, obesity, poor posture, rickets, or tuberculosis of the spine. A lateral projection of the spine will best demonstrate the extent of lordosis.

Metastases are primary malignant neoplasms that spread to distant sites via blood and lymphatics. The vertebrae are common sites of metastatic lesions, which may be characterized and visualized on the image as follows:
- **Osteolytic**—destructive lesions with irregular margins
- **Osteoblastic**—proliferative bony lesions of increased density
- **Combination osteolytic and osteoblastic**—moth-eaten appearance of bone resulting from the mix of destructive and blastic lesions

Scoliosis is lateral curvature of the vertebral column that usually occurs with some rotation of the vertebra. It involves the thoracic and lumbar regions. Dextroscoliosis is the exaggerated curvature to the right. Levoscoliosis is the exaggerated curvature to the left.

Spina bifida is a congenital condition in which the posterior aspects of the vertebrae fail to develop, thus exposing part of the spinal cord. This condition varies greatly in severity and occurs most often at L5 (see clinical indications in Chapter 16).

Spondylolisthesis involves the forward movement of one vertebra in relation to another. It is commonly due to a developmental defect in the pars interarticularis or may result from spondylolysis or severe osteoarthritis. It is most common at L5–S1 but also occurs at L4–L5. Severe cases require a spinal fusion.

Spondylolysis is the dissolution of a vertebra, such as from aplasia (lack of development) of the vertebral arch and **separation of the pars interarticularis** of the vertebra. On the oblique projection, the neck of the Scottie dog appears broken. It is most common at L4 or L5.

See Table 9.3 for a summary of clinical indications.

TABLE 9.3 SUMMARY OF CLINICAL INDICATIONS

CONDITION OR DISEASE	MOST COMMON RADIOGRAPHIC EXAMINATION	POSSIBLE RADIOGRAPHIC APPEARANCE	EXPOSURE FACTOR ADJUSTMENT[a]
Ankylosing spondylitis	AP, lateral lumbar spine, sacroiliac joints; nuclear medicine bone scan	Vertebral column becoming fused, appearance of piece of bamboo; anterior longitudinal ligaments calcifying	None
Fractures			
Compression	AP, lateral lumbar spine, CT	Anterior wedging of vertebrae; loss of body height	None or slight decrease (−), depending on severity
Chance	AP, lateral lumbar spine, CT	Fracture through vertebral body and posterior elements	None
Herniated nucleus pulposus (HNP) (herniated lumbar disk)	AP, lateral lumbar spine, CT, MRI	Possible narrowing of intervertebral disk spaces	None
Lordosis	Lateral lumbar spine, scoliosis series, including erect PA-AP and lateral	Normal concave lumbar curvature or abnormal or exaggerated lumbar curvature	None
Metastases	Bone scan, AP, lateral of spine	Dependent on lesion type: • Destructive—irregular margins and decreased density • Osteoblastic lesions—increased density • Combination—moth-eaten appearance	None or increase (+) or decrease (−), depending on type of lesion and stage of pathologic process
Scoliosis	Erect PA and lateral spine	Lateral curvature of vertebral column	None
Spina bifida	Prenatal ultrasound, PA and lateral spine, CT or MRI	Open posterior vertebra, exposure of part of spinal cord	None
Spondylolisthesis	AP, lateral lumbar spine, CT	Forward slipping of one vertebra in relation to another	None
Spondylolysis	AP, lateral, oblique views of spine, CT	Defect in the pars interarticularis (Scottie dog appearing to wear a collar)	None

[a]Depends on stage or severity of disease or condition.

Routine and Special Positioning

Protocols and positioning routines vary among facilities, depending on factors such as administrative structures and liabilities. Technologists should become familiar with current standards of practice, protocols, and routine or special projections for any facility in which they work.

AP (OR PA) PROJECTION—LUMBAR SPINE

Clinical Indications
- Pathology of the lumbar vertebrae, including fractures, scoliosis, and neoplastic processes

Lumbar Spine
ROUTINE
- AP (or PA)
- Oblique—anterior or posterior
- Lateral
- Lateral L5–S1

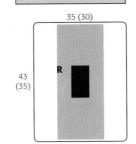

Technical Factors
- Minimum SID—40 inches (100 cm)
- IR size—14 × 17 inches (35 × 43 cm), portrait
- Grid
- kVp range: 75–90

Shielding Shield radiosensitive tissues outside region of interest.

Patient Position—Supine Position Position patient supine with arms at side and head on pillow (also may be done in prone or erect position; see NOTES).

Part Position
- Align midsagittal plane to CR and midline of table and/or grid (Fig. 9.28).
- **Flex knees and hips** to reduce lordotic curvature.
- Ensure that **no rotation** of thorax or pelvis exists.

CR
- CR perpendicular to IR.
  - **More open collimation 14 × 17 inches (35 × 43 cm):** Direct CR to **level of iliac crest** (L4–L5). This larger IR will include lumbar vertebrae, sacrum, and possibly coccyx.
  - **Tighter collimation 11 × 14 inches (30 × 35 cm):** Direct CR to **level of L3,** which may be localized by palpation of the lower costal margin (1.5 inches [4 cm] above iliac crest). This tighter collimation will include primarily the five lumbar vertebrae.
- Center IR to CR.

Recommended Collimation Collimate on four sides to anatomy of interest.

Respiration Suspend respiration on **expiration.**

NOTES: Partial flexion of knees as shown straightens the spine, which helps open intervertebral disk spaces.

Radiograph may be done prone as a PA projection, which places the intervertebral spaces more closely parallel to the diverging rays.

The erect position may be useful for demonstrating the natural weight-bearing stance of the spine.

Evaluation Criteria
Anatomy Demonstrated • Lumbar vertebral bodies, intervertebral joints, spinous and transverse processes, SI joints, and sacrum are shown. • 14 × 17 inch (35 × 43 cm) collimation—approximately T11 to the distal sacrum included. • 11 × 14 inch (35 × 43 cm) collimation—T12 to S1 included (Figs. 9.29 and 9.30).

Position • **No patient rotation** indicated by SI joints equidistant from spinous processes, spinous processes in midline of vertebral column, and transverse processes of equal length. Open intervertebral joint spaces. • Collimation to **area of interest.**

Exposure • Clear demonstration of bony margins and trabecular markings of lumbar vertebrae. • **No motion.**

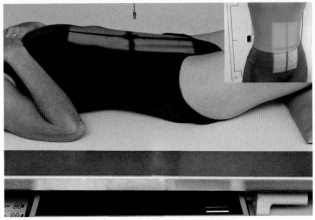

Fig. 9.28 AP projection (centered for 14 × 17-inch [35 × 43-cm] IR). *Inset,* Alternative PA projection.

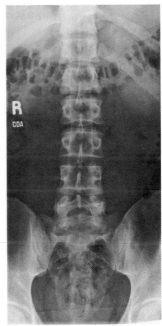

Fig. 9.29 AP lumbar projection (centered for 14 × 17-inch [35 × 43-cm] IR).

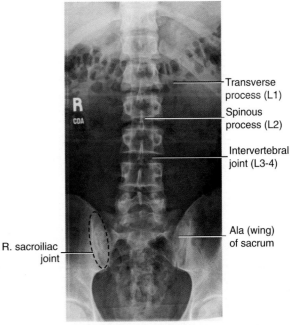

Transverse process (L1)
Spinous process (L2)
Intervertebral joint (L3-4)
Ala (wing) of sacrum
R. sacroiliac joint

Fig. 9.30 AP lumbar projection.

POSTERIOR (OR ANTERIOR) OBLIQUE POSITIONS—LUMBAR SPINE

Clinical Indications
- Defects of the pars interarticularis (e.g., spondylolysis)

  Both right and left oblique projections are obtained.

Lumbar Spine
ROUTINE
• AP (or PA)
• Oblique—posterior or anterior
• Lateral
• Lateral L5–S1

Technical Factors
- Minimum SID—40 inches (100 cm)
- IR size—10 × 12 inches (24 × 30 cm), portrait
- Grid
- kVp range: 75–90

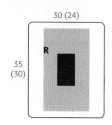

30 (24)

R

35 (30)

Shielding Shield radiosensitive tissues outside region of interest.

Patient Position—Posterior or Anterior Oblique Positions
Position patient semisupine (RPO and left posterior oblique [LPO]) or semiprone (RAO and left anterior oblique [LAO]), with arms extended and head on pillow.

Part Position
- **Rotate body 45° and align** spinal column to midline of table and/or IR; 50° oblique is best for L1–L2 zygapophyseal joints, and 30° for L5–S1.
- Ensure equal rotation of shoulders and pelvis. Flex knee for stability and bring arm furthest from IR across chest (Fig. 9.31).
- Support shoulders and pelvis with radiolucent sponges to maintain position. This support is strongly recommended to prevent patients from grasping the edge of the table, which may result in their fingers being pinched.

CR
- CR perpendicular to IR.
- Direct CR to **L3 at the level of the lower costal margin** (1 to 2 inches [2.5 to 5 cm]) **above iliac crest** and 2 inches (5 cm) medial to upside ASIS.
- Center IR to CR.

Recommended Collimation Collimate on four sides to anatomy of interest.

Respiration Suspend respiration on expiration.

Evaluation Criteria
Anatomy Demonstrated • Visualization of zygapophyseal joints (RPO and LPO show downside; RAO and LAO show upside) (Figs. 9.32 and 9.33).

Position • Accurate 45° patient rotation as indicated by open zygapophyseal joints and the pedicle (eye of the Scottie dog) between the midline and lateral aspect of the vertebral border. • If the pedicle is demonstrated closer to the midline of the vertebral border and less of the pedicle is seen, this indicates over-rotation. If the pedicle is demonstrated laterally on the vertebral body border with more of the lamina (body of Scottie dog) demonstrated, this indicates under-rotation.[2] • Collimation to **area of interest**.

Exposure • Clear demonstration of bony margins and trabecular markings of lumbar vertebrae. • No motion.

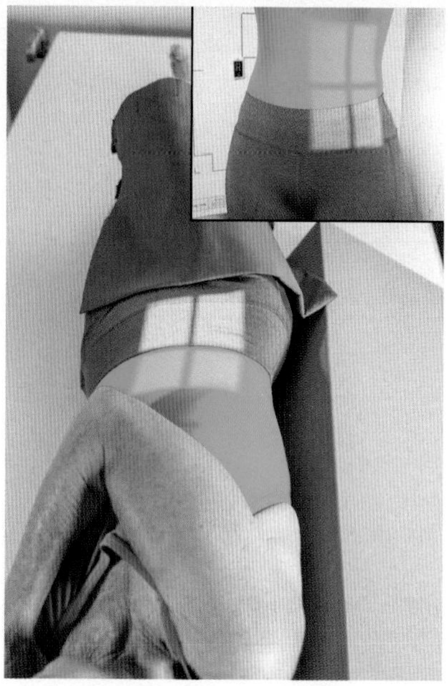

Fig. 9.31 45° RPO of lumbar spine, visualizing right (downside) zygapophyseal joints. Alternative anterior oblique, LAO—right joints.

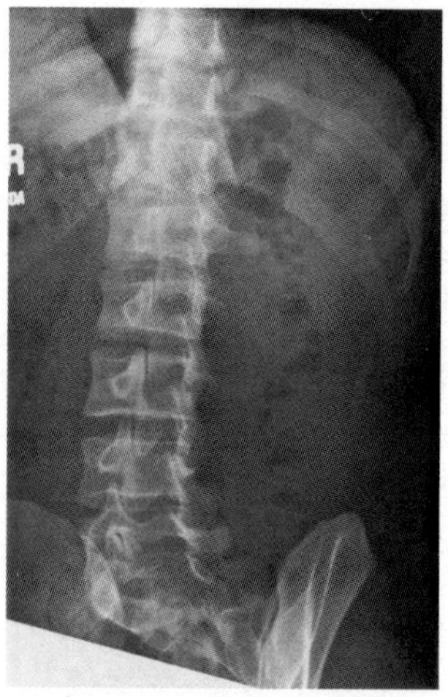

Fig. 9.32 45° RPO of lumbar spine.

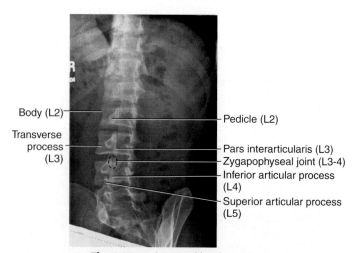

Body (L2)
Transverse process (L3)
Pedicle (L2)
Pars interarticularis (L3)
Zygapophyseal joint (L3-4)
Inferior articular process (L4)
Superior articular process (L5)

Fig. 9.33 45° RPO of lumbar spine.

LATERAL POSITION—LUMBAR SPINE

Clinical Indications
- **Pathology** of the lumbar vertebrae including fractures, spondylolisthesis, neoplastic processes, and osteoporosis

Lumbar Spine
ROUTINE
• AP (or PA)
• Oblique—posterior or anterior
• Lateral
• Lateral L5–S1

Technical Factors
- Minimum SID—40 inches (100 cm)
- IR size—14 × 17 inches (35 × 43 cm), portrait
- Grid
- kVp range: 80–90
- Lead masking on tabletop behind patient

35 (30)

43 (35)   L

Shielding Shield radiosensitive tissues outside region of interest.

Patient Position—Lateral Position
Place patient in the lateral recumbent position, with head on pillow, knees flexed, with support between knees and ankles to better maintain a true lateral position and ensure patient comfort.

Part Position
- Align midcoronal plane to CR and midline of table and/or IR (Fig. 9.34).
- Place radiolucent support under waist as needed to place the long axis of the spine near parallel to the table (palpating spinous processes to determine; see NOTES).
- Ensure that **no rotation** of thorax or pelvis exists.

CR
- CR perpendicular to IR (see NOTES).
  More open collimation 14 × 17 inches (35 × 43): Center to level of iliac crest (L4–L5). This projection includes lumbar vertebrae, sacrum, and possibly coccyx.
  Tighter collimation 11 × 14 inches (30 × 35): Center to L3 at the level of the lower costal margin (1.5 inches [4 cm] above iliac crest). This includes the five lumbar vertebrae. Center IR to CR.

Recommended Collimation Collimate on four sides to anatomy of interest.

Respiration
Suspend respiration on **expiration.**

NOTES: Although the average male patient (and some female patients) requires no CR angle, a patient with a wider pelvis and a narrow thorax may require a 5° to 8° caudad angle even with support, as shown in Fig. 9.35.

If patient has a lateral curvature (scoliosis) of the spine (as determined by viewing the spine from the back, with the patient in the erect position and with hospital gown open), patient should be placed in whichever lateral position **places the sag, or convexity of the spine, down** to open the intervertebral spaces better.

Evaluation Criteria
Anatomy Demonstrated • Intervertebral foramina L1–L4, vertebral bodies, intervertebral joints, spinous processes, and L5–S1 junction. • Depending on the IR size used, the entire sacrum also may be included (Figs. 9.36 and 9.37).

Position • Spinal column aligned parallel to the IR, as indicated by open intervertebral foramina and open intervertebral joint spaces. • **No rotation** is indicated by superimposed greater sciatic notches and posterior vertebral bodies. • Collimation to **area of interest.**

Exposure • Clear demonstration of bony margins and trabecular markings of lumbar vertebrae. **No motion.**

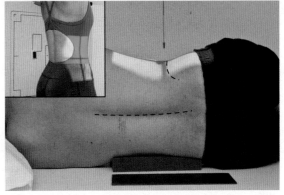

Fig. 9.34 Left lateral lumbar (CR perpendicular to IR).

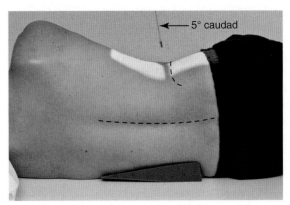

5° caudad

Fig. 9.35 Left lateral lumbar (CR 5° caudad).

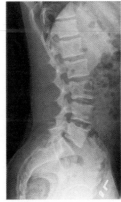

Fig. 9.36 Lateral lumbar.

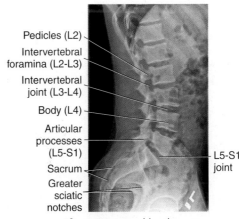

Pedicles (L2)
Intervertebral foramina (L2-L3)
Intervertebral joint (L3-L4)
Body (L4)
Articular processes (L5-S1)
Sacrum
Greater sciatic notches
L5-S1 joint

Fig. 9.37 Lateral lumbar.

LATERAL L5–S1 POSITION–LUMBAR SPINE

Clinical Indications
- Spondylolisthesis involving L4–L5 or L5–S1 and other L5–S1 pathologies

Lumbar Spine
ROUTINE
• AP (or PA)
• Oblique–posterior or anterior
• Lateral
• Lateral L5-S1

Technical Factors
- Minimum SID—40 inches (100 cm)
- IR size—8 × 10 inches (18 × 24 cm), portrait
- Grid
- kVp range: 85–95
- Lead masking on tabletop behind patient

Shielding Shield radiosensitive tissues outside region of interest.

Patient Position–Lateral Position Place patient in the lateral recumbent position, with head on pillow, knees flexed, with support between knees and ankles to maintain a true lateral position better and ensure patient comfort.

Part Position
- Align midcoronal plane to CR and midline of table and/or IR (Fig. 9.38).
- Place radiolucent support under waist as needed to place the long axis of the spine near parallel to the table (palpating spinous processes to determine; see NOTES later).
- Ensure that **no rotation** of thorax or pelvis exists.

CR
- CR **perpendicular** to IR with sufficient waist support, or angle **5° to 8° caudad** with less support (see NOTES).
- Direct CR **1.5 inches (4 cm) inferior to iliac crest and 2 inches (5 cm) posterior to ASIS.**
- Center IR to CR.

Recommended Collimation Collimate on four sides to anatomy of interest.

Respiration Suspend respiration to limit patient motion.

NOTES: If waist is not supported sufficiently, resulting in sagging of the vertebral column, the CR must be angled 5° to 8° caudad to be **parallel to the interiliac line**[3] (imaginary line between iliac crests [Fig. 9.39]).

High amounts of secondary or scatter radiation are generated as the result of the part thickness. Close collimation is essential, along with placement of lead masking on tabletop behind patient. This is especially important with digital imaging.

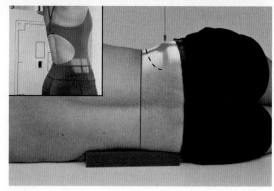

Fig. 9.38 Left lateral L5–S1 with sufficient support; 0° CR angle.

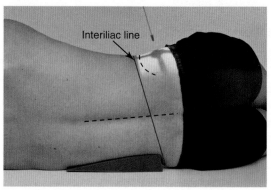

Interiliac line

Fig. 9.39 Left lateral L5–S1 with less support; CR 5° to 8° caudad (CR parallel to interiliac line).

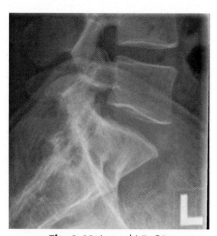

Fig. 9.40 Lateral L5–S1.

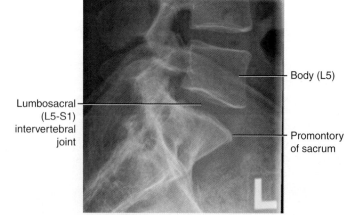

Lumbosacral (L5-S1) intervertebral joint

Body (L5)

Promontory of sacrum

Fig. 9.41 Lateral L5–S1.

Evaluation Criteria
Anatomy Demonstrated • L5 vertebral body, first and second sacral segments and L5–S1 joint space (Figs. 9.40 and 9.41).

Position • **No rotation** of patient evidenced by superimposition of greater sciatic notches and posterior borders of the vertebral bodies. • Correct alignment of the vertebral column and CR indicated by open L5–S1 joint space. • Collimation to **area of interest.**

Exposure • Clear demonstration of bony margins and trabecular markings of L5–S1 region. • **No motion.**

AP AXIAL L5–S1 PROJECTION—LUMBAR SPINE

Clinical Indications
- Pathology of L5–S1 and the sacroiliac joints

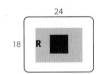

Lumbar Spine
SPECIAL
- AP axial L5–S1

Technical Factors
- Minimum SID—40 inches (100 cm)
- IR size—8 × 10 inches (18 × 24 cm), landscape
- Grid
- kVp range: 80–90

Shielding Shield radiosensitive tissues outside region of interest.

Patient Position—Supine Position Position patient supine with arms at side and head on pillow, and legs extended, with support under knees for comfort.

Part Position
- Align midsagittal plane to CR and midline of table and/or IR (Fig. 9.42).
- Ensure that **no rotation** of thorax or pelvis exists.

CR
- Angle CR cephalad, 30° (male patients) and 35° (female patients).
- Direct CR to the level of the ASIS at the midline of the body.
- Center IR to CR.

Recommended Collimation Collimate on four sides to anatomy of interest.

Respiration Suspend respiration to limit patient motion.

NOTES: Angled AP projection "opens" L5–S1 joint.

Lateral view of L5–S1 generally provides more information than the AP projection.

This projection also may be performed **prone** with **caudal** angle of CR (increases object–image receptor distance [OID]).

Evaluation Criteria
Anatomy Demonstrated • L5–S1 joint space and sacroiliac joints (Figs. 9.43 and 9.44).

Position • Sacroiliac joints demonstrate equal distance from spine, indicating no pelvic rotation. • Correct alignment of CR and L5–S1 evidenced by an open joint space. • Collimation to **area of interest**.

Exposure • Clear demonstration of bony margins and trabecular markings of L5–S1 region. • **No motion.**

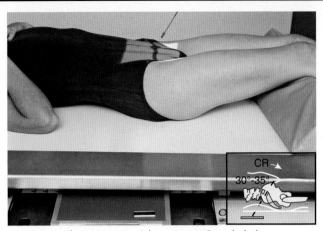

Fig. 9.42 AP axial L5–S1—35° cephalad.

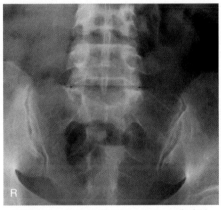

Fig. 9.43 AP axial L5–S1—35° cephalad.

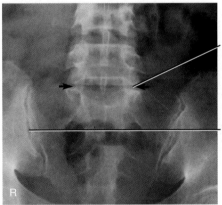

Lumbosacral (L5-S1) intervertebral joint

Sacroiliac joint

Fig. 9.44 AP axial L5–S1.

9

PA PROJECTION: SCOLIOSIS SERIES

Clinical Indications

- To determine the degree and severity of scoliosis

A scoliosis series may include **two PA projections** taken for comparison, one erect and one recumbent (see NOTES).

Scoliosis Series
ROUTINE
• PA erect and/or recumbent
• Erect lateral

Technical Factors

- SID—40 to 60 inches (100 to 150 cm); longer SID required with larger IR to obtain required collimation
- IR size—14 × 17 inches (35 × 43 cm), portrait; taller patients, 14 × 36 inches (35 × 90 cm), if available
- Grid
- Compensating filters to obtain a more uniform density along the vertebral column
- kVp range: 75–90
- Erect marker for erect position

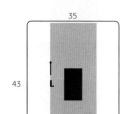

Shielding Shield radiosensitive tissues outside region of interest.

Patient Position—Erect and Recumbent Position
Place patient in the erect and recumbent position with arms at side. Distribute weight evenly on both feet for the erect position.

Part Position
- Align midsagittal plane to CR and midline of table and/or IR (Fig. 9.45).
- Ensure that **no rotation** of thorax or pelvis exists, if possible. Scoliosis may result in twisting and rotation of vertebrae, making some rotation unavoidable.
- Place **lower margin of IR** a **minimum** of 1 to 2 inches (3 to 5 cm) below iliac crest (centering height determined by IR size and/or area of scoliosis).

CR
- CR perpendicular to IR.
- Center IR to CR.

Recommended Collimation Collimate on four sides to anatomy of interest.

Respiration Suspend respiration on **expiration**.

Evaluation Criteria

Anatomy Demonstrated • Thoracic and lumbar vertebrae, including 1 to 2 inches (3 to 5 cm) of the iliac crests (Fig. 9.48).

Position • **No patient rotation** indicated by thoracic and lumbar vertebrae with spinous processes aligned with the vertebral midline and symmetry of iliac alae/wings and upper sacrum. • However, scoliosis is often accompanied by twisting or rotation of involved vertebrae. • Collimation to **area of interest**.

Exposure • Clear demonstration of bony margins and trabecular markings of thoracic and lumbar vertebrae. • **No motion.**

NOTES: A PA rather than an AP projection is highly recommended because of the significantly reduced dose to radiation-sensitive areas, such as the female breasts and thyroid gland. Studies have shown that this projection results in approximately 90% reduction in dosage to the breasts.[4]

Scoliosis generally requires repeat examinations over several years, especially for pediatric patients. Measures should be taken to provide careful shielding. Fig. 9.46 demonstrates an example of shielding that can be used during a scoliosis series. Fig. 9.47 demonstrates the radiographic appearance with the use of shielding.

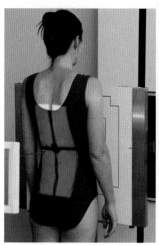

Fig. 9.45 PA erect.

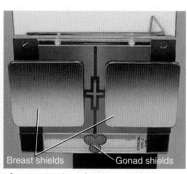

Breast shields   Gonad shields

Fig. 9.46 Clear, lead-equivalent, compensating filters with breast and gonadal shields attached to bottom of collimator with magnets. (Courtesy Nuclear Associates, Carle Place, NY.)

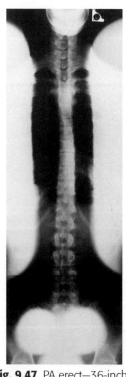

Fig. 9.47 PA erect—36-inch (90-cm) IR, shadow shields in place. (Courtesy Nuclear Associates, Carle Place, NY.)

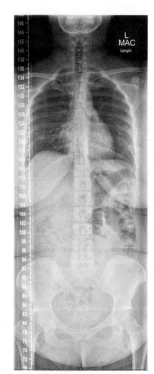

Fig. 9.48 PA erect—14 × 17-inch (35 × 43-cm) IR.

LATERAL POSITION (ERECT): SCOLIOSIS SERIES

Clinical Indications
- Spondylolisthesis, degree of kyphosis, or lordosis

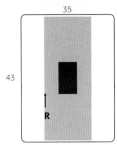

Scoliosis Series
ROUTINE
- PA erect and/or recumbent
- Erect lateral

Technical Factors
- SID—40 to 60 inches (100 to 150 cm); longer SID required with larger IR to obtain required collimation
- IR size—14 × 17 inches (35 × 43 cm), portrait, or 14 × 36 inches (35 × 90 cm) on taller patients, if available
- Grid
- Erect marker for erect position
- Use of compensating filters to help obtain a more uniform density along the vertebral column
- kVp range: 85–95

Shielding Shield radiosensitive tissues outside region of interest. Fig. 9.49 demonstrates the radiographic appearance with the use of breast shielding.

Patient Position—Erect Lateral Position Place patient in an erect lateral position with arms elevated, or, if unsteady, grasping a support in front. Place the convex side of the curve against the IR.

Part Position
- Align midcoronal plane to CR and midline of table and/or IR (Fig. 9.50).
- Ensure that **no rotation** of thorax or pelvis exists.
- Place lower margin of IR a **minimum of 1 to 2 inches (2.5 to 5 cm) below level of iliac crests** (centering determined by IR size and patient size).

CR
- CR perpendicular to IR.
- Center IR to CR.

Recommended Collimation Collimate on four sides to anatomy of interest.

Respiration Suspend respiration on **expiration**.

Evaluation Criteria
Anatomy Demonstrated • Thoracic and lumbar vertebrae including 1 to 2 inches (2.5 to 5 cm) of the iliac crests (Fig. 9.51).

Position • Thoracic and lumbar vertebrae aligned parallel to the IR, as indicated by open intervertebral foramina and open intervertebral joint spaces. • **No rotation** indicated by superimposed greater sciatic notches and posterior vertebral bodies. However, scoliosis is often accompanied by twisting or rotation of involved vertebrae. • Collimation to **area of interest**.

Exposure • Clear demonstration of bony margins and trabecular markings of thoracic and lumbar vertebrae. • **No motion**.

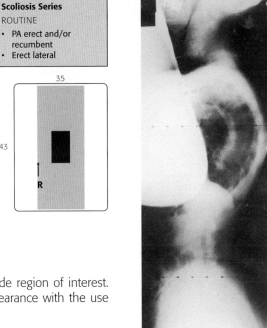

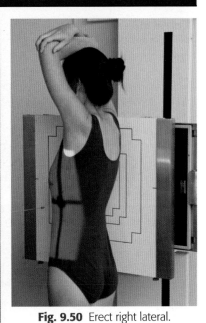

Fig. 9.50 Erect right lateral.

Fig. 9.49 Erect lateral. Clear Pb lateral thoracic compensating filter and breast shadow shield in place.

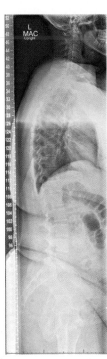

Fig. 9.51 Erect left lateral.

9

PA PROJECTION (FERGUSON METHOD): SCOLIOSIS SERIES

Clinical Indications This method assists in differentiating deforming (primary) curve from compensatory curve.

Two images are obtained—one standard erect PA and one with the foot or hip on the **convex side** of the curve elevated.

> **Scoliosis Series**
> SPECIAL
> • PA—Ferguson method
> • AP—R and L bending

Technical Factors

- SID—40 to 60 inches (100 to 150 cm); longer SID is required to obtain adequate collimation if a 14 × 36-inch (35 × 90-cm) IR is used
- IR size—14 × 17 inches (35 × 43 cm), portrait, or 14 × 36 inches (35 × 90 cm)
- Grid
- Erect marker for erect position
- Use of compensating filters to help obtain a more uniform density along the vertebral column
- kVp range: 80–90

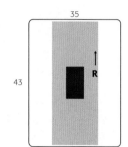

Shielding Shield radiosensitive tissues outside region of interest.

Patient Position—Erect

- Place patient in an erect (seated or standing) position facing the table, with arms at side (Fig. 9.52).
- For second image, place a block under foot (or hip if seated) on **convex side** of curve so that the patient can barely maintain position **without assistance**. A 3 to 4-inch (8 to 10-cm) block of some type may be used under the buttocks if sitting or under the foot if standing (Fig. 9.53).

Part Position

- Align midsagittal plane to CR and midline of table and/or IR.
- Ensure that **no rotation** of thorax or pelvis exists, if possible.
- Place IR to include a minimum 1 to 2 inches (2.5 to 5 cm) below the iliac crest.

CR

- Direct CR perpendicular to IR.
- Center IR to CR.

Recommended Collimation Collimate on four sides to anatomy of interest.

Respiration Suspend respiration on **expiration**.

NOTES: No form of support (e.g., compression band) is to be used in this examination. For second image, patient should stand or sit with block under one side, unassisted.

Perform PA projections to reduce dosage to radiation-sensitive areas of thyroid and breast.

Evaluation Criteria

Anatomy Demonstrated • Thoracic and lumbar vertebrae including 1 to 2 inches (2.5 to 5 cm) of the iliac crests (Figs. 9.54 and 9.55).

Position • **No patient rotation** indicated by thoracic and lumbar vertebrae with spinous processes aligned with the vertebral midline and symmetry of iliac alae/wings and upper sacrum. • Collimation to **area of interest**.

Exposure • Clear demonstration of bony margins and trabecular markings of thoracic and lumbar vertebrae. • **No motion**.

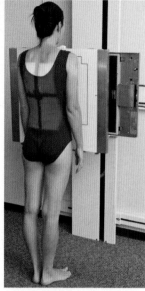

Fig. 9.52 PA erect.

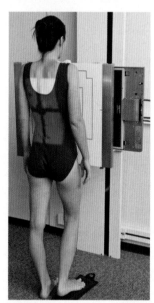

Fig. 9.53 PA with block under foot on convex side of curve.

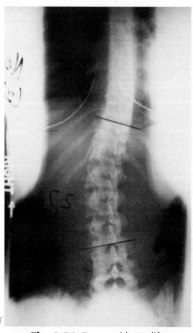

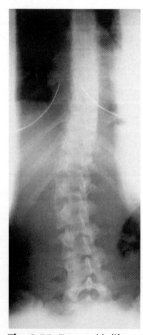

Fig. 9.54 Erect, with no lift.

Fig. 9.55 Erect, with lift on right.

PA (AP) PROJECTION—RIGHT AND LEFT BENDING: SCOLIOSIS SERIES

Clinical Indications
- Assessment of the range of motion of the vertebral column

Scoliosis Series
SPECIAL
• PA —Ferguson method
• PA —R and L bending

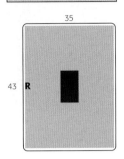

Technical Factors
- SID—40 to 60 inches (100 to 150 cm); longer SID required to obtain adequate collimation if a 14 × 36-inch (35 × 90-cm) IR is used
- IR size—14 × 17 inches (35 × 43 cm) or 14 × 36 inches (35 × 90 cm), portrait
- Grid
- Erect marker for erect position
- Use of compensating filters to help obtain a more uniform density along the vertebral column
- kVp range: 80–95

Shielding Shield radiosensitive tissues outside region of interest.

Patient Position—Erect or Recumbent Position Position patient erect (preferred) or recumbent (in supine position), with arms at side (see NOTES).

Part Position ⊞
- Align midsagittal plane to CR and midline of table and/or IR.
- Ensure that **no rotation** of thorax or pelvis exists, if possible.
- Place bottom edge of IR **1 to 2 inches (2.5 to 5 cm) below iliac crest.**
- With the pelvis acting as a fulcrum, ask patient to bend laterally (lateral flexion) **as far as possible** to either side (Figs. 9.56 and 9.57).
- If recumbent, move both the upper torso and legs to achieve maximum lateral flexion.
- Repeat above steps for opposite side.

CR
- CR perpendicular to IR.
- Center IR to CR.

Recommended Collimation Collimate on four sides to anatomy of interest.

Respiration Suspend respiration on **expiration.**

NOTES: The pelvis must remain as stationary as possible during positioning. The pelvis acts as a fulcrum (pivot point) during changes in position.

PA projections are recommended when performed erect to reduce exposure significantly to radiation-sensitive organs.

Evaluation Criteria
Anatomy Demonstrated • Thoracic and lumbar vertebrae including 1 to 2 inches (2.5 to 5 cm) of the iliac crests (Figs. 9.58 and 9.59).

Position • Spinal column aligned parallel to the IR, as indicated by open intervertebral foramina and open intervertebral joint spaces. • **No rotation** indicated by superimposed greater sciatic notches and posterior vertebral bodies. • Collimation to **area of interest.**

Exposure • Clear demonstration of bony margins and trabecular markings of thoracic and lumbar vertebrae. • **No motion.**

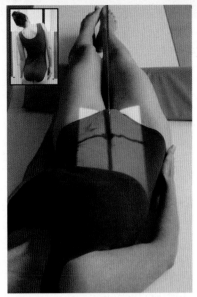

Fig. 9.56 AP supine—L bending. *Inset,* PA erect—L bending.

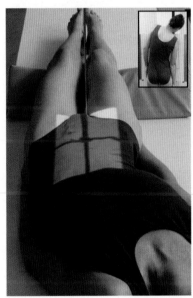

Fig. 9.57 AP supine—R bending. *Inset,* PA erect—R bending.

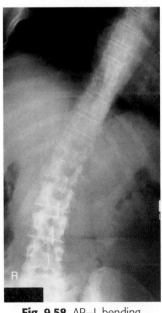

Fig. 9.58 AP—L bending.

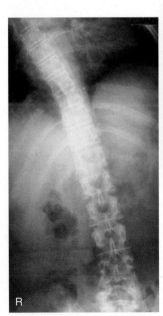

Fig. 9.59 AP—R bending.

LATERAL POSITIONS—HYPEREXTENSION AND HYPERFLEXION: SPINAL FUSION SERIES

Clinical Indications

* Assessment of mobility at a spinal fusion site

> **Spinal Fusion Series**
> ROUTINE
> * PA—R and L bending
> * Lateral—hyperextension and hyperflexion

Two images are obtained with the patient in the lateral position (one in hyperflexion and one in hyperextension).

Right- and left-bending positions also are generally part of a spinal fusion series and are the same as for the scoliosis series on pp. 346 and 347..

Technical Factors

* Minimum SID—40 inches (100 cm)
* IR size—14 × 17 inches (35 × 43 cm), portrait
* Grid
* kVp range: 80–95
* Extension and flexion markers

Shielding Shield radiosensitive tissues outside region of interest.

Patient Position—Lateral Position

* Place patient in erect (preferred) or lateral recumbent position. (see NOTES).
* Place lower edge of IR 1 to 2 inches (2.5 to 5 cm) below iliac crest.

Part Position

* Align midcoronal plane to CR and midline of table and/or IR.

Hyperflexion

* Using pelvis as fulcrum, ask patient to assume hyperflexed position while remaining within collimation field (Fig. 9.60).

Hyperextension

* Using pelvis as fulcrum, ask patient to move torso posteriorly **as far as possible** to hyperextend long axis of body (Fig. 9.61).
* Ensure that no rotation of thorax or pelvis exists.

CR

* CR perpendicular to IR.
* Direct CR to **site of fusion** if known or to center of IR.

Recommended Collimation Collimate on four sides to anatomy of interest.

Respiration Suspend respiration on **expiration**.

NOTES: Projection is frequently performed with patient standing erect or sitting on a stool, first leaning forward as far as possible, gripping the stool legs, and then leaning backward as far as possible, gripping the back of the stool to maintain this position.

The pelvis must remain as stationary as possible during positioning. The pelvis acts as a fulcrum (pivot point) during changes in position.

> **Evaluation Criteria**
>
> **Anatomy Demonstrated** • Thoracic and lumbar vertebra including 1 to 2 inches (2.5 to 5 cm) of the iliac crests (Figs. 9.62 and 9.63).
> **Position** • Spinal column aligned parallel to the IR, as indicated by open intervertebral foramina and open intervertebral joint spaces. **No rotation** indicated by superimposed greater sciatic notches and posterior vertebral bodies. • Collimation to **area of interest**.
> **Exposure** • Clear demonstration of bony margins and trabecular markings of thoracic and lumbar vertebrae. • **No motion**.

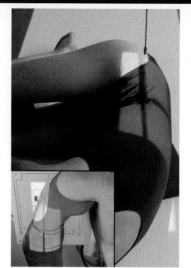

Fig. 9.60 Lateral—hyperflexion.

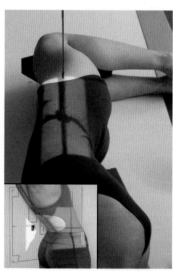

Fig. 9.61 Lateral—hyperextension.

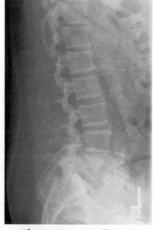

Fig. 9.62 Hyperflexion.

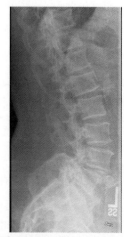

Fig. 9.63 Hyperextension.

AP AXIAL PROJECTION—SACRUM

Clinical Indications
- Pathology of the sacrum, including fracture

NOTE: The urinary bladder should be emptied before this procedure begins. It is also desirable to have the lower colon free of gas and fecal material, which may require a cleansing enema, as ordered by a physician.

Sacrum and Coccyx
ROUTINE
• AP axial sacrum
• AP axial coccyx
• Lateral

Technical Factors
- Minimum SID—40 inches (100 cm)
- IR size—10 × 12 inches (24 × 30 cm), portrait
- Grid
- kVp range: 75–90

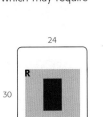

Shielding Shield radiosensitive tissues outside region of interest.

Patient Position—Supine Position
Position patient supine with arms at side, head on pillow, and legs extended with support under knees for comfort.

Part Position
- Align midsagittal plane to CR and midline of table and/or IR (Fig. 9.64).
- Ensure that no rotation of the pelvis exists.

CR
- Angle CR 15° cephalad. Direct CR 2 inches (5 cm) superior to pubic symphysis.
- Center IR to CR.

Recommended Collimation Collimate on four sides to anatomy of interest.

Respiration Suspend respiration to limit patient motion.

NOTES: Technologist may have to increase CR angle to 20° cephalad for patients with an apparent greater posterior curvature or tilt of the sacrum and pelvis.

Female sacrum is generally shorter and wider than male sacrum (a consideration in close four-sided collimation).

This projection also may be performed **prone** (angle **15° caudad**) if necessary for patient's condition.

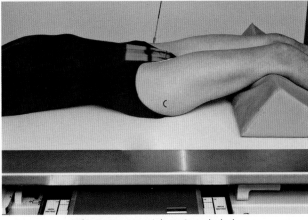
Fig. 9.64 AP axial—15° cephalad.

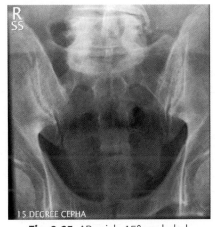
Fig. 9.65 AP axial—15° cephalad.

Evaluation Criteria
Anatomy Demonstrated • Sacrum, SI joints, and L5–S1 intervertebral joint space (Figs. 9.65 and 9.66).
Position • No rotation indicated by alignment of the median sagittal crests and coccyx with the symphysis pubis. • Correct alignment of the sacrum and CR demonstrates the sacrum free of foreshortening and the pubis and sacral foramina are not superimposed. • Collimation to **area of interest.**
Exposure • Clear demonstration of bony margins and trabecular markings of sacrum. • **No motion.**

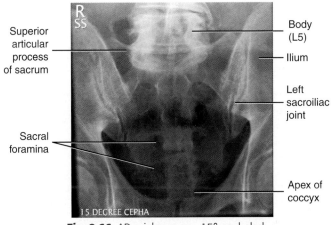

Superior articular process of sacrum

Sacral foramina

Body (L5)

Ilium

Left sacroiliac joint

Apex of coccyx

Fig. 9.66 AP axial sacrum—15° cephalad.

9

AP AXIAL PROJECTION—COCCYX

Clinical Indications
- Pathology of the coccyx including fracture

Sacrum and Coccyx
ROUTINE
• AP axial sacrum
• AP axial coccyx
• Lateral

NOTE: The urinary bladder should be emptied before this procedure begins. It is also desirable to have the lower colon free of gas and fecal material, which may require a cleansing enema, as ordered by a physician.

Technical Factors
- Minimum SID—40 inches (100 cm)
- IR size—8 × 10 inches (18 × 24 cm), portrait
- Grid
- kVp range: 75–85
- Cautious use of AEC

Shielding Shield radiosensitive tissues outside region of interest.

Patient Position—Supine Position Position patient supine with arms at side and head on pillow and legs extended with support under knees for comfort.

Part Position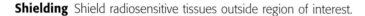
- Align midsagittal plane to midline of table and/or IR (Fig. 9.67).
- Ensure that **no rotation** of the pelvis exists.

CR
- Angle CR 10° caudad. Direct CR 2 inches (5 cm) superior to symphysis pubis.
- Center IR to CR.

Recommended Collimation Collimate on four sides to anatomy of interest.

Respiration Suspend respiration to limit patient motion.

NOTES: Technologist may have to increase CR angle to 15° caudad with a greater anterior curvature of the coccyx if apparent by palpation or as evidenced on the lateral.

This projection also may be performed **prone** (angle **10° cephalad**) if necessary for patient's condition, with CR centered to the coccyx, which can be localized using the greater trochanter.

Fig. 9.67 AP axial coccyx—10° caudad.

Fig. 9.68 AP axial coccyx—10° caudad.

Evaluation Criteria
Anatomy Demonstrated • Coccyx (Fig. 9.68)

Position • Correct coccyx and CR alignment demonstrates coccyx free of superimposition and projected superior to pubis. • Coccygeal segments should appear open. If not, they may be fused or CR angle may have to be increased (greater curvature of the coccyx requires greater CR angle). • Coccyx should appear equidistant from the lateral walls of the pelvic opening, indicating no patient rotation. • Collimation to **area of interest.**

Exposure • Clear demonstration of bony margins and trabecular markings of coccyx. • **No motion.**

LATERAL POSITION—SACRUM AND COCCYX

Clinical Indications

- Pathology of the sacrum and coccyx, including fracture

Sacrum and Coccyx
ROUTINE
• AP axial sacrum
• AP axial coccyx
• Lateral sacrum and coccyx

NOTE: The sacrum and coccyx are commonly imaged together. Separate AP projections are required because of different CR angles, **but the lateral projection can be obtained with one exposure** centering to include both the sacrum and coccyx. This projection is recommended to decrease gonadal doses.

Technical Factors

- Minimum SID—40 inches (100 cm)
- IR size—10 × 12 inches (24 × 30 cm), portrait
- Grid
- kVp range: 85–95
- Lead masking on table behind patient to reduce scatter to IR
- If coccyx is to be included, a boomerang-type filter is useful to ensure optimal density

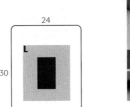

Shielding Shield radiosensitive tissues outside region of interest.

Patient Position—Lateral Position Place patient in the lateral recumbent position, with head on pillow, and knees flexed.

Part Position

- Align long axis of sacrum and coccyx to CR and midline of table and/or IR (Figs. 9.69 and 9.70).
- Ensure that no rotation of thorax or pelvis exists.

CR

- CR perpendicular to IR.
- Direct CR 3 to 4 inches (8 to 10 cm) **posterior to ASIS** (centering for sacrum).
- Center IR to CR.

Recommended Collimation Collimate on four sides to anatomy of interest.

Respiration Suspend respiration to limit patient motion.

NOTE: High amounts of secondary and scatter radiation are generated. Close collimation is essential to reduce patient dose and obtain a high-quality image.

Evaluation Criteria

Anatomy Demonstrated • Sacrum, L5–S1 joint, and coccyx (Fig. 9.71).
Position • **No rotation** indicated by superimposed greater sciatic notches and femoral heads. • Collimation to **area of interest.**
Exposure • Clear demonstration of bony margins and trabecular markings of sacrum and coccyx. • **No motion.**

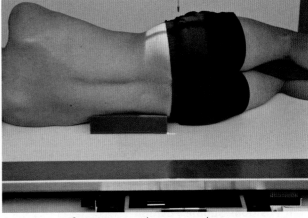

Fig. 9.69 Lateral sacrum and coccyx.

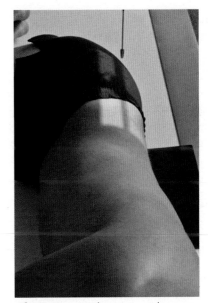

Fig. 9.70 Lateral sacrum and coccyx.

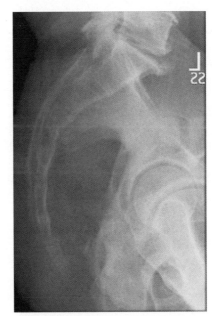

Fig. 9.71 Lateral sacrum and coccyx.

9

AP AXIAL PROJECTION—SACROILIAC JOINTS

Clinical Indications
- **Pathology** of the SI joint, including fracture and joint dislocation or subluxation

Sacroiliac Joints
ROUTINE
- AP axial
- Posterior oblique projections

Technical Factors
- Minimum SID—40 inches (100 cm)
- IR size—10 × 12 inches (24 × 30 cm), portrait
- Grid
- kVp range: 80–95

Shielding Shield radiosensitive tissues outside region of interest.

Patient Position—Supine Position
Position patient supine with arms at side, head on pillow, and legs extended with support under knees for comfort.

Part Position
- Align midsagittal plane to CR and midline of table and/or IR (Fig. 9.72).
- Ensure that **no rotation** of pelvis exists.

CR
- Angle CR **30° to 35° cephalad** (generally, males require about 30° and females 35°, with an increase in the lumbosacral curve).
- Direct CR to midline **about 2 inches (5 cm) below level of ASIS**.
- Center IR to CR.

Recommended Collimation Collimate on four sides to anatomy of interest.

Respiration Suspend respiration to limit patient motion.

Alternative PA axial projection If patient cannot assume the supine position, this image can be obtained as a PA projection with patient prone, using a 30° to 35° **caudad** angle. The CR would be centered to the level of L4 or slightly above the iliac crest.

Evaluation Criteria
Anatomy Demonstrated • Sacroiliac joints and L5–S1 intervertebral joint space (Figs. 9.73 and 9.74).

Position • **No rotation** as evidenced by spinous process of L5 in center of vertebral body and symmetric appearance of bilateral alae/wings of sacrum (with SI joints equally distant from midline of vertebrae). • Collimation to **area of interest.**

Exposure • Clear demonstration of bony margins and trabecular markings of sacrum. • **No motion.**

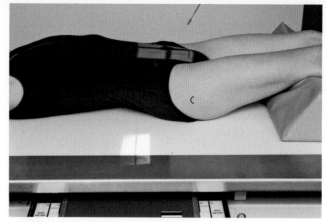
Fig. 9.72 AP axial of SI joints—CR 30° to 35° cephalad.

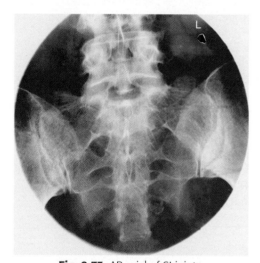
Fig. 9.73 AP axial of SI joints.

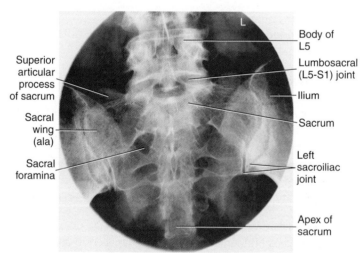

Body of L5

Lumbosacral (L5-S1) joint

Ilium

Sacrum

Left sacroiliac joint

Apex of sacrum

Superior articular process of sacrum

Sacral wing (ala)

Sacral foramina

Fig. 9.74 AP axial of SI joints.

POSTERIOR OBLIQUE POSITIONS (LPO AND RPO)—SACROILIAC JOINTS

Clinical Indications
- **Pathology** of the SI joint, including dislocation or subluxation
- Bilateral study for comparison

Sacroiliac Joints
ROUTINE
- AP axial
- Posterior oblique projections

Technical Factors
- Minimum SID—40 inches (100 cm)
- IR size—10 × 12 inches (24 × 30 cm), portrait
- Grid
- kVp range: 80–95

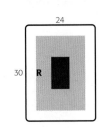

Shielding Shield radiosensitive tissues outside region of interest.

Patient Position—Supine Position
Position patient supine with arms at side and head on pillow.

Part Position
- Rotate body into 25° to 30° posterior oblique, with side of interest elevated (LPO for right joint and RPO for left joint) (Figs. 9.75 and 9.76).
- Align joint of interest to CR and midline of table and/or IR.
- Use an angle-measuring device to ensure correct and consistent angles on both oblique positions.
- Place support under elevated hip and flex elevated knee.

CR
- CR perpendicular to IR (Fig. 9.77).
- Direct CR 1 inch (2.5 cm) medial to upside ASIS (see NOTE for optional cephalad angle).
- Center IR to CR.

Recommended Collimation Collimate on four sides to anatomy of interest.

Respiration Suspend respiration to limit patient motion.

NOTE: To demonstrate the inferior or distal part of the joint more clearly, the CR may be angled 15° to 20° **cephalad.**

Evaluation Criteria
Anatomy Demonstrated • Sacroiliac joint farthest from IR (Fig. 9.78).
Position • Accurate rotation of the patient indicated by no superimposition of the ala of the ilium and sacrum with the open SI joint. • Collimation to **area of interest.**
Exposure • Clear demonstration of bony margins and trabecular markings of sacrum. • **No motion.**

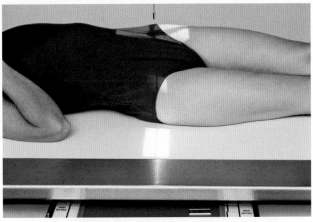
Fig. 9.75 RPO for left side (upside) SI joints.

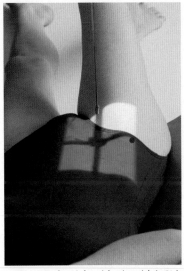
Fig. 9.76 LPO for right side (upside) SI joints.

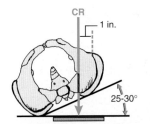
Fig. 9.77 LPO of SI joints.

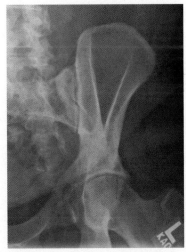
Fig. 9.78 RPO projection for left (upside) SI joints.

RADIOGRAPHS FOR CRITIQUE

This section consists of an ideal projection (Image A) along with one or more projections that may demonstrate positioning and/or technical errors. Critique Figs. C9.79 through C9.83 Compare Image A to the other projections and identify the errors. While examining each image, consider the following questions:

1. Is all essential anatomy demonstrated on the image?
2. What positioning errors are present that compromise image quality?

3. Are technical factors optimal?
4. Is there evidence of collimation and are pre-exposure anatomic side markers visible on the image?
5. Do these errors require a repeat exposure?
   Feedback for each set of images is located on the faculty Evolve site.

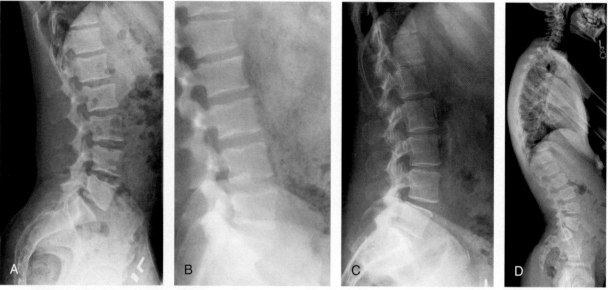

Fig. 9.79 Lateral lumbar spine.

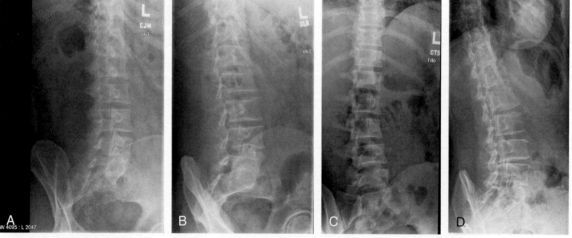

Fig. 9.80 Left posterior oblique (LPO).

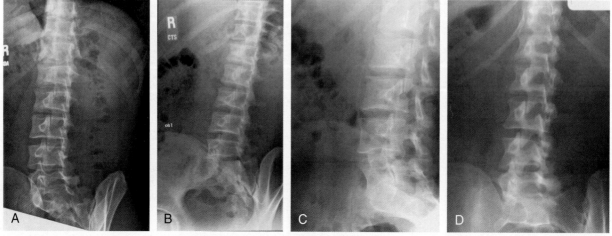

Fig. 9.81 Right posterior oblique (RPO).

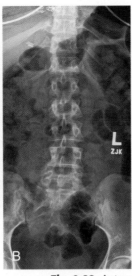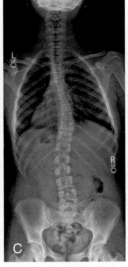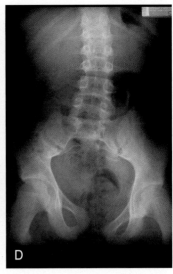

Fig. 9.82 Anteroposterior projection (AP).

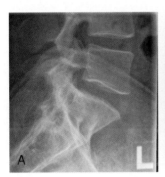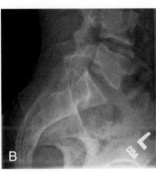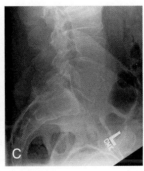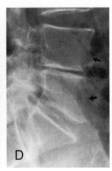

Fig. 9.83 Lateral L5–S1 projection.

9

CHAPTER 10

Bony Thorax—Sternum and Ribs

CONTRIBUTIONS BY **Katrina Lynn Steinsultz,** RT (R)(M), M.Adm, MPH

CONTRIBUTORS TO PAST EDITIONS John P. Lampignano, MEd, RT(R)(CT), Patti Ward, PhD, RT(R), Cindy Murphy, BHSc, RT(R), ACR

CONTENTS

RADIOGRAPHIC ANATOMY

Bony Thorax

The main function of the bony thorax is to serve as an expandable, bellows-like chamber, wherein the interior capacity expands during inspiration and contracts during expiration. These acts of respiration are created by the synchronous work of muscles attached to the rib cage and atmospheric pressure, resulting in air moving into and out of the lungs during respiration.

The bony thorax consists of the **sternum** anteriorly, the **thoracic vertebrae** posteriorly, and the **12 pairs of ribs** that connect the sternum to the vertebral column. This chapter focuses on the sternum and the ribs; details for the thoracic vertebrae are discussed in Chapter 8. The bony thorax also serves to protect important organs of the respiratory system and vital structures within the mediastinum, such as the heart and great vessels.

Fig. 10.1 demonstrates the relationship of the sternum to the 12 pairs of ribs and the 12 thoracic vertebrae. The thin sternum is superimposed by the structures within the mediastinum and the dense thoracic spine in a direct frontal position. Therefore, any anteroposterior (AP) or posteroanterior (PA) projection radiograph would demonstrate the thoracic spine but would show the sternum minimally, if at all.

STERNUM

The adult sternum is a thin, narrow, flat bone with three divisions, the manubrium, body, and xiphoid process (Fig. 10.2). The total length of the adult sternum is approximately 7 inches (18 cm). It is composed of highly vascular cancellous tissue covered by a thin layer of compact bone. This vascular cancellous tissue allows for the sternum to be a common site for marrow biopsy, in which, under local anesthesia, a needle is inserted into the medullary cavity of the sternum to withdraw a sample of red bone marrow.

The upper portion is the **manubrium** *(mah-nu'-bre-um)*. The adult manubrium averages 2 inches (5 cm) in length. The longest part of the sternum is the **body,** which is about 4 inches (10 cm) long. At birth, the body of the sternum is in four separate segments. The union of these four segments begins during puberty and may not be complete until about the age of 25 years.

The most inferior portion of the sternum is the **xiphoid** *(zi'-foid)* **process.** This is composed of cartilage during infancy and youth. It does not become totally ossified until about the age of 40 years. The xiphoid process generally is rather small; however, it can vary in size, shape, and degree of ossification.

RIBS

Each rib is numbered according to the thoracic vertebra to which it attaches; therefore, the ribs are numbered from the top down. The first seven pairs of ribs are considered **true ribs.** True ribs are those ribs that connect directly to the sternum with a short piece of cartilage, called *costocartilage.* The term **false ribs** applies to the last five pairs of ribs, numbered 8 through 12. All of the false ribs, except rib pairs 11 and 12, have costalcartilage that join together at the costocartilage of rib 7. The combined costocartilage at rib 7 connects to the sternum. Rib pairs 11 and 12 do not have costocartilage and therefore do not connect to the sternum. The term **floating ribs** can be used to designate these two pairs of ribs.

The drawing in Fig. 10.3 again clearly shows that, although ribs 8 through 10 have costocartilages, they connect to the costocartilage of the seventh rib.

The last two pairs of false ribs (11 and 12) are unique because they do not possess costocartilage.

Typical Rib

Inferior View A typical rib viewed from its inferior surface is illustrated in Fig. 10.4. A central rib is used to show the common

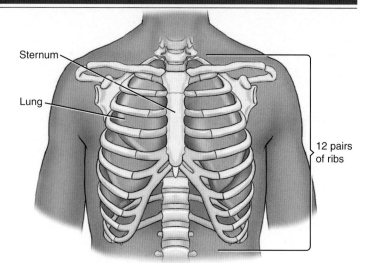

Fig. 10.1 Bony thorax, expandable enclosure for lungs.

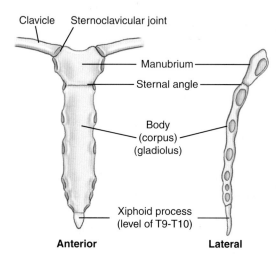

Fig. 10.2 Sternum.

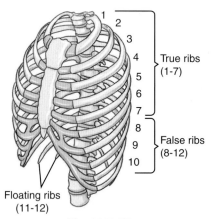

Fig. 10.3 Ribs.

characteristics of a typical rib. Each rib has two ends, a posterior or **vertebral end, which articulates with the thoracic vertebrae** and an anterior or **sternal end, which articulates with the costocartilage.** Between the two ends is the **shaft,** or body, of the rib.

The vertebral end consists of a **head,** which articulates with one or two thoracic vertebral bodies, and a flattened **neck.** Lateral to the neck is an elevated **tubercle** that articulates with the transverse process of a vertebra and allows for attachment of a ligament. The body extends laterally from the tubercle and then angles forward and downward. The area of forward angulation is termed the **angle** of the rib (Fig. 10.5).

Posterior view Fig. 10.5 demonstrates a posterior view of a typical central rib. Seen on this posterior view are the **articular facets of the head, the neck,** and the articular facets of the **tubercle** at the vertebral end of the rib. Progressing laterally, the angle of the rib is that part at which the shaft curves forward and downward toward the sternal end.

The posterior or vertebral end of a typical rib is 3 to 5 inches (8 to 13 cm) **higher** than the anterior or sternal end. Therefore, when viewing a radiograph of a chest or ribs, remember the part of a rib most superior is the posterior end, or the end nearest the vertebrae. The anterior end is more inferior.

The lower inside margin of each rib protects an **artery,** a **vein,** and a **nerve;** therefore, rib injuries are very painful and may be associated with substantial hemorrhage. This inside margin, which contains the blood vessels and nerves, is termed the **costal groove.**

RIB CAGE

Fig. 10.6 illustrates the bony thorax with the sternum and costocartilage removed. The **fifth ribs have been shaded to illustrate the downward angulation of the ribs better.**

Not all ribs have the same appearance. The first ribs are short and broad and are the most vertical of all the ribs. Counting downward from the short first pair, the ribs get longer and longer down to the seventh ribs. From the seventh ribs down, they get shorter and shorter through the fairly short twelfth, or last, pair of ribs. The first ribs are the most sharply curved. The bony thorax is typically **widest** at the lateral margins of the **eighth or ninth ribs.**

Palpable Landmarks and Articulations of Bony Thorax

PALPABLE LANDMARKS

The anterior location and relatively easy palpability of the sternum provide the technologist the ability to locate thoracic and rib structures. The uppermost border of the manubrium has a slightly notched area between the two clavicles, and is easy to visualize and palpate. This area is termed the *jugular notch;* however, the terms *suprasternal notch* and *manubrial notch* are also used. The jugular notch is at the level of T2–T3.

The lower end of the manubrium joins the body of the sternum to form a palpable prominence, the sternal angle (manubriosternal joint). This is also an easily palpated landmark that may be used to locate other structures of the bony thorax. The sternal angle is at the level of the intervertebral disk space between T4 and T5 for an average adult. The xiphoid process corresponds to the level of T9–T10. The inferior rib (costal) angle (inferior costal margin) corresponds to the level of L2–L3 (see Fig. 10.7).

STERNOCLAVICULAR ARTICULATION

Each clavicle articulates medially with the manubrium of the sternum at the clavicular notch; this is called the *sternoclavicular joint.* It is the only bony connection between each shoulder girdle and the bony thorax.

STERNAL RIB ARTICULATIONS

The first seven pairs of ribs connect anteriorly to the sternum through individual sections of costocartilage. The sternum has seven pair of facets, or depressions, located laterally along the manubrium and body to accept the costocartilage. The first pair of facets is located just below the clavicular notch. In Fig. 10.8, the costocartilage and ribs have been added to one side of the drawing to show this relationship.

The second costocartilage connects to the sternum at the level of the sternal angle. An easy way to locate the anterior end of the second rib is to locate the sternal angle first and then feel laterally along the cartilage and the bone of the rib.

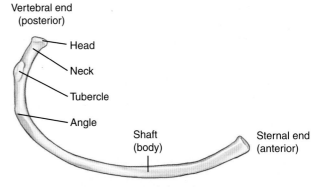

Fig. 10.4 Typical rib—inferior view.

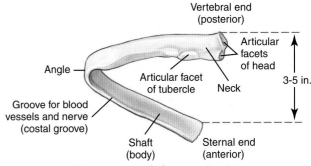

Fig. 10.5 Typical rib—posterior view.

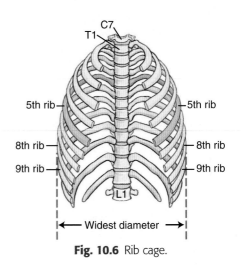

Fig. 10.6 Rib cage.

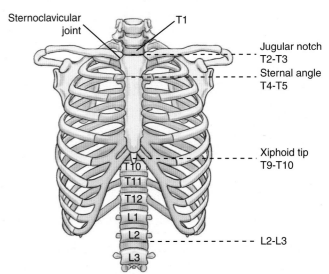

Fig. 10.7 Bony thorax—sternum, ribs, thoracic vertebrae (landmarks and associated vertebrae).

The third through the seventh costocartilages connect directly to the body of the sternum.

Ribs 8, 9, and 10 also possess costocartilage, but these connect to costocartilage 7, which then connects to the sternum.

JOINT CLASSIFICATIONS OF BONY THORAX

A frontal view of an articulated thorax is illustrated in Fig. 10.9. The joints or articulations of the anterior bony thorax are identified on this drawing. The joint classifications and types of motion allowed are described as follows (also see Table 10.1):

Part A demonstrates an example of a costochondral union, or junction, which is a joint between the costocartilage and the sternal end of a rib (shown on left side at the fourth rib). Costochondral unions, found on ribs 1 through 10, are classified as a unique type of union, wherein the cartilage and bone are bound together by the periosteum of the bone itself. This joint permits **no motion;** therefore, they are termed **synarthrodial.**

Part B demonstrates an example of one **sternoclavicular joint,** which occurs between a clavicle and the manubrium of the sternum. The sternoclavicular joints are **synovial** joints, containing articular capsules that permit a plane motion, or **gliding motion,** and are therefore termed **diarthrodial** joints.

Part C illustrates the **sternocostal joint** of the first rib. The cartilage of the first rib attaches directly to the manubrium with no synovial capsule (unlike the sternocostal joints of ribs 2 through 7) and allows **no motion** (termed **synarthrodial**). Therefore, this is a **cartilaginous** class joint of the **synchondrosis** type.

Part D demonstrates an example of a **sternocostal joint,** typical of the second through seventh joints between costocartilage and sternum. These are **synovial** joints, which allow a slight **plane (gliding) motion,** making them what is termed **diarthrodial** joints.

Part E represents the continuous borders of the **interchondral joints** between the costal cartilages of the anterior sixth through ninth ribs. These are all interconnected by a **synovial** type of joint, with a long, thin, articular capsule lined by synovial membrane. These allow a slight **plane (gliding) type** of movement (diarthrodial), facilitating movement of the bony thorax during the breathing process. Interchondral joints between the ninth and tenth cartilages are not synovial and are classified as fibrous syndesmosis.

POSTERIOR ARTICULATIONS

The posterior types of joints in the bony thorax, **parts F and G,** are illustrated in Fig. 10.10. The joints between the ribs and the vertebral column, the **costotransverse joints** (F) and the **costovertebral joints** (G), are **synovial** joints with articular capsules lined by synovial membrane, which allow a plane or **gliding motion,** and are therefore **diarthrodial.** Costotransverse joints are found on the first through the tenth ribs. The eleventh and twelfth ribs lack this joint (see Table 10.1).

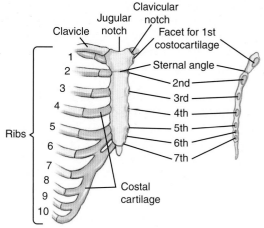

Fig. 10.8 Sternal rib articulations.

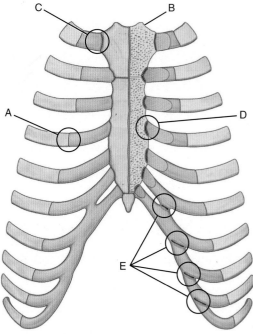

Fig. 10.9 Articulated thorax.

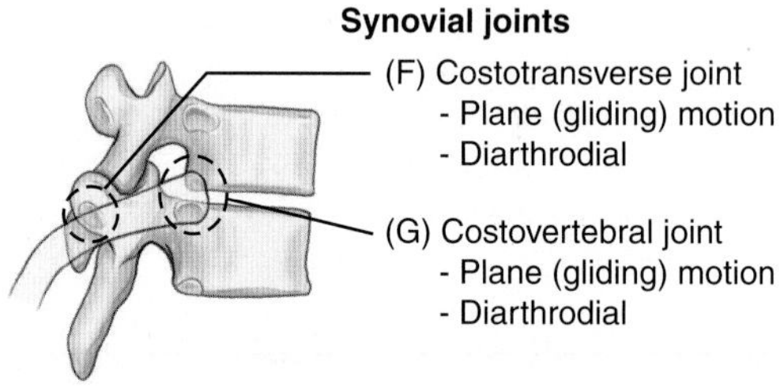

Synovial joints
- (F) Costotransverse joint
  - Plane (gliding) motion
  - Diarthrodial
- (G) Costovertebral joint
  - Plane (gliding) motion
  - Diarthrodial

Fig. 10.10 Posterior articulations.

TABLE 10.1 **SUMMARY OF JOINT CLASSIFICATIONS OF THORAX**			
JOINTS	**CLASSIFICATION**	**MOBILITY TYPE**	**MOVEMENT TYPE**
First to tenth costochondral unions (between costocartilage and ribs)	Unique type of union	Synarthrodial (immovable)	N/A
Sternoclavicular joints (between clavicles and sternum)	Synovial	Diarthrodial	Plane (gliding)
First sternocostal joint (between first rib and sternum)	Cartilaginous (synchondrosis)	Synarthrodial (immovable)	N/A
Second to seventh sternocostal joints (between second and seventh ribs and sternum)	Synovial	Diarthrodial	Plane (gliding)
Sixth to ninth interchondral joints (between anterior sixth and ninth costal cartilages)	Synovial	Diarthrodial	Plane (gliding)
First to tenth costotransverse joints (between ribs and transverse processes of thoracic vertebrae)	Synovial	Diarthrodial	Plane (gliding)
First to twelfth costovertebral joints (between heads of ribs and thoracic vertebrae)	Synovial	Diarthrodial	Plane (gliding)

RADIOGRAPHIC POSITIONING

Positioning Considerations for the Sternum

The sternum is difficult to radiograph because of its thin bony cortex and position within the thorax. It is an anterior midline structure that is in the same plane as the thoracic spine. Because the thoracic spine is more dense than the sternum, it is almost impossible to see the sternum in a true AP or PA projection. Therefore, the patient is rotated in a 15° to 20° right anterior oblique (RAO) position to shift the sternum just to the left of the thoracic vertebrae and over the homogeneously dense heart (Fig. 10.11). By rotating the patient and superimposing the sternum over the heart, the outline of the sternum is more easily recognized.

The degree of obliquity required is dependent on the size of the thoracic cavity. A patient with a shallow or thin chest requires more rotation than a patient with a deep chest to cast the sternum away from the thoracic spine. For example, a patient with a large, barrel-chested thorax with a greater AP measurement requires less rotation (≈15°), whereas a thin-chested patient requires more rotation (≈20°). This principle is illustrated in Figs. 10.11 and 10.12.

EXPOSURE FACTORS

It is difficult to obtain an optimally uniform radiographic appearance of brightness and contrast on sternum images. The sternum is made up primarily of spongy bone with a thin layer of hard compact bone surrounding it. This feature, combined with the close proximity of the easy-to-penetrate lungs and the harder-to-penetrate mediastinum-heart, makes exposure factor selection a challenge. A kVp range of 70 to 85 is recommended for adult sthenic patients to achieve acceptable contrast on the image. Even with optimal exposure factors and patient positioning, the sternum examination results in a low-contrast image making the sternum difficult to visualize (Fig. 10.13).

A breathing technique may be used for radiographic examination of the sternum. A breathing technique involves the patient taking **shallow breaths** during the exposure. This technique is also referred to as an **orthostatic technique.** If performed properly, the lung markings overlying the sternum will become blurred, whereas the image of the sternum will remain sharp and well defined (see Fig. 10.13). This requires a medium kVp range (70 to 80) range, a low mA, and a long exposure time, from 3 to 4 seconds. The technologist must be sure the thorax in general is not moving during the exposure, other than from the gentle breathing motion.

SOURCE–IMAGE RECEPTOR DISTANCE (SID)

A minimum SID for sternum radiography is 40 inches (100 cm). In the past, a common practice was to lower the SID to create magnification of the overlying posterior ribs and sternum with resultant unsharpness (blurring). Although this produced a more visible but distorted image of the sternum, it also resulted in an increase in radiation exposure to the patient. Therefore, this practice is not recommended. To minimize dose to the patient, the patient's skin should be at least 15 inches (40 cm) from the surface of the collimator.[1]

COLLIMATION

Proper collimation is important when imaging the sternum. Because this examination typically results in low-contrast images, scatter must be eliminated as much as possible. Collimation to the sternum will reduce the amount of scattered radiation produced, thereby improving image contrast.

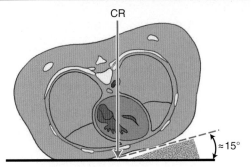

Fig. 10.11 RAO; large, barrel-chested thorax, ≈15°.

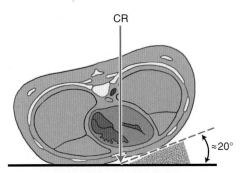

Fig. 10.12 RAO; thin-chested thorax, ≈20°.

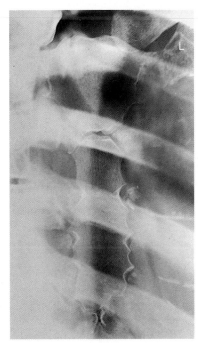

Fig. 10.13 RAO sternum, orthostatic (breathing) technique.

Positioning Considerations for the Sternoclavicular Joints

PA VERSUS AP
Sternoclavicular joint projections are typically performed PA, rather than AP, which can be challenging for the technologist. In the AP projection, the sternoclavicular joints are more easily located. However, PA projections provide the least amount of magnification distortion and reduce the amount of radiation reaching the patient's thyroid.

Positioning Considerations for the Ribs
Specific projections performed in a radiographic examination of the ribs are determined by the patient's clinical history and department protocol. If the patient's history is not provided by the referring physician, the technologist must obtain a complete clinical history that includes the following:

1. The nature of the patient's complaint (acute versus chronic pain or how the injury occurred)
2. The location of the rib pain or injury
3. Whether the injury was caused by trauma to the thoracic cavity (Does the patient have difficulty in breathing?)
4. Whether the patient is able to stand.

The following positioning guidelines will enable the technologist to produce a diagnostic radiologic examination of the ribs.

ABOVE OR BELOW DIAPHRAGM
The location of the trauma and/or patient complaint determines which region of the ribs is to be imaged. Ribs above the diaphragm require different exposure factors, different breathing instructions, and generally different body positions than ribs located below the diaphragm.

The **upper nine posterior ribs** generally represent the minimum number of ribs above the dome or central portion of the diaphragm on full inspiration, as described in Chapter 2. However, with painful rib injuries, the patient may not be able to take as deep an inspiration; thus, only eight posterior ribs may be seen above the diaphragm on inspiration.

SID
A minimum SID of 40 inches (100 cm) should be used for all rib studies. Some departments require a 72-inch (180-cm) SID for rib studies to minimize magnification (distortion) of the thorax and reduce skin dose.

EXPOSURE FACTORS
A medium kVp range is optimal for rib images and allows for penetration of the more dense aspects of the bony thorax while preserving the proper radiographic contrast needed. Use of automatic exposure control (AEC) is not recommended due to the lack of uniformity of tissue density within the bony thorax region.

Above Diaphragm
To demonstrate the above-diaphragm ribs best, the technologist should do the following:

1. Take the radiographs **erect** (Fig. 10.14), if the patient is able to stand or sit. Gravity assists in lowering the diaphragm when the patient is in the erect position. This position also allows a deeper inspiration, which depresses the diaphragm to its lowest position. Also, rib injuries are very painful and body movement that creates pressure against the rib cage, such as movement on the x-ray table, can cause severe pain and discomfort.
2. Suspend respiration and expose on deep **inspiration.** This should project the diaphragm below the ninth or tenth ribs on full inspiration.
3. Select **optimal kVp** range (70 to 85 kVp). Because the upper ribs are surrounded by lung tissue, a lower kVp will preserve radiographic contrast and will allow visualization of the ribs through the air-filled lungs. However, if the site of injury is over the heart area, a higher kVp may be used to obtain a longer scale contrast to visualize ribs through the heart shadow and through the lung fields.

Below Diaphragm
To demonstrate these ribs below the diaphragm best, the technologist should do the following:

1. Take the radiographs with the patient **recumbent** (supine) (Fig. 10.15). This allows the diaphragm to rise to the highest position and results in a less thick abdomen (especially on hypersthenic patients, because the abdomen flattens when recumbent). This provides better visualization of the lower ribs through abdominal structures.
2. Suspend respiration and expose on **expiration.** This should allow the diaphragm to rise to the level of the seventh or eighth posterior ribs, again providing a uniform density for below-diaphragm ribs.
3. Select an **optimal kVp** (75 to 85). Because the lower ribs are surrounded by the muscular diaphragm and dense abdominal structures, a medium kVp will ensure proper penetration of these tissues.

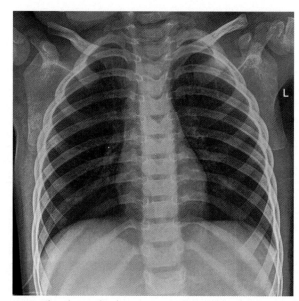

Fig. 10.14 Ribs above diaphragm—erect if possible; inspiration; lower kVp (70 to 75).

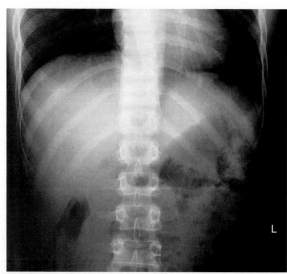

Fig. 10.15 Ribs below diaphragm—recumbent; expiration; medium kVp (75 to 85).

RECOMMENDED PROJECTIONS

Departmental routines for ribs may vary depending on the preference of radiologists. One recommended routine is as follows.

Select the two projections that will place the **area of interest closest to the image receptor** and **rotate the spine away from the area of interest** (prevents the spine from superimposing the region of interest and better demonstrates the axillary portion of the involved region of ribs). For example, if a patient has a history of trauma to the **left posterior ribs,** the two preferred projections with this routine are a straight **AP** and a **left posterior oblique (LPO).** (An above- or below-diaphragm technique would be determined by the level of the injured ribs.) The LPO (Fig. 10.16) will move the spinous processes **away from** the left side. The left posterior ribs are closest and parallel to the IR to increase visibility of this portion of the ribs.

A second example is a patient who has trauma to the **right anterior ribs.** Two preferred projections are a straight **PA** and a **left anterior oblique (LAO).** The **PA** will place the site of injury closest to the image receptor (IR), and the **LAO** will rotate the spinous process **away from** the site of trauma while demonstrating the axillary portion of the right ribs better.

MARKING THE SITE OF INJURY

Some department protocols request the technologist tape a small metallic BB or some other **small** type of radiopaque marker over the site of injury before obtaining the images. This ensures that the radiologist is aware of the location of the trauma or pathology as indicated by the patient.

NOTE: Each technologist should determine department protocol on this practice before using this method of identifying the potential site of injury.

CHEST RADIOGRAPHY

Departmental protocols also differ concerning the inclusion of a chest study as part of a rib examination. Trauma to the bony thorax may result in injury to the respiratory system, and patients with a history of rib injuries may require **erect PA and lateral** projections of the chest and/or inspiration/expiration projections to rule out a possible pneumothorax, hemothorax, pulmonary contusion, or other chest pathology (Fig. 10.17). If the patient cannot assume an erect position and the presence of air-fluid levels must be ruled out, an image obtained with a horizontal beam with the patient in a **decubitus position** should be included. This is described in Chapter 2.

Special Patient Considerations

PEDIATRIC APPLICATIONS

Two primary concerns in pediatric radiography are **patient motion** and **safety.** A clear explanation of the procedure is required to obtain maximal trust and cooperation from the patient and guardian.

Careful immobilization is important to achieve proper positioning and to reduce patient motion. A short exposure time with optimal mA and kVp help reduce patient motion. To secure their safety, ensure that pediatric patients are continuously watched and cared for.

Communication

A clear explanation of the procedure is required to obtain maximum trust and cooperation from the patient and guardian. Distraction techniques that use, for example, toys or stuffed animals are also effective in maintaining patient cooperation.

Immobilization

Pediatric patients (depending on age and condition) are often unable to maintain the required position. Use of an immobilization device to support the patient is recommended to reduce the need for the patient to be held, thus reducing radiation exposure. (Chapter 16 provides an in-depth description of these devices.) If the patient must be held by the guardian, the technologist must provide a lead apron and/or gloves and, if the guardian is female, must ensure no possibility of pregnancy.

Exposure Factors

Exposure factors will vary as a result of various patient sizes. Use of short exposure times (associated with the use of high mA) is recommended to reduce the risk for patient motion. A breathing technique is not indicated for the young pediatric patient.

Collimation

When possible, collimate to the involved region and reduce exposure to the thyroid gland and other radiosensitive structures.

GERIATRIC APPLICATIONS

Communication and Comfort

Sensory losses (e.g., eyesight, hearing) associated with aging may result in the need for additional assistance, time, and patience in helping the older patient achieve the required positions for the sternum and ribs. Decreased position awareness may cause these patients to fear falling off the radiography table when they are imaged in the recumbent position. Reassurance and additional care from the technologist will enable the patient to feel secure and comfortable.

If the examination is performed with the patient in the recumbent position, a radiolucent mattress or pad placed on the examination table will provide comfort. Extra blankets also may be required to keep the patient warm.

Exposure Factors

Because of the high incidence of osteoporosis in older patients, the kVp or mAs may require a decrease if manual exposure factors are used with analog imaging. Older patients may have tremors or difficulty holding steady. Use of short exposure times (associated with the use of high mA) is recommended to reduce the risk for motion.

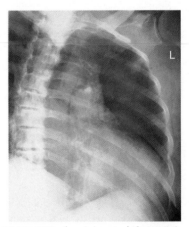

Fig. 10.16 LPO ribs—injury to left posterior ribs.

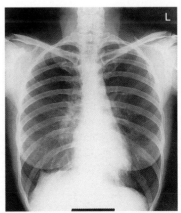

Fig. 10.17 PA erect chest to rule out a possible pneumothorax and/or hemothorax.

BARIATRIC PATIENT CONSIDERATIONS

The bariatric patient does present some unique challenges in imaging of the bony thorax. Landmarks such as the xiphoid process, sternal angle, and vertebra prominens (spinous process of C7) may be difficult to palpate. The easiest landmark to locate through palpation is the jugular notch. Use this landmark for sternum and rib positioning to determine the upper border of the sternum, SC joints, and ribs. The iliac crest or lower costal angle can be used as a landmark to indicate the lower margin of the ribs.

Although the thorax region looks larger in the bariatric patient than in the sthenic patient, it is important to remember the thoracic structures are often the same dimensions. Maintain the same degree of collimation for sternum and rib projections as with other body sizes. Do not set the field size larger than the size of the IR being used. The sternum and SC joint projections can still be performed with a 10 × 12-inch (24 × 30-cm) IR.

Because of the thickness of the anatomy, it is important to use a grid (bucky) for all procedures to decrease scatter radiation reaching the image receptor. This is especially important when performing mobile procedures for studies of the bony thorax. Manual exposure factors may need to be adjusted because of the size of the patient. However, the kVp should be set as high as appropriate while keeping the mAs low to minimize radiation dose to the patient.

Digital Imaging Considerations

Guidelines for digital imaging (computed radiography and digital radiography [DR]) of the bony thorax, sternum, and ribs are similar to those described in previous chapters. These include the following:

1. Correct study and projections selected.
2. Centering and **four-sided** collimation (especially for sternum projections).
3. Apply **ALARA** principle (as low as reasonably achievable) in determining exposure factors (may be desirable to increase kVp and decrease mAs for reducing patient exposure.)
4. Post-processing evaluation of exposure indicator (for highest quality image with least amount of radiation to the patient). Based on the exposure indicator and department standards, this determines whether a reduction in mAs is possible for future and repeat exposures.

Alternative Modalities and Procedures

COMPUTED TOMOGRAPHY

Computed tomography (CT) provides sectional images of the bony thorax. Skeletal detail and associated soft tissues may be evaluated with CT when clinically indicated. CT is useful for visualizing pathology involving the sternum (Fig. 10.18) and/or sternoclavicular joints without obstruction by overlying dense structures (Fig. 10.19).

NUCLEAR MEDICINE

Nuclear medicine (NM) provides a sensitive diagnostic procedure (radionuclide bone scan) for detection of skeletal pathologies of the thoracic cage (e.g., metastases, occult fractures). A radiopharmaceutical-tagged tracer element is injected, which will concentrate in areas of increased bone activity, demonstrating a hot spot on the nuclear medicine image. Any abnormal area then is investigated further with radiography.

It is common practice for patients who are at risk of or symptomatic for skeletal metastases to undergo a bone scan; patients with multiple myeloma are exceptions to this.

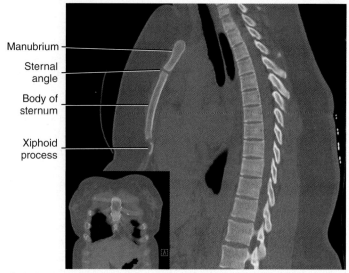

Fig. 10.18 CT of the sternum—sagittal reconstruction. *Inset,* Coronal reconstruction.

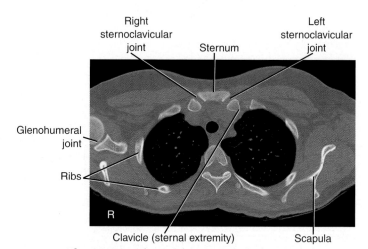

Fig. 10.19 Axial CT of the sternoclavicular joints.

Clinical Indications

Fractures: The word *fracture* refers to a break in the structure of a bone. Fractures of the bony thorax can be particularly dangerous because of the proximity of the lungs, heart, and great vessels. Areas of common fracture include the following:

- **Ribs:** Rib fractures are most commonly caused by trauma or underlying pathology. Any rib fracture may cause injury to the lung or cardiovascular structures (e.g., pneumothorax, pulmonary or cardiac contusion). In particular, fractures to the first rib often are associated with injury to the underlying arteries or veins, whereas fractures to the lower ribs (9 to 12) may be associated with injury to adjacent organs such as the spleen, liver, or kidney.
- **Flail chest:** This fracture of adjacent ribs in two or more places is caused by blunt trauma and is associated with underlying pulmonary injury. This type of injury can lead to instability of the chest wall. If the technologist suspects a flail chest injury, perform rib studies erect if the patient's condition permits it for best visualization.
- **Sternum:** Typically caused by blunt trauma, fractures of the sternum are associated with underlying cardiac injury.

Congenital anomalies: Congenital anomalies are conditions present from birth that may become more evident as a child ages.

- **Pectus carinatum (pigeon breast):** This defect is characterized by anterior protrusion of the lower sternum and xiphoid process. It is usually a benign condition but could lead to cardiopulmonary complications in rare cases.
- **Pectus excavatum:** Also referred to as **funnel chest,** this deformity is characterized by a depressed sternum. This condition rarely interferes with respiration but often is corrected surgically for cosmetic reasons.

Metastases: These primary malignant neoplasms spread to distant sites via blood and lymphatics. The ribs are common sites of metastatic lesions, which may be characterized and visualized on the image as follows:

- **Osteolytic**—destructive lesions with irregular margins
- **Osteoblastic**—proliferative bony lesions of increased density
- **Combination osteolytic and osteoblastic**—moth-eaten appearance of bone resulting from the mix of destructive and blastic lesions

Osteomyelitis: This localized or generalized infection of bone and marrow can be associated with postoperative complications of open heart surgery, which requires the sternum to be split. The most common cause of osteomyelitis is a bacterial infection. See Table 10.2 for a summary of clinical indications.

Routine and Special Projections

Protocols and positioning routines vary among facilities, depending on administrative structures, liabilities, and other factors. All technologists should become familiar with the current standards of practice, protocols, and routine or basic and special projections for any facility in which they are working.

Certain routine and special projections for the sternum, sternoclavicular joints, and ribs are demonstrated and described on the following pages as suggested standard routine and special departmental routines or procedures.

TABLE 10.2 SUMMARY OF CLINICAL INDICATIONS

CONDITION OR DISEASE	MOST COMMON RADIOGRAPHIC EXAMINATION	POSSIBLE RADIOGRAPHIC APPEARANCE	EXPOSURE FACTOR ADJUSTMENT[a]
Fractures			
Ribs—flail chest	Routine radiographic views of the ribs and chest. Perform study erect when possible	Disruption of bony cortex of the rib; linear lucency through the rib	None
Sternum	Routine radiographic sternum views, computed tomography	Disruption of bony cortex of the sternum; linear lucency or a displaced sternal segment	None
Congenital Anomalies			
Pectus carinatum (pigeon breast)	Routine chest and possible lateral sternum	Anterior protrusion of lower sternum	None
Pectus excavatum (funnel chest)	Routine chest and possible lateral sternum	Depressed sternum	None
Metastases	Routine radiographic views, nuclear medicine bone scan	Depends on lesion type: • Osteolytic: irregular margins and decreased density • Osteoblastic lesions: increased density • Combination—moth-eaten appearance	Lesion type: • Osteolytic: decrease (−) • Osteoblastic: increase (+) • Combination: none
Osteomyelitis	Routine sternum views, nuclear medicine bone scan	Erosion of bony margins	None

[a]Dependent on stage or severity of disease or condition.

RAO POSITION—STERNUM

Clinical Indications
- Pathology of the sternum, including fractures and inflammatory processes

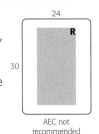

Sternum
ROUTINE
- RAO
- Lateral

Technical Factors
- Minimum SID—40 inches (100 cm)
- IR size—10 × 12 inches (24 × 30 cm), portrait
- Grid
- 3- to 4-second exposure if breathing technique is used
- kVp range: 70–85

24

R

30

AEC not recommended

Shielding
Shield radiosensitive tissues outside region of interest.

Patient Position
Erect (preferred) or semiprone position with slight rotation, right arm down by side, and left arm up.

Part Position ⊞
- Position patient oblique, **15° to 20°** toward the right side, RAO (see NOTE 1).
- Align long axis of sternum to CR and to midline of table/upright bucky.
- Place top of IR approximately 1½ inches (4 cm) superior to the jugular notch.

CR
- CR perpendicular to IR
- CR directed to **center of sternum** (1 inch [2.5 cm] to left of midline and midway between the jugular notch and xiphoid process) (Fig. 10.20)

Recommended Collimation
Long, narrow collimation field to region of sternum

Respiration
Orthostatic (shallow breathing) technique can be performed if patient can cooperate. If breathing technique is not possible, suspend respiration on expiration. Orthostatic breathing technique requires a minimum of a 3-second exposure time and a low mA to produce blurring of overlying vascular structures. The orthostatic technique for the RAO sternum projection is most effective for the recumbent patient in whom the sternum is less likely to move during the long exposure. There is a risk of unintentional movement of the body thorax when the position is performed erect.

NOTE 1—Rotation: A large, deep-chested thorax requires less rotation than a thin-chested thorax to shift the sternum just to the left of the vertebral column superimposed over the homogeneous heart shadow. The amount of required rotation also can be determined by placing one hand on the sternum and the other on the spinous processes and determining that these two points are not superimposed, as viewed from the position of the x-ray tube (see Figs 10.11 and 10.12).

NOTE 2—Adaptation: This can be obtained in an LPO position if the patient's condition does not permit an RAO position. (See Chapter 15 for trauma positions of the sternum.) If the patient cannot be rotated, an oblique image may be obtained by angling the CR 15° to 20° across the right side of the patient to project the sternum lateral to the vertebral column, onto the heart shadow (see Fig. 10.20, inset). A portable grid would be required and should be placed crosswise on the stretcher or tabletop to prevent grid cutoff.

Evaluation Criteria
Anatomy Demonstrated: • Sternum is visualized, superimposed on heart shadow (Figs. 10.21 and 10.22).

Position: • Correct patient rotation is demonstrated by visualizing sternum alongside vertebral column with no superimposition by vertebrae. No distortion of sternum due to excessive rotation of the thorax. • **Collimation** to area of interest.

Exposure: • Optimal contrast and density (brightness) demonstrate outline of sternum through overlying ribs, lung, and heart. • Bony margins of the sternum appear sharp, but lung markings are blurred if breathing technique was used. • **No motion** (with suspended respiration).

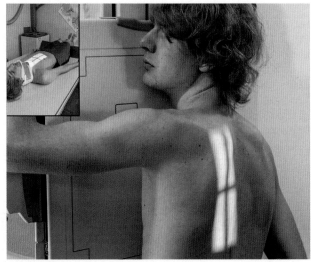

Fig. 10.20 Erect—RAO sternum. *Inset,* 15° to 20° cross-angle, grid crosswise.

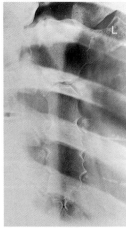

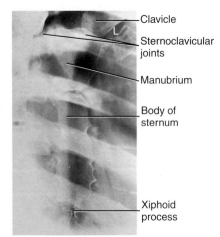

Clavicle

Sternoclavicular joints

Manubrium

Body of sternum

Xiphoid process

Fig. 10.21 RAO sternum.

Fig. 10.22 RAO sternum.

LATERAL POSITION: R OR L LATERAL—STERNUM

Clinical Indications
- Pathology of the sternum, including fractures and inflammatory processes
- Depressed sternal fractures

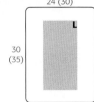

Sternum
ROUTINE
• RAO
• Lateral

24 (30)

30 (35)

L

AEC not recommended

Technical Factors
- Minimum SID—40 inches (100 cm) (see NOTE 1)
- IR size—10 × 12 inches (24 × 30 cm), or 14 × 14 inches (35 × 35 cm), portrait
- Grid
- kVp range: 75–85

Shielding Shield radiosensitive tissue outside region of interest.

Patient Position Erect (preferred) or lateral recumbent

Part Position
Erect
- Position patient standing or seated with shoulders and arms **drawn back** (Fig. 10.23).

Lateral Recumbent
- Position patient lying on side with arms up above head and keeping shoulders back (see NOTE 2).
- Place top of IR 1½ inches (4 cm) above the jugular notch.
- Align long axis of sternum to CR and midline of grid or table/upright bucky.
- Ensure a true lateral, with **no rotation.**

CR
- CR is perpendicular to IR.
- CR is directed to **center of sternum** (midway between the jugular notch and xiphoid process).
- Center IR to CR.

Recommended Collimation Long, narrow collimation field, to region of sternum.

Respiration Suspend respiration on **inspiration.**

NOTE 1: SID of 60 to 72 inches (150 to 180 cm) is recommended to reduce magnification of sternum caused by increased OID. (If unable to obtain this SID and if a minimum of 40 inches [100 cm] is used, a larger IR of 14 × 14 inches [35 × 35 cm] is recommended to compensate for the magnification.)

NOTE 2: Large, pendulous breasts of female patients may be drawn to the sides and held in position with a wide bandage if necessary.

Adaptation The lateral image can be obtained with the use of a horizontal x-ray beam with patient in the supine position if patient's condition warrants this modification (Fig. 10.24).

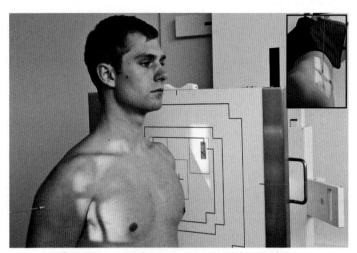

Fig. 10.23 Lateral—erect. *Inset,* Lateral recumbent.

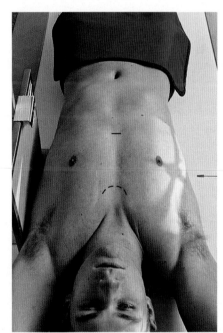

Fig. 10.24 Horizontal beam lateral.

Evaluation Criteria
Anatomy Demonstrated: • Entire sternum with minimal overlap of soft tissues (Figs. 10.25 and 10.26).

Position: • Correct patient position with **no rotation** demonstrates the following: • Entire sternum with no superimposition of the ribs. • Lower aspect of sternum not obscured by breasts of female patient. • **Collimation** to area of interest.

Exposure: • Optimal contrast and density (brightness) to visualize the entire sternum. • **No motion,** indicated by sharp bony margins.

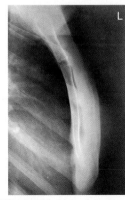

Fig. 10.25 Lateral sternum.

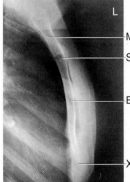

Manubrium

Sternal angle

Body

Xiphoid process

Fig. 10.26 Lateral sternum.

10

PA PROJECTION—STERNOCLAVICULAR JOINTS

Clinical Indications

- Joint subluxation or other pathology of the sternoclavicular joints

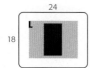

Sternoclavicular Joints
ROUTINE
• PA
• Anterior oblique

Technical Factors

- Minimum SID—40 inches (100 cm)
- IR size—8 × 10 inches (18 × 24 cm), landscape
- Grid
- kVp range: 75–85

Shielding Shield radiosensitive tissues outside region of interest.

Patient Position Patient prone, chin resting on radiolucent positioning sponge, arms up beside head or down by side (Fig. 10.27). Projection may also be taken erect.

Part Position

- Align midsagittal plane to CR and to midline of grid or table/upright bucky.
- Allow **no rotation** of shoulders or thorax.
- Center IR to CR (3 inches [7 cm] distal to vertebra prominens at level of T2–T3).

CR

- CR perpendicular, centered to midsagittal plane at the level of T2–T3, or 3 inches (7 cm) distal to vertebra prominens (spinous process of C7)

Recommended Collimation Collimate to region of sternoclavicular joints (approximately 2 inches (5 cm) on either side of the thoracic spine).

Respiration Suspend on **expiration** for a more uniform density.

Evaluation Criteria

Anatomy Demonstrated: • Bilateral right and left sternoclavicular joints. Lateral aspect of manubrium and medial portion of the clavicles visualized lateral to vertebral column through superimposing ribs and lungs. (Figs. 10.28 and 10.29).

Position: • No rotation of patient, as demonstrated by equal distance of sternoclavicular joints from vertebral column on both sides. • Collimation to area of interest.

Exposure: • Optimal contrast and density (brightness) to visualize the manubrium and medial portion of the clavicles through superimposing ribs and lungs. • No motion, as indicated by sharp bony margins.

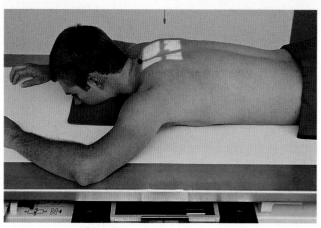

Fig. 10.27 PA bilateral, SC joints.

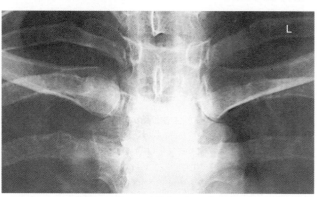

Fig. 10.28 PA bilateral, SC joints.

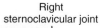

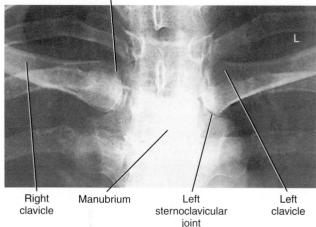

Right sternoclavicular joint

Right clavicle   Manubrium   Left sternoclavicular joint   Left clavicle

Fig. 10.29 PA bilateral, SC joints.

ANTERIOR OBLIQUE POSITIONS: RAO AND LAO— STERNOCLAVICULAR JOINTS

IMAGES OF THE RIGHT AND LEFT JOINTS ARE OBTAINED

Clinical Indications

- Joint separation, subluxation, or other pathology of the sternoclavicular joints
  Best visualizes the sternoclavicular joint on **downside**, which also is demonstrated closest to the spine on the radiograph (see NOTE 1; see NOTE 2 for less obliquity to visualize upside joint).

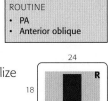

Sternoclavicular Joints
ROUTINE
• PA
• Anterior oblique

Technical Factors

- Minimum SID—40 inches (100 cm)
- IR size—8 × 10 inches (18 × 24 cm), landscape
- Grid
- kVp range: 75–85

Shielding Shield radiosensitive tissues outside region of interest.

Patient Position Prone or erect with slight rotation (10° to 15°) of thorax with upside elbow flexed and hand placed adjacent to head

Part Position

- With patient rotated 10° to 15°, align and center spinous process 1 to 2 inches (3 to 5 cm) lateral (toward upside) to CR and midline of grid or table/upright bucky (Fig. 10.30).
- Center IR to CR

CR

- CR perpendicular to level of T2 to T3, or 3 inches (7.5 cm) distal to vertebra prominens, and 1 to 2 inches (2.5 to 5 cm) lateral (toward upside) to midsagittal plane

Recommended Collimation Collimate to region of sternoclavicular joints.

Respiration Suspend on expiration for a more uniform density (brightness).

NOTE 1: A 10° to 15° rotation in an anterior oblique position will rotate the SC joint across the spine to the opposite lung field, thus demonstrating the downside SC joint. An RAO best demonstrates the right SC joint in the left lung field (Fig. 10.31), whereas the LAO position best demonstrates the left SC joint in the right lung field.

NOTE 2: With less obliquity (5° to 10°), the opposite SC joint (the upside joint) would be visualized next to the vertebral column.

Evaluation Criteria

Anatomy Demonstrated: • The manubrium, medial portion of clavicles, and sternoclavicular joint are best demonstrated on the downside (Figs. 10.31 and 10.32). • The SC joint on the upside will be foreshortened.

Position: • Correct patient rotation demonstrates the downside sternoclavicular joint visualized with no superimposition of the vertebral column or manubrium.

Exposure: • Optimal contrast and density (brightness) to visualize the sternoclavicular joints through overlying ribs and lungs. • **No motion**, as indicated by sharp bony margins.

Adaptation (1) If the patient's condition requires this, oblique images may be obtained by using posterior oblique with 10° to 15° rotation with the CR 1 to 2 inches (2.5 to 5 cm) lateral to midsagittal (toward downside). The upside SC joint would be best visualized in this projection. (2) Oblique images may also be obtained by angling the CR 15° across the patient to project the SC joint lateral to the vertebrae. A portable grid would be required and should be placed crosswise on the stretcher or tabletop to prevent grid cutoff.

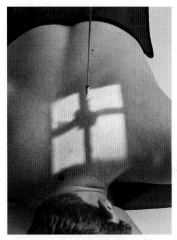

Fig. 10.30 10° to 15° RAO, for right SC joints.

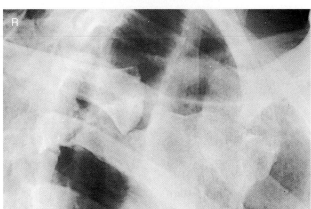

Fig. 10.31 10° to 15° RAO, best demonstrates right (downside) SC joint.

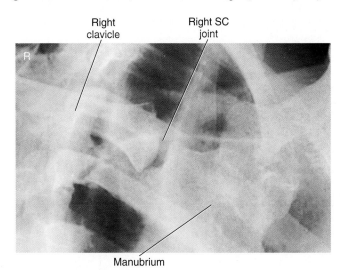

Fig. 10.32 10° to 15° RAO, right SC joint.

AP PROJECTION—BILATERAL POSTERIOR RIBS

ABOVE OR BELOW DIAPHRAGM

Clinical Indications
- Pathology of the ribs posterior ribs, including fracture and neoplastic processes

Technical Factors
- Minimum SID—40 inches (100 cm). When performing a bilateral rib examination, a 72-inch (180-cm) SID can be used to minimize magnification of the anatomy.
- IR size—14 × 17 inches (35 × 43 cm), landscape (see NOTE)
- Grid
- kVp range (above or below diaphragm): 75–85

Ribs
ROUTINE
• Posterior ribs (AP) or anterior ribs (PA)— bilateral study
• Unilateral rib (AP/PA) study
• Axillary ribs (anterior or posterior oblique)
• PA chest (see Chapter 2)

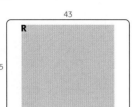

Shielding Shield radiosensitive tissues outside region of interest.

Patient Position Erect position is preferred for above diaphragm if patient's condition allows and supine for below diaphragm (Fig. 10.33).

Part Position
- Align midsagittal plane to CR and to midline of grid or table/upright bucky.
- **Raise chin** to prevent it from superimposing the upper ribs; look straight ahead.
- Rotate shoulders anteriorly to remove scapulae from lung fields.
- Allow **no rotation** of thorax or pelvis.

CR
Above diaphragm
- CR **perpendicular** to IR, centered to the midsagittal plane, at a level **3 or 4 inches** (8 to 10 cm) **below jugular notch** (level of T7)

Below diaphragm
- CR perpendicular to IR, centered to the midsagittal plane, at a level midway between the xiphoid process and the lower rib margin.

Recommended Collimation Collimate to region of interest. Below-diaphragm rib images allow for increased collimation.

Respiration Suspend respiration on **deep inspiration** for ribs **above** the diaphragm and on **full expiration** for ribs **below** the diaphragm.

Evaluation Criteria
Anatomy Demonstrated: • Above diaphragm: Ribs 1 through 9 should be visualized (Fig. 10.34). • **Below diaphragm:** Ribs 10 through 12 (minimum) should be visualized (Fig. 10.35).

Position: • Rotation of the thorax should not be evident. • **Collimation** to area of interest.

Exposure: • Optimal contrast and density (brightness) to visualize ribs through the lungs and heart shadow or through the dense abdominal organs if below the diaphragm. • **No motion**, as demonstrated by sharp bony markings.

NOTE: When performing a bilateral rib examination, place IR landscape for 40-inch (100-cm) SID and/or for large patients for both above- and below-diaphragm ribs to ensure that lateral rib margins are not cut off. A 72-inch (180-cm) SID also can be used to minimize magnification of the anatomy and may allow the IR to be positioned portrait.

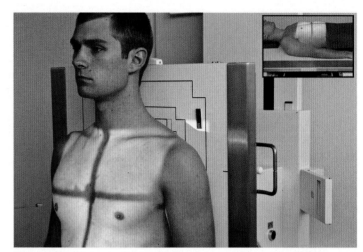

Fig. 10.33 AP erect—above diaphragm. *Inset,* AP supine—below diaphragm.

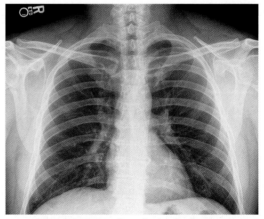

Fig. 10.34 AP ribs—above diaphragm.

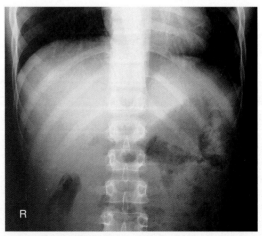

Fig. 10.35 AP ribs—below diaphragm.

PA PROJECTION—BILATERAL ANTERIOR RIBS

ABOVE DIAPHRAGM

Clinical Indications
- Pathology of the anterior ribs, including fracture or neoplastic processes

Injuries to ribs below the diaphragm are generally to posterior ribs; therefore, AP projections are indicated.

Technical Factors
- Minimum SID—40 inches (100 cm). When performing a bilateral rib examination, 72-inch (180-cm) SID can be used to minimize magnification of the anatomy.
- IR size—14 × 17 inches (35 × 43 cm), landscape or 14 × 14 inches (35 × 35 cm), portrait (see NOTE)
- Grid
- kVp range: 75–85

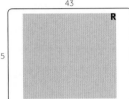

Ribs

ROUTINE
- Posterior ribs (AP) or anterior ribs (PA)— bilateral study
- Unilateral rib (AP/PA) study
- Axillary ribs (anterior or posterior oblique)
- PA chest (see Chapter 2)

Shielding Shield radiosensitive tissues outside region of interest.

Patient Position Erect preferred or prone if necessary, with arms down to the side (Fig. 10.36)

Part Position
- Align midsagittal plane to CR and to midline of grid or table/ upright bucky.
- Rotate shoulders anteriorly to remove scapulae from lung fields.
- Allow **no rotation** of thorax or pelvis.

CR
- CR **perpendicular** to IR, centered to midsagittal plane, at the level of **T7** (7 to 8 inches [18 to 20 cm] below vertebra prominens as for PA chest)

Recommended Collimation Collimate to region of interest.

Respiration Suspend respiration on **inspiration.**

NOTE: Use of a 72-inch (180-cm) SID and/or narrow chest dimensions may allow the IR to be positioned portrait.

PA erect and lateral chest study A common rib routine series typically includes an erect PA and (sometimes) lateral chest projections with lung exposure techniques to rule out respiratory trauma or dysfunctions such as pneumothorax (white arrows) or hemothorax (black arrows), which may accompany rib injuries (Fig. 10.37).

Evaluation Criteria
Anatomy Demonstrated: • Ribs 1 through 9 visualized above the diaphragm (Fig. 10.38).

Position: • No rotation of the thorax. • **Collimation** to area of interest.

Exposure: • Optimal contrast and density (brightness) to visualize ribs through the lungs and heart. • **No motion,** as demonstrated by sharp bony markings.

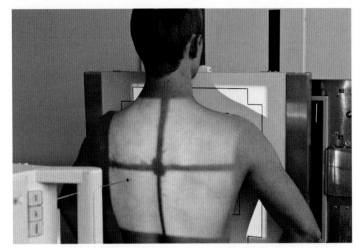

Fig. 10.36 Bilateral PA ribs—above diaphragm.

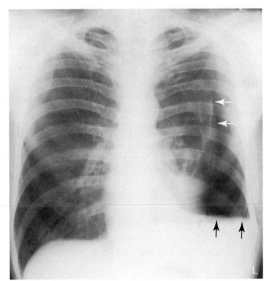

Fig. 10.37 PA erect chest (chest technique). This demonstrates a combination hemothorax *(black arrows)* and pneumothorax *(white arrows)* on the left side.

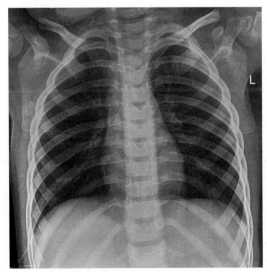

Fig. 10.38 Bilateral PA ribs—above diaphragm.

10

AP PROJECTION: UNILATERAL RIB STUDY—POSTERIOR RIBS

ABOVE OR BELOW DIAPHRAGM

NOTE: This projection is taken to demonstrate specific trauma to posterior ribs along one side of the thoracic cavity.

Technical Factors

- Minimum SID—40 inches (100 cm)
- IR sizes: Above diaphragm—14 × 17 inches (35 × 43 cm), portrait, or below diaphragm—14 × 14 inches (35 × 35 cm), portrait
- Grid
- kVp range (above or below diaphragm): 75–85

Shielding Shield radiosensitive tissues outside region of interest.

Patient Position Erect position is preferred for above diaphragm (Fig. 10.39) if patient's condition allows or supine for below diaphragm.

Part Position ⊞

- Align left or right side of thorax to CR and to midline of grid or table/upright bucky.
- **Raise chin** to prevent it from superimposing upper ribs; look straight ahead.
- Allow **no rotation** of thorax or pelvis.

CR
Above diaphragm

- CR **perpendicular** to IR, centered midway between midsagittal plane and lateral margin of thorax at a level **3 to 4 inches** (8 to 10 cm) **below the jugular notch**

Below diaphragm

- CR **perpendicular** to IR, centered midway between midsagittal plane and lateral margin of thorax at a level midway between the xiphoid process and the lower rib margin
- Align left or right side of thorax to CR and to midline of grid or table/upright bucky.
- IR centered to CR (bottom of IR at iliac crest)

Recommended Collimation Collimate to region of interest.

Respiration Suspend respiration on **deep inspiration** for ribs **above** the diaphragm and on **full expiration** for ribs **below** the diaphragm.

Ribs
ROUTINE
- Posterior ribs (AP) or anterior ribs (PA)—bilateral study
- Unilateral rib (AP/PA) study
- Axillary ribs (anterior or posterior oblique)
- PA chest (see Chapter 2)

35 / 43 / R

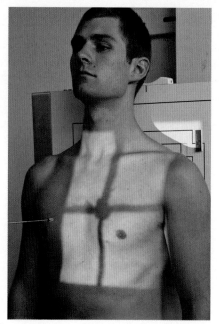

Fig. 10.39 Erect AP projection of unilateral ribs.

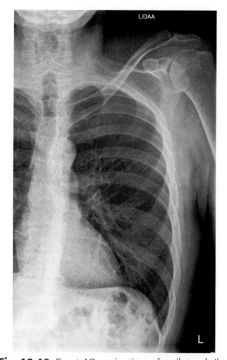

Fig. 10.40 Erect AP projection of unilateral ribs.

Evaluation Criteria

Anatomy Demonstrated: • Above diaphragm: Ribs 1 through 9 should be visualized (Fig. 10.40). • Below diaphragm: Ribs 10 through 12 (minimum) should be visualized.

Position: • Rotation of the thorax should not be evident. • Collimation to area of interest.

Exposure: • Optimal contrast and density (brightness) to visualize ribs through the lungs and heart shadow or through the dense abdominal organs if below the diaphragm. • **No motion,** as demonstrated by sharp bony markings.

ANTERIOR OBLIQUE POSITIONS—AXILLARY RIBS

ABOVE OR BELOW DIAPHRAGM

Clinical Indications
- Pathology of the ribs, including fracture and neoplastic processes

Oblique positions will demonstrate the axillary portion of the ribs that is not well seen on the AP-PA projections.

Posterior–lateral injury: Posterior oblique positions, affected side toward IR

Anterior–lateral injury: Anterior oblique positions, affected side away from IR (see NOTE)

Ribs
ROUTINE
• Posterior ribs (AP) or anterior ribs (PA)
• Axillary ribs (anterior or posterior oblique)
• PA chest (see Chapter 2)

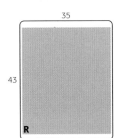

Technical Factors
- Minimum SID—40 inches (100 cm). A 72-inch (180 cm) SID can be used to minimize magnification of the anatomy.
- IR size—14 × 17 inches (35 × 43 cm) or 14 × 14 inches (35 × 35 cm), landscape (see NOTE 1)
- Grid
- kVp range (above or below diaphragm): 75–85

Shielding Shield radiosensitive tissues outside region of interest.

Patient Position Erect position is preferred for above diaphragm if patient's condition allows or supine for below diaphragm.

Part Position
- Rotate patient into 45° posterior or anterior oblique, with **affected side closest to IR** on **posterior** oblique and **affected side away from IR** on **anterior** oblique. Fig. 10.41 is an RPO, which will demonstrate the axillary portion of the **right** ribs. Fig. 10.42 is an RAO, which demonstrates the axillary portion of the **left** ribs. (Hint: rotate spine **away** from site of injury.)
- Raise elevated side arm above head; extend opposite arm down and behind patient away from thorax.
- If recumbent, flex knee of elevated side to help maintain this position.
- Support body with positioning sponges if needed.
- Align a plane of the thorax midway between the spine and the lateral margin of thorax on side of interest to CR and to midline of the grid or table/bucky. (Ensure that side of interest is **not** cut off.)

CR
- CR perpendicular to IR

Above diaphragm
- CR to level 3 or 4 inches (8 to 10 cm) below jugular notch **(T7)** for posterior oblique or 7 to 8 inches [18 to 20 cm] below vertebra prominens (T7) for anterior oblique projections

Below diaphragm
- CR to level midway between xiphoid process and lower rib margin (bottom of IR at about level of iliac crest) (Fig. 10.43)

Recommended Collimation Collimate to region of interest.

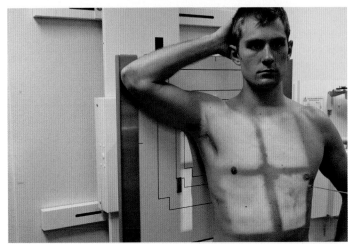

Fig. 10.41 RPO—injury to the right posterior ribs, above diaphragm.

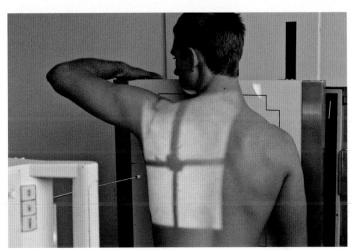

Fig. 10.42 RAO—injury to left anterior ribs, above diaphragm.

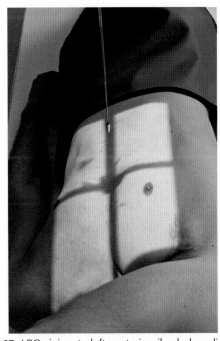

Fig. 10.43 LPO—injury to left posterior ribs, below diaphragm.

10

Respiration Suspend respiration on **inspiration** for above-diaphragm ribs and on **expiration** for below-diaphragm ribs.

NOTE: To demonstrate the axillary portion of the right ribs, perform an RPO or LAO position. To demonstrate the axillary portion of the left ribs, perform an LPO or RAO position (Figs. 10.44 and 10.45)

Additional collimated projection Some departmental routines include one well-collimated projection of the region of injury taken on a smaller IR (Fig. 10.46).

Evaluation Criteria

Anatomy Demonstrated: • Above-diaphragm ribs: Ribs 1 through 9 should be included and seen above the diaphragm. • Below-diaphragm ribs: Ribs 10 through 12 (minimum) should be included and seen below the diaphragm; the axillary portion of the ribs under examination is projected without self-superimposition.

Position: • An accurate 45° oblique position should demonstrate the axillary ribs in profile with the spine shifted away from the area of interest. • **Collimation** to area of interest.

Exposure: • Optimal contrast and density (brightness) to visualize ribs through the lungs and heart shadow or through the dense abdominal organs if below the diaphragm. • **No motion**, as demonstrated by sharp bony markings.

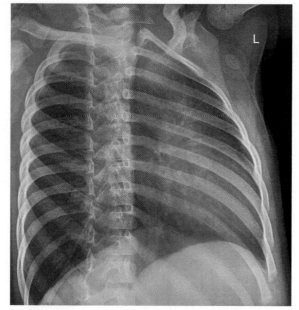

Fig. 10.44 LPO—above diaphragm, left axillary ribs.

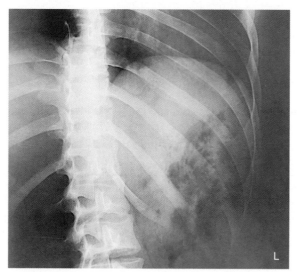

Fig. 10.45 LPO—below diaphragm, left axillary ribs.

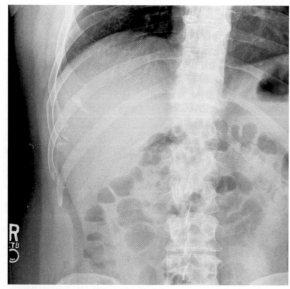

Fig. 10.46 AP below diaphragm, centered for right ribs.

RADIOGRAPHS FOR CRITIQUE

This section consists of an ideal projection (Image A) along with one or more projections that may demonstrate positioning and/or technical errors. Critique Figures C10.47 through C10.50. Compare Image A to the other projections and identify the errors. While examining each image, consider the following questions:

1. Is all essential anatomy demonstrated on the image?
2. What positioning errors are present that compromise image quality?

3. Are technical factors optimal?
4. Is there evidence of collimation and are pre-exposure anatomic side markers visible on the image?
5. Do these errors require a repeat exposure?

Feedback for each set of images is located on the faculty Evolve site.

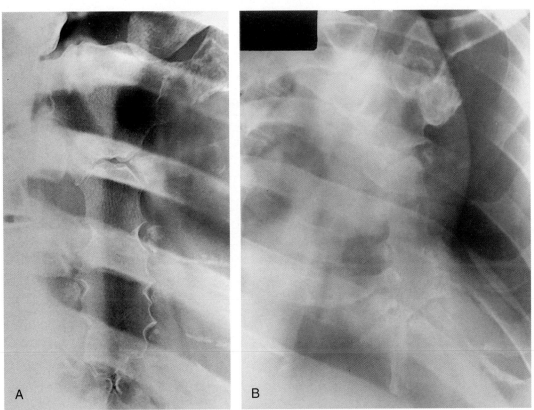

Fig. C10.47 Oblique sternum.

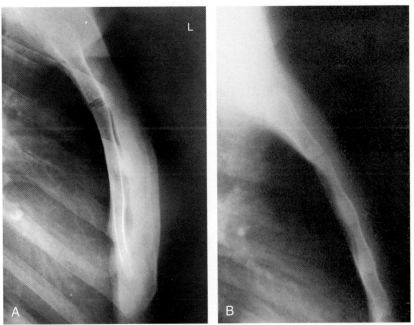

Fig. C10.48 Lateral sternum.

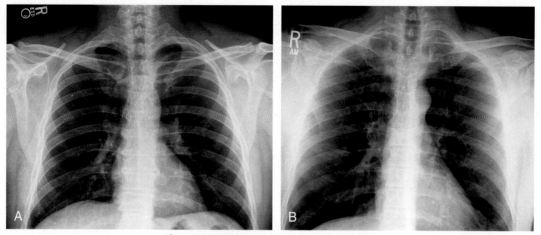

Fig. C10.49 Bilateral ribs above diaphragm.

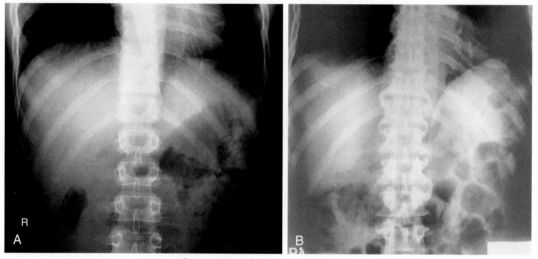

Fig. C10.50 Ribs—below diaphragm.

CHAPTER 11

Cranium, Facial Bones, and Paranasal Sinuses

CONTRIBUTIONS BY **Michele L. Gray-Murphy,** M.Ed., RT(R)(M)(ARRT)

CONTRIBUTORS TO PAST EDITIONS   Kathy M. Martensen, BS, RT(R), Barry T. Anthony, RT(R), Cindy Murphy, BHSc, RT(R), ACR, Renee F. Tossell, PhD, RT(R)(M)(CV), Mindy S. Shapiro, RT(R)(CT)

CONTENTS

RADIOGRAPHIC ANATOMY

11

Skull

As with other body parts, radiography of the skull requires a good understanding of all related anatomy. The anatomy of the skull is very complex, and specific attention to detail is required of the technologist.

The **skull,** or bony skeleton of the head, rests on the superior end of the vertebral column and is divided into two main sets of bones—**8 cranial bones** and **14 facial bones** (Fig. 11.1). Anatomy and positioning for the cranial and facial bones are described in this chapter.

CRANIAL BONES

The eight bones of the cranium are divided into the calvarium (skullcap) and the floor. Each of these two areas primarily consists of four bones.

Calvarium (Skullcap)

1. Frontal
2. Right parietal *(pah-ri′-e-tal)*
3. Left parietal
4. Occipital *(ok-sip′-i-tal)*

Floor

1. Right temporal
2. Left temporal
3. Sphenoid *(sfe′-noid)*
4. Ethmoid *(eth′-moid)*

The eight bones that make up the calvarium (skullcap) and the floor or base of the cranium are demonstrated on these frontal, lateral, and superior cutaway view drawings (Figs. 11.2, 11.3, and 11.4). These cranial bones are fused in an adult to form a protective enclosure for the brain. Each of these cranial bones is demonstrated and described individually in the pages that follow.

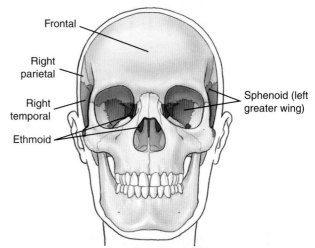

Fig. 11.2 Cranium—frontal view.

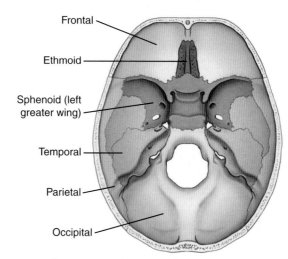

Fig. 11.3 Cranium—superior cutaway view.

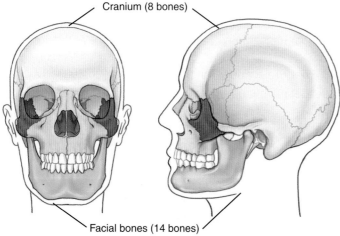

Fig. 11.1 Skull—bony skeleton of head (cranial and facial bones).

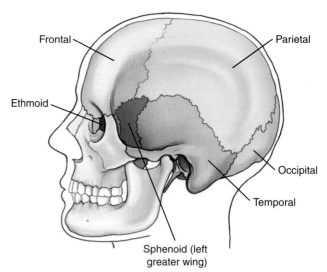

Fig. 11.4 Cranium—lateral view.

Frontal Bone As viewed from the front, the bone of the calvarium that is most readily visible is the **frontal bone.** This bone contributes to the formation of the forehead and the superior part of each orbit. It consists of two main parts: the **squamous** or **vertical portion,** which forms the forehead, and the **orbital** or **horizontal portion,** which forms the superior part of the orbit.

Squamous or vertical portion The **glabella** is the smooth, raised prominence between the eyebrows just above the bridge of the nose (Figs. 11.5 and 11.6).

The **supraorbital groove (SOG)** is the slight depression above each eyebrow. The SOG becomes an important landmark because it corresponds to the floor of the anterior fossa of the cranial vault, which is also at the level of the orbital plate or at the highest level of the facial bone mass (Fig. 11.7).

NOTE: You can locate the SOG on yourself by placing your finger against the length of your eyebrow and feeling the raised arch of bone, then allowing your finger to slide upward and drop slightly into the SOG.

The superior rim of each orbit is the **supraorbital margin (SOM).** The **supraorbital notch** (foramen) is a small hole or opening within the SOM slightly medial to its midpoint. The supraorbital nerve and artery pass through this small opening.

On each side of the squamous portion of the frontal bone above the SOG is a larger, rounded prominence termed the **frontal tuberosity** (eminence).

Orbital or horizontal portion As can be seen from the inferior aspect, the frontal bone shows primarily the horizontal or orbital portion (see Fig. 11.7), which consists of the **SOMs, superciliary ridges, glabella,** and **frontal tuberosities.**

The **orbital plate** on each side forms the superior part of each orbit. Below the orbital plates lie facial bones, and above the orbital plates is the anterior part of the floor of the brain case.

Each orbital plate is separated from the other by the **ethmoidal notch.** The ethmoid bone, one of the bones of the floor of the cranium, fits into this notch.

Articulations The frontal bone articulates with **four** cranial bones: right and left parietals, sphenoid, and ethmoid. These can be identified on frontal, lateral, and superior cutaway drawings in Figs. 11.3 and 11.4. (The frontal bone also articulates with eight facial bones.)

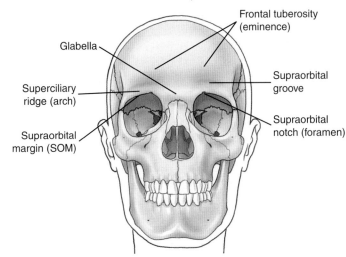

Fig. 11.5 Frontal bone—frontal view.

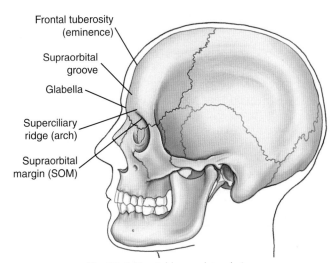

Fig. 11.6 Frontal bone—lateral view.

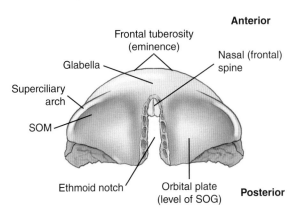

Fig. 11.7 Orbital portion of frontal bone—inferior view.

11

Parietal Bones The paired **right** and **left parietal bones** are well demonstrated on the lateral and superior view drawings of Figs. 11.8 and 11.9. The lateral walls of the cranium and part of the roof are formed by the two parietal bones. The parietal bones are roughly square and have a concave internal surface.

The widest portion of the entire skull is located between the **parietal tubercles (eminences)** of the two parietal bones. The frontal bone is primarily anterior to the parietals; the occipital bone is posterior; the temporal bones are inferior; and the greater wings of the sphenoid are inferior and anterior.

Articulations Each parietal bone articulates with five cranial bones: frontal, occipital, temporal, sphenoid, and opposite parietal bones.

Occipital Bone The inferoposterior portion of the calvarium (skullcap) is formed by the single occipital bone. The external surface of the occipital bone presents a rounded part called the **squamous portion**. The squamous portion forms most of the back of the head and is the part of the occipital bone that is superior to the **external occipital protuberance, or inion,** which is the prominent bump or protuberance at the inferoposterior portion of the skull (Fig. 11.10).

The large opening at the base of the occipital bone through which the spinal cord passes as it leaves the brain is called the **foramen magnum** (literally meaning "great hole").

The two lateral **condylar portions (occipital condyles)** are oval processes with convex surfaces, with one on each side of the foramen magnum. These articulate with depressions on the first cervical vertebra, called the *atlas*. This two-part articulation between the skull and the cervical spine is called the **atlantoccipital joint.** They form a pair of ellipsoid joints that permits flexion, extension and a limited amount of lateral flexion and rotation.

Articulations The occipital bone articulates with **six** bones: two parietals, two temporals, sphenoid, and atlas (first cervical vertebra).

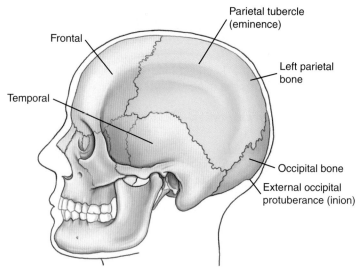

Fig. 11.8 Parietal and occipital bones—lateral view.

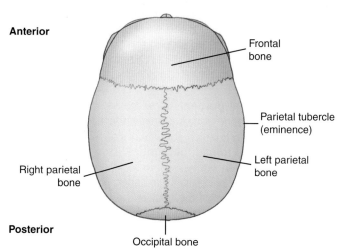

Fig. 11.9 Parietal and occipital bones—superior view.

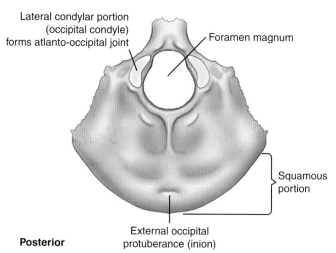

Fig. 11.10 Occipital bone—inferior view.

Temporal Bones

Lateral view The paired **right** and **left temporal bones** are complex structures that house the delicate organs of hearing and balance. As seen from this lateral view drawing (Fig. 11.11), the left temporal bone is situated between the greater wing of the sphenoid bone anteriorly and the occipital bone posteriorly.

Extending anteriorly from the squamous portion of the temporal bone is an arch of bone termed the **zygomatic** *(zi″-go-mat′-ik)* **process.** This process meets the temporal process of the zygomatic bone (one of the facial bones) to form the easily palpated **zygomatic arch.**

Inferior to the zygomatic process and just anterior to the **external acoustic (auditory) meatus (EAM)** is the **temporomandibular (TM) fossa,** into which the mandible fits to form the **temporomandibular joint (TMJ).**

Projecting inferior to the mandible and anterior to the EAM is a slender bony projection called the **styloid process.**

Frontal cutaway view Each temporal bone is divided into **three primary parts** (Fig. 11.12). First is the thin upper portion that forms part of the wall of the skull, the **squamous portion.** This part of the skull is quite thin and is the most vulnerable portion of the entire skull to fracture.

The second portion is the area posterior to the EAM, the **mastoid portion,** with a prominent **mastoid process,** or **tip.** Many air cells are located within the mastoid process.

The third main portion is the dense **petrous** *(pet′-rus)* **portion,** which also is called the **petrous pyramid,** or **pars petrosa;** it houses the organs of hearing and equilibrium, including the mastoid air cells, as described later in this chapter. Sometimes this is also called the **petromastoid portion** of the temporal bone because internally it includes the mastoid portion. The upper border or ridge of the petrous pyramids is commonly called the **petrous ridge,** or petrous apex.

Superior view The floor of the cranium is well visualized in this drawing (Fig. 11.13). The single occipital bone resides between the paired temporal bones. The third main portion of each temporal bone, the **petrous portion,** again is shown in this superior view. This pyramid-shaped portion of the temporal bone is the thickest and densest bone in the cranium. The **petrous pyramids** project anteriorly and toward the midline from the area of the **EAM.**

The **petrous ridge** of these pyramids **corresponds to the level of an important external landmark,** the **TEA** (top of the ear attachment). Near the center of the petrous pyramid on the posterior surface just superior to the **jugular foramen** is an opening or orifice called the **internal acoustic meatus,** which serves to transmit the nerves of hearing and equilibrium. The bilateral jugular foramina are located in the base of the cranium and are where the internal jugular veins are formed and three cranial nerves (IX, X, and XI) pass.[1]

NOTE: The openings of the external and internal acoustic meatus cannot be visualized on this superior view drawing (Fig. 11.13) because they are located on the posteroinferior aspect of the petrous pyramid.

Articulations Each temporal bone articulates with **three** cranial bones: parietal, occipital, and sphenoid. (Each temporal bone also articulates with two facial bones.)

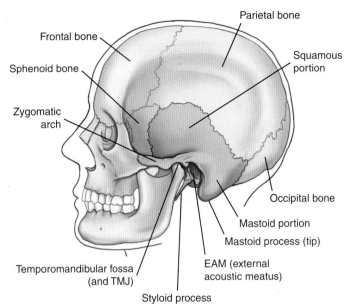

Fig. 11.11 Temporal bone—lateral view.

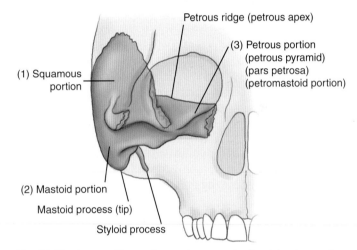

Fig. 11.12 Temporal bone, three primary parts—frontal cutaway view.

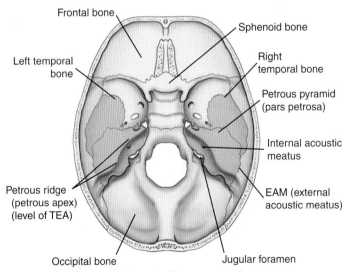

Fig. 11.13 Temporal bones—superior view.

Sphenoid Bone

Superior view The single centrally located **sphenoid bone** forms the anchor for the other seven cranial bones. The central portion of the sphenoid is the body, which lies in the midline of the floor of the cranium and contains the sphenoid sinus, as is best shown on a sagittal sectional drawing (see Fig. 11.18).

The central depression on the body is termed the **sella turcica** (*sel'-a tur'-si-ka*). This depression looks like a saddle from the side (see Fig. 11.16), and it derives its name from words meaning "Turkish saddle." The sella turcica partially surrounds and protects a major gland of the body, the **hypophysis cerebri**, or **pituitary gland**. Posterior to the sella turcica is the back of the saddle, the **dorsum sellae** (*dor'-sum sel'-e*) (also best seen in Fig. 11.16).

The **clivus** (*kli'-vus*) is a shallow depression that begins on the posteroinferior aspect of the dorsum sellae of the sphenoid bone and extends posteriorly to the foramen magnum at the base of the occipital bone (Fig. 11.14; also see Fig. 11.16). This slightly depressed area forms a base of support for the pons (a portion of the brainstem) and for the basilar artery.

Extending laterally from the body to either side are two pairs of wings. The smaller pair, termed the **lesser wings**, are triangular and are nearly horizontal, ending medially in the two **anterior clinoid processes.** They project laterally from the superoanterior portion of the body and extend to the middle of each orbit. The **greater wings** extend laterally from the sides of the body and form a portion of the floor of the cranium and a portion of the sides of the cranium.

Three pairs of small openings or foramina exist in the greater wings for passage of certain cranial nerves (see Fig. 11.14). Lesions that can cause erosion of these foramina can be detected radiographically. The **foramen rotundum** (*ro-tun'-dum*) and the **foramen ovale** (*o-va'-le*) are seen as small openings on superior and oblique view drawings (Figs. 11.14 and 11.15). The small rounded **foramen spinosum** (*spi-no'-sum*) (one of a pair) is also labeled on the superior view drawing (see Fig. 11.14).

Oblique view An oblique drawing of the sphenoid bone demonstrates the complexity of this bone. The shape of the sphenoid has been compared with a bat with its wings and legs extended as in flight. The centrally located depression, the **sella turcica**, again is seen on this view (see Fig. 11.15).

Arising from the posterior aspect of the **lesser wings** are two bony projections termed **anterior clinoid processes.** The anterior clinoid processes are larger and are spread farther apart than the **posterior clinoid processes** that extend superiorly from the **dorsum sellae,** which is best seen on the lateral drawing (Fig. 11.16).

Between the anterior body and the lesser wings on each side are groovelike canals through which the optic nerve and certain arteries pass into the orbital cavity. These canals begin in the center as the **chiasmatic** (*ki-az-mat'-ik*) or **optic groove,** which leads on each side to an **optic canal,** which ends at the **optic foramen,** or the opening into the orbit. The optic foramina can be demonstrated radiographically with the parieto-orbital oblique projection (Rhese method) described later in this chapter. Slightly lateral and posterior to the optic foramina on each side are irregularly shaped openings, which are seen best on this oblique view, called **superior orbital fissures.** These openings provide additional communication with the orbits for numerous cranial nerves and blood vessels. The foramen rotundum and the foramen ovale are seen again on this oblique view (Fig. 11.15).

Projecting downward from the inferior surface of the body are four processes that correspond to the legs of the imaginary bat. The more lateral, flat extensions are called the **lateral pterygoid** (*ter'-i-goyd*) **processes,** which sometimes are called *plates.* Directly medial to these are two **medial pterygoid processes** or plates, which end inferiorly in small hooklike processes, called the **pterygoid hamuli.** The pterygoid processes or plates form part of the lateral walls of the nasal cavities.

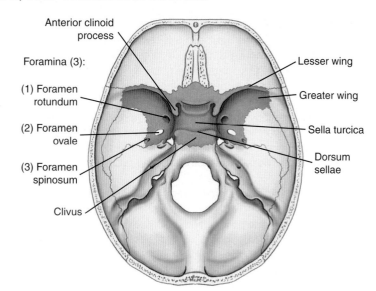

Fig. 11.14 Sphenoid bone—superior view.

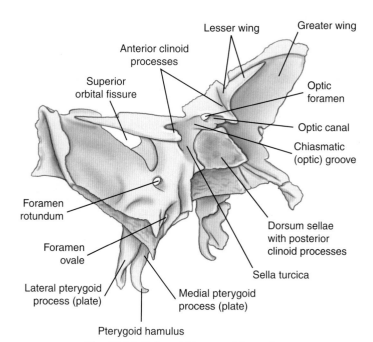

Fig. 11.15 Sphenoid bone—oblique view.

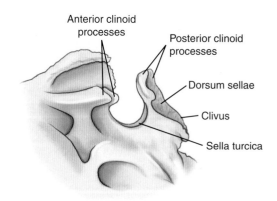

Fig. 11.16 Sella turcica of sphenoid bone—lateral view.

Sella turcica–lateral view A true lateral view of the sella turcica would look similar to the image in Fig. 11.16. Deformity of the sella turcica is often an indication that a lesion exists intracranially as seen radiographically. Computed tomography (CT) and magnetic resonance imaging (MRI) of the **sella turcica** may be performed to detect such deformities. The **sella turcica** and the **dorsum sellae** are also demonstrated best on a lateral projection of the cranium.

Articulations Because of its central location, the sphenoid articulates with the other **seven** cranial bones. The sphenoid also articulates with five facial bones.

Ethmoid Bone

The eighth and last cranial bone to be studied is the **ethmoid bone.** The single ethmoid bone lies primarily below the floor of the cranium. Only the top of the ethmoid is shown on a superior view situated in the ethmoidal notch of the frontal bone (Fig. 11.17).

A magnified coronal view of the entire ethmoid is shown on the right in Fig. 11.17. The small upper horizontal portion of the bone, termed the **cribriform plate,** contains many small openings or foramina through which segmental branches of the olfactory nerves (or the nerves of smell) pass. Projecting superiorly from the cribriform plate is the **crista galli** *(kris'-ta gal'-le),* which is derived from words meaning "rooster's comb."

The major portion of the ethmoid bone lies beneath the floor of the cranium. Projecting downward in the midline is the **perpendicular plate,** which helps to form the bony nasal septum. The two **lateral labyrinths** (masses) are suspended from the undersurface of the cribriform plate on each side of the perpendicular plate. The lateral masses contain the ethmoid air cells or sinuses and help to form the medial walls of the orbits and the lateral walls of the nasal cavity. Extending medially and downward from the medial wall of each labyrinth are thin, scroll-shaped projections of bone. These projections are termed the **superior** and **middle nasal conchae** *(kong'-ha)* or **turbinates;** they are best shown on facial bone drawings in Figs. 11.46 and 11.47.

Articulations The ethmoid articulates with **two** cranial bones: frontal and sphenoid. The ethmoid bone also articulates with 11 facial bones.

Cranium–Sagittal View

Fig. 11.18 represents the right half of the skull, which is sectioned near the midsagittal plane (MSP). The centrally located **sphenoid** and **ethmoid** bones are well demonstrated, showing their relationship to each other and to the other cranial bones.

The **ethmoid bone** is located anterior to the sphenoid bone. The smaller **crista galli** and **cribriform plate** project superiorly, and the larger **perpendicular plate** extends inferiorly. The perpendicular plate forms the upper portion of the bony nasal septum.

The **sphenoid bone,** which contains the saddle-shaped sella turcica, is located directly posterior to the ethmoid bone. Shown again is one of the two long, slender **pterygoid processes** or plates extending down and forward and ending with the small pointed process called the **pterygoid hamulus.** Inferior and slightly anterior to the sella turcica of the sphenoid bone in this sagittal view is a hollow-like body area of the sphenoid, which houses the **sphenoid sinus.**

The larger **frontal bone** also demonstrates a cavity directly posterior to the glabella that contains the **frontal sinus.** The vomer (a facial bone) is shown as a midline structure between parts of the sphenoid and parts of the ethmoid, as is seen in Fig. 11.18.

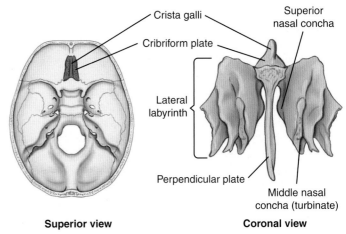

Superior view   **Coronal view**

Fig. 11.17 Ethmoid bone.

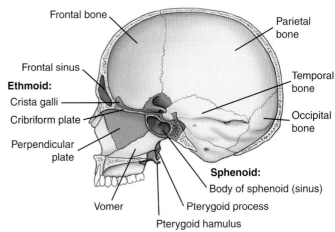

Fig. 11.18 Cranium—midsagittal view of sphenoid and ethmoid bones.

11

JOINTS OF THE CRANIUM—SUTURES

Adult Cranium
The articulations or joints of the cranium are called **sutures** and are classified as **fibrous joints.** In an adult, these are immovable and therefore are **synarthrodial-type joints.** They are demonstrated in Fig. 11.19 in lateral, superior oblique, and posterior views.

The **coronal** *(ko-ro'-nal)* **suture** separates the frontal bone from the two parietal bones. Separating the two parietal bones in the midline is the **sagittal suture.** Posteriorly, the **lambdoidal** *(lam'-doy-dal)* **suture** separates the two parietal bones from the occipital bone. The **squamosal** *(skwa-mo'-sal)* **sutures** are formed by the inferior junctions of the two parietal bones with their respective temporal bones.

Each end of the sagittal suture is identified as a point or area with a specific name as labeled. The anterior end of the sagittal suture is termed the **bregma** *(breg'-mah),* and the posterior end is called the **lambda** *(lam'-dah).* The right and left **pterions** *(ter'-re-ons)* are points at the junction of the frontal, parietals, temporals, and the greater wings of the sphenoid. (The pterions are at the **posterior** end of the sphenoparietal suture.[1])

The right and left **asterions** *(as-te'-re-ons)* are points posterior to the ear where the squamosal and lambdoidal sutures meet. These six recognizable bony points are used in surgery or other cases in which specific reference points for cranial measurements are necessary.

Infant Cranium
The calvarium (skullcap) on an infant is very large in proportion to the rest of the body, but the facial bones are quite small, as can be seen on these drawings (Fig. 11.20). Ossification of the individual cranial bones is incomplete at birth, and the sutures are membrane-covered spaces that fill in soon after birth. However, certain regions where sutures join are slower in their ossification, and these are called **fontanels** *(fon"-tah-nels').* The cranial sutures themselves generally do not ossify completely until the mid-to-late 20s, and some may not completely close until the fifth decade of life.[2]

Fontanels Early in life, the bregma and the lambda are not bony but are membrane-covered openings or "soft spots." These soft spots are termed the **anterior** and **posterior fontanels** in an infant. The anterior fontanel is the largest and at birth measures approximately 1 inch (2.5 cm) wide and 1½ inches (4 cm) long. It does not completely close until about 18 months of age.

Two smaller lateral fontanels that close soon after birth are the **sphenoid** (pterion in an adult) and **mastoid** (asterion in an adult) **fontanels,** which are located at the sphenoid and mastoid angles of the parietal bones on each side of the head. **Six fontanels** occur in an infant as follows:

INFANT	ADULT
Anterior fontanel	Bregma
Posterior fontanel	Lambda
Right sphenoid fontanel	Right pterion
Left sphenoid fontanel	Left pterion
Right mastoid fontanel	Right asterion
Left mastoid fontanel	Left asterion

Sutural, or Wormian, Bones
Certain small, irregular bones called *sutural,* or *wormian, bones* sometimes develop in adult skull sutures. These isolated bones most often are found in the lambdoidal suture but occasionally also are found in the region of the fontanels, especially the posterior fontanel. In the adult skull, these are completely ossified and are visible only by the sutural lines around their borders.

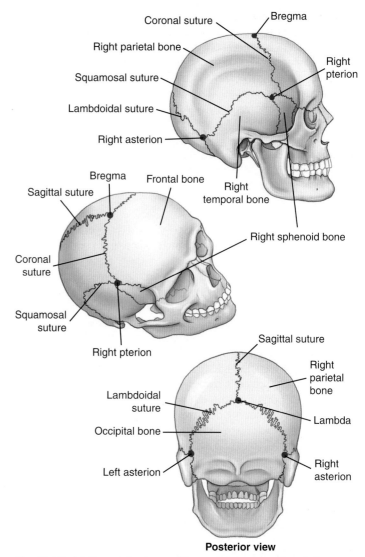

Fig. 11.19 Adult cranial sutures—**fibrous joints, synarthrodial** (immovable).

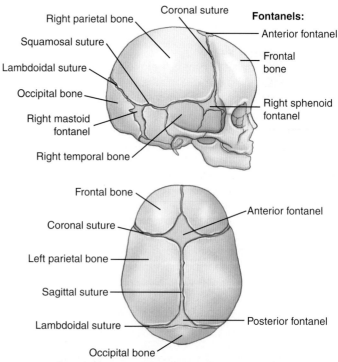

Fig. 11.20 Infant cranial sutures and **fontanels.**

ANATOMY REVIEW WITH RADIOGRAPHS

The following review exercises focus on the anatomy of the eight cranial bones as labeled on the radiographs on the right. A recommended method of review and reinforcement is to cover the answers and first try to identify each of the labeled parts from memory. Specific anatomic parts may be more difficult to recognize on radiographs compared with drawings, but knowing locations and relationships to surrounding structures and bones should aid in identifying these parts.

Cranial Bones—PA Axial Caldwell Projection, 15° caudad (Fig. 11.21)

A. Supraorbital margin of right orbit
B. Crista galli of ethmoid
C. Sagittal suture (posterior skull)
D. Lambdoidal suture (posterior skull)
E. Petrous ridge

Cranial Bones—AP Axial Projection (Fig. 11.22)

A. Dorsum sellae of sphenoid
B. Posterior clinoid processes
C. Petrous ridge or petrous pyramid
D. Parietal bone
E. Occipital bone
F. Foramen magnum

Cranial Bones—Lateral Projection (Fig. 11.23)

A. EAM
B. Mastoid portion of temporal bone
C. Occipital bone
D. Lambdoidal suture
E. Clivus
F. Dorsum sellae
G. Posterior clinoid processes
H. Anterior clinoid processes
I. Vertex of cranium
J. Coronal suture
K. Frontal bone
L. Orbital plates
M. Cribriform plate
N. Sella turcica
O. Body of sphenoid (sphenoid sinus)
P. Petrous portion of temporal bone

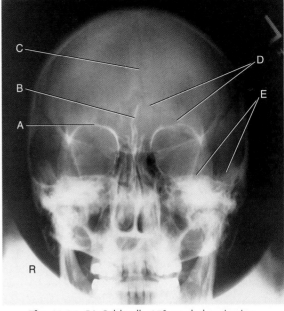

Fig. 11.21 PA Caldwell—15° caudad projection.

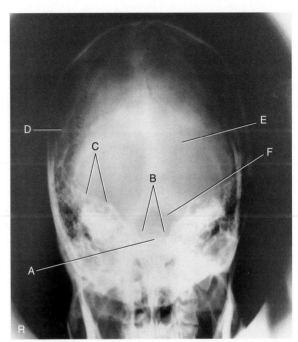

Fig. 11.22 AP axial projection.

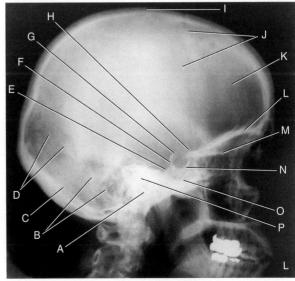

Fig. 11.23 Lateral projection.

11

Anatomy of Organs of Hearing and Equilibrium

Because of the density (brightness) and relative location of the temporal bones, the mastoids and petrous portions are difficult to visualize with conventional radiography. CT and MRI have largely replaced conventional radiography for imaging of these regions. However, a knowledge of temporal bone anatomy is critical whether performing conventional radiography, CT, or MRI.

The organs of hearing and equilibrium are the main structures found within the petrous portion of the temporal bones. The three divisions of the ear—**external, middle,** and **internal portions**—are illustrated in Fig. 11.24.

EXTERNAL EAR

The **external ear** begins with the **auricle** or **pinna** on each side of the head. The **tragus** is part of this external structure. It is the small liplike structure located anterior to the EAM that acts as a partial shield to the ear opening.

The **EAM** is the opening or canal of the external ear. The external acoustic canal or meatus is approximately 1 inch (2.5 cm) long; half is bony in structure, and half is cartilaginous (Fig. 11.25).

The **mastoid process** and **mastoid tip** of the temporal bone are posterior and inferior to the EAM, whereas the **styloid process** is inferior and slightly anterior. The meatus narrows as it meets the **tympanic membrane** or **eardrum.** The eardrum is situated at an oblique angle, forming a depression, or well, at the lower medial end of the meatus.

MIDDLE EAR

The **middle ear** is an irregularly shaped, air-containing cavity located between the external and internal ear portions. The three main parts of the middle ear are the **tympanic membrane,** the three small bones called **auditory ossicles,** and the **tympanic cavity** (Fig. 11.26). The tympanic membrane is considered part of the middle ear even though it serves as a partition between the external and middle ears.

The tympanic cavity is divided further into two parts. The larger cavity opposite the eardrum is called the **tympanic cavity proper.** The area above the level of the EAM and the eardrum is called the **attic,** or **epitympanic recess.** The **drum crest,** or **spur,** is a structure that is important radiographically. The tympanic membrane is attached to this sharp, bony projection. The drum crest or spur separates the EAM from the epitympanic recess.

The tympanic cavity communicates anteriorly with the nasopharynx by way of the **eustachian tube,** or **auditory tube.**

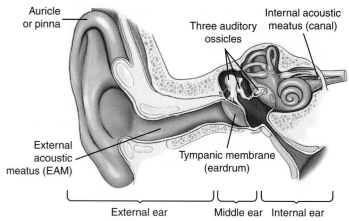

Fig. 11.24 Ear.

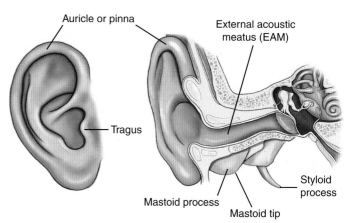

Fig. 11.25 External ear.

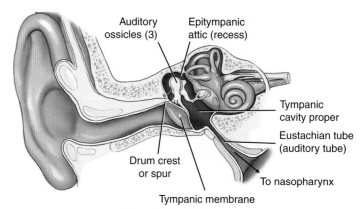

Fig. 11.26 Middle ear.

COMPUTED TOMOGRAPHY OF THE TEMPORAL BONE

Fig. 11.27 demonstrates select organs of hearing and equilibrium of the middle and inner ear as seen on this CT of the temporal bone.

Eustachian Tube

The **eustachian tube** is the passageway between the middle ear and the nasopharynx. This tube is approximately 1½ inches (4 cm) long and serves to equalize the pressure within the middle ear to the outside atmospheric air pressure through the nasopharynx (Fig. 11.28). The sensation of one's ears popping is caused by pressure being adjusted internally in the middle ear to prevent damage to the eardrum.

A problem associated with this direct communication between the middle ear and the nasopharynx is that disease organisms have a direct passageway from the throat to the middle ear. Therefore, ear infections often accompany sore throats, especially in children whose immune system is still developing.

Internal Acoustic Meatus

Fig. 11.29 illustrates the ear structures as they would appear in a **modified posteroanterior (PA) projection.** A 5° to 10° central ray (CR) caudad angle to the orbitomeatal line projects the petrous ridges to the **midorbital level,** as is shown in this drawing. This results in a special transorbital view, which may be taken to demonstrate the **internal acoustic meatus.** The opening to the internal acoustic meatus is an oblique aperture that is smaller in diameter than the opening to the EAM and is very difficult to demonstrate clearly on any conventional radiographic projection. It is best demonstrated with CT (for bony erosion) and MRI (for demonstration of acoustic neuromas).

In the drawing of a PA axial projection (see Fig. 11.29), the internal acoustic meatus is projected into the orbital shadow slightly below the petrous ridge, allowing it to be visualized on radiographs taken in this position. The lateral portions of the petrous ridges are at approximately the level of the **TEA.**

Mastoids

A second direct communication into the middle ear occurs posteriorly to the **mastoid air cells.** The schematic drawing in Fig. 11.30 is a sagittal section that shows the relationships of the mastoid air cells to the **attic,** or **epitympanic recess,** and the **tympanic cavity proper.** The **aditus** is the opening between the epitympanic recess and the mastoid portion of the temporal bone.

The aditus connects directly to a large chamber within the mastoid portion termed the **antrum.** The antrum connects to the various **mastoid air cells.** This communication allows infection in the middle ear, which may have originated in the throat, to pass into the mastoid area. Infection within the mastoid area is separated from brain tissue only by thin bone. Before effective antibiotics were commonly used, this was often a pathway for **encephalitis,** a serious infection of the brain. The thin plate of bone that forms the roof of the antrum, aditus, and attic area of the tympanic cavity is called the **tegmen tympani.**

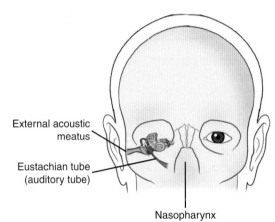

Fig. 11.28 Middle ear.

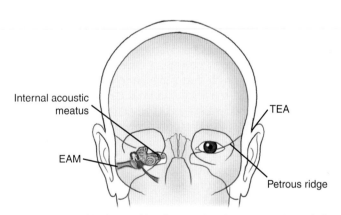

Fig. 11.29 Modified PA Caldwell projection (CR 5° to 10° caudad).

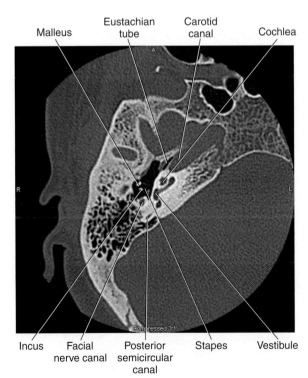

Fig. 11.27 CT of temporal bone.

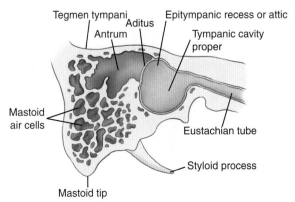

Fig. 11.30 Mastoid connection.

Auditory Ossicles

The **auditory ossicles** are three small bones that are prominent structures within the middle ear. Figs. 11.31 and 11.32 show that these three small bones are articulated to permit vibratory motion. The three auditory ossicles are located partly in the attic, or epitympanic recess, and partly in the tympanic cavity proper. These delicate bones bridge the middle ear cavity to transmit sound vibrations from the tympanic membrane to the oval window of the internal ear.

Vibrations are first picked up by the **malleus**, meaning "hammer," which is attached directly to the inside surface of the tympanic membrane. The head of the malleus articulates with the central ossicle, the **incus**. The incus receives its name from a supposed resemblance to an anvil, but it actually looks more like a premolar tooth with a body and two roots. The incus connects to the stirrup-shaped **stapes**, which is the smallest of the three auditory ossicles. The footplate of the stapes is attached to another membrane called the **oval window**, which leads into the inner ear.

Auditory Ossicles—Frontal and Lateral View

Fig. 11.32 illustrates the relationship of the auditory ossicles to one another in a close-up frontal view and a lateral view. As can be seen from the front, the most lateral of the three bones is the **malleus**, whereas the most medial of the three bones is the **stapes**. The lateral view drawing demonstrates how the ossicles would appear if one looked through the **EAM** to see the bony ossicles of the middle ear. The malleus, with its attachment to the eardrum, is located slightly anterior to the other two bones.

The resemblance of the **incus** to a premolar tooth with a body and two roots is well visualized in the lateral drawing. The longer root of the incus connects to the stapes, which connects to the oval window of the cochlea, resulting in the sense of hearing.

INTERNAL EAR

The complex **internal ear** contains the essential sensory apparatus of both **hearing** and **equilibrium.** Lying within the densest portion of the petrous pyramid, it can be divided into two main parts—the **osseous,** or **bony, labyrinth,** which is important radiographically, and the **membranous labyrinth.** The osseous labyrinth is a bony chamber that houses the membranous labyrinth, a series of intercommunicating ducts and sacs. One such duct is the **endolymphatic duct,** a blind pouch or closed duct contained in a small, canal-like, bony structure. The canal of the endolymphatic duct arises from the medial wall of the vestibule and extends to the posterior wall of the petrous pyramid, located both posterior and lateral to the **internal acoustic meatus.**

Osseous (Bony) Labyrinth

The osseous, or bony, labyrinth is divided into **three** distinctly shaped parts: the **cochlea** (meaning "snail shell"), the **vestibule,** and the **semicircular canals.** The osseous labyrinth completely surrounds and encloses the ducts and sacs of the membranous

labyrinth. As is illustrated on the frontal cutaway view in Fig. 11.33, the snail-shaped, bony cochlea houses a long, coiled, tubelike duct of the membranous labyrinth.

The **cochlea** is the most anterior of the three parts of the osseous labyrinth. This is best shown on the lateral view of the osseous labyrinth in Fig. 11.34. The **round window,** sometimes called the **cochlear window,** is shown to be at the base of the cochlea.

The **vestibule,** the central portion of the bony labyrinth, contains the **oval window,** sometimes called the **vestibular window.**

Semicircular Canals

The **three semicircular canals** are located posterior to the other inner ear structures and are named according to their position: **superior, posterior,** and **lateral semicircular canals.** Each is located at a right angle to the other two, allowing a sense of equilibrium in addition to a sense of direction. The **semicircular canals relate to the sense of direction or equilibrium,** and the **cochlea relates to the sense of hearing** because of its connection to the stapes through the oval window.

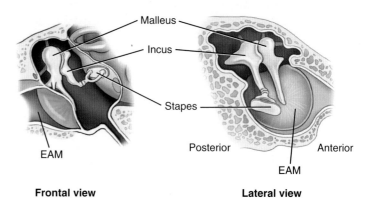

Frontal view   **Lateral view**

Fig. 11.32 Auditory ossicles.

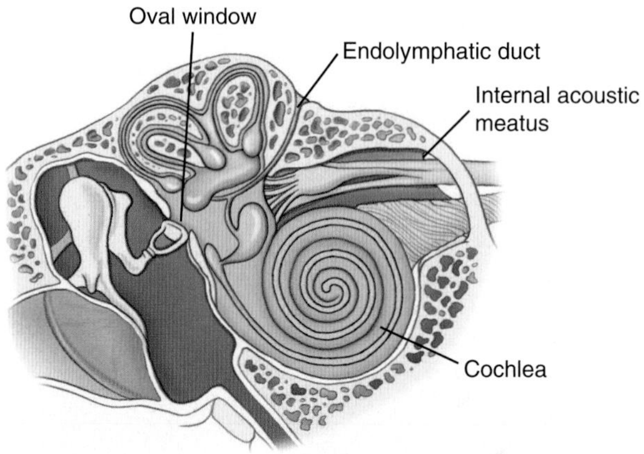

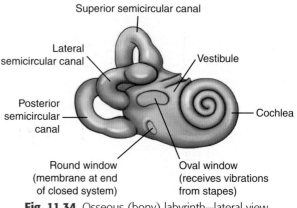

Fig. 11.33 Internal ear, osseous labyrinth—frontal view.

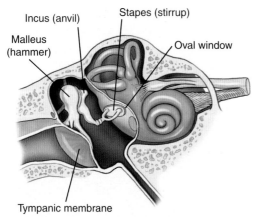

Fig. 11.31 Auditory ossicles—malleus, incus, and stapes.

Fig. 11.34 Osseous (bony) labyrinth—lateral view.

"Windows" of the Internal Ear

The two openings into the internal ear are covered by membranes (see Fig. 11.34). The **oval,** or **vestibular, window** receives vibrations from the external ear through the distal aspect of the stapes of the middle ear and transmits these vibrations into the **vestibule** of the internal ear. The vestibule is the structure that houses the semicircular canals. The **round,** or **cochlear, window** is located at the base of the first coil of the cochlea. The round window is a membrane that allows movement of fluid within the closed duct system of the membranous labyrinth. As the oval window moves slightly inward with a vibration, the round window moves outward because this is a closed system and fluid does not compress. Vibrations and associated slight fluid movements within the cochlea produce impulses that are transmitted to the auditory nerve within the internal acoustic meatus, creating the sense of hearing.

ANATOMY REVIEW WITH RADIOGRAPHS

Specific anatomy of the temporal bone is difficult to recognize on conventional radiographs. Conventional positioning for mastoids is rarely performed today, but these two projections are provided to review the anatomy of the inner ear and mastoids.

Axiolateral Projection (Fig. 11.35)

A. EAM
B. Mastoid antrum
C. Mastoid air cells
D. Downside mandibular condyle (just anterior to EAM)
E. Upside (magnified) mandibular condyle

Posterior Profile Position (Fig. 11.36)

A. Petrous ridge
B. Bony (osseous) labyrinth (semicircular canals)
C. EAM
D. Region of internal acoustic canal

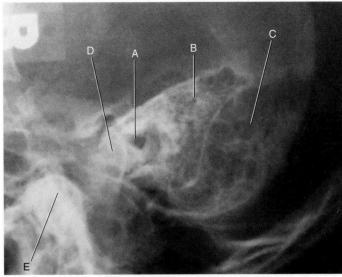

Fig. 11.35 Axiolateral projection for mastoids.

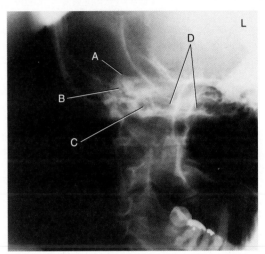

Fig. 11.36 Posterior profile projection for mastoids.

Facial Bones

Each of the facial bones can be identified on frontal and lateral drawings (Figs. 11.37 and 11.38) except for the two palatine bones and the vomer, both of which are located internally and are not visible on a dry skeleton from the exterior. These bones are identified on sectional drawings later in this chapter.

The 14 facial bones contribute to the shape and form of a person's face. In addition, the cavities of the orbits, nose, and mouth are largely constructed from the bones of the face. Of the 14 bones that make up the facial skeleton, only 2 bones are unpaired, the vomer and mandible. The remaining 12 consist of six pairs of bones, with similar bones on each side of the face.

2	Maxillae *(mak-sil′-e)* (upper jaw), or maxillary bones
2	Zygomatic *(zi″-go-mat′-ik)* bones
2	Lacrimal *(lak′-ri-mal)* bones
2	Nasal bones
2	Inferior nasal conchae *(kong′-ke)*
2	Palatine *(pal′-ah-tin)* bones
1	Vomer *(vo′-mer)*
1	Mandible (lower jaw)
14	*Total*

Each of the facial bones is studied individually or in pairs. After the description of each in the figures is a listing of the specific adjoining bones with which they articulate. Knowledge of these anatomic relationships aids in understanding the structure of the bony skeleton of the head.

RIGHT AND LEFT MAXILLARY BONES

The two maxillae, or maxillary bones, are the largest immovable bones of the face (Fig. 11.39). The only facial bone larger than the maxilla is the movable lower jaw, or mandible. All the other bones of the upper facial area are closely associated with the two maxillae; they are structurally the most important bones of the upper face. The right and left maxillary bones are solidly united at the midline below the nasal septum. Each maxilla assists in the formation of three cavities of the face: (1) the mouth, (2) the nasal cavity, and (3) one orbit.

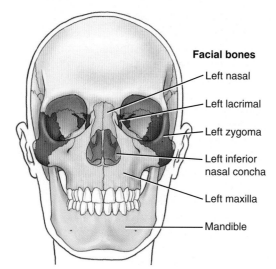

Facial bones
Left nasal
Left lacrimal
Left zygoma
Left inferior nasal concha
Left maxilla
Mandible

Fig. 11.37 Facial bones—frontal view.

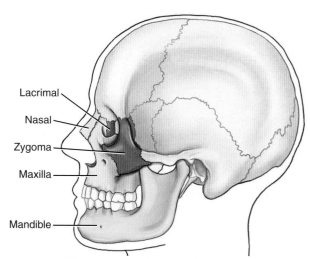

Lacrimal
Nasal
Zygoma
Maxilla
Mandible

Fig. 11.38 Facial bones—lateral view.

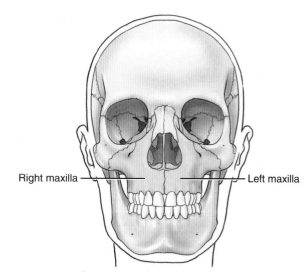

Right maxilla
Left maxilla

Fig. 11.39 Right and left maxillae.

Lateral View of Left Maxilla

Each maxilla consists of a centrally located **body** and **four processes** that project from that body. Three processes are more obvious and are visible on lateral and frontal drawings (Figs. 11.40 and 11.41). The fourth process, described later, is the palatine process, which is part of the hard palate.

The **body** of each maxilla is the centrally located portion that lies lateral to the nose. One of the three processes is the **frontal process,** which projects upward along the lateral border of the nose toward the frontal bone. The **zygomatic process** projects laterally to unite with the zygoma. The third process, the **alveolar process,** is the inferior aspect of the body of each maxilla. Eight upper teeth occur along the inferior margin of each alveolar process.

The two maxillae are solidly united in the midline anteriorly. At the upper part of this union is the **anterior nasal spine.** A blow to the nose sometimes results in separation of the nasal spine from the maxillae.

A point at the superior aspect of the anterior nasal spine is the **acanthion,** which is described later in this chapter as a surface landmark at the midline point where the nose and the upper lip meet.

Frontal View

The relationship of the two maxillary bones to the remainder of the bones of the skull is well demonstrated in the frontal view (see Fig. 11.41). Note again **three processes,** as seen in the frontal view of the skull. Extending upward toward the frontal bone is the **frontal process.** Extending laterally toward the zygoma is the **zygomatic process,** and supporting the upper teeth is the **alveolar process.**

The body of each maxillary bone contains a large, air-filled cavity known as a **maxillary sinus.** Several of these air-filled cavities are found in certain bones of the skull. These sinuses communicate with the nasal cavity and are collectively termed *paranasal sinuses;* they are described further later on in this chapter.

Hard Palate (Inferior Surface)

The **fourth process** of each maxillary bone is the palatine process, which can be demonstrated only on an inferior view of the two maxillae (Fig. 11.42). The two palatine processes form the anterior portion of the roof of the mouth, called the *hard* or *bony palate.* The two palatine processes are solidly united at the midline to form a synarthrodial (immovable) joint. A common congenital defect called a *cleft palate* is an opening between the palatine processes that is caused by incomplete joining of the two bones.

The horizontal portion of two other facial bones, the **palatine bones,** forms the posterior part of the hard palate. Only the horizontal portions of the L-shaped palatine bones are visible on this view. The vertical portions are demonstrated later on a cutaway drawing (see Fig. 11.47).

Note the differences between the palatine process of the maxillary bone and the separate palatine facial bones.

The two small inferior portions of the sphenoid bone of the cranium also are shown on this inferior view of the hard palate. These two processes, the **pterygoid hamuli,** are similar to the feet of the outstretched legs of a bat, as described in an earlier drawing in the chapter (also see Fig. 11.15, p. 384).

Articulations

Each maxilla articulates with **two cranial bones** (frontal and ethmoid) and with **seven facial bones** (zygoma, lacrimal, nasal, palatine, inferior nasal concha, vomer, and adjacent maxilla).

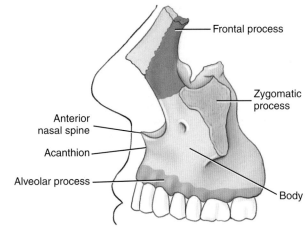

Fig. 11.40 Left maxilla—lateral view.

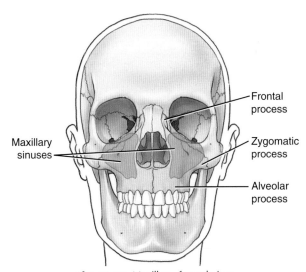

Fig. 11.41 Maxillae—frontal view.

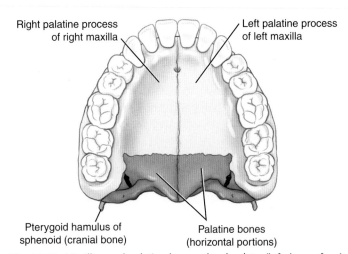

Fig. 11.42 Maxillae and palatine bones—hard palate (inferior surface).

11

RIGHT AND LEFT ZYGOMATIC BONES

One **zygoma** is located lateral to the zygomatic process of each maxilla. These bones (sometimes termed *malar bones*) form the prominence of the cheeks and make up the lower outer portion of the orbits.

Projecting posteriorly from the zygoma is a slender process that connects with the zygomatic process of the temporal bone to form the **zygomatic arch.** The zygomatic arch is a delicate structure that sometimes is fractured or "caved in" by a blow to the cheek. The anterior portion of the arch is formed by the zygoma, and the posterior portion is formed by the zygomatic process of the temporal bone. The **zygomatic prominence** is a positioning landmark, and the term refers to this prominent portion of the zygoma (Fig. 11.43).

Articulations

Each zygoma articulates with **three cranial bones** (frontal, sphenoid, and temporal) and with **one facial bone** (maxilla).

RIGHT AND LEFT NASAL AND LACRIMAL BONES

The lacrimal and nasal bones are the thinnest and most fragile bones in the entire body.

Lacrimal Bones

The two small and delicate lacrimal bones (about the size and shape of a fingernail) lie anteriorly on the medial side of each orbit just posterior to the frontal process of the maxilla (Fig. 11.44). *Lacrimal,* derived from a word meaning "tear," is an appropriate term because the lacrimal bones are closely associated with the tear ducts.

Nasal Bones

The two fused nasal bones form the bridge of the nose and are variable in size. Some people have very prominent nasal bones, whereas nasal bones are quite small in other people. Much of the nose is made up of cartilage, and only the two nasal bones form the bridge of the nose. The nasal bones lie anterior and superomedial to the frontal process of the maxillae and inferior to the frontal bone. The point of junction of the two nasal bones with the frontal bone is a surface landmark called the *nasion* (Fig. 11.45).

Articulations

Lacrimal Each lacrimal bone articulates with **two cranial bones** (frontal and ethmoid) and with **two facial bones** (maxilla and inferior nasal concha).

Nasal Each nasal bone articulates with **two cranial bones** (frontal and ethmoid) and with **two facial bones** (maxilla and adjacent nasal bone) (see Fig. 11.45).

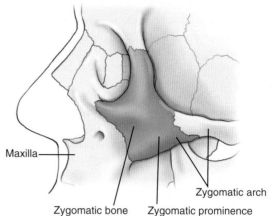

Fig. 11.43 Zygomatic bone—lateral view.

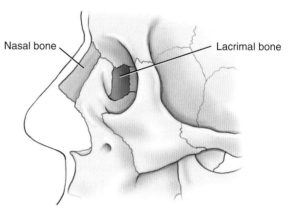

Fig. 11.44 Nasal and lacrimal bones—lateral view.

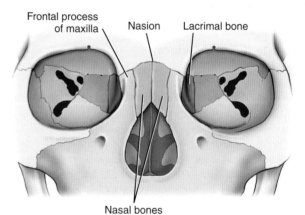

Fig. 11.45 Nasal and lacrimal bones—frontal view.

RIGHT AND LEFT INFERIOR NASAL CONCHAE

Within the nasal cavity are two platelike, curved (or scroll-shaped) facial bones called the **inferior nasal conchae** *(turbinates)*. These two bones project from the lateral walls of the nasal cavity on each side and extend medially (Fig. 11.46).

There are three pairs of nasal conchae. The superior and middle pairs are parts of the ethmoid bone, and the inferior pair consists of separate facial bones.

The effect of the three pairs of nasal conchae is to divide the nasal cavities into various compartments. These irregular compartments tend to break up or mix the flow of air coming into the nasal cavities before it reaches the lungs. In this way, incoming air is warmed and cleaned as it comes in contact with the mucous membrane that covers the conchae.

Sectional Drawing

Inferior Nasal Conchae The relationship between the various nasal conchae and the lateral wall of one nasal cavity is illustrated in this sectional drawing (Fig. 11.47). The midline structures that make up the nasal septum have been removed so that the lateral portion of the right nasal cavity can be seen. The **superior and middle conchae** are part of the ethmoid bone, and the **inferior nasal conchae** are separate facial bones. The **cribriform plate** and the **crista galli** of the ethmoid bone help to separate the cranium from the facial bone mass. The **palatine process** of the maxilla is shown again.

RIGHT AND LEFT PALATINE BONES

The two **palatine bones** are difficult to visualize in the study of a dry skeleton because they are located internally and are not visible from the outside. Each palatine bone is roughly L-shaped (see Fig. 11.47). The vertical portion of the "L" extends upward between one maxilla and one pterygoid plate of the sphenoid bone. The horizontal portion of each "L" helps to make up the posterior portion of the hard palate, as shown in an earlier drawing (see Fig. 11.42). Additionally, the most superior small tip of the palatine can be seen in the posterior aspect of the orbit (see Fig. 11.71, p. 401).

Articulations

Inferior Nasal Conchae Each inferior nasal concha articulates with **one cranial bone** (ethmoid) and with **three facial bones** (maxilla, lacrimal, and palatine).

Palatine Each palatine articulates with **two cranial bones** (sphenoid and ethmoid) and **four facial bones** (maxilla, inferior nasal conchae, vomer, and adjacent palatine).

NASAL SEPTUM

The midline structures of the nasal cavity, including the **bony nasal septum,** are shown on this sagittal view drawing (Fig. 11.48). Two bones—the **ethmoid** and the **vomer**—form the bony nasal septum. Specifically, the septum is formed superiorly by the **perpendicular plate** of the ethmoid bone and inferiorly by the single vomer bone, which can be demonstrated radiographically. Anteriorly, the nasal septum is cartilaginous and is termed the **septal cartilage.**

Vomer

The single **vomer** (meaning "plowshare") bone is a thin, triangular bone that forms the inferoposterior part of the nasal septum. The surfaces of the vomer are marked by small, furrow-like depressions for blood vessels, a source of nosebleed with trauma to the nasal area. A deviated nasal septum describes the clinical condition wherein the nasal septum is deflected or displaced laterally from the midline of the nose. This deviation usually occurs at the site of junction between the septal cartilage and the vomer. A severe deviation can entirely block the nasal passageway, making breathing through the nose impossible.

Articulations The vomer articulates with **two cranial bones** (sphenoid and ethmoid) and with **four facial bones** (right and left palatine bones and right and left maxillae). The vomer also articulates with the septal cartilage.

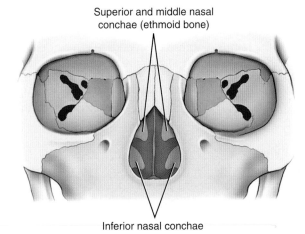

Fig. 11.46 Inferior nasal conchae.

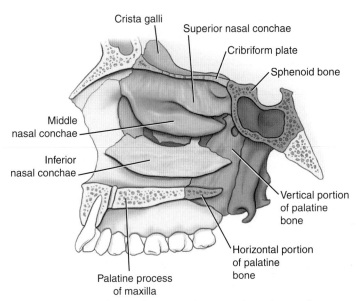

Fig. 11.47 Sectional view drawing—inferior nasal conchae and palatine bones.

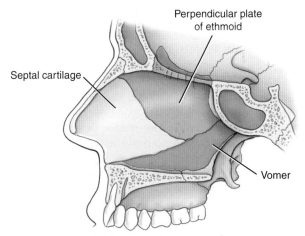

Fig. 11.48 Bony nasal septum and vomer.

MANDIBLE

The last and largest facial bone is the lower jaw, or **mandible.** It is the only movable bone in the adult skull. This large facial bone, which is a single bone in the adult, originates from two separate bones. The two bones in the infant join to become one at approximately 1 year of age.

Lateral View

The **angle** (gonion) of the mandible divides each half of the mandible into two main parts. That area anterior to the angle is termed the **body** of the mandible, whereas the area superior to each angle is termed the **ramus.** Because the mandible is a single bone, the body extends from the left angle around to the right angle (Fig. 11.49).

The lower teeth are rooted in the mandible. An **alveolar process,** or ridge, extends along the entire superior portion of the body of the mandible.

Frontal View

The anterior aspect of the adult mandible is best seen on a frontal view. The single body forms from each lateral half and unites at the anterior midline. This union is called the **symphysis** of the mandible, or the **symphysis menti.** The flat triangular area below the symphysis, marked by two knoblike protuberances that project forward, is called the **mental protuberance.** The center of the mental protuberance is described as the **mental point.** *Mentum* and *mental* are Latin words that refer to the general area known as the chin. The mental point is a specific point on the chin, whereas the mentum is the entire area.

Located on each half of the body of the mandible is a **mental foramen.** The mental foramina serve as passageways for the mental artery and vein and mental nerve (branch of inferior alveolar nerve) that innervates the lower lip and chin.

Ramus

The upper portion of each **ramus** terminates in a U-shaped notch termed the **mandibular notch.** At each end of the mandibular notch is a process. The process at the anterior end of the mandibular notch is termed the **coronoid process** (Fig. 11.50). This process does not articulate with another bone and cannot be palpated easily because it lies just inferior to the zygomatic arch and serves as a site for muscle attachment.

The **coronoid process** of the mandible must not be confused with the **coronoid process** of the proximal ulna of the forearm or the **coracoid process** of the scapula.

The posterior process of the upper ramus is termed the **condyloid process** and consists of two parts. The rounded end of the condyloid process is the **condyle** or **head,** whereas the constricted area directly below the condyle is the **neck.** The condyle of the condyloid process fits into the TM fossa of the temporal bone to form the **TMJ.**

Submentovertical Projection

The horseshoe shape of the mandible is well visualized on a **submentovertical** (SMV) projection (Fig. 11.51). The mandible is a thin structure, which explains why it is susceptible to fracture. The area of the **mentum** is well demonstrated, as are the **body, ramus,** and **gonion** of the mandible. The relative position of the upper ramus and its associated **coronoid process** and **condyle** are also demonstrated with this projection. The condyle projects medial and the coronoid process slightly lateral on this view.

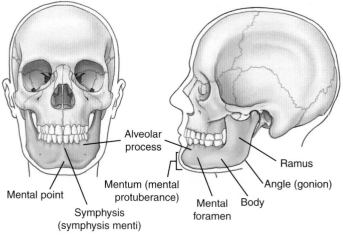

Fig. 11.49 Mandible—lateral and frontal views.

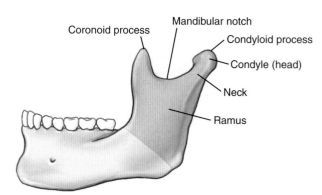

Fig. 11.50 Ramus of mandible—lateral view.

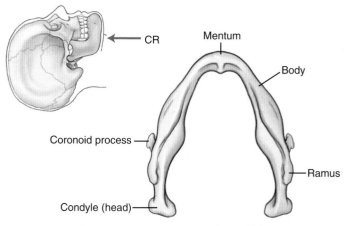

Fig. 11.51 SMV projection of mandible.

TEMPOROMANDIBULAR JOINT

The TMJ, the only movable joint in the skull, is shown on this lateral drawing (Fig. 11.52) and on the lateral view photograph of the skull (Fig. 11.53). The relationship of the mandible to the temporal bone of the cranium is well demonstrated. The TMJ is located just anterior and slightly superior to the **EAM.**

Joint Classifications (Mandible and Skull)
SYNOVIAL JOINTS (DIARTHRODIAL)
The complex TMJ is classified as a **synovial type** of joint divided into upper and lower synovial cavities by a single articular fibrous disk (Table 11.1). A series of strong ligaments join the condylar neck, ramus, and gonion of the mandible to the lower borders of the zygomatic process of the temporal bone.

This complete two-part synovial joint, along with its fibrous articular disk, allows for not only a hinge-type motion but also a gliding movement. The action of this type of joint is very complex. Two movements are predominant. When the mouth opens, the condyle and the fibrocartilage move forward, and at the same time, the condyle revolves around the fibrocartilage. The TMJ is classified as a bicondylar joint similar to the knee.[3]

FIBROUS JOINTS (SYNARTHRODIAL)
Two types of fibrous joints involve the skull, both of which are **synarthrodial,** or immovable. First are the **sutures** between cranial bones, as described earlier. Second is a unique type of fibrous joint involving the teeth with the mandible and maxillae. This is a **gomphosis** *(gom-fo'-sis)* subclass type of fibrous joint that is found between the roots of the teeth and the alveolar processes of both the maxillae and the mandible.

TMJ Motion

The drawings and radiographs illustrate the TMJ in both **open-mouth** and **closed-mouth** positions (Fig. 11.54). When the mouth is opened widely, the condyle moves forward to the front edge of the fossa. If the condyle slips too far anteriorly, the joint may dislocate. If the TMJ dislocates, either by force or by jaw motion, it may be difficult or impossible to close the mouth, which returns the condyle to its normal position.

Radiographs (Open and Closed Mouth)

Two axiolateral projections (Schuller method) of the TMJ are shown in closed-mouth and open-mouth positions (Figs. 11.55 and 11.56). The range of anterior movement of the condyle in relationship to the TM fossa is clearly demonstrated.

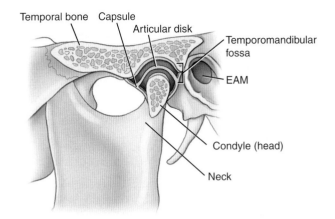

Fig. 11.52 Temporomandibular joint.

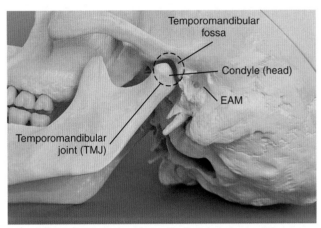

Fig. 11.53 Temporomandibular joint of mandible.

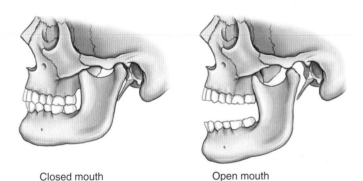

Closed mouth   Open mouth

Fig. 11.54 TMJ movements.

TABLE 11.1 **JOINTS OF MANDIBLE**	
TEMPOROMANDIBULAR JOINT	**ALVEOLI AND ROOTS OF TEETH**
Classification Synovial (diarthrodial)	**Classification** Fibrous (synarthrodial)
Movement Types Bicondylar	**Subclass** Gomphosis
Plane (gliding)	

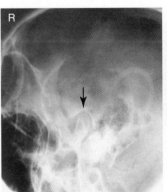

Fig. 11.55 Closed mouth.

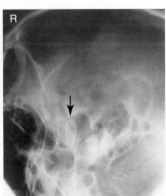

Fig. 11.56 Open mouth.

Paranasal Sinuses

The large, air-filled cavities of the **paranasal sinuses** are sometimes called the accessory nasal sinuses because they are lined with mucous membrane, which is continuous with the nasal cavity. These sinuses are divided into four groups, according to the bones that contain them:

Maxillary (?)	Maxillary (facial) bones
Frontal (usually 2)	Frontal (cranial) bones
Ethmoid (many)	Ethmoid (cranial) bones
Sphenoid (1 or 2)	Sphenoid (cranial) bone

Only the **maxillary sinuses** are part of the **facial bone** structure. The **frontal, ethmoid,** and **sphenoid** sinuses are contained within their respective **cranial bones** (Fig. 11.57).

PURPOSE

The purpose of the paranasal sinuses is subject to speculation. Various sources suggest they assist in vocal resonance, lighten the weight of the skull, and produce mucus to moisten the nasal passageways and air entering the nasal airway.

The paranasal sinuses begin to develop in the fetus, but only the maxillary sinuses exhibit a definite cavity at birth. The frontal and sphenoid sinuses begin to be visible on radiographs at age 6 or 7. The ethmoid sinuses develop last. All the paranasal sinuses generally are fully developed by the late teenage years.

Each of these groups of sinuses is studied, beginning with the largest, the maxillary sinuses.

MAXILLARY SINUSES

The large **maxillary sinuses** are paired structures, one of which is located within the body of each maxillary bone. An older term for maxillary sinus is **antrum**, an abbreviation for **antrum of Highmore.**

Each maxillary sinus is shaped like a pyramid on a frontal view. Laterally, the maxillary sinuses appear more cubic. The average total vertical dimension is 1 to 1½ inches (2.5 to 4 cm), and the other dimensions are approximately 1 inch (2.5 cm).

The bony walls of the maxillary sinuses are thin. The floor of each maxillary sinus is slightly below the level of the floor of each nasal fossa. The two maxillary sinuses vary in size from one person to another and sometimes from one side to the other. Projecting into the floor of each maxillary sinus are several conic elevations related to roots of the first and second upper molar teeth (Fig. 11.58). Occasionally, one or more of these roots can allow infection that originates in the teeth, particularly in the molars and premolars, to travel upward into the maxillary sinus.

All the paranasal sinus cavities communicate with one another and with the **nasal cavity,** which is divided into two equal chambers, or **fossae.** In the case of the maxillary sinuses, this site of communication is the opening into the middle nasal meatus passageway located at the superior medial aspect of the sinus cavity itself, as demonstrated in Fig. 11.59. (The osteomeatal complex is illustrated in greater detail later in Figs. 11.63 and 11.64.) When a person is erect, any mucus or fluid trapped within the sinus tends to remain there and layer out, forming an air-fluid level. Therefore, radiographic positioning of the paranasal sinuses should be accomplished with the patient in the **erect position,** if possible, to delineate any possible air-fluid levels.

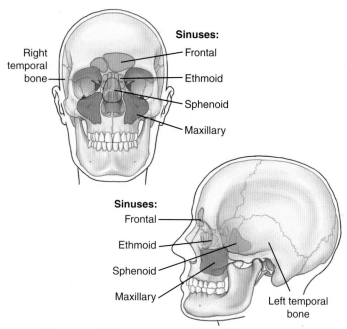

Fig. 11.57 Skull—paranasal sinuses and temporal bone.

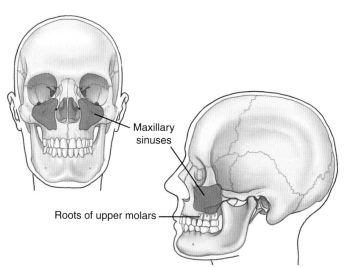

Fig. 11.58 Maxillary sinuses (2).

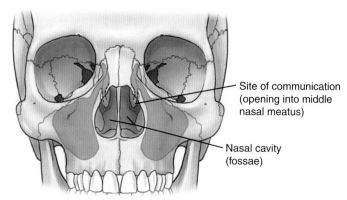

Fig. 11.59 Maxillary sinuses.

FRONTAL SINUSES

The **frontal sinuses** are located between the inner and outer tables of the skull, posterior to the glabella; they **rarely become aerated before age 6.** Whereas the maxillary sinuses are always paired and are usually fairly symmetric in size and shape, the frontal sinuses are rarely symmetric (Fig. 11.60). The frontal sinuses usually are separated by a septum, which deviates from one side to the other or may be absent entirely, resulting in a single cavity. However, two cavities generally exist, which vary in terms of size and shape. They generally are larger in men than in women. They may be singular on the right or the left side, they may be paired as shown, or they may be absent.

ETHMOID SINUSES

The **ethmoid sinuses** are contained within the lateral masses or labyrinths of the ethmoid bone. These air cells are grouped into **anterior, middle,** and **posterior collections,** but they all intercommunicate (Fig. 11.61).

When viewed from the side, the anterior ethmoid sinuses appear to fill the orbits. This occurs because portions of the ethmoid sinuses are contained in the lateral masses of the ethmoid bone, which helps to form the medial wall of each orbit.

SPHENOID SINUSES

The **sphenoid sinuses** lie in the body of the sphenoid bone directly below the sella turcica (Fig. 11.62). The body of the sphenoid that contains these sinuses is cubic and frequently is divided by a thin septum to form two cavities. This septum may be incomplete or absent entirely, resulting in only one cavity.

Because the sphenoid sinuses are so close to the base or floor of the cranium, sometimes pathologic processes make their presence known by their effect on these sinuses. An example is the demonstration of an air-fluid level within the sphenoid sinuses after skull trauma. This air-fluid level may provide evidence that the patient has a basal skull fracture and that either blood or cerebrospinal fluid is leaking through the fracture into the sphenoid sinuses, a condition referred to as **sphenoid effusion.**

Osteomeatal Complex

The drainage pathways of the frontal, maxillary, and ethmoid sinuses make up the **osteomeatal complex,** which can become obstructed, leading to infection of these sinuses, a condition termed **sinusitis.** The osteomeatal complex, sometimes called the osteomeatal unit (OMU), can be imaged with CT to evaluate for obstructions.

Figs. 11.63 and 11.64 illustrate **two key passageways** (infundibulum and middle nasal meatus) and their associated structures identified on coronal CT. The **large maxillary sinus** drains through the **infundibulum** passageway down through the **middle nasal meatus** into the **inferior nasal meatus.** The **uncinate process** of the ethmoid bone makes up the medial wall of the infundibulum passageway. The **ethmoid bulla** receives drainage from the frontal and ethmoid sinus cells, which drains down through the middle nasal meatus into the inferior nasal meatus, where it exits the body through the exterior nasal orifice.

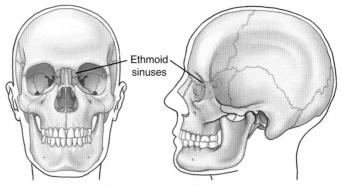

Fig. 11.61 Ethmoid sinuses.

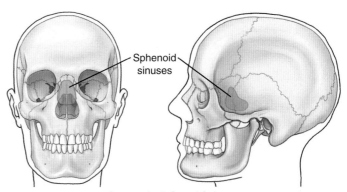

Fig. 11.62 Sphenoid sinuses.

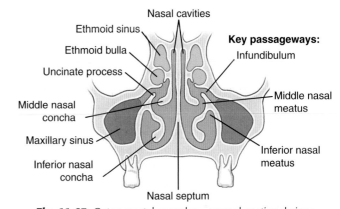

Fig. 11.63 Osteomeatal complex—coronal sectional view.

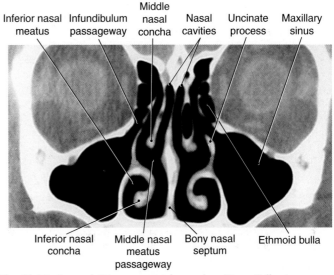

Fig. 11.64 Coronal CT, osteomeatal complex. (From Kelley L, Petersen C: *Sectional anatomy for imaging professionals,* ed 4, St. Louis, 2018, Elsevier.)

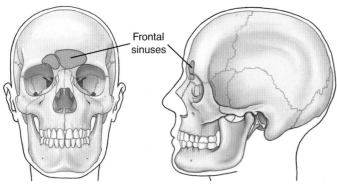

Fig. 11.60 Frontal sinuses.

11

RADIOGRAPHS—PARANASAL SINUSES

Drawings of the sinuses on preceding pages revealed definite sizes and shapes of the sinuses with clear-cut borders. On actual radiographs, these borders are not nearly as defined because various sinuses overlap and superimpose each other, as can be seen on these radiographs of four common sinus projections. The labeled radiographs clearly demonstrate the relative locations and relationships of each of these sinuses. (Note the following abbreviations: **F**—frontal sinuses; **E**—ethmoid sinuses; **M**—maxillary sinuses; and **S**—sphenoid sinuses.)

Lateral Position

The frontal sinuses are clearly visualized between the inner and outer tables of the skull (Fig. 11.65).

The sphenoid sinuses appear to be continuous with the ethmoid sinuses anteriorly.

The large maxillary sinuses are clearly visualized. The roots of the molars and premolars of the upper teeth appear to extend up through the floor of the maxillary sinuses.

PA (Caldwell) Projection

The frontal, ethmoid, and maxillary sinuses are clearly illustrated on this PA axial projection radiograph (Fig. 11.66). The sphenoid sinuses are not demonstrated specifically because they are located directly posterior to the ethmoid sinuses. This relationship is demonstrated on the lateral view (see Fig. 11.65) and the SMV projection (see Fig. 11.68).

Parietoacanthial Transoral Projection (Open-Mouth Waters)

All four groups of sinuses are clearly demonstrated on this projection taken with the mouth open and the head tipped back to separate and project the sphenoid sinuses inferior to the ethmoid sinuses (Fig. 11.67). The open mouth also removes the upper teeth from direct superimposition of the sphenoid sinuses. The pyramid-shaped maxillary sinuses are clearly seen.

SMV Projection

The SMV projection is obtained with the head tipped back so that the top of the head (vertex) is touching the table/upright imaging device surface and the CR is directed inferior to the chin (mentum) (Fig. 11.68).

The centrally located sphenoid sinuses are anterior to the large opening, the foramen magnum. The multiple clusters of ethmoid air cells extend to each side of the nasal septum. The mandible and teeth superimpose the maxillary sinuses. Portions of the maxillary sinuses are visualized laterally.

Fig. 11.68 demonstrates these air-filled mastoids (labeled A) and the dense petrous portions of the temporal bones (labeled B).

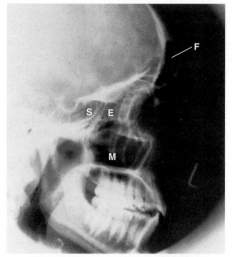
Fig. 11.65 Lateral sinuses projection.

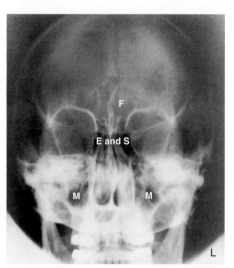
Fig. 11.66 PA axial—Caldwell projection.

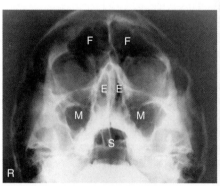
Fig. 11.67 Parietoacanthial transoral projection (open-mouth Waters method).

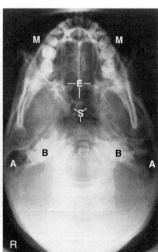
Fig. 11.68 SMV projection.

Orbits

The complex anatomy of the 14 facial bones helps to form several facial cavities. These cavities, which are formed in total or in part by the facial bones, include the mouth (oral cavity), the nasal cavities, and the orbits. The mouth and nasal cavities are primarily passageways and are rarely imaged. However, the orbits that contain the vital organs of sight and associated nerves and blood vessels are imaged more frequently. The structure and shape of the orbits are illustrated in this simplified drawing (Fig. 11.69). Each orbit is a **cone-shaped,** bony-walled structure, as is shown in the drawing.

The rim of the orbit, which corresponds to the outer circular portion of the cone, is called the **base.** However, the base of the orbit is not a true circle and may even look like a figure with four definite sides. The posterior portion of the cone, the **apex,** corresponds to the **optic foramen,** through which the optic nerve passes.

The long axis of the orbits projects both upward and toward the midline. With the head placed in an upright frontal or lateral position with the orbitomeatal line adjusted parallel to the floor, each orbit would project superiorly at an angle of **30°** and toward the MSP at an angle of **37°.** These two angles are important for radiographic positioning of the optic foramina. Each optic foramen is located at the apex of its respective orbit. To radiograph either optic foramen, it is necessary both to extend the patient's chin by 30° and to rotate the head 37°. The CR projects through the base of the orbit along the long axis of the cone-shaped orbit.

BONY COMPOSITION OF ORBITS

Each orbit is composed of parts of **seven bones.** The circumference or circular base of each orbit is composed of parts of **three bones—** the **frontal bone (orbital plate)** from the cranium and the **maxilla** and the **zygoma** from the facial bones (Fig. 11.70). A roof, a floor, and two walls, parts of which also are formed by these three bones, are found inside each orbital cavity. The orbital plate of the frontal bone forms most of the roof of the orbit. The zygoma forms much of the lateral wall and some of the floor of the orbit, whereas a portion of the maxilla helps to form the floor.

The slightly oblique frontal view in Fig. 11.71 demonstrates all seven bones that form each orbit. The **frontal bone, zygoma,** and **maxilla,** which form the base of the orbit, are shown again. A portion of the medial wall of the orbit is formed by the thin **lacrimal bone.** The **sphenoid** and **ethmoid** bones make up most of the posterior orbit, whereas only a small bit of the **palatine** bone contributes to the innermost posterior portion of the floor of each orbit.

The **seven** bones that make up each orbit include **three cranial bones** and **four facial bones,** as shown in Box 11.1.

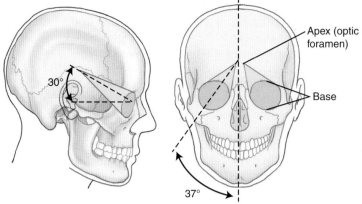

Fig. 11.69 Orbits (cone shaped).

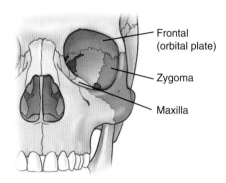

Fig. 11.70 Base of orbit—**three bones** (direct frontal view).

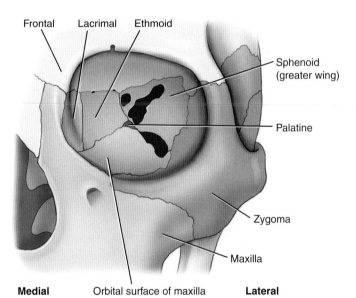

Fig. 11.71 Orbit—seven bones (slightly oblique frontal view).

BOX 11.1 **BONES OF ORBITS**	
CRANIAL BONES	**FACIAL BONES**
Frontal	Maxilla
Sphenoid	Zygoma
Ethmoid	Lacrimal
	Palatine

OPENINGS IN POSTERIOR ORBIT

Each orbit also contains three holes or openings in the posterior portion, as shown in Fig. 11.72. These openings provide for passage of specific cranial nerves (**CN**). (The 12 pairs of cranial nerves are listed and described in the anatomy section of Chapter 18.)

The **optic foramen** is a small hole in the sphenoid bone that is located posteriorly at the apex of the cone-shaped orbit. The optic foramen allows for passage of the optic nerve (CN II), which is a continuation of the retina.

The **superior orbital fissure** is a cleft or opening between the greater and lesser wings of the sphenoid bone, located lateral to the optic foramen. It allows transmission of four primary cranial nerves (CN III to CN VI), which control movement of the eye and eyelid.

A third opening is the **inferior orbital fissure,** which is located between the maxilla, zygomatic bone, and greater wing of the sphenoid. It allows for transmission of the maxillary branch of CN V, which permits entry of sensory innervation for the cheek, nose, upper lip, and teeth.

The small root of bone that separates the superior orbital fissure from the optic canal is known as the **sphenoid strut.** The optic canal is a small canal into which the optic foramen opens. Any abnormal enlargement of the optic nerve could cause erosion of the sphenoid strut, which is actually a portion of the lateral wall of the optic canal.

Anatomy Review

Review exercises for anatomy of the cranial and facial bones follow. Anatomy can be demonstrated on a dry skull or on radiographs. Some anatomic parts identified on the dry skull are not visualized on these radiographs. The parts that are identifiable are labeled as such. A good learning or review exercise is to study both the skull illustrations and the radiographs carefully and identify each part before looking at the answers listed next.

Seven Bones of Left Orbit (Fig. 11.73)

A. Frontal bone (orbital plate)
B. Sphenoid bone
C. Small portion of palatine bone
D. Zygomatic bone
E. Maxillary bone
F. Ethmoid bone
G. Lacrimal bone

Openings and Structures of Left Orbit (Fig. 11.74)

A. Optic foramen
B. Sphenoid strut
C. Superior orbital fissure
D. Inferior orbital fissure

Parieto-Orbital Oblique (Rhese method) Projection of Orbits (Fig. 11.75)

A. Orbital plate of frontal bone
B. Sphenoid bone
C. Optic foramen and canal
D. Superior orbital fissure
E. Infraorbital margin (IOM)
F. Sphenoid strut (part of inferior and lateral wall of optic canal)
G. Lateral orbital margin
H. Supraorbital margin

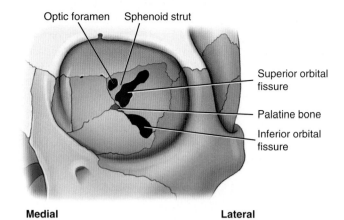

Fig. 11.72 Orbits—posterior openings (slightly oblique frontal view).

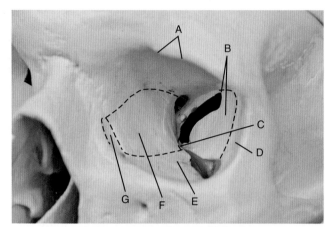

Fig. 11.73 Seven bones of left orbit.

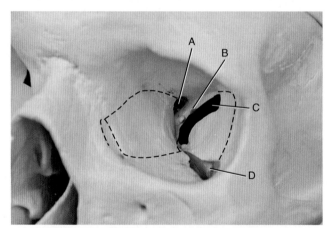

Fig. 11.74 Openings and structures of left orbit.

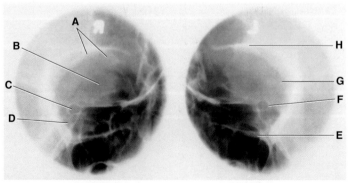

Fig. 11.75 Parieto-orbital oblique projection of orbits (optic foramina).

Facial Bones—Lateral (Figs. 11.76 and 11.77)

A. Zygomatic arch
B. Right zygomatic bone
C. Right nasal bone
D. Frontal process of right maxilla
E. Anterior nasal spine
F. Alveolar process of maxilla
G. Alveolar process of mandible
H. Mentum or mental protuberance
 I. Mental foramen
J. Body of mandible
K. Angle (gonion)
 L. Ramus of mandible
M. Coronoid process
N. Mandibular notch
O. Neck of mandibular condyle
P. Condyle or head of mandible
Q. EAM
R. TM fossa of temporal bone
S. Greater wings of sphenoid
T. Lesser wings of sphenoid with anterior clinoid processes
U. Ethmoid sinuses between orbits
V. Body of maxilla containing maxillary sinuses

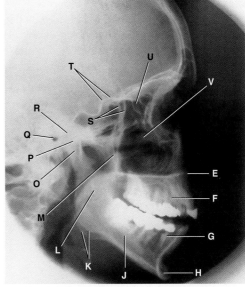

Fig. 11.77 Facial bones—lateral projection.

Facial Bones—Parietoacanthial (Waters)

The photograph (Fig. 11.78) and the radiograph (Fig. 11.79) represent the skull in a parietoacanthial projection (Waters method), with the head tilted back. This is one of the more common projections used to visualize the facial bones, as follows:

A. Zygomatic prominence
B. Body of maxilla (contains maxillary sinuses)
C. Bony nasal septum (perpendicular plate of ethmoid and vomer bone)
D. Anterior nasal spine
E. Zygomatic arch
F. Coronoid process of mandible (Fig. 11.78 only)
G. Condyle (head) of mandible
H. Mastoid process of temporal bone
 I. Angle of mandible
J. Foramen magnum (Fig. 11.79, which demonstrates the dens or odontoid process within the foramen magnum)

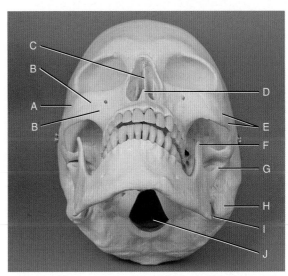

Fig. 11.78 Facial bones—parietoacanthial projection (Waters method).

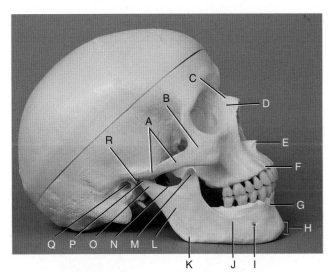

Fig. 11.76 Facial bones—lateral.

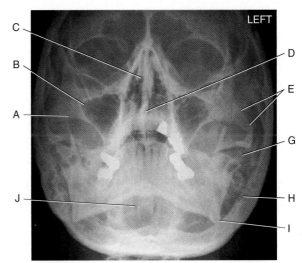

Fig. 11.79 Facial bones—parietoacanthial projection (Waters method).

Facial Bones—SMV (Inferior View)

Fig. 11.80 shows an inferior view of the dry skull with the mandible removed. The SMV projection radiograph in Fig. 11.81 demonstrates positioning whereby the top of the head (vertex) is placed against the image receptor (IR), and the CR enters under the chin (mentum).

Skull (Fig. 11.80)

A. Zygomatic arch
B. Palatine process of maxilla
C. Horizontal process of palatine bone
D. Pterygoid hamulus of sphenoid

Radiograph (Fig. 11.81)

E. Foramen ovale of sphenoid
F. Foramen spinosum of sphenoid
G. Foramen magnum
H. Petrous pyramid of temporal bone
I. Mastoid portion of temporal bone
J. Sphenoid sinus in body of sphenoid
K. Condyle (head) of mandible
L. Posterior border (vertical portion) of palatine bone
M. Vomer or bony nasal septum
N. Right maxillary sinuses
O. Ethmoid sinuses

Facial Bones—Frontal View (Fig. 11.82)

A. Left nasal bone
B. Frontal process of left maxilla
C. Optic foramen
D. Superior orbital fissure
E. Inferior orbital fissure
F. Superior and middle nasal conchae of ethmoid bone
G. Vomer bone (lower portion of bony nasal septum)
H. Left inferior nasal conchae
I. Anterior nasal spine
J. Alveolar process of left maxilla
K. Alveolar process of left mandible
L. Mental foramen
M. Mentum or mental protuberance
N. Body of right mandible
O. Angle (gonion) of right mandible
P. Ramus of right mandible
Q. Body of right maxilla (contains maxillary sinuses)
R. Zygomatic prominence of right zygomatic bone
S. Outer orbit portion of right zygomatic bone
T. Sphenoid bone (cranial bone)

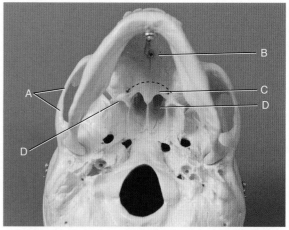

Fig. 11.80 Facial bones—inferior view.

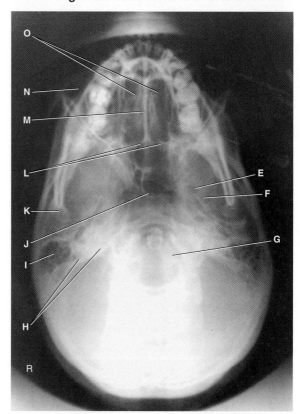

Fig. 11.81 SMV projection.

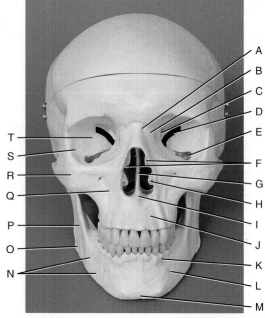

Fig. 11.82 Facial bones—frontal view.

Clinical Indications: Cranium

SKULL AND CRANIAL PATHOLOGY

Indications for skull and cranial radiographic procedures have markedly decreased because CT or MRI is increasingly available. However, smaller hospitals, clinics, and rural centers may still perform these procedures.

Skull fractures are disruptions in the continuity of **bones** of the skull.

NOTE: Although radiographic images of the skull provide excellent spatial resolution of bone, the presence or absence of a fracture is in no way an indication of underlying brain injury. Additional imaging procedures (i.e., CT or MRI) must be performed if brain tissue is to be fully assessed.

- **Linear fractures** are fractures of the skull that may appear as jagged or irregular lucent lines that lie at right angles to the axis of the bone.
- **Depressed fractures** are sometimes called *ping-pong fractures.* A fragment of bone that is separated and depressed into the cranial cavity can occur. A tangential view may be used to determine the degree of depression if CT is unavailable.
- **Basal skull fractures** are fractures through the dense inner structures of the temporal bone. These fractures are very difficult to visualize because of the complexity of the anatomy in this area. If bleeding occurs, radiographic images may reveal an air-fluid level in the sphenoid sinus if a horizontal ray is used for the lateral skull projection. CT is the modality of choice to differentiate between epidural and subdural hemorrhage.

Gunshot wounds can be visualized by radiographic images typically performed to localize bullets in gunshot victims in an antemortem or postmortem examination. The bullet is easily recognizable because of lead content.

Neoplasms are new and abnormal growths.

- **Metastases** are primary malignant neoplasms that spread to distant sites via blood and the lymphatic system. The skull is a common site of metastatic lesions, which may be characterized and visualized on the image as follows:
  - **Osteolytic** lesions are destructive lesions with irregular margins.
  - **Osteoblastic** lesions are proliferative bony lesions of increased density (brightness).
  - **Combination osteolytic and osteoblastic** lesions have a "moth-eaten" appearance of bone because of the mix of destructive and blastic lesions.

Multiple myeloma is a condition in which one or more bone tumors originate in the bone marrow. The skull is a commonly affected site.

Pituitary adenomas are investigated primarily by CT or MRI. Radiographic images may demonstrate enlargement of the sella turcica and erosion of the dorsum sellae, often as an incidental finding.

Paget disease (osteitis deformans) is a disease of unknown origin that begins as a stage of bony destruction followed by bony repair. It involves many bony sites, including the skull, pelvis, spine, and lower limbs. Radiographically, areas of lucency demonstrate the destructive stage, and a "cotton-wool" appearance with irregular areas of increased density (sclerosis) shows the reparative stage. Often these regions of bone become fragile and deformed. Nuclear medicine scans can demonstrate both regions of no (cold) and increased (hot) uptake of the radionuclide based on the stage of the disease.

TEMPORAL BONE PATHOLOGY

Common pathologic indications for temporal bone radiographic procedures include the following.

Acute mastoiditis *(mas"-toid-i'-tis)* is a bacterial infection of the mastoid process that can destroy the inner part of the mastoid process. It often results from middle ear infections. Bacteria in the middle ear can migrate to the mastoids. Mastoid air cells are replaced with a fluid-filled abscess, which can lead to progressive hearing loss. A CT scan demonstrates a fluid-filled abscess that replaces air-filled mastoid air cells.

Neoplasms are new and abnormal growths (tumors).

- **Acoustic neuroma** (vestibular schwannoma) refers to a benign, usually slow-growing tumor of the auditory nerve sheath that originates in the internal auditory canal. Symptoms include hearing loss, dizziness, and loss of balance. It typically is diagnosed with the use of CT or MRI (preferred modality), but it may be visualized on radiographic images in advanced cases with expansion and asymmetry of the affected internal acoustic canal.
- **Cholesteatoma** *(ko"-le-ste"-a-to'-ma)* is a benign, cystic mass or tumor that is most common in the middle ear. It occurs due to a congenital defect or chronic otitis media. It may destroy surrounding bone, which can lead to serious complications, including hearing loss. Surgery is required to remove a cholesteatoma.[4]

A **polyp** is a growth that arises from a mucous membrane and projects into a cavity (sinus). It may cause chronic sinusitis.

Otosclerosis *(o"-to-skle-ro'-sis)* is a hereditary disease that involves irregular ossification of the auditory ossicles of the middle ear. One common finding is fixation of the stapes to the oval window (eardrum). This leads to an impediment of sound transmission. It is the most common cause of hearing loss in adults without eardrum damage. Symptoms first become evident between the ages of 11 and 30 years. Otosclerosis is more common in women.[5] It is best demonstrated on CT imaging. See Table 11.2 for a summary of clinical indications related to the cranium.

TABLE 11.2 SUMMARY OF CLINICAL INDICATIONS: CRANIUM[A]

CONDITION OR DISEASE	MOST COMMON RADIOGRAPHIC EXAMINATION	POSSIBLE RADIOGRAPHIC APPEARANCE	EXPOSURE FACTOR ADJUSTMENT[B]
Fractures	CT, routine skull series		None
Linear	Routine skull series, CT	Jagged or irregular lucent line with sharp borders	None
Depressed	Tangential projection sometimes helpful, CT	Bone fragment depressed into cranial cavity	None
Basal	Horizontal beam lateral for potential air-fluid level in sphenoid sinuses and SMV projection if patient's condition allows, CT	Fracture visualized in dense inner structures of temporal bone	None
Gunshot wound	Routine skull series, CT	High-density object in cranial cavity if bullet has not exited; skull fracture also present because of entrance of projectile	None
Metastases	Routine skull series, bone scan	Depends on lesion type: destructive lesions with decreased density or osteoblastic lesions with increased density or a combination with a moth-eaten appearance	(+) or (−) depending on type of lesion and stage of pathology
Multiple myeloma	Routine skull series, MRI	Osteolytic (radiolucent) areas scattered throughout skull	(−) or none depending on severity
Pituitary adenoma	CT, MRI, collimated AP axial (Towne), and lateral	Enlarged, eroded aspects of sella turcica	(+) because of decreased field size
Paget disease (osteitis deformans)	Routine skull series, nuclear medicine scan	Depends on stage of disease; mixed areas of sclerotic (radiodense) and lytic (radiolucent); cotton-wool appearance; "cold" and "hot" regions of skull on nuclear medicine scan	(+) if in advanced sclerotic stage
Mastoiditis	CT, MRI	Increased densities (fluid-filled) replace mastoid air cells	None
Neoplasia			
Acoustic neuroma	MRI, CT	Widened internal auditory canal	None
Cholesteatoma	CT, MRI	Bone destruction involving middle ear	None
Polyp	Routine radiographic sinus views, CT, MRI	Increased density in affected sinus, typically with rounded borders	None
Otosclerosis	CT, MRI	Excessive bone formation involving middle and inner ear	None

[a]For the purpose of this table, a routine skull series is considered to be PA axial (Caldwell), AP axial (Towne), and lateral projections.
[b]Depends on stage or severity of disease or condition.

Clinical Indications: Facial Bones and Paranasal Sinuses

In addition to CT or MRI procedures, conventional radiographic examinations for the facial bones and paranasal sinuses still are commonly performed in smaller hospitals and clinics. For paranasal sinuses, radiographs are performed to demonstrate pathologies such as mucosal thickening, air-fluid levels, or erosion of bony margins of the sinuses.

Common clinical indications for various types of radiographic examinations for the facial bones and sinuses include the following:

Fracture is a break in the structure of a bone caused by a direct or indirect force. Examples of specific fractures involving the facial bones include the following:

*   **Blowout fracture** is a fracture of the floor of the orbit caused by an object striking the eyes straight on (Fig. 11.83). As the floor of the orbit ruptures, the inferior rectus muscle is forced through the fracture into the maxillary sinus, causing entrapment and diplopia (perception of two images). A blowout fracture may also involve the medial walls of the orbit. CT is an effective imaging modality in demonstrating blowout fractures (Fig. 11.84).
*   **Tripod fracture** is caused by a blow to the cheek, resulting in fracture of the zygoma in three places—orbital process, maxillary process, and arch. The result is a "free-floating" zygomatic bone, or a tripod fracture (Fig. 11.85).
*   **Le Fort fractures** are severe bilateral horizontal fractures of the maxillae that may result in an unstable detached fragment.
*   **Contrecoup fracture** is a fracture to one side of a structure that is caused by an impact on the opposite side. For example, a blow to one side of the mandible results in a fracture on the opposite side.

Foreign body of the eye refers to metal or other types of fragments in the eye, a relatively common industrial mishap. Radiographic images are taken to detect the presence of a metallic foreign object but are limited in their ability to demonstrate damage to tissues caused by these objects.

The patient interview before an MRI procedure includes questions regarding the history of a foreign object in the eye. Because the magnetic field causes the metal, ferrous fragments to move, injury occurs to the soft tissues (even blindness may occur if the optic nerve is damaged). Radiographic images may be obtained before MRI to confirm the presence of a foreign object.

Neoplasm describes a new and abnormal growth (tumor) that may occur in the skeletal structures of the face.

Osteomyelitis is a localized infection of bone or bone marrow. This infection may be caused by bacteria from a penetrating trauma or postoperative or fracture complications. It also may be spread by blood from a distant site.

Sinusitis (si-nu-si'-tis) is an infection of the sinus mucosa that may be acute or chronic. The patient complains of headache, pain, swelling over the affected sinus, and possibly a low-grade fever.

Secondary osteomyelitis, an infection of the bone and marrow secondary to sinusitis, results in erosion of the bony margins of the sinus.

TMJ syndrome describes a set of symptoms, which may include pain and clicking, that indicate dysfunction of the TMJ. This condition may be caused by malocclusion, stress, muscle spasm, or inflammation.

See Table 11.3 for a summary of clinical indications related to facial bones and sinuses.

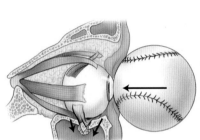

Fig. 11.83 Blowout fracture.

Fig. 11.84 Blowout fracture of the orbit.

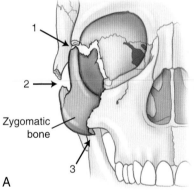

Zygomatic bone

A

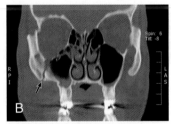

B

Fig. 11.85 A, Tripod fracture. B, Coronal CT of tripod fracture involving right lateral orbital wall and zygoma.

TABLE 11.3 **SUMMARY OF CLINICAL INDICATIONS: FACIAL BONES AND SINUSES**			
CONDITION OR DISEASE	**MOST COMMON RADIOGRAPHIC EXAMINATION**	**POSSIBLE RADIOGRAPHIC APPEARANCE**	**EXPOSURE FACTOR ADJUSTMENT**
Fractures	Routine radiographic projections of affected area, CT	Disruption of bony cortex	None
Foreign body of eye	Routine facial bone (orbits) projections, including modified parietoacanthial projection	Increased density if foreign body is metallic	None
Neoplasms	Routine radiographic projections of affected area, CT/MRI	Possible increase or decrease in density, depending on lesion type	None
Osteomyelitis	Nuclear medicine bone scan, routine radiographic projections of affected area	Soft tissue swelling; loss of cortical margins	None
Sinusitis	Routine radiographic sinus projections, CT, MRI	Sinus mucosal thickening, air-fluid levels, opacified sinus	None
Secondary osteomyelitis	Routine radiographic sinus projections, CT	Erosion of bony margins of sinus	None
TMJ syndrome	Axiolateral projections of TMJ (open- and closed-mouth position), CT/MRI	Abnormal relationship or range of motion between condyle and TM fossa	None

11

RADIOGRAPHIC POSITIONING CONSIDERATIONS: CRANIUM

Traditionally, the cranium has been one of the most difficult and challenging parts of the body to image. A good understanding of the anatomy and relationships of bones and structures of the skull as described in this chapter is essential before a study of radiographic positioning of the cranium is begun. Conventional radiography of certain parts of the cranium, such as the denser temporal bone regions, is less common today because of advances in other imaging modalities such as CT and MRI. However, these imaging modalities may be unavailable in remote areas, and every technologist should be able to perform conventional skull radiography as described in this chapter.

Skull Morphology (Classifications by Shape and Size)

MESOCEPHALIC SKULL

The shape of the average head is termed **mesocephalic** *(mes″-o-se-fal′-ik)*. The average caliper measurements of the adult skull are 6 inches (15 cm) between the parietal eminences (lateral), 7½ inches (19 cm) from frontal eminence to external occipital protuberance (anteroposterior [AP] or PA), and 9 inches (23 cm) from vertex to beneath the chin (SMV projection) (Fig. 11.86). Although most adults have a skull of average size and shape, exceptions to this rule exist.

A general rule for describing skull type is to compare the width of the skull at the parietal eminence with the length measured from the frontal eminence to the external occipital protuberance. For an average mesocephalic skull, the **width is 75% to 80% of the length.**[6]

BRACHYCEPHALIC AND DOLICHOCEPHALIC SKULLS

Variations of the average-shaped or mesocephalic skull include **brachycephalic** *(brak″-e-se-fal′-ik)* and **dolichocephalic** *(dol″-i-ko-se-fal′-ik)* designations. A short, broad head is termed *brachycephalic,* and a long, narrow head is called *dolichocephalic.*

The width of the brachycephalic type is **80% or greater** than the length. The width of the long, narrow dolichocephalic type is **less than 75%** of the length.[6]

A second variation is the **angle difference** between the petrous pyramids and the MSP. In the average-shaped, mesocephalic head, the petrous pyramids form an angle of **47°.** In the brachycephalic skull, the angle is **greater than 47°** (approximately 54°), and in the dolichocephalic skull, the angle is **less than 47°** (approximately 40°) (Fig. 11.87).

POSITIONING CONSIDERATIONS RELATED TO SKULL MORPHOLOGY

The positioning descriptions, including CR angles and head rotations, as described in this text are based on the average-shaped mesocephalic skull. For example, the axiolateral oblique projection (Law method) for TMJs requires 15° of head rotation. A long, narrow, dolichocephalic head requires slightly more than 15° of rotation, and a short, broad, brachycephalic type requires less than 15°.

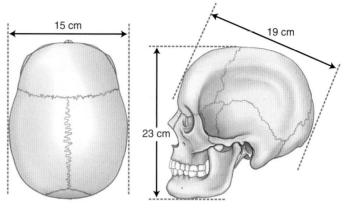

Fig. 11.86 Average skull (mesocephalic).

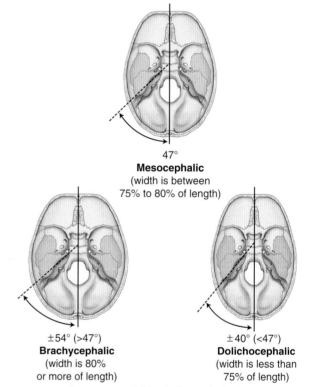

47°
Mesocephalic
(width is between
75% to 80% of length)

±54° (>47°)
Brachycephalic
(width is 80%
or more of length)

±40° (<47°)
Dolichocephalic
(width is less than
75% of length)

Fig. 11.87 Variable skull morphologies.

Cranial Topography (Surface Landmarks)

Certain surface landmarks and localizing lines must be used for accurate positioning of the cranium. Each of the following topographic structures can be seen or palpated.

BODY PLANES (FIG. 11.88)

The **midsagittal**, or **median, plane (MSP)** divides the body into left and right halves. This plane is important for accurate positioning of the cranium because for every AP and PA or lateral projection, the MSP is perpendicular to or parallel to the plane of the IR.

ANTERIOR AND LATERAL VIEW LANDMARKS (FIGS. 11.89 AND 11.90)

The **superciliary ridge (arch)** is the ridge or arch of bone that extends across the forehead directly above each eye. Slightly above this ridge is a slight groove or depression, the **SOG** (see Fig. 11.88).

NOTE: The SOG is important because it corresponds to the highest level of the facial bone mass, which is also the level of the **floor of the anterior fossa** of the cranial vault.

The **glabella** *(glah-bel'-ah)* is the smooth, slightly raised triangular area between and slightly superior to the eyebrows and above the bridge of the nose.

The **nasion** *(na'-ze-on)* is located at the junction of the two nasal bones and the frontal bone.

The **acanthion** *(ah-kan'-the-on)* ("little thorn") is the midline point at the junction of the upper lip and the nasal septum. This is the point where the nose and the upper lip meet.

The **angle**, or **gonion** *(go'-ne-on)*, refers to the lower posterior angle on each side of the jaw or mandible.

A flat triangular area projects forward as the **chin**, or **mentum**, in humans. Imagine the base of a triangle formed between the two mental protuberances and the two sides extending between the two innermost medial incisors to form the apex. The midpoint of this triangular area of the chin as it appears from the front is termed the **mental point.**

Ear

Parts of the ear that may be used as positioning landmarks are the **auricle**, or **pinna** (external portion of ear), the large flap of ear made of cartilage, and the **tragus**, the small cartilaginous flap that covers the opening of the ear. **TEA** refers to the superior attachment of the auricle, or the part where the side frames of eyeglasses rest. This is an important landmark because it corresponds to the highest level of the **petrous ridge** on each side.

Eye

The junctions of the upper and lower eyelids are termed **canthi** *(kan'-thi)*. The **inner canthus** *(kan'-thus)* is where the eyelids meet near the nose; the more lateral junction of the eyelids is termed the **outer canthus.**

The superior rim of the bony orbit of the eye is the **SOM**, and the inferior rim is the **IOM**. Another landmark is the **midlateral orbital margin**, which is the portion of the lateral rim that is near the outer canthus of the eye. These three landmarks contribute to the base of the orbit.

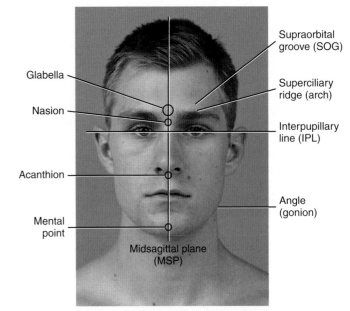

Fig. 11.88 Body planes and landmarks.

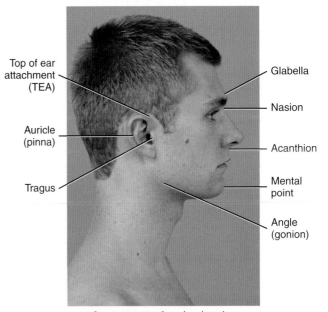

Fig. 11.89 Surface landmarks.

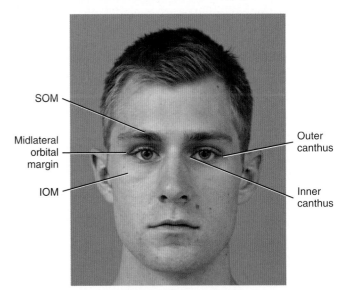

Fig. 11.90 Orbital landmarks.

CRANIAL POSITIONING LINES (FIG. 11.91)

Certain positioning lines are important in cranial radiography. These lines are formed by connecting certain facial landmarks to the midpoint of the **EAM.** The EAM is the opening of the external ear canal. The center point of this opening is called the **auricular point.**

The most superior of these positioning lines is the **glabellomeatal line (GML),** which is not as precise as the other lines because the glabella is an area and not a specific point. The GML refers to a line between the glabella and the EAM.

The **orbitomeatal line (OML)** is a frequently used positioning line that is located between the outer canthus (midlateral orbital margin) and EAM.

The **infraorbitomeatal line (IOML)** is formed by connecting the IOM to the EAM. Two older terms identify this same line as **Reid's base line** or the **anthropologic base line.** An average difference of **7° to 8°** exists between the angles of the OML and IOML. There is also an approximate 7° to 8° average angle difference between the OML and GML. Knowing the angle differences between these three lines is helpful in making positioning adjustments for specific projections of the cranium and facial bones.

The **acanthiomeatal line (AML)** and **mentomeatal line (MML)** are important in radiography of the facial bones. Connecting the acanthion (for the AML) or the mental point (for the MML) to the EAM forms the AML or MML.

A line from the junction of the lips to the EAM, called the **lips-meatal line (LML),** is a positioning line used in this textbook to position for a specific projection of the facial bones called a modified parietoacanthial (modified Waters) projection.

The **glabelloalveolar line (GAL)** connects the glabella to a point at the anterior aspect of the alveolar process of the maxilla. This line is used for positioning a tangential projection for the nasal bones and the lateral position of the cranium.

The **interpupillary,** or **interorbital, line (IPL)** is a line that connects the pupils or the outer canthi of the patient's eyes. When the head is placed in a **true lateral** position, the PL must be exactly perpendicular to the plane of IR (see Fig. 11.88).

The **inion** *(in'-e-on)* is the most prominent point of the external occipital protuberance. It corresponds to the highest "nuchal" line of the occipital bone and allows insertion of the occipitofrontalis muscle. A posterior extension of the IOML approximates the location of the inion.

SKULL POSITIONING AIDS

Two simple devices may be used to ensure accurate placement of a cranial positioning line. A straightedge can be used to illustrate that a cranial line is perpendicular (Fig. 11.92); an angle ruler can also be used and is often the preferred tool. The angle ruler or goniometer (Fig. 11.93) has the advantage of allowing the technologist to determine how many degrees the cranial line is from perpendicular or horizontal so that the patient position or CR angle may be accurately adjusted.

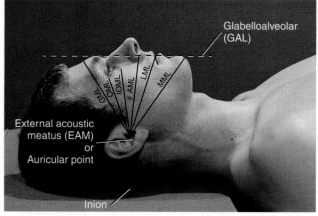

- Glabellomeatal line (GML)
- Orbitomeatal line (OML)
- Infraorbitomeatal line (IOML) (Reid's base line)
- Acanthiomeatal line (AML)
- Lips-meatal line (LML)
- Mentomeatal line (MML)

Fig. 11.91 Positioning lines.

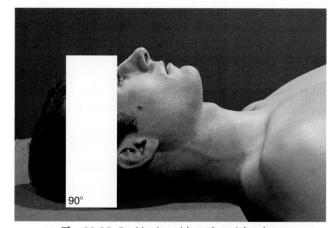

Fig. 11.92 Positioning aid—90° straightedge.

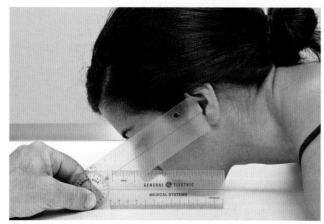

Fig. 11.93 Positioning aid—angle ruler demonstrating degrees of IOML to IR.

Positioning Considerations
ERECT VERSUS RECUMBENT
Projections of the cranium may be taken with the patient in the recumbent or erect position, depending on the patient's condition (Figs. 11.94 and 11.95). Images can be obtained in the erect position with the use of a standard x-ray table in the vertical position or an upright imaging device. The erect position allows the patient to be positioned quickly and easily and permits the use of a horizontal x-ray beam. A horizontal beam is necessary to visualize any existing air-fluid levels within the cranial or sinus cavities.

When positioning for facial bone projections, an **erect position is preferred** if the patient's condition allows for it. This positioning can be done with an erect table or an upright imaging device (see Fig. 11.94). Moving the patient's entire body in the erect position (to adjust the various planes and positioning lines) often is easier for accurate skull positioning; this is especially true with hypersthenic patients. In addition, air-fluid levels in the sinuses or other cranial cavities may indicate certain pathologic conditions that are visible only in the erect position or with the use of horizontal beam radiography.

PATIENT COMFORT
Patient motion almost always results in an unsatisfactory image. During cranial, facial bone, and sinus radiography, the patient's head must be placed in precise positions and held motionless long enough for an exposure to be obtained. Always remember a patient is attached to the skull that is being manipulated. Every effort should be made to make the patient as comfortable as possible and positioning aids such as sponges, sandbags, and pillows should be used if needed.

Except in cases of severe trauma, respiration should be suspended during the exposure to help prevent blurring of the image caused by breathing movements of the thorax. Suspending respiration is especially important when the patient is in a prone position.

Hygiene
Cranial, facial bone and sinus radiography may require the patient's face to be in direct contact with the technologist's hands and the table/upright imaging surface. In the case of infectious diseases or skin conditions, the technologist must wear gloves while positioning. It is important that proper handwashing techniques and surface disinfectants be used before and after the examination.

EXPOSURE FACTORS
Principal exposure factors for radiography of the cranium and facial bones include the following:
- Medium kVp (75 to 95)
- Small focal spot for improved sharpness (if equipment allows)
- Short exposure time

Paranasal Sinuses
EXPOSURE FACTORS
- A medium kVp range of 75 to 90 is commonly used to provide sufficient contrast of the air-filled paranasal sinuses.
- Optimum exposure as controlled by the mAs is especially important for sinus radiography to visualize pathology within the sinus cavities.
- A small focal spot should be used for improved sharpness.
- As with cranial and facial bone imaging, shielding of radiosensitive organs is recommended.
- Close collimation and elimination of unnecessary repeats are the best measures for reducing radiation dose in sinus radiography.

SOURCE–IMAGE RECEPTOR DISTANCE
The minimum source–image receptor distance (SID) with the image receptor (IR) in the table or upright imaging device is 40 inches (100 cm).

RADIATION PROTECTION
The best techniques for minimizing radiation exposure to the patient in cranial, facial bone, and paranasal sinus radiography are to (1) use **close collimation;** (2) immobilize the head when necessary, **minimizing repeats;** and (3) **center properly.**

PATIENT SHIELDING
Along with close collimation, shielding of radiosensitive organs is recommended unless it interferes with the radiographic study.

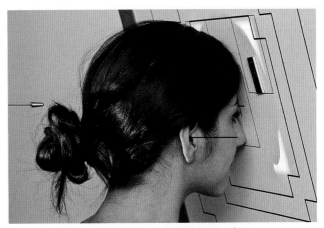
Fig. 11.94 Erect—upright imaging device.

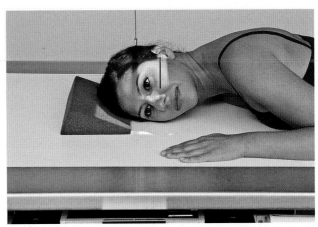
Fig. 11.95 Recumbent—table-imaging device.

11

CAUSES OF POSITIONING ERRORS

When positioning a patient's head, look at various facial features and palpate anatomic landmarks to place the appropriate body plane precisely in relation to the plane of the IR. Although the human body is expected to be symmetric bilaterally (i.e., the right half is anticipated to be identical to the left half), this is not always true. The ears, nose, and jaw are often asymmetric. The nose frequently deviates to one side of the MSP, and the ears are not necessarily in the same place or of the same size on each side.

The lower jaw or mandible is also often asymmetric. Bony parts, such as the mastoid tips and the orbital margins, are safer landmarks to use. Although the patient's eyes are often used as landmarks during positioning, the nose, which may not be straight, should not be used. As a rule of thumb, use the relationship of the eye to the EAM when deciding on the use of the OML or IOML for certain positions of the skull.

FIVE COMMON POSITIONING ERRORS

Five potential positioning errors related to cranial, facial bone, and paranasal sinus positioning are as follows:

1. Rotation
2. Tilt
3. Excessive neck flexion
4. Excessive neck extension
5. Incorrect CR angle

Rotation and **tilt** are two very common positioning errors, as demonstrated by the drawings on the right. Rotation of the skull almost always results in a retake; therefore, the body planes should be correctly aligned (e.g., MSP is parallel to the IR in a lateral position) (Fig. 11.96).

Tilt is a tipping or slanting of the MSP laterally, even though rotation may not be present (Fig. 11.97).

Incorrect flexion or **extension** of the cervical spine, along with an **incorrect CR angle,** must be avoided (Fig. 11.98).

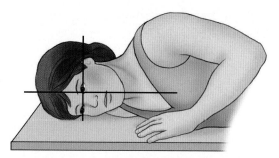

Fig. 11.96 Rotation—MSP is rotated, not parallel to tabletop and IR.

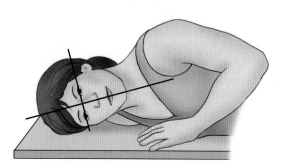

Fig. 11.97 Tilt—MSP is tipped or slanted, not parallel to tabletop or IR.

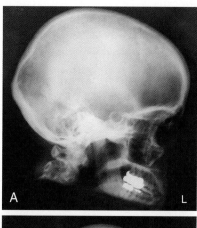

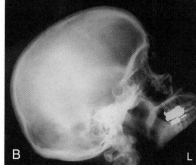

Fig. 11.98 A, Excessive flexion. B, Excessive extension.

RADIOGRAPHIC POSITIONING CONSIDERATIONS: FACIAL BONES AND PARANASAL SINUSES

Special Projections and Anatomic Relationships

Unobstructed radiographic images of various aspects of the facial bones and paranasal sinuses may be difficult to obtain because of the overall shape and structures of the skull. For example, dense internal bony structures of the skull superimpose the delicate facial bones on a routine AP or PA projection. Therefore, very specific CR angles and head positions are required, as described and illustrated subsequently.

PA Skull Projection

The PA skull projection in Fig. 11.99 was obtained with no tube angulation and with the OML (dotted line in Fig. 11.100) perpendicular to the plane of the IR. The CR is parallel to the OML. This position causes the **petrous pyramids to be projected directly into the orbits.** Drawn on both images (Figs. 11.99 and 11.100) is a line through the roof of the orbits and through the petrous ridges. With the orbits superimposed by the petrous pyramids, very little facial bone detail can be demonstrated radiographically. With the head in this position, the PA projection with a perpendicular CR has limited value for visualizing the facial bones.

Parietoacanthial (Waters Method) Projection

To visualize the facial bone mass with conventional radiography, the petrous pyramids must be removed from the facial bone area of interest. This can be done either by tube angulation or by extension of the neck. The radiographs in Figs. 11.101 and 11.102 demonstrate the result. The neck is extended by raising the chin so that the **petrous pyramids are projected just below the maxillary sinuses.** The CR is parallel to the MML. The radiograph on the right (Fig. 11.102; Waters method), if done correctly as described later in this chapter, demonstrates the petrous ridges (see arrows) projected below the maxillae and the maxillary sinuses. Except for the mandible, the **facial bones are now projected superior to** the dense petrous pyramids and are **not superimposed by** them. As stated previously, erect projections are preferred for facial bones and sinuses to demonstrate any possible air-fluid levels (Fig. 11.103). In the case of possible cervical spine injury, cranial and facial bone studies must be performed recumbent to prevent further injury (Fig. 11.104).

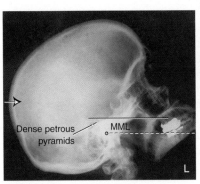

Fig. 11.101 Lateral skull for comparison of bony relationships—CR parallel to MML.

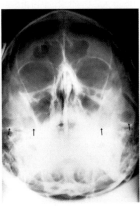

Fig. 11.102 Facial bones— parietoacanthial (Waters method) projection.

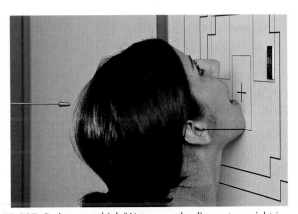

Fig. 11.103 Parietoacanthial (Waters method) erect—upright imaging device.

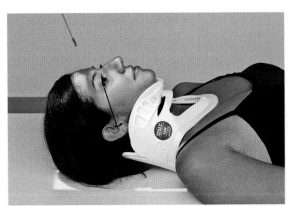

Fig. 11.104 AP, supine—trauma patient.

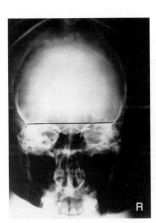

Fig. 11.99 Skull—PA projection.

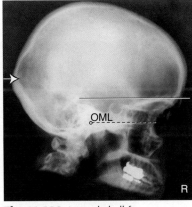

Fig. 11.100 Lateral skull for comparison of bony relationships—CR parallel to OML.

Special Patient Considerations
PEDIATRIC APPLICATIONS
Communication
A clear explanation of the procedure is required to obtain the trust and cooperation of the patient and guardian. Distraction techniques using toys, stuffed animals, and other items are also effective in maintaining patient cooperation.

Immobilization
Pediatric patients (depending on age and condition) are often unable to maintain the required positions. Use of immobilization devices to support the patient is recommended to reduce the need for the patient to be held, reducing radiation exposure. (Chapter 16 provides a detailed description of such devices.) If it is necessary for the guardian to hold the patient, the technologist must provide a lead apron or gloves or both. If the guardian is female, the technologist must ensure that no possibility of pregnancy exists.

Exposure Factors
Exposure factors vary because of various patient sizes and pathologies. Use of short exposure times (associated with the use of high mA) is recommended to reduce the risk of patient motion.

GERIATRIC APPLICATIONS
Communication and Comfort
Sensory loss (e.g., poor eyesight, hearing) associated with aging may result in the need for additional assistance, time, and patience in obtaining the required positions for cranial, facial bone, and paranasal sinus radiography in geriatric patients.

If the examination is performed with the patient in the recumbent position, decreased position awareness may cause the patient to fear falling off the radiography table. A radiolucent mattress or pad placed on the examination table provides comfort, and extra blankets may be required for warmth. Reassurance and attention from the technologist help the patient feel secure and comfortable.

If the patient is able, attaining the required positions in the erect position (sitting) at an upright imaging device may be more comfortable (Fig. 11.105), especially if he or she has an increased kyphosis. Lateral images obtained with a horizontal ray often are indicated for elderly patients who have limited movement.

Exposure Factors
Because of the high incidence of osteoporosis in geriatric patients, the kVp may require a 15% decrease.

Older patients may have tremors or signs of unsteadiness; use of short exposure times (associated with the use of high mA) is recommended to reduce the risk for motion.

BARIATRIC PATIENT CONSIDERATIONS
Positioning for cranial and facial bone projections on the bariatric patient is far more comfortable and easier to assume when performed erect. Unless the patient's health and safety prevents it, perform skull and facial bone positions erect.

If you are unable to place the OML perpendicular to the plane of the IR because of the thickness of the shoulders and restricted flexion of the neck, most cranial projections allow the technologist to use the IOML to perform the relatively same position. Please remember there is approximately 7° to 8° difference between the OML and IOML. In the case of the AP axial projection for the cranium, the technologist would increase the CR angle from 30° to 37°.

Alternative Modalities
COMPUTED TOMOGRAPHY (CT)
CT is the most commonly performed neuroimaging procedure. CT provides sectional images of the brain and bones of the cranium in axial, sagittal, or coronal planes, whereas analog and digital images provide a two-dimensional image of the bony skull only.

Because injury and pathology of the head often involve the brain and associated soft tissues, CT is a vital tool in the full evaluation of the patient. It can distinguish between blood clots, white and gray matter, cerebrospinal fluid, cerebral edema, and neoplasms.

CT provides sectional images of the facial bones, orbits, mandible, and TMJs in axial, sagittal, or coronal planes. CT assists in the full evaluation of these structures because both skeletal detail and associated soft tissues may be visualized with CT.

CT sinus studies may be performed in the prone position, which allows for coronal scans to be created. Coronal CT scans demonstrate any air-fluid levels that are present. CT also allows visualization of the soft tissue planes of the sinuses and evaluation of related bony structures. If the patient cannot be examined prone, the study can be performed supine. In the supine position, axial images are obtained in which sagittal and coronal reconstructed images can be created (Fig. 11.106). These images assist the radiologist in determining the presence of any pathology.

Intravenous contrast medium is not given for most CT sinus examinations. The most common clinical indications for a CT sinus study are sinusitis and possible masses within the sinuses. Three-dimensional reconstruction of CT scans often is useful when facial reconstructive surgery is required.

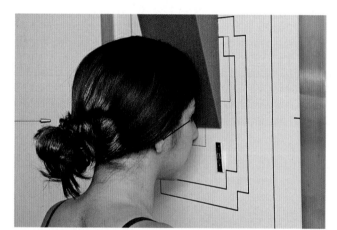

Fig. 11.105 Modified PA projection—**horizontal CR,** OML tilted 15° from perpendicular (**routine** projection for sinuses).

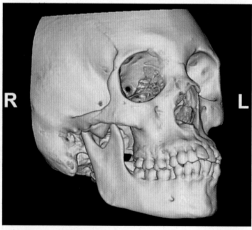

Fig. 11.106 3D CT reconstruction of skull and facial bones.

MAGNETIC RESONANCE IMAGING (MRI)

MRI also provides images of the brain in axial, sagittal, and coronal planes. MRI provides increased sensitivity in detecting differences between normal and abnormal tissues in the brain and associated soft tissues. MRI has limited usefulness in evaluation of bone; however, it is superior to other methods in evaluation of soft tissues.

The magnetic fields used in MRI are thought to be harmless, which means that the patient is spared exposure to ionizing radiation. MRI is useful for evaluating TMJ syndrome to diagnose possible damage to the articular disk of the glenoid cavity of the TM fossa.

SONOGRAPHY

Sonography of the brain of the neonate (through the fontanels) is an integral part of treatment in the intensive care unit. It allows for rapid evaluation and screening of premature infants for intracranial hemorrhage. It is preferred over CT and MRI for this purpose because it is highly portable and less expensive, requires no sedation of the patient, and provides no ionizing radiation.

Sonography can also be valuable in the investigation and follow-up of hydrocephalus. Cranial sutures also may be evaluated, assisting in the diagnosis of premature suture closure (craniosynostosis).

Research is ongoing regarding the use of sonography as a screening tool for maxillary sinusitis. Because it does not involve ionizing radiation exposure, this method would be advantageous for pediatric and pregnant patients.

NUCLEAR MEDICINE (NM)

NM provides a sensitive screening procedure (radionuclide bone scan) for detection of skeletal metastases, of which the cranium is a common site. A bone scan is ordered frequently for patients who are at risk or symptomatic for metastases. Any focal abnormality on the bone scan is investigated radiographically to examine the pathology further. Patients with a history of multiple myeloma are often exceptions to this protocol.

Brain tissue also may be studied with the use of nuclear medicine technology. New radiopharmaceuticals allow perfusion studies of the brain to be performed, typically on patients with Alzheimer disease, seizure disorders, or dementia. Tumor response to treatment also may be assessed with this modality.

Radionuclide bone scan is a sensitive diagnostic procedure for detection of osteomyelitis and occult fractures that may not be demonstrated on radiographic images.

Routine and Special Projections

Projections or positions for the cranium (skull series), facial bones, and paranasal sinuses are demonstrated and described on the following pages as suggested standard routine and special departmental procedures.

11

AP AXIAL PROJECTION—SKULL SERIES

TOWNE METHOD

Clinical Indications
- Skull fractures (medial and lateral displacement), neoplastic processes, and Paget disease

Skull Series
ROUTINE
- AP axial (Towne method)
- Lateral
- PA axial 15° (Caldwell method) or PA axial 25° to 30°
- PA

Technical Factors
- Minimum SID—40 inches (100 cm)
- IR size—10 × 12 inches (24 × 30 cm), portrait
- Grid
- kVp range: 75–90

```
       24
  ┌──────────┐
  │          │
30 │   ▮      │
  │          │
  │ R        │
  └──────────┘
```

Shielding Shield radiosensitive tissues outside region of interest.

Patient Position Remove all metal, plastic, or other removable objects from the patient's head. Take radiograph with the patient in the erect or supine position.

Part Position ⊞
- Depress chin, bringing **OML perpendicular** to IR. For patients unable to flex the neck to this extent, align **IOML** perpendicular to IR. Add radiolucent support under the head if needed (see NOTE).
- Align MSP to CR and to midline of the grid or the table/imaging device surface.
- Ensure that no head rotation or tilt exists.
- Ensure that the vertex of the skull is within collimation field.

CR
- Angle CR 30° caudad to OML or 37° caudad to IOM (Fig. 11.107) (see NOTE).
- Center at MSP 2½ inches (6.5 cm) above the glabella to pass through the foramen magnum at the level of the base of the occiput.
- Center IR to projected CR.

Recommended Collimation Collimate on four sides to anatomy of interest.

Respiration Suspend respiration.

NOTE: If patient is unable to depress the chin sufficiently to bring **OML** perpendicular to IR even with a small sponge under the head, **IOML** can be placed perpendicular instead and the CR angle increased to **37°** caudad. This maintains the **30° angle between OML and CR** and demonstrates the same anatomic relationships. (A 7° to 8° difference exists between OML and IOML.)

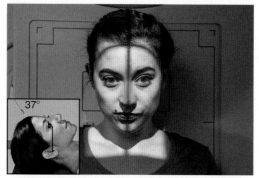
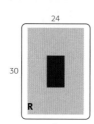

Fig. 11.107 Erect and supine (*inset*)—AP axial.

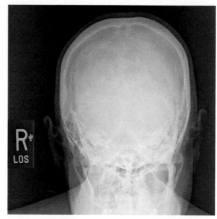

Fig. 11.108 AP axial.

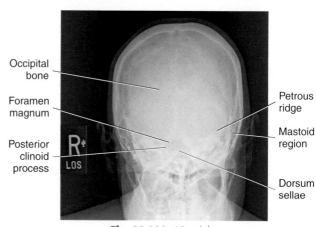

Occipital bone

Foramen magnum

Posterior clinoid process

Petrous ridge

Mastoid region

Dorsum sellae

Fig. 11.109 AP axial.

Evaluation Criteria
Anatomy Demonstrated: • Occipital bone, petrous pyramids, and foramen magnum are demonstrated with the dorsum sellae and posterior clinoid processes visualized in the shadow of the foramen magnum (Figs. 11.108 and 11.109).
Position: • Petrous ridges should be symmetric, indicating **no rotation** (petrous ridge will appear narrowed in the direction of rotation). • Dorsum sellae and posterior clinoid processes visualized in the foramen magnum indicate **correct CR angle and proper neck flexion/extension.** • Underangulation of CR or insufficient flexion of neck projects the dorsum sellae superior to **the foramen magnum. Overangulation** of CR or excessive neck flexion superimposes the **posterior arch of C1 over the dorsum sellae** within the foramen magnum and produces foreshortening of the dorsum sellae. • Shifting of the anterior or posterior clinoid processes laterally within the foramen magnum indicates tilt.[7] • Collimation to area of interest.
Exposure: • Density (brightness) and contrast are sufficient to visualize occipital bone and sellar structures within foramen magnum. • Sharp bony margins indicate **no motion.**

LATERAL POSITION: RIGHT OR LEFT LATERAL—SKULL SERIES

Clinical Indications
- Skull fractures, neoplastic processes, and Paget's disease

Trauma Routine A horizontal beam projection is required to obtain a lateral perspective for trauma patients. This may demonstrate air-fluid levels in the sphenoid sinus—a sign of a basal skull fracture if intracranial bleeding occurs. See Chapter 15 for details on trauma skull projections.

> **Skull Series**
> ROUTINE
> - AP axial (Towne method)
> - Lateral
> - PA axial 15° (Caldwell method) or PA axial 25° to 30°
> - PA

Technical Factors
- Minimum SID—40 inches (100 cm)
- IR size—10 × 12 inches (24 × 30 cm), landscape
- Grid
- kVp range: 70–85

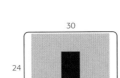

Shielding Shield radiosensitive tissues outside region of interest.

Patient Position Remove all metal, plastic, or other removable objects from patient's head. Take radiograph with patient in the erect or recumbent semiprone position.

Part Position
- Place the head in a **true lateral position,** with the side of interest closest to IR and the patient's body in a semiprone or erect position as needed for comfort. Align **MSP parallel** to IR, ensuring **no rotation or tilt.**
- Align **IPL perpendicular** to IR, ensuring no tilt of head (Fig. 11.110) (see NOTE).
- Adjust neck flexion to align **IOML perpendicular** to front edge of IR. (GAL is parallel to front edge of IR.)

CR
- Align CR **perpendicular** to IR.
- Center to a point 2 inches (5 cm) superior to EAM or halfway between the glabella and the inion for other types of skull morphologies.
- Center IR to CR.

Recommended Collimation Collimate on four sides to anatomy of interest.

Respiration Suspend respiration.

NOTE: For patients in the recumbent position, a radiolucent support placed under the chin helps in maintaining a true lateral position. A patient with a broad chest may require a radiolucent sponge under the entire head to prevent tilt, and a thin patient may require support under the upper thorax.

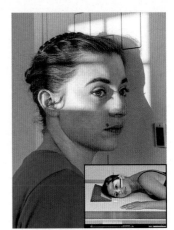

Fig. 11.110 Lateral skull—erect and recumbent (*inset*).

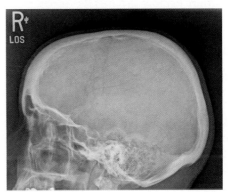

Fig. 11.111 Lateral.

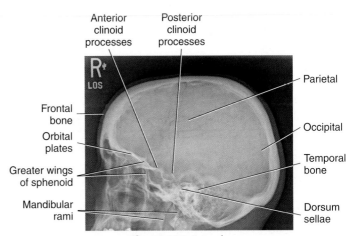

Anterior clinoid processes — Posterior clinoid processes — Parietal — Frontal bone — Orbital plates — Greater wings of sphenoid — Mandibular rami — Occipital — Temporal bone — Dorsum sellae

Fig. 11.112 Lateral.

Evaluation Criteria
Anatomy Demonstrated: • Entire cranium visualized and superimposed parietal bones of cranium. • The entire sella turcica, including anterior and posterior clinoid processes and dorsum sellae, is also demonstrated. • The sella turcica and clivus are demonstrated in profile (Figs. 11.111 and 11.112).
Position: • No rotation or tilt of the cranium is evident. • Rotation is evident by anterior and posterior separation of symmetric vertical bilateral structures such as the mandibular rami, and greater wings of the sphenoid. • Tilt is evident by **superior and inferior separation** of symmetric horizontal structures such as the orbital plates **and greater wings of sphenoid bone.** • Collimation to area of interest.
Exposure: • Density (brightness) and contrast are sufficient to visualize bony detail of bony structures and surrounding skull. • Sharp bony margins indicate **no motion.**

PA AXIAL PROJECTION–SKULL SERIES
15° CR (CALDWELL METHOD) OR 25° TO 30° CR

Clinical Indications
- Skull fractures, neoplastic processes, and Paget disease

Technical Factors
- Minimum SID—40 inches (100 cm)
- IR size—10 × 12 inches (24 × 30 cm), portrait
- Grid
- kVp range: 75–85

Skull Series
ROUTINE
• AP axial (Towne method)
• Lateral
• PA axial 15° (Caldwell method) or PA axial 25° to 30°
• PA

Shielding Shield radiosensitive tissues outside region of interest.

Patient Position Remove all metallic or plastic objects from the patient's head and neck. Take radiograph with patient in the erect or prone position.

Part Position
- Rest patient's nose and forehead against table/imaging device surface.
- Flex neck as needed to align **OML perpendicular** to IR.
- Align the **MSP perpendicular** to the IR to **prevent rotation and/or tilt.**
- Center IR to CR.

CR
- Angle CR 15° caudad, and center to exit at nasion (Fig. 11.113).
- Alternative with CR 25° to 30° caudad, and center to exit at nasion.

Recommended Collimation Collimate on four sides to anatomy of interest.

Respiration Suspend respiration.

Alternative 25° to 30° An alternative projection is a **25° to 30° caudad** tube angle (Fig. 11.114) that allows better visualization of the superior orbital fissures (black arrows), the foramen rotundum (small white arrows) (Fig. 11.114), and the inferior orbital rim region. CR exits at level of mid orbit.

NOTE: Decreased caudal angulation of the CR to 15° and/or increased neck flexion (chin down) will result in projection of the petrous pyramids to the lower third of the orbits.

Alternative AP Axial Projection For patients who are unable to be positioned for a PA projection (e.g., trauma patients), an AP axial projection may be obtained with the use of a 15° cephalic angle, with OML positioned perpendicular to IR (see Chapter 15).

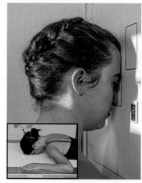

Fig. 11.113 PA axial—CR 15° caudad, OML perpendicular; *inset - (solid arrow),* and alternative CR 30° caudad *(dotted arrow).*

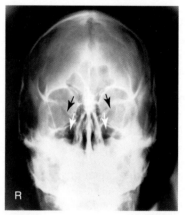

Fig. 11.114 Alternative PA axial—30° caudad.

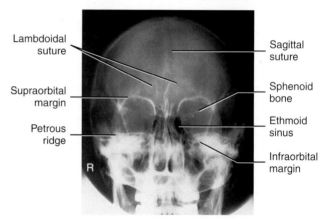

Fig. 11.115 PA axial—15° caudad (Caldwell method).

Evaluation Criteria
Anatomy Demonstrated: • Frontal bone, greater and lesser sphenoid wings, superior orbital fissures, frontal and anterior ethmoid sinuses, supraorbital margins, and crista galli are demonstrated (Fig. 11.115).
PA Axial 25° to 30° Caudad Angle • In addition to the structures mentioned previously, the foramen rotundum adjacent to each IOM is visualized, and the superior orbital fissures (see Fig. 11.114, white and black arrows) are visualized within the orbits.
Position: • No rotation as assessed by equal distance from the midlateral orbital margins to the lateral cortex of the cranium on each side and the superior orbital fissures symmetric within the orbits, correct extension of neck (OML alignment). • **Example:** If the distance between the right lateral orbit and lateral cranial cortex is greater than the left side, the face is rotated toward the left side. • **No tilt with the MSP perpendicular to IR.**
PA Axial 15° Caudad Angle: • Petrous pyramids are projected into the lower one-third of the orbits. • Supraorbital margin is visualized without superimposition. CR angle and OML alignment will impact location of petrous ridges within the orbits.
PA Axial 25° to 30° Caudad Angle: • Petrous pyramids are projected at or just below the IOM to allow visualization of the entire orbital base. CR angle and OML alignment will impact location of petrous ridges within the orbits. • Collimation to area of interest.
Exposure: • Density (brightness) and contrast are sufficient to visualize the frontal bone and sellar structures without overexposure to perimeter regions of skull. • Sharp bony margins indicate **no motion.**

PA PROJECTION—SKULL SERIES

Clinical Indications
- Skull fractures (medial and lateral displacement), neoplastic processes, and Paget disease. This projection is intended to demonstrate the frontal bone with minimal distortion.

Skull Series
ROUTINE
- AP axial (Towne method)
- Lateral
- PA axial 15° (Caldwell method) or PA axial 25° to 30°
- PA

Technical Factors
- Minimum SID—40 inches (100 cm)
- IR size—10 × 12 inches (24 × 30 cm), portrait
- Grid
- kVp range: 75–85

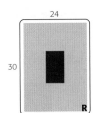

Shielding Shield radiosensitive tissues outside region of interest.

Patient Position Remove all metallic or plastic objects from patient's head and neck. Exposure is taken with patient in the erect or prone position.

Part Position
- Rest patient's nose and forehead against table/imaging surface.
- Flex neck, aligning **OML perpendicular** to IR.
- Align **MSP perpendicular** to midline of table/imaging device to prevent head rotation or tilt (EAM same distance from table/imaging device surface).
- Center IR to CR.

CR
- CR is perpendicular to IR (parallel to OML) and is centered to exit at glabella (Fig. 11.116).

Recommended Collimation Collimate on four sides to anatomy of interest.

Respiration Suspend respiration.

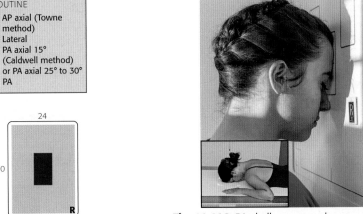
Fig. 11.116 PA skull - erect and prone (*inset*).

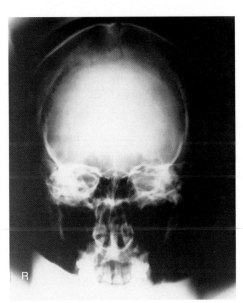
Fig. 11.117 PA skull.

Evaluation Criteria
Anatomy Demonstrated: • Frontal bone, crista galli, internal auditory canals, frontal and anterior ethmoid sinuses, petrous ridges, greater and lesser wings of sphenoid, and dorsum sellae are demonstrated (Figs. 11.117 and 11.118).
Position: • **No rotation** is evident, as indicated by equal distance bilaterally from lateral orbital margin to lateral cortex of skull. • Petrous portion of temporal bone fills the orbits with the petrous ridges at the level of the supraorbital margin. • Posterior and anterior clinoid processes are visualized just superior to ethmoid sinuses. • Collimation to area of interest.
Exposure: • Density (brightness) and contrast are sufficient to visualize frontal bone and surrounding bony structures. • Sharp bony margins indicate **no motion.**

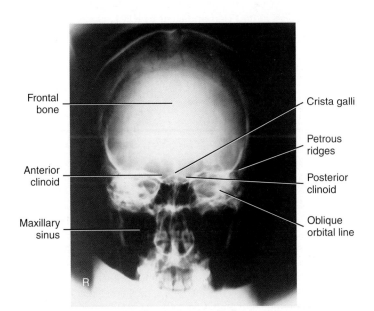
Fig. 11.118 PA skull.

SUBMENTOVERTICAL (SMV) PROJECTION—SKULL SERIES

WARNING: Rule out cervical spine fracture or subluxation on trauma patient before attempting this projection.

Clinical Indications
- Advanced bony pathology of the inner temporal bone structures (skull base)
- Possible basal skull fracture

Skull Series
SPECIAL
• SMV

Technical Factors
- Minimum SID—40 inches (100 cm)
- IR size—10 × 12 inches (24 × 30 cm), portrait
- Grid
- kVp range: 75–85

Shielding Shield radiosensitive tissues outside region of interest.

Patient Position Remove all metal, plastic, and other removable objects from patient's head. Take radiograph with patient in an erect or supine position.

The erect position is recommended using an erect table or an upright imaging device (Fig. 11.119, inset). A wheelchair can also be used. A wheelchair offers support for the back and provides greater stability in maintaining the position. (Ensure wheels are locked before positioning patient.)

Part Position
- Raise patient's chin and hyperextend the neck if possible until **IOML is parallel to IR** (see NOTE).
- Rest patient's head on vertex.
- Align **MSP perpendicular** to the midline of the grid or table/imaging device surface, **avoiding tilt or rotation.**

Supine With patient in the supine position, extend patient's head over end of table and support grid cassette and head as shown in Fig. 11.119, keeping **IOML parallel to IR** and **perpendicular to CR.** Place a positioning sponge/pillow under the patient's back to support neck extension.

Erect If patient is unable to extend the neck sufficiently, compensate by angling CR to remain **perpendicular to IOML.** Depending on the equipment used, IR also may be angled to maintain the perpendicular relationship with CR (e.g., with an adjustable upright imaging device).

NOTE: This position is very uncomfortable for patients in the erect or the supine position; perform it as quickly as possible.

CR
- CR is perpendicular to infraorbitomeatal line.
- Center 1½ inch (4 cm) inferior to mandibular symphysis, or midway between the gonions (approximately ¾ inch [2 cm] anterior to level of EAM).
- Center IR to CR.

Recommended Collimation Collimate on four sides to anatomy of interest.

Respiration Suspend respiration.

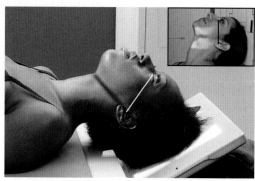

Fig. 11.119 SMV tabletop with grid cassette (*inset* demonstrates use of upright imaging device). CR perpendicular to IOML.

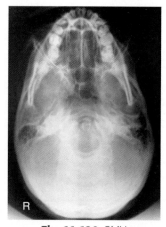

Fig. 11.120 SMV.

Evaluation Criteria
Anatomy Demonstrated: • Foramen ovale and spinosum, mandible, sphenoid and posterior ethmoid sinuses, mastoid processes, petrous ridges, hard palate, foramen magnum, and occipital bone are demonstrated (Figs. 11.120 and 11.121).
Position: • Correct extension of neck and relationship between IOML and CR as indicated by mandibular mentum anterior to the ethmoid sinuses. • **No rotation** evidenced by the MSP parallel to edge of IR. • **No tilt** evidenced by equal distance between mandibular ramus and lateral cranial cortex. • **Example:** If the distance on the left side between the ramus and lateral cranium is greater on the left than the right, the cranial vertex is tilted to the left. • Collimation to area of interest.
Exposure: • Density (brightness) and contrast are sufficient to visualize clearly outline of ethmoid and sphenoid sinuses and cranial foramen. • Sharp bony margins indicate **no motion.**

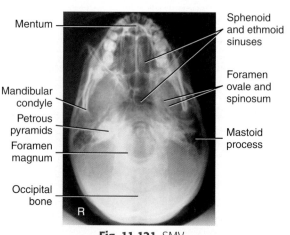

Mentum — Sphenoid and ethmoid sinuses

Mandibular condyle — Foramen ovale and spinosum

Petrous pyramids

Foramen magnum — Mastoid process

Occipital bone

Fig. 11.121 SMV.

PA AXIAL PROJECTION—SKULL SERIES

HAAS METHOD

Clinical Indications

- Skull fractures (medial and lateral displacement), neoplastic processes, and Paget disease

This is an **alternative projection** for patients who cannot flex the neck sufficiently for AP axial (Towne). It can also be performed for hypersthenic and bariatric patients with limited range of cervical motion. It results in magnification of the occipital area but in lower doses to facial structures and the thyroid gland.

This projection is not recommended when the occipital bone is the area of interest because of excessive magnification.

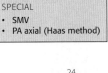

Skull Series
SPECIAL
• SMV
• PA axial (Haas method)

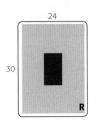

Technical Factors

- Minimum SID—40 inches (100 cm)
- IR size—10 × 12 inches (24 × 30 cm), portrait
- Grid
- kVp range: 75–90

Shielding Shield radiosensitive tissues outside region of interest.

Patient Position Remove all metallic or plastic objects from patient's head and neck. Take radiograph with patient in the erect or prone position.

Part Position ⊞

- Rest patient's nose and forehead against the table/imaging device surface.
- Flex neck, bringing **OML perpendicular** to IR (Fig. 11.122).
- Align MSP to CR and to the midline of the grid or table/imaging device surface.
- Ensure that **no rotation or tilt** exists (MSP perpendicular to IR).

CR

- Angle CR 25° cephalad to OML.
- Center CR to MSP and 1½ inches (4 cm) inferior to the inion and exit 1½ inches (4 cm) superior to nasion.
- Center IR to projected CR.

Recommended Collimation Collimate on four sides to anatomy of interest.

Respiration Suspend respiration.

Evaluation Criteria
Anatomy Demonstrated: • Occipital bone, petrous pyramids, and foramen magnum are demonstrated, with the dorsum sellae and posterior clinoid processes visualized in the shadow of the foramen magnum (Figs. 11.123 and 11.124).
Position: • No rotation is evident, as indicated by bilateral symmetric petrous ridges. • Dorsum sellae and posterior clinoid processes are visualized in the foramen magnum, which indicates correct CR angle and proper neck flexion and extension. • No tilt as evidenced by correct placement of anterior clinoid processes within the middle of the foramen magnum • Collimation to area of interest.
Exposure: • Density (brightness) and contrast are sufficient to visualize occipital bone and sellar structures within foramen magnum. • Sharp bony margins indicate **no motion**.

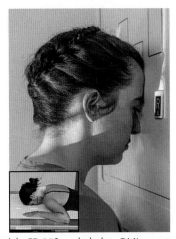

Fig. 11.122 PA axial—CR 25° cephalad to OML, erect and prone (*inset*).

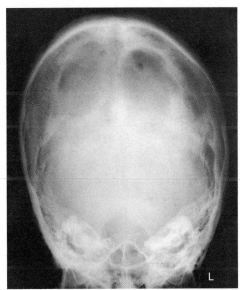

Fig. 11.123 PA axial.

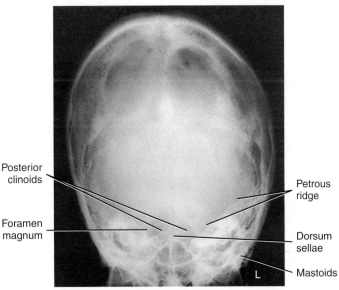

Posterior clinoids

Foramen magnum

Petrous ridge

Dorsum sellae

Mastoids

Fig. 11.124 PA axial.

LATERAL POSITION: RIGHT OR LEFT LATERAL—FACIAL BONES

Clinical Indications
- Fractures and neoplastic or inflammatory processes of the facial bones, orbits, and mandible

Facial Bones
ROUTINE
• Lateral
• Parietoacanthial (Waters method)
• PA axial (Caldwell method)

Technical Factors
- Minimum SID—40 inches (100 cm)
- IR size—8 × 10 inches (18 × 24 cm), portrait
- Grid
- kVp range: 70–85

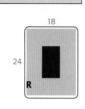

Shielding Shield radiosensitive tissues outside region of interest.

Patient Position Remove all metallic or plastic objects from head and neck. Patient position is erect or recumbent semiprone.

Part Position
- Rest lateral aspect of head against table or upright imaging device surface, **with side of interest closest to IR.**
- Adjust head into a **true lateral position** and oblique body as needed for patient's comfort. (Palpate external occipital protuberance posteriorly and nasion or glabella anteriorly to ensure that these two points are equidistant from IR [Fig. 11.125].)
- Align **MSP parallel** to IR.
- Align IPL perpendicular to IR.
- Adjust chin to bring **IOML perpendicular** to front edge of IR.

CR
- Align CR **perpendicular** to IR.
- Center CR to **zygoma (prominence of the cheek)**, midway between outer canthus and EAM (Fig. 11.126).
- Center IR to CR.

Recommended Collimation Collimate on four sides to anatomy of interest.

Respiration Suspend respiration.

NOTE: Use radiolucent support under the head if needed to bring IPL perpendicular to tabletop on patient with a large chest.

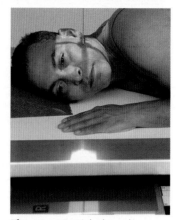

Fig. 11.125 Right lateral—erect.   **Fig. 11.126** Right lateral—recumbent semiprone.

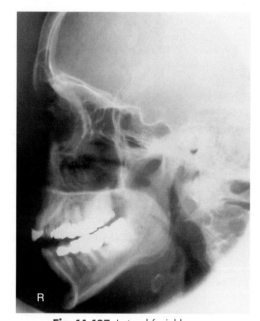

Fig. 11.127 Lateral facial bones.

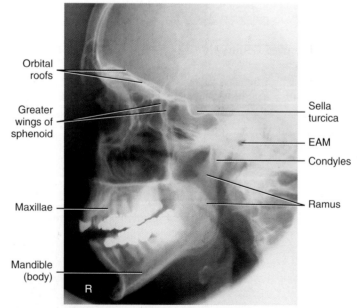

Orbital roofs
Greater wings of sphenoid
Maxillae
Mandible (body)
Sella turcica
EAM
Condyles
Ramus

Fig. 11.128 Lateral facial bones.

PARIETOACANTHIAL PROJECTION—FACIAL BONES

WATERS METHOD

Clinical Indications
- Fractures (particularly tripod and Le Fort fractures) and neoplastic or inflammatory processes
- Foreign bodies in the eye

Facial Bones
ROUTINE
• Lateral
• Parietoacanthial (Waters method)
• PA axial (Caldwell method)

Technical Factors
- Minimum SID—40 inches (100 cm)
- IR size—8 × 10 inches (18 × 24 cm) or 10 × 12 inches (24 × 30 cm), portrait
- Grid
- kVp range: 70–85

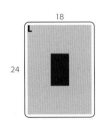

Shielding Shield radiosensitive tissues outside region of interest.

Patient Position Remove all metallic or plastic objects from head and neck. Patient position is erect or prone (erect is preferred if patient's condition allows).

Part Position
- Extend neck, resting chin against table/upright imaging device surface.
- Adjust head until **MML is perpendicular to plane of IR.** OML forms a 37° angle with the table/upright imaging device surface (Fig. 11.129).
- Position **MSP perpendicular** to midline of grid or table/imaging device surface, preventing rotation or tilting of head. (One way to check for rotation is to palpate the mastoid processes on each side and the lateral orbital margins with the thumb and fingertips to ensure that these lines are equidistant from the IR.)

CR
- Align CR perpendicular to IR, to exit at acanthion.
- Center IR to CR.

Recommended Collimation Collimate on four sides to anatomy of interest.

Respiration Suspend respiration.

Evaluation Criteria
Anatomy Demonstrated: • IOMs, maxillae, nasal septum, zygomatic bones, zygomatic arches, and anterior nasal spine.
Position: • Correct neck extension demonstrates petrous ridges (black arrows) just inferior to the maxillary sinuses (Figs. 11.130 and 11.131). • **No** patient **rotation** exists, as indicated by equal distance from the midlateral orbital margin to the lateral cortex of cranium on each side. • Collimation to area of interest.
Exposure: • Contrast and density (brightness) are sufficient to visualize maxillary region. • Sharp bony margins indicate **no motion.**

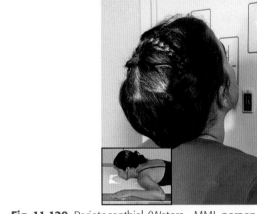

Fig. 11.129 Parietocanthial (Waters - MML perpendicular (OML 37° to IR) - erect and recumbent (*inset*).

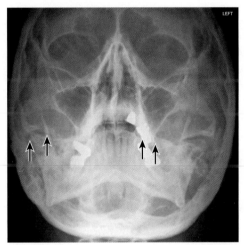

Fig. 11.130 Parietoacanthial (Waters) projection.

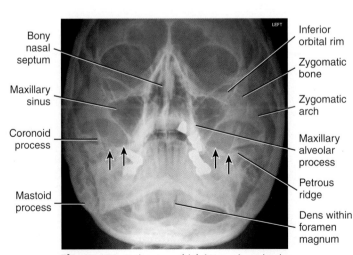

Bony nasal septum

Maxillary sinus

Coronoid process

Mastoid process

Inferior orbital rim

Zygomatic bone

Zygomatic arch

Maxillary alveolar process

Petrous ridge

Dens within foramen magnum

Fig. 11.131 Parietoacanthial (Waters) projection.

11

PA AXIAL PROJECTION—FACIAL BONES

CALDWELL METHOD

Clinical Indications
- Fractures and neoplastic or inflammatory processes of the facial bones

Facial Bones
ROUTINE
• Lateral
• Parietoacanthial (Waters method)
• PA axial (Caldwell method)

Technical Factors
- Minimum SID—40 inches (100 cm)
- IR size—8 × 10 inches (18 × 24 cm) or 10 × 12 inches (24 × 30 cm), portrait
- Grid
- kVp range: 70–85

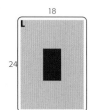

Shielding Shield radiosensitive tissues outside region of interest.

Patient Position Remove all metallic or plastic objects from head and neck. Patient position is erect or prone (erect is preferred if patient's condition permits it).

Part Position
- Rest patient's nose and forehead against the imaging device.
- Tuck chin, bringing **OML perpendicular** to IR.
- Align **MSP perpendicular** to midline of grid or table/imaging device surface. Ensure **no rotation or tilt** of head (Fig. 11.132).

CR
- Angle CR 15° caudad, to exit at nasion (see NOTE).
- Center CR to IR.

Recommended Collimation Collimate on four sides to anatomy of interest.

Respiration Suspend respiration.

NOTE: If area of interest is the orbital margins, use a **30° caudad angle** to project the petrous ridges below the IOM. CR will exit level of midorbits.

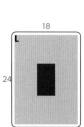

Fig. 11.132 PA axial Caldwell—OML perpendicular, CR 15° caudad, erect and prone (*inset*).

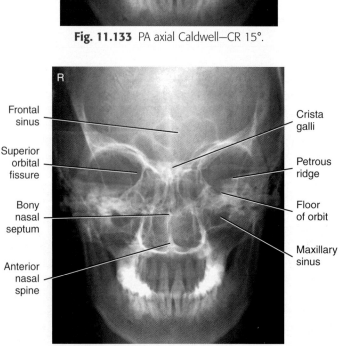

Fig. 11.133 PA axial Caldwell—CR 15°.

Evaluation Criteria
Anatomy Demonstrated: • Superior orbital margins, maxillae, nasal septum, zygomatic bones, and anterior nasal spine (Figs. 11.133 and 11.134).
Position: • Correct patient position/CR angulation is indicated by petrous ridges projected into the **lower one-third of orbits** with 15° caudad CR. If the inferior orbital margins are the area of interest, 30° caudad angle projects the petrous ridges below the IOMs. • **No rotation** of cranium is indicated by equal distance from midlateral orbital margin to the lateral cortex of the cranium (a narrower distance would indicate rotation towards the IR); superior orbital fissures are symmetric. • Collimation to area of interest.
Exposure: • Contrast and density (brightness) are sufficient to visualize maxillary region and superior orbital margins. • Sharp bony margins indicate **no motion.**

Frontal sinus

Crista galli

Superior orbital fissure

Petrous ridge

Bony nasal septum

Floor of orbit

Anterior nasal spine

Maxillary sinus

Fig. 11.134 PA axial Caldwell—CR 15°.

MODIFIED PARIETOACANTHIAL PROJECTION—FACIAL BONES

MODIFIED WATERS METHOD

Clinical Indications
- Orbital fractures (e.g., blowout) and neoplastic or inflammatory processes
- Foreign bodies in the eye

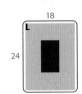

> **Facial Bones**
> SPECIAL
> - Modified parietoacanthial (modified Waters method)

Technical Factors
- Minimum SID—40 inches (100 cm)
- IR size—8 × 10 inches (18 × 24 cm) or 10 × 12 inches (24 × 30 cm), portrait
- Grid
- kVp range: 70–85

Shielding Shield radiosensitive tissues outside region of interest.

Patient Position Remove all metallic or plastic objects from the head and neck. Patient position is erect or prone (erect is preferred if patient's condition allows).

Part Position
- Extend neck, resting chin and nose against table/upright imaging device surface.
- Adjust head until **LML is perpendicular**; OML forms a **55°** angle with IR (Fig. 11.135).
- Position **MSP perpendicular** to midline of grid or table/upright imaging device surface. Ensure **no rotation or tilt** of head.

CR
- Align CR perpendicular, centered to exit at acanthion.
- Center IR to CR.

Recommended Collimation Collimate on four sides to anatomy of interest.

Respiration Suspend respiration.

> ### Evaluation Criteria
> **Anatomy Demonstrated:** • Inferior orbital margins are perpendicular to IR, which also provides a less distorted view of the orbital base than a parietoacanthial (Waters) projection (Figs. 11.136 and 11.137).
> **Position:** • Correct position/CR angulation is indicated by petrous ridges projected into the lower half of the maxillary sinuses, below the IOMs. • **No rotation** of the cranium is indicated by equal distance from the midlateral orbital margin to the lateral cortex of the cranium. • Collimation to area of interest.
> **Exposure:** • Contrast and density (brightness) are sufficient to visualize the inferior orbital margins. • Sharp bony margins indicate **no motion**.

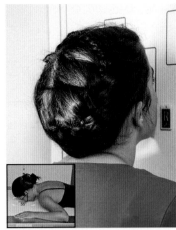

Fig. 11.135 Modified parietoacanthial (Waters)—**LML perpendicular (OML 55°).** (Prone shown in *inset*.)

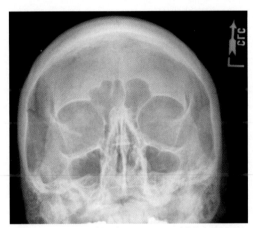

Fig. 11.136 Modified parietoacanthial (Waters).

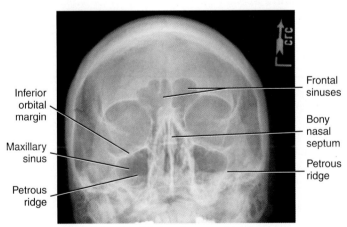

Inferior orbital margin

Maxillary sinus

Petrous ridge

Frontal sinuses

Bony nasal septum

Petrous ridge

Fig. 11.137 Modified parietoacanthial (Waters).

11

LATERAL POSITION—NASAL BONES

Clinical Indications

- Nasal bone fractures
  Both sides should be examined for comparison, with side closest to IR best demonstrated.

Nasal Bones
ROUTINE
• Lateral
• Parietoacanthial (Waters method)

Technical Factors

- Minimum SID—40 inches (100 cm)
- IR size—8 × 10 inches (18 × 24 cm), landscape
- Nongrid
- kVp range: 65–80

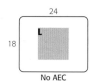

24

L

18

No AEC

Shielding Shield radiosensitive tissues outside region of interest.

Patient Position Remove all metallic or plastic objects from head and neck. Patient position is recumbent semiprone or erect.

Part Position

- Rest lateral aspect of head against the table/upright imaging device surface, with side of interest closest to IR.
- Position nasal bones to center of IR.
- Adjust head into a **true lateral position** and oblique body as needed for patient's comfort (place sponge block under chin if needed) (Fig. 11.138).
- Align **MSP parallel** with a table/upright imaging device surface.
- Align **IPL perpendicular** to table/upright imaging device surface.
- Position **IOML perpendicular** to front edge of IR.

CR

- Align CR perpendicular to IR.
- Center CR to ½ inch (1.25 cm) inferior to nasion.

Recommended Collimation Collimate on all sides to within 2 inches (5 cm) of nasal bone.

Respiration Suspend respiration.

Fig. 11.138 Left lateral nasal bones—recumbent semiprone and erect (*inset*).

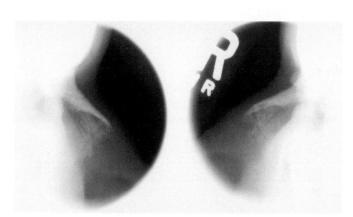

Fig. 11.139 Lateral (L and R).

Evaluation Criteria
Anatomy Demonstrated: • Nasal bones with soft tissue nasal structures, the region of the frontonasal suture, and the anterior nasal spine are demonstrated (Fig. 11.139).
Position: • Nasal bones are demonstrated **without rotation.** • Collimation to area of interest.
Exposure: • Contrast and density (brightness) are sufficient to visualize nasal bone and soft tissue structures. • Sharp bony structures indicate **no motion.**

SUPEROINFERIOR TANGENTIAL (AXIAL) PROJECTION—NASAL BONES

Clinical Indications
- Fractures of the nasal bones (medial-lateral displacement)

Nasal Bones
SPECIAL
• Superoinferior tangential (axial)

Technical Factors
- Minimum SID—40 inches (100 cm)
- IR size—8 × 10 inches (18 × 24 cm), landscape
- Nongrid
- kVp range: 65–80

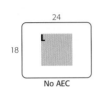

No AEC

Shielding Shield radiosensitive tissues outside region of interest.

Patient Position Patient is seated erect in a chair at end of table or in the prone position on table.

Part Position (insert part position icon here)
- Extend and rest chin on IR. Place angled support under IR, as demonstrated, to **place IR perpendicular to GAL** (Fig. 11.140).
- Align **MSP** perpendicular to CR and to IR midline.

CR
- Center CR to nasion and angle as needed to ensure that it is **parallel to GAL.** (CR must just skim glabella and anterior upper front teeth.)

Recommended Collimation Collimate on all sides to nasal bones.

Respiration Suspend respiration.

Evaluation Criteria
Anatomy Demonstrated: • Tangential projection of midnasal and distal nasal bones (with minimal superimposition of the glabella or alveolar ridge) and nasal soft tissue (Figs. 11.141 and 11.142). Petrous ridges are inferior to maxillary sinuses.
Position: • No patient **rotation** is evident, as indicated by equal distance from anterior nasal spine to outer soft tissue borders on each side. • Incorrect neck position is indicated by visualization of alveolar ridge (excessive extension) or visualization of too much glabella (excessive flexion).
Exposure: • Contrast and density (brightness) are sufficient to visualize nasal bones and nasal soft tissue. • Sharp bony margins indicate **no motion.**

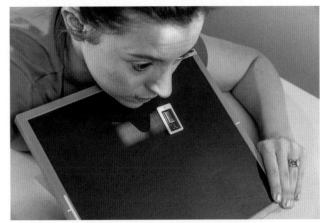

Fig. 11.140 Superoinferior tangential (axial) projection.

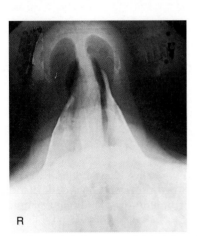

R

Fig. 11.141 Superoinferior tangential (axial) projection.

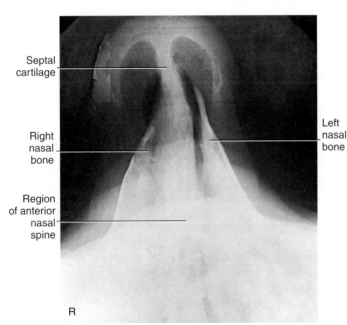

Septal cartilage

Right nasal bone

Region of anterior nasal spine

Left nasal bone

R

Fig. 11.142 Superoinferior tangential (axial) projection.

SUBMENTOVERTICAL (SMV) PROJECTION—ZYGOMATIC ARCHES

11

Clinical Indications
- Fractures of zygomatic arch
- Neoplastic or inflammatory processes

Technical Factors
- Minimum SID—40 inches (100 cm)
- IR size—8 × 10inches (18 × 24 cm), landscape
- Grid or nongrid
- kVp range: 75–85

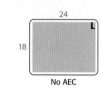

Zygomatic Arches
ROUTINE
• SMV
• Oblique inferosuperior (tangential)
• AP axial (modified Towne method)

24 / 18 / L / No AEC

Shielding Shield radiosensitive tissues outside region of interest.

Patient Position
Remove all metallic or plastic objects from head and neck. This projection may be taken with the patient erect or supine.

Part Position
- Raise chin, hyperextend neck until **IOML is parallel** to IR (see NOTE 1).
- Rest head on vertex of skull.
- Align **MSP perpendicular** to midline of the grid or the table/upright imaging device surface, **avoiding all tilt or rotation.**

CR
- Align CR **perpendicular** to IR (see NOTE 2).
- Center CR **midway between zygomatic arches**, at a **level 1½ inches (4 cm) inferior to mandibular symphysis.**
- Center IR to CR, with plane of IR parallel to IOML.

Recommended Collimation Collimate to outer margins of zygomatic arches.

Respiration Suspend respiration.

NOTE 1: This position is very uncomfortable for patients; complete the projection as quickly as possible.

NOTE 2: If patient is unable to extend neck adequately, angle CR **perpendicular to IOML.** If equipment allows, IR should be angled to maintain CR/IR perpendicular relationship (Fig. 11.143, inset).

Evaluation Criteria
Anatomy Demonstrated: • Zygomatic arches are demonstrated laterally from each mandibular ramus (Figs. 11.144 and 11.145).
Position: • Correct IOML/CR relationship, as indicated by superimposition of mandibular symphysis on frontal bone. • No patient **rotation**, as indicated by zygomatic arches visualized symmetrically. • Collimation to area of interest.
Exposure: • Sufficient contrast and density (brightness) to visualize zygomatic arches. • Sharp bony margins indicate **no motion.**

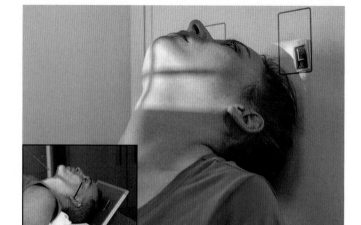

Fig. 11.143 SMV projection, erect and supine (*inset*)—IOML parallel to IR; CR perpendicular to IOML.

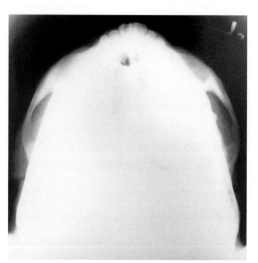

Fig. 11.144 SMV projection.

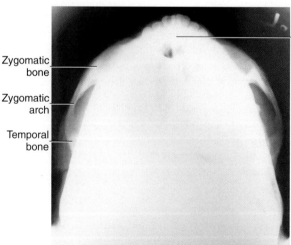

Zygomatic bone

Zygomatic arch

Temporal bone

Mandibular symphysis over frontal bone

Fig. 11.145 SMV projection.

OBLIQUE INFEROSUPERIOR (TANGENTIAL) PROJECTION—ZYGOMATIC ARCHES

Clinical Indications
- Fractures of zygomatic arch
- Especially useful for depressed zygomatic arches caused by trauma or skull morphology

  Radiographs of both sides generally are taken for comparison.

Zygomatic Arches
ROUTINE
• SMV
• Oblique inferosuperior (tangential)
• AP axial (modified Towne method)

Technical Factors
- Minimum SID—40 inches (100 cm)
- IR size—8 × 10 inches (18 × 24 cm), portrait
- Grid or nongrid
- kVp range: 70–85
- AEC not recommended

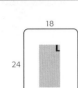
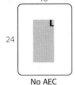

18

24

L

No AEC

Shielding Shield radiosensitive tissues outside region of interest.

Patient Position Remove all metallic or plastic objects from head and neck. Patient position is erect or supine. Erect, which is easier for the patient, may be done with erect table or upright imaging device.

Part Position
- Raise chin, hyperextending neck until **IOML is parallel** to IR (see NOTE 1).
- Rest head on vertex of skull.
- Rotate head 15° toward side to be examined; also tilt chin 15° toward side of interest (Fig. 11.146).

CR
- Align CR perpendicular to IR and IOML (see NOTE 2).
- Center CR to zygomatic arch of interest (CR skims mandibular ramus, passes through arch, and skims parietal eminence on the downside).
- Adjust IR so it is parallel to IOML and perpendicular to CR.

Recommended Collimation Collimate closely to zygomatic bone and arch.

Respiration Suspend respiration.

NOTE 1: This position is very uncomfortable for the patient; complete the projection as quickly as possible.

NOTE 2: If patient is unable to extend neck sufficiently, angle CR **perpendicular to IOML**. If equipment allows, IR should be angled to maintain CR/IR perpendicular relationship.

Evaluation Criteria
Anatomy Demonstrated: • Single zygomatic arch, free of superimposition, is demonstrated (Figs. 11.147 and 11.148).
Position: • Correct patient position provides for demonstration of zygomatic arch without superimposition of parietal bone or mandible. • Collimation to area of interest.
Exposure: • Contrast and density (brightness) are sufficient to visualize zygomatic arch. • Sharp bony margins indicate **no motion.**

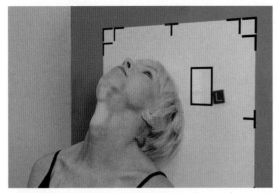

Fig. 11.146 Oblique inferosuperior (tangential), upright imaging device (15° tilt, 15° rotation, CR perpendicular to IOML).

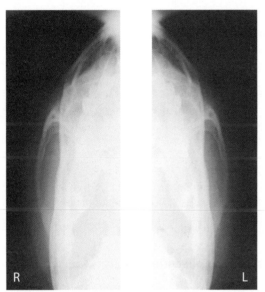

R   L

Fig. 11.147 Oblique inferosuperior (tangential).

Right and left zygomatic arches

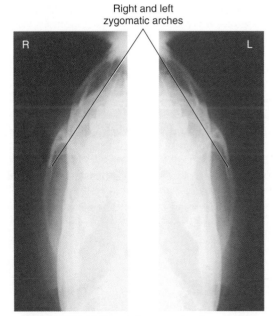

R   L

Fig. 11.148 Oblique inferosuperior (tangential).

11

AP AXIAL PROJECTION—ZYGOMATIC ARCHES

MODIFIED TOWNE METHOD

Clinical Indications
- Fractures and neoplastic or inflammatory processes of zygomatic arch

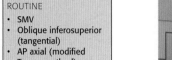

Zygomatic Arches
ROUTINE
- SMV
- Oblique inferosuperior (tangential)
- AP axial (modified Towne method)

Technical Factors
- Minimum SID—40 inches (100 cm)
- IR size—8 × 10 inches (18 × 24 cm), landscape
- Grid
- kVp range: 70–85
- AEC not recommended

Shielding
Shield radiosensitive tissues outside region of interest

Patient Position
Remove all metallic or plastic objects from head and neck. Patient position is erect or supine.

Part Position
- Rest patient's posterior skull against table/upright imaging device surface.
- Tuck chin, bringing **OML (or IOML) perpendicular** to IR (see NOTE).
- Align **MSP perpendicular** to midline of grid or table/upright imaging device surface to **prevent head rotation or tilt** (Fig. 11.149).

CR
- Angle CR 30° caudad to OML or 37° to IOML (see NOTE).
- Center CR to 1 inch (2.5 cm) superior to nasion (to pass through midarches) at level of the gonion.
- Center IR to projected CR.

Recommended Collimation
Collimate to outer margins of zygomatic arches.

Respiration
Suspend respiration.

NOTE: If patient is unable to depress the chin sufficiently to bring OML perpendicular to IR, **IOML** can be placed perpendicular instead and CR angle increased to 37° caudad. This positioning maintains the 30° angle between OML and CR and demonstrates the same anatomic relationships. (A 7° to 8° difference is noted between OML and IOML.)

Evaluation Criteria
Anatomy Demonstrated: • Bilateral zygomatic arches, free of superimposition, are demonstrated (Figs. 11.150 and 11.151).
Position: • Zygomatic arches are visualized **without** patient **rotation** as indicated by symmetric appearance of arches bilaterally. • Collimation to area of interest.
Exposure: • Contrast and density (brightness) are sufficient to visualize zygomatic arches. • Sharp bony margins indicate **no motion.**

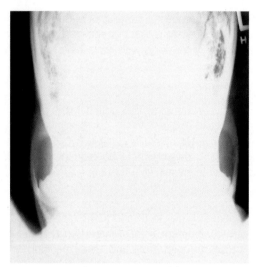

Fig. 11.149 AP axial—zygomatic arches—**CR 30° to OML** (37° to IOML), erect and supine (*inset*).

Fig. 11.150 AP axial.

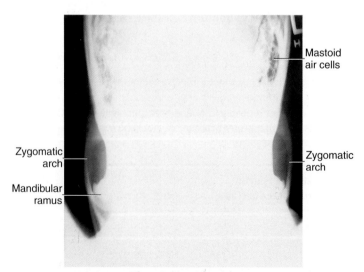

Mastoid air cells

Zygomatic arch

Zygomatic arch

Mandibular ramus

Fig. 11.151 AP axial.

PARIETO-ORBITAL OBLIQUE PROJECTION—OPTIC FORAMINA

RHESE METHOD

Clinical Indications

- Bony abnormalities of the optic foramen
- Demonstrate lateral margins of orbits and foreign bodies within eye

CT is the preferred modality for a detailed investigation of the optic foramina. Radiographs of both sides generally are taken for comparison. This projection can also provide an excellent image of the mid-lateral and inferior orbital margins.

Optic Foramina
ROUTINE
• Parieto-orbital oblique (Rhese method)
• Parietoacanthial (Waters method)
SPECIAL
• Modified parietoacanthial (modified Waters method)

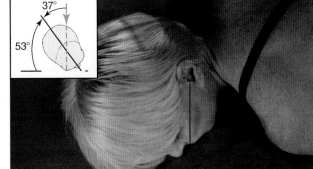

Fig. 11.152 Parieto-orbital oblique projection—53° rotation; AML perpendicular; CR perpendicular.

Technical Factors

- Minimum SID—40 inches (100 cm)
- IR size—8 × 10 inches (18 × 24 cm), landscape
- Grid
- kVp range: 70–85
- AEC not recommended

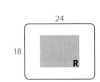

No AEC

Shielding Shield radiosensitive tissues outside region of interest.

Patient Position Remove all metallic or plastic objects from head and neck. Position patient erect or supine.

Part Position

- As a starting reference, position patient's head in a prone position with MSP perpendicular to IR. Adjust flexion and extension so that AML is perpendicular to IR. Adjust the patient's head so that the chin, cheek, and nose touch the table/upright imaging device surface (this position is historically known as the "3 point landing").
- Rotate the head 37° toward the affected side. The angle formed between MSP and plane of IR measures 53° (Fig. 11.152). (An angle indicator should be used to obtain an accurate angle of 37° from CR to MSP.)

CR

- Align CR **perpendicular** to IR at the midportion of the **downside orbit.**

Recommended Collimation Collimate on all sides to yield a field size of approximately 3 inches (7.5 cm) square.

Respiration Suspend respiration during exposure.

Evaluation Criteria

Anatomy Demonstrated: • Bilateral, nondistorted view of the optic foramen. • Lateral orbital margins are demonstrated (Figs. 11.153 and 11.154).
Position: • Accurate positioning projects the optic foramen into the lower outer quadrant of the orbit. • Proper positioning results when AML is correctly placed perpendicular to IR and correct rotation of skull. • Collimation to area of interest.
Exposure: • Contrast and density (brightness) are sufficient to visualize the optic foramen. • Sharp bony margins indicate **no motion.**

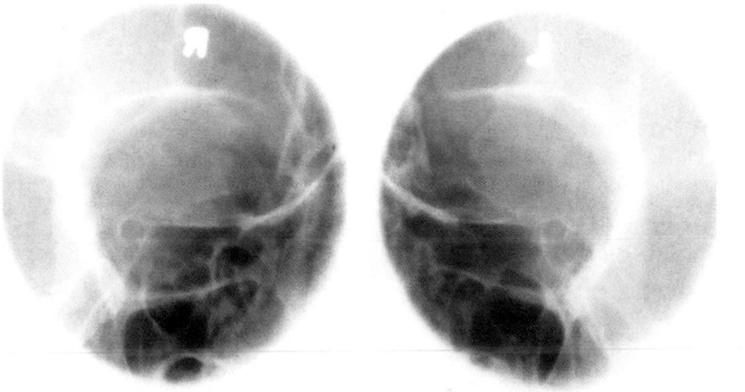

Fig. 11.153 Bilateral parieto-orbital oblique projection.

Frontal sinus

Lateral orbital margin

Optical foramen and canal   Inferior orbital rim

Maxillary sinus   Optic foramen and canal

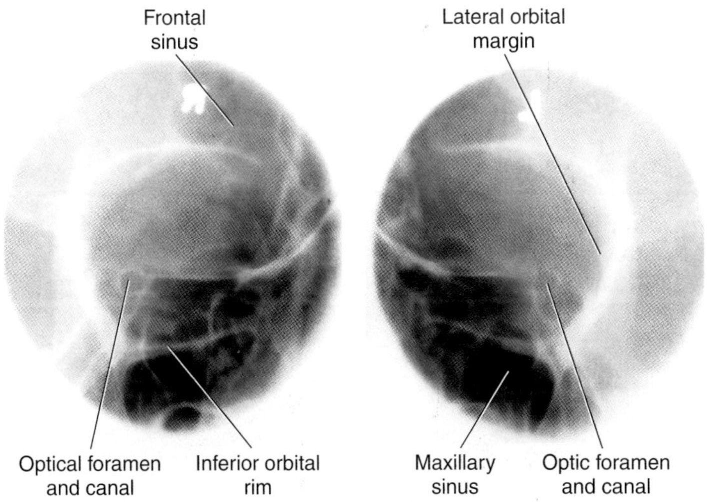

Fig. 11.154 Bilateral parieto-orbital oblique projection.

AXIOLATERAL OR AXIOLATERAL OBLIQUE PROJECTION—MANDIBLE

Clinical Indications
- Fractures and neoplastic or inflammatory processes of mandible
  Both sides of mandible are examined for comparison.

Mandible
ROUTINE
• Axiolateral or axiolateral oblique
• PA (or PA axial)
• AP axial (Towne method)

Technical Factors
- Minimum SID—40 inches (100 cm)
- IR size—8 × 10 inches (18 × 24 cm) or 10 × 12 inches (24 × 30 cm) landscape
- Grid (often performed nongrid)
- kVp range: 70–85
- AEC not used

24
18
R
No AEC

Shielding Shield radiosensitive tissues outside region of interest.

Patient Position Remove all metallic or plastic objects from head and neck. Patient position is erect or recumbent. If performed recumbent, place IR on wedge sponge to minimize OID (Fig. 11.155). For erect position, place region of interest against wall bucky and parallel to IR (Fig. 11.156). For horizontal beam trauma position, place IR (and grid if used) parallel to mandible (Fig. 11.157).

Part Position
- Place head in a true lateral position, with side of interest against IR.
- If possible, have patient close mouth and bring teeth together.
- Extend neck slightly to prevent superimposition of the gonion over the cervical spine.
- Rotate head toward IR (for axiolateral oblique) to place the mandibular area of interest parallel to IR. The degree of rotation/obliquity depends on which section of the mandible is of interest.
- Head in **true lateral** position best demonstrates **ramus.**
- **10° to 15°** rotation best provides a **general survey** of the mandible.
- **30°** rotation toward IR best demonstrates **body.**
- **45°** rotation best demonstrates **mentum.**

CR
- Three methods are suggested for demonstrating the specific region of the mandible of interest (side closest to IR) without superimposing the opposite side:
  1. Angle CR 25° cephalad from IPL; for horizontal beam trauma position.
  2. Use a combination of head tilt and CR angle that does not exceed 25° cephalad (e.g., angle the tube 10° cephalad and add 15° of head tilt toward the IR).
  3. Use 25° of head tilt toward IR and use perpendicular CR.
- Direct CR to exit mandibular region of interest.
- Center IR to projected CR.

Recommended Collimation Collimate on four sides to anatomy of interest.

Respiration Suspend respiration.

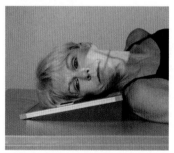

Fig. 11.155 Semisupine—15° wedge sponge and 10° cephalad CR angle.

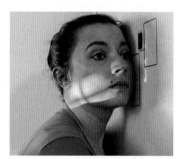

Fig. 11.156 Erect 10°–15° head rotation toward IR and 10° cephalad CR angle.

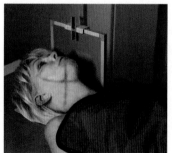

Fig. 11.157 Horizontal beam trauma projection—**25° cephalad** CR angle; left lateral.

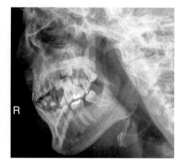

Fig. 11.158 Axiolateral oblique (general survey).

Evaluation Criteria
Anatomy Demonstrated: • Ramus, condyloid, and coronoid processes, body, and mentum of mandible nearest the IR are demonstrated (Figs. 11.158 and 11.159).
Position: • The appearance of the image/position of the patient depends on the structures under examination. • For the ramus and body, the ramus of interest is demonstrated with **no superimposition** from the opposite mandible (indicating correct CR angulation). • **No superimposition** of the cervical spine by the ramus should occur (indicating sufficient extension of neck). • The ramus and body should be demonstrated without foreshortening (indicating correct rotation of head). • The area of interest is demonstrated with minimal superimposition and minimal foreshortening. • **Collimation** to area of interest.
Exposure: • Contrast and density (brightness) are sufficient to visualize the mandibular area of interest. • Sharp bony margins indicate **no motion.**

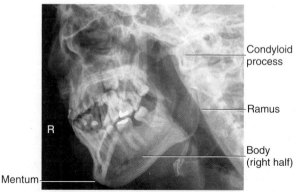

Condyloid process

Ramus

Body (right half)

Mentum

Fig. 11.159 Axiolateral oblique (general survey).

PA OR PA AXIAL PROJECTION—MANDIBLE

Clinical Indications
- Fractures
- Neoplastic or inflammatory processes of mandible

Optional PA axial best demonstrates proximal rami and elongated view of condyloid processes.

Mandible
ROUTINE
• Axiolateral oblique
• PA (or PA axial)
• AP axial (Towne method)

Technical Factors
- Minimum SID—40 inches (100 cm)
- IR size—8 × 10 inches (18 × 24 cm) or 10 × 12 inches (24 × 30 cm) portrait
- Grid
- kVp range: 75–90

18
24
L
No AEC

Shielding Shield radiosensitive tissues outside region of interest.

Patient Position Remove all metallic or plastic objects from head and neck. Patient position is erect or prone.

Part Position
- Rest patient's forehead and nose against table/upright imaging device surface (Fig. 11.160).
- Tuck chin, bringing **OML perpendicular** to IR (see NOTE).
- Align **MSP perpendicular** to midline of grid or table/imaging device surface (ensuring **no rotation or tilt** of head).
- Center IR to projected CR (to junction of lips).

CR
- PA: Align CR perpendicular to IR, centered to exit at junction of lips. For trauma patients, this position is best performed supine.
- Optional PA axial: Angle CR 20° to 25° cephalad, centered to exit at acanthion.

Recommended Collimation Collimate on four sides to anatomy of interest.

Respiration Suspend respiration.

NOTE: For a true PA projection of the body (if this is area of interest), raise chin to bring AML perpendicular to IR.

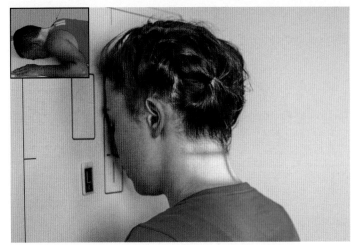

Fig. 11.160 PA—CR perpendicular, exit at junction of lips. *Inset,* Optional PA axial—CR 20° to 25° cephalad, exit at acanthion.

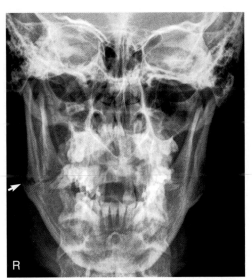

Fig. 11.161 PA; fracture through left ramus.

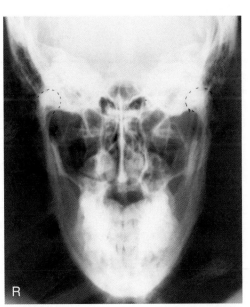

Fig. 11.162 Optional PA axial—CR 20° to 25° cephalad.

Evaluation Criteria
Anatomy Demonstrated: • **PA:** Mandibular rami and lateral portion of body are visible (Fig. 11.161). • **Optional PA axial:** TMJ region and heads of condyles are visible through mastoid processes; condyloid processes are well visualized (slightly elongated) (Fig. 11.162).
Position: • No patient **rotation** exists, as indicated by mandibular rami visualized symmetrically, lateral to the cervical spine. • Midbody and mentum are faintly visualized, superimposed on cervical spine. • Collimation to area of interest.
Exposure: • Contrast and density (brightness) are sufficient to visualize mandibular body and rami. • Sharp bony margins indicate **no motion.**

11

AP AXIAL PROJECTION—MANDIBLE

TOWNE METHOD

Clinical Indications

- Fractures
- Neoplastic or inflammatory processes of condyloid processes of mandible

Mandible
SPECIAL
• SMV
• Orthopantomography (mandible or TMJs or both)

Technical Factors

- Minimum SID—40 inches (100 cm)
- IR size—8 × 10 inches (18 × 24 cm) or 10 × 12 inches (24 × 30 cm), portrait
- Grid
- kVp range: 75–90

Shielding Shield radiosensitive tissues outside region of interest.

Patient Position Remove all metallic or plastic objects from head and neck. Patient position is erect or supine.

Part Position

- Rest patient's posterior skull against table/upright imaging device surface.
- Tuck chin, aligning **OML perpendicular** to IR or place IOML perpendicular and adjust the CR angle accordingly (see NOTE).
- Align **MSP perpendicular** to midline of grid or table/upright imaging device surface to prevent head rotation or tilt.

CR

- Angle CR 35° caudad if OML is perpendicular to IR, or 42° caudad if IOML is perpendicular to IR (see NOTE).
- Center CR 1 inch (2.5 cm) superior to glabella.
- Center IR to CR.

Recommended Collimation Collimate on four sides to anatomy of interest.

Respiration Suspend respiration.

NOTE: If patient is unable to bring OML perpendicular to IR, align IOML perpendicular and increase the 35° CR angle by 7° to 42° caudad (Fig. 11.163). If area of interest is the TM fossae, increase CR angle to 40° to OML to reduce superimposition of TM fossae and mastoid portions of the temporal bone.

Evaluation Criteria

Anatomy Demonstrated: • Condyloid processes of mandible and TM fossae.

Position: • A correctly positioned image with **no rotation** demonstrates the following: condyloid processes visualized symmetrically, lateral to the cervical spine; clear visualization of condyle/TM fossae relationship, with minimal superimposition of the TM fossae and mastoid portions (Figs. 11.164 and 11.165). • Collimation to area of interest.

Exposure: • Contrast and density (brightness) are sufficient to visualize condyloid process and TM fossa. • **No motion** exists, as indicated by sharp bony margins.

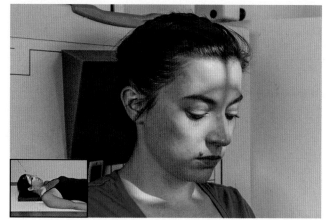

Fig. 11.163 AP axial—CR 35° to 40° to OML, erect and supine (*inset*).

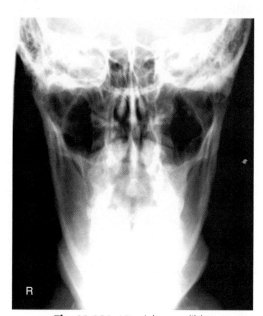

Fig. 11.164 AP axial—mandible.

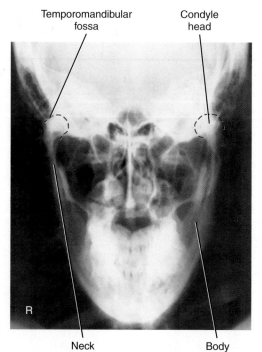

Temporomandibular fossa · Condyle head · Neck · Body

Fig. 11.165 AP axial—mandible.

SUBMENTOVERTICAL (SMV) PROJECTION—MANDIBLE

Clinical Indications
- Fractures and neoplastic or inflammatory process of mandible

Mandible
SPECIAL
• SMV
• Orthopantomography (mandible or TMJs or both)

Technical Factors
- Minimum SID—40 inches (100 cm)
- IR size—8 × 10 inches (18 × 24 cm) or 10 × 12 inches (24 × 30 cm), portrait
- Grid
- kVp range: 80–95

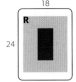

Shielding Shield radiosensitive tissues outside region of interest.

Patient Position Remove all metallic or plastic objects from head and neck. Patient position is erect or supine (erect preferred, if patient's condition allows). Erect may be done with an upright imaging device (Fig. 11.166).

Part Position
- Hyperextend neck until **IOML is parallel** to IR.
- Rest head on vertex of skull.
- Align **MSP perpendicular** to midline of grid or table/upright imaging device surface to prevent head rotation or tilt.

CR
- Align CR perpendicular to IR or IOML (see NOTE).
- Center CR to a point midway between angles of mandible or at a level 1 ½ inches (4 cm) inferior to mandibular symphysis.
- Center IR to projected CR.

Recommended Collimation Collimate on four sides to anatomy of interest.

Respiration Suspend respiration.

NOTE: If patient is unable to extend the neck sufficiently, angle tube to align CR **perpendicular to IOML**. This position is very uncomfortable for the patient; complete the projection as quickly as possible.

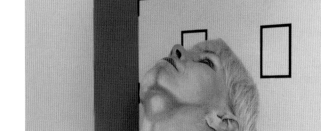

Fig. 11.166 SMV—mandible.

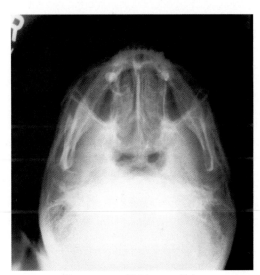

Fig. 11.167 SMV—mandible.

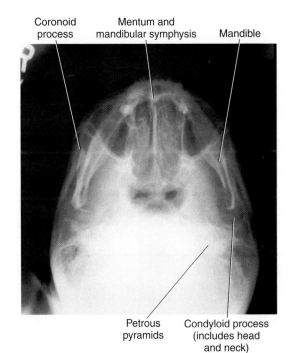

Coronoid process   Mentum and mandibular symphysis   Mandible

Petrous pyramids   Condyloid process (includes head and neck)

Fig. 11.168 SMV—mandible.

Evaluation Criteria
Anatomy Demonstrated: • Entire mandible and coronoid and condyloid processes are demonstrated (Figs. 11.167 and 11.168).

Position: • Correct neck extension is indicated by the following: mandibular symphysis superimposing frontal bone; mandibular condyles projected anterior to petrous ridges. • No patient **rotation or tilt** is indicated by the following: no tilt as evidenced by equal distance from mandible to lateral border of skull; no rotation as evidenced by symmetric mandibular condyles. • **Collimation** to area of interest.

Exposure: • Contrast and density (brightness) are sufficient to visualize the mandible superimposed on the skull. • Sharp bony margins indicate **no motion.**

ORTHOPANTOMOGRAPHY: PANORAMIC TOMOGRAPHY—MANDIBLE

11

Clinical Indications
- Fractures or infectious processes of mandible
- Pre-surgical assessment before bone marrow transplants

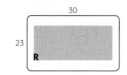

Mandible
ROUTINE
• Axiolateral oblique
• PA (or PA axial)
• AP axial (Towne method)

Technical Factors (Conventional Radiographic Systems)
- IR size—9 × 12 inches (23 × 30 cm), landscape
- Curved nongrid cassette or digital detector
- kVp range: 70–85

Unit Preparation
- Attach IR to panoramic unit.
- Position tube and IR at starting position.
- Raise chin rest to approximately same level as patient's chin.

Shielding Wrap vest-type lead apron around patient.

Patient Position
- Remove all metal, plastic, and other removable objects from head and neck.
- Explain to patient how tube and IR rotate and the time span needed for exposure.
- Guide patient into unit, resting patient's chin on bite-block (Fig. 11.169).
- Position patient's body, head, and neck as demonstrated in Figs. 11.170 and 11.171. Do not allow head and neck to stretch forward (Fig. 11.172); have patient stand with spine straight and hips forward.

Part Position
- Adjust height of chin rest until **IOML is aligned parallel with floor.** The occlusal plane (plane of biting surface of teeth) declines 10° from posterior to anterior.
- Align **MSP** with vertical center line of chin rest.
- Position bite-block between patient's front teeth (see NOTE).
- Instruct patient to place lips together and position tongue on roof of mouth.

CR
- CR is fixed and directed slightly cephalic to project anatomic structures, positioned at the same height, on top of one another.
- Fixed SID, per panoramic unit.

Recommended Collimation A narrow, vertical-slit diaphragm is attached to tube, providing collimation.

NOTE: When TMJs are of interest, a second panoramic image is taken with the mouth open. This requires placement of a larger bite-block between the patient's teeth.

Digital Orthopantomography The first digital **orthopantomography** system was developed in 1995. Since 1997, digital orthopantomography systems have been replacing the analog systems. These systems do not require a cassette or chemical processing of images. They use a digital detector or a photostimulable phosphor to convert the analog signal into a digitized image. A key advantage of digital orthopantomography over film-based systems is increased exposure latitude and fewer repeat studies. This leads to reduced costs and patient exposure (see Figs. 11.169 and 11.171).

Advantages of Orthopantomography Compared with Conventional Mandible Positioning
- More comprehensive image of the mandible, TMJs, surrounding facial bones, and teeth
- Low patient radiation dose (slit collimation reduces exposure to eyes and thyroid gland)
- Convenience of examination for patient (one position provides the panoramic view of entire mandible)
- Ability to image the teeth in a patient who cannot open the mouth or when the oral cavity is restricted
- Shorter examination time

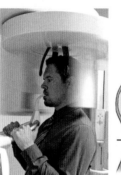
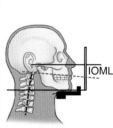
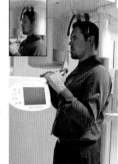

Fig. 11.169 Digital orthopantomography head correctly positioned.

Fig. 11.170 Correct position.

Fig. 11.171 Digital orthopantomography—correct body position.

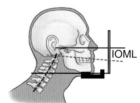
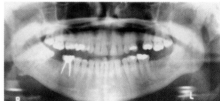

Fig. 11.172 Incorrect position.

Fig. 11.173 Orthopantomogram.

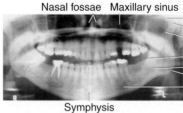

Nasal fossae   Maxillary sinus

Zygomatic arch
Condyle
Mandibular notch
Occlusal plane
Ramus
Angle (gonion)
Body

Symphysis

Fig. 11.174 Orthopantomogram.

AP AXIAL PROJECTION—TEMPOROMANDIBULAR JOINTS

MODIFIED TOWNE METHOD

WARNING: Opening the mouth should not be attempted with possible fracture.

Clinical Indications
- Fractures and abnormal relationship or range of motion between condyle and TM fossa.

See NOTE 1 on open-mouth and closed-mouth comparisons.

> **Temporomandibular Joints**
> ROUTINE
> - AP axial (modified Towne method)
>
> SPECIAL
> - Axiolateral oblique (modified Law method)
> - Axiolateral (Schuller method)
> - Orthopantomography

Technical Factors
- Minimum SID—40 inches (100 cm)
- IR size—8 × 10 inches (18 × 24 cm), landscape
- Grid
- kVp range: 75–85

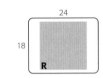

Shielding Shield radiosensitive tissues outside region of interest.

Patient Position
Remove all metallic or plastic objects from head and neck. Position patient erect or supine.

Part Position
- Rest patient's posterior skull against table/upright imaging device surface.
- Tuck chin, bringing **OML perpendicular** to table/imaging device surface or bringing IOML perpendicular and increasing CR angle by 7° (Fig. 11.175).
- Align **MSP perpendicular** to midline of the grid or the table/upright imaging device surface to prevent head rotation or tilt.

CR
- Angle CR 35° caudad from OML or 42° from IOML (see NOTE 2).
- Direct CR 3 inches (7.5 cm) superior to the nasion. Center IR to projected CR.

Recommended Collimation
Collimate on four sides to anatomy of interest.

Respiration
Suspend respiration.

NOTE 1: Some departmental protocols indicate that these projections should be taken in both closed-mouth and open-mouth positions for comparison purposes when patient's condition allows.

NOTE 2: An additional 5° increase in CR may best demonstrate the TM fossae and TMJs.

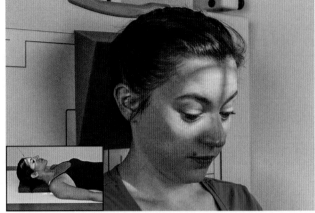

Fig. 11.175 AP axial—CR 35° to OML (closed-mouth position) or 42° to the IOML *(inset).*

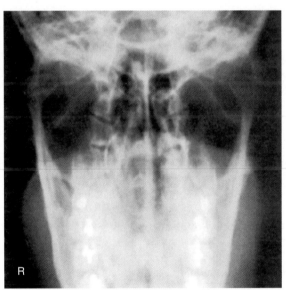

Fig. 11.176 AP axial (closed-mouth position).

Evaluation Criteria
Anatomy Demonstrated: • Condyloid processes of mandible and TM fossae are demonstrated (Fig. 11.176).
Position: • Correctly positioned patient, with **no rotation**, is indicated by the following: condyloid processes visualized symmetrically, lateral to the cervical spine; clear visualization of condyle and TM fossae relationship. • Collimation to area of interest.
Exposure: • Contrast and density (brightness) are sufficient to visualize condyloid process and TM fossa. • Sharp bony margins indicate **no motion.**

AXIOLATERAL OBLIQUE PROJECTION—TEMPOROMANDIBULAR JOINT

MODIFIED LAW METHOD

Clinical Indications
- Abnormal relationship or range of motion between condyle and TM fossa

Technical Factors
- Minimum SID—40 inches (100 cm)
- IR size—8 × 10 inches (18 × 24 cm), portrait
- Grid
- kVp range: 75–85
- AEC not recommended

Temporomandibular Joints
ROUTINE
- AP axial (modified Towne method)

SPECIAL
- Axiolateral 15° oblique (modified Law method)
- Axiolateral (Schuller)
- Orthopantomography

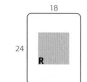

Shielding Shield radiosensitive tissues outside region of interest.

Patient Position Patient position is erect or semiprone (erect is preferred if patient's condition allows). Rest lateral aspect of head against table/upright imaging device surface, with side of interest closest to IR.

Part Position
- Prevent tilt by maintaining **IPL perpendicular** to IR. MSP is parallel to IR to start.
- Align **IOML perpendicular** to front edge of IR (Fig. 11.177).
- From lateral position, **rotate face toward IR 15°** (with MSP of head rotated 15° from plane of IR).
- Closed- and open-mouth projections are often taken to demonstrate range of motion of the TMJ (Fig. 11.178).

CR
- Angle CR **15° caudad,** centered to 1 ½ **inches (4 cm) superior to upside EAM** (to pass through downside TMJ).
- Center IR to projected CR.

Recommended Collimation Collimate on four sides to anatomy of interest.

Respiration Suspend respiration.

Evaluation Criteria
Anatomy Demonstrated: • TMJ nearest IR is visible. • Closed-mouth image demonstrates condyle within mandibular fossa; the condyle moves to the anterior margin (articular tubercle) of the mandibular fossa in the open-mouth position (Figs. 11.179 and 11.180).
Position: • Correctly positioned images demonstrate TMJ closest to IR clearly, **without superimposition** of opposite TMJ (15° rotation prevents superimposition). • TMJ of interest is **not superimposed** by cervical spine. • **Collimation** to area of interest.
Exposure: • Contrast and density (brightness) are sufficient to visualize TMJ. • Sharp bony margins indicate **no motion.**

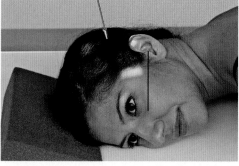

Fig. 11.177 Right TMJ—closed mouth; 15° oblique; CR 15° caudad.

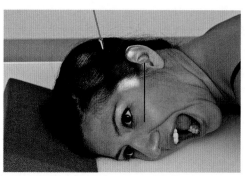

Fig. 11.178 Right TMJ—open mouth; 15° oblique; CR 15° caudad.

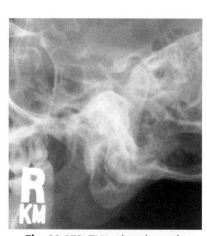

Fig. 11.179 TMJ—closed mouth.

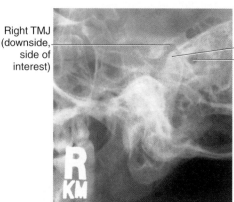

Right TMJ (downside, side of interest)

Right condyle
Right EAM

Fig. 11.180 TMJ—closed mouth.

AXIOLATERAL PROJECTION—TEMPOROMANDIBULAR JOINT

SCHULLER METHOD

Clinical Indications
- Abnormal relationship or range of motion between condyle and TM fossa

Technical Factors
- Minimum SID—40 inches (100 cm)
- IR size—8 × 10 inches (18 × 24 cm), portrait
- Grid
- kVp range: 75–85
- AEC not recommended

Shielding Shield radiosensitive tissues outside region of interest.

Patient Position Position patient erect or semiprone. Place the head in a true lateral position, with side of interest nearest IR.

Part Position
- Adjust head into **true lateral position** and move patient's body in an oblique direction, as needed for patient's comfort.
- Align IPL perpendicular to IR.
- Align **MSP parallel** with table/imaging device surface.
- Position **IOML perpendicular** to front edge of IR (Fig. 11.181). Closed- and open-mouth projections are often taken to demonstrate range of motion of the TMJ (Fig. 11.182).

CR
- Angle CR **25° to 30° caudad,** centered to ½ inch (1.3 cm) anterior and 2 inches (5 cm) superior to upside EAM.
- Center IR to projected TMJ.

Recommended Collimation Collimate on four sides to anatomy of interest.

Respiration Suspend respiration.

Temporomandibular Joints
ROUTINE
- AP axial (modified Towne method)

SPECIAL
- Axiolateral 15° oblique (modified Law method)
- Axiolateral (Schuller method)
- Orthopantomography

Evaluation Criteria
Anatomy Demonstrated: • TMJ nearest IR is visible. • Closed-mouth image (Figs. 11.183 and 11.184) demonstrates the condyle within the mandibular fossa; the condyle moves to the anterior margin (articular tubercle) of fossa in the open-mouth position (Fig. 11.185).
Position: • TMJs are demonstrated **without rotation,** as evidenced by superimposed lateral margins. • **Collimation** to area of interest.
Exposure: • Contrast and density (brightness) are sufficient to visualize TMJ. • Sharp bony margins indicate **no motion.**

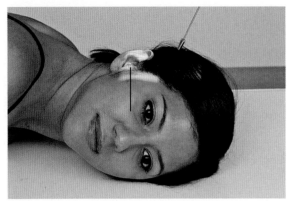

Fig. 11.181 Left TMJ—closed mouth; true lateral, CR 25° to 30° caudad angle.

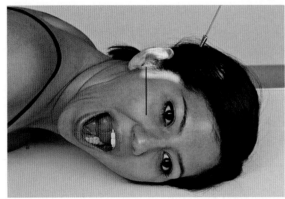

Fig. 11.182 Left TMJ—open mouth; true lateral, CR 25° to 30° caudad angle.

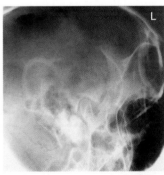

Fig. 11.183 Closed mouth.

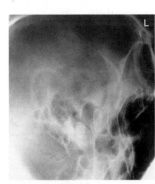

Fig. 11.185 Open mouth.

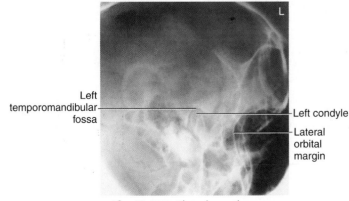

Left temporomandibular fossa

Left condyle

Lateral orbital margin

Fig. 11.184 Closed mouth.

LATERAL POSITION: RIGHT OR LEFT LATERAL—SINUSES

Clinical Indications
- Inflammatory conditions (sinusitis, secondary osteomyelitis)
- Sinus polyps or cysts

Sinuses
ROUTINE
• Lateral
• PA (Caldwell method)
• Parietoacanthial (Waters method)

Technical Factors
- Minimum SID—40 inches (100 cm)
- IR size—8× 10 inches (18 × 24 cm), portrait
- Grid
- kVp range: 75–85
- AEC not recommended

Shielding Shield radiosensitive tissues outside region of interest.

Patient Position Remove all metal, plastic, and other removable objects from head. Position patient **erect** (see NOTE).

Part Position
- Place lateral aspect of head against table/upright imaging device surface, with side of interest closest to IR (Fig. 11.186).
- Adjust head into **true lateral** position, moving body in an oblique direction as needed for patient's comfort (MSP parallel to IR).
- Align **IPL perpendicular to IR** (ensures no tilt).
- Adjust chin to align IOML perpendicular to front edge of IR.

CR
- Align **horizontal CR** perpendicular to IR.
- Center CR to a point midway between outer canthus and EAM.
- Center IR to CR.

Recommended Collimation Collimate on four sides to anatomy of interest.

Respiration Suspend respiration.

NOTE: To visualize air-fluid levels, an erect position with a horizontal beam is required. Fluid within the paranasal sinus cavities is thick and gelatinous, causing it to cling to the cavity walls. To visualize this fluid, allow a short time (at least 5 minutes) for the fluid to settle after patient's position has been changed (i.e., from recumbent to erect). If patient is unable to be placed in the upright position, the image may be obtained with the use of a horizontal beam, similar to trauma lateral facial bones, as described in Chapter 15.

Evaluation Criteria
Anatomy Demonstrated: • All four paranasal sinus groups are demonstrated (Figs. 11.187 and 11.188).
Position: • Accurately positioned cranium without rotation or tilt. • **Rotation** is evident by **anterior and posterior separation** of symmetric bilateral vertical structures such as the mandibular rami and greater wings of the sphenoid. • **Tilt** is evident by **superior and inferior separation** of symmetric horizontal structures such as the orbital plates **and greater wings of sphenoid** • Collimation to area of interest.
Exposure: • Density (brightness) and contrast are sufficient to visualize the sphenoid sinuses through the cranium without overexposing the maxillary and frontal sinuses. • Sharp bony margins indicate **no motion.**

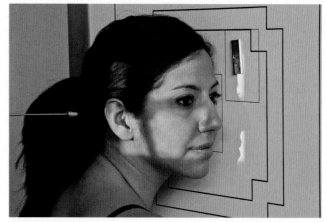

Fig. 11.186 Erect left lateral—sinuses (upright imaging device).

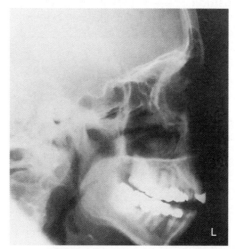

Fig. 11.187 Lateral sinuses.

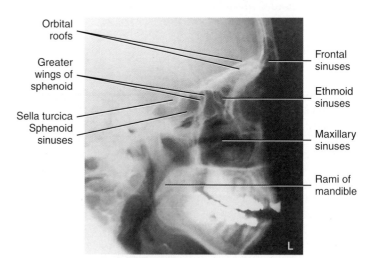

Fig. 11.188 Lateral sinuses.

Orbital roofs
Greater wings of sphenoid
Sella turcica
Sphenoid sinuses
Frontal sinuses
Ethmoid sinuses
Maxillary sinuses
Rami of mandible

PA PROJECTION—SINUSES

CALDWELL METHOD

Clinical Indications
- Inflammatory conditions (sinusitis, secondary osteomyelitis)
- Sinus polyps or cysts

Sinuses
ROUTINE
• Lateral
• PA (Caldwell method)
• Parietoacanthial (Waters method)

Technical Factors
- Minimum SID—40 inches (100 cm)
- IR size—8 × 10 inches (18 × 24 cm), portrait
- Grid
- kVp range: 75–85
- Upright imaging device angled 15° if possible, CR horizontal (see NOTE)
- AEC not recommended

Shielding Shield radiosensitive tissues outside region of interest.

Patient Position Remove all metallic or plastic objects from head and neck. Position patient erect (see NOTE).

Part Position
- Place patient's nose and forehead against upright imaging device or table with neck extended to elevate **OML 15° from horizontal.** A radiolucent support between forehead and upright imaging device or table may be used to maintain this position (Fig. 11.189). **CR remains horizontal.** (See alternative method if imaging device can be tilted 15°.)
- Align **MSP perpendicular to midline** of grid or upright imaging device surface.
- Center IR to CR and to nasion, ensuring **no rotation.**

CR
- Align **CR horizontal,** parallel with floor (see NOTE).
- Center CR to **exit at nasion.**

Recommended Collimation Collimate on four sides to anatomy of interest.

Respiration Suspend respiration.

NOTE: To assess air-fluid levels accurately, **CR must be horizontal,** and the **patient must be erect.**

Alternative Method An alternative method if the **imaging device can be tilted 15°** is shown (see Fig. 11.189, inset). The patient's forehead and nose can be supported directly against the imaging device with **OML perpendicular to imaging device surface** and **15° to horizontal CR.**

Evaluation Criteria
Anatomy Demonstrated: • Frontal sinuses projected above the frontonasal suture are demonstrated. • Anterior ethmoid air cells are visualized lateral to each nasal bone, directly below the frontal sinuses (Figs. 11.190 and 11.191).
Position: • Accurately positioned cranium with **no rotation or tilt** is indicated by the following: equal distance from the lateral margin of the orbit to the lateral cortex of the cranium on both sides; equal distance from the MSP (identified by the crista galli) to the lateral orbital margin on both sides; superior orbital fissures symmetrically visualized within the orbits. • Correct alignment of OML and CR projects petrous ridges into lower one-third of orbits (black arrows). • Collimation to area of interest.
Exposure: • Density (brightness) and contrast are sufficient to visualize the frontal and ethmoid sinuses. • Sharp bony margins indicate **no motion.**

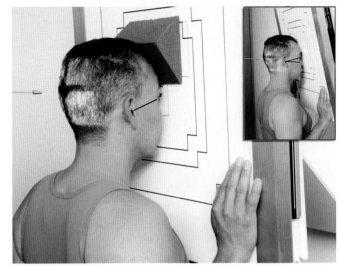

Fig. 11.189 CR horizontal, OML 15° to CR (if cannot be tilted). *Inset,* If upright, imaging device can be tilted 15°.

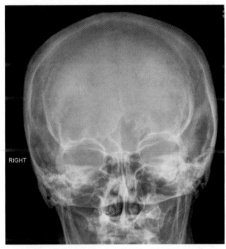

Fig. 11.190 PA projection—sinuses.

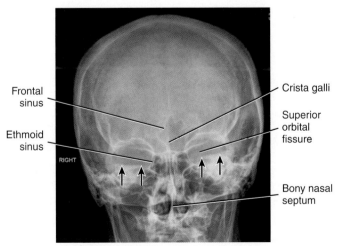

Frontal sinus — Crista galli — Superior orbital fissure — Ethmoid sinus — Bony nasal septum

Fig. 11.191 PA projection—sinuses.

PARIETOACANTHIAL PROJECTION—SINUSES

WATERS METHOD

Clinical Indications
- Inflammatory conditions (sinusitis, secondary osteomyelitis)
- Sinus polyps and cysts

Sinuses
ROUTINE
• Lateral
• PA (Caldwell method)
• Parietoacanthial (Waters method)

Technical Factors
- Minimum SID—40 inches (100 cm)
- IR size—8 × 10 inches (18 × 24 cm) or 10 × 12 inches (24 × 30 cm), portrait
- Grid
- kVp range: 75–85
- AEC not recommended

Shielding Shield radiosensitive tissues outside region of interest.

Patient Position Remove all metallic or plastic objects from head and neck. Position patient erect (see NOTE).

Part Position

- Extend neck, placing chin and nose against table/upright imaging device surface.
- Adjust head until **MML is perpendicular** to IR; OML forms a 37° angle with plane of IR (Fig. 11.192).
- Position **MSP perpendicular** to midline of grid.
- Ensure that **no rotation or tilt** exists.
- Center IR to CR and to acanthion.

CR
- Align horizontal CR perpendicular to IR centered to exit at acanthion.

Recommended Collimation Collimate on four sides to anatomy of interest.

Respiration Suspend respiration.

NOTE: CR must be horizontal, and patient must be erect to demonstrate air-fluid levels within the paranasal sinus cavities.

Evaluation Criteria
Anatomy Demonstrated: • Maxillary sinuses with the inferior aspect visualized free from superimposing alveolar processes and petrous ridges, the inferior orbital margin, and an oblique view of the frontal sinuses (Figs. 11.193 and 11.194).
Position: • No rotation of the cranium is indicated by the following: equal distance from MSP (identified by the bony nasal septum) to lateral orbital margin on both sides; equal distance from the lateral orbital margin to the lateral cortex of the cranium on both sides. • Adequate extension of neck demonstrates petrous ridges just inferior to the maxillary sinuses. • Collimation to area of interest.
Exposure: • Density (brightness) and contrast are sufficient to visualize maxillary sinuses. • Sharp bony margins indicate **no motion.**

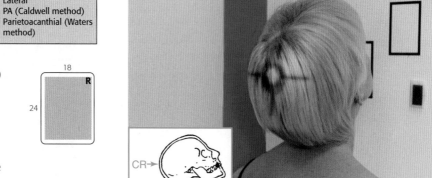

Fig. 11.192 Parietoacanthial projection (upright imaging device/table)—CR and MML perpendicular (OML 37° to IR).

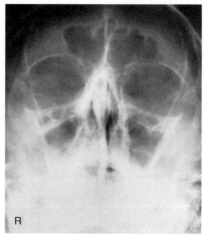

Fig. 11.193 Parietoacanthial projection—sinuses.

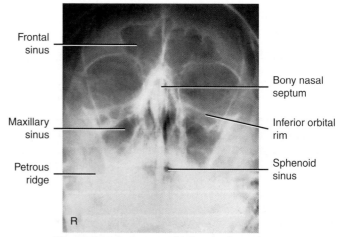

Frontal sinus

Maxillary sinus

Petrous ridge

Bony nasal septum

Inferior orbital rim

Sphenoid sinus

Fig. 11.194 Parietoacanthial projection—sinuses.

SUBMENTOVERTICAL (SMV) PROJECTION—SINUSES

Clinical Indications
- Inflammatory conditions (sinusitis, secondary osteomyelitis)
- Sinus polyps and cysts

Sinuses
SPECIAL
- Submentovertical (SMV)

Technical Factors
- Minimum SID—40 inches (100 cm)
- IR size—8 × 10 inches (18 × 24 cm) or 10 × 12 inches (24 × 30 cm), portrait
- Grid
- kVp range: 75–85
- AEC not recommended

Shielding Shield radiosensitive tissues outside region of interest.

Patient Position Remove all metallic or plastic objects from head and neck. Position patient erect, if possible, to show air-fluid levels.

Part Position
- Raise chin, hyperextend neck if possible until **IOML is parallel** to table/upright imaging device surface (see NOTE 1).
- Head rests on vertex of skull.
- Align **MSP perpendicular** to midline of the grid; ensure **no rotation or tilt.**

CR
- CR directed perpendicular to IOML (see NOTE 2).
- CR centered midway between angles of mandible, at a level 1½ to 2 inches (4 to 5 cm) inferior to mandibular symphysis (Fig. 11.195).
- CR centered to IR

Recommended Collimation Collimate on four sides to anatomy of interest.

Respiration Suspend respiration.

NOTE 1: This position is very uncomfortable for the patient; have all factors set before positioning the patient, and complete the projection as quickly as possible.

NOTE 2: If patient is unable to extend neck sufficiently, angle the tube from horizontal as needed to align CR perpendicular to IOML.

Evaluation Criteria
Anatomy Demonstrated: • Sphenoid sinuses, ethmoid sinuses, nasal fossae, and maxillary sinuses are demonstrated (Figs. 11.196 and 11.197).
Position: • Accurate IOML and CR relationship is demonstrated by the following: correct extension of neck and relationship between IOML and CR as indicated by **mandibular mentum anterior to** ethmoid sinuses. • **No rotation** evidenced by MSP parallel to edge of IR. • **No tilt** evidenced by equal distance between mandibular ramus and lateral cranial cortex. • Collimation to area of interest.
Exposure: • Density (brightness) and contrast are sufficient to visualize sphenoid and ethmoid sinuses. • Sharp bony margins indicate **no motion.**

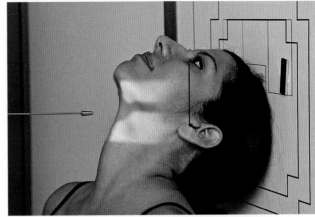

Fig. 11.195 SMV projection (upright imaging device/table).

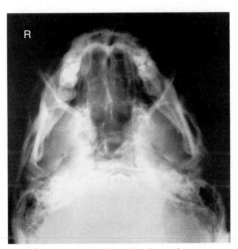

Fig. 11.196 SMV projection—sinuses.

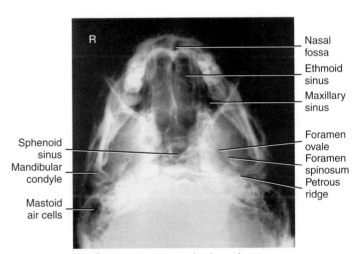

Nasal fossa
Ethmoid sinus
Maxillary sinus
Foramen ovale
Foramen spinosum
Petrous ridge
Sphenoid sinus
Mandibular condyle
Mastoid air cells

Fig. 11.197 SMV projection—sinuses.

PARIETOACANTHIAL TRANSORAL PROJECTION—SINUSES

OPEN-MOUTH WATERS METHOD

11

Clinical Indications

• Inflammatory conditions (sinusitis, secondary osteomyelitis)
• Sinus polyps and cysts

NOTE: This projection is a good alternative to demonstrate the sphenoid sinuses for patients who cannot perform the submentovertex (SMV) position.

> **Sinuses**
> SPECIAL
> • Submentovertical (SMV)
> • Parietoacanthial transoral (open-mouth Waters method)

Technical Factors

• Minimum SID—40 inches (100 cm)
• IR size—8 × 10 inches (18 × 24 cm) or 10 × 12 inches (24 × 30 cm), portrait
• Grid
• kVp range: 75–85
• AEC not recommended

Shielding Shield radiosensitive tissues outside region of interest.

Patient Position Remove all metallic or plastic objects from head and neck. Position patient **erect**.

Part Position

• Extend neck, placing chin and nose against table/upright imaging device surface.
• Adjust head until **OML forms 37° angle** with IR (**MML is perpendicular** with mouth closed) (Fig. 11.198).
• Position **MSP perpendicular** to the midline of grid; ensure **no rotation or tilt.**
• Instruct patient to open mouth (i.e., "drop your jaw without moving your head"); MML may not be perpendicular.
• Center IR to CR and to **acanthion.**

CR

• Align horizontal CR perpendicular to IR.
• Center CR to exit at acanthion.

Recommended Collimation Collimate on four sides to anatomy of interest.

Respiration Suspend respiration.

NOTE: Remember, the CR must be horizontal and the patient erect to demonstrate air-fluid levels within the paranasal sinuses.

Evaluation Criteria

Anatomy Demonstrated: • Maxillary sinuses with the inferior aspect visualized, free from superimposing alveolar processes and petrous ridges; the inferior orbital margin, an oblique view of the frontal sinuses, and the sphenoid sinuses visualized through the open mouth (Figs. 11.199 and 11.200).

Position: • No rotation of the cranium is indicated by the following: equal distance from the MSP (identified by the bony nasal septum) to the lateral orbital margin on both sides; equal distance from the lateral orbital margin to the lateral cortex of the cranium on both sides; accurate extension of the neck demonstrating petrous ridges just inferior to the maxillary sinuses. • Collimation to area of interest.

Exposure: • Density (brightness) and contrast are sufficient to visualize the maxillary and sphenoid sinuses. • Sharp bony margins indicate **no motion.**

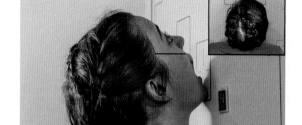

Fig. 11.198 Parietoacanthial transoral projection (upright imaging device/table).

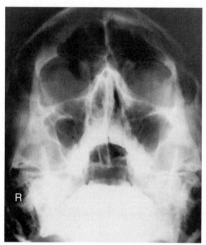

Fig. 11.199 Parietoacanthial transoral projection.

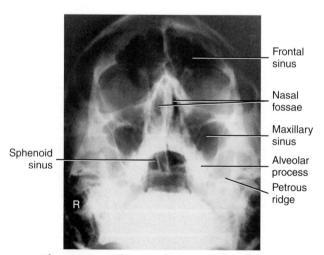

Frontal sinus

Nasal fossae

Maxillary sinus

Sphenoid sinus

Alveolar process

Petrous ridge

Fig. 11.200 Parietoacanthial transoral projection.

RADIOGRAPHS FOR CRITIQUE—CRANIUM

This section consists of an ideal projection (Image A) along with one or more projections that may demonstrate positioning and/or technical errors. Critique Figures C11.201 through C11.203. Compare Image A to the other projections and identify the errors. While examining each image, consider the following questions:

1. Is all essential anatomy demonstrated on the image?
2. What positioning errors are present that compromise image quality?
3. Are technical factors optimal?
4. Is there evidence of collimation and are pre-exposure anatomic side markers visible on the image?
5. Do these errors require a repeat exposure?

Feedback for each set of images is located on the faculty Evolve site.

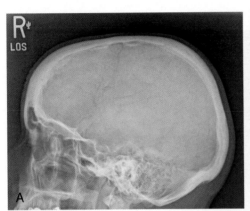
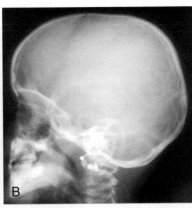
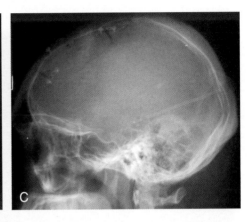

Fig. C11.201 Lateral cranium.

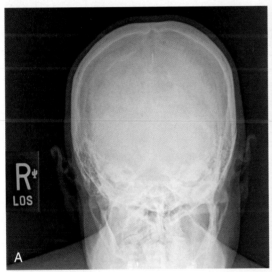
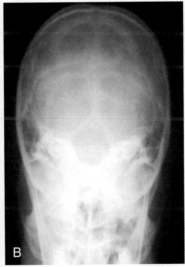
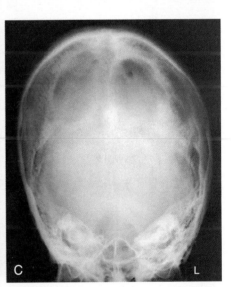

Fig. C11.202 AP axial cranium.

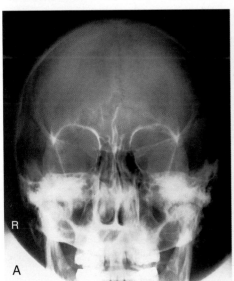
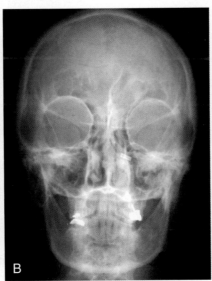
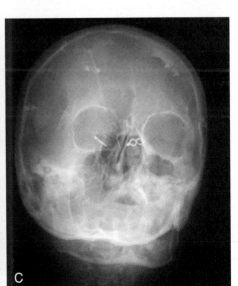

Fig. C11.203 PA Axial (Caldwell method) cranium.

RADIOGRAPHS FOR CRITIQUE—FACIAL BONES

This section consists of an ideal projection (Image A) along with one or more projections that may demonstrate positioning and/or technical errors. Critique Figures C11.204 through C11.206. Compare Image A to the other projections and identify the errors. While examining each image, consider the following questions:

1. Is all essential anatomy demonstrated on the image?
2. What positioning errors are present that compromise image quality?
3. Are technical factors optimal?
4. Is there evidence of collimation and are pre-exposure anatomic side markers visible on the image?
5. Do these errors require a repeat exposure?

Feedback for each set of images is located on the faculty Evolve site.

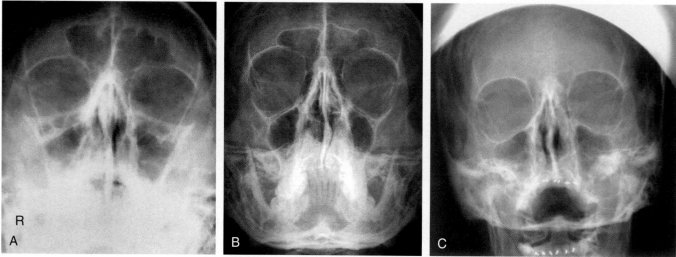

Fig. C11.204 Parietoacanthial projection—facial bones (Waters method).

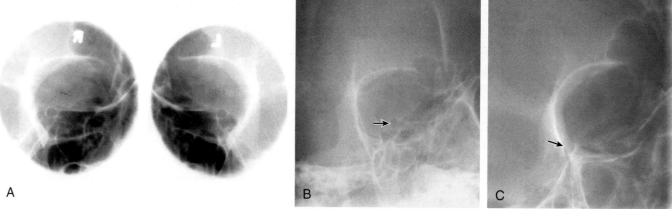

Fig. C11.205 Parieto-orbital oblique (Rhese method)—optic foramen.

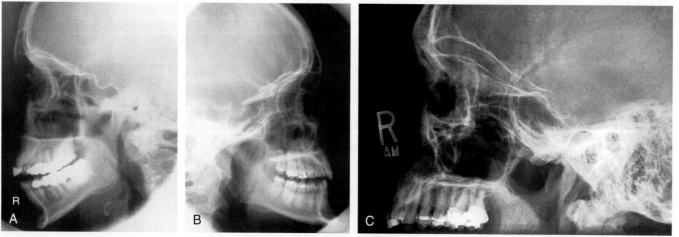

Fig. C11.206 Lateral facial bones.

RADIOGRAPHS FOR CRITIQUE—PARANASAL SINUSES

This section consists of an ideal projection (Image A) along with one or more projections that may demonstrate positioning and/or technical errors. Critique Figure C11.207. Compare Image A to the other projections and identify the errors. While examining each image, consider the following questions:

1. Is all essential anatomy demonstrated on the image?
2. What positioning errors are present that compromise image quality?

3. Are technical factors optimal?
4. Is there evidence of collimation and are pre-exposure anatomic side markers visible on the image?
5. Do these errors require a repeat exposure?

Feedback for each set of images is located on the faculty Evolve site.

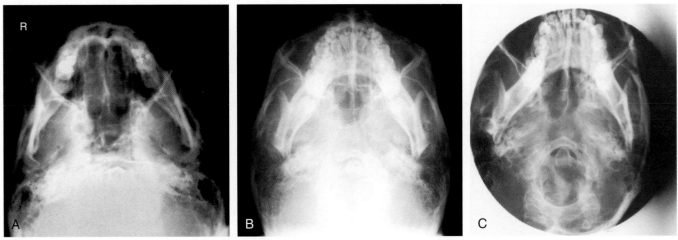

Fig. C11.207 SMV projection—paranasal sinuses.

CHAPTER 12

Biliary Tract and Upper Gastrointestinal System

CONTRIBUTIONS BY **Michele Patrícia Müller Mansur Vieira, MSc, TCNL-CRTR-PR (Brazil)**

CONTRIBUTORS TO PAST EDITIONS Leslie E. Kendrick, MS, RT(R)(CT)(MR), Barry T. Anthony, RT(R)

CONTENTS

RADIOGRAPHIC ANATOMY

Liver

Radiographic examination of the biliary system involves studying the manufacture, transport, and storage of bile. Bile is manufactured by the liver, transported by various ducts, and stored in the gallbladder. Understanding the radiographic examination of the biliary system requires knowledge of the basic anatomy and physiology of the liver, gallbladder, and connecting ducts.

The liver is the largest solid organ in the human body and weighs 3 to 4 lb (about 1.5 to 2 kg). It occupies most of the **right upper quadrant.** Of the nine abdominal regions, the liver occupies almost all of the right hypochondrium, a major part of the epigastrium, and a significant part of the left hypochondrium.

As viewed from the front in Fig. 12.1, the liver is triangular in shape. The superior border is the widest portion of the liver, approximately 8 to 9 inches (20 to 23 cm) and is convex to conform to the inferior surface of the right hemidiaphragm.

The right border of the liver is its greatest vertical dimension, approximately 6 to 7 inches (15 to 17.5 cm). In the average person, the right border extends from the diaphragm to just below the body of the tenth rib. The liver is protected by the lower right rib cage. Because the liver is highly vascular and easily lacerated, protection by the ribs is necessary.

The gallbladder is typically nestled centrally in the posterior inferior region of the liver. The distal end of the gallbladder extends slightly below the posterior inferior margin of the liver (Fig. 12.2). The axial abdominal computed tomography (CT) image (Fig. 12.3) demonstrates this typical orientation of the gallbladder in relation to the posterior inferior aspect of the right lobe of the liver.

LOBES OF THE LIVER

The liver is partially divided into two major lobes and two minor lobes. As viewed from the front in Fig. 12.4, only the two major lobes can be seen. A much larger **right lobe** is separated from the smaller **left lobe** by the **falciform** *(fal'-si-form)* **ligament.**

The two minor lobes of the liver can be found on the posterior aspect of the right lobe (see Fig. 12.2). The first of these is the small **quadrate lobe,** which is located on the inferior surface of the right lobe between the gallbladder and the falciform ligament. Just posterior to the quadrate lobe is the **caudate lobe,** which extends **superiorly** to the diaphragmatic surface. The large **inferior vena cava** contours over the surface of this caudate lobe. The midinferior surface includes the hepatic bile ducts, which are described and illustrated on the following page.

FUNCTION OF THE LIVER

The liver is a complex organ that is essential to life. The liver performs more than 100 different functions, but the function most applicable to radiographic study is the **production of large amounts of bile.** It secretes about 1 quart, or 800 to 1000 mL, of bile per day.

The major functions of bile are to aid in the digestion of fats by emulsifying (breaking down) fat globules and in the absorption of fat following its digestion. Bile also contains cholesterol, which is made soluble in the bile by the bile salts.

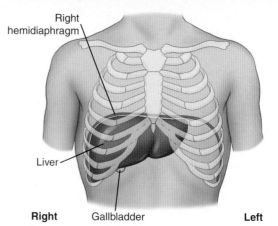

Fig. 12.1 Liver and gallbladder—anterior view.

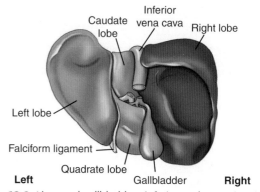

Fig. 12.2 Liver and gallbladder—inferior and posterior view.

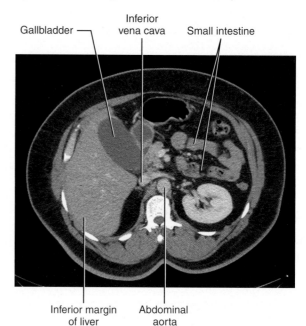

Fig. 12.3 Axial abdominal CT—liver and gallbladder.

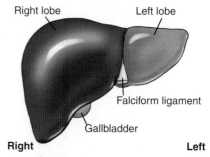

Fig. 12.4 Liver—anterior view.

Gallbladder and Biliary Ducts

The gallbladder and the extrahepatic biliary ducts (located outside of the liver) are shown in Fig. 12.5. Bile is formed in small lobules of the liver and travels by small ducts to the larger **right** or **left hepatic ducts.** The right and left hepatic ducts join to continue as the **common hepatic duct.** Bile is carried to the **gallbladder** via the **cystic duct** for temporary storage, or it may be secreted directly into the **duodenum** via the **common bile duct.** The common bile duct is joined by the **pancreatic duct** at the **hepatopancreatic sphincter,** which empties into the duodenum via the **duodenal papilla.**

The **gallbladder** is a pear-shaped sac composed of three parts: **fundus, body,** and **neck** (Fig. 12.6). The fundus is the distal end and the broadest part of the gallbladder. The body is the main section of the gallbladder. The neck is the narrow proximal end, which continues as the **cystic duct.** The cystic duct is 1 to 1½ inches (3 to 4 cm) long and contains several membranous folds along its length. These folds are called the **spiral valve,** which functions to prevent distention or collapse of the cystic duct.

The normal gallbladder is 2½ to 4 inches (7 to 10 cm) long and approximately 1 inch (2.5 cm) wide. It generally holds 2 to 2½ tablespoons (30 to 40 mL) of bile.

FUNCTIONS OF THE GALLBLADDER

The **three** primary functions of the gallbladder are (1) to **store** bile, (2) to **concentrate** bile, and (3) to **contract when stimulated.**
1. If bile is not needed for digestive purposes, it is **stored** for future use in the gallbladder.
2. Bile is **concentrated** within the gallbladder as a result of hydrolysis (removal of water). In an abnormal situation, when too much water is absorbed or the cholesterol becomes too concentrated, gallstones (choleliths) may form in the gallbladder. (Cholesterol forms the most common type of gallstones.[1])
3. The gallbladder normally **contracts** when foods, such as fats or fatty acids, are in the duodenum. These foods stimulate the duodenal mucosa to secrete the hormone **cholecystokinin (CCK).** Increased levels of CCK in the blood cause the gallbladder to contract and the terminal opening of the common bile duct to relax. In addition, CCK causes increased exocrine activity by the pancreas.

COMMON BILE DUCT

The **common bile duct** averages approximately 3 inches (7.5 cm) in length and has an internal diameter about the size of a drinking straw. The common bile duct descends behind the superior portion of the duodenum and the head of the pancreas to enter the second or **descending portion of the duodenum.**

The terminal end of the common bile duct is closely associated with the terminal end of the **pancreatic duct (duct of Wirsung)** *(ver'-soong),* as shown in Fig. 12.7.

In about 40% of individuals, these ducts pass into the duodenum as two separate ducts with separate openings. In the remaining 60%, the common bile duct joins the pancreatic duct to form one common passageway through the single papilla into the duodenum.[1] In these individuals, this short, single channel becomes narrower as it passes into the duodenum and is a common site for impaction of gallstones.[1] Some references identify this common passageway as an ampulla, the **hepatopancreatic ampulla,** or the older term, **ampulla of Vater.**

Near the terminal opening of this passageway into the duodenum, the duct walls contain circular muscle fiber, termed the **hepatopancreatic sphincter,** or **sphincter of Oddi** *(od'-e).* This sphincter relaxes when levels of CCK increase in the bloodstream. The presence of this ring of muscle causes a protrusion into the lumen of the duodenum termed the **duodenal papilla (papilla of Vater).**

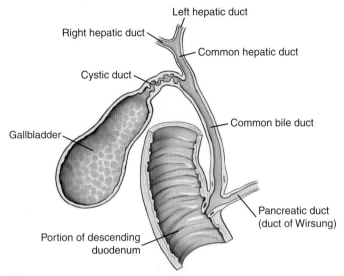

Fig. 12.5 Gallbladder and extrahepatic biliary ducts.

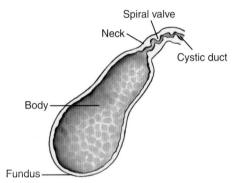

Fig. 12.6 Gallbladder and cystic duct.

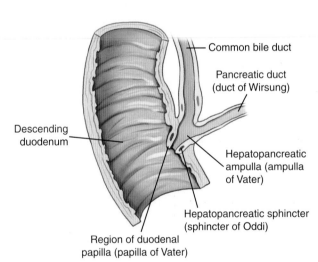

Fig. 12.7 Common bile duct.

GALLBLADDER AND BILIARY DUCTS (LATERAL VIEW)

The simplified lateral view drawing in Fig. 12.8 illustrates the relationship of the **liver, gallbladder,** and **biliary ducts** as seen from the right side. The gallbladder is **anterior** to the midcoronal plane, whereas the duct system is more midline. This spatial relationship influences optimal positioning of the gallbladder or the biliary ducts. If it is necessary to place the gallbladder as close to the image receptor (IR) as possible, the prone position would be more appropriate than the supine position. If the primary purpose is to **drain the gallbladder** into the duct system, the patient would be placed **supine** to assist this drainage.

Anatomy Review

RADIOGRAPH OF GALLBLADDER

The left anterior oblique (LAO) position of the gallbladder in Fig. 12.9 demonstrates the cystic duct and the three major divisions of the gallbladder:

A. Cystic duct
B. Neck
C. Body
D. Fundus

MEDICAL SONOGRAPHY

Sonography (ultrasound) of the gallbladder provides a noninvasive means of studying the gallbladder and the biliary ducts (Fig. 12.10). Sonography offers four advantages:

1. **No ionizing radiation:** Sonography is a non–ionizing radiation imaging modality that eliminates radiation exposure to the patient, radiologist, and technologist.
2. **Detection of small calculi:** Sonography can detect small calculi in the gallbladder and biliary ducts.
3. **No contrast medium:** No contrast medium is required with sonography. Therefore, this is an ideal alternative for patients who are sensitive to iodinated contrast agents.
4. **Less patient preparation:** Patient preparation with sonography is greatly reduced compared with other modalities. For sonography, the patient should be **NPO** (*nil per os,* meaning "nothing by mouth") 8 hours before the examination. Sonography provides a quick diagnosis for gallbladder disease, and the physician can make a surgical decision in hours.

Clinical Indications

GALLBLADDER AND BILIARY DUCT RADIOGRAPHY

Clinical indications for gallbladder diseases include nausea, heartburn, premature full feeling when eating, right upper quadrant (RUQ) discomfort and vomiting. Many abnormal conditions may be demonstrated using various imaging modalities, including the following. It is important for technologists to be familiar with biliary terminology (Table 12.1).

TABLE 12.1 BILIARY TERMINOLOGY

TERM	MEANING
Chole- *(ko´-le)*	Prefix denoting relationship to bile
Cysto- *(sis´-to)*	Prefix denoting sac or bladder
Choleliths *(ko´-le-liths)*	Gallstones
Cholelithiasis *(ko´-le-li-thi´-ah-sis)*	Condition of having gallstones
Cholecystitis *(ko´-le-sis-ti´-tis)*	Inflammation of the gallbladder
Cholecystectomy *(ko´-le-sis-tek´-ta-me)*	Surgical removal of the gallbladder

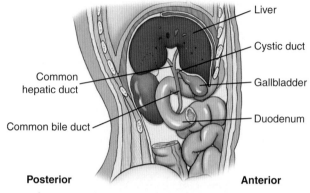

Fig. 12.8 Side view of gallbladder and biliary ducts.

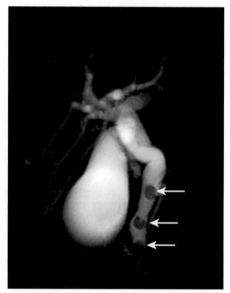

Fig. 12.9 Choledocholithiasis. The thick-slab MRCP image yields a more comprehensive appraisal of the biliary tree, showing choledocholithiasis *(arrows)* and the full extent of intrahepatic and extrahepatic biliary dilation. (From Roth CG, Deshmukh S. *Fundamentals of body MRI,* ed 2, Philadelphia, 2017, Elsevier.)

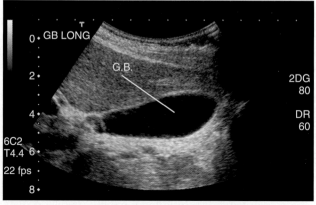

Fig. 12.10 Sonography of gallbladder.

Biliary Calculi (Gallstones)

Choledocholithiasis is the presence of stones in the biliary ducts. Biliary stones may form in the biliary ducts or migrate from the gallbladder. These stones often produce a blockage in the ducts. Symptoms include pain, tenderness in the right upper quadrant, jaundice, and sometimes pancreatitis.

Cholelithiasis is the condition of having abnormal calcifications or stones in the gallbladder. Increased levels of bilirubin, calcium, or cholesterol may lead to the formation of gallstones. There are two types of stones, cholesterol and pigment stones; 75% of stones that occur are the cholesterol type. Risk factors for developing gallstones include family history, excessive weight, being over 40 years of age, and being female.[2] Symptoms of cholelithiasis include right upper quadrant pain usually after a meal, nausea, and possibly vomiting. Patients with complete blockage of the biliary ducts may develop jaundice.

Gallstones are primarily composed of cholesterol, making them highly radiolucent; another 25% to 30% are primarily cholesterol and crystalline salts, which also are radiolucent. This leaves a smaller percentage (approximately 20%) of gallstones that are composed of crystalline calcium salts, which are often visible on an abdominal radiographic image without contrast media.[2]

Milk calcium bile is the emulsion of biliary stones in the gallbladder. This emulsion buildup of calcium deposits within the gallbladder may be difficult to diagnose during cholangiography. It is seen as a diffuse collection of sandlike calcifications or sediment.

Although drugs have been developed that dissolve these stones, most patients have the gallbladder removed. A laparoscopic technique for removing the gallbladder (cholecystectomy) has greatly reduced the convalescence of the patient.

With sonography, stones within the gallbladder or biliary ducts produce a "shadowing" effect. The shadowing effect is created by the partial blockage of the sound wave as it passes by.

Cholecystitis

Acute or chronic cholecystitis is inflammation of the gallbladder. In acute cholecystitis, often a blockage of the cystic duct restricts the flow of bile from the gallbladder into the common bile duct. The blockage is frequently (95% of cases[2]) due to a stone lodged in the neck of the gallbladder. Over time, the bile begins to irritate the inner lining of the gallbladder, and it becomes inflamed. Symptoms of acute cholecystitis include abdominal pain, tenderness in the right upper quadrant, and fever. Bacterial infection and ischemia (obstruction of blood supply) of the gallbladder may also produce acute cholecystitis. Gas-producing bacteria may lead to a gangrenous gallbladder.

Chronic cholecystitis is almost always associated with gallstones but may also be an outcome of pancreatitis or carcinoma of the gallbladder. Symptoms of right upper quadrant pain, heartburn, and nausea may occur after a meal. Calcified plaques, thickening or calcification of the wall of the gallbladder, may be related to chronic cholecystitis. Chronic cholecystitis may produce repetitive attacks following meals that typically subside in 1 to 4 hours.

Neoplasms

Neoplasms are new growths, which may be benign or malignant. Malignant or cancerous tumors of the gallbladder can be aggressive and spread to the liver, pancreas, or gastrointestinal tract. Neoplasms of the gallbladder are rare. Of the malignant tumors of the gallbladder, 85% are adenocarcinomas, and 15% are squamous cell carcinomas.[3] Common benign tumors of the gallbladder include adenomas and cholesterol polyps.

Approximately 80% of patients with carcinoma of the gallbladder have stones. As the tumor grows, it may obstruct the biliary system. Patients may experience pain, vomiting, and jaundice. Sonography and CT are the best modalities to demonstrate neoplasms of the gallbladder. A stent or drain sometimes needs to be inserted within the common bile duct to provide a pathway to the buildup of bile resulting from obstruction.

Biliary Stenosis

Biliary stenosis is a narrowing of one of the biliary ducts. The flow of bile may be restricted by this condition. In the case of gallstones, the stenosis may prevent the passage of the small gallstones into the duodenum, leading to obstruction of the duct. Cholecystitis and jaundice may result from biliary stenosis. During cholangiography, the common bile duct may appear elongated, tapered, and narrowed. A gallstone lodged at the distal common bile duct often presents a filling defect with a small channel of contrast media passing around it.

Table 12.2 presents a summary of clinical indications for gallbladder and biliary tract radiography.

TABLE 12.2 SUMMARY OF CLINICAL INDICATIONS: GALLBLADDER AND BILIARY TRACT			
CONDITION OR DISEASE	**MOST COMMON RADIOGRAPHIC EXAMINATION**	**POSSIBLE RADIOGRAPHIC APPEARANCE**	**EXPOSURE FACTOR ADJUSTMENT[a]**
Choledocholithiasis (stones in biliary ducts)	Sonography MRI ERCP Operative cholangiography	Enlargement or narrowing of biliary ducts owing to presence of stones	None
Cholelithiasis (stones in gallbladder)	Sonography MRI Cholescintigraphy (radionuclide studies)[2]	Both radiolucent and radiopaque densities seen in the region of the gallbladder; "shadowing" effect with ultrasound; failure to accumulate radionuclide within gallbladder[2]	None
Acute cholecystitis	Sonography MRI Cholescintigraphy (radionuclide studies)[2]	Thickened wall of gallbladder with ultrasound; failure to accumulate radionuclide within gallbladder[2]	None
Chronic cholecystitis	Sonography MRI	Calcified plaques or calcification of wall of gallbladder	None
Neoplasms	Sonography MRI CT	Mass seen within gallbladder, liver, or biliary ducts; extensive calcification of gallbladder wall	None
Biliary stenosis	Operative cholangiogram ERCP	Elongation, tapering, and narrowing of common bile duct	None

[a]Dependent on stage or severity of condition.
ERCP, Endoscopic retrograde cholangiopancreatogram.

Digestive System

The digestive system includes the entire **alimentary canal** and several **accessory organs** (Fig. 12.11).

ALIMENTARY CANAL

The alimentary canal begins at the (1) oral cavity (mouth) and continues as the (2) pharynx, (3) esophagus, (4) stomach, and (5) small intestine; it ends as the (6) large intestine, which terminates as the (7) anus. Anatomy and positioning of (1) the oral cavity through (5) the duodenum are covered in this chapter. The remainder of the small intestine, (6) the large intestine, and (7) the anus are discussed in Chapter 13.

ACCESSORY ORGANS

Accessory organs of digestion include the **salivary glands, pancreas, liver,** and **gallbladder.**

FUNCTIONS

The digestive system performs the following **three primary functions:**

1. The first primary function is the **intake or digestion** of food, water, vitamins, and minerals. Food is ingested in the form of carbohydrates, lipids, and proteins. These complex food groups must be broken down, or digested, so that absorption can occur.
2. The second function of the digestive system is to **absorb** digested food particles, along with water, vitamins, and essential elements from the alimentary canal, into the blood or lymphatic capillaries.
3. The third function is to **eliminate** any unused material in the form of semisolid waste products.

COMMON RADIOGRAPHIC PROCEDURES

Two common radiographic procedures involving the upper gastrointestinal (UGI) system are presented in this chapter. These radiographic examinations involve the administration of a contrast medium.

Esophagography (Study of Pharynx and Esophagus)

Radiographic examination specifically of the pharynx and esophagus is termed **esophagography.** This procedure studies the form and function of the swallowing aspect of the pharynx and esophagus.

Upper Gastrointestinal Series (Study of Distal Esophagus, Stomach, and Duodenum)

The procedure designed to study the distal esophagus, stomach, and duodenum in one examination is termed an **upper gastrointestinal series (UGI, upper GI).** A posteroanterior (PA) radiograph from an upper GI series is shown in Fig. 12.12.

Barium sulfate mixed with water is the preferred contrast medium for the entire alimentary canal. The negative density area (appearing white) on the radiograph indicates the stomach and duodenal area filled with barium sulfate contrast medium.

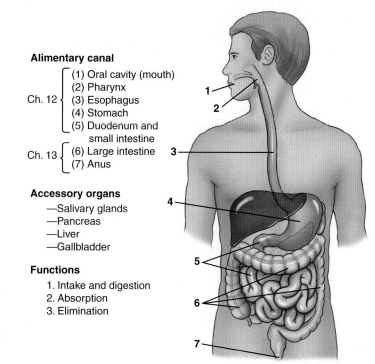

Alimentary canal

Ch. 12
- (1) Oral cavity (mouth)
- (2) Pharynx
- (3) Esophagus
- (4) Stomach
- (5) Duodenum and small intestine

Ch. 13
- (6) Large intestine
- (7) Anus

Accessory organs
- —Salivary glands
- —Pancreas
- —Liver
- —Gallbladder

Functions
1. Intake and digestion
2. Absorption
3. Elimination

Fig. 12.11 Digestive system.

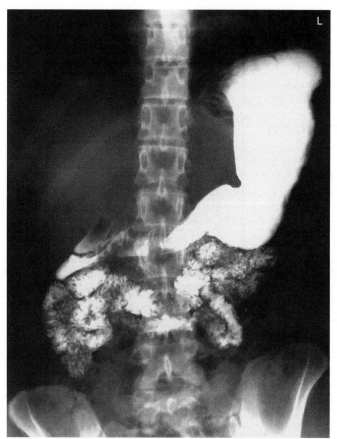

Fig. 12.12 PA—upper GI series (barium in stomach and duodenum).

Mouth (Oral Cavity)

The alimentary canal is a continuous hollow tube, beginning with the **oral cavity** (mouth). The oral cavity and surrounding structures are visualized in the midsagittal plane in Fig. 12.13.

The oral cavity is bordered anteriorly and bilaterally by the inner surfaces of the **upper** and **lower teeth.** The roof of the oral cavity is formed by the **hard** and **soft palates.** Hanging from the mid-posterior aspect of the soft palate is a small conical process termed the **palatine uvula,** commonly referred to simply as the **uvula** *(u'-vu-lah).* Most of the floor of the oral cavity is formed by the **tongue.** The oral cavity connects posteriorly with the **pharynx** *(far'-inks),* as described subsequently.

ACCESSORY ORGANS IN ORAL CAVITY

The **salivary glands** are accessory organs of digestion associated with the mouth. The teeth and tongue cooperate in chewing movements to reduce the size of food particles and mix food with saliva. These chewing movements, termed **mastication** *(mas"-ti-ka'-shun),* initiate the mechanical part of digestion.

Three pairs of glands secrete most of the saliva in the oral cavity (Fig. 12.14). These glands are the (1) **parotid** *(pah-rot'-id),* meaning "near the ear," which is the largest of the salivary glands located just anterior to the external ear; (2) **submandibular,** sometimes called *submaxillary,* meaning "below the mandible or maxilla"; and (3) **sublingual** *(sub-ling'-gwal),* meaning "below the tongue."

Saliva is 99.5% water and 0.5% solutes or salts and certain digestive enzymes. The salivary glands secrete 1000 to 1500 mL of saliva daily. Saliva dissolves foods to begin the digestion process. It also contains the enzyme amylase *(am'-i-lays),* which breaks down starches.

Specific salivary glands secrete a thickened fluid that contains mucus. Mucus lubricates food as it is being chewed so that the food can form into a ball, or bolus, for swallowing. The act of swallowing is termed **deglutition** *(deg"-loo-tish'-un).*

NOTE: The salivary glands, especially the parotid glands, may be the site of infection. **Mumps** is an inflammation and enlargement of the parotid glands caused by a paramyxovirus, which can result in inflammation of the testes in approximately 30% of infected males.

Pharynx

The alimentary canal continues as the pharynx posterior to the oral cavity. The **pharynx** is about 5 inches (12.5 cm) long and is the part of the digestive tube found posterior to the nasal cavity, mouth, and larynx. Midsagittal and coronal sections of the pharynx, as seen from the side and posterior views, are shown in Fig. 12.15. The three parts of the pharynx are named according to their locations.

The **nasopharynx** is posterior to the bony nasal septum, nasal cavities, and soft palate. This portion of the pharynx is not part of the digestive system.

The **oropharynx** is directly posterior to the oral cavity proper. The oropharynx extends from the **soft palate** to the **epiglottis** *(ep"-i-glot'-is).* The epiglottis is a membrane-covered cartilage that moves down to cover the opening of the larynx during swallowing.

The third portion of the pharynx is called the **laryngopharynx,** or *hypopharynx.* The laryngopharynx extends from the level of the epiglottis to the level of the lower border of the larynx (level of C6, as described in Chapter 2). From this point, it continues as the **esophagus.** The **trachea** is seen anterior to the esophagus.

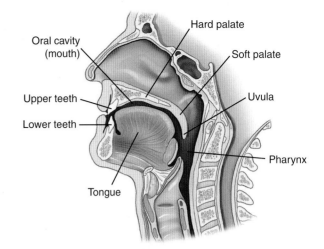

Fig. 12.13 Midsagittal section of mouth (oral or buccal cavity).

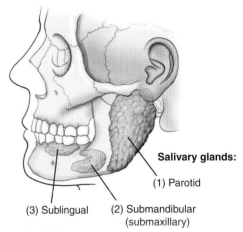

Salivary glands:
(1) Parotid
(2) Submandibular (submaxillary)
(3) Sublingual

Fig. 12.14 Accessory organs in the mouth.

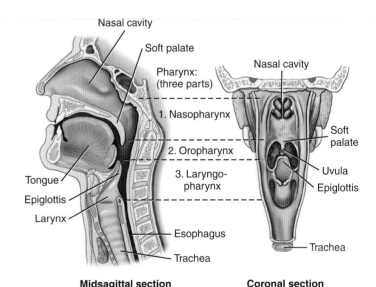

Midsagittal section   Coronal section
Fig. 12.15 Pharynx.

CAVITIES THAT COMMUNICATE WITH PHARYNX

The drawing in Fig. 12.16 illustrates **seven cavities**, or **openings**, that communicate with the three portions of the pharynx. The two **nasal cavities** and the two **tympanic cavities** connect to the **nasopharynx.** The tympanic cavities of the middle ears connect to the nasopharynx via the **auditory** or **eustachian tubes** (not shown in the drawing).

The **oral cavity** (mouth) connects posteriorly to the **oropharynx.** Inferiorly, the **laryngopharynx** connects to the openings of both the **larynx** and the **esophagus.**

DEGLUTITION (SWALLOWING)

Food and fluid travel from the oral cavity directly to the esophagus during the act of swallowing, or **deglutition.** During swallowing, the **soft palate closes off the nasopharynx** to prevent swallowed substances from regurgitating into the nose. The tongue prevents this material from reentering the mouth.

During swallowing, the **epiglottis is depressed to cover the laryngeal opening** like a lid. The vocal folds, or cords, also come together to close off the epiglottis. These actions combine to prevent food and fluid from being aspirated (entering the larynx, trachea, and bronchi).

Respiration is inhibited during deglutition to prevent swallowed substances from entering the trachea and lungs. Occasionally, bits of material pass into the larynx and trachea during deglutition, causing a forceful episode of reflex coughing.

Esophagus

The third part of the alimentary canal is the **esophagus.** The esophagus is a muscular canal, about 10 inches (25 cm) long and about ½ inch (1 to 2 cm) in diameter, extending from the laryngopharynx to the stomach. The esophagus begins posterior to the level of the lower border of the **cricoid cartilage of the larynx** (C5 to C6), which is at the level of the upper margin of the thyroid cartilage. The esophagus terminates at its connection to the stomach, at the level of the **eleventh thoracic vertebra** (T11).

In Fig. 12.17, the esophagus is shown to be located **posterior to the larynx and trachea.** The spatial relationship of the esophagus to both the trachea and the thoracic vertebrae is an important relationship to remember. The esophagus is posterior to the trachea and just anterior to the cervical and thoracic vertebral bodies.

The descending **thoracic aorta** is between the distal esophagus and the lower thoracic spine. The **heart,** within its pericardial sac, is immediately posterior to the sternum, anterior to the esophagus, and superior to the diaphragm.

The esophagus is essentially vertical as it descends to the stomach. This swallowing tube is the narrowest part of the entire alimentary canal. The esophagus is most constricted first at its proximal end, where it enters the thorax, and second where it passes through the diaphragm at the esophageal hiatus, or opening. The esophagus pierces the diaphragm at the **level of T10.** Just before passing through the diaphragm, the esophagus presents a distinct dilation, as shown in Fig. 12.18.

As the esophagus descends within the posterior aspect of the mediastinum, **two indentations** are present. One indentation occurs at the **aortic arch,** and the second is found where the esophagus crosses the **left primary bronchus.**

The lower portion of the esophagus lies close to the posterior aspects of the heart.

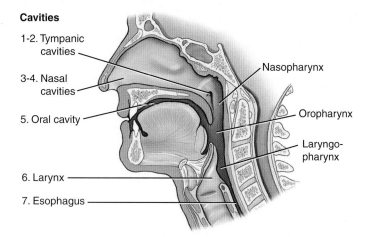

Fig. 12.16 Seven cavities, or openings, communicate with the pharynx.

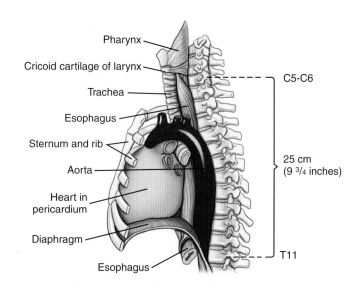

Fig. 12.17 Esophagus in mediastinum—lateral view.

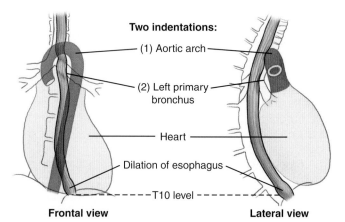

Fig. 12.18 Esophagus in mediastinum, demonstrating two indentations.

DIAPHRAGMATIC OPENINGS

The **esophagus** passes through the **diaphragm** slightly to the left and posterior to the midpoint of the diaphragm. Fig. 12.19 represents the inferior surface of the diaphragm and indicates the relative positions of the **esophagus, inferior vena cava,** and **aorta.**

The lateral view drawing on the right shows the short abdominal portion of the esophagus below the diaphragm. The **abdominal segment of the esophagus,** termed the **cardiac antrum,** measures about ½ inch (1 to 2 cm) in length. The cardiac antrum curves sharply to the left after passing through the diaphragm to attach to the stomach.

The opening between the esophagus and the stomach is termed the **esophagogastric junction** *(cardiac orifice)* (see Fig. 12.23). *Cardiac* is an adjective that denotes a relationship to the heart; the cardiac antrum and the cardiac orifice are located near the heart.

The junction of the stomach and the esophagus normally is securely attached to the diaphragm; thus, the upper stomach tends to follow the respiratory movements of the diaphragm.

SWALLOWING AND PERISTALSIS

The esophagus contains well-developed skeletal muscle layers (circular and longitudinal) in its upper third, skeletal and smooth muscle in its middle third, and smooth muscle in its lower third. In contrast to the trachea, the esophagus is a collapsible tube that opens only when swallowing occurs. The process of deglutition continues in the esophagus after originating in the mouth and pharynx. Fluids tend to pass from the mouth and pharynx to the stomach, primarily by gravity. A bolus of solid material tends to pass both by gravity and by peristalsis.

Peristalsis is a wavelike series of involuntary muscular contractions that propel solid and semisolid materials through the tubular alimentary canal. A solid bolus of barium sulfate filling the entire esophagus is seen in Fig. 12.20 descending to the stomach both by gravity and peristalsis. Accumulation of barium in the stomach is seen in this right anterior oblique (RAO) radiograph.

Spot radiographs in an RAO position in Fig. 12.21 demonstrate the esophagus partially filled with barium, with normal peristaltic constrictions most evident in midportions and upper portions of the esophagus.

The relationship of the esophagus to the heart is seen on these radiographs. The esophagus is located immediately adjacent to the right and posterior heart borders.

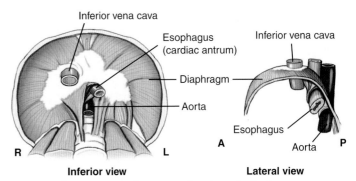

Fig. 12.19 Esophagus passing through diaphragm.

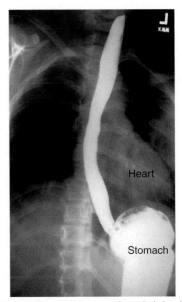

Fig. 12.20 RAO esophagography (slightly oblique).

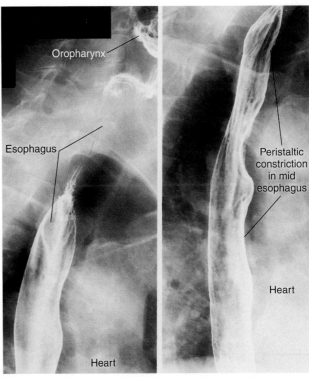

Fig. 12.21 RAO esophagography—upper esophagus. Midesophagus and lower esophagus are just above diaphragm.

Stomach

The Greek word *gaster* means "stomach," and *gastro* is a common term denoting stomach—hence the term *gastrointestinal* tract.

The **stomach**, which is located between the **esophagus** and the **small intestine**, is the most dilated portion of the alimentary canal (Fig. 12.22). When empty, the stomach tends to collapse. When the stomach must serve as a reservoir for swallowed food and fluid, it is remarkably expandable. After a full meal, the stomach stretches to what would appear to be almost the point of rupture.

Because the shape and position of the stomach are highly variable, the average shape and location are used in the following illustrations, with variations to follow later in this chapter.

STOMACH OPENINGS AND CURVATURES

The **esophagogastric junction** (cardiac orifice) is the aperture, or opening, between the esophagus and the stomach (Fig. 12.23). A small, circular muscle, called the *cardiac sphincter,* allows food and fluid to pass through the cardiac orifice. This opening (esophagogastric junction) is commonly called the **cardiac orifice,** which refers to the relationship of this orifice to the portion of the diaphragm near the heart, on which the heart rests.

Directly superior to this orifice is a notch called the **cardiac notch** *(incisura cardiaca).* This distal abdominal portion of the esophagus curves sharply into a slightly expanded portion of the terminal esophagus called the **cardiac antrum.**

The opening, or orifice, of the distal stomach is termed the **pyloric orifice, or pylorus.** The pyloric sphincter at this orifice is a thickened muscular ring that relaxes periodically during digestion to allow stomach or gastric contents to move into the first part of the small intestine, the duodenum.

The **lesser curvature,** which is found along the medial border of the stomach, forms a concave border as it extends between the cardiac and pyloric orifices.

The **greater curvature** is found along the lateral border of the stomach. This greater curvature is four to five times longer than the lesser curvature. It extends from the cardiac notch and the pylorus.

STOMACH SUBDIVISIONS

The stomach is composed of three main subdivisions: (1) the **fundus,** (2) the **body,** and (3) the **pylorus** (see Fig. 12.23). The fundus is the ballooned portion that lies lateral and superior to the cardiac orifice. The upper portion of the stomach, including the cardiac antrum of the esophagus, is relatively fixed to the diaphragm and tends to move with motion of the diaphragm. In the upright, or erect, position, the fundus is usually filled by a bubble of swallowed air; this is referred to as a *gastric bubble.*

The lower end of the large body of the stomach has a partially constricted area that separates the body from the pyloric portion of the stomach. This "notch," or constricted ringlike area, is called the **angular notch** *(incisura angularis).*

The smaller terminal portion of the stomach to the right of, or medial to, the angular notch is the pyloric portion of the stomach. The pyloric portion of the stomach frequently is divided into two parts: the **pyloric antrum,** shown as a slight dilation immediately distal to the angular notch, and the narrowed **pyloric canal,** which ends at the pyloric sphincter.

The barium-filled stomach in Fig. 12.24 demonstrates the actual appearance and shape of the stomach, as seen on a PA projection of the stomach and duodenum as part of an upper GI series. Review the labeled parts and compare them with the drawings in Figs. 12.22 and 12.23.

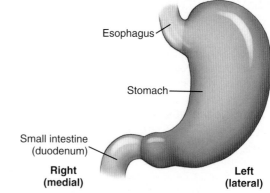

Fig. 12.22 Stomach—frontal view.

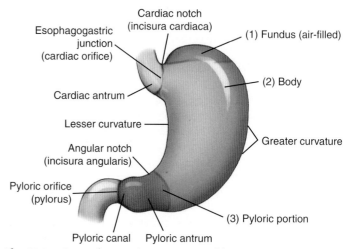

Fig. 12.23 Stomach—openings, greater and lesser curvatures, and subdivisions.

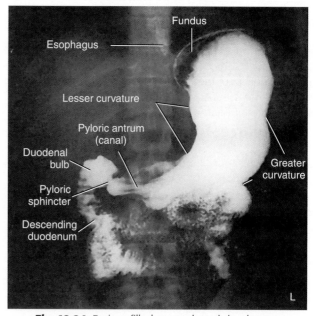

Fig. 12.24 Barium-filled stomach and duodenum.

MUCOSAL FOLDS WITHIN THE STOMACH—RUGAE

When the stomach is empty, the internal lining is thrown into numerous longitudinal mucosal folds termed **rugae** (*[roo'-je]*; singular, ruga *[roo'-gah]*). Rugae are most evident in the lower body of the stomach along the greater curvature. These folds are shown in the drawing in Fig. 12.25 (they also are demonstrated by the streaklike folds of the air/barium-filled stomach radiograph in Fig. 12.28). The rugae assist with mechanical digestion of food within the stomach.

A **gastric canal,** formed by rugae along the lesser curvature (see Fig. 12.25), funnels fluids directly from the body of the stomach to the pylorus.

STOMACH POSITION

The illustration in Fig. 12.26 shows the typical orientation of an average, partially filled stomach in anterior and lateral views. The **fundus,** in addition to being the most superior portion of the stomach in general, is located posterior to the **body** of the stomach, as can be seen on the lateral view. The body can be seen to curve inferior and anterior from the fundus.

The **pylorus** is directed posteriorly. The pyloric valve (sphincter) and the first part of the small bowel are very near the posterior abdominal wall. The relationships of these components of the stomach affect the distribution of air and barium within the stomach during specific body positions.

AIR/GAS-BARIUM DISTRIBUTION IN STOMACH

If an individual swallows a barium sulfate and water mixture, along with gas-producing crystals, as seen in Figs. 12.27 and 12.28, the position of the person's body determines the distribution of barium and air/carbon dioxide (CO_2) gas within the stomach.

In the supine **position,** the fundus of the stomach is the most posterior portion and is where the heavy barium settles (see Fig. 12.27). Note the collection of gas in the body and pylorus of the stomach.

In the **RAO, prone position,** the fundus is in the highest position, causing the **gas** to fill this portion of the stomach, as can be seen in Fig. 12.28. The barium settles in the more anterior body and pylorus portions of the stomach.

This appearance is also shown in the three position drawings in Fig. 12.29, in which the air/gas is shown as black and the barium as white, similar to the appearance of air and barium in a radiographic image.

The drawing on the left depicts the stomach of a person in **supine** position. The middle drawing shows the stomach of a person in **prone** position. The drawing on the right depicts the stomach of a person who is in an **erect** position. In the erect position, air/gas rises to fill the fundus, whereas barium descends by gravity to fill the pyloric portion of the stomach. The air-barium line tends to be a straight line in the erect position compared with the prone and supine positions.

When studying radiographic images of a stomach that contains both air/gas and barium, you can determine the patient's position by the relative locations of air versus barium within the stomach.

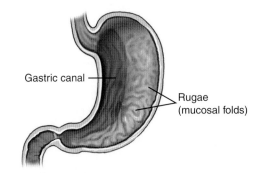

Fig. 12.25 Stomach—coronal section.

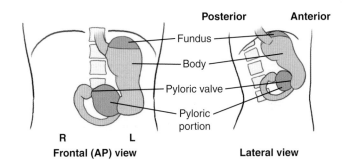

Fig. 12.26 Average empty stomach orientation.

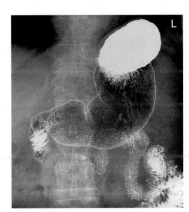

Fig. 12.27 AP stomach—supine position (barium in fundus).

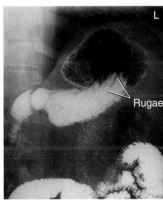

Fig. 12.28 RAO stomach—prone position (air in fundus).

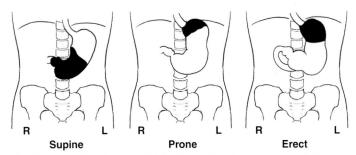

Fig. 12.29 Air/gas-barium distribution in the stomach—frontal views in various body positions. Black areas indicate air/gas; white areas indicate barium.

Duodenum

The fifth and final part of the upper GI system to be studied in this chapter is the **duodenum** *(du″-o-de′-num),* which is the first portion of the small intestine, commonly called the *small bowel.* Because the duodenum is examined radiographically during a routine upper GI series, the duodenum is studied in this chapter; the remainder of the small bowel is studied in Chapter 13 with the lower gastrointestinal system.

The duodenum is about 7½ to 9 inches (20 to 24 cm) long and is the shortest, widest, and most fixed portion of the small intestine. The drawing in Fig. 12.30 demonstrates that the C-shaped duodenum is closely related to the **head of the pancreas.** The head of the pancreas, nestled in the C-loop of the duodenum, has been affectionately labeled the "romance of the abdomen" by some authors.

The C-loop of the duodenum and the pancreas are **retroperitoneal** structures; that is, they are located **posterior to the parietal peritoneum,** as described in Chapter 3.

FOUR PARTS OF DUODENUM

The duodenum is shaped like the letter C and consists of **four parts** (Fig. 12.31). The **first (superior) portion** begins at the pylorus of the stomach. The first part of the superior portion is termed the **duodenal bulb,** or **cap.** The duodenal bulb is easily located during barium studies of the upper gastrointestinal tract and must be carefully studied because this area is a common site of ulcer disease. This portion of the duodenum is intraperitoneal; the remainder of the duodenum is retroperitoneal.

The next part of the duodenum is the **second (descending) portion,** the longest segment. The descending portion of the duodenum possesses the **duodenal papilla,** which is the opening for the common bile and pancreatic ducts into the duodenum.

The **third** part of the duodenum is the **horizontal portion.** This portion curves back to the left to join the final segment, the **fourth (ascending) portion** of the duodenum.

The junction of the duodenum with the second portion of the small intestine, the **jejunum** *(je-joo′-num),* is termed the **duodenojejunal flexure.** This portion is relatively fixed and is held in place by a fibrous muscular band, the **ligament of Treitz (suspensory muscle of the duodenum).** This structure is a significant reference point in certain radiographic small bowel studies.

Anatomy Review

RADIOGRAPH OF STOMACH AND DUODENUM

The PA radiograph of the stomach and duodenum in Fig. 12.32 provides a good review of important radiographic anatomy. Identify the structures labeled on the radiograph, and then compare your answers with the following list.

A. Distal esophagus
B. Area of esophagogastric junction (cardiac orifice)
C. Lesser curvature of stomach
D. Angular notch (incisura angularis) of stomach
E. Pylorus of stomach
F. Pyloric valve or sphincter
G. Duodenal bulb (cap)
H. Second (descending) portion of duodenum
I. Body of stomach
J. Greater curvature of stomach
K. Mucosal folds, or rugae, of stomach
L. Fundus of stomach

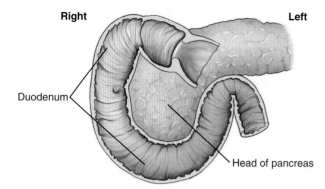

Right   Left

Fig. 12.30 Duodenum and pancreas.

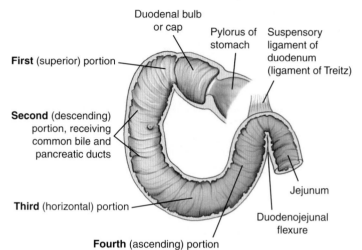

Fig. 12.31 Duodenum (four parts).

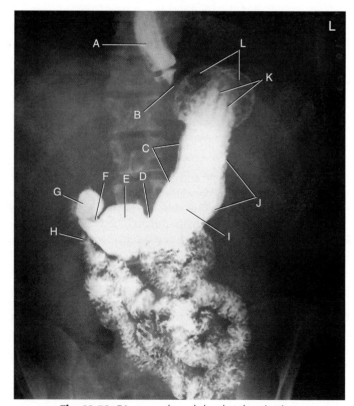

Fig. 12.32 PA stomach and duodenal projection.

Digestion

MECHANICAL DIGESTION

Digestion can be divided into a **mechanical process** and a **chemical component.** Mechanical digestion includes all movements of the gastrointestinal tract, beginning in the oral cavity (mouth) with chewing, or **mastication** *(mas"-ti-ka'-shun),* and continuing in the pharynx and esophagus with swallowing, or **deglutition** (Table 12.3).

Peristaltic activity can be detected in the lower esophagus and in the remainder of the alimentary canal. The passage of solid or semisolid food from the mouth to the stomach takes 4 to 8 seconds, whereas liquids pass in about 1 second.

The stomach, acting as a reservoir for food and fluid, also acts as a large mixing bowl. Peristalsis moves the gastric contents toward the pyloric valve, but this valve opens selectively. If it is closed, the stomach contents are churned or mixed with stomach fluids into a semifluid mass termed **chyme.** When the valve opens, small amounts of chyme are passed into the duodenum by **stomach peristalsis.** Gastric emptying is a slow process, taking 2 to 6 hours for the stomach to empty totally after an average meal. Food with high carbohydrate content leaves the stomach in several hours, whereas food with high protein or fat content moves through much more slowly.

The small intestine (small bowel) continues mechanical digestion with a churning motion within segments of the small bowel. This churning or mixing activity is termed **rhythmic segmentation.** Rhythmic segmentation is intended to mix food and digestive juices thoroughly. The digested food is also brought into contact with the intestinal lining, or mucosa, to facilitate absorption. **Peristalsis** is again present to propel intestinal contents along the alimentary canal. However, peristaltic contractions in the small intestine are much weaker and slower than contractions in the esophagus and stomach. Chyme moves through the small intestine at about 1 cm/min. Chyme normally takes 3 to 5 hours to pass through the entire small intestine.

CHEMICAL DIGESTION

Chemical digestion includes all the chemical changes that food undergoes as it travels through the alimentary canal (Box 12.1). Six different classes of substances are ingested: (1) **carbohydrates,** or complex sugars; (2) **proteins;** (3) **lipids** *(lip'-idz),* or **fats;** (4) **vitamins;** (5) **minerals;** and (6) **water.** Only carbohydrates, proteins, and lipids must be chemically digested to be absorbed. Vitamins, minerals, and water are useful in the form in which the body absorbs them.

Chemical digestion is sped up by various **enzymes.** Enzymes are **biologic catalysts** found in various digestive juices produced by salivary glands in the mouth and by the stomach, small bowel, and pancreas. These various enzymes are organic compounds, which are proteins. They accelerate chemical changes in other substances without appearing in the final products of the reaction.

Digested Substances and Resultant By-Products

1. **Carbohydrate** digestion of starches begins in the mouth and stomach and is completed in the small intestine. The end products of digestion of these complex sugars are **simple sugars.**
2. **Protein** digestion begins in the stomach and is completed in the small intestine. The end products of protein digestion are **amino acids.**
3. **Lipid,** or fat, digestion essentially occurs only in the small bowel, although small amounts of the enzyme necessary for fat digestion are found in the stomach. The end products of lipid digestion are **fatty acids** and **glycerol** *(glis'-er-ol).*

Bile, manufactured by the liver and stored in the gallbladder, is released into the duodenum to assist in the breakdown of lipids (fats). Bile contains no enzymes, but it does emulsify fats. During emulsification, large fat droplets are broken down to small fat droplets, which have greater surface area (to volume) and give enzymes greater access for the breakdown of lipids. The end products of fat (or lipids) during digestion are **fatty acids** and **glycerol.**

Most of the absorption of digestive end products occurs in the small intestine. Simple sugars, amino acids, fatty acids, glycerol, water, and most salts and vitamins are absorbed into the bloodstream or the lymphatic system through the lining of the small intestine. Limited absorption takes place in the stomach and may include some water, alcohol, vitamins, and certain drugs but no nutrients. Any residues of digestion or unabsorbed digestive products are eliminated from the large bowel as a component of feces.

TABLE 12.3 SUMMARY OF MECHANICAL DIGESTION

Oral cavity (teeth and tongue)	Mastication (chewing)
	Deglutition (swallowing)
Pharynx	Deglutition
Esophagus	Deglutition
	Peristalsis (waves of muscular contraction) (1–8 sec)
Stomach	Mixing (chyme)
	Peristalsis (2–6 hr)
Small intestine (small bowel)	Rhythmic segmentation (churning)
	Peristalsis (3–5 hr)

BOX 12.1 SUMMARY OF CHEMICAL DIGESTION

SUBSTANCES INGESTED, DIGESTED, AND ABSORBED

1. Carbohydrates (complex sugars) × simple sugars (mouth and stomach)
2. Proteins × amino acids (stomach and small bowel)
3. Lipids (fats) × fatty acids and glycerol (small bowel only)

SUBSTANCES INGESTED BUT NOT DIGESTED

4. Vitamins
5. Minerals
6. Water

ENZYMES (DIGESTIVE JUICES)

Biologic catalysts

BILE (FROM GALLBLADDER)

Emulsification of fats

SUMMARY

Three primary functions of the digestive system are accomplished within the alimentary canal (Box 12.2).

1. **Ingestion** or **digestion** takes place in the oral cavity, pharynx, esophagus, stomach, and small intestine.
2. Digestive end products, along with water, vitamins, and minerals, are **absorbed** primarily by the small intestine and to a very small degree by the stomach and are transported into the circulatory system.
3. Unused or unnecessary solid material is **eliminated** by the large intestine. (Digestive functions of the large intestine are described in Chapter 13.)

Body Habitus

The type of body habitus has a major impact on the location of gastrointestinal organs within the abdominal cavity. To position for gastrointestinal procedures accurately and consistently, one must know and understand the characteristics of each of these classes of body habitus. The four general classes of body habitus are shown in Fig. 12.33.

BODY TYPE CLASSIFICATIONS

Hypersthenic Body Type

In the hypersthenic body type (Fig. 12.34), the chest and abdomen are quite broad and deep from front to back. The lungs are short, and the diaphragm is high. The transverse colon is also quite high, and the entire **large intestine** extends to the periphery of the abdominal cavity. This body type generally requires two radiographs placed landscape to include the entire large intestine.

The location of the **gallbladder** is associated with the duodenal bulb and pylorus region of the stomach. For a hypersthenic patient, the gallbladder is high and almost transverse. It lies well to the right of midline in the upper abdominal cavity. The **stomach** is also very high and assumes a transverse position. The level of the stomach extends from approximately T9 to T12, with the center of the stomach about 1 inch (2.5 cm) distal to the xiphoid process. The duodenal bulb is at the approximate level of **T11 or T12**, to the right of midline.

Hyposthenic/Asthenic Body Type

The hyposthenic/asthenic body type is more slender and typically has long, narrow lungs, with a low diaphragm. This pushes the **large intestine** down into the low abdominal and pelvic cavities.

The **stomach** is J shaped and low in the abdominal cavity, extending from approximately T11 down to L5 or lower. The vertical portion of the stomach is to the left of midline, with the duodenal bulb near the midline at the level of **L3 or L4.**

The **gallbladder** is near the midline, at the level of the iliac crest, approximately at L3 to L4.

Sthenic Body Type

The sthenic body type (Fig. 12.35) is a more slender version of the hypersthenic classification. The **stomach** is also J shaped and is located lower within the abdominal cavity than in the hypersthenic body type. It generally extends from T11 down to L2. The duodenal bulb is at the approximate level of **L1 to L2,** to the right of the midline. The **gallbladder** is less transverse and lies midway between the lateral abdominal wall and midline. The **left colic (splenic) flexure** of the **large intestine** is often quite high, resting under the left diaphragm.

ADDITIONAL FACTORS

In addition to body habitus, other factors that may affect the position of the stomach include **stomach contents, respiration, body position** (erect versus recumbent), **previous abdominal surgeries,** and **age.** Because the upper stomach is attached to the diaphragm, whether one is in full inspiration or expiration affects the superior extent of the stomach. All abdominal organs tend to drop

1 to 2 inches (2.5 to 5 cm) in an erect position, or even farther with age and loss of muscle tone. As a technologist, correct localization of the stomach and other organs for different body types in various positions comes with positioning practice.

BOX 12.2 SUMMARY OF PRIMARY FUNCTIONS OF DIGESTIVE SYSTEM

1. INGESTION AND DIGESTION

Oral cavity
Pharynx
Esophagus
Stomach
Small intestine

2. ABSORPTION

Small intestine (and stomach)

3. ELIMINATION

Large intestine

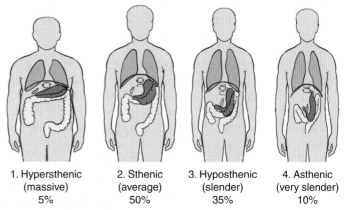

1. Hypersthenic (massive) 5%
2. Sthenic (average) 50%
3. Hyposthenic (slender) 35%
4. Asthenic (very slender) 10%

Fig. 12.33 Body habitus—four body types.

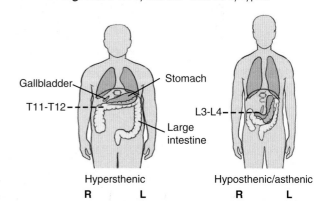

Gallbladder
Stomach
T11-T12
L3-L4
Large intestine

Hypersthenic
R   L

Hyposthenic/asthenic
R   L

Fig. 12.34 Hypersthenic body type compared with hyposthenic/asthenic type.

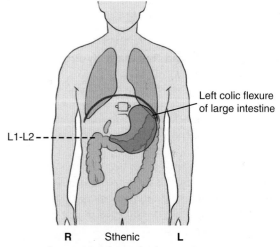

Left colic flexure of large intestine

L1-L2

R   Sthenic   L

Fig. 12.35 Sthenic body type (average).

Radiographs of Upper Gastrointestinal Tract Demonstrating Body Types

Most people do not fall clearly into one of the distinct three body types but are a combination of these types. The technologist must be able to evaluate each patient for probable stomach and gallbladder locations.

The radiographic and photographic body type examples demonstrate the position and location of the stomach on the three most common body types (Figs. 12.36 to 12.41). The location of the stomach and duodenal bulb in relation to specific vertebrae should be noted, in addition to the iliac crest and lower costal margin positioning landmarks.

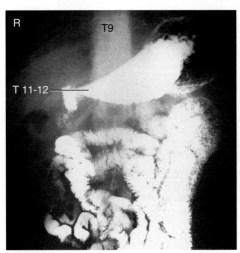

Fig. 12.36 Hypersthenic body type. **General stomach**—high and transverse, level T9 to T12. **Pyloric portion**—level T11 to T12, at midline. **Duodenal bulb location**—level T11 to T12, to right of midline.

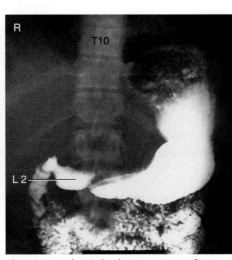

Fig. 12.37 Sthenic body type. **General stomach**—level T10 to L2. **Pyloric portion**—level L2, near midline. **Duodenal bulb location**—level L1 to L2, near midline.

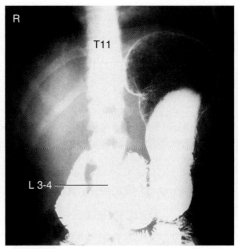

Fig. 12.38 Hyposthenic/asthenic body type. **General stomach**—low and vertical, level T11 to L5. **Pyloric portion**—level L3 to L4, to left of midline. **Duodenal bulb location**—level L3 to L4, at midline.

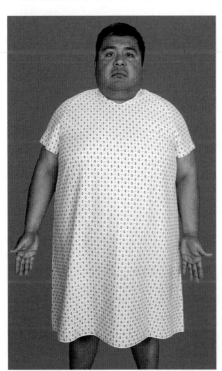

Fig. 12.39 Hypersthenic body type. Generally more in the broad shoulders and hips and potentially a short torso (less distance between lower rib cage and iliac crest). Abdominal cavity is widest at upper margin.

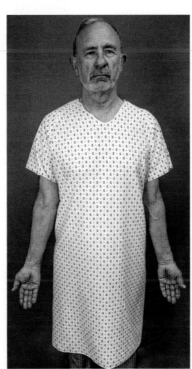

Fig. 12.40 Sthenic body type. Near average in weight and length of torso (may be heavier than average, with some hypersthenic characteristics).

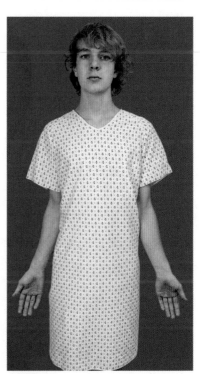

Fig. 12.41 Hyposthenic/asthenic body type. Generally thin with potentially a long torso. (This example is between hyposthenic and asthenic.) Abdominal cavity is widest at lower margin for a true asthenic.

RADIOGRAPHIC PROCEDURES

Similarities

Radiographic procedures or examinations of the entire alimentary canal are similar in three general aspects.

First, because most parts of the gastrointestinal tract are comparable in density with the tissues surrounding them, some type of **contrast medium** must be added to visualize these structures. Ordinarily, the only parts of the alimentary canal that can be easily identified on plain radiographs are the fundus of the stomach (in the upright position), because of the gastric air bubble, and parts of the large intestine, because of pockets of gas and collections of fecal matter.

Most of the alimentary canal simply blends in with the surrounding structures and cannot be visualized without the use of contrast media. This fact is illustrated by comparison of a noncontrast abdominal radiograph (Fig. 12.42) with an upper GI series radiograph with barium sulfate used as a contrast medium (Fig. 12.43).

A **second** similarity is that the initial stage of each radiographic examination of the alimentary canal is carried out with **fluoroscopy** (Fig. 12.44). Fluoroscopy allows the radiologist to (1) observe the gastrointestinal tract in motion, (2) produce radiographic images during the course of the examination, and (3) determine the most appropriate course of action for a complete radiographic examination. Radiographic examination of the upper gastrointestinal tract requires dynamic viewing of organs in motion. The structures in this area assume a wide variety of shapes and sizes, depending on body habitus, age, and other individual differences.

In addition, the functional activity of the alimentary canal exhibits a wide range of differences that are considered within normal limits. In addition to these variations, numerous abnormal conditions exist, making it important that these organs be viewed directly by fluoroscopy.

A **third** similarity is that **radiographic images are recorded during and after the fluoroscopic examination** to provide a permanent record of the normal or abnormal findings. In Fig. 12.45, the patient has been positioned for a postfluoroscopic radiograph following fluoroscopic evaluation of the upper gastrointestinal tract. The positioning section of this chapter describes the most common postfluoroscopy routine projections for esophagogram and upper GI procedures.

With increased use of **digital fluoroscopy,** the number of postfluoroscopy radiographs has diminished greatly. Most departments rely strictly on the digital images produced during the fluoroscopy examination rather than additional postfluoroscopy radiographs. Digital fluoroscopy is described in greater detail later in this chapter.

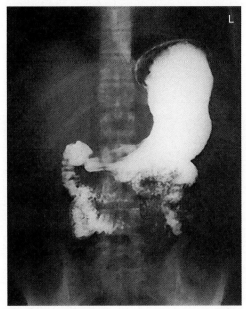

Fig. 12.43 Upper GI image demonstrating barium in the stomach.

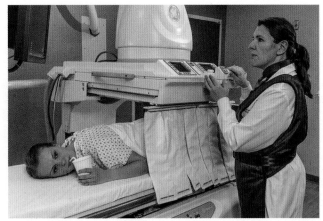

Fig. 12.44 Patient and radiologist ready to begin upper GI fluoroscopy procedure. (Combination digital/spot film system.)

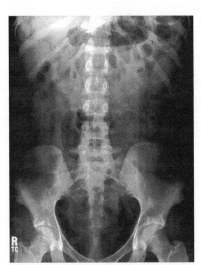

Fig. 12.42 Noncontrast abdominal radiograph.

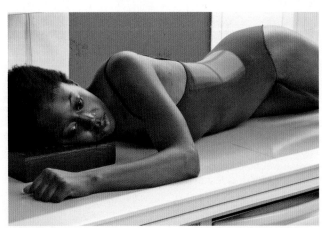

Fig. 12.45 Patient in RAO position for postfluoroscopy imaging.

Contrast Media

Radiolucent and radiopaque contrast media are used to render the gastrointestinal tract visible radiographically.

Radiolucent, or **negative, contrast** media include **swallowed air, CO_2 gas crystals,** and the normally present **gas bubble** in the stomach. Calcium and magnesium citrate carbonate crystals are frequently used to produce CO_2 gas.

BARIUM SULFATE

The most common positive, or radiopaque, contrast medium used to visualize the gastrointestinal system is barium sulfate ($BaSO_4$), which is also referred to simply as *barium*. As illustrated in Fig. 12.46, barium sulfate is a powdered, chalklike substance. The powdered barium sulfate is mixed with water before ingestion by the patient.

This particular compound, which is a salt of barium, is relatively inert because of its extreme insolubility in water and other aqueous solutions, such as acids. All other salts of barium tend to be toxic or poisonous to the human system. Therefore, the barium sulfate used in radiology departments must be chemically pure. Because it does not interact chemically with the body, it rarely produces an allergic reaction. Barium sulfate eventually is expelled rectally after the radiographic procedure.

A mixture of barium sulfate and water forms a **colloidal suspension,** not a solution. For a solution, the molecules of the substance added to water must actually dissolve in the water. **Barium sulfate never dissolves in water.** In a colloidal suspension, the particles suspended in water tend to settle over time when allowed to sit.

Fig. 12.47 shows four cups of different brands of barium that were mixed at a ratio by volume of 1 part water to 1 part barium sulfate. The cups were then allowed to sit for 24 hours. Because different brands of barium sulfate were used, some cups exhibit greater separation or settling than others. This settling demonstrates the need to mix the barium sulfate and water thoroughly just before use.

Most barium sulfate preparations are prepackaged; water is added to the cup followed by mixing. Some barium sulfate preparations come in a liquid form, which does not require water to be added but must still be shaken thoroughly before the procedure is performed. Most of these preparations contain finely divided barium sulfate in a special suspending agent, so they resist settling and stay in suspension longer. However, no matter the manufacturer or packaging, all barium suspensions must be mixed well just before use.

Each brand may come in a variety of smells and flavors, such as apple, chocolate, chocolate malt, vanilla, lemon, lime, or strawberry. This is in an effort to make the barium sulfate more palatable for the patient during the procedure.

Thin Barium

Barium sulfate may be prepared or purchased in a relatively thin or thick mixture. The thin barium sulfate and water mixture contained in a cup, as illustrated in Fig. 12.48, contains **1 part $BaSO_4$ to 1 part water.** Thin barium has the consistency of a thin milkshake and is used to study the entire gastrointestinal tract. Thin barium mixtures, on average, consist of 60% weight-to-volume (w/v) of barium sulfate to water.

The motility, or speed, with which barium sulfate passes through the gastrointestinal tract depends on the suspending medium and additives, the temperature, and the consistency of the preparation, in addition to the general condition of the patient and the gastrointestinal tract. Mixing the preparation exactly according to radiologist preferences and departmental protocol is most important. When the mixture is cold, the chalky taste is much less objectionable.

Thick Barium

Thick barium contains **3 or 4 parts $BaSO_4$ to 1 part water** and should have the consistency of cooked cereal (Fig. 12.49). Thick

barium is more difficult to swallow but is well suited for use in the esophagus because it descends slowly and tends to coat the mucosal lining. Some commercially prepared thick barium sulfate may possess a 98% w/v of barium to water.

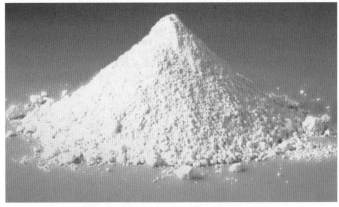

Fig. 12.46 Barium sulfate ($BaSO_4$).

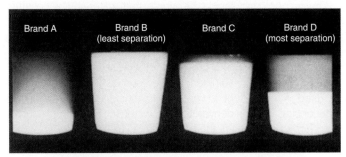

Fig. 12.47 Cups of barium.

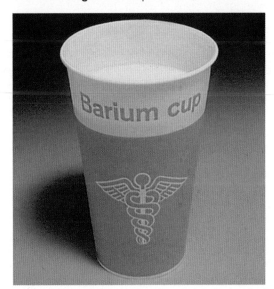

Fig. 12.48 Thin barium sulfate and water mixture (1 part barium to 1 part water).

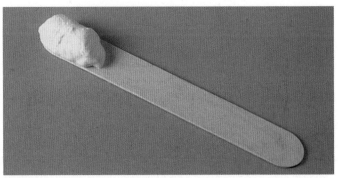

Fig. 12.49 Thick barium sulfate mixture (3 or 4 parts barium to 1 part water).

12

Contraindications to Barium Sulfate

Barium sulfate mixtures are contraindicated if **there is any chance that the mixture might escape into the peritoneal cavity.** If large amounts of barium sulfate escape into the peritoneal cavity, this can lead to intestinal infarcts or peritonitis. This escape may occur through a perforated viscus or during surgery that follows the radiographic procedure. In either of these two cases, **water-soluble, iodinated contrast media** should be used. One example of this type of contrast media is MD-Gastroview, which is shown in Fig. 12.50. This water-soluble contrast agent contains 37% organically bound iodine, which opacifies the gastrointestinal tract. It can be removed easily by aspiration before or during surgery. If any of this water-soluble material escapes into the peritoneal cavity, the body can readily absorb it. Barium sulfate is not absorbed.

One drawback to the water-soluble materials is their bitter taste. Although these iodinated contrast media sometimes are mixed with carbonated soft drinks to mask the taste, they often are used "as is" or diluted with water. The patient should be forewarned that the taste may be slightly bitter.

The technologist should be aware that water-soluble contrast agents travel through the gastrointestinal tract faster than barium sulfate. The shorter transit time of water-soluble contrast agents should be kept in mind if delayed images of the stomach or duodenum are ordered.

WARNING: Water-soluble iodinated contrast media **should not be used** if the patient is sensitive to iodine, or if the patient is experiencing severe dehydration. A water-soluble contrast agent often further dehydrates the patient. It has also been reported that a small number of patients are hypersensitive to barium sulfate or the additives. Although this is a rare occurrence, the patient should be observed for any signs of allergic reaction.

DOUBLE CONTRAST

Double-contrast techniques have been used widely to enhance the diagnosis of certain diseases and conditions during upper GI series. Some departments also perform double-contrast esophagograms. Double-contrast procedures using both radiolucent and radiopaque contrast media were developed in Japan, where a high incidence of stomach carcinoma exists.

The **radiopaque** contrast medium is **barium sulfate.** High-density barium is used to coat the stomach mucosa. A premeasured, commercially produced cup of barium is a common choice for departments to supply. The technologist needs only to add water and mix thoroughly.

The **radiolucent** contrast medium is either **room air** or **CO_2 gas.** To introduce room air, small pinprick holes are placed in the patient's straw. As the patient drinks the barium mixture, air is drawn in with it.

CO_2 gas is created when the patient ingests gas-producing crystals. Two common forms of these crystals are **calcium and magnesium citrate.** On reaching the stomach, these crystals **form a large gas bubble.** The gas mixes with the barium and forces the barium sulfate against the stomach mucosa, providing better coating and visibility of the mucosa and its patterns (Fig. 12.51). Longitudinal mucosal folds (rugae) of the stomach are indicated by the arrows in Fig. 12.52. Potential polyps, diverticula, and ulcers are better demonstrated with a double-contrast technique.

POSTEXAMINATION ELIMINATION (DEFECATION)

One of the functions of the large intestine is to absorb water. Any barium sulfate mixture remaining in the large intestine after an upper GI series or barium enema may become solidified. Consequently, the barium may be difficult to evacuate. Some patients may require a laxative after these examinations to help remove the barium sulfate. If laxatives are contraindicated, the patient should increase fluid or fiber intake until stools are free from all traces of the white barium.

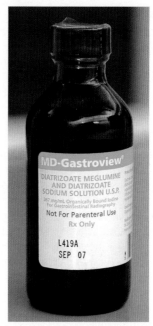

Fig. 12.50 Example of water-soluble iodinated contrast medium.

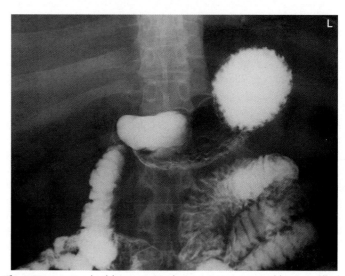

Fig. 12.51 UGI—double contrast; demonstrates gas and barium-filled stomach.

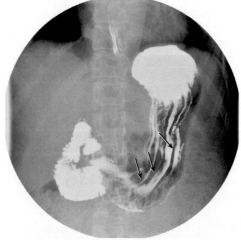

Fig. 12.52 UGI—double contrast; demonstrates gas and barium-filled stomach, with mucosal folds lined with barium.

Digital Fluoroscopy

A **C-arm digital fluoroscopy unit** is shown in Fig. 12.53. In this position, the x-ray tube is on the lower portion of the C-arm, and the image intensifier is on the upper portion. This type of digital fluoroscopy unit is very versatile. It can be rotated around the patient in any position for various types of special procedures, including invasive angiography studies, as described in Chapter 17.

DIGITAL RADIOGRAPHY-FLUOROSCOPY

A digital radiography-fluoroscopy (R/F) system is shown in Fig. 12.54. This type of combination radiography-fluoroscopy system is commonly used for gastrointestinal procedures. The digital R/F system incorporates digital fluoroscopy capabilities with a conventional type of x-ray table and an "under-the-table" fluoroscopy x-tube. It also includes a separate **radiography tube** for conventional "overhead" radiography applications.

Digital fluoroscopy is similar to conventional fluoroscopy with the addition of a **flat panel detector** and a **computer** for image manipulation and storage. A thin film transistor is incorporated within the system to convert the x-ray energy into a digital signal. From there, the image information is transferred to a computer for manipulation and storage. The system's hard drive stores a limited number of images. When the examination is completed, these images are sent to a Picture Archiving and Communication System (PACS) or are printed via a laser printer.

A computer workstation provides software capabilities for image manipulations. Images can be displayed on high-resolution monitors for evaluation or interpretation. The use of digital fluoroscopy permits gastrointestinal studies to remain in a digital format that can be sent to various locations inside and outside the hospital. Digital fluoroscopy has led to the expanded use of PACS, which is a digital imaging network that provides the ability to store, retrieve, manipulate, and print specific examinations at various locations. As described in greater detail in Chapter 1, PACS ties together all digital imaging modalities, such as ultrasound, nuclear medicine, magnetic resonance imaging (MRI), and radiography, into a digital community where radiologists, technologists, and referring physicians can access these images. The concept of the "film room" is becoming obsolete.

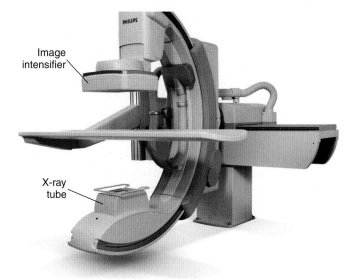

Fig. 12.53 C-arm digital fluoroscopy unit. (Courtesy Philips Medical Systems.)

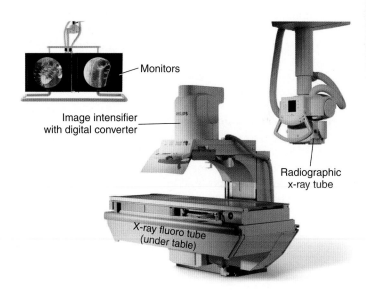

Fig. 12.54 Combination digital R/F system. (Courtesy Philips Medical Systems.)

Optional Postfluoroscopy Images

The question of whether to take images routinely after fluoroscopy is decided by the radiologist or by departmental protocol. Frequently, sufficient digital images are recorded of the entire gastrointestinal tract in various positions during fluoroscopy that no postfluoroscopy images are required. Elimination of these images can result in decreased examination times and patient exposure for upper and lower GI series procedures.

Multiple Frame Formatting and Multiple "Original" Films

If requested, multiple images can be formatted and printed on one piece of laser film. This format can be 4 on 1 (Fig. 12.55), 6 on 1, 9 on 1, or 12 on 1. "Hard copy" films can be printed at any time and as often as desired. If radiographs are lost or misplaced or if duplicates are needed, additional "original" films can be reprinted at any time.

Cine Loop Capability

Individual images also can be recorded in rapid succession and displayed as moving or cine images. This feature is beneficial for certain studies, such as an esophagogram for possible esophageal reflux or impaired swallowing mechanisms. This capability has replaced the need for spot film cameras or video recording. When the study has been completed, the technologist can play back the cine loop to demonstrate the dynamic flow of barium through the esophagus or stomach. The radiologist can interpret the study from a monitor located in an office or reading room.

Image Enhancement and Manipulation

Digital fluoroscopy images can be enhanced and manipulated with the use of post-processing tools (Figs. 12.56 and 12.57). These image enhancement and manipulation features include edge enhancement, window and leveling, dynamic range control, and dual energy subtraction. Other options include inverting the image contrast, motion artifact control, and smoothing. With the study saved on the hard disk, the technologist or radiologist has the ability to alter these imaging parameters at will.

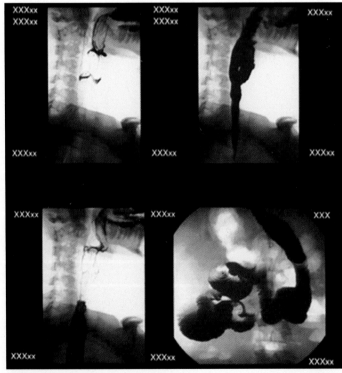

Fig. 12.55 Multiple-frame upper GI images—four images on one 14 × 17-inch (35 × 43-cm) film.

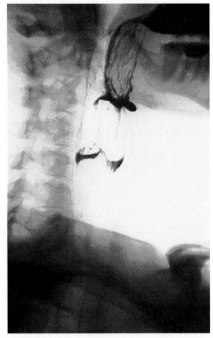

Fig. 12.56 Digital fluoroscopy of upper GI image without equalization filter.

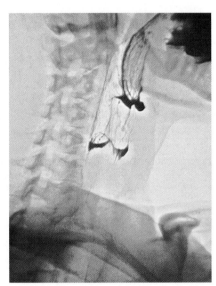

Fig. 12.57 Digital fluoroscopy of upper GI image with equalization filter.

WORKER PROTECTION DURING FLUOROSCOPY

Radiation protection practices during fluoroscopy are described in Chapter 1.

Exposure Patterns

Exposure patterns and related doses within the fluoroscopy room, indicating where one should stand or not stand in the room during fluoroscopy, also are provided in Chapter 1. Fig. 12.58 demonstrates these exposure patterns, which remind the assisting technologist *not* to stand close to the table on either side of the radiologist, but rather to **stay back** from the **higher scatter fields** as much as possible throughout the fluoroscopy procedure.

Lead Drape Shield

The flexible **lead tower drape shield** attached to the front of the fluoroscopic and spot film device is very important and should be inspected regularly to ensure it is not damaged or improperly placed (see Fig. 12.68).

Bucky Slot Shield

The technologist should always ensure the **bucky is all the way to the end of the table** before beginning a fluoroscopic procedure, which then brings out the metal **bucky slot shield** to cover the approximately 2 inches (5 cm) of space directly under the tabletop (Fig. 12.59). This shield significantly reduces scatter radiation resulting from the fluoroscopy x-ray tube located under the table. Leakage or scatter rays can escape through this waist-high bucky space if the bucky shield is not completely out on this type of system.

The requirement of the bucky at the end of the table during fluoroscopy not only is important for worker protection but also is necessary to keep the bucky mechanism from the path of the fluoroscopy x-ray tube under the table.

Lead Aprons

Protective aprons of 0.5-mm lead equivalency (Pb/Eq) must always be worn during fluoroscopy. Some technologists and radiologists may also choose to wear **lead-equivalent (Pb-Eq) protective eyewear** and **thyroid shields** (Fig. 12.60).

Before the radiologist or technologist places a hand into the fluoroscopy beam, a **leaded glove** must always be worn, and the beam must be first attenuated by the patient's body. The use of a **compression paddle** (see Fig. 12.70) is an even better alternative when compression of the patient's abdomen is required.

Cardinal Principles of Radiation Protection

One of the best ways to reduce worker dose during fluoroscopy is to apply the following three "cardinal principles of radiation protection." If these principles are applied correctly, dose to both the fluoroscopist and the technologist can be greatly reduced.

1. **Time:** Reduce the amount of time the fluoroscopy tube is energized. Although most procedures are performed by radiologists and the amount of fluoroscopy time is controlled by them, the technologist should also keep track of fluoroscopy time. If fluoroscopy time becomes excessive, the situation should be discussed with a supervisor. The use of "intermittent fluoroscopy" reduces dose to the patient and workers. With digital fluoroscopy, the "image freeze" function should be used, which allows the last energized image to remain visible on the monitor. Then the fluoroscopy tube is activated only when a new image is required.
2. **Shielding:** Follow all shielding precautions described previously, including correct use of the **lead drape shield,** the **bucky slot shield,** and **lead gloves.**
3. **Distance:** The most effective method of reducing dose during fluoroscopy procedures is to increase the distance between the x-ray tube and the technologist. By applying the inverse square law, technologists can significantly reduce dose to themselves. Doubling the distance between the x-ray tube and the worker can reduce dose by a factor of 4. Technologists should maximize their distance from the x-ray tube when not assisting the radiologist or managing the patient. See Table 12.4 for a summary of technologist protection devices.[4]

TABLE 12.4 **TECHNOLOGIST PROTECTION SUMMARY CHART**	
PROTECTIVE DEVICES4	**BENEFIT**
Fluoroscopy leaded tower drape (0.25 mm Pb/Eq minimum)	Greatly reduces exposure to fluoroscopy personnel
Protective lead apron (0.5 mm Pb/Eq minimum)	Reduces exposure to torso during fluoroscopy
Lead gloves (0.25 mm Pb/Eq minimum)	Reduces exposure to hands and wrists
Bucky slot shield (0.25 mm Pb/Eq minimum)	Reduces exposure to gonadal region
Protective eyewear (0.35 mm Pb/Eq minimum)	Reduces exposure to lenses of the eye
Thyroid shield (0.5 mm Pb/Eq minimum)	Reduces exposure to thyroid gland
Compression paddle	Reduces exposure to arm and hand of fluoroscopist

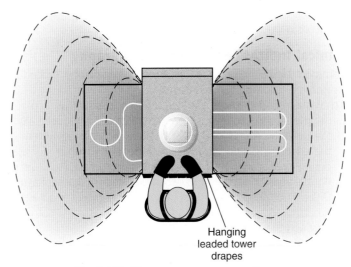

Fig. 12.58 Fluoroscopy exposure patterns.

Hanging leaded tower drapes

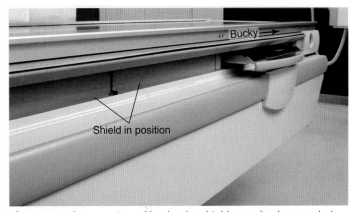

Fig. 12.59 Close-up view of bucky slot shield completely extended with bucky tray at far end of table.

Bucky

Shield in position

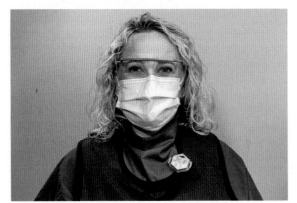

Fig. 12.60 Lead apron, with thyroid shield, and lead glasses.

Esophagography Procedure

Two common radiographic procedures of the upper gastrointestinal system involving the administration of contrast media are the **esophagography** and the **upper GI series.** Each of these procedures is described in detail, beginning with the esophagography

DEFINITION AND PURPOSE

Esophagography is the common radiographic procedure or examination of the **pharynx** and **esophagus** in which a radiopaque contrast medium is used. Occasionally, a negative or radiolucent contrast medium may be used.

The purpose of an esophagography is to demonstrate radiographically the form and function of the pharynx and esophagus.

CONTRAINDICATIONS

No major contraindications exist for esophagography except possible sensitivity to the contrast media used. The technologist should determine whether the patient has a history of sensitivity to barium sulfate or water-soluble contrast media.

Clinical Indications for Esophagography

Common clinical indications for an esophagography procedure include the following conditions.

Achalasia *(ak″-a-la′-zha),* also termed *cardiospasm,* is a motor disorder of the esophagus in which peristalsis is reduced along the distal two-thirds of the esophagus. Achalasis is evident at the esophagogastric sphincter because of its inability to relax during swallowing. The thoracic esophagus may also lose its normal peristaltic activity and become dilated (megaesophagus). Digital fluoroscopy is most helpful in the diagnosis of achalasia. It occurs equally in males and females and is most common between the ages of 20 and 40 years.[3]

Anatomic anomalies may be congenital or may be caused by disease, such as cancer of the esophagus. Patients who have a stroke often develop impaired swallowing mechanisms. Certain foods and contrast agents are administered during the examination for evaluation of swallowing patterns. A speech pathologist may perform the study to understand better the speech and swallowing patterns of the patient. Digital fluoroscopy is used during these studies.

Barrett esophagus, or *Barrett syndrome,* is the replacement of the normal squamous epithelium with columnar-lined epithelium ulcer tissue in the mid-to-lower esophagus (Fig. 12.61). This replacement may produce a stricture in the distal esophagus. In advanced cases, a peptic ulcer may develop in the distal esophagus. The esophagogram may demonstrate subtle tissue changes in the esophagus, but **nuclear medicine** is the modality of choice for this condition. The patient is injected with technetium-99m pertechnetate to demonstrate the shift in tissue types in the esophagus.

Carcinoma of the esophagus includes one of the most common malignancies of the esophagus, **adenocarcinoma** (Fig. 12.62). Advanced symptoms include dysphagia (difficulty in swallowing), localized pain during meals, and bleeding. Other tumors of the esophagus include **carcinosarcoma,** which often produces a large, irregular polyp, and **pseudocarcinoma.** An esophagography and endoscopy are performed to detect these tumors. The esophagography may demonstrate atrophic changes in the mucosa caused by invasion of the tumor and stricture. CT may be performed in staging of the tumor and determining whether it has extended beyond the inner layer of mucosa of the esophagus.

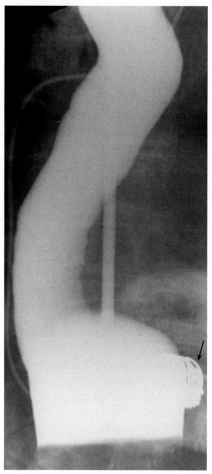

Fig. 12.61 Barrett esophagus. Ulcerations *(arrow)* have developed at some distance from esophagogastric junction.

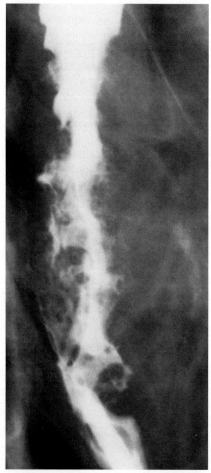

Fig. 12.62 Esophagography—carcinoma of esophagus. (From Eisenberg RL, Johnson NM. *Comprehensive radiographic pathology,* ed 7, St. Louis, 2021, Elsevier.)

Dysphagia *(dis-fa'-je-a)* is difficulty swallowing. This difficulty may be due to a congenital or acquired condition, a trapped bolus of food, paralysis of the pharyngeal or esophageal muscles, or inflammation. Narrowing or an enlarged, flaccid appearance of the esophagus may be seen during the esophagography, depending on the cause of the dysphagia. Digital fluoroscopy is the modality of choice.

Esophageal varices are characterized by dilation of the veins in the wall of the distal esophagus (Fig. 12.63). This condition is often seen with acute liver disease, such as cirrhosis secondary to increased portal hypertension. With restriction in venous flow through the liver, the coronary veins in the distal esophagus become dilated, tortuous, and engorged with blood. In advanced cases, the veins may begin to bleed. Advanced esophageal varices manifest with narrowing of the distal third of the esophagus and a "wormlike" or "cobblestone" appearance caused by enlarged veins during an esophagogram.

Foreign bodies that patients may ingest include a bolus of food, metallic objects, and other materials that lodge in the esophagus (Fig. 12.64). Locations and dimensions may be determined during an esophagography. Radiolucent foreign bodies, such as fish bones, may require the use of additional materials and techniques for detection. Cotton may be shredded and placed in a cup of barium and then swallowed by the patient. The intent of this technique is to cause a tuft of the cotton to be caught by the radiolucent foreign body and show its location under fluoroscopy. Although this technique has been used for decades, most gastroenterologists prefer the use of endoscopy to isolate and remove these foreign bodies.

Gastroesophageal reflux disease (GERD), or **esophageal reflux,** is the entry of gastric contents into the esophagus, irritating the lining of the esophagus. Esophageal reflux is reported as heartburn by most patients. This condition may lead to **esophagitis** demonstrated by an irregular or ulcerative appearance of the mucosa of the esophagus. Although specific causes for GERD or esophageal reflux have not been confirmed, cigarette smoking and excessive intake of aspirin, alcohol, and caffeine increase the incidence of reflux. It is also common in newborns up to 3 months but often resolves on its own.[3]

Specific methods used to demonstrate esophageal reflux during fluoroscopy are discussed later in this chapter. In advanced cases, the distal esophagus demonstrates longitudinal streaks during an esophagography because of changes in the mucosa. Endoscopy is often performed to detect early signs of GERD.

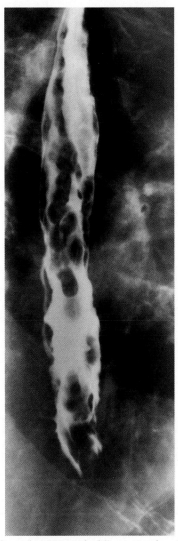

Fig. 12.63 Esophageal varices with diffuse round and oval filling defects. (From Eisenberg RL, Johnson NM. *Comprehensive radiographic pathology,* ed 7, St. Louis, 2021, Elsevier.)

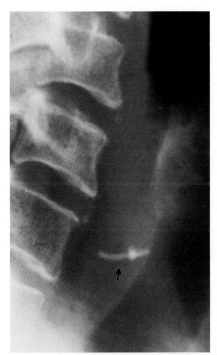

Fig. 12.64 Fish bone *(arrow)* in lower cervical portion of esophagus. (From Eisenberg RL, Johnson NM. *Comprehensive radiographic pathology,* ed 7, St. Louis, 2021, Elsevier.)

Zenker diverticulum is characterized by a large outpouching of the esophagus just above the upper esophageal sphincter (Fig. 12.65). It is believed to be caused by weakening of the muscle wall. Because of the size of the diverticulum, the patient may experience dysphagia, aspiration, and regurgitation of food eaten hours earlier. Although medication can reduce the symptoms of Zenker diverticulum, surgery may be required.

See Table 12.5 for a summary of clinical indications for esophagography.

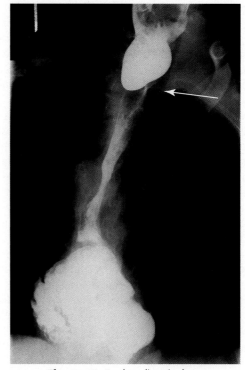

Fig. 12.65 Zenker diverticulum.

TABLE 12.5 SUMMARY OF CLINICAL INDICATIONS: ESOPHAGOGRAPHY

CONDITION OR DISEASE	MOST COMMON RADIOGRAPHIC EXAMINATION	POSSIBLE RADIOGRAPHIC APPEARANCE	EXPOSURE FACTOR ADJUSTMENT[a]
Achalasia	Esophagography with digital fluoroscopy	Stricture or narrowing of esophagus	None
Anatomic anomalies (including foreign bodies)	Esophagography with digital fluoroscopy (functional study) endoscopy employed for foreign bodies	Abnormal peristaltic patterns	None
		Various radiopaque and radiolucent foreign bodies	None
Barrett esophagus	Esophagography or NM scan	Stricture or "streaked" appearance of distal esophagus	None
Carcinoma	Esophagography MRI, and CT scan	Point of stricture, narrowing, or atrophic changes in mucosa	None
Dysphagia	Esophagography with digital fluoroscopy (functional study)	Narrowing or enlargement of esophagus, depending on cause	None
Esophageal varices	Esophagography (and endoscopy)	Narrowing and "wormlike" appearance of esophagus	None
Zenker diverticulum	Esophagography (and endoscopy)	Enlarged recess or cavity in proximal esophagus	None

[a]Dependent on stage or severity of disease or condition.

PATIENT AND ROOM PREPARATION FOR ESOPHAGOGRAM

Because the esophagus is empty most of the time, **patients need no preparation for an esophagography unless an upper GI series is to follow.** When combined with an upper GI, or if the primary interest is the lower esophagus, preparation for the UGI takes precedence.

For an esophagography only, all clothing and anything metallic between the mouth and the waist should be removed, and the patient should wear a hospital gown. Before the fluoroscopic procedure is performed, a pertinent history should be taken, and each step of the examination should be carefully explained to the patient (Figs. 12.66).

The first part of an esophagus study involves fluoroscopy with a positive-contrast medium. The examination room should be clean, tidy, and appropriately stocked before the patient is escorted to the room. The appropriate amount and type of contrast medium should be ready. Esophagography generally use **both thin and thick barium.** Additional items useful in the detection of a radiolucent foreign body are (1) cotton balls soaked in thin barium, (2) barium pills or gelatin capsules filled with $BaSO_4$, and (3) marshmallows. After swallowing any one of these three substances, the patient is asked to swallow an additional thin barium mixture.

Because the esophagography begins with the table in the vertical position, the footboard should be in place and tested for security. Lead aprons, compression paddle, and lead gloves should be provided for the radiologist, in addition to lead aprons for all other personnel in the room. Proper radiation protection methods must be observed at all times during fluoroscopy.

GENERAL PROCEDURE

Fluoroscopy

With the room prepared and the patient ready, the patient and the radiologist are introduced, and the patient's history and the reason for the examination are discussed (Fig, 12.67). The fluoroscopic examination usually begins with a general survey of the patient's chest, including heart, lungs, diaphragm, and abdomen.

During fluoroscopy, the technologist's duties generally are to follow the radiologist's instructions, assist the patient as needed, and expedite the procedure in any manner possible. Because the examination is begun with the patient in the upright or erect position, a cup of thin barium is placed in the patient's left hand close to the left shoulder. The patient is instructed to follow the radiologist's instructions concerning how much to drink and when. The radiologist observes the flow of barium with the fluoroscope.

Swallowing (deglutition) of thin barium is observed with the patient in various positions. Similar positions may be used while the patient swallows thick barium. The use of thick barium allows better visualization of mucosal patterns and any lesion within the esophagus. The type of barium mixture to be used is determined by the radiologist.

After upright studies have been completed, horizontal and Trendelenburg positions with thick and thin barium may follow. Fig. 12.68 shows a patient in position for an **RAO projection** with a cup of thin barium. The pharynx and the cervical esophagus usually are studied fluoroscopically with spot images, whereas the main portion of the esophagus down to the stomach is studied both with fluoroscopy and with postfluoroscopy imaging.

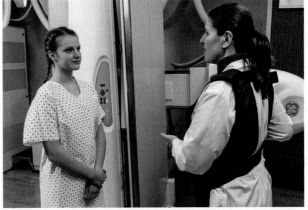

Fig. 12.66 Prepare patient; explain procedure to patient.

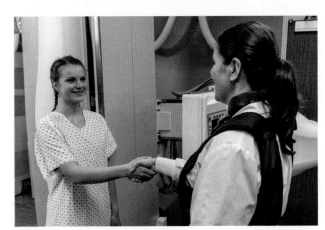

Fig. 12.67 Introduce yourself to the patient and assist the radiologist during the procedure.

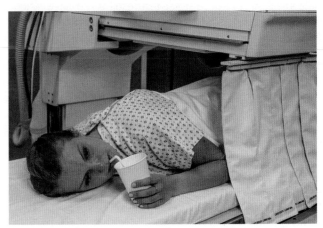

Fig. 12.68 RAO, with cup of thin barium.

DEMONSTRATION OF ESOPHAGEAL REFLUX

The diagnosis of possible esophageal reflux or regurgitation of gastric contents may occur during fluoroscopy or an esophagography. One or more of the following procedures may be performed to detect esophageal reflux:

1. Breathing exercises
2. Water test
3. Compression paddle technique
4. Toe-touch maneuver

Breathing Exercises

Various breathing exercises are designed to increase both intrathoracic and intra-abdominal pressures. The most common breathing exercise is the **Valsalva maneuver.** The patient is asked to take a deep breath and, while holding the breath in, to bear down as though trying to move the bowels. This maneuver forces air against the closed glottis. A modified Valsalva maneuver is accomplished as the patient pinches off the nose, closes the mouth, and tries to blow the nose. The cheeks should expand outward as though the patient were blowing up a balloon.

A **Mueller maneuver** also can be performed as the patient exhales and then tries to inhale against a closed glottis.

With both methods, the increase in intra-abdominal pressure may produce the reflux of ingested barium that would confirm the presence of esophageal reflux. The radiologist carefully observes the esophagogastric junction during these maneuvers.

Water Test

The water test (Fig. 12.69) is done with the patient in the supine position and turned up slightly on the left side. This slight left posterior oblique (LPO) position fills the fundus with barium. The patient is asked to swallow a mouthful of water through a straw. Under fluoroscopy, the radiologist closely observes the esophagogastric junction. A positive water test result is indicated when significant amounts of barium regurgitate into the esophagus from the stomach.

Compression Technique

A compression paddle (Fig. 12.70) can be placed under the patient in the prone position and inflated as needed to provide pressure to the stomach region. The radiologist can demonstrate the obscure esophagogastric junction during this process to detect possible esophageal reflux.

Toe-Touch Maneuver

The toe-touch maneuver (Fig. 12.71) also is performed to study possible regurgitation into the esophagus from the stomach. Under fluoroscopy, the cardiac orifice is observed as the patient bends over and touches the toes. Esophageal reflux and hiatal hernias sometimes are demonstrated with the toe-touch maneuver.

Although the procedures described above still are performed, most cases of esophageal reflux are confirmed through endoscopy.

Postfluoroscopy Imaging

After the fluoroscopy portion of the esophagography, radiographs of the entire barium-filled esophagus are obtained. Positioning routines and descriptions for postfluoroscopy imaging are described in detail in the positioning section of this chapter.

The need for postfluoroscopy imaging for esophagography has been greatly reduced with the use of digital fluoroscopy.

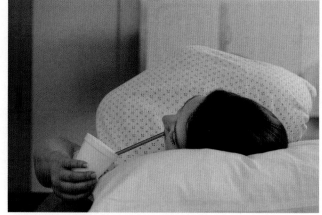

Fig. 12.69 Water test—LPO position.

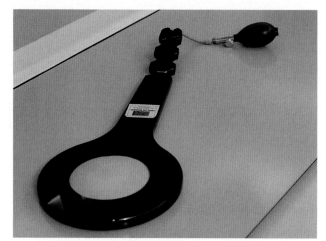

Fig. 12.70 Compression paddle.

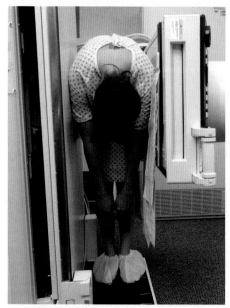

Fig. 12.71 Toe-touch maneuver.

Upper GI Series Procedure

In addition to the esophagography, the second and very common radiographic procedure for examination of the upper GI system involving contrast media is the **upper GI series**.

DEFINITION AND PURPOSE

Radiographic examination of the **distal esophagus, stomach,** and **duodenum** is called an upper GI or UGI.

The purposes of the upper GI are to study radiographically the form and function of the distal esophagus, stomach, and duodenum and to detect abnormal anatomic and functional conditions.

CONTRAINDICATIONS

Contraindications to upper GI examinations apply primarily to the type of contrast media used. If the patient has a history of bowel perforation, laceration, or rupture of the viscus, the use of barium sulfate may be contraindicated. An oral, water-soluble, iodinated contrast medium may be used in place of barium sulfate.

Clinical Indications for Upper GI Series

Common clinical indications for an upper GI series include the following conditions.

Bezoar describes a mass of **undigested material** that becomes trapped in the stomach. This mass usually is made up of hair, certain vegetable fibers, or wood products. The material builds up over time and may form an obstruction in the stomach.

> Specific terms for bezoars include **trichobezoar,** made up of ingested hair, and **phytobezoar,** which is ingested vegetable fiber or seeds.[5] Some patients are unable to break down or process certain vegetable fibers or seeds.
> The upper GI demonstrates the bezoar. Radiographic appearances include a mass defined as a filling defect within the stomach. The bezoar retains a light coating of barium even after the stomach has emptied most of the barium (Fig. 12.72).

Diverticula are pouchlike herniations of a portion of the mucosal wall. They can occur in the stomach or small intestine. Gastric diverticula are generally about ½ inch (1 to 2 cm) but may be as large as 3 inches (8 cm) in diameter. Of gastric diverticula, 70% to 90% arise in the posterior aspect of the fundus. Consequently, the lateral position taken during an upper GI study may be the only projection that demonstrates gastric diverticula. Most gastric diverticula are asymptomatic and are discovered accidentally.

> Although benign, diverticula can lead to perforation if untreated.[5] Other complications include inflammation and ulceration at the site of neoplasm formation. A double-contrast upper GI is recommended to diagnose any tumors or diverticula. An air-filled, barium-lined diverticulum of the duodenal bulb is shown in Fig. 12.73.

Emesis *(em'-e-sis)* is the act of vomiting. Blood in vomit is called **hematemesis** and may indicate that other forms of pathologic processes are present in the gastrointestinal tract.

Gastric carcinomas account for more than 70% of all stomach neoplasms, and 95% of them are adenocarcinomas.[3] Radiographic signs include a large, irregular filling defect within the stomach, marked or nodular edges of the stomach lining, rigidity of the stomach, and associated ulceration of the mucosa.

> The double-contrast upper GI remains the gold standard for the detection of gastric carcinoma. CT or endoscopy may be performed to determine the degree of invasion of the tumor into tissues surrounding the stomach.

Gastritis is an inflammation of the lining or mucosa of the stomach (Fig. 12.74). Gastritis may develop in response to various physiologic and environmental conditions. **Acute gastritis** manifests with severe symptoms of pain and discomfort. **Chronic gastritis** is an intermittent condition that may be brought on by changes in diet, stress, or other factors.

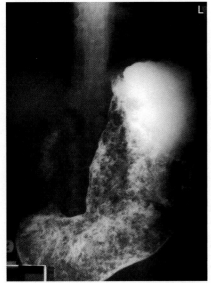

Fig. 12.72 AP stomach projection— very large trichobezoar.

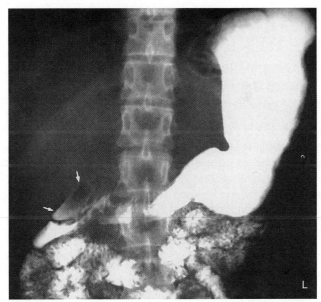

Fig. 12.73 PA stomach projection—diverticulum in duodenum *(arrows)*.

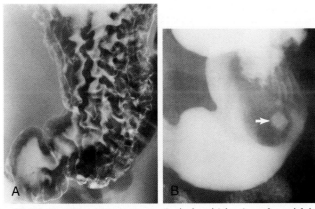

Fig. 12.74 Gastritis. A, Appearance includes thickening of rugal folds throughout stomach. B, Appearance includes some absence of rugal folds. (From Eisenberg RL, Johnson NM. *Comprehensive radiographic pathology,* ed 7, St. Louis, 2021, Elsevier.)

Gastritis is best demonstrated with a double-contrast upper GI. The fine coating of barium demonstrates subtle changes to the mucosal lining. Specific radiographic appearances may include, but are not restricted to, absence of rugae, a thin gastric wall, and "speckled" appearance of the mucosa. Endoscopy also may be performed to inspect the mucosa visually for signs of gastritis.

Hiatal hernia is a condition in which a portion of the stomach herniates through the diaphragmatic opening. The herniation may be slight, but in severe cases, most of the stomach is found within the thoracic cavity above the diaphragm.

Hiatal hernia may be due to a congenitally short esophagus or weakening of the muscle that surrounds the diaphragmatic opening, allowing passage of the esophagus.[5] These hernias are common in 50% of the U.S. population over the age of 50 years.[3] This form of hiatal hernia may occur in both pediatric and adult patients. An adult moderate-size hiatal hernia is shown in Fig. 12.75, in which a portion of the stomach containing air and barium is seen above the diaphragm.

Sliding hiatal hernia is a second type of hiatal hernia that is caused by weakening of a small muscle (esophageal sphincter) located between the terminal esophagus and the diaphragm. The purposes of the esophageal sphincter are to keep the cardiac portion of the stomach below the diaphragm and to produce a high-pressure zone to prevent esophageal reflux. As a result of aging or other factors, this sphincter may weaken and permit a portion of the stomach to herniate through the esophageal hiatus. Because the degree of herniation may vary from time to time, it is termed a *sliding hiatal hernia.* The condition is frequently present at birth, but symptoms of difficulty in swallowing usually do not begin until young adulthood.

NOTE: A sliding hiatal hernia may produce a radiographic sign termed *Schatzki ring,* which is a ring of mucosal tissue (which lines the distal esophagus) that protrudes into the lumen of the esophagus[3,5] (Fig. 12.76).

Hypertrophic pyloric stenosis (HPS) is the most common type of gastric obstruction in infants. It is caused by hypertrophy of the antral muscle at the orifice of the pylorus. Hypertrophy of this muscle produces an obstruction at the pylorus. Symptoms of HPS include projectile vomiting after feedings, acute pain, and possible distention of the abdomen. HPS can be diagnosed during an upper GI. HPS often manifests as distention of the stomach with a small channel (if any at all) of barium passing through the pylorus into the duodenum. Sonography has become the modality of choice in diagnosing HPS. Sonography can measure the diameter and length of the antral muscle to determine whether it is larger (hypertrophic) than normal. It is reported that a muscle thickness greater than 4 mm is a positive sign of HPS.[6] In addition, sonography does not require radiation exposure to the infant or use of contrast media.

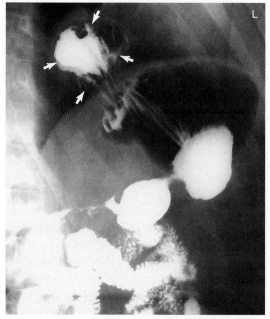

Fig. 12.75 Upper GI—demonstrating hiatal hernia *(arrows).*

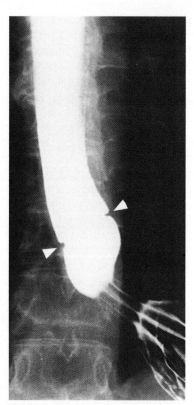

Fig. 12.76 Schatzki ring demonstrated in the case of a sliding hiatal hernia *(arrows).* (The Ohio State University Wexner Medical Center, Columbus, Ohio. In Kowalczyk N. *Radiographic pathology for technologists,* ed 6, St. Louis, 2014, Mosby.)

Ulcers are erosions of the stomach or duodenal mucosa that are caused by various physiologic or environmental conditions, such as excessive gastric secretions, stress, diet, and smoking. Some more recent studies suggest that ulcers may be caused by bacteria and can be treated with antibiotics. If untreated, an ulcer may lead to perforation of the stomach or duodenum.

During an upper GI study, the ulcer appears as a punctate barium collection that may appear to be surrounded by a lucent halo. A small peptic ulcer filled with barium is seen in Fig. 12.77. A double-contrast upper GI is recommended for most ulcer studies. It may be preceded or followed by endoscopy of the upper gastrointestinal tract. Types of ulcers include the following:

- **Duodenal ulcer** is a peptic ulcer situated in the duodenum. These ulcers frequently are located in the second or third aspect of the duodenum. Duodenal ulcers are rarely malignant.[6]
- **Peptic ulcer** describes ulceration of the mucous membrane of the esophagus, stomach, or duodenum, caused by the action of acid gastric juice. The term *peptic ulcer* can be synonymous with *gastric ulcer* or *duodenal ulcer*. Peptic ulcer disease often is preceded by gastritis and is secondary to hyperacidity.
- **Gastric ulcer** is an ulcer of the gastric mucosa.
- **Perforating ulcer** is an ulcer that involves the entire thickness of the wall of the stomach or intestine, creating an opening on both surfaces. Only 5% of all ulcers lead to perforation.[6] If an ulcer becomes perforated, it creates an opening between the intestine and the peritoneal cavity. Radiographic signs include the presence of free air under the diaphragm, as seen with an erect abdomen radiograph. If untreated, this type of ulcer may lead to peritonitis and eventual death.

See Table 12.6 for a summary of clinical indications for the upper GI series.

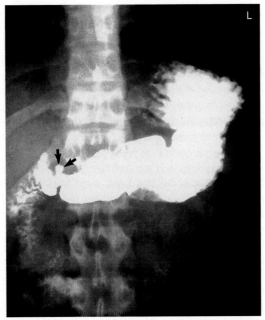

Fig. 12.77 PA stomach projection—peptic ulcer *(arrows)*.

TABLE 12.6 SUMMARY OF CLINICAL INDICATIONS: UPPER GI SERIES

CONDITION OR DISEASE	MOST COMMON RADIOGRAPHIC EXAMINATION	POSSIBLE RADIOGRAPHIC APPEARANCE	EXPOSURE FACTOR ADJUSTMENT[a]
Bezoar Phytobezoar Trichobezoar	Upper GI or endoscopy	Filling defect or ill-defined mass within stomach	None
Diverticula	Double-contrast upper GI	Outpouching of mucosal wall	None
Gastric carcinoma	Double-contrast upper GI	Irregular filling defect within stomach	None
Gastritis	Double-contrast upper GI	Absence of rugae, thin gastric wall, and "speckled" appearance of mucosa with acute cases of gastritis	None
Hiatal hernia (sliding hiatal hernia)	Single-contrast or double-contrast upper GI	Gastric bubble or protruding aspect of stomach above diaphragm or Schatzki ring	None
Hypertrophic pyloric stenosis	Upper GI or sonography	Distention of stomach owing to obstruction of pylorus	None
Ulcer	Double-contrast upper GI	Punctate collection of barium and "halo" sign	None

[a]Dependent on stage or severity of disease or condition.

PATIENT PREPARATION FOR UPPER GI SERIES

The goal of patient preparation for an upper GI series is for the patient to arrive in the radiology department with a completely empty stomach. For an examination scheduled during the morning hours, the patient should be **NPO** from midnight until the time of the examination. Food and fluids should be withheld for at least 8 hours before the examination. **The patient also is instructed not to smoke cigarettes or chew gum during the NPO period.** These activities tend to increase gastric secretions and salivation, which prevents proper coating of barium to the gastric mucosa.

The upper GI series is often a time-consuming procedure, so the patient should be forewarned about the time the examination may take when the appointment is made. This is especially true if the UGI is to be followed by a small bowel series. The importance of an empty stomach also should be stressed when the appointment is made so that the patient arrives properly prepared both physically and psychologically.

PREGNANCY PRECAUTIONS

If the patient is female, a menstrual history must be obtained. Irradiation of an early pregnancy is one of the most hazardous situations in diagnostic radiography.

Radiographic examinations such as the upper GI series that include the pelvis and the uterus in the primary beam, in addition to fluoroscopy, should be done on pregnant women only when absolutely necessary.

In general, abdominal radiographs of a known pregnancy should be delayed at least until the third trimester or, if the patient's condition allows (as determined by the physician), until after the pregnancy. This waiting period is especially important when fluoroscopy, which greatly increases patient exposure, is involved.

ROOM PREPARATION AND FLUOROSCOPY PROCEDURE

Room setup for a UGI series is very similar to that for an esophagogram. The thin barium sulfate mixture is the typical contrast medium of choice for an upper GI series. Occasionally, thick barium may be used in addition to some type of gas-forming preparation. Rarely, water-soluble contrast media are used in preference to the barium sulfate mixture.

The fluoroscopy table is raised to the vertical position, although with some very ill patients, the examination must be started with the table horizontal. Therefore, the footboard should be placed at the end of the table. The room should be clean and tidy, and the control panel should be set up for fluoroscopy. If conventional fluoroscopy is being used, the spot film mechanism should be properly loaded and in working condition. All image receptors for the entire examination should be set aside for easy access. Lead aprons, lead gloves, and the compression paddle should be available for radiologist as well as lead aprons for all other personnel in the room.

Before introduction of the patient and the radiologist, the patient's history must be obtained, and the examination procedure must be carefully explained to the patient.

General duties during fluoroscopy for an upper GI series are similar to those for an esophagogram. The technologist should follow the radiologist's instructions, assist the patient as needed, and expedite the procedure in any manner possible.

The fluoroscopic routine followed by fluoroscopists varies greatly but usually begins with the patient in the upright position (Fig. 12.78). A wide variety of table movements, patient positions, and special maneuvers follow until the fluoroscopy portion of the procedure is complete.

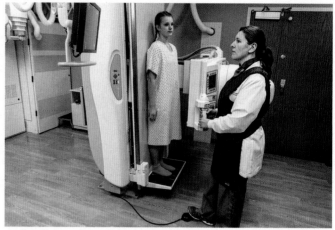

Fig. 12.78 Fluoroscopy— patient positioned for upper GI tract procedure.

PATIENT AND TABLE MOVEMENTS

Various patient positions combined with table movements are used during the fluoroscopic procedure (Fig. 12.79). The technologist must help the patient with the barium cup, provide a pillow when the patient is lying down, and keep the patient adequately covered at all times. The barium cup should be held by the patient in the left hand near the left shoulder whenever the patient is upright. The cup must be taken from the patient when the table is tilted up or down.

Part of the technologist's responsibility is to watch the patient's hands and fingers during table movements. Sometimes, holding onto the edge of the table can result in pinched fingers. The radiologist is occupied by watching the fluoroscopy screen or the monitor during these moves and may not be able to see the patient's hands.

The RAO position, illustrated in Fig. 12.80, allows barium to migrate toward the pyloric portion or distal stomach, whereas any air in the stomach shifts toward the fundus.

POSTFLUOROSCOPY ROUTINES

After fluoroscopy, routine positions or projections may be obtained to document further any tentative diagnosis concluded fluoroscopically. These radiographs, such as the RAO shown in Fig. 12.80, must be obtained immediately after fluoroscopy, before too much of the barium has passed into the jejunum.

With **digital fluoroscopy,** routine postfluoroscopy radiographs may not be requested by the radiologist, as described earlier in this chapter.

Special Patient Considerations

PEDIATRIC APPLICATIONS

Refer to Chapter 16 for further details.

Pediatric Patient Preparation for Upper GI

The following guidelines are suggested, but department protocol should be followed:
- Infant younger than 1 year: NPO for 4 hours
- Children older than 1 year: NPO for 6 hours

Barium Preparation

Dilution of the barium may be required if the child will be fed through a bottle. A larger hole in the nipple may be required to ensure a smooth flow of barium. Some suggested barium volume guidelines are listed next, but specific department protocol should be followed.
- Newborn to 1 year: 2 to 4 oz
- 1 to 3 years: 4 to 6 oz
- 3 to 10 years: 6 to 12 oz
- Older than 10 years: 12 to 16 oz

Room Preparation

Most upper GI series for pediatric patients are performed with the table in the horizontal position. Protective aprons must be provided for all persons in the fluoroscopy room (Fig. 12.81). Individuals who feed or restrain the child during fluoroscopy should wear protective gloves and should be instructed *not* to stand at the head or foot of the table, where radiation exposure is greatest. Pulsed, grid-controlled fluoroscopy should be used to reduce doses for all patients, especially children.

GERIATRIC APPLICATIONS

The risk of dehydration during GI studies is a concern for geriatric patients. These patients may require additional attention and monitoring with the normal patient preparation of withholding fluids and ingesting barium. The use of water-soluble contrast agents such as

Gastrografin or MD-Gastroview may increase the risk of dehydration further. Geriatric patients should be scheduled for GI studies early in the morning to permit a return to normal fluid and dietary intake after the procedure.

Geriatric patients may require additional time and assistance while changing positions on the table. Geriatric patients may feel nervous and express fear of falling off the examination table.

A decrease in exposure factors is required for geriatric patients with lower tissue density and asthenic-type body habitus.

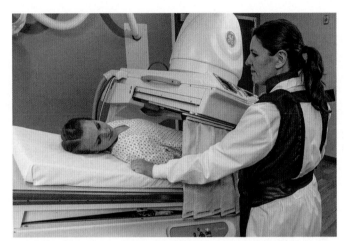

Fig. 12.79 Assisting the patient during the procedure with table movements.

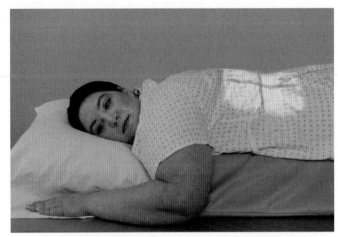

Fig. 12.80 Postfluoroscopy RAO position.

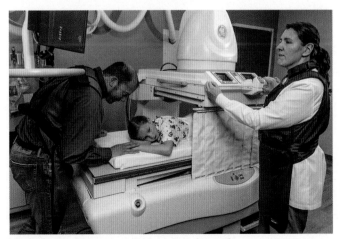

Fig. 12.81 Preparing a pediatric patient for GI fluoroscopy. Parent must step back before fluoroscopy begins.

BARIATRIC PATIENT CONSIDERATIONS

Preliminary scout and post-contrast introduction images of the stomach and duodenum on bariatric patients may require multiple images be taken to ensure all of the anatomy has been covered. Regardless of the number of images taken to cover the entire stomach and duodenum in the various positions, be sure there is sufficient but not excessive overlap to verify that no anatomic regions are missed.

Very hypersthenic patients may require assistance moving into the necessary positions during the fluoroscopic and postfluoroscopic imaging. Clear instructions are necessary to help the patient successfully move within the confined space under the fluoroscopic tower.

SUMMARY OF POSITIONING TIPS FOR UPPER GI EXAMINATIONS

Clinical History

Obtain a clinical history from the patient, and record the clinical indications for the study. Note any past or recent abdominal surgery, especially surgeries involving the gastrointestinal tract. Surgery or resection of the bowel or stomach may alter its normal position. Pay close attention to the fluoroscopy monitor to detect such differences, which may affect positioning and centering on postfluoroscopy imaging.

Review the patient's chart to ensure that the correct procedure has been ordered. Also identify specific allergies and other pertinent information.

Body Habitus

Consider the body habitus of the patient. The stomach is high and transverse with a hypersthenic patient but low and vertical with a hyposthenic patient. In a sthenic or average patient the duodenum bulb is near the L2 region. Usually L2 is located 1 to 2 inches (2.5 to 5 cm) above the lower margin of the lateral rib cage. Centering points in this text are designed for the average, sthenic patient.

Fluoroscopy

During fluoroscopy, identify the stomach on the fluoroscopy monitor. Pinpoint surrounding structures to gain clues about the location of the stomach and duodenum. For example, if the body of the stomach is adjacent to the iliac wing, center lower than the average or sthenic patient.

High kVp and Short Exposure Time

A high kVp of 110 to 125 is required to penetrate adequately and increase visibility of barium-filled structures. A kVp less than 100 would not provide visibility of the mucosa of the esophagus, stomach, or duodenum. Short exposure times are needed to control peristaltic motion. With double contrast, reduction of the kVp to 90 to 100 is common to provide higher contrast images without over-penetrating the anatomy (determine departmental kVp preferences). Iodinated, water-soluble contrast studies often require a kVp range of 80 to 90 kVp.

Digital Imaging Considerations

With the use of digital fluoroscopy, postfluoroscopy projections are taken less frequently during esophagography and upper GI procedures. If such projections are requested and digital imaging equipment is used, the following technical considerations should be kept in mind:

1. **Collimation:** To ensure the digital image is recognized correctly by the imaging system and a diagnostic image is produced, **close collimation is essential.** Because of the proximity of the spine, without accurate collimation the imaging system may rescale the image to display a longer than optimal scale of contrast. This could lead to certain soft tissue structures and pathology being obscured during the image reconstruction process. Careful collimation to the organs of interest minimizes this possibility.

2. **Accurate centering:** Careful analysis of body habitus is crucial during an esophagogram and upper GI procedure. Keep in mind how the position of the stomach varies between a hypersthenic and an asthenic patient. If the stomach is not centered to the IR, the image will not be displayed correctly. It is important to ensure that the **central ray, body part,** and **IR are aligned** for correct centering of the anatomy of interest.

3. **Exposure factors:** With digital imaging systems, minimum kVp and mAs must be used to create an acceptable image. Inadequate kVp or mAs produces a "mottled" image; however, the technologist must not increase mAs needlessly because this would increase patient dose. Departments should have established technical charts to ensure that adequate kVp and mAs are used for these procedures. After images have been produced, the exposure index should be verified to determine whether it is within the acceptable range to ensure that sufficient exposure factors were used without needless overexposure of the patient.

Alternative Modalities and Procedures

COMPUTED TOMOGRAPHY (CT)

CT is an excellent modality that may be used to demonstrate tumors of the gastrointestinal tract, liver, spleen, and pancreas. With the use of diluted oral contrast media, CT can demonstrate diverticula, hiatal hernia, and bowel perforation.

CT has become the modality of choice for demonstrating trauma and tumors of the gastrointestinal tract and accessory organs.

MAGNETIC RESONANCE IMAGING (MRI)

Tumor and vascular disease of the liver and esophageal varices are demonstrated well on MRI with the use of a flow-sensitive, short flip angle pulse sequence. Magnetic resonance cholangiopancreatography (MRCP) is a procedure specific for demonstration of the hepatobiliary and pancreatic systems.

Hemochromatosis, or iron overload, may be a genetic condition or may be due to multiple blood transfusions and is well visualized with MRI. This condition leads to deposition of an abnormal amount of iron within the liver parenchyma. Excessive iron deposited in the tissue produces a strong signal on MRI.

MEDICAL SONOGRAPHY

Intraesophageal sonography for esophageal varices and carcinoma of the esophagus is becoming an alternative to the esophagography. With passage of a small transducer into the esophagus, detailed images of the inner mucosal layer can be acquired. Small varices and polyps of the esophagus and upper stomach can be evaluated. As stated earlier, ultrasound has become an effective diagnostic tool for HPS in infants.

Doppler ultrasound can be used to detect vascular flow to specific accessory organs in the gastrointestinal tract.

NUCLEAR MEDICINE (NM)

With the use of specific radionuclides, NM scans demonstrate cirrhosis of the liver, splenic tumors, gastrointestinal bleeding, and gastric emptying studies. Gastric emptying studies are performed to determine the rate of emptying of food from the stomach.

Also, esophageal reflux can be diagnosed by the addition of a radionuclide to a drink, such as milk. With a compression band placed along the upper abdomen, the nuclear medicine camera can measure any return of gastric contents through the esophagogastric junction. NM is also very effective in demonstrating Barrett esophagus.

Routine and Special Projections

The three routine postfluoroscopy projections for **esophagography** are described in the following positioning section, along with one special oblique position. The five projections for the **upper GI series** are listed in order of suggested clinical usefulness when postfluoroscopy projections are requested. With the increased use of digital fluoroscopy, these postfluoroscopy projections are not as common as in the past, but technologists should be able to perform them when requested.

RAO POSITION—ESOPHAGOGRAPHY

Clinical Indications
- Strictures, foreign bodies, anatomic anomalies, and neoplasms of the esophagus

Esophagography
ROUTINE
• RAO (35° to 40°)
• Lateral
• AP (PA)

Technical Factors
- Minimum SID—40 inches (100 cm) or 72 inches (180 cm) if patient is erect
- IR size—14 × 17 inches (35 × 43 cm), portrait
- Grid
- kVp range: 110–125

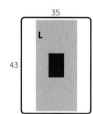

Shielding
Shield all radiosensitive tissues outside region of interest.

Patient Position
Position patient recumbent or erect. Recumbent is preferred because of more complete filling of the esophagus (caused by the gravity factor with the erect position).

Part Position
- Rotate **35° to 40°** from a prone position, with the right anterior body against the IR or table (Fig. 12.82).
- Place right arm down with left arm flexed at elbow and up by the patient's head, holding cup of barium, with a straw in patient's mouth.
- Flex left knee for support.
- Align midline of thorax in the oblique position to midline of IR or table.
- Place top of IR about 2 inches (5 cm) above level of shoulders to place center of IR at CR.

CR
- CR perpendicular to IR
- CR to center of IR at level of T6 (2 to 3 inches [5 to 8 cm] inferior to jugular notch)

Recommended Collimation
Collimate the lateral borders to create two-sided collimation about 5 to 6 inches (12 to 15 cm) wide. L or R marker should be placed within collimation field.

Respiration
Suspend respiration (see NOTES).

Evaluation Criteria
Anatomy Demonstrated: • Esophagus should be visible between the vertebral column and heart (Figs. 12.83 and 12.84). • RAO provides better visibility of esophagus between vertebrae and heart than LAO.
Position: • Adequate rotation of body projects esophagus between vertebral column and heart. • If esophagus is situated over the spine, more rotation of the body is required. • Entire esophagus is filled or lined with contrast media. • Upper limbs should not superimpose esophagus. • Proper collimation is applied. • CR is centered at level of T5 and T6 to include entire esophagus.
Exposure: • Appropriate technique is used to visualize clearly borders of the contrast media–filled esophagus. • Sharp structural margins indicate **no motion.**

NOTE 1: **Thick barium:** Two or three spoonfuls of thick barium should be ingested, and the exposure should be made immediately after the last bolus is swallowed. (The patient generally does not breathe immediately after a swallow.)

NOTE 2: **Thin barium:** For complete filling of the esophagus with thin barium, the patient may have to drink through a straw, with continuous swallowing and exposure made after three or four swallows without suspending respiration (using as short an exposure time as possible).

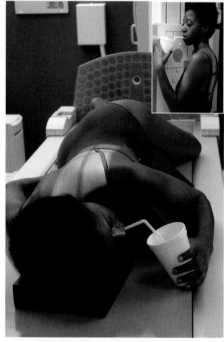

Fig. 12.82 35° to 40° RAO—recumbent or erect (*inset*).

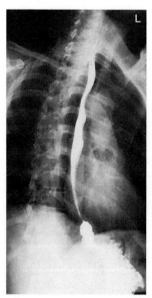

Fig. 12.83 RAO esophagus.

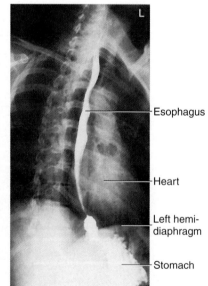

Fig. 12.84 RAO esophagus.

— Esophagus

— Heart

— Left hemidiaphragm

— Stomach

LATERAL POSITION—ESOPHAGOGRAPHY

Clinical Indications
- Strictures, foreign bodies, anatomic anomalies, and neoplasms of the esophagus

Esophagography
ROUTINE
• RAO (35° to 40°)
• Lateral
• AP (PA)

Technical Factors
- Minimum SID—40 inches (100 cm) or 72 inches (180 cm) if erect
- IR size—14 × 17 inches (35 × 43 cm), portrait
- Grid
- kVp range: 110–125

Shielding Shield all radiosensitive tissues outside region of interest.

Patient Position Position patient recumbent or erect (recumbent preferred) (Fig. 12.85).

Part Position
- Place patient's arms near the head, with the elbows flexed and superimposed.
- Align **midcoronal plane to midline** of IR or table.
- Place shoulders and hips in a true lateral position.
- Place top of IR about 2 inches (5 cm) above level of shoulders, to place center of IR at CR.

CR
- CR perpendicular to IR
- CR to level of T6 (2 to 3 inches [5 to 8 cm] inferior to jugular notch)

Recommended Collimation Collimate along the lateral borders to create two-sided collimation about 5 to 6 inches (12 to 15 cm) wide. L or R marker should be placed within collimation field.

Respiration Suspend respiration.

NOTE: See preceding page for barium swallow instructions.

Optional Swimmer's Lateral Position This position (Fig. 12.86) allows for better demonstration of the upper esophagus without superimposition of arms and shoulders.

Position hips and shoulders in true lateral position; separate shoulders from esophageal region by placing upside shoulder down and back, with arm behind back. Place downside shoulder and arm up and in front to hold cup of barium.

> **Evaluation Criteria**
> **Anatomy Demonstrated:** • Entire esophagus is seen between thoracic spine and heart (Fig. 12.87).
> **Position:** • True lateral is indicated by direct superimposition of posterior ribs. • Patient's arms should not superimpose esophagus. • Entire esophagus is filled or lined with contrast media. • Proper collimation is applied.
> **Exposure:** • Appropriate technique is used to visualize clearly borders of the contrast media–filled esophagus. • Sharp structural margins indicate **no motion.**

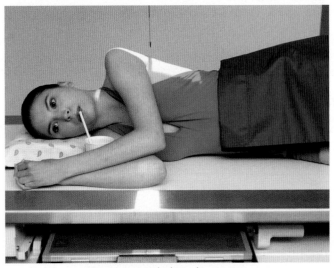

Fig. 12.85 Right lateral—arms up.

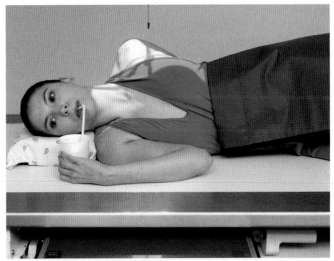

Fig. 12.86 Optional—swimmer's lateral for better visualization of upper esophagus.

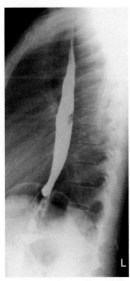

Fig. 12.87 Lateral esophagus—arms up.

AP (PA) PROJECTION —ESOPHAGOGRAPHY

Clinical Indications
- Strictures, foreign bodies, anatomic anomalies, and neoplasms of the esophagus

This projection may not be as diagnostic as the RAO or lateral position.

Esophagography
ROUTINE
• RAO (35° to 40°)
• Lateral
• AP (PA)

Technical Factors
- Minimum SID—40 inches (100 cm) or 72 inches (180 cm) if erect
- IR size—14 × 17 inches (35 × 43 cm), portrait
- Grid
- kVp range: 110–125

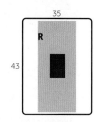

Shielding Shield all radiosensitive tissues outside region of interest.

Patient Position Position patient recumbent or erect (recumbent preferred) (Fig. 12.88).

Part Position
- Align **MSP to midline** of IR or table.
- Ensure that shoulders and hips are **not rotated.**
- Place right arm up to hold cup of barium.
- Place top of IR about 2 inches (5 cm) above top of shoulder, to place CR at center of IR.

CR
- CR perpendicular to IR
- CR to MSP, 1 inch (2.5 cm) inferior to sternal angle (T5–T6) or approximately 3 inches (8 cm) inferior to jugular notch

Recommended Collimation Use tight side collimation to result in a collimation field that is about 5 to 6 inches (12 to 15 cm) wide. L or R marker should be placed within collimation field.

Respiration Suspend respiration and expose on **expiration.**

Alternative PA This image also can be taken as a PA projection with similar positioning, centering, and CR locations.

NOTES: Two or three spoonfuls of thick barium should be ingested, and the exposure should be made immediately after the last bolus is swallowed. (Patient generally does not breathe immediately after a swallow.)

For complete filling of the esophagus with thin barium, the patient may have to drink through a straw, with continuous swallowing and exposure made after three or four swallows without suspending respiration.

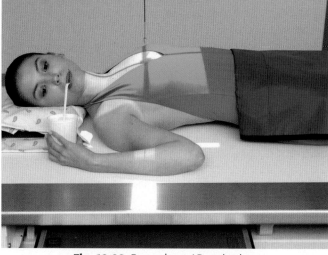

Fig. 12.88 Recumbent AP projection.

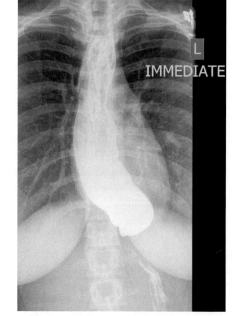

Fig. 12.89 AP esophageal projection.

Evaluation Criteria
Anatomy Demonstrated: • Entire esophagus is filled with barium (Fig. 12.89).
Position: • **No rotation** of the patient's body is evidenced by symmetry of sternoclavicular joints. • Proper collimation is applied.
Exposure: • Appropriate technique is used to visualize the esophagus through the superimposed thoracic vertebrae. • Sharp structural margins indicate **no motion.**

LAO POSITION—ESOPHAGOGRAPHY

Clinical Indications
- Strictures, foreign bodies, anatomic anomalies, and neoplasms of the esophagus

Esophagography
SPECIAL
• LAO

Technical Factors
- Minimum SID—40 inches (100 cm) or 72 inches (180 cm) if erect
- IR size—14 × 17 inches (35 × 43 cm), portrait
- Grid
- kVp range: 110–125

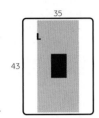

Shielding Shield all radiosensitive tissues outside the region of interest.

Patient Position Position patient recumbent or erect (recumbent preferred) (Fig. 12.90).

Part Position
- Rotate **35° to 40°** from a PA, with the left anterior body against IR or table.
- Place left arm down by patient's side, with right arm flexed at elbow and up by patient's head.
- Flex right knee for support.
- Place top of IR about 2 inches (5 cm) above level of shoulders, to place CR at center of IR.

CR
- CR perpendicular to IR
- CR to level of T5 or T6 (2 to 3 inches [5 to 7.5 cm] inferior to jugular notch)

Recommended Collimation Collimate lateral borders to create two-sided collimation about 5 to 6 inches (12 to 15 cm) wide. L or R marker should be placed within collimation field.

Respiration Suspend respiration and expose on expiration.

NOTE 1: Thick barium: Two or three spoonfuls of thick barium should be ingested, and the exposure should be made immediately after the last bolus is swallowed. (Patient generally does not breathe immediately after a swallow.)

NOTE 2: Thin barium: For complete filling of the esophagus with thin barium, the patient may have to drink through a straw, with continuous swallowing and exposure made after three or four swallows without suspending respiration (using as short an exposure time as possible).

Evaluation Criteria

Anatomy Demonstrated: • Esophagus is seen between hilar region of lungs and thoracic spine (Figs. 12.91 and 12.92). • Entire esophagus is filled with contrast medium.

Position: • The patient's upper limbs should not superimpose the esophagus. • Proper collimation is applied.

Exposure: • Appropriate technique is used to visualize clearly borders of contrast media–filled esophagus through the heart shadow. • Sharp structural margins indicate **no motion.**

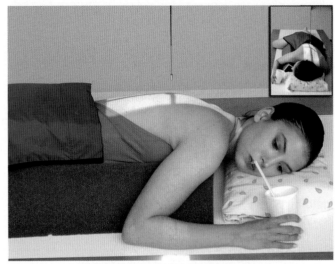

Fig. 12.90 Recumbent LAO position.

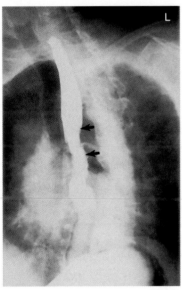

Fig. 12.91 LAO esophagus—demonstrating a constricted area of esophagus, probably carcinoma *(arrows)*.

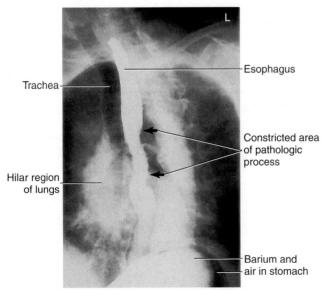

Fig. 12.92 LAO esophageal position.

RAO POSITION—UPPER GI SERIES

Clinical Indications
- Ideal position for demonstrating polyps and ulcers of the pylorus, duodenal bulb, and C-loop of the duodenum

Upper GI Series
ROUTINE
• RAO
• PA
• Right lateral
• LPO
• AP

Technical Factors
- Minimum SID—40 inches (100 cm)
- IR size—10 × 12 inches (24 × 30 cm), portrait
- Grid
- kVp range: 110–125; 90–100 for double-contrast study; 80–90 for water-soluble contrast media

Shielding
Shield all radiosensitive tissues outside region of interest.

Patient Position
Position patient recumbent, with body partially rotated into an RAO position; provide a support for patient's head and upper torso (Fig. 12.93).

Part Position
- From a prone position, rotate **40° to 70°,** with right anterior body against IR or table (more rotation is often required for hypersthenic patients, and less is required for asthenic patients). Place right arm down and left **arm flexed** at elbow and up by the patient's head.
- Flex left knee for support.

CR
- Direct CR **perpendicular** to IR
- **Sthenic body type:** Center CR and IR to duodenal bulb at **level of L1** (1 to 2 inches [2.5 to 5 cm] above lower lateral rib margin), **midway between spine and upside lateral border of abdomen,** 45° to 55° oblique
- **Asthenic body type:** Center about 2 inches (5 cm) below level of L1, 40° oblique
- **Hypersthenic body type:** Center about 2 inches (5 cm) above level of L1 and nearer midline, 70° oblique
- Center IR to CR

Recommended Collimation
Collimate on four sides to outer margins of IR or to area of interest on larger IR. L or R marker should be placed within collimation field.

Respiration
Suspend respiration and expose on **expiration.**

Evaluation Criteria
Anatomy Demonstrated: • Entire stomach and C-loop of duodenum are visible (Figs. 12.94 and 12.95).
Position: • Duodenal bulb is in profile. • Proper collimation is applied. • CR is centered to level of L1, with body of stomach and C-loop centered on radiograph.
Exposure: • Appropriate technique is used to visualize clearly the gastric folds without overexposing other pertinent anatomy. • Sharp structural margins indicate **no motion.**

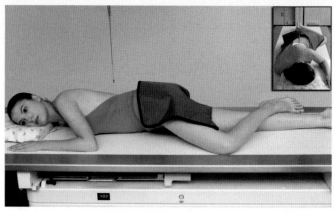

Fig. 12.93 RAO position.

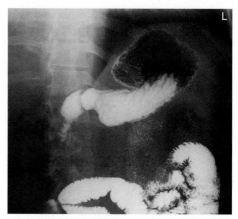

Fig. 12.94 RAO upper GI position.

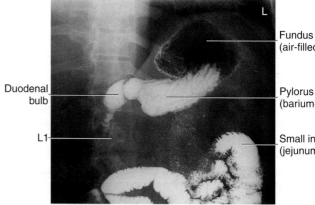

Duodenal bulb

L1

Fundus (air-filled)

Pylorus (barium-filled)

Small intestine (jejunum)

Fig. 12.95 RAO upper GI position.

PA PROJECTION—UPPER GI SERIES

Clinical Indications
- Polyps, diverticula, bezoars, and signs of gastritis in the body and pylorus of the stomach

Upper GI Series
ROUTINE
• RAO
• PA
• Right lateral
• LPO
• AP

Technical Factors
- Minimum SID—40 inches (100 cm)
- IR size—10 × 12 inches (24 × 30 cm) or 14 × 17 inches (35 × 43 cm) portrait if small bowel is to be included
- Grid
- kVp range: 110–125; 90–100 for double-contrast study; 80–90 for water-soluble contrast media

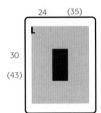

Shielding Shield all radiosensitive tissues outside region of interest.

Patient Position Position patient prone, with arms up beside head; provide a support for patient's head (Fig. 12.96).

Part Position
- Align MSP to CR and to table.
- Ensure that the **body is not rotated.**

CR
- Direct CR **perpendicular** to IR.
- **Sthenic body type:** Center CR and IR to level of pylorus and duodenal bulb at **level of L1** (1 to 2 inches [2.5 to 5 cm] above lower lateral rib margin) and about **1 inch (2.5 cm) left of the vertebral column.**
- **Asthenic body type:** Center about 2 inches (5 cm) below level of L1.
- **Hypersthenic body type:** Center about 2 inches (5 cm) above level of L1 and nearer midline.
- Center IR to CR.

Recommended Collimation Collimate on four sides to outer margins of IR or to area of interest on a larger IR. L or R marker should be placed within collimation field.

Respiration Suspend respiration and expose on **expiration.**

Evaluation Criteria
Anatomy Demonstrated: • Entire stomach and duodenum are visible.
Position: • Body and pylorus of the stomach are filled with barium. • Proper collimation is applied.
Exposure: • Appropriate technique is used to visualize the gastric folds without overexposing other pertinent anatomy. • Sharp structural margins indicate **no motion.**

Alternate PA Axial The position of the high transverse stomach on a **hypersthenic** patient causes almost an end-on view, with much overlapping of the pyloric region of the stomach and the duodenal bulb with a PA projection (Fig. 12.97). Therefore, a **35° to 45° cephalic angle** of the CR separates these areas for better visualization. The greater and lesser curvatures of the stomach also are better visualized in profile.

For **infants,** a **20° to 25° cephalic CR angle** is recommended to open the body and pylorus of stomach.

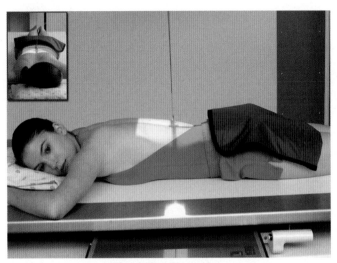
Fig. 12.96 PA position.

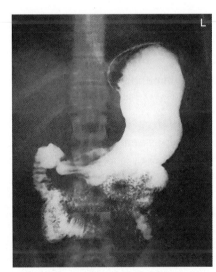
Fig. 12.97 PA projection.

RIGHT LATERAL POSITION—UPPER GI SERIES

Clinical Indications
- Pathologic processes of the **retrogastric space** (space behind the stomach)
- Diverticula, tumors, gastric ulcers, and trauma to the stomach may be demonstrated along posterior margin of stomach

Upper GI Series
ROUTINE
• RAO
• PA
• Right lateral
• LPO
• AP

Technical Factors
- Minimum SID—40 inches (100 cm)
- IR size—10 × 12 inches (24 × 30 cm), portrait
- kVp range: 110–125; 90–100 for double-contrast study; 80–90 for water-soluble contrast media

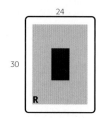

Shielding
Shield all radiosensitive tissues outside region of interest.

Patient Position
Position patient recumbent in a right lateral position (Fig. 12.98). Provide a support for patient's head. Place arms up near patient's head and flex knees.

Part Position
- Ensure that shoulders and hips are in a true lateral position.
- Center IR at CR (bottom of IR about at level of iliac crest).

CR
- Direct CR **perpendicular** to IR
- **Sthenic body type:** Center CR and IR to duodenal bulb at level of **L1** (level of lower lateral margin of the ribs) and **1 to 1½ inches (2.5 to 4 cm) anterior to midcoronal plane** (near midway between anterior border of vertebrae and anterior abdomen)
- **Hypersthenic body type:** Center about 2 inches (5 cm) above L1
- **Asthenic body type:** Center about 2 inches (5 cm) below L1

Recommended Collimation
Collimate on four sides to outer margins of IR or to area of interest on larger IR. L or R should be placed within collimation field.

Respiration
Suspend respiration and expose on expiration.

NOTE: The stomach generally is located about one vertebra higher in this position than in the PA or oblique position.

Evaluation Criteria
Anatomy Demonstrated: • Entire stomach and duodenum are visible (Figs. 12.99 and 12.100). • Retrogastric space is demonstrated. • Pylorus of stomach and C-loop of duodenum should be visualized well on hypersthenic patients.
Position: • No rotation should be present. • Vertebral bodies should be seen for reference purposes. • Intervertebral foramen should be open, indicating a true lateral position. • Proper collimation is applied. • CR is centered to duodenal bulb at level of L1.
Exposure: • Appropriate technique is used to visualize the gastric folds without overexposing other pertinent anatomy. • Sharp structural margins indicate **no motion.**

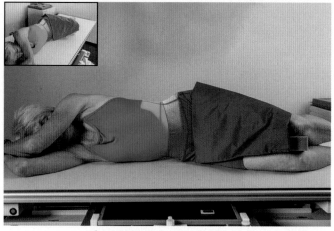

Fig. 12.98 Right lateral position.

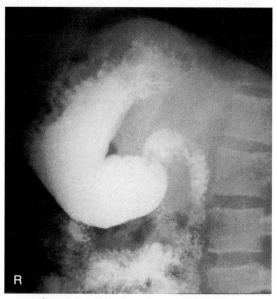

Fig. 12.99 Right lateral upper GI position.

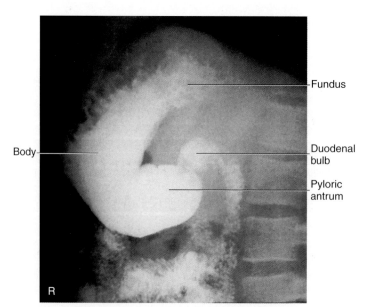

Fundus

Body

Duodenal bulb

Pyloric antrum

Fig. 12.100 Right lateral upper GI position.

LPO POSITION—UPPER GI SERIES

Clinical Indications

- When a double-contrast technique is used, the air-filled pylorus and duodenal bulb may better demonstrate signs of gastritis and ulcers.

Upper GI Series
ROUTINE
• RAO
• PA
• Right lateral
• LPO
• AP

Technical Factors

- Minimum SID—40 inches (100 cm)
- IR size—10 × 12 inches (24 × 30 cm), portrait
- Grid
- kVp range: 110–125; 90–100 for double-contrast study; 80–90 for water-soluble contrast media

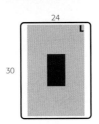

Shielding Shield all radiosensitive tissues outside region of interest.

Patient Position Position patient recumbent, with the body partially rotated into an LPO position; provide support for patient's head and upper torso (Fig. 12.101).

Part Position

- Rotate **30° to 60°** from supine position, with left posterior against IR or table (more rotation (up to 60°) is often required for hypersthenic body habitus and less rotation (30°) for asthenic body habitus[7]).
- Flex right knee for support.
- Extend left arm from body and raise right arm high across chest to grasp end of table for support. (Do not pinch fingers when moving bucky.)
- Center IR at CR (bottom of IR at level of iliac crest).

CR

- Direct CR **perpendicular** to IR
- **Sthenic body type:** Center CR and IR to **level of L1** (about midway between xiphoid tip and lower lateral margin of ribs) and **midway between midline of body** and **left lateral margin** of abdomen, 45° oblique
- **Hypersthenic body type:** Center about 2 inches (5 cm) above L1, 60° oblique
- **Asthenic body type:** Center about 2 inches (5 cm) below L1 and nearer to midline, 30° oblique

Recommended Collimation Collimate on four sides to outer margins of IR or to area of interest on larger IR.

Respiration Suspend respiration and expose on **expiration**.

NOTE: The stomach generally is located higher in this position than in the lateral; therefore, center one vertebra higher than on PA or RAO position.

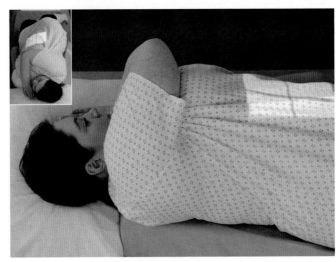

Fig. 12.101 LPO position.

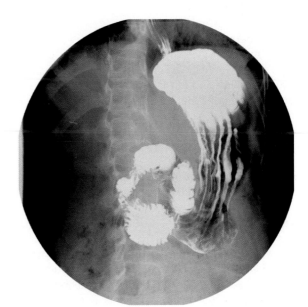

Fig. 12.102 LPO position.

Evaluation Criteria

Anatomy Demonstrated: • Entire stomach and duodenum are visible (Fig. 12.102). • Unobstructed view of duodenal bulb should be provided, without superimposition by the pylorus of the stomach.

Position: • Fundus should be filled with barium. • With a double-contrast procedure, body and pylorus and occasionally duodenal bulb are air filled. • Proper collimation is applied. • CR is centered level to the duodenal bulb.

Exposure: • Appropriate technique is used to visualize gastric folds without overexposing other pertinent anatomy. • Sharp structural margins indicate **no motion**.

AP PROJECTION—UPPER GI SERIES

Clinical Indications
- Possible hiatal hernia may be demonstrated in Trendelenburg position

Upper GI Series
ROUTINE
- RAO
- PA
- Right lateral
- LPO
- AP

Technical Factors
- Minimum SID—40 inches (100 cm).
- IR size—14 × 17 inches (35 × 43 cm) portrait
- Grid
- kVp range: 110–125; 90–100 for double-contrast study; 80–90 for water-soluble contrast media

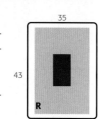

Shielding Shield all radiosensitive tissues outside region of interest.

Patient Position Position patient supine, arms at sides; provide a support for patient's head and knees (Fig. 12.103).

Part Position
- Align MSP to midline of table.
- Ensure that body is not rotated.
- Center IR to CR.
- Bottom of 14 × 17-inch (35 × 43-cm) IR should be about at level of iliac crest.

CR
- Center CR **perpendicular** to IR
- **Sthenic body type:** Center CR and IR to **level of L1** (about midway between xiphoid tip and lower margin of ribs), **midway between midline and left lateral margin** of abdomen
- **Hypersthenic body type:** Center about 2 inches (5 cm) above L1
- **Asthenic body type:** Position CR about 2 inches (5 cm) below and nearer to midline

Recommended Collimation Collimate on four sides to outer margins of IR or to area of interest if larger IR is used.

Respiration Suspend respiration and expose on **expiration**.

Alternative AP: Partial Trendelenburg Position A partial Trendelenburg (head-down) position may be necessary to fill the fundus on a thin asthenic patient. A full Trendelenburg angulation facilitates the demonstration of hiatal hernia. (Install shoulder brace for patient safety.)

Evaluation Criteria
Anatomy Demonstrated: • Entire stomach and duodenum are visible (Figs. 12.104 and 12.105). • Diaphragm and lower lung fields are included for demonstration of possible hiatal hernia.
Position: • Fundus of stomach is filled with barium and is near center of IR. • Proper collimation is applied. • CR is centered to duodenal bulb at level of L1.
Exposure: • Appropriate technique is used to visualize the gastric folds without overexposing other pertinent anatomy. • Sharp structural margins indicate no motion.

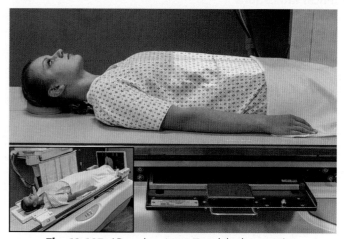

Fig. 12.103 AP supine. *Inset,* Trendelenburg option.

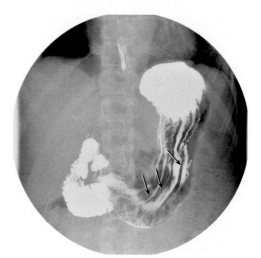

Fig. 12.104 AP—supine.

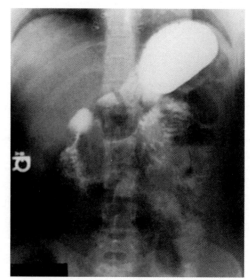

Fig. 12.105 AP—Trendelenburg position.

CHAPTER 13

Lower Gastrointestinal System

CONTRIBUTIONS BY **Michele Patrícia Müller Mansur Vieira,** MSc, TCNL-CRTR-PR (BRAZIL)

CONTRIBUTORS TO PAST EDITIONS Leslie E. Kendrick, MS, RT(R)(CT)(MR), Barry T. Anthony, RT(R)

CONTENTS

RADIOGRAPHIC ANATOMY

Digestive System

The first five parts of the alimentary canal (through the stomach and first part of the small intestine, the duodenum) are described in Chapter 12 (Fig. 13.1).

This chapter continues with the alimentary canal of the digestive system beyond the stomach, beginning with the **small intestine** (small bowel). If the entire small intestine were removed from the body at autopsy, separated from its mesenteric attachment, uncoiled, and stretched out, it would average 23 feet (7 m) in length. During life, with good muscle tone, the actual length of the small intestine is shorter, measuring 15 to 18 feet (4.5 to 5.5 m). However, tremendous individual variation exists. In one series of 100 autopsies, the small bowel ranged in length from 15 to 31 feet. The diameter varies from 1½ inches (3.8 cm) at the proximal aspect to about 1 inch (2.5 cm) at the distal end.

The **large intestine** (large bowel) begins in the right lower quadrant (RLQ) with its connection to the small intestine. The large intestine extends around the periphery of the abdominal cavity to end at the **anus.** The large intestine is about 5 feet (1.5 m) long and about 2½ inches (6 cm) in diameter.

COMMON RADIOGRAPHIC PROCEDURES

Two common radiographic procedures involving the lower gastrointestinal system are presented in this chapter. Both procedures involve administration of a contrast medium.

'Small Bowel Series—Study of Small Intestine

Radiographic examination specifically of the small intestine is called a **small bowel series (SBS).** This examination often is combined with an upper gastrointestinal (GI) series, and under these conditions may be termed a *small bowel follow-through.* A radiograph of the barium-filled small bowel is shown in Fig. 13.2.

Barium Enema (Lower GI Series, Colon)—Study of Large Intestine

The radiographic procedure designed to study the large intestine is most commonly termed a **barium enema.** Alternative designations include *BE, BaE,* and *lower GI series.* Fig. 13.3 shows a large bowel or colon filled with a combination of air and barium, referred to as a *double-contrast barium enema.* This patient has **situs inversus,** in which abdominal and thoracic organs are reversed from their normal orientation within the body.

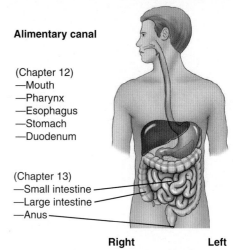

Alimentary canal

(Chapter 12)
—Mouth
—Pharynx
—Esophagus
—Stomach
—Duodenum

(Chapter 13)
—Small intestine
—Large intestine
—Anus

Right   Left

Fig. 13.1 Digestive system.

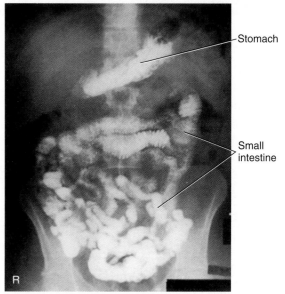

Stomach

Small intestine

R

Fig. 13.2 PA—small bowel series.

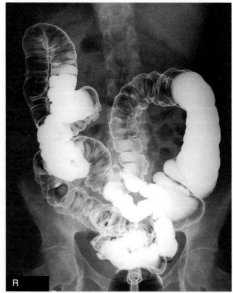

R

Fig. 13.3 AP—double-contrast barium enema; patient with situs inversus.

Small Intestine

Beginning at the pyloric valve of the stomach, the three parts of the small intestine, in order, are the **duodenum, jejunum,** and **ileum.** The relative location of the three parts of the small intestine in relation to the four abdominal quadrants (right upper quadrant [RUQ], RLQ, left upper quadrant [LUQ], left lower quadrant [LLQ]) is demonstrated.

DUODENUM (RUQ AND LUQ)

The **duodenum** is the first part of the small intestine, as described in detail in Chapter 12. It is the shortest, widest, and most 'fixed portion of the small bowel. It is located primarily in the RUQ. It also extends into the LUQ, where it joins the jejunum at a point called the *duodenojejunal flexure*. It represents the shortest aspect of the small intestine and averages about 8 to 10 inches (20 to 25 cm) in length.[1]

JEJUNUM (LUQ AND LLQ)

The **jejunum** is located primarily to the left of midline in the LUQ and LLQ, making up about **two-fifths** of the remaining aspect of the small intestine. Its inner diameter is approximately 1 inch (2.5 cm). The jejunum contains numerous mucosal folds (plicae circulares), which increase the surface area to aid with absorption of nutrients. These numerous mucosal folds produce the feathery appearance of the jejunum.[1]

The jejunum begins at the site of the duodenojejunal flexure, slightly to the left of midline in the LUQ (under the transverse colon, as seen in Fig. 13.4). This relatively fixed site of the small bowel may become a radiographic reference point during a small bowel study.

ILEUM (RLQ AND LLQ)

The **ileum** is located primarily in the RUQ, RLQ, and LLQ. The ileum makes up the distal **three-fifths** of the remaining aspect of the small intestine and is the longest portion of the small intestine. The terminal ileum joins the large intestine at the **ileocecal valve (sphincter or fold)** in the RLQ, as shown in Fig. 13.4. Although it is longer than the jejunum, the ileum possesses a thinner wall and has fewer mucosal folds (plicae circulares). At the point of the ileocecal valve (sphincter), the inner lumen of the ileum is nearly smooth.[1]

SECTIONAL DIFFERENCES

Various sections of the small intestine can be identified radiographically by their **location** and by their **appearance.** The C-shaped duodenum is fairly fixed in position immediately distal to the stomach and is recognized easily on radiographs. The internal lining of the second and third (descending and horizontal) portions of the duodenum is gathered into tight circular folds formed by the mucosa of the small intestine, which contains numerous small, fingerlike projections termed **villi,** resulting in a feathery appearance when filled with barium.

Jejunum

The mucosal folds of the distal duodenum also are found in the jejunum. Although there is no abrupt end to the circular feathery folds, the ileum tends not to have this appearance. This difference in appearance between the jejunum and the ileum can be seen in the barium-filled small bowel radiograph in Fig. 13.5 and the coronal abdominal computed tomography (CT) image in Fig. 13.6.

Ileum

The internal lining of the ileum appears on a radiograph as smoother, with fewer indentations and a less feathery appearance. Another observable difference in the three sections of small intestine is that the internal diameter gets progressively smaller from duodenum to ileum.

CT Cross-Sectional Image

A CT axial or sectional image through the level of the second portion of the duodenum is seen in Fig. 13.7. This image shows the

relative positions of the stomach and duodenum in relation to the head of the pancreas. A portion of jejunal loops is also shown on the patient's left, along with a small aspect of the left colic flexure, seen lateral to the stomach.

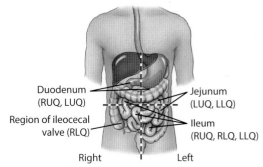

Fig. 13.4 Small intestines—four quadrants.

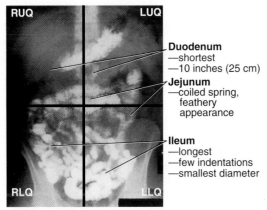

Fig. 13.5 Barium-filled stomach and small intestine (four quadrants).

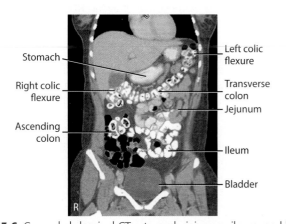

Fig. 13.6 Coronal abdominal CT—stomach, jejunum, ileum, and large intestine.

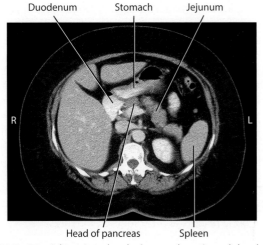

Fig. 13.7 CT axial section—level of second portion of duodenum.

Large Intestine

The large intestine begins in the RLQ, just lateral to the ileocecal valve. The large intestine consists of four major parts: **cecum, colon, rectum,** and **anal canal** (Fig. 13.8).

The final segment of the large intestine is the **rectum.** The distal rectum contains the **anal canal,** which ends at the **anus.**

COLON VERSUS LARGE INTESTINE

Large intestine and *colon* are *not* synonyms, although many technologists use these terms interchangeably. The **colon** consists of **four sections** and **two flexures** and does *not* include the cecum and rectum. The four sections of the colon are (1) the **ascending colon,** (2) the **transverse colon,** (3) the **descending colon,** and (4) the **sigmoid colon.** The **right** (hepatic) and **left** (splenic) **colic flexures** are included as part of the colon.

The transverse colon has a wide range of motion and normally loops down farther than is shown on the drawing in Fig. 13.8.

CECUM

At the proximal end of the large intestine is the **cecum,** a large blind pouch located inferior to the level of the ileocecal valve. The vermiform **appendix** (commonly referred to as just the appendix) is attached to the cecum. The internal appearance of the cecum and **terminal ileum** is shown in Fig. 13.9. The most distal part of the small intestine, the ileum, joins the cecum at the **ileocecal valve.** The ileocecal valve consists of two lips that extend into the large bowel.

The ileocecal valve acts as a sphincter to prevent the contents of the ileum from passing too quickly into the cecum. A second function of the ileocecal valve is to prevent reflux, or a backward flow of large-intestine contents, into the ileum. The ileocecal valve does only a fair job of preventing reflux because some barium can almost always be refluxed into the terminal ileum when a barium enema is performed. The **cecum,** the widest portion of the large intestine, is fairly free to move about in the RLQ.

Appendix

The **vermiform appendix** (appendix) is a long (½ to 8-inch [2 to 20-cm]), narrow, worm-shaped tube that extends from the cecum. The term *vermiform* means "wormlike." The appendix usually is attached to the posteromedial aspect of the cecum and commonly extends toward the pelvis. However, it may pass posterior to the cecum. Because the appendix has a blind ending, infectious agents may enter the appendix, which cannot empty itself. Also, obstruction of the opening into the vermiform appendix caused by a small fecal mass may lead to narrowing of the blood vessels that feed it. The result is an inflamed appendix, or **appendicitis.** Appendicitis may require surgical removal, which is termed an **appendectomy,** before the diseased structure ruptures, causing peritonitis. Acute appendicitis accounts for about 50% of all emergency abdominal surgeries and is 1.5 times more common in men than in women.

Occasionally, fecal matter or barium sulfate from a gastrointestinal tract study may fill the appendix and remain there indefinitely.

LARGE INTESTINE—BARIUM FILLED

The radiograph shown in Fig. 13.10 demonstrates the four parts of the colon—**ascending, transverse, descending,** and **sigmoid;** and the two flexures—the **right colic** (hepatic) **flexure** and the **left colic** (splenic) **flexure.** The remaining three parts of the large intestine—**cecum, rectum,** and **anal canal**—are also shown. As is shown by this radiograph, these various parts are not as neatly arranged around the periphery of the abdomen as they are on drawings. There is a wide range of structural locations and relative sizes for these various portions of the large intestine, depending on the individual body habitus and contents of the intestine.

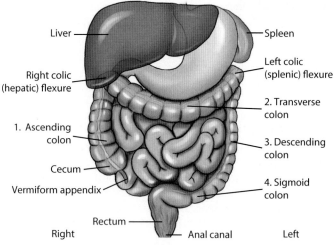

Fig. 13.8 Large intestine (includes colon).

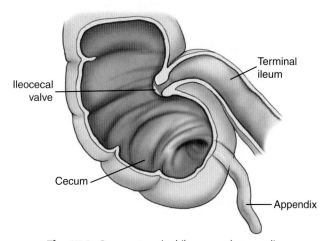

Fig. 13.9 Cecum, terminal ileum, and appendix.

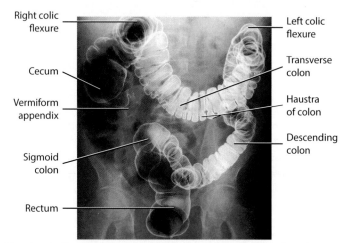

Fig. 13.10 Double-contrast barium enema of large intestine. (From Hombach-Klonisch S, Klonisch T, Peeler J (eds.). *Sobotta clinical atlas of human anatomy,* Munich, 2019, Elsevier GmbH.)

Rectum and Anal Canal

The **rectum** extends from the sigmoid colon to the **anus.** The rectum begins at the level of S3 (third sacral segment) and is about 4½ inches (12 cm) long. The final 1 to 1½ inches (2.5 to 4 cm) of large intestine is constricted to form the **anal canal.** The anal canal terminates as an opening to the exterior, the **anus.** The rectum closely follows the sacrococcygeal curve, as demonstrated in the lateral view in Fig. 13.11.

The **rectal ampulla** is a dilated portion of the rectum located anterior to the coccyx. The initial direction of the rectum along the **sacrum** is inferior and posterior. However, in the region of the rectal ampulla, the direction changes to inferior and anterior. A second abrupt change in direction occurs in the region of the anal canal, which is directed again inferiorly and posteriorly. Therefore, the rectum presents **two anteroposterior curves.** This fact must be remembered when the technologist inserts a rectal tube or enema tip into the lower gastrointestinal tract for a barium enema procedure. Serious injury can occur if the enema tip is forced at the wrong angle into the anus and anal canal.

LARGE VERSUS SMALL INTESTINE

Three characteristics readily differentiate the large intestine from the small intestine.

1. The **internal diameter** of the large intestine is usually greater than the diameter of the small bowel.
2. The muscular portion of the intestinal wall contains three external bands of longitudinal muscle fibers of the large bowel that form three bands of muscle called **taeniae coli,** which tend to pull the large intestine into pouches. Each of these pouches, or sacculations, is termed a **haustrum. Most of the large intestine except for the rectum possesses haustra.** Therefore, a second primary identifying characteristic of the large bowel is the presence of multiple haustra. This characteristic can be seen in the enlarged drawing of the proximal large intestine in Fig. 13.12.
3. The third differentiation is the **relative positions** of the two structures. The **large intestine** extends around the **periphery** of the abdominal cavity, whereas the **small intestine** is more **centrally** located.

RELATIVE LOCATIONS OF AIR AND BARIUM IN LARGE INTESTINE

The distribution of air and barium is influenced most often by the location of each portion of the large intestine in relation to the peritoneum. Aspects of the large intestine are more anterior or more posterior in relation to the peritoneum. The cecum, transverse colon, and sigmoid colon are more anterior than other aspects of the large intestine.

The simplified drawings in Fig. 13.13 represent the large intestine in **supine** and **prone** positions. If the large intestine contained both air and barium sulfate, the air would tend to rise and the barium would tend to sink because of gravity. Displacement and the ultimate location of **air** are shown as **black,** and displacement and the ultimate location of the **barium** are shown as **white.**

When a person is **supine,** air rises to fill the structures that are most anterior—that is, the transverse colon and loops of the sigmoid colon. The barium sinks to fill primarily the ascending and descending colon and aspects of the sigmoid colon.

When a patient is **prone,** barium and air reverse positions. The drawing on the right illustrates the prone position—air has risen to fill the rectum, ascending colon, and descending colon.

Recognizing these spatial relationships is important during fluoroscopy and during radiography when barium enema examinations are performed.

See Table 13.1 for differences in peritoneal location of the large intestine structures.

TABLE 13.1 LOCATION OF LARGE INTESTINE STRUCTURES IN RELATION TO PERITONEUM

STRUCTURE	LOCATION
Cecum	Intraperitoneal
Ascending colon	Retroperitoneal
Transverse colon	Intraperitoneal
Descending colon	Retroperitoneal
Sigmoid colon	Intraperitoneal
Upper rectum	Retroperitoneal
Lower rectum	Infraperitoneal

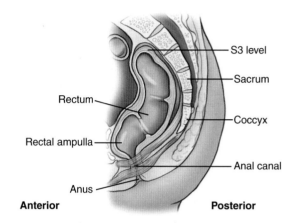

Fig. 13.11 Rectum—lateral view.

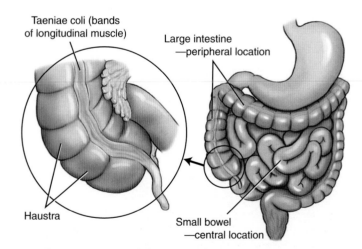

Fig. 13.12 Intestinal differences—large versus small intestine.

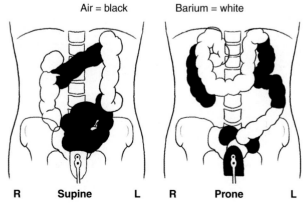

Fig. 13.13 Barium *(white)* versus air *(black)* in the large intestine.

Anatomy Review
SMALL BOWEL RADIOGRAPHS

Three parts of the small bowel can be seen in these 30-minute and 2-hour small bowel radiographs, taken 30 minutes and 2 hours after ingestion of barium (Figs. 13.14 to 13.16). Note the characteristic feathery sections of duodenum (A) and jejunum (C). The smoother appearance of the ileum is also evident (D).

The terminal portion of the ileum (D), the ileocecal valve (E), and the cecum of the large intestine are best shown on a spot film of this area (see Fig. 13.16). A spot image of the ileocecal valve area such as this, obtained with a compression cone, frequently is taken at the end of a small bowel series to visualize this region best. These figures illustrate the following labeled parts of the small intestine:

A. Duodenum
B. Region of the ligament of Treitz (suspensory ligament of the duodenum), site of duodenojejunal flexure (superimposed by stomach on these radiographs)
C. Jejunum
D. Ileum
E. Area of ileocecal valve

BARIUM ENEMA

Anteroposterior (AP), lateral rectum, and left anterior oblique (LAO) radiographs of a barium enema examination (Figs. 13.17 to 13.19) illustrate the key anatomy of the large intestine, labeled as follows:

a. Cecum
b. Ascending colon
c. Right colic (hepatic) flexure (usually located lower than the left colic flexure because of the presence of the liver)
d. Transverse colon
e. Left colic (splenic) flexure
f. Descending colon
g. Sigmoid colon
h. Rectum

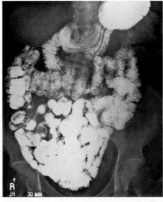

Fig. 13.14 PA—30-minute small bowel.   **Fig. 13.15** PA—2-hour small bowel.

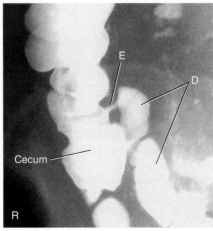

Fig. 13.16 Spot image of ileocecal valve. (Courtesy J. Sanderson, RT.)

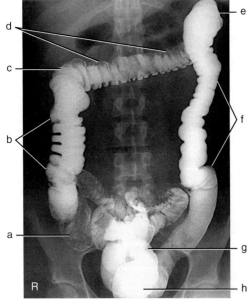

Fig. 13.17 AP—barium enema.

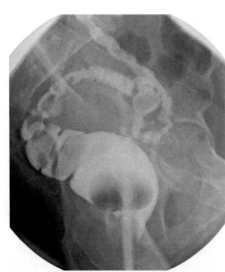

Fig. 13.18 Lateral rectum—Gastrografin

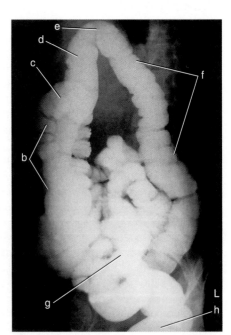

Fig. 13.19 LAO—barium enema (single-contrast study).

Digestive Functions
DIGESTIVE FUNCTIONS OF THE INTESTINES
The following four primary digestive functions are accomplished largely by the small and large intestines (Table 13.2):
1. **Digestion** (chemical and mechanical)
2. **Absorption**
3. **Reabsorption** of water, inorganic salts, vitamin K, and amino acids
4. **Elimination** (defecation)

Most **digestion** and **absorption** take place within the **small intestine.** Also, most **salts** and approximately **95% of water are reabsorbed** in the small intestine. Minimal reabsorption of water and inorganic salts occurs in the large intestine, as does the elimination of unused or unnecessary materials.

The primary function of the **large intestine** is the **elimination of feces** (defecation). Feces consist normally of 65% water and 35% solid matter, such as food residues, digestive secretions, and bacteria. Other specific functions of the large intestine include absorption of water, inorganic salt, vitamin K, and certain amino acids. These vitamins and amino acids are produced by a large collection of naturally occurring microorganisms (bacteria) found in the large intestine.

The last stage of digestion occurs in the large intestine through **bacterial action,** which converts the remaining proteins into amino acids. Some vitamins, such as B and K, are synthesized by bacteria and absorbed by the large intestine. A by-product of this bacterial action is the release of hydrogen, carbon dioxide, and methane gas. These gases, called **flatus** *(fla'-tus),* help to break down remaining proteins to amino acids.

MOVEMENTS OF DIGESTIVE TRACT
Of the various digestive functions of the intestine, digestive movements, sometimes referred to as *mechanical digestion,* are best demonstrated and evident on radiographic studies (Table 13.3).

Small Intestine
Digestive movements throughout the length of the small bowel consist of (1) **peristalsis** *(per″-i-stal'-sis)* and (2) **rhythmic segmentation.** Peristalsis describes wavelike contractions that propel food from the stomach through the small and large intestines and eventually expel it from the body. Barium sulfate enters the stomach and reaches the ileocecal valve 2 to 3 hours after ingestion.

Rhythmic segmentation describes localized contractions in areas or regions that contain food. For example, food within a specific aspect of the small intestine is contracted to produce segments of a particular column of food. Through rhythmic segmentation, digestion and reabsorption of select nutrients are more effective.

Large Intestine
In the large intestine, digestive movements continue as (1) **peristalsis,** (2) **haustral** *(haws'-tral)* **churning,** (3) **mass peristalsis,** and (4) **defecation** *(def″-e-ka'-shun).* Haustral churning produces movement of material within the large intestine. During this process, a particular group of haustra (bands of muscle) remains relaxed and distended while the bands are filling up with material. When distention reaches a certain level, the intestinal walls contract or "churn" to squeeze the contents into the next group of haustra. Mass peristalsis tends to move the entire large bowel contents into the sigmoid colon and rectum, usually once every 24 hours. Defecation is a so-called bowel movement, or emptying of the rectum.

TABLE 13.2 SUMMARY OF LOWER DIGESTIVE SYSTEM FUNCTIONS

RESPONSIBLE COMPONENT OF INTESTINE	FUNCTION
Small intestine	**Digestion:** Chemical and mechanical
Duodenum and jejunum (primarily)	**Absorption:** Nutrients, H_2O, salts, and proteins
	Reabsorption: H_2O and salts
Large intestine	Some reabsorption of H_2O and inorganic salts; vitamins B and K; amino acids
	Elimination (**defecation**)

TABLE 13.3 SUMMARY OF DIGESTIVE MOVEMENTS AND ELIMINATION

RESPONSIBLE COMPONENT OF INTESTINE	FUNCTION
Small intestine	Peristalsis
	Rhythmic segmentation
Large intestine	Peristalsis
	Haustral churning
	Mass peristalsis
	Defecation

RADIOGRAPHIC PROCEDURES

Small Bowel Series

The plain abdominal radiograph (KUB) shown in Fig. 13.20 is from a healthy, ambulatory adult. The many meters of small intestine are generally not visible in the central portion of the abdomen. In the average ambulatory adult, a large collection of gas in the small intestine is considered abnormal. With no gas present, the small bowel simply blends in with other soft tissue structures. Therefore, radiographic examination of the alimentary canal requires the introduction of contrast media for visualization.

DEFINITION

A radiographic study specifically of the small intestine is termed a **small bowel series.** Upper GI and small bowel series are frequently combined. Under these circumstances, the small bowel portion of the examination may be called a *small bowel follow-through.* Radiopaque contrast media are required for this study.

PURPOSE

The purposes of the small bowel series are to study the form and function of the three components of the small bowel and to detect any abnormal conditions.

Because this study also examines **function** of the small bowel, the procedure **must be timed.** The time when the patient has ingested a substantial amount (at least 8 oz) of contrast medium should be noted.

CONTRAINDICATIONS

Two strict contraindications to contrast media studies of the intestinal tract are known.

First, presurgical patients and patients suspected to have a **perforated hollow viscus** (intestine or organ) should *not* receive barium sulfate. Water-soluble, iodinated contrast media should be used instead. With young or dehydrated patients, care must be taken when a water-soluble contrast medium is used. Because of the hypertonic nature of these patients, water tends to be drawn into the bowel, leading to increased dehydration.

Second, barium sulfate by mouth is contraindicated in patients with a possible **large bowel obstruction.** An obstructed large bowel should be ruled out first with an acute abdominal series and a barium enema.

CLINICAL INDICATIONS

Common clinical indications for a small bowel series include the following (Table 13.4).

Enteritis *(en″-ter-i′-tis)* describes inflammation of the intestine, primarily of the small intestine. Enteritis may be caused by bacterial or protozoan organisms and other environmental factors. When the stomach is also involved, the condition is known as **gastroenteritis.** Chronic irritation may cause the lumen of the intestine to become thickened, irregular, and narrowed.

Regional enteritis (segmental enteritis or Crohn disease) is a form of inflammatory bowel disease of unknown origin, involving any part of the gastrointestinal tract but commonly involving the terminal ileum. This condition leads to scarring and thickening of the bowel wall. This scarring produces the "cobblestone" appearance visible during a small bowel series, or enteroclysis. Radiographically, these lesions resemble gastric erosions or ulcers seen in barium studies as minor variations in barium

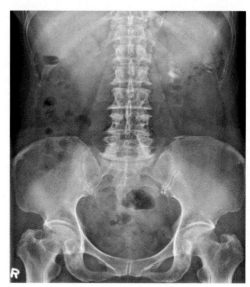

Fig. 13.20 Unenhanced abdominal radiograph—normal (some gas seen in large intestine). (From Partin AW et al. *Campbell-Walsh urology,* ed 12, Philadelphia, 2021, Elsevier.)

CONDITION OR DISEASE	MOST COMMON RADIOGRAPHIC EXAMINATION	POSSIBLE RADIOGRAPHIC APPEARANCE	EXPOSURE FACTOR ADJUSTMENT[a]
Enteritis	Small bowel series, enteroclysis	Thickening of mucosal folds and poor definition of circular folds	None
Regional enteritis (Crohn disease)	Small bowel series, enteroclysis	Segments of lumen narrowed and irregular; "cobblestone" appearance and "string sign" common	None
Giardiasis	Small bowel series, enteroclysis	Dilation of intestine, with thickening of circular folds	None
Ileus (obstruction) Adynamic Mechanical	Acute abdomen series, small bowel series, enteroclysis	Abnormal gas patterns, dilated loops of bowel, "circular staircase" or "herringbone" pattern	(−) Decrease if large segments of intestine are gas filled
Malabsorption syndromes (sprue)	Small bowel series, enteroclysis, or CT of abdomen	Thickening of mucosal folds and poor definition of normal feathery appearance	None
Meckel diverticulum	Nuclear medicine scan, small bowel series, enteroclysis	Large diverticulum of ileum, proximal to ileocecal valve; rarely seen on barium studies	None
Neoplasm	Small bowel series, enteroclysis, or CT of abdomen	Narrowed segments of intestine; "apple core" or "napkin ring sign"; partial or complete obstruction	None
Whipple disease	Small bowel series	Dilation and distorted loops of small bowel	None

[a]Dependent on stage or severity of disease or condition.

coating (Fig. 13.21). In advanced cases, segments of the intestine become narrowed as the result of chronic spasm, producing the "string sign" evident during a small bowel series. Regional enteritis frequently leads to intestinal obstruction, fistula, and abscess formation. This disorder also has a high rate of recurrence after treatment.

Giardiasis *(je″-ahr-di′-a-sis)* is a common infection of the lumen of the small intestine that is caused by the flagellate protozoan *Giardia lamblia* (Fig. 13.22). It is often spread by contaminated food and water. It can also be spread via person-to-person contact. Symptoms of giardiasis include nonspecific gastrointestinal discomfort, mild to profuse diarrhea, nausea, anorexia, and weight loss. The presence of this organism usually affects the duodenum and jejunum with spasms, irritability, and increased secretions. A small bowel series typically demonstrates giardiasis as dilation of the intestine, with thickening of the circular folds. Laboratory analysis of a stool specimen can confirm the presence of the *Giardia* organism.

Ileus *(il′-e-us)* is an **obstruction of the small intestine,** as shown in Fig. 13.23, wherein the proximal jejunum is markedly expanded with air. Two types of ileus have been identified: (1) **adynamic,** or **paralytic,** and (2) **mechanical.**

> **Adynamic,** or **paralytic,** ileus is due to the **cessation of peristalsis.** Without these involuntary, wavelike contractions, the bowel is flaccid and is unable to propel its contents forward. Causes for adynamic ileus include infection, such as peritonitis or appendicitis; the use of certain drugs; and postsurgical complications. Adynamic ileus usually involves the entire gastrointestinal tract. With adynamic ileus, usually no fluid levels are demonstrated on the erect abdomen projection. However, the intestine is distended with a thin bowel wall.

> A **mechanical obstruction** is a physical blockage of the bowel that may be caused by tumors, adhesions, or hernia. The loops of intestine proximal to the site of obstruction are markedly dilated with gas. This dilation produces the radiographic sign commonly called the "circular staircase" or "herringbone" pattern, which is evident on an erect or decubitus abdomen projection. Air-fluid levels usually are present, as can be seen on these projections.

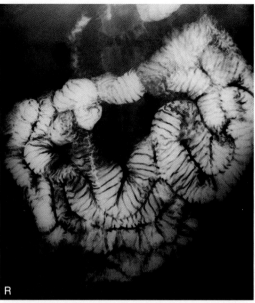

Fig. 13.22 Giardiasis of small intestine, jejunum, and ileum. (Dilation of intestine, with thick circular folds, is visible.)

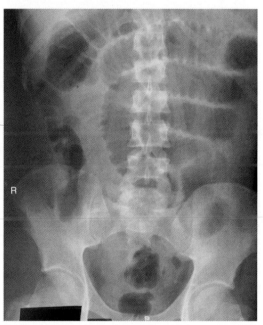

Fig. 13.23 Ileus (obstruction) of small bowel demonstrated by greatly extended air-filled loops of small bowel.

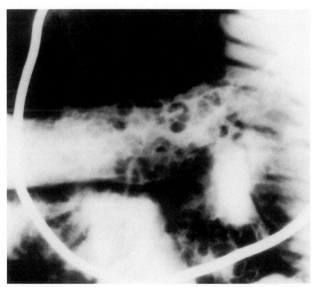

Fig. 13.21 Crohn disease involving ileum, cobblestone appearance. (From Eisenberg RL, Johnson NM. *Comprehensive radiographic pathology,* ed 7, St. Louis, 2021, Elsevier.)

Meckel diverticulum[2] is a common birth defect caused by the persistence of the yolk sac (umbilical vesicle), resulting in a saclike outpouching of the intestinal wall. This outpouching is seen in the ileum of the small bowel. It may measure 4 to 4½ inches (10 to 12 cm) in diameter and is usually 1½ to 3 feet (50 to 100 cm) proximal to the ileocecal valve. Meckel diverticulum is found incidentally in approximately 3% of adults. The condition does not typically cause symptoms unless inflammation (diverticulitis) or bowel obstruction develops. Pain may mimic acute appendicitis. Surgical removal is often recommended to prevent possible diverticulitis, obstruction, or blood loss. Meckel diverticulum is rarely seen on barium studies of the small bowel because of rapid emptying during a barium study. It is best diagnosed with a radionuclide (nuclear medicine) scan (Fig. 13.24).

Neoplasm *(ne'-o-plazm)* is a term that means "new growth." This growth may be benign or malignant (cancerous). Common benign tumors of the small intestine include **adenomas** and **leiomyomas.** Most benign tumors are found in the jejunum and ileum.

Carcinoid tumors, the most common tumors of the small bowel, have a benign appearance, although they have the potential to become malignant. These small lesions tend to grow submucosally and frequently are missed radiographically.

Lymphoma and **adenocarcinoma** are malignant tumors of the small intestine. Lymphomas are demonstrated during a small bowel series as the "stacked coin" sign. This sign is caused by thickening, coarsening, and possible hemorrhage of the mucosal wall. Other segments of the intestine may become narrowed and ulcerative. Adenocarcinomas produce short and sharp "napkin-ring" defects within the lumen, which may lead to complete obstruction. These radiographic signs of neoplasm are demonstrated during a barium enema procedure. The most frequent sites for adenocarcinoma are the duodenum and the proximal jejunum.

The small bowel series, or **enteroclysis,** may demonstrate stricture or blockage caused by the neoplasm. CT of the abdomen may further ascertain the location and size of the tumor.

Sprue *(spru)* and **malabsorption syndromes**[3] are conditions in which the gastrointestinal tract is unable to process and absorb certain nutrients. Sprue consists of a group of intestinal malabsorption diseases that involve an inability to absorb certain proteins and dietary fat. The malabsorption may be due to an intraluminal (digestive) defect, a mucosal abnormality, or a lymphatic obstruction. Malabsorption syndrome is often experienced by patients with lactose and sucrose sensitivities. Deficiency syndromes may result from excessive loss of vitamins, electrolytes, iron, or calcium. During a small bowel series, the mucosa may appear thickened as a result of constant irritation.

Celiac disease is a form of sprue or malabsorption disease that affects the proximal small bowel, especially the proximal duodenum. It commonly involves the insoluble protein (gluten) found in cereal grains.

Whipple disease[3] is a rare disorder of the proximal small bowel whose cause is unknown. Symptoms include dilation of the intestine, edema, malabsorption, deposits of fat in the bowel wall, and mesenteric nodules. Whipple disease is best diagnosed with a small bowel series, which shows distorted loops of small intestine.

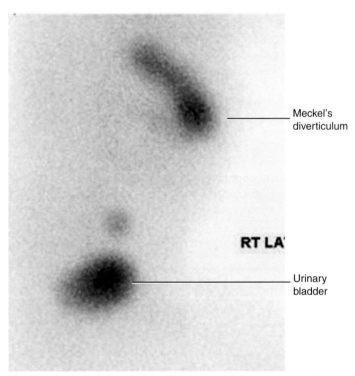

Meckel's diverticulum

RT LA

Urinary bladder

Fig. 13.24 Meckel diverticulum. Nuclear medicine scan—lateral view. (Courtesy Jeanne Dial, MEd, CNMT.)

Small Bowel Procedures

Four methods are used to study the small intestine radiographically. Methods 1 and 2 are the more common methods. Methods 3 and 4 are special small bowel studies that are performed only when methods 1 and 2 are unsatisfactory or contraindicated.
1. Upper GI–small bowel combination (Box 13.1)
2. Small bowel–only series (Box 13.2)
3. Enteroclysis (Box 13.3)
4. Intubation method (Box 13.4)

CONTRAST MEDIA

A thin mixture of barium sulfate is used for most small bowel series. When perforated bowel is suspected or when surgery is scheduled to follow the small bowel series, a water-soluble, iodinated contrast medium may be given. If the patient exhibits hypomotility of the bowel, ice water or another stimulant may be provided to promote the transit of barium. Also, water-soluble, iodinated contrast medium can be added to the barium to increase peristalsis and transit time of contrast media through the small intestine.

UPPER GI–SMALL BOWEL COMBINATION

For an upper GI–small bowel combination procedure, a routine upper GI series is performed first. After the routine stomach study is completed, progress of the barium is followed through the entire small bowel. During a routine upper GI series, the patient generally should ingest one full cup, or 8 oz, of barium sulfate mixture. For any small bowel examination, the time the patient ingested this barium should be noted for timing of sequential radiographs. However, some departments begin timing after ingestion of the second cup.

After completion of fluoroscopy and routine radiography of the stomach, the patient is given one additional cup of barium to ingest. The time this is finished should be noted. A posteroanterior (PA) radiograph of the proximal small bowel is obtained 30 minutes following the initial barium ingestion. The PA projection is preferred over the AP to allow for compression of the abdomen, which will produce some separation of the loops of intestine. This first radiograph of the small bowel series (marked "30 minutes") is commonly obtained about 15 minutes after the upper GI series has been completed.

Radiographs are obtained at specific intervals throughout the small bowel series until the barium sulfate column passes through the ileocecal valve and progresses into the ascending colon. For the first 2 hours in the small bowel series, radiographs are usually obtained at 15-minute to 30-minute intervals. If the examination needs to be continued beyond the 2-hour time frame, radiographs are usually obtained every hour until barium passes through the ileocecal valve.

Review of Images

As soon as each radiograph in the small bowel series is processed, it should be reviewed by the radiologist. The physician may wish to examine any suspicious area with fluoroscopy or may request additional radiographs.

BOX 13.1 PROCEDURE SUMMARY: UPPER GI–SMALL BOWEL COMBINATION

ROUTINE
- Routine upper GI first
- Notation of time patient ingested first cup (8 oz) of barium
- Ingestion of second cup of barium
- 30-minute PA radiograph (centering high for proximal small bowel)
- Half-hour interval radiographs, centered to iliac crest, until barium reaches large bowel (usually 2 hours)
- 1-hour interval radiographs, if more time is needed after 2 hours

OPTIONAL
- Fluoroscopy and spot imaging of ileocecal valve and terminal ileum (compression cone may be used)

BOX 13.2 PROCEDURE SUMMARY: SMALL BOWEL–ONLY SERIES

ROUTINE
- Plain abdomen radiograph (scout)
- 2 cups (16 oz) of barium ingested (noting time)
- 15- to 30-minute radiograph (centered high for proximal small bowel)
- Half-hour interval radiographs (centered to crest) until barium reaches large bowel (usually 2 hours)
- 1-hour interval radiographs, if more time is needed (some routines including continuous half-hour intervals)

OPTIONAL
- Fluoroscopy with compression sometimes required

BOX 13.3 PROCEDURE SUMMARY: ENTEROCLYSIS (DOUBLE-CONTRAST SMALL BOWEL SERIES)

PROCEDURE
- Special guidewire and catheter advanced to duodenojejunal junction
- Thin mixture of barium sulfate instilled
- Air or methylcellulose instilled
- Fluoroscopic spot images and conventional radiographs taken

OPTIONAL
- Patient may have CT scan of gastrointestinal tract
- On successful completion of examination, intubation tube removed

---

BOX 13.4 PROCEDURE SUMMARY: INTUBATION METHOD (SINGLE-CONTRAST SMALL BOWEL SERIES)

PROCEDURE
- Single-lumen catheter advanced to proximal jejunum (double-lumen catheter used for therapeutic intubation)
- Water-soluble iodinated agent or thin mixture of barium sulfate instilled
- Time at which contrast medium is instilled noted
- Conventional radiographs or optional fluoroscopic spot films taken at specific time intervals

OPTIONAL
- Patient may have CT scan of gastrointestinal tract following the small bowel series. In those cases, an iodinated contrast medium or dilute barium sulfate (e.g., VoLumen®) must be given.

13

Fluoroscopic Study

The region of the terminal ileum and the ileocecal valve generally is studied fluoroscopically. Spot filming of the terminal ileum usually indicates completion of the examination.

The patient shown in Fig. 13.25 is in position under the compression cone, which, when lowered against the abdomen, spreads out loops of ileum to visualize the ileocecal valve better.

Delayed Radiographs

The radiologist may request delayed radiographs to follow the barium through the entire large bowel. A barium meal given by mouth usually reaches the rectum within 24 hours.

SMALL BOWEL–ONLY SERIES

The second possibility for study of the small intestine is the small bowel–only series, as summarized on the right. For every contrast medium examination, including the small bowel series, a radiograph of the abdomen should be obtained before the contrast medium is introduced.

For the small bowel–only series, the patient generally ingests two cups (16 oz) of barium, and the time is noted. Depending on departmental protocol, the first radiograph is taken 15 minutes or 30 minutes after completion of barium ingestion. This first radiograph requires high centering to include the diaphragm. From this point on, the examination is exactly the same as the follow-up series of the upper GI. Radiographs generally are taken every half-hour for 2 hours followed by radiographs every hour thereafter until barium reaches the cecum or ascending colon.

NOTES: Some routines may include continuous half-hour imaging until the barium reaches the cecum.

In the routine small bowel series, regular barium sulfate ordinarily reaches the large intestine within 2 or 3 hours, but this time varies greatly among patients.

Fluoroscopy with spot imaging and use of a compression cone may provide options for better visualization of the ileocecal valve.

ENTEROCLYSIS–DOUBLE-CONTRAST SMALL BOWEL PROCEDURE

A third method of small bowel study is the **enteroclysis** *(en″-ter-ok′-li-sis)* procedure, which is a **double-contrast method** that is used to evaluate the small bowel.

Enteroclysis describes the injection of a nutrient or medicinal liquid into the bowel. In the context of a radiographic small bowel procedure, it refers to a study wherein the patient is intubated under fluoroscopic control using a guidewire with a special **enteroclysis catheter** passed over it. This catheter is passed through the stomach into the duodenojejunal junction (ligament of Treitz). With fluoroscopy guidance, a duodenojejunal tube is placed into the terminal duodenum. It is held in the correct location with a retention balloon.

First, a high-density suspension of **barium** is injected through this catheter at a rate of 100 mL/min. Fluoroscopic and conventional radiographs may be taken at this time. **Air** or **methylcellulose** is injected into the bowel to distend it, which provides a double-contrast effect. Methylcellulose is preferred because it adheres to the bowel while distending it. This double-contrast effect dilates the loops of small bowel while enhancing visibility of the mucosa. This action leads to increased accuracy of the study. If a CT study is to follow the enteroclysis, iodinated contrast media or water may be used in place of the barium.

Disadvantages of enteroclysis include increased patient discomfort and the possibility of bowel perforation during catheter placement.

Enteroclysis is indicated for patients with clinical histories of **small bowel ileus, regional enteritis (Crohn disease)**, or **malabsorption syndrome.**

When the small bowel has been successfully filled with contrast medium, the radiologist typically takes fluoroscopy spot images. The technologist may be asked to produce various projections of the small bowel, including AP, PA, oblique, and possibly erect projections.

When the procedure has been completed, the catheter is removed, and the patient is encouraged to increase his or her water intake for the day. Laxatives may also be recommended to promote evacuation of the barium sulfate.

The radiograph seen in Fig. 13.26 is an example of an enteroclysis. The end of the catheter (small arrows) is seen in the distal duodenum, not yet reaching the duodenojejunal junction (ligament of Treitz; large upper arrow). The introduction of methylcellulose dilates the lumen of the bowel, and barium coats the mucosa.

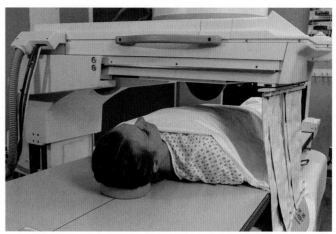

Fig. 13.25 Fluoroscopy of ileocecal region with compression cone.

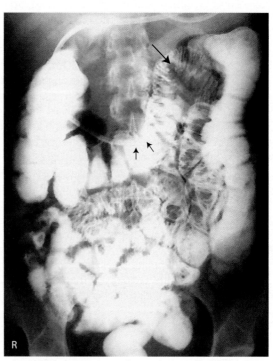

Fig. 13.26 PA radiograph—enteroclysis.

Many departments perform a dual-modality procedure in which the duodenojejunal tube is inserted and contrast medium is instilled under fluoroscopic guidance. After the initial fluoroscopy has been performed, the patient undergoes a CT scan of the gastrointestinal tract to detect any obstructions or adhesions (Fig. 13.27).

INTUBATION METHOD—SINGLE-CONTRAST STUDY

The fourth and final method of small bowel study is gastrointestinal **intubation** *(in″-tu-ba′-shun)*, sometimes referred to as a *small bowel enema*. With this technique, a **nasogastric tube** is passed through the patient's nose, through the esophagus, stomach, and duodenum, and into the jejunum (Fig. 13.28). This radiograph shows the end of the tube (small arrows) still looped in the lower part of the stomach, having not yet passed into the duodenum. The distended air-filled loops of small bowel demonstrating air-fluid levels indicate some type of small bowel obstruction.

This procedure is performed for both diagnostic and therapeutic purposes. The **diagnostic intubation** procedure may be referred to as a **small bowel enema**. A **single-lumen tube** is passed into the proximal jejunum. Placing the patient into a right anterior oblique (RAO) position may aid in passage of the tube from the stomach into the duodenum by gastric peristaltic action. A water-soluble iodinated agent or a thin barium sulfate suspension is injected through the tube. Radiographs are taken at timed intervals similar to those in a standard small bowel series.

The **therapeutic intubation** procedure is performed often to relieve postoperative distention or to decompress a small bowel obstruction. A **double-lumen** catheter, termed a **Miller-Abbott (M-A) tube,** is advanced into the stomach. Radiopaque materials often are incorporated into the design of the catheter to assist during fluoroscopy-guided placement. Through peristalsis, the catheter is advanced into the jejunum. The technologist may be asked to take radiographs at timed intervals to determine whether the catheter is advancing. Gas and excessive fluids can be withdrawn through the catheter.

An optional part of this study may include fluoroscopy, whereby the tube can be guided into the duodenum through the use of compression and manual manipulation.

PATIENT PREPARATION

Patient preparation for a small bowel series is identical to preparation for an upper GI series. The most common method of small bowel study consists of a combination of the two examinations into one long examination, with the small bowel series following the upper GI series.

The goal of patient preparation for the upper GI series or the small bowel series is an **empty stomach.** Food and fluid must be withheld for at least **8 hours** before these examinations are performed. Ideally, the patient should be on a low-residue diet 48 hours before the small bowel series is conducted. In addition, the patient should not use any type of tobacco or nicotine products or chew gum during the NPO period. Before the procedure is performed, the patient should be asked to void, so as not to cause displacement of the ileum secondary to a distended bladder.

PREGNANCY PRECAUTIONS

If the patient is female, a menstrual history must be obtained. Irradiation of an early pregnancy is one of the most hazardous situations in diagnostic radiography. X-ray examinations such as the small bowel series or the barium enema that include the pelvis and uterus in the primary beam **should not be performed on pregnant women unless absolutely necessary.** If the patient is unsure whether she may be pregnant, the technologist should bring this to the attention of the radiologist. A pregnancy test may be ordered before the procedure.

METHOD OF IMAGING

An image receptor (IR) of 14 × 17 inches (35 × 43 cm) is commonly used to visualize as much of the small intestine as possible

on the radiographs. Spot imaging of selected portions of the small bowel may use smaller IRs.

The prone position is most appropriate for a small bowel series unless the patient is unable to assume that position. The **prone position** allows abdominal compression **to separate the various loops of bowel, creating a higher degree of visibility.** Asthenic patients may be placed in the Trendelenburg position to separate overlapping loops of ileum.

For the 30-minute image, the IR is placed high enough to include the stomach on the radiograph. This placement often requires longitudinal centering to the duodenal bulb and side-to-side centering to the midsagittal plane. Approximately three-fourths of the IR should extend above the iliac crest. Because most of the barium is in the stomach and proximal small bowel, a high-kVp (110 to 125) technique should be used on this initial radiograph.

All radiographs after the initial 30-minute exposure should be centered to the iliac crest. For the 1-hour and later radiographs, 90 to 100 kVp settings may be used because the barium is spread through more of the alimentary canal and is not concentrated in the stomach. Fluoroscopic spot imaging of the terminal ileum usually completes the examination.

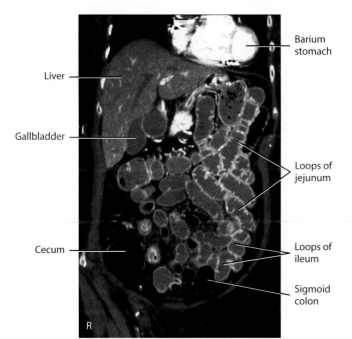

Fig. 13.27 CT enteroclysis.

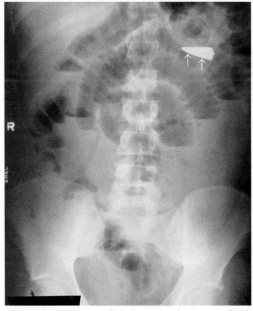

Fig. 13.28 AP erect abdomen—intubation method.

Barium Enema (Lower GI Series)
DEFINITION
The radiographic study of the large intestine is commonly termed a **barium enema.** It requires the use of contrast media to demonstrate the large intestine and its components. Alternative names include **BE (BaE)** and **lower GI series.**

PURPOSE
The purpose of the barium enema is to demonstrate radiographically the form and function of the large intestine to detect any abnormal conditions. Both the single-contrast and the double-contrast barium enema (Fig. 13.29) involve study of the entire large intestine.

CONTRAINDICATIONS
The two strict contraindications for the barium enema are similar to the contraindications described for the small bowel series. These have been described as a **possible perforated hollow viscus** and a **possible large bowel obstruction.** These patients should not be given barium as a contrast medium. Although not as radiopaque as barium sulfate, water-soluble contrast media can be used for these conditions.

Careful review of the patient's chart and clinical history may help to prevent problems during the procedure. The radiologist should be informed of any conditions or disease processes noted in the patient's chart. This information may dictate the type of study performed.

It is also important to review the patient's chart to determine whether the patient has had a recent **sigmoidoscopy** or a **colonoscopy** before undergoing the barium enema. If a **biopsy of the colon** was performed during these procedures, the involved section of the colon wall may be weakened. This may lead to perforation during the barium enema. The **radiologist must be informed** of this situation before beginning the procedure.

Appendicitis
The barium enema generally is not performed in cases of acute appendicitis because of the danger of perforation.

When clinical indications are unclear, high-resolution **ultrasound** with graded compression and CT have become the modalities of choice for the diagnosis of acute appendicitis.

CLINICAL INDICATIONS FOR BARIUM ENEMA
Common clinical indications for barium enema include the following (Table 13.5).

Colitis *(ko-li'-tis)* is an **inflammatory condition of the large intestine** that may be caused by many factors, including bacterial infection, diet, stress, and other environmental conditions. The intestinal mucosa may appear rigid and thick and lack haustral markings along the involved segment. Because of chronic inflammation and spasm, the intestinal wall has a "saw-tooth" or jagged appearance.

Ulcerative colitis is a severe form of colitis that is most common among young adults. It is a chronic condition that often leads to development of coinlike ulcers within the mucosal wall. Along with Crohn disease, it is one of the most common forms of inflammatory bowel disease. These ulcers may be seen during a barium enema as multiple ring-shaped filling defects that create a "cobblestone" appearance along the mucosa. Patients with long-term bouts of ulcerative colitis may develop "stovepipe" colon, in which haustral markings and flexures are absent (Fig. 13.30).

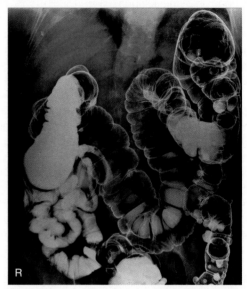

Fig. 13.29 Barium enema—double-contrast study.

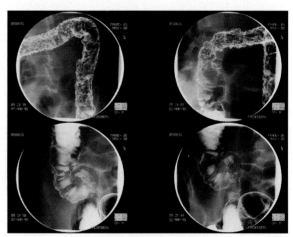

Fig. 13.30 Ulcerative colitis.

TABLE 13.5 **SUMMARY OF CLINICAL INDICATIONS: LARGE INTESTINE**			
CONDITION OR DISEASE	**MOST COMMON RADIOGRAPHIC EXAMINATION**	**POSSIBLE RADIOGRAPHIC APPEARANCE**	**EXPOSURE FACTOR ADJUSTMENT[a]**
Colitis	Single-contrast and double-contrast (preferred) barium enema	Thickening of mucosal wall with loss of haustral markings	None
Ulcerative colitis	Single-contrast and double-contrast (preferred) barium enema	"Cobblestone" and possible "stovepipe" appearance with severe forms	None
Diverticula (diverticulosis/ diverticulitis)	Double-contrast barium enema recommended	Barium-filled circular defects projecting outward from colon wall; jagged or "sawtooth" appearance of mucosa	None
Intussusception	Single-contrast or air/gas contrast enema recommended	"Mushroom-shaped" dilation at distal aspect of intussusception, with very little barium or gas passing beyond it	None
Neoplasm	Double-contrast barium enema recommended to detect small polyps; CT; colonography	Filling defects; narrowness or tapering of lumen; "apple-core" or "napkin-ring" lesions	None
Polyps	Double-contrast barium enema recommended; CT; colonography	Barium-filled, saclike projections projecting inward into the lumen of the bowel	None
Volvulus	Single-contrast barium enema	Tapered or beak appearance, with air-filled distended region of intestine	None

[a]Dependent on stage or severity of disease or condition.

A **diverticulum** *(di″-ver-tik′-u-lum)* is an **outpouching of the mucosal wall** that may result from herniation of the inner wall of the colon. Although this is a relatively benign condition, it may become widespread throughout the colon, specifically the sigmoid colon. It is most common among adults older than 40 years of age.

Diverticulosis is the condition of having numerous diverticula. If these diverticula become infected, the condition is referred to as **diverticulitis.** Inflamed diverticula may become a source of bleeding, in which case surgical removal may be necessary. A patient may develop peritonitis if a diverticulum perforates the mucosal wall, permitting fecal matter to escape.

Diverticula appear as small, barium-filled, circular defects that project **outward** from the colon wall during a barium enema (see small arrows in Fig. 13.31). The double-contrast barium enema provides an excellent view of the intestinal mucosa, revealing small diverticula. A double-contrast barium enema clearly demonstrates the presence of most diverticula.

Intussusception *(in″-ta-sa-sep′-shan)* is a telescoping or invagination of one part of the intestine into another. It is most common in infants younger than 2 years of age but can occur in adults. A barium enema or an air/gas enema may play a therapeutic role in re-expanding the involved bowel. Radiographically, progression of the barium through the colon terminates at a "mushroom-shaped" dilation; very little barium/gas, if any, passes beyond this area. The dilation marks the point of obstruction. Intussusception must be resolved quickly so that it does not lead to obstruction and necrosis of the bowel (see Chapter 16). If the condition recurs, surgery may be necessary.

Neoplasms are common in the large intestine. Although benign tumors do occur, carcinoma of the large intestine is a leading cause of death among both men and women. Most carcinomas of the large intestine occur in the rectum and sigmoid colon. These cancerous tumors often encircle the lumen of the colon, producing an irregular channel through it. The radiographic appearance of these tumors, as demonstrated during a barium enema, has led to the use of descriptive terms such as "apple-core" or "napkin-ring" lesions (Fig. 13.32). Both benign and malignant tumors may begin as **polyps.**

Annular carcinoma (adenocarcinoma), one of the most typical forms of colon cancer, may form an "apple-core" or "napkin-ring" appearance as the tumor grows and infiltrates the bowel walls. It frequently results in large bowel obstruction.

Polyps are saclike projections similar to diverticula except that they project **inward** into the lumen rather than outward, as do diverticula. Similar to diverticula, polyps can become inflamed and may be a source of bleeding. In this case, they may have to be surgically removed. Barium enema, endoscopy, and CT colonography are the most effective modalities used to demonstrate neoplasms in the large intestine (Fig. 13.33).

Volvulus *(vol′-vu-lus)* is a twisting of a portion of the intestine on its own mesentery, leading to a mechanical type of obstruction. Blood supply to the twisted portion is compromised, leading to obstruction and localized death of tissue. A volvulus may be found in portions of the jejunum or ileum. This can also occur in the cecum and sigmoid colon. Volvulus is more likely to occur in men than in women and is most common in adults 20 to 50 years old. The classic sign is a "beak" sign—a tapered narrowing at the volvulus site as demonstrated during a barium enema. A volvulus produces an air-fluid level, which is well demonstrated on an erect abdomen projection.

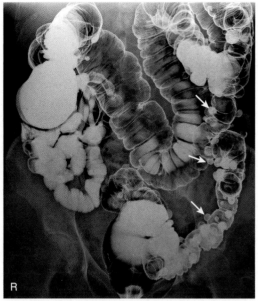

Fig. 13.31 Diverticulosis primarily in descending colon

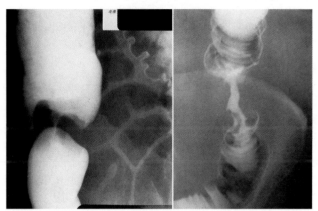

Fig. 13.32 *Left,* Neoplasm—colon cancer with "apple-core" lesion. *Right,* Advanced carcinoma of the colon.

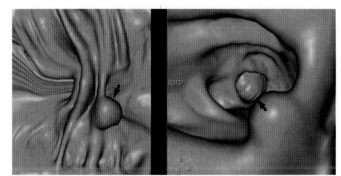

Fig. 13.33 CT colonography—images demonstrating a polyp. (Courtesy Philips Medical Systems.)

Cecal volvulus describes the ascending colon and the cecum as having a long mesentery, which makes them more susceptible to a volvulus (Fig. 13.34).

Barium Enema Procedure

PATIENT PREPARATION

Preparation of the patient for a barium enema is more involved than preparation of the stomach and small bowel. However, the final objective is the same. The section of alimentary canal to be examined must be empty. Thorough cleansing of the entire large bowel is of paramount importance for a satisfactory contrast media study of the large intestine.

CONTRAINDICATIONS TO LAXATIVES (CATHARTICS)

Certain conditions contraindicate the use of the very effective cathartics or purgatives needed to cleanse the large bowel thoroughly. These conditions include (1) gross bleeding, (2) severe diarrhea, (3) obstruction, and (4) inflammatory conditions such as appendicitis.

A laxative is a substance that produces frequent soft or liquid bowel movements. These substances increase peristalsis in the large bowel and occasionally in the small bowel as well by irritating sensory nerve endings in the intestinal mucosa. This increased peristalsis dramatically accelerates the passage of intestinal contents through the digestive system.

TWO CLASSES OF LAXATIVES

Two different classes of laxatives may be prescribed. First are irritant laxatives, such as castor oil; second are saline laxatives, such as magnesium citrate or magnesium sulfate. The use of irritant laxatives is rare today. For best results, bowel-cleansing procedures should be specified on patient instruction sheets for both inpatients and outpatients. The technologist should be completely familiar with the type of preparation used in each radiology department. The importance of a clean large intestine for a barium enema, especially for a double-contrast barium enema, cannot be overstated. Any retained fecal matter may obscure the normal anatomy or may yield false diagnostic information, leading to rescheduling of the procedure after the large intestine has been properly cleaned.

RADIOGRAPHIC ROOM PREPARATION

The radiographic room should be prepared in advance of the patient's arrival. The fluoroscopy room and the examination table should be clean and tidy for each patient (Fig. 13.35). The control panel should be set for fluoroscopy, with the appropriate technical factors selected. The fluoroscopy timer may be set up to its maximum time, which is usually 5 minutes. If conventional fluoroscopy is used, the photo-spot mechanism should be in proper working order, and a supply of spot film cassettes should be handy. The anticipated number of needed IRs for postprocedure images should be set aside. Protective lead aprons and lead gloves should be available for the radiologist, and lead aprons should be available for all other personnel present in the room. The fluoroscopic table should be placed in the horizontal position, with waterproof backing or disposable pads placed on the tabletop. Waterproof protection is essential in cases of premature evacuation of the contrast material.

The bucky tray must be positioned at the foot end of the table, if the fluoroscopy tube is located beneath the tabletop. This expands the bucky slot shield, reducing gonadal dose to the fluoroscopist, as described in Chapter 12 (see Fig. 12.59). The foot control switch should be placed appropriately for the radiologist, or the remote control area should be prepared. Tissues, towels, replacement linen, bedpan, extra gowns, a room air freshener, and a waste receptacle should be readily available. The appropriate contrast medium or media, container, tubing, and enema tip should be prepared. A proper lubricant should be provided for the enema tip. The type of barium sulfate used and the concentration of the mixture vary considerably, depending on radiologist preferences and the type of examination to be performed. Refer to the five safety consideration for all barium enema procedures before initiating one of these procedures (Box 13.5).

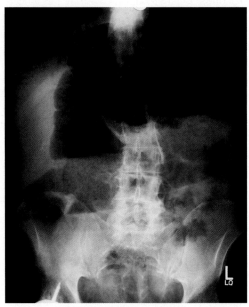

Fig. 13.34 Cecal volvulus.

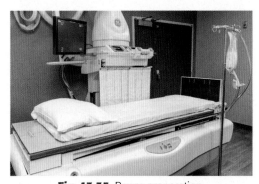

Fig. 13.35 Room preparation.

BOX 13.5 SUMMARY OF SAFETY CONCERNS DURING BARIUM ENEMA PROCEDURES

Safety during any barium enema procedure is of utmost importance. Five important safety concerns are as follows:

1. **Review patient's chart:** Note any pertinent clinical history on the examination requisition, and inform the radiologist about whether the patient underwent a sigmoidoscopy or colonoscopy before the barium enema was given, especially if a biopsy was performed. Determine whether the patient has any known allergies to the contrast media or natural latex products. Diabetic patients should not be given glucagon before or during a procedure unless ordered by physician.
2. **Never force enema tip into rectum:** This action may lead to a perforated rectum. The radiologist inserts the enema tip under fluoroscopic guidance, if needed.
3. **Ensure height of enema bag does not exceed 24 inches (60 cm) above table:** This distance should be maintained before the procedure is begun. The radiologist may wish to raise the bag height during the procedure based on the rate of flow of the contrast medium.
4. **Verify water temperature of contrast medium:** Water that is too hot or too cold may injure the patient or compromise the procedure.
5. **Escort patient to restroom after completion of the study:** A barium enema can be stressful for some patients. Patients have been known to faint during or after evacuation.

EQUIPMENT AND SUPPLIES
Barium Enema Containers

A closed-system enema container is used to administer barium sulfate or an air and barium sulfate combination during the barium enema. This closed-type, disposable barium enema bag system has replaced the older open-type system for convenience and for reducing the risk of cross-infection.

This system (see Fig. 13.36) includes the disposable enema bag with a premeasured amount of barium sulfate. Once mixed, the suspension travels down its own connective tubing. Flow is controlled by a plastic stopcock. An enema tip is placed on the end of the tubing and is inserted into the patient's rectum.

After the examination has been completed, much of the barium can be drained back into the bag by lowering the system to below tabletop level. The entire bag and tubing are disposed of after a single use.

Enema Tips

Various types and sizes of enema tips are available (Fig. 13.37). The three most common types are plastic disposable (A), rectal retention (B), and air-contrast retention (C) enema tips. All are considered single-use, disposable enema tips.

Rectal disposable retention tips (B and C), sometimes called *retention catheters,* are used with patients who have relaxed anal sphincters or who cannot for whatever reason retain the contrast material. Rectal retention catheters consist of a double-lumen tube with a thin rubber balloon at the distal end. After rectal insertion, this balloon is carefully inflated with air through a small tube to assist the patient in retaining the barium enema. These retention catheters should be **fully inflated only under fluoroscopic guidance provided by the radiologist** because of the potential danger of intestinal rupture. To prevent discomfort for the patient, the balloon should not be fully inflated until the fluoroscopic procedure begins.

A special type of rectal tip (C) is needed to inject air through a separate tube into the colon. The air mixes with the barium to produce a **double-contrast barium enema examination.**

LATEX ALLERGIES

Today, most products are primarily latex free, but identifying whether the patient is sensitive to natural latex products is still important. Patients with sensitivity to latex experience anaphylactoid-type reactions that include sneezing, redness, rash, difficulty in breathing, and even death.

If the patient has a history of latex sensitivity, the technologist must ensure that the enema tip, tubing, and gloves are latex free. Even dust produced from removal of latex gloves can introduce latex protein into the air, which may be inhaled by the patient.

Technologists with latex sensitivity must be keenly aware of the types of gloves, catheters, and other latex devices found in the department. If a rash develops while technologists are wearing gloves or handling certain objects, they should consult a physician to explore the possibility of latex sensitivity.

CONTRAST MEDIA

Barium sulfate is the most common type of positive-contrast medium used for the barium enema. The concentration of the barium sulfate suspension varies according to the study performed. A standard mixture used for single-contrast barium enemas is between 15% and 25% weight-to-volume (w/v). The thicker barium used for double-contrast barium enemas has a weight-to-volume concentration between 75% and 95% or greater. The barium sulfate solution introduced during a CT scan of the large intestine possesses a low w/v to prevent artifacts that may obscure anatomy from being produced. The evacuative proctogram (discussed later in the chapter) requires a contrast medium with a minimum w/v of 100%.

Negative-Contrast Agent

The double-contrast study uses numerous negative-contrast agents, in addition to barium sulfate. Room air, nitrogen, and carbon dioxide are the most common forms of negative-contrast media used. Carbon dioxide is gaining wide use because it is well tolerated by the large intestine and is absorbed rapidly after the procedure. Carbon dioxide and nitrogen gas are stored in a small tank and can be introduced into the rectum through an air-contrast retention enema tip.

An iodinated, water-soluble contrast medium may be used in the case of a perforated or lacerated intestinal wall. It may also be used when the patient is scheduled for surgery after the imaging procedure. A kVp range of 85 to 95 should be used with a water-soluble, negative-contrast agent.

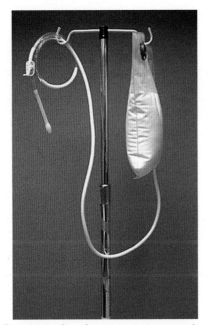

Fig. 13.36 Closed-system enema container.

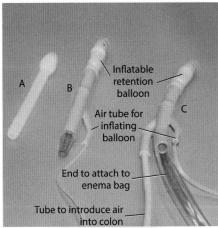

A   B   Inflatable retention balloon

Air tube for inflating balloon   C

End to attach to enema bag

Tube to introduce air into colon

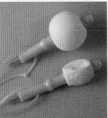

Inflated and un-inflated retention enema tips.

Fig. 13.37 Enema tips. A, Plastic disposable. B, Rectal retention tip. C, Contrast retention tip.

Contrast Media Preparation

The mixing instructions as supplied by the manufacturer should be followed precisely.

A debate has evolved over the temperature of the water used to prepare the barium sulfate suspension. Some experts recommend the use of cold water (40° to 45° F) in the preparation of contrast media. Cold water is reported to have an anesthetic effect on the colon and to increase the retention of contrast media. Critics have stated that the use of cold water may lead to colonic spasm.

Tepid water (85° to 90° F) is recommended by most experts for completion of a more successful examination with maximal patient comfort. The technologist should *never* use hot water to prepare contrast media. Hot water may scald the mucosal lining of the colon.

Because barium sulfate produces a colloidal suspension, shaking the enema bag before tip insertion is important for preventing separation of barium sulfate from water.

Spasm during the barium enema is a common side effect. Patient anxiety, overexpansion of the intestinal wall, discomfort, and related disease processes all may lead to colonic spasm. To minimize the possibility of spasm, a topical anesthetic such as lidocaine may be added to the contrast medium. If spasm does occur during the study, glucagon can be given intravenously and should be kept in the department for these situations.

PROCEDURE PREPARATION

Sims Position

Sims position is shown in Fig. 13.38. The patient is asked to roll onto the left side and lean forward. The right leg is flexed at the knee and hip and is placed in front of the left leg. The left knee is comfortably flexed. Sims position relaxes the abdominal muscles and decreases pressure within the abdomen.

Each phase of the rectal tube insertion must be explained to the patient. Before insertion, the barium sulfate solution should be well mixed and a little of the barium mixture run into a waste receptacle to ensure no air remains in the tubing or enema tip.

PROCEDURE

A patient undergoing a barium enema should be dressed in an appropriate hospital gown (Fig. 13.39). A cotton gown with the opening and ties in the back is preferable. The type of gown that must be pulled over the patient's head for removal should never be used. Sometimes the gown becomes soiled during the examination and must be changed. An outpatient should be instructed to remove all clothing, including shoes and socks or pantyhose. Disposable slippers should be provided in case some barium is lost on the way to the restroom.

After the fluoroscopic room and the contrast media have been completely prepared, the patient is escorted to the examination room. First, the patient history should be taken, and the examination should be carefully explained. Because complete cooperation is essential and this examination can be embarrassing, extra effort should be made to communicate thoroughly with the patient at every stage of the examination.

Previous barium enema studies should be made available to the fluoroscopist.

Preparation for Rectal Tip Insertion

The patient is placed in **Sims position** before the enema tip is inserted. The technologist must put on protective gloves. The rectal tip must be well lubricated with a water-soluble lubricant.

Before the rectal tip is inserted, the patient should be instructed (1) not to push the tip out of the rectum by bearing down once the

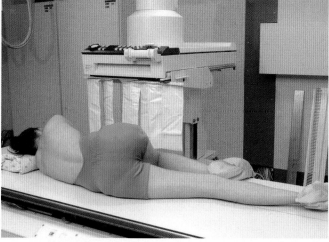

Fig. 13.38 Sims position (for rectal tip insertion).

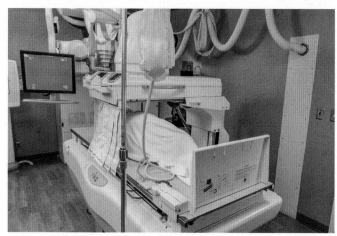

Fig. 13.39 Procedure preparation.

tip is inserted, (2) to relax the abdominal muscles to prevent increased intra-abdominal pressure, and (3) to concentrate on breathing by mouth to reduce spasms and cramping. The patient must be assured that the barium flow will be stopped if cramping occurs.

ENEMA TIP INSERTION

Before the enema tip is inserted, the opening in the back of the patient's gown should be adjusted to expose only the anal region. The rest of the patient should be well covered when the rectal tube is inserted. The patient's modesty should be protected in every way possible during the barium enema examination. The right buttock should be raised to open the gluteal fold and expose the anus. The patient should take in a few deep breaths before actual insertion of the enema tip. If the tip will not enter with gentle pressure, the patient should be asked to relax and assist if possible. The tip should *never* be forced in a manner that could cause injury to the patient. If resistance is felt during tip insertion, it should be performed under physician supervision. Because the abdominal muscles relax on expiration, the tip should be inserted during the exhalation phase of respiration.

The rectum and anal canal present a double curvature; the tube is inserted first in a forward direction approximately 1 to 4 inches (2.5 to 4 cm). This initial insertion should be **aimed toward the umbilicus.** After the initial insertion, the rectal tube is directed **superiorly and slightly anteriorly** to follow the normal curvature of the rectum (Fig. 13.40). The total insertion of the tip should **not exceed 3 to 4 inches (7.5 to 10 cm)** to prevent possible injury to the wall of the rectum. The rectal tube may be taped in place or held to prevent it from slipping out while the patient turns back into a supine position for the start of fluoroscopy. This position is usually supine but may be prone, depending on the preference of the radiologist.

If the retention-type tip is necessary, most departments allow the technologist to instill one or two puffs of air into the balloon end to help hold it in place. However, the bulb should be **filled to its maximum only under fluoroscopic control** as the fluoroscopy procedure begins. As the procedure begins, the intravenous pole supporting the enema bag should be **no higher than 24 inches (60 cm)** above the radiographic table. Box 13.6 lists the steps of enema tip insertion.

FLUOROSCOPY ROUTINE

NOTE: The following routine may differ for countries or facilities in which the expanded scope of technologists includes barium enema fluoroscopy.

The fluoroscopist is summoned to the radiographic room after all room and patient preparations have been completed (Fig. 13.41). Following introduction of the physician and the patient, the patient's history and the reason for the examination are discussed.

During barium enema fluoroscopy, the general duties of the technologist are to follow the radiologist's instructions, assist the patient as needed, and expedite the procedure in any way possible. The technologist also must control the flow of barium or air and must change fluoroscopy spot cassettes (when used). The flow of barium is started and stopped several times during the barium enema. Each time the fluoroscopist asks that the flow be started, the technologist should say "barium on" after the clamp or hemostat is released. Each time the fluoroscopist requests that the flow be stopped, the technologist should say "barium off" after the tubing is clamped.

Many changes in patient position are made during fluoroscopy. These positional changes are made to visualize superimposed sections of bowel better and aid in advancement of the barium column. The technologist may have to assist the patient with positional moves and ensure that the tubing is not kinked or accidentally pulled out during the examination.

The fluoroscopic procedure begins with a general survey of the patient's abdomen and pelvis. For some departmental routines, if the retention-type enema tip is required, the air balloon may be inflated under fluoroscopic control at this point.

Various spot radiographs of selected portions of the large intestine are obtained as the barium column proceeds in retrograde fashion from rectum to cecum. At the end of the fluoroscopic procedure, a little barium is refluxed through the ileocecal valve, and fluoroscopy images of that area are obtained. Moderate discomfort usually is experienced when the large bowel is totally filled, so the examination must be concluded as rapidly as possible.

Routine radiographs may be requested with the bowel filled.

BOX 13.6 PROCEDURE SUMMARY: ENEMA TIP INSERTION

1. Describe the tip insertion procedure to the patient. Answer any questions before, during and after the procedure.
2. Place the patient in Sims position. The patient should lie on the left side, with the right leg flexed at the knee and hip.
3. Shake the enema bag once more to ensure proper mixing of barium sulfate suspension. Allow barium to flow through the tubing and from the tip to remove any air in the system.
4. Wearing gloves, coat the enema tip well with water-soluble lubricant.
5. On expiration, insert the enema tip in the rectum by directing it toward the umbilicus approximately 1 to 1½ inches (2.5 to 4 cm).
6. After initial insertion, advance up superiorly and slightly anteriorly. The total insertion should not exceed 3 to 4 inches (7.5 to 10 cm). Do *not* force enema tip.
7. Tape tubing in place to prevent slippage. Do *not* inflate retention tip unless directed by the fluoroscopist.
8. Ensure that the intravenous pole/enema bag is no more than 24 inches (60 cm) above the table. Ensure that the tubing stopcock is in the closed position, and no barium flows into the patient.

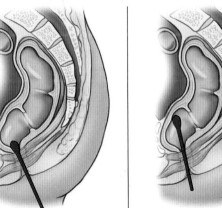
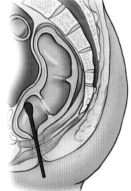

Initial insertion
(toward umbilicus)

Final placement
(slightly anterior,
then superior)

Fig. 13.40 Enema tip insertion.

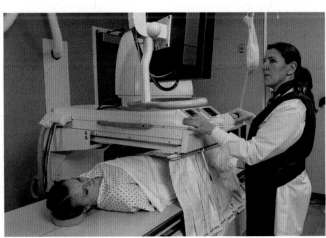

Fig. 13.41 Barium enema fluoroscopy.

TYPES OF LOWER GI EXAMINATIONS (PROCEDURES)

Three specific types of lower GI radiographic examinations or procedures are described in this chapter:

1. Single-contrast barium enema
2. Double-contrast barium enema
3. Evacuative proctography (defecogram)

Single-Contrast Barium Enema Procedure

The **single-contrast barium enema** is a procedure in which only positive-contrast media are used. In most cases, the contrast material is barium sulfate in a thin mixture. Occasionally, the contrast media must be a water-soluble contrast material. For example, if the patient is scheduled for surgery after undergoing the single-contrast enema procedure, a water-soluble contrast medium must be used.

An example of a single-contrast barium enema in which barium sulfate was used as the contrast medium is shown in Fig. 13.42.

Double-Contrast Barium Enema Procedure

A second common type of barium enema procedure is the **double-contrast type.** Double-contrast studies are more effective in demonstrating polyps and diverticula than single-contrast studies. Radiographic and fluoroscopic procedures for a double-contrast barium enema are different in that both air and barium must be introduced into the large bowel. Fig. 13.43 shows a double-contrast barium enema radiograph taken in the left lateral decubitus position. An absolutely **clean large bowel is essential** for a double-contrast study, and a **much thicker barium mixture is required.** Although exact ratios depend on the commercial preparations used, the ratio approaches a 1:1 mix, so that the final product is like heavy cream.

Two-stage Procedure One preferred method used to coat the bowel is a two-stage, double-contrast procedure. Initially, the thick barium is allowed to fill the left side of the intestine, including the left colic flexure. (The purpose of the thick barium mixture is to facilitate adherence to the mucosal lining.) Air is instilled into the bowel, pushing the barium through to the right side. At this time, the radiologist may ask that the enema bag be lowered below the table to allow any excess barium to be drained from the large intestine to provide better visualization of the intestinal mucosa.

The second stage consists of inflation of the bowel with a large amount of air/gas. This air/gas moves the main bolus of barium forward, leaving behind only the barium adhering to the mucosal wall. These steps are carried out under fluoroscopic control because the air bolus should not be pushed in front of the barium bolus.

This procedure demonstrates neoplasms or polyps that may be forming on the inner surface of the bowel and projecting into the lumen or opening of the bowel. These formations generally would not be visible during a single-contrast barium enema study.

Single-stage Procedure A single-stage, double-contrast procedure, wherein barium and air are instilled in a single procedure that reduces time and radiation exposure to the patient, also may be used. With this method, high-density barium is instilled into the rectum first with the patient in a slight Trendelenburg position. The barium tube is then clamped. With the table in a horizontal position, the patient is placed into various oblique and lateral positions after various amounts of air are added through the double-contrast procedure.

Spot Images (During Fluoroscopy) With both single-contrast and double-contrast studies, "spot" radiographs may be obtained to document any suspicious area. The patient may be asked to rotate several times to distribute the barium and air better during a double-contrast procedure.

Digital fluoroscopy With **digital fluoroscopy,** these "spot" images are obtained digitally rather than with separate IRs. Images taken during the study are stored in the memory of the computer. Once the images have undergone quality assurance, they are transferred to the picture archiving and communications system (PACS) for interpretation. The radiologist can review all recorded images and print only the images that have diagnostic importance. With PACS, images can be reviewed, read, and stored within the database system without the need for hard-copy prints.

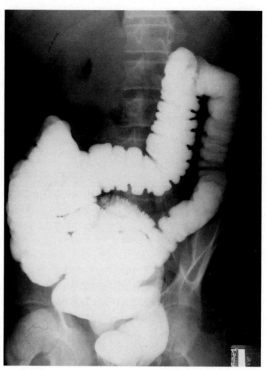

Fig. 13.42 Single-contrast barium enema.

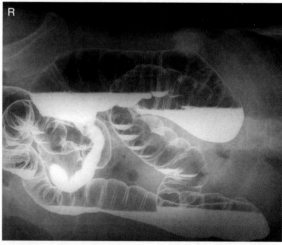

Fig. 13.43 Double-contrast barium enema (left lateral decubitus).

Postfluoroscopy Radiographs After fluoroscopy and before the patient is permitted to empty the large bowel, additional radiographs of the filled intestine may be obtained. The standard enema tip can be removed before these radiographs are taken when removal promotes retention of the contrast material, although some department protocols are to keep the enema tip in during the postfluoroscopy imaging. The retention-type tip is generally not removed until the large bowel is ready to be emptied and the patient is placed on a bedpan or sent to the bathroom.

Fig. 13.44 demonstrates the most common position for a routine barium enema. This is the **PA projection** with a full-sized 14 × 17-inch (35 × 43-cm) IR centered to the iliac crest. The PA projection with the patient in a prone position is preferred over the AP projection (Fig. 13.45) in a supine position because compression of the abdomen in the prone position results in more uniform radiographic density of the entire abdomen.

The IR should be centered to include the rectal ampulla on the bottom of the image. This positioning usually includes the entire large intestine with the exception of the left colic flexure. Clipping the left colic flexure off the radiographs may be acceptable if this area is well demonstrated on a previously obtained spot film. However, some departmental routines may include a second image centered higher to include this area on larger patients, or two images, with IR placed landscape.

Other projections are also obtained before evacuation of the barium. Double-contrast procedures generally require right and left lateral decubitus AP or PA projections, with a horizontal x-ray beam to demonstrate better the upside or air-filled portions of the large intestine.

NOTE: Because of the vast difference in density between the air-filled and barium-filled aspects of the large intestine, a tendency to overexpose the air-filled region may be noted. The recommendation is that the technologist consider using a compensating filter for the decubitus and ventral lateral projections taken during an air-contrast study. One version of a compensating filter that works well attaches to the face of the collimator with two small magnetic disks. The disks can be adjusted to place the filter over the air-filled portion of the large intestine.

All postfluoroscopy radiographs must be obtained as quickly as possible because the patient may have difficulty retaining the barium.

After the routine pre-evacuation radiographs and any supplemental radiographs have been obtained, the patient is allowed to expel the barium. For the patient who has had the enema tip removed, a quick trip to a nearby restroom is necessary. For the patient who cannot make such a trip, a bedpan should be provided. For the patient who is still connected to a closed system, simple lowering of the plastic bag to floor level to allow most of the barium to drain back into the bag is helpful. Department protocol determines how a retention tip should be removed. One way is first to clamp off the retention tip and then disconnect it from the enema tubing and container. When the patient is safely on a bedpan or commode, air is released from the bulb and the tip is removed.

Postevacuation Radiograph After most of the barium has been expelled, a postevacuation radiograph is obtained (Fig. 13.46). The postevacuation radiograph usually is taken in the prone position but may be taken supine if needed. Most of the barium should have been evacuated. If too much barium is retained, the patient is given more time for evacuation, and a second postevacuation image is obtained.

Postprocedure instructions to patients should include increased fluid intake and a high-fiber diet because of the possibility of constipation from the barium (most important for geriatric patients).

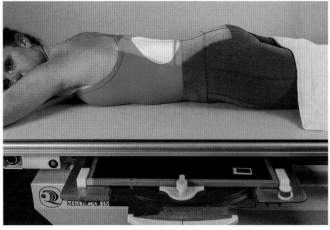
Fig. 13.44 PA projection—postfluoroscopy radiography.

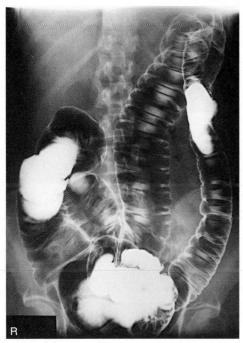
Fig. 13.45 AP—double-contrast barium enema.

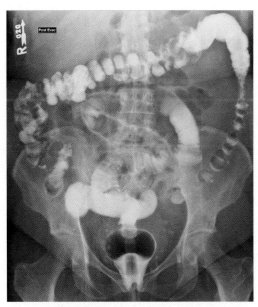
Fig. 13.46 AP—postevacuation.

Evacuative Proctography—Defecography

A third, less common type of radiographic study involving the lower gastrointestinal tract is **evacuative proctography,** sometimes called **defecography.** This study is a more specialized procedure that is performed in some departments, especially on children or younger adult patients.

Definition and Purpose Evacuative proctography is a functional study of the anus and rectum that is conducted during the evacuation and rest phases of defecation (bowel movement).

Clinical Indications Clinical indications for evacuative proctography include **rectoceles, rectal intussusception,** and **prolapse** of the rectum. A rectocele, a common form of the pathologic process, is a blind pouch of the rectum that is caused by weakening of the anterior or posterior wall. Rectoceles may retain fecal material even after evacuation.

Special Equipment A special commode is required for this study (Fig. 13.47). It consists of a toilet seat built onto a frame that contains a waste receptacle or a disposable plastic bag (A). The commode shown has wheels or casters (B) so that it can be rolled into position over the extended footboard and platform (C) attached to the table-top (D). The entire commode with the patient can be raised or lowered by raising the tabletop with the attached footboard and commode during the procedure (arrows). Clamps (not shown in these photographs) should be used to secure the commode to the footboard platform for stability during the procedure. These clamps allow the commode to be attached to the footboard and raised as needed for use of the bucky table and fluoroscopy unit. The seat often is cushioned (E) for patient comfort. The filters found beneath the seat (not shown) compensate for tissue differences and help maintain acceptable levels of density and contrast.

Contrast Media To study the process of evacuation, a very-high-density barium sulfate mixture is required. Some departments produce their own contrast media by mixing barium sulfate with potato starch or commercially produced additives. The potato starch thickens the barium sulfate to produce a mashed-potato consistency. The normal barium sulfate suspension evacuates too quickly to allow detection of any pathologic processes.

A ready-to-use contrast medium, **Anatrast,** is available (Fig. 13.48). This contrast medium is premixed and packaged in a single-use tube. Some departments also introduce thick liquid barium, such as **Polibar Plus** or **EZ-HD,** before using Anatrast to evaluate the sigmoid colon and the rectum.

Applicator The mechanical applicator (see Fig. 13.48) resembles a caulking gun used in the building industry. The premixed and prepackaged tube of Anatrast is inserted into the applicator, and a flexible tube with an enema tip is attached to the opened tip of the tube (B-1).

The thick liquid barium is drawn into a syringe and is inserted through a rectal tube and tip. In this example, an inner plastic tube (C) is being used after insertion into an outer rectal tube (D), to which the enema tip is attached. The syringe is used to instill the thick liquid contrast medium. The inner plastic tube is attached to the syringe filled with the liquid Polibar Plus or equivalent and is inserted within the rectal tube, to which is attached a standard enema tip for insertion into the rectum.

Labeled parts are as follows:
A. Mechanical applicator
B. Tube of Anatrast (B-1 tip to be opened)
C. Inner plastic tube (for insertion of syringe or tube of Anatrast)
D. Rectal tube (to which enema tip is attached, D-1)
E. Syringe

EVACUATIVE PROCTOGRAM PROCEDURE

With the patient in a lateral recumbent position on a cart, the contrast medium is instilled into the rectum with the applicator. A nipple marker (small BB) may be placed at the anal orifice.

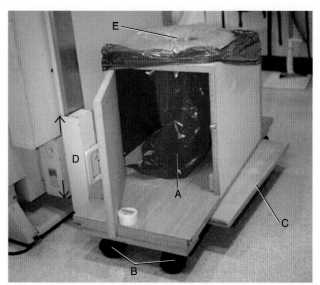

Fig. 13.47 Commode for defecogram.

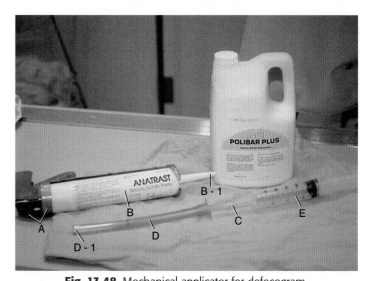

Fig. 13.48 Mechanical applicator for defecogram.

The patient is quickly placed on the commode for filming during defecation (Fig. 13.49). Lateral fluoroscopy images and standard radiographic projections are taken during the study. The lateral rectum position is preferred by most radiologists.

The anorectal angle or junction must be demonstrated during the procedure. This angle represents alignment between the anus and the rectum that shifts between the straining and evacuating phases (Fig. 13.50 and 13.51A). The radiologist measures this angle during these phases to determine whether any abnormalities exist.

A lateral recumbent postevacuation (resting) radiograph is taken as the final part of this procedure (Fig. 13.51B). Box 13.7 lists the steps for evacuative proctogram.

Colostomy Barium Enema

A colostomy *(ka-los'-ta-me)* is the surgical formation of an artificial or a surgical connection between two portions of the large intestine.

In the case of disease, tumor, or inflammatory processes, a section of the large intestine may have been removed or altered. Often, because of a tumor in the sigmoid colon or rectum, this part of the lower intestine is removed. The terminal end of the intestine is brought to the anterior surface of the abdomen, where an artificial opening is created. This artificial opening is termed a **stoma.**

In some cases, a temporary colostomy is performed to allow healing of the involved section of large intestine. The involved region is bypassed through the use of the colostomy. Once healing is complete, the two sections of the large intestine are reconnected. Fecal matter is discharged from the body via the stoma into a special appliance bag that is attached to the skin over the stoma. When healing is complete, an anastomosis (reconnection) of the two sections of the large intestine is performed surgically. For select patients, the colostomy is permanent because of the amount of large intestine removed or other factors.

CLINICAL INDICATION AND PURPOSE

The clinical indication or purpose for the colostomy barium enema is to **assess for proper healing, obstruction, or leakage or to perform a presurgical evaluation.** Sometimes, in addition to the colostomy barium enema, another enema may be given rectally at the same time. This type of study evaluates the terminal large intestine before it is reconnected surgically.

BOX 13.7 PROCEDURE SUMMARY: EVACUATIVE PROCTOGRAM

1. Place radiographic table vertical and attach commode with clamps.
2. Prepare the appropriate contrast medium according to department specifications.
3. Set up imaging equipment (fluoroscopy or digital recorder), or use digital fluoroscopy.
4. Ask patient to remove all clothing and change into a hospital gown.
5. Take a scout image using a conventional x-ray tube. (Scout image must include the region of the anorectal angle.)
6. Place patient in a lateral recumbent position on a cart and instill contrast medium.
7. Position patient on the commode and take radiographs in the strain and evacuation phases, with patient in a lateral position.
8. Using fluoroscopy imaging devices or digital recorder, image patient during defecation.
9. Assist in taking of postevacuation (resting) radiograph.

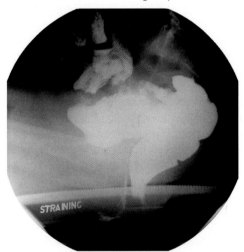

Fig. 13.50 Lateral defecogram (during strain phase).

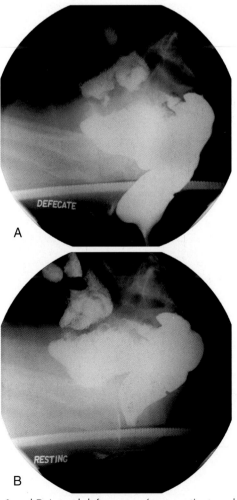

A

B

Fig. 13.51 A and B, Lateral defecogram (same patient as shown in Fig. 13.50), defecation and resting phase.

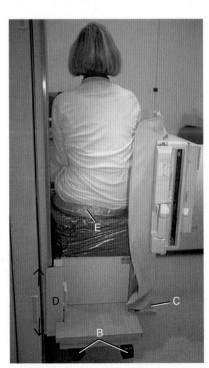

Fig. 13.49 Patient in position for defecogram.

SPECIAL SUPPLIES FOR COLOSTOMY BARIUM ENEMA

Ready-to-use colostomy barium enema kits (Fig. 13.52) are available that contain stoma tips, tubing, a premeasured barium enema bag, adhesive disks, lubricant, and gauze. Because the stoma has no sphincter with which to retain the barium, a tapered irrigation tip is inserted into the stoma. Once the irrigation tip has been inserted, a special adhesive pad holds it in place. The enema bag tubing is attached directly to the irrigation tip.

Small balloon retention catheters (Fig. 13.53) can be used instead of the tapered irrigation tip. Care must be taken during insertion and inflation of these catheters. The stoma is delicate and can be perforated if too much pressure is applied. Most departments require the radiologist to perform this task.

PATIENT PREPARATION

If the barium enema is used for nonacute reasons, the patient is asked to irrigate the ostomy before undergoing the procedure. The patient may be asked to bring an irrigation device and additional appliance bags. The patient should follow the same dietary restrictions required for the standard barium enema.

PROCEDURE

Barium sulfate remains the contrast medium of choice. A single-contrast or double-contrast media procedure may be performed, as with any routine barium enema. Iodinated, water-soluble contrast media may be used if indicated. The colostomy barium enema requires the contrast media to take a different route through the stoma. As a result of bowel resection, anatomic structures and landmarks are often altered. The technologist must observe the anatomy during fluoroscopy to plan for alterations in the positioning routine. Before the resected bowel is reattached (eliminating the need for the colostomy), barium may be delivered through both the stoma and the rectum to ensure that healing is complete. Finally, the technologist should have a clean appliance bag available for the postevacuation phase of the study. Some patients are unable to use the restroom. Box 13.8 lists the steps for a colostomy barium enema.

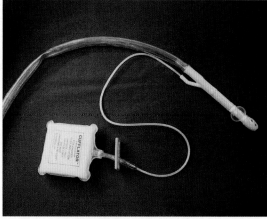

Fig. 13.53 Colostomy tip.

BOX 13.8 PROCEDURE SUMMARY: COLOSTOMY BARIUM ENEMA

1. Dress the patient in a hospital gown. Depending on the location of the stoma, leave gown open in front or back.
2. Prepare fluoroscopic room, open tray, and lay out contents.
3. Mix contrast medium according to department specifications.
4. Take a preliminary scout image using conventional x-ray tube.
5. Wearing gloves, remove and discard dressings that cover the stoma.
6. Once the radiologist has inserted an irrigation tip into the stoma, tape enema tubing in place.
7. Assist during fluoroscopic phase of study.
8. Take postfluoroscopic radiographic images as requested.
9. After imaging, lower enema bag, allowing contrast medium to flow back into enema bag.
10. Once the intestine is drained, assist in taking a postevacuation image.
11. Assist patient with cleanup and in securing the appliance bag over the stoma.

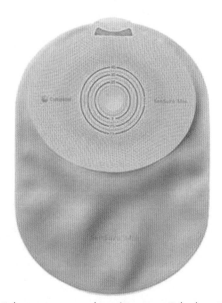

Fig. 13.52 Colostomy enema bag. (Courtesy Coloplast, Minneapolis, MN.)

Special Patient Considerations
PEDIATRIC APPLICATIONS
Small Bowel Series and Barium Enema
The pediatric small bowel series and the barium enema are similar in many ways to the procedures in adults. However, the transit time of barium from the stomach to the ileocecal region is faster in children compared with adults. During the small bowel series, images should be taken **every 20 to 30 minutes** to avoid missing crucial anatomy and possible pathology during the study. Often the barium reaches the ileocecal valve within 1 hour.

For the barium enema, care must be taken when inserting the enema tip into the rectum. For an infant, often a 10F, flexible silicone catheter is used. For an older child, a flexible enema tip is recommended to minimize injury to the rectum during insertion.

For both the small bowel series and the barium enema, these procedures should be scheduled early in the morning to permit the child to return to normal fluid intake and diet. See Chapter 16 for specific information on bowel and procedure preparation for the small bowel series and the barium enema.

GERIATRIC APPLICATIONS
Lower GI procedures such as the barium enema and the evacuative proctogram are especially stressful for geriatric patients. The technologist must exhibit patience and explain the procedure completely. As with all patients, the technologist should provide every opportunity to maintain the modesty of the patient during the procedure. Extra care and patience are frequently required as geriatric patients are turned and moved around on the radiographic table. Because of space disorientation, these patients may experience a fear of falling off the table. Escort the patient to the restroom after the procedure.

Because many geriatric patients have limited sphincter control, the retention balloon enema tip is recommended.

After the procedure, instructions for increased intake of liquids and a high-fiber diet are important for geriatric patients to prevent or minimize possible impaction of the barium. These recommendations apply to upper GI studies, lower GI studies, and small bowel series whenever large amounts of barium are orally ingested or given retrograde, as with the barium enema.

BARIATRIC PATIENT CONSIDERATIONS
Preliminary scout and post–contrast introduction images of bariatric patients may require multiple images to be taken to cover all of the large intestine. Two landscape-oriented images may cover the entire colon, or it may be required that images be taken as quadrants of the colon. Regardless of the number of images taken to cover the entire large bowel in the various positions, be sure there is sufficient but not excessive overlap to verify that no anatomic regions are missed. This is especially important for the oblique projections taken during the barium enema procedure. The left colic flexure is frequently more superior than in the sthenic patient.

Digital Imaging Considerations
With the use of digital fluoroscopy, postfluoroscopy projections may not be required. However, when postfluoroscopy projections are requested, technical considerations regarding **collimation, accurate centering, exposure factors,** and postprocessing **verification of exposure indicators** all are important, as described in preceding chapters.
1. **Collimation: Correct collimation is essential** to ensure that the image is identified correctly by the imaging system. By eliminating extraneous tissue or signal from the IR, the system is better able to produce a quality image without artifact.

2. **Accurate centering:** Careful analysis of body habitus is crucial during a small bowel series or a barium enema procedure. Keep in mind how the positions of the small and large bowels vary between hypersthenic and asthenic patients. If specific regions of the small or large bowel are not centered to the IR, the imaging system will not reproduce them correctly. It is important to ensure that the **central ray (CR), body part,** and **IR are aligned** to permit correct centering of the anatomy of interest.
3. **Exposure factors:** With any digital imaging system, adequate radiation must reach the IR to form a diagnostic image. With most imaging systems, minimum kVp and mAs must be used to create an acceptable image. Inadequate kVp or mAs produces a mottled image. However, the technologist must not increase mAs needlessly; this increases patient dose. Departments should have established technical charts to ensure that adequate kVp and mAs are used for these procedures. Once each image is produced, the exposure index should be reviewed to ensure that the technologist is using the correct exposure factors and not needlessly overexposing the patient.

Alternative Modalities and Procedures
COMPUTED TOMOGRAPHY (CT)
CT provides a comprehensive evaluation of the lower gastrointestinal tract for tumors, gastrointestinal bleeds, and abscesses caused by infection. Although most CT studies of the abdomen use intravenous contrast media, the use of rectal contrast media continues to be debated. Some experts state that the use of rectal contrast media during CT of the abdomen obscures subtle types of pathologic processes within the intestine. Others argue that a fully distended large intestine may pinpoint the location of tumors and abscesses adjacent to the large intestine.

The use of CT has become a common means of diagnosing acute appendicitis. Thin, consecutive slices taken in the region of the cecum may demonstrate a coprolith or abscess surrounding the vermiform appendix. To delineate the vermiform appendix better, rectal contrast media often are required.

CT ENTEROCLYSIS
The use of CT enteroclysis is growing in frequency. Often, the duodenojejunal tube is inserted under fluoroscopic guidance. Very thin barium (e.g., VoLumen®, which contains a 0.1% barium sulfate suspension) or water is instilled. The patient is scanned for detection of obstructions, adhesions, or narrowing of the intestinal lumen.

CT COLONOGRAPHY (CTC)
CT colonography, or "virtual colonoscopy," is a scan of the large intestine. This procedure was made possible with the advent of multidetector CT scanners and three-dimensional software with which a virtual tour through the entire large intestine is created. CT colonography is reported to be an effective diagnostic tool in detecting polyps, tumors, diverticula, defects, and strictures within the large intestine. It is considered an alternative to endoscopic colonoscopy.

Following a CT scan of the abdomen, two-dimensional scan data are processed through a special computer application that creates a virtual "fly-through" of the large intestine.

Patient Preparation
To ensure no fecal debris is present in the large intestine to obscure anatomy or possible pathology, the patient should undergo a cleansing bowel preparation. On the morning of the procedure, food intake should be limited to clear liquids such as tea, water, or simple broth. The patient should wear loose-fitting clothing with no metal snaps or clips.

Procedure

A small rectal tube is inserted through which air or carbon dioxide gas is instilled into the large intestine. The purpose of the gas is to distend the large intestine so that the intestinal wall is completely visualized. In some cases, oral contrast material may be given to mark or "tag" fecal matter.[4]

The patient is first scanned supine, then rolled over and scanned prone. Scan data are processed through special software to create three-dimensional images and virtual fly-through of the anatomy (see Fig. 13.33, page 505).

The scan itself takes approximately 10 minutes to complete. Because no sedation is required in most cases, the patient is able to leave and resume normal diet and activities.

Advantages of CT Colonography[4]

- Three-dimensional images that clearly demonstrate possible polyps and lesions are created.
- The risk of perforating the intestinal wall is less than with endoscopic colonoscopy.
- No sedation is required in most cases, which makes CT colonography a better option for elderly or frail patients.
- It is ideal for an intestine that has been narrowed by stricture or a tumor in such a way that the endoscopic device cannot pass through the region.
- It provides a more detailed assessment of the large intestine compared with the barium enema procedure; CT colonography can reveal pathology outside of the intestinal wall that may be missed during endoscopic colonoscopy.
- It is a less expensive procedure compared with endoscopic colonoscopy.

Disadvantages of CT Colonography

- The chief disadvantage is that a biopsy cannot be performed or polyps removed during CT colonography. The patient has to undergo endoscopic colonoscopy for a biopsy to be performed or for polyps to be removed.
- Inflating the large intestine with air or gas may rupture a weakened area of the intestinal wall.
- Radiation dose to the patient is high.

- The procedure is contraindicated in pregnant patients.
- There is a small possibility of a false-positive reading, in which a fecal artifact would be classified as a polyp.[4]

NUCLEAR MEDICINE (NM)

Several NM procedures can be performed for various lower gastrointestinal conditions and diseases. The use of radionuclides can assist in the diagnosis of Meckel diverticulum or gastrointestinal bleeding and is useful for gastric emptying motility studies.

MAGNETIC RESONANCE IMAGING (MRI)

Although MRI is not the gold standard for imaging of the gastrointestinal tract, it has been used in limited applications. MRI cannot detect mucosal lesions, but it can demonstrate primary tumors of the bowel and adjacent structures. It also can prove helpful in the planning stages of surgical excision of these tumors. Abscesses in the mesentery or retroperitoneum can be demonstrated easily on T2-weighted MRI.

SONOGRAPHY (ULTRASOUND)

Although the large intestine is too gaseous for ultrasound, the detection of tumors and collections of fluid and cysts is feasible. A filled urinary bladder provides an acoustic window for the study of structures and regions that surround the large intestine. Sonography with graded compression may be useful, along with clinical evaluation, in the diagnosis of appendicitis.

Routine and Special Projections

Certain routine and special projections of the small and large intestine are demonstrated and described on the following pages. The radiologist and the technologist must closely coordinate their efforts during both the small bowel series and the barium enema. A great deal of individual variation is noted among radiologists. The routine projections listed may vary from hospital to hospital. The radiographic routine for the barium enema, in particular, must be thoroughly understood by the technologist before the examination because any radiographs needed must be obtained as rapidly as possible.

PA PROJECTION—SMALL BOWEL SERIES

Clinical Indications
- Inflammatory processes, neoplasms, and obstructions of the small intestine
- **Upper GI–small bowel combination:** Commonly performed; additional barium is ingested after completion of the upper GI (see p. 501)
- **Small bowel–only series:** Includes a scout abdomen radiograph followed by ingestion of barium and timed-interval radiographs (see p. 502)
- **Enteroclysis and intubation procedures:** See descriptions on pp. 502 and 503.

Small Bowel Series
ROUTINE
• PA (every 15 to 30 minutes) enteroclysis and intubation

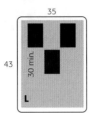

Technical Factors
- Minimum SID—40 inches (100 cm)
- IR size—14 × 17 inches (35 × 43 cm), portrait
- Grid
- kVp range—110–125
- Time markers to be used

Shielding Shield all radiosensitive tissues outside region of interest.

Patient Position Patient is prone (or supine if patient cannot lie in prone position) with a support for the head.

Part Position
- Align midsagittal plane (MSP) to midline of table/grid or CR.
- Place arms up beside head with legs extended and support provided under the ankles.
- Ensure that **no rotation** occurs.

CR
- CR is **perpendicular** to IR.
  - **15 or 30 minutes:** Center to about 2 inches (5 cm) above iliac crest (see NOTES) (Fig. 13.54).
  - **Hourly:** Center CR and midpoint of IR to iliac crest (Fig. 13.55).
- Center IR to CR.

Recommended Collimation Collimate on four sides to anatomy of interest.

Respiration Suspend respiration and expose on expiration.

NOTES: Timing begins with ingestion of barium. Timed intervals of radiographs depend on transit time of the specific barium preparation used and on department protocol. **For the first 30-minute radiograph,** center high to include the entire stomach.

Subsequent 30-minute interval radiographs are taken until barium reaches the large bowel (usually 2 hours). The study is generally completed when the contrast medium reaches the cecum or the ascending colon.

Fluoroscopy and spot imaging of the **ileocecal valve** and terminal ileum after barium reaches this area are commonly included in the routine small bowel series. This procedure is determined by the fluoroscopist's preference and by department protocols.

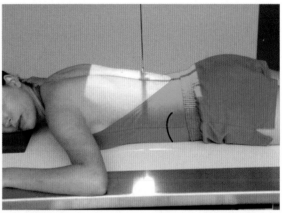

Fig. 13.54 PA—15 or 30 minutes—centered approximately 2 inches (5 cm) above iliac crest.

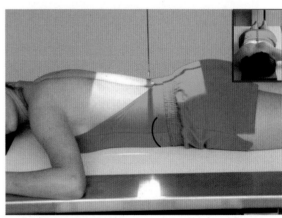

Fig. 13.55 PA—hourly, centered to iliac crest.

13

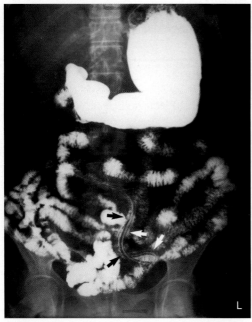

Fig. 13.56 PA small bowel series—30 minutes (most barium located in stomach and jejunum). The linear object seen in this view is a large (12-inch [approximately 30-cm]) parasitic roundworm (*Ascaris* sp.) in the jejunum.

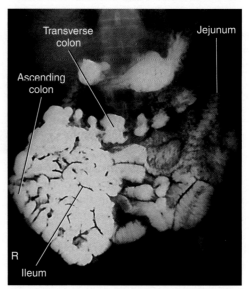

Fig. 13.58 PA—2 hours (most barium located in ileum and proximal colon).

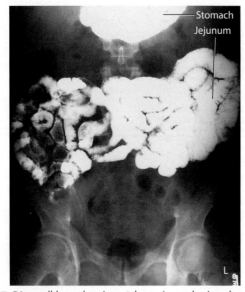

Fig. 13.57 PA small bowel series—1 hour (most barium located in jejunum).

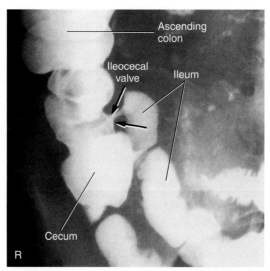

Fig. 13.59 PA (ileocecal spot). (Courtesy J. Sanderson, RT.)

PA OR AP PROJECTION—BARIUM ENEMA

Clinical Indications
- Obstructions, including ileus, volvulus, and intussusception
  Double-contrast media barium enema is ideal for demonstrating diverticulosis, polyps, and mucosal changes.

Barium Enema
ROUTINE
• PA or AP

Technical Factors
- Minimum SID—40 inches (100 cm)
- IR size—14 × 17 inches (35 × 43 cm), portrait
- Grid
- kVp range—110–125 (single contrast); 90–100 (double contrast); 80–90 (iodinated, water-soluble contrast)

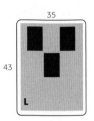

Shielding Shield all radiosensitive tissues outside the region of interest.

Patient Position Patient is prone or supine, with a support for the head (Fig. 13.60).

Part Position
- Align MSP to midline of table.
- Ensure that **no** body **rotation** occurs.

CR
- CR is perpendicular to IR.
- Center CR to level of iliac crest.
- Center IR to CR.

Recommended Collimation Collimate on four sides to anatomy of interest.

Respiration Suspend respiration and expose on expiration.

NOTES: For most patients, the enema tip can be removed before radiographs are obtained, unless a retention-type tip is used. This type generally should not be removed until the patient is ready to evacuate.

Include rectal ampulla at lower margin of radiograph. Determine department policy regarding inclusion of the left colic flexure on all patients if this area is adequately included in spot images during fluoroscopy. (Most adult patients require two images if this area is to be included.)

For hypersthenic patients, use two 14 × 17-inch (35 × 43-cm) image receptors placed landscape to include the entire large intestine.

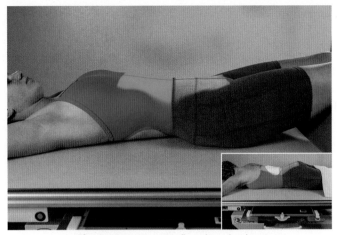

Fig. 13.60 AP or PA *(inset)* projection.

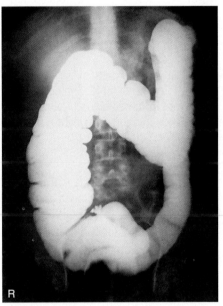

Fig. 13.61 PA projection—single-contrast barium enema.

Evaluation Criteria
Anatomy Demonstrated: • The transverse colon should be primarily barium filled on the PA and air filled on the AP with a double-contrast study (Fig. 13.61). • Entire large intestine, including the left colic flexure, should be visible (see NOTES).
Position: • No rotation should occur. • The ala of the ilium and the lumbar vertebrae are symmetric. • Proper collimation is applied.
Exposure: • Appropriate technique should visualize the entire air-filled and barium-filled large intestine without overexposing the mucosal outlines of the sections of primarily air-filled bowel on a double-contrast study. • Sharp structural margins indicate no motion.

13

RAO POSITION—BARIUM ENEMA

Clinical Indications
- Obstructions, including ileus, volvulus, and intussusception
  Double-contrast media barium enema is ideal for demonstrating diverticulosis, polyps, and mucosal changes.

Barium Enema
ROUTINE
• PA or AP
• RAO

Technical Factors
- Minimum SID—40 inches (100 cm)
- IR size—14 × 17 inches (35 × 43 cm), portrait
- Grid
- kVp range—110–125 (single contrast); 90–100 (double contrast); 80–90 (iodinated, water-soluble contrast)

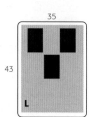

Shielding Shield all radiosensitive tissues outside region of interest.

Patient Position Patient is semiprone, rotated into a 35° to 45° RAO; a positioning sponge can be used to help align the upper body into the correct position; patient also is offered a support for the head (Fig. 13.62).

Part Position
- Align MSP along long axis of table, with right and left abdominal margins equidistant from centerline of table or CR.
- Place left arm up on support, with right arm down behind the patient and left knee partially flexed.
- Check posterior pelvis and trunk for **35° to 45° rotation.**

CR
- Direct CR **perpendicular** to IR to a point about **1 inch** (2.5 cm) **to the left** of the MSP.
- Center CR and IR to **level of iliac crest** (see NOTE).

Recommended Collimation Collimate on four sides to anatomy of interest.

Respiration Suspend respiration and expose on expiration.

NOTE: Ensure that rectal ampulla is included on lower margin of IR. This action may require centering 1 to 2 inches (2.5 to 5 cm) below the iliac crest on larger patients and taking a second image centered 1 to 2 inches (2.5 to 5 cm) above the crest to include the right colic flexure (Figs. 13.63 to 13.65).

Evaluation Criteria
Anatomy Demonstrated: • The right colic flexure and the ascending and sigmoid colon are seen "open" without significant superimposition. • The entire large intestine is included, with the possible exception of the left colic flexure, which is best demonstrated in LAO position (or may require a second image centered higher). • The rectal ampulla should be included on the lower margin of the radiograph.
Position: • The spine is parallel to the edge of the radiograph (unless scoliosis is present). • The ala of the right ilium is foreshortened, and the left side is elongated; the right colic flexure is seen in profile if included. • Proper collimation is applied.
Exposure: • Appropriate technique should visualize the entire air-filled and barium-filled large intestine without overexposing the mucosal outlines of the sections of primarily air-filled bowel on a double-contrast study. • Sharp structural margins indicate **no motion.**

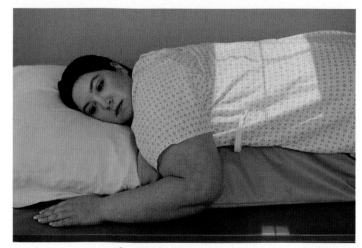

Fig. 13.62 RAO—35° to 45°.

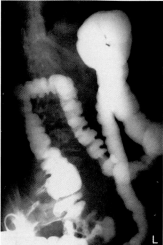

Fig. 13.63 RAO (centered high to include R and L colic flexures).

Fig. 13.64 RAO (centered low to include rectal ampulla).

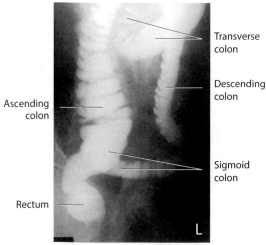

Transverse colon

Descending colon

Ascending colon

Sigmoid colon

Rectum

Fig. 13.65 RAO (to include rectal ampulla).

LAO POSITION—BARIUM ENEMA

Clinical Indications
- Obstructions, including ileus, volvulus, and intussusception

  Double-contrast media barium enema is ideal for demonstrating diverticulosis, polyps, and mucosal changes.

Barium Enema
ROUTINE
• PA or AP
• RAO
• LAO

Technical Factors
- Minimum SID—40 inches (100 cm)
- IR size—14 × 17 inches (35 × 43 cm), portrait
- Grid
- kVp range—110–125 (single contrast); 90–100 (double contrast); 80–90 (iodinated, water-soluble contrast)

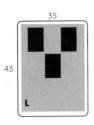

Shielding
- Shield all radiosensitive tissues outside region of interest.

Patient Position
Patient is semiprone, rotated into a 35° to 45° LAO, with a support for the head (Fig. 13.66).

Part Position
- Align MSP along long axis of table, with right and left abdominal margins equidistant from centerline of table or CR.
- Place right arm up on pillow, with left arm down behind patient and right knee partially flexed.
- Check posterior pelvis and trunk for **35° to 45° rotation.**

CR
- CR is **perpendicular** to IR, directed to a point about 1 inch (2.5 cm) **to the right** of MSP.
- Center CR and IR to **1 to 2 inches** (2.5 to 5 cm) **above iliac crest** (see NOTE).
- Center cassette to CR.

Recommended Collimation
Collimate on four sides to anatomy of interest.

Respiration
Suspend respiration and expose on expiration.

NOTE: Most adult patients require about 2 inches (5 cm) higher centering to include the **left colic flexure,** which generally cuts off the lower large bowel; a second image centered 2 or 3 inches (5 to 7.5 cm) lower is required to include the rectal area.

Evaluation Criteria
Anatomy Demonstrated: • The left colic flexure should be seen as "open" without significant superimposition. • The descending colon should be well demonstrated. • The entire large intestine should be included (see NOTE) (Figs. 13.67 and 13.68).
Position: • Spine is parallel to the edge of the radiograph (unless scoliosis is present). • The ala of the right ilium is elongated (if visible), whereas the left side is foreshortened; the left colic flexure is seen in profile. • Proper collimation is applied.
Exposure: • Appropriate technique should visualize the contrast-filled large intestine without significant overexposure of any portion. • Sharp structural margins indicate **no motion.**

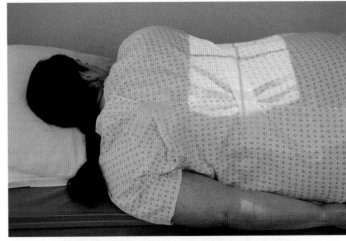

Fig. 13.66 LAO position.

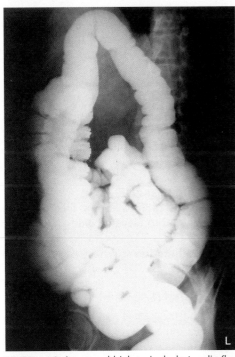

Fig. 13.67 LAO (centered high to include L colic flexure).

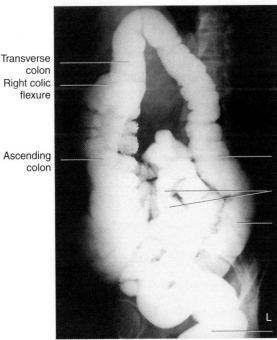

Transverse colon
Right colic flexure
Ascending colon
Descending colon
Sigmoid colon
Descending colon
Rectum

Fig. 13.68 LAO position.

LPO AND RPO POSITIONS —BARIUM ENEMA

Clinical Indications

- Obstructions, including ileus, volvulus, and intussusception
  Double-contrast barium enema is ideal for demonstrating diverticulosis, polyps, and mucosal changes.

Barium Enema
ROUTINE
• PA or AP
• RAO
• LAO
• LPO or RPO

Technical Factors

- Minimum SID—40 inches (100 cm)
- IR size—14 × 17 inches (35 × 43 cm), portrait
- Grid
- kVp range—110–125 (single contrast); 90–100 (double contrast); 80–90 (iodinated, water-soluble contrast)

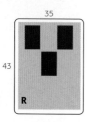

Shielding Shield all radiosensitive tissues outside region of interest.

Patient Position Patient is semisupine, rotated 35° to 45° into right and left posterior obliques, with a support for the head.

Part Position

- Flex elevated-side elbow and place in front of head; place opposite arm down by patient's side (Fig. 13.69).
- Partially flex elevated-side knee to maintain this position.
- Align **MSP along long axis of table,** with right and left abdominal margins equidistant from centerline of table.

CR

- Direct CR **perpendicular** to IR.
- Angle CR and center of IR to level of **iliac crests** and about **1 inch** (2.5 cm) **lateral to elevated side** of MSP (see NOTE).

Recommended Collimation Collimate on four sides to anatomy of interest.

Respiration Expose on expiration.

NOTE: Ensure that rectal ampulla is included. Most adult patients require a second IR centered 2 to 3 inches (5 to 7.5 cm) higher on the **RPO** if the left colic (splenic) flexure is to be included (see Fig. 13.71).

Evaluation Criteria

Anatomy Demonstrated: • LPO: The **right colic** (hepatic) **flexure** and the ascending and rectosigmoid portions should appear "open" without significant superimposition (Fig. 13.70). • RPO: The **left colic** (splenic) **flexure** and the descending portions should appear "open" without significant superimposition (Fig. 13.71). (A second IR centered lower to include the rectal area is required on most adult patients if this area is to be included on these postfluoroscopy radiographs). • The rectal ampulla should be included on the lower margins of the radiograph. • Entire contrast-filled large intestine, including the rectal ampulla, should be included (see NOTE).
Position: • LPO: No tilt is evident, and spine is parallel to the edge of the radiograph. • The ala of the left ilium is elongated, and the right side is foreshortened. • RPO: No tilt is present; spine is parallel to the edge of the radiograph. • The ala of the right ilium is elongated, and the left side is foreshortened. • Proper collimation is applied.
Exposure: • Appropriate technique should visualize the contrast-filled large intestine without significant overexposure of any portion. • Sharp structural margins indicate **no motion.**

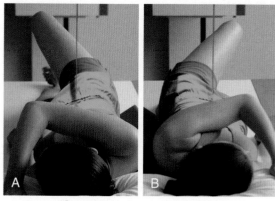

Fig. 13.69 *Left,* LPO. *Right,* RPO.

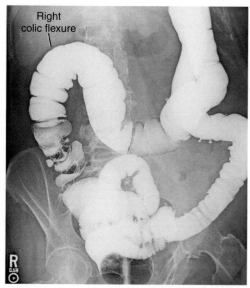

Fig. 13.70 LPO—for right colic flexure. (Image centered low to demonstrate the right flexure and rectum)

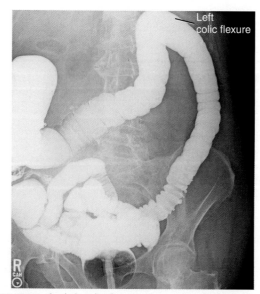

Fig. 13.71 RPO—for left colic flexure. (Image centered to demonstrate left colic flexure.)

LATERAL RECTUM POSITION OR VENTRAL DECUBITUS LATERAL—BARIUM ENEMA

Clinical Indications
- Lateral position for demonstrating polyps, strictures, and fistulas between rectum and bladder/uterus
  The ventral decubitus position is best for double-contrast study.

Technical Factors
- Minimum SID—40 inches (100 cm)
- IR size—10 × 12 inches (24 × 30 cm), portrait
- Grid
- kVp range—110 –125
- Compensating or wedge filter for more uniform density on ventral decubitus lateral

Barium Enema
ROUTINE
• PA or AP
• RAO
• LAO
• LPO or RPO
• Lateral rectum

Shielding Shield all radiosensitive tissues outside region of interest.

Patient Position Patient position is lateral recumbent, with a support for the head.

Part Position (Lateral Position)
- Align midaxillary plane to midline of table or IR.
- Flex and superimpose knees; place arms up in front of the head (Fig. 13.72).
- Ensure that **no rotation** occurs; superimpose shoulders and hips.

CR
- CR is **perpendicular** to IR (CR is **horizontal** for ventral decubitus).
- Center CR to level of **anterior superior iliac spine (ASIS)** and **midcoronal plane** (midway between ASIS and posterior sacrum).
- Center IR to CR.
  Alternative ventral decubitus lateral horizontal beam positions are beneficial for double-contrast studies. Centering for the ventral decubitus is similar to the lateral rectum position (Fig. 13.73).

Recommended Collimation Collimate on four sides to anatomy of interest.

Respiration Suspend respiration and expose on expiration.

Evaluation Criteria
Anatomy Demonstrated: • Contrast-filled rectosigmoid region is demonstrated (Fig. 13.74).
Position: • No rotation is evident; femoral heads are superimposed. • Proper collimation is applied.
Exposure: • Appropriate technique is used to visualize both the contrast-filled rectum and the sigmoid regions, with adequate penetration to demonstrate these areas through the superimposed pelvis and hips. • Sharp structural margins indicate **no motion.**

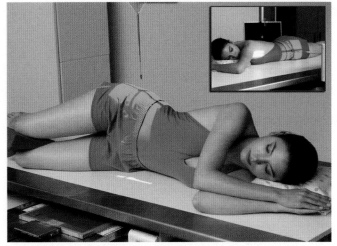

Fig. 13.72 Left lateral rectum. *Inset,* Ventral decubitus (double-contrast study).

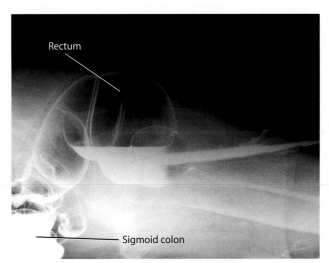

Fig. 13.73 Ventral decubitus—lateral rectum.

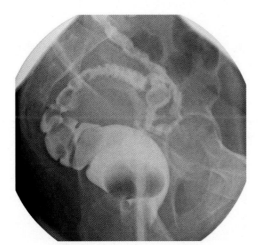

Fig. 13.74 Left lateral rectum.

13

RIGHT LATERAL DECUBITUS POSITION (AP OR PA PROJECTION)—BARIUM ENEMA: DOUBLE CONTRAST

Clinical Indications
- Demonstrating polyps of the left side or air-filled portions of the large intestine
  Both right and left decubitus positions generally are taken with the double-contrast study.

Barium Enema
ROUTINE
• PA or AP
• RAO
• LAO
• LPO or RPO
• Lateral rectum
• R and L lateral decubitus (double-contrast study)

Technical Factors
- Minimum SID—40 inches (100 cm)
- IR size—14 × 17 inches (35 × 43 cm), portrait to patient
- Bucky or grid cassette
- kVp range—90–100 (double-contrast study)
- Compensating filter placed on upside of abdomen (attached to collimator face with magnets)

Shielding Shield all radiosensitive tissues outside region of interest.

Patient Position Patient is in lateral recumbent position, with a support for the head and lying on the **right** side on a radiolucent pad, with a portable grid placed behind the patient's back for an AP projection. The patient also can be facing the portable grid or the vertical table for a PA projection. (If patient is on a cart, **lock wheels** or secure cart to prevent patient from falling.)

Part Position
- Position patient or IR so that iliac crest is placed to center of IR and CR.
- Place arms up, with knees flexed (Fig. 13.75).
- Ensure that **no rotation** occurs; superimpose shoulders and hips from above.

CR
- Direct CR **horizontal,** perpendicular to IR.
- Center CR to **level of iliac crest** and **MSP.**

Recommended Collimation Collimate on four sides to anatomy of interest.

Respiration Suspend respiration and expose on expiration.

NOTES: Proceed as rapidly as possible.
For hypersthenic patients, use two 14 × 17-inch (35 × 43-cm) IRs placed landscape to include all of the large intestine.

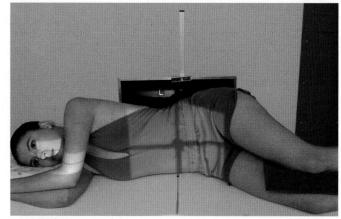

Fig. 13.75 Right lateral decubitus—AP (with portable grid).

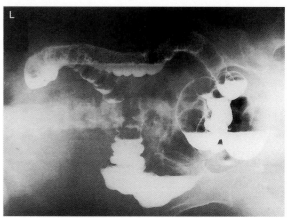

Fig. 13.76 Right lateral decubitus.

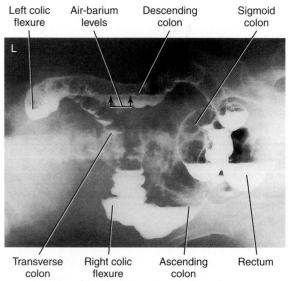

Left colic flexure   Air-barium levels   Descending colon   Sigmoid colon

Transverse colon   Right colic flexure   Ascending colon   Rectum

Fig. 13.77 Right lateral decubitus.

Evaluation Criteria
Anatomy Demonstrated: • Entire large intestine is demonstrated to include air-filled left colic flexure and descending colon (Figs. 13.76 and 13.77).
Position: • No rotation is evident by symmetric appearance of pelvis and ribcage. • Proper collimation is applied.
Exposure: • Appropriate technique is used to visualize the borders of the entire large intestine, including barium-filled portions, but to avoid overpenetration of the air-filled portion of the large intestine. • Mucosal patterns of air-filled colon should be clearly visible. • If the air-filled portion of the large intestine is overpenetrated consistently, a compensating filter should be considered. • Sharp structural margins indicate **no motion.**

LEFT LATERAL DECUBITUS POSITION (AP OR PA PROJECTION)— BARIUM ENEMA

Clinical Indications

- Demonstrate the entire contrast-filled large intestine, especially helpful in identifying polyps
- **Right side** is demonstrated best, which includes air-filled portions of the large intestine

Both right and left decubitus positions (AP or PA) generally are taken with the double-contrast study.

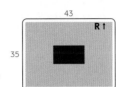

Barium Enema
ROUTINE
• PA or AP
• RAO
• LAO
• LPO or RPO
• Lateral rectum
• R and L lateral decubitus (double-contrast study)

Technical Factors

- Minimum SID—40 inches (100 cm)
- IR size—14 × 17 inches (35 × 43 cm), portrait with patient
- Bucky or grid cassette
- kVp range—90–100 (double-contrast study)
- Compensating filter placed on upside of abdomen (attached to collimator face with magnets)

Shielding Shield all radiosensitive tissues outside region of interest.

Patient Position Position patient lateral recumbent, with a support for the head, and lying on the **left** side on a radiolucent pad. (If on a cart, **lock wheels** or secure cart to prevent patient from falling.)

Part Position

- Position patient or IR so that iliac crest is placed to center of IR and CR (Fig. 13.78).
- Place arms up, with knees flexed.
- Ensure that **no rotation** occurs; superimpose shoulders and hips from above.

CR

- Direct CR **horizontal**, perpendicular to IR.
- Center CR to **level of iliac crest** and MSP.

Recommended Collimation Collimate on four sides to anatomy of interest.

Respiration Suspend respiration and expose on expiration.

NOTES: Because most double-contrast barium enema studies include both right and left lateral decubitus positions, it generally is easier to take one projection with the back against the table or cassette holder and then have the patient roll over on the other side and move the cart around, with the

patient's head at the other end of the table. This task may be easier than sitting the patient up and turning the patient end-to-end on the cart or table.

For hypersthenic patients, use two IRs (each 14 × 17 inches [35 × 43 cm]) placed landscape to include all of the large intestine.

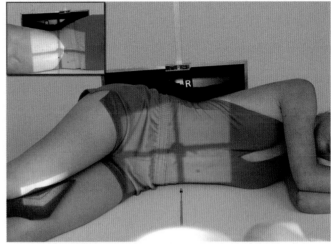

Fig. 13.78 Left lateral decubitus—AP projection. *Inset,* PA projection.

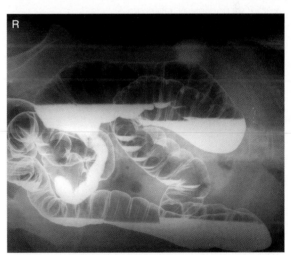

Fig. 13.79 Left lateral decubitus.

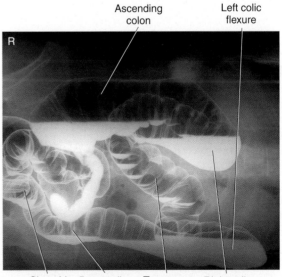

Ascending colon | Left colic flexure

Sigmoid colon | Descending colon | Transverse colon | Right colic flexure

Fig. 13.80 Left lateral decubitus.

13

PA (AP) PROJECTION—POSTEVACUATION: BARIUM ENEMA

Clinical Indications
- Demonstrates mucosal pattern of the large intestine with residual contrast media for identifying small polyps and defects

This projection is most commonly taken prone as a PA but may be taken with the patient supine as an AP, if necessary.

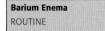

Barium Enema
ROUTINE
• PA or AP
• RAO
• LAO
• LPO or RPO
• Lateral rectum
• R and L lateral decubitus (double-contrast study)
• PA postevacuation

Technical Factors
- Minimum SID—40 inches (100 cm)
- IR size—14 × 17 inches (35 × 43 cm), portrait
- Grid
- kVp range—90–100

Use postevacuation marker

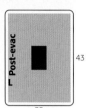

Shielding Shield all radiosensitive tissues outside region of interest.

Patient Position Patient is prone or supine, with a support for the head (Fig. 13.81).

Part Position
- Align MSP to midline of table or CR.
- Ensure that **no** body **rotation** occurs.

CR
- CR is perpendicular to IR.
- Center CR and center of IR to iliac crest.

Recommended Collimation Collimate on four sides to anatomy of interest.

Respiration Suspend respiration and expose on expiration.

NOTES: Image should be taken after patient has had sufficient time for adequate evacuation. If radiograph shows insufficient evacuation to visualize the mucosal pattern clearly, a second radiograph should be obtained after further evacuation. Coffee or tea sometimes can be given as a stimulant for this purpose. Include the rectal ampulla on the lower margin of the radiograph.

Use lower kVp to prevent overpenetration, with only the residual contrast media remaining in the large intestine.

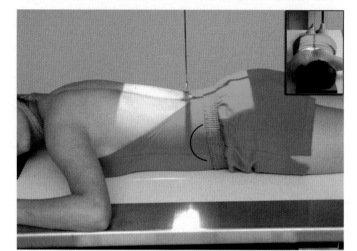

Fig. 13.81 PA postevacuation.

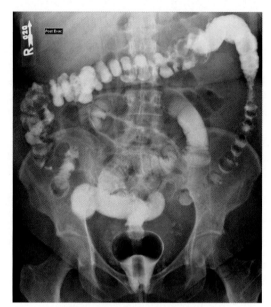

Fig. 13.82 PA postevacuation.

Evaluation Criteria
Anatomy Demonstrated:
Entire large intestine should be visualized with only a residual amount of contrast media (Fig. 13.82).
Position:
Spine is parallel to the edge of the radiograph (unless scoliosis is present). • **No rotation** occurs; the ala of the ilium and the lumbar vertebrae are symmetric. • Proper collimation is applied.
Exposure:
Appropriate technique is used to visualize the outline of entire mucosal pattern of the large intestine without overexposure of any parts. • Sharp structural margins indicate **no motion**. • Postevacuation and R or L markers should be visible.

AP AXIAL OR AP AXIAL OBLIQUE (LPO) PROJECTIONS—BARIUM ENEMA

Clinical Indications
- Polyps or other pathologic processes in the rectosigmoid aspect of the large intestine

Barium Enema
SPECIAL
• AP or LPO axial

Technical Factors
- Minimum SID—40 inches (100 cm)
- IR size—14 × 17 inches (35 × 43 cm)portrait
- Grid
- kVp range—110 –125 (single contrast); 90–100 (double contrast); 80–90 (iodinated, water-soluble contrast)

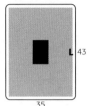

Shielding Shield all radiosensitive tissues outside region of interest.

Patient Position Position patient supine or partially rotated into an LPO position, with a support for the head (Fig. 13.83).

Part Position
AP Axial
- Position patient supine and align MSP to midline of table.
- Extend legs; place arms down by patient's side or up across chest; ensure **no rotation.**

LPO
- Rotate patient **30° to 40°** into LPO (left posterior side down).
- Raise right arm, with left arm extended and right knee partially flexed.

CR
- Angle CR 30° to 40° cephalad.

AP
- Direct CR 2 inches (5 cm) inferior to level of ASIS and to MSP.

LPO
- Direct CR 2 inches (5 cm) inferior and 2 inches (5 cm) medial to right ASIS.
- Center IR to CR.

Recommended Collimation
Use 14 × 17-inch (35 × 43-cm) field of view or collimate on four sides to anatomy of interest.

Respiration
Suspend respiration and expose on expiration.

Evaluation Criteria
Anatomy Demonstrated:
Elongated views of the rectosigmoid segments should be visible with less overlapping of sigmoid loops than with a 90° AP projection.
Position:
AP axial: Adequate CR angulation is evidenced by elongation of rectosigmoid segments of large intestine (Fig. 13.84).
• **LPO axial:** Adequate CR angulation and patient obliquity are evidenced by elongation and less superimposition of rectosigmoid segments of large intestine (Fig. 13.85).
• Proper collimation is applied.
Exposure:
Appropriate technique is used to visualize outlines of all rectosigmoid segments of large intestine. • Sharp structural margins indicate **no motion.**

NOTE: Proceed as rapidly as possible. Similar views can be obtained with a PA axial and an RAO with a 30° to 40° caudad CR angle (see following page).

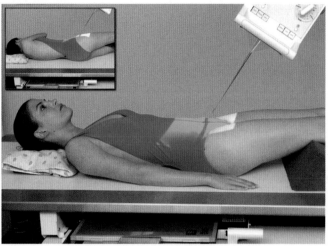

Fig. 13.83 AP axial—CR 30° to 40° cephalad. *Inset,* 30° to 40° LPO.

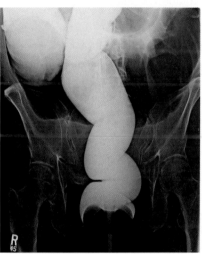

Fig. 13.84 AP axial.

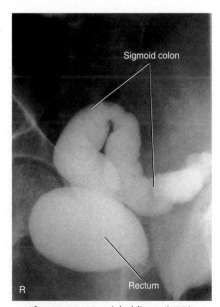

Sigmoid colon

Rectum

Fig. 13.85 AP axial oblique (LPO).

PA AXIAL OR PA AXIAL OBLIQUE (RAO) PROJECTIONS—BARIUM ENEMA

Clinical Indications
- Polyps or other pathologic processes in the rectosigmoid aspect of the large intestine

Barium Enema
SPECIAL
- AP or LPO axial
- PA or RAO axial

Technical Factors
- Minimum SID—40 inches (100 cm)
- IR size— 14 × 17 inches (35 × 43 cm), portrait
- Grid
- kVp range—110 –125 (single contrast); 90–100 (double contrast); 80–90 (iodinated, water-soluble contrast)

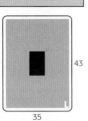

Shielding
Shield all radiosensitive tissues outside region of interest.

Patient Position
Position patient prone or partially rotated into an RAO position, with a support for the head (Fig. 13.86).

Part Position
PA
- Position patient prone and align MSP to midline of table.
- Place arms up beside head or down by sides away from body.
- Ensure **no rotation** of pelvis or trunk.

RAO
- Rotate patient **35° to 45°** into **RAO** (right anterior side down).
- Place left arm up, with right arm down by side and left knee partially flexed.

CR
- Angle CR 30° to 40° caudad.

PA
- Align CR to exit at level of ASIS and MSP.

RAO
- Align CR to exit at level of ASIS and 2 inches (5 cm) to left of lumbar spinous processes.
- Center film holder to CR.

Recommended Collimation
Collimate on four sides to anatomy of interest.

Respiration
Suspend respiration and expose on expiration.

NOTES: Proceed as rapidly as possible.

Evaluation Criteria
Anatomy Demonstrated:
Elongated views of rectosigmoid segments of the large intestine are shown without excessive superimposition (Fig. 13.87). • The double-contrast study best visualizes this region of overlapping loops of bowel (Fig. 13.88).

Position:
Adequate CR angulation and patient obliquity on the oblique are evidenced by elongation and less superimposition of rectosigmoid segments of large intestine. • Proper collimation is applied.

Exposure:
Appropriate technique is used to visualize outlines of all rectosigmoid segments of the large intestine without overpenetrating the air-filled outlines of these segments of large intestine with air-contrast study. • Sharp structural margins indicate **no motion**.

Similar views of rectosigmoid region—AP and LPO with 30° to 40° cephalad angle—are described on the preceding pages.

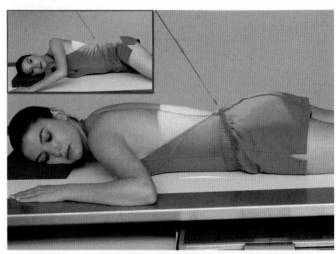

Fig. 13.86 PA axial—CR 30° to 40° caudad. *Inset,* RAO axial.

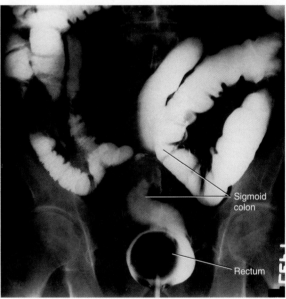

Fig. 13.87 PA axial (single-contrast study).

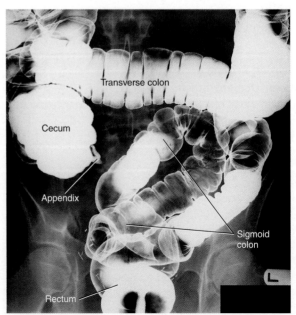

Fig. 13.88 PA axial (double-contrast study).

CHAPTER 14

Urinary System and Venipuncture

CONTRIBUTIONS BY **Chad Hensley,** PhD, RT(R)(MR)

CONTRIBUTORS TO PAST EDITIONS Leslie E. Kendrick, MS, RT(R)(CT)(MR), Jenny A. Kellstrom, MEd, RT(R), Barry T. Anthony, RT(R)

CONTENTS

RADIOGRAPHIC ANATOMY

Urinary System

Radiographic examinations of the urinary system are among the common contrast medium procedures performed in radiology departments. The urinary system consists of **two kidneys, two ureters** *(u-re'-ter[1] or yoo-ret'-er[2])*, **one urinary bladder,** and **one urethra** *(u-re'-thrah[1] or yoo-re'-thra[2])* (Fig. 14.1).

NOTE: Determine which of the possible pronunciations of these terms is (are) most common in your region.

The two kidneys and the ureters are organs that lie in the retroperitoneal space. These two bean-shaped organs lie on either side of the vertebral column in the most posterior part of the abdominal cavity. The right kidney is generally slightly lower or more inferior than the left because of the presence of the liver. Superior and medial to each kidney is a **suprarenal** (adrenal) **gland.** These important glands of the endocrine system are located in the fatty capsule that surrounds each kidney.

Each kidney is connected to the single urinary bladder by its own ureter. Waste material, in the form of urine, travels from the kidneys to the bladder via the *ureters.* The saclike urinary bladder serves as a reservoir that stores urine until it can be eliminated from the body via the **urethra.**

The Latin designation for kidney is *ren,* and *renal* is an adjective that is commonly used to refer to the kidney.

KIDNEYS

The various organs of the urinary system and their relationship to the bony skeleton are shown from the back in Fig. 14.2 and from the left side in Fig. 14.3. The posteriorly placed **kidneys** lie in the upper posterior abdomen on either side of the vertebral column. The right kidney is positioned posterior to the lower portion of the **liver.** The left kidney is positioned posterior to the inferior border of the **spleen** (see Fig. 14.2). The lower rib cage thus forms a protective enclosure for the kidneys.

URETERS

Most of each **ureter** lies anterior to its respective kidney. The ureters follow the natural curve of the vertebral column. Each ureter initially curves anteriorly, following the lumbar lordotic curvature, and then curves posteriorly on entering the pelvis. After passing into the pelvis, each ureter follows the sacrococcygeal curve before entering the posterolateral aspect of the bladder.

URETHRA

The **urethra** connects the bladder to the exterior. The urethra exits from the body inferior to the symphysis pubis.

The entire urinary system is posterior to or below the peritoneum. The kidneys and ureters are retroperitoneal structures, whereas the bladder and urethra are infraperitoneal structures.

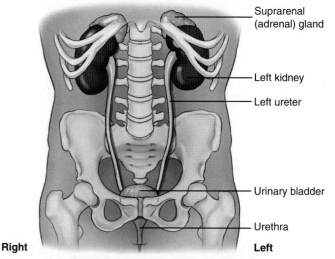

Fig. 14.1 Urinary system, anterior view.

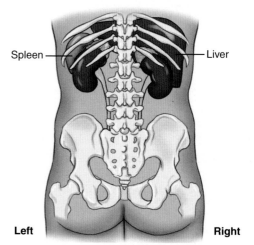

Fig. 14.2 Urinary system, posterior view.

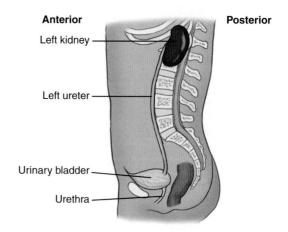

Fig. 14.3 Urinary system, lateral view.

14

Kidneys

The average adult kidney is fairly small, weighing about 5¼ oz (150 g). The measurements are 4 to 5 inches (10 to 12 cm) long, 2 to 3 inches (5 to 7.5 cm) wide, and 1 inch (2.5 cm) thick. The left kidney is a little longer, but more narrow than the right. Despite its small size, at least one functional kidney is absolutely essential for normal health. Failure of both kidneys, unless corrected, means inevitable death.

KIDNEY ORIENTATION

The usual orientation of the kidneys in the supine individual is shown in Fig. 14.4. The large muscles on either side of the vertebral column cause the longitudinal plane of the kidneys to form a vertical angle of about 20° with the midsagittal plane. These large muscles include the two **psoas** *(so'-es)* **major muscles.** These muscle masses grow larger as they progress inferiorly from the upper lumbar vertebrae. This gradual enlargement produces the 20° angle, wherein the upper pole of each kidney is closer to the midline than its lower pole (see Fig. 14.4).

These large posterior abdominal muscles also cause the kidneys to rotate backward within the retroperitoneal space. As a result, the medial border of each kidney is more anterior than the lateral border (Fig. 14.5).

The **aorta** and **inferior vena cava** are also indicated to show their relationship to the kidneys.

CROSS-SECTIONAL VIEW

Transverse cross-sectional views through the level of L2 illustrate the usual amount of backward rotation of the kidneys (Figs. 14.5 and 14.6). The normal kidney rotation of about **30°** is due to the midline location of the vertebral column and the large **psoas major muscles** on either side. The **quadratus lumborum muscles** are also shown on each side just posterior to the kidneys. The deep muscles of the back include the group of **erector spinae muscles** on each side of the spine.

When posterior oblique projections are used during radiographic studies of the urinary system, each kidney in turn is placed parallel to the plane of the image receptor. The body is rotated about **30° in each direction** to place one kidney, and then the other, parallel to the image receptor (IR) plane. A 30° left posterior oblique (LPO) positions the right kidney parallel to the IR, and a 30° right posterior oblique (RPO) positions the left kidney parallel.

Each kidney is surrounded by a mass of fatty tissue termed the *adipose capsule,* or **perirenal fat.** The presence of these fatty capsules around the kidneys permits radiographic visualization of the kidneys on plain abdominal radiographs. A sufficient density difference between fat and muscle allows visualization of the outline of each kidney on most technically satisfactory abdominal radiographs.

CT Axial Section

Fig. 14.6 represents a computed tomography (CT) axial section through the level of the midkidneys at L2. This section demonstrates the anatomic relationships of the kidneys to adjoining organs and structures. The anatomy that should be recognizable is as follows:

A. Pancreas
B. Gallbladder
C. Right lobe of the liver
D. Right kidney
E. Right crus of the diaphragm
F. Erector spinae muscles
G. L2 vertebra
H. Quadratus lumborum muscle
I. Renal pelvis—proximal ureter of left kidney
J. Descending colon
K. Abdominal aorta
L. Inferior vena cava (IVC)
M. Small intestine (jejunum)

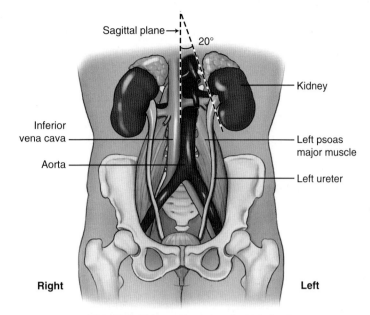
Fig. 14.4 Kidney orientation, frontal view.

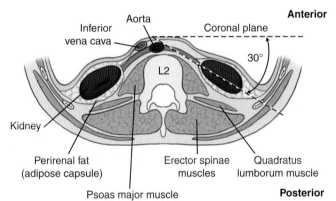
Fig. 14.5 Kidney orientation, cross-sectional view.

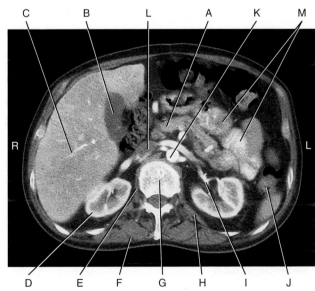
Fig. 14.6 CT axial section at level of L2.

14

ᴺᴏᴿMAL KIDNEY LOCATION

Most abdominal radiographs are performed on expiration with the patient supine. The combined effect of expiration and a supine position allows the kidneys to lie slightly higher in the abdominal cavity. Under these conditions, the kidneys normally lie about **halfway between the xiphoid process and the iliac crest.** The left kidney normally lies about 1 cm more superior than the right one. The top of the left kidney is usually at the level of the **T11–T12 interspace.** The bottom of the right kidney is most often level with the superior endplate of **L3** (Fig. 14.7).

Kidney Movement

Because the kidneys are only loosely attached within their fatty capsule, they tend to move up and down with movements of the diaphragm and position changes. When one inhales deeply, the kidneys normally drop about 1 inch (2.5 cm). When one stands upright, the kidneys normally drop about one lumbar vertebra, or 2 inches (5 cm). If the kidneys drop farther than this, a condition termed *nephroptosis (nef"-rop-to'-sis)* is said to exist. With some very thin and older patients in particular, the kidneys may drop dramatically and end up within the pelvis, which may create problems caused by "kinking" or twisting of the ureters.

FUNCTIONS OF URINARY SYSTEM

The primary function of the urinary system is the **production of urine and its elimination** from the body. During urine production, the kidneys perform the following functions:

1. Remove nitrogenous wastes
2. Regulate water levels in the body
3. Regulate acid-base balance and electrolyte levels of the blood

Nitrogenous waste products such as urea and creatinine are formed during the normal metabolism of proteins. Buildup of these nitrogenous wastes in the blood results in the clinical condition termed *uremia* and may indicate renal dysfunction.

RENAL BLOOD VESSELS

Large blood vessels are needed to handle the vast quantities of blood flowing through the kidneys daily. At rest, about 25% of the blood pumped from the heart with each beat passes through the kidneys. Arterial blood is received by the kidneys directly from the **abdominal aorta** via the left and right renal arteries. Each **renal artery** branches and rebranches until a vast capillary network is formed within each kidney.

Because most of the blood volume that enters the kidneys is returned to the circulatory system, the **renal veins** must be large vessels. The renal veins connect directly to the **inferior vena cava** to return the blood to the right side of the heart. The renal veins are anterior to the renal arteries (Fig. 14.8).

Along the medial border of each kidney is a centrally located, longitudinal fissure termed the **hilum** *(hi'-lum).* The hilum serves to transmit the renal artery, renal vein, lymphatics, nerves, and ureter. Each kidney is generally divided into an upper part and a lower part, called the **upper pole** and the **lower pole,** respectively.

Urine Production

The average water intake for humans during a 24-hour period is approximately 2.5 L (2500 mL). This water comes from ingested liquids, foods, and from the end products of metabolism. This

2.5 L of water eventually ends up in the bloodstream. Vast quantities of blood are filtered through the kidneys. At rest, more than 1 L of blood flows through the kidneys every 60 seconds, which results in removal of about 180 L of filtrate from the blood every 24 hours. More than 99% of this filtrate volume is reabsorbed by the kidneys and returned to the bloodstream. During the reabsorption process, the blood pH and quantities of various electrolytes, such as sodium, potassium, and chloride, are regulated (Fig. 14.9).

From the large amount of blood that flows through the kidneys each day, an average of approximately **1.5 L (1500 mL)** of urine is formed. This amount varies greatly, depending on fluid intake, amount of perspiration, and other factors.

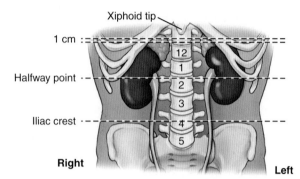

Fig. 14.7 Normal kidney location.

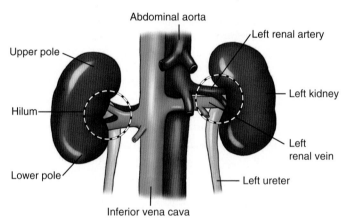

Fig. 14.8 Renal blood vessels.

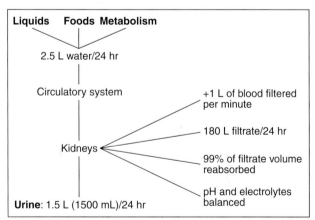

Fig. 14.9 Urine production.

MACROSCOPIC STRUCTURE

The macroscopic internal structure of the kidney is shown in Fig. 14.10. The outer covering of the kidney is termed the **renal (fibrous) capsule.** Directly under the renal capsule, surrounding each kidney, is the **cortex.** This forms the peripheral, or outer, portion of the kidney. Under the cortex is the internal structure termed the *medulla,* which is composed of 8 to 18 conical masses termed **renal pyramids.** The cortex periodically dips between the pyramids to form the **renal columns,** which extend to the **renal sinus.**

The renal pyramids are primarily a collection of tubules that converge at an opening called the **renal papilla** (apex). This renal papilla drains into the **minor calyx** (*kal'-lis* or *ka'-liks*[2]). Calyces appear as hollowed flattened tubes. From 4 to 13 minor calyces unite to form two to three **major calyces.** The major calyces unite to form the **renal pelvis,** which appears in the shape of a larger flattened funnel. Each expanded renal pelvis narrows to continue as the **ureter.** Thus, urine formed in the microscopic or nephron portion of the kidney finally reaches the ureter by passing through the various collecting tubules, a minor calyx, and a major calyx, and finally to the renal pelvis.

The general term *renal parenchyma (par-eng'-ki-mah)* is used to describe the total functional portions of the kidneys, such as those visualized during an early phase of an intravenous (IV) urographic procedure.

The structural and functional unit of the kidney is the microscopic **nephron.** Approximately 1 million nephrons exist within each kidney. One such nephron is shown in Fig. 14.11, a greatly magnified but very small cutaway section of the kidney. A more detailed view of a single nephron and its collecting ducts is shown in Fig. 14.12. Small arteries in the renal **cortex** form tiny capillary tufts, termed *glomeruli (glo-mer'-u-li).* Blood initially is filtered through the many glomeruli.

Afferent arterioles supply blood **to** the glomeruli. **Efferent arterioles** take blood **away** to a secondary capillary network in close relation to the straight and convoluted tubules. Each glomerulus is surrounded by a **glomerular capsule** (Bowman capsule), which is the proximal portion of each nephron collecting filtrate. (The glomerulus is also part of the **nephron,** which is made up of the glomerulus and the long tubules.) The glomerular filtrate travels from the **glomerular capsule** to a **proximal convoluted tubule,** to the **descending** and **ascending limbs** of the **loop of Henle**[a]*(Hen'-le),* to a **distal convoluted tubule,** to a **collecting tubule** and, finally, into a **minor calyx.** The filtrate is termed *urine* by the time it reaches the minor calyx. Between the Bowman capsule and the minor calyces, more than 99% of the filtrate is reabsorbed into the kidney's venous system.

Microscopically, the glomeruli, glomerular capsules, and proximal and distal convoluted tubules of the many nephrons are located within the **cortex** of the kidney. The loop of Henle and the collecting tubules are located primarily within the **medulla.** The renal pyramids within the medulla are primarily a collection of tubules. The major calyces unite to form the renal pelvises.

[a] Named for Friedrich Gustav Jakob Henle, German anatomist, 1809–1885.

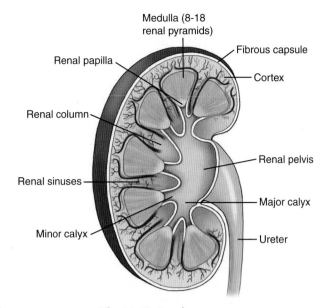

Fig. 14.10 Renal structure.

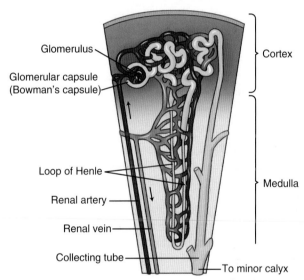

Fig. 14.11 Microscopic structure (nephron).

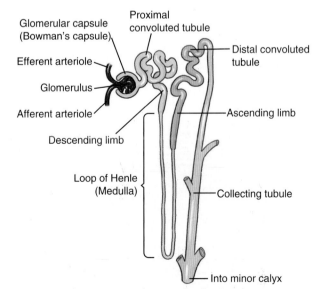

Fig. 14.12 Nephron and collecting duct.

eters

The **ureters** transport urine from the kidneys to the urinary bladder. Slow peristaltic waves and gravity force urine down the ureters into the bladder, as demonstrated in Fig. 14.13. This is a radiographic image taken 10 minutes after injection of contrast medium into the bloodstream. It was performed as part of an IV urographic procedure.

The **renal pelvis** leaves each kidney at the hilum to become the **ureter.** The ureters vary in length from about 11 to 13 inches (28 to 34 cm), with the right one being slightly shorter than the left.

As the ureters pass inferiorly, they **lie on the anterior surface of each psoas major muscle** (Fig. 14.14). Continuing to follow the curvature of the vertebral column, the ureters eventually enter the posterolateral portion of each side of the **urinary bladder.**

URETER SIZE AND POINTS OF CONSTRICTION

The ureters vary in diameter from 1 mm to almost 1 cm. Normally, **three constricted points** exist along the course of each ureter. If a kidney stone attempts to pass from the kidney to the bladder, it may have trouble passing through these three regions (see Fig. 14.14).

The **first** point is the **ureteropelvic** *(u-re″-ter-o-pel′-vic)* **(UP) junction,** at which the renal pelvis funnels down into the small ureter. This section is best seen on the radiograph in Fig. 14.13.

The **second** is near the **brim of the pelvis,** where the iliac blood vessels cross over the ureters (see Fig. 14.14).

The **third** is where the ureter joins the bladder, termed the **ureterovesical** *(u-re″-ter-o-ves′-i-kal)* **junction,** or UV junction. Most kidney stones that pass down the ureter tend to hang up at the third site, the UV junction. Once the stone passes this point and moves into the bladder, it generally has little trouble passing from the bladder through the urethra to the exterior.

Urinary Bladder

The urinary bladder is a musculomembranous sac that serves as a reservoir for urine. The empty bladder is somewhat flattened and assumes the more oval shape seen only when partially or fully distended (Fig. 14.13).

The triangular portion of the bladder along the inner, posterior surface is termed the **trigone** *(tri′-gon).* The trigone is the muscular area formed by the entrance of the two **ureters** from behind and the exit site of the **urethra** (see Fig. 14.15A). The trigone is firmly attached to the floor of the pelvis. The mucosa of the trigone is smooth, whereas the remaining aspect of the inner mucosa of the bladder has numerous folds termed *rugae.* As the bladder fills, the top of the bladder expands upward and forward toward the abdominal cavity.

In the male anatomy, the gland that surrounds the proximal urethra is the **prostate gland.** It is situated inferior to the bladder and measures approximately 1½ inches (3.8 cm) in diameter and

1 inch (2.5 cm) in height. Fig. 14.15B represents a male bladder, although the internal structure of the bladder is similar in both genders. The prostate produces a fluid that improves the motility of sperm during reproduction.

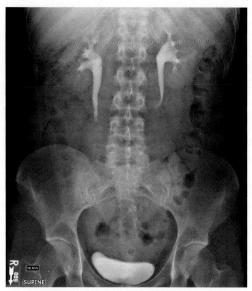

Fig. 14.13 IVU radiograph demonstrating kidneys, ureters, and bladder.

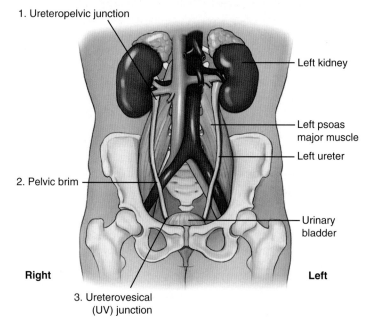

1. Ureteropelvic junction

Left kidney

Left psoas major muscle

Left ureter

2. Pelvic brim

Urinary bladder

Right **Left**

3. Ureterovesical (UV) junction

Fig. 14.14 Three possible points of constriction in the ureters (possible sites for lodging of renal calculi).

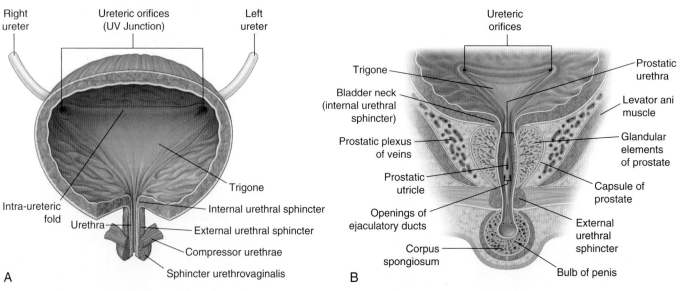

Right ureter — Ureteric orifices (UV Junction) — Left ureter

Trigone
Intra-ureteric fold
Urethra
Internal urethral sphincter
External urethral sphincter
Compressor urethrae
Sphincter urethrovaginalis

A

Ureteric orifices

Trigone
Bladder neck (internal urethral sphincter)
Prostatic plexus of veins
Prostatic utricle
Openings of ejaculatory ducts
Corpus spongiosum

Prostatic urethra
Levator ani muscle
Glandular elements of prostate
Capsule of prostate
External urethral sphincter
Bulb of penis

B

Fig. 14.15 A, Female bladder, coronal view. B, Male bladder, coronal view. (From Drake RL et.al. *Gray's atlas of anatomy*, ed 3, Philadelphia, 2021, Elsevier.)

BLADDER FUNCTIONS

The **bladder** functions as a reservoir for urine and, aided by the urethra, expels urine from the body. Normally, some urine is in the bladder at all times, but as the amount reaches 250 mL, the desire to void arises. Retention of urine in the bladder is maintained through the involuntarily controlled internal urethral sphincter (IUS) and the voluntarily controlled external urethral sphincter (EUS). The IUS is located at the junction of the bladder to the urethra (neck of bladder); the EUS is more distal. In males the EUS is distal to the prostate. The female EUS is more elaborate than males and composed of 3 areas that include: 1) Urethral sphincter 2) Compressor urethrae 3) Urethrovaginalis sphincter (Fig. 14.15A). The act of voiding (urination/micturation) is normally under voluntary control through relaxation of the EUS, and the desire to void may pass if the bladder cannot be emptied right away. The total capacity of the bladder varies from **350 to 500 mL.** As the bladder becomes fuller, the desire to void becomes more urgent. If the internal bladder pressure rises too high, involuntary urination occurs. Weakening or damage to the EUS can also lead to involuntary urination called **incontinence.**

SIZE AND POSITION OF THE BLADDER

The size, position, and functional status of the bladder depend somewhat on surrounding organs and the amount of urine within the bladder. When the rectum contains fecal matter, the bladder is pushed upward and forward. During pregnancy, as shown in Fig. 14.16, the fetus can exert tremendous downward pressure on the bladder.

NOTE: This drawing is provided only to show the anatomy and location of the urinary bladder in relation to the symphysis pubis and fetus. Remember, **no** radiographic urinary system examinations or procedures are performed during pregnancy, except in rare cases in which the benefits outweigh the risks, as determined by a physician.

FEMALE PELVIC ORGANS

The female pelvic organs are shown in the midsagittal section in Fig. 14.17. The **urinary bladder** lies posterior to and just superior to the upper margin of the **symphysis pubis,** depending on the amount of bladder distention. The female **urethra** is a narrow canal, about 1½ inches (4 cm) long, which extends from the internal urethral orifice to the external urethral orifice. The single function of the female urethra is the passage of urine to the exterior.

Female Reproductive Organs

The female reproductive organs include the paired **ovaries** (female gonads), the **uterine** (fallopian) **tubes,** and the **vagina** (see Fig. 14.17).

A close relationship exists between the urethra and bladder and the uterus and vagina. The urethra is embedded in the anterior wall of the vagina. The spatial relationship of the three external openings becomes important during certain radiographic procedures. The anal opening is most posterior, the urethral opening is most anterior, and the vaginal opening is in between.

Retroperitoneal and Infraperitoneal Organs

The **kidneys** and **ureters** are shown to be **retroperitoneal organs** located posterior to the peritoneal cavity in both males and females. The **urinary bladder, urethra,** and **male reproductive organs** are **infraperitoneal** (inferior to the peritoneal cavity).

As described in Chapter 3, the female **uterus, uterine tubes,** and **ovaries** pass **into** the peritoneal cavity. The male reproductive organs, however, are located totally **below** the peritoneum and are separated completely from organs within the peritoneal cavity. Thus the lower aspect of the peritoneum is a **closed sac in the male but not in the female.**

MALE PELVIC ORGANS

The male pelvic organs are shown in the midsagittal section in Fig. 14.18. When the **urinary bladder** is empty, most of the bladder lies directly posterior to the superior margin of the **symphysis pubis.** As the bladder distends, as it would during cystography, the radiographic study of the bladder, more and more of the bladder lies above the level of the symphysis pubis.

Male Reproductive Organs

The male reproductive organs include the **testes** (male gonads), **seminal vesicles and related ducts, ejaculatory ducts** and **ductus deferens** (vas deferens), **penis,** and **scrotum,** which contains the testes. The relative location of these organs is shown in Fig. 14.18.

The male **urethra** extends from the internal urethral orifice to the external urethral orifice at the end of the penis. The urethra extends through the **prostate gland** and the entire length of the penis. The male urethra averages 6½ to 7½ inches (17.5 to 20 cm) in length and has two functions—to eliminate urine stored in the bladder and to serve as a passageway for semen.

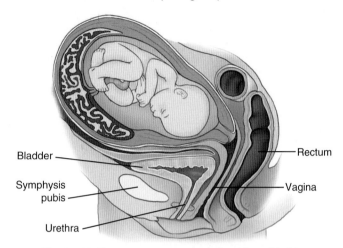

Fig. 14.16 Term pregnancy and relationship to bladder.

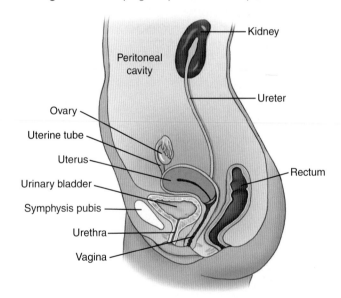

Fig. 14.17 Female pelvic organs.

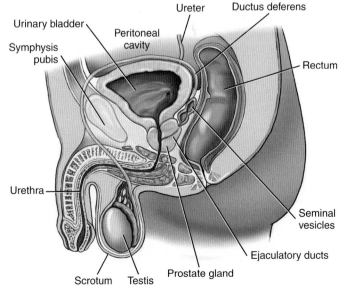

Fig. 14.18 Male pelvic organs.

Anatomy Review

RETROGRADE PYELOGRAM

Identify the following anatomic structures as labeled on this retrograde pyelogram (Fig. 14.19) in which contrast medium is being injected through a catheter inserted (retrograde) through the urethra, bladder, and ureter to the level of the renal pelvis:

A. Minor calyces
B. Major calyces .
C. Renal pelvis
D. Ureteropelvic junction (UPJ)
E. Proximal ureter
F. Distal ureter
G. Urinary bladder

VOIDING CYSTOURETHROGRAM

Identify the following anatomic structures labeled on this radiograph of the urinary bladder and urethra (Fig. 14.20), taken as a young male patient is voiding the contrast medium (patient with **vesicoureteral reflux;** see p. 547 for explanation):

A. Distal ureters
B. Urinary bladder
C. Trigone area of bladder
D. Area of prostate gland
E. Urethra

COMPUTED TOMOGRAPHY AXIAL SECTION

Anatomic structures of the abdomen are seen in a sectional view of an axial CT image (Fig. 14.21). Identifying the following abdominal organs and structures provides a good review of all abdominal anatomic structures and their relative relationships to one another:

A. Liver (lower portion of right lobe)
B. Gallbladder
C. Small intestine
D. Spleen
E. Left kidney
F. Left renal cortex
G. Abdominal aorta
H. Right psoas muscle
I. Right ureter
J. Right kidney

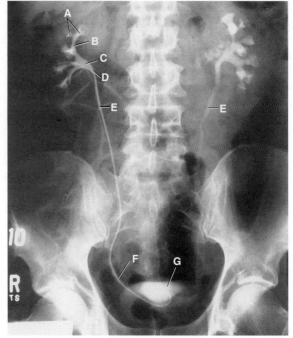

Fig. 14.19 Retrograde pyelogram (catheter in right ureter).

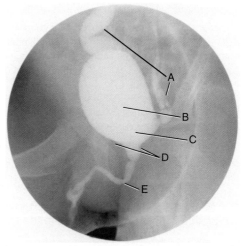

Fig. 14.20 Voiding cystourethrogram, RPO (male).

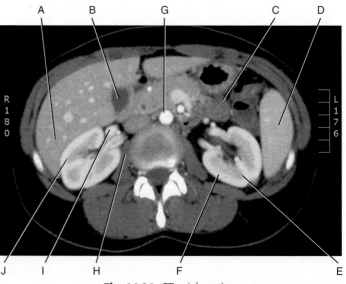

Fig. 14.21 CT axial section.

14

VENIPUNCTURE

Introduction

Venipuncture is defined as **the percutaneous puncture of a vein for withdrawal of blood or injection of a solution** such as contrast medium for urographic procedures. In the past, venipuncture for urography was performed by physicians, laboratory staff, or nursing personnel. However, venipuncture is part of the scope of practice for the diagnostic imaging professional. Although it is within the technologist's scope of practice, it is important to be aware of local laws and institutional policies that may require an additional certification in venipuncture.

Preparation for Administration of Contrast Agents

Before contrast medium is withdrawn from any vial or bottle, confirmation of the correct contents of the container, route of administration, amount to be administered, and expiration date is imperative (Fig. 14.22).

Water-soluble, iodinated contrast medium is used for radiographic examinations of the urinary system. This type of contrast medium can be administered by **bolus injection** or **drip infusion**.

BOLUS INJECTION

A bolus injection is one in which the entire dose of contrast medium is injected into the venous system at one time (Fig. 14.23). This method of administration is typically used for maximum contrast enhancement. Hand injection or the use of a power injector are both acceptable methods.

The **rate** of bolus injection is controlled by the following:
- Gauge of needle or connecting tubing
- Amount of contrast medium injected
- Viscosity of contrast medium
- Stability of vein
- Force applied by the individual who is performing the injection or determined by the rate set on the power injector.

DRIP INFUSION

Drip infusion is a method whereby contrast medium is introduced into the venous system via connective tubing attached to the IV site. A specified amount of contrast medium is introduced over a specified period. This method is used most frequently when the drip infusion catheter is already in place for repeated or continuous infusions.

The contrast medium is contained in an IV solution bag or bottle that is inverted and connected to the tubing (Fig. 14.24). The rate of infusion, which may be gradual or rapid, depending on the needs of the study, is controlled by a clamp device located below the drip chamber on the IV tubing.

EQUIPMENT AND SUPPLIES

In preparation for this procedure, the technologist must gather all necessary supplies (Fig. 14.25). These supplies should include access to an emergency cart stocked with epinephrine or Benadryl® for emergency injection in the event of an adverse contrast reaction.

The following is a list of supplies needed for performance of venipuncture:
- Sharps container
- Tourniquets
- Alcohol wipe
- Various sizes of butterfly and over-the-needle catheters
- Disposable or prefilled syringes
- IV infusion tubing
- Arm board
- Cotton balls or 2 × 2-inch (5 × 5-cm) gauze
- Tape or securing device (e.g., Tegaderm)
- Gloves (latex-free recommended)
- Water-soluble, iodinated contrast medium

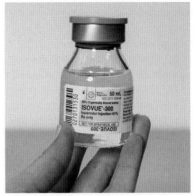
Fig. 14.22 Confirm contents and expiration date.

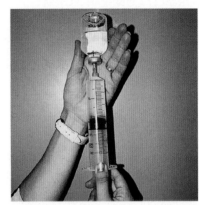
Fig. 14.23 Drawing into syringe for bolus injection.

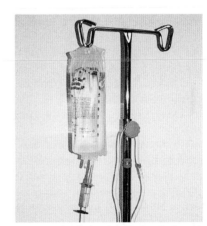
Fig. 14.24 Inverted solution bag or bottle for drip infusion.

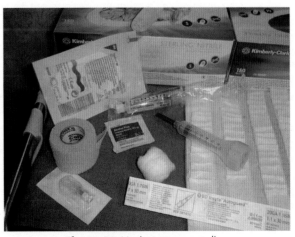
Fig. 14.25 Venipuncture supplies.

14

Patient Preparation

During **introductions, identification of the patient,** and explanation of the procedure, the mental and emotional status of the patient must be assessed. This assessment may confirm the patient is more comfortable lying down, especially if syncope (temporary loss of consciousness) is a concern.

When assessing a child, the technologist must determine the child's ability to cooperate during the procedure. If the technologist believes the child may become combative or move suddenly during needle insertion, the guardian or other personnel should be asked to help keep the child calm and immobilize the limb. However, attempts to gain the cooperation of the child through proper therapeutic communication are always preferable. The technologist should not mislead a child in terms of the discomforts of the procedure, but should instead be truthful. The technologist should be open to questions and recognize a child's concerns.

SIGNING INFORMED CONSENT FORM

Venipuncture is an invasive procedure that carries risks for complications, especially when contrast medium is injected. Before beginning the procedure, the technologist must ensure the patient is fully aware of these potential risks and has signed an **informed consent form.** If a child is undergoing venipuncture, the procedure should be explained to the child and guardian. The guardian must sign the informed consent form.

Selection of Vein

For most IV urograms, veins found within the **antecubital fossa** are ideal. Veins in this region are generally large, easy to access, and typically sufficiently durable to withstand a bolus injection of contrast medium without extravasation (leaking of the contrast medium from a blood vessel into the surrounding tissues).

Veins found within the antecubital fossa commonly used during venipuncture include the **median cubital, cephalic,** and **basilic veins.** Because these typically are easily accessible veins, they may become overused from frequent phlebotomy and IV access. Other access sites might have to be investigated if the antecubital fossa veins are damaged or inaccessible. Other common IV access sites include the **cephalic vein** of the lateral wrist and veins on the posterior hand or lower forearm, such as the **cephalic** or **basilic veins** (Fig. 14.26).

The technologist should avoid veins that are sclerotic (hardened), tortuous (twisted), rolling, or overused. Areas of vein bifurcation or veins that lie directly over an artery should not be used. **Do not** inject directly into a shunt, central line, or vascular catheter unless it has been manufactured for contrast injections or under the direction of a physician.

ENSURE VESSEL IS A VEIN AND NOT AN ARTERY

When selecting an injection site, ensure the vessel is **not an artery.** The vessel should not be pulsatile and most likely will be close to the skin's surface.

Type and Size of Needle

For bolus injections of 50 to 100 mL of contrast medium into adults, an **18- to 22-gauge needle** is generally used. Some technologists prefer the butterfly needle and claim this type of needle provides greater control during venipuncture because of the two side flaps (Fig. 14.27). The size of the needle is determined by the size of the vein. The length of the needle may vary between 1 and 1 ½ inches (2.5 to 3.75 cm). For pediatric patients, a smaller 23- to 25-gauge needle is often used. The technologist may choose to use an **over-the-needle catheter** instead of the butterfly.

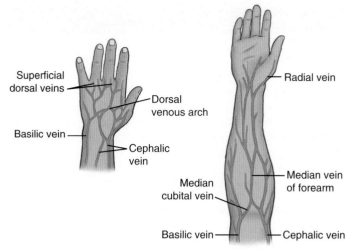

Fig. 14.26 Possible veins for venipuncture.

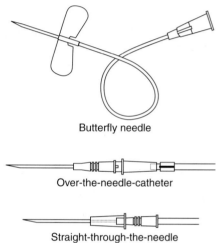

Butterfly needle

Over-the-needle-catheter

Straight-through-the-needle

Fig. 14.27 Three types of needles.

NOTE: It is recommended that IV access be maintained until the imaging procedure is completed in the event that treatment for an adverse contrast reaction becomes necessary.

Venipuncture Procedure

Step 1: Wash Hands and Put On Gloves (Figs. 14.28 and 14.29)

After making introductions, checking the patient's ID, explaining the procedure, and obtaining a signature for the consent form, the technologist proceeds with the following:

A. Wash the hands thoroughly.

B. Put on non-sterile gloves. (Avoid latex gloves if possible because of possible allergies in the technologist or patient.)

Step 2: Apply Tourniquet, Select Site, and Cleanse the Site (Figs. 14.30 to 14.32)

A. Ensure patient comfort by having the person sit or lie down. Support the arm of interest by using a hard surface such as a table. Adjust the height of the arm to match the appropriate working level of the technologist. Select the injection site by using the technologist's finger of the nondominant hand and place the tourniquet **3 to 4 inches (7.5 to 10 cm)** above the site. Tighten the tourniquet sufficiently to dilate the veins. Check for the radial artery pulse to verify the tourniquet is sufficiently tight to compress the veins but still allow blood flow to the distal regions. Verify the resilience of the selected vein and then release the tourniquet.

B. Cleanse the selected site with an alcohol (70% isopropyl) wipe, using a circular motion from the center outward 2 to 3 inches (5 to 7.5 cm) for a minimum of 30 seconds. Never lift the wipe from the skin until the cleansing process has been completed.

C. Allow just a moment for the alcohol to dry before inserting the needle.

Step 3: Initiate Puncture (Fig. 14.33)

A. Retighten the tourniquet.

B. Using the nondominant hand, anchor the vein by making the skin taut just below the puncture site.

C. With the **bevel** of the needle **facing upward,** approach the vein at an angle between 20° and 45°. Advance the needle through the skin just superior to the vein of interest until venous access is obtained. Access can be verified by visualizing blood in the tubing (butterfly) or the flashback chamber (over the needle catheter). Care should be taken to not go through both walls of the vein.

D. Decrease the angle of the needle to run parallel with the vein while advancing the needle slightly farther into the vein, approximately ¼ inch (0.6 cm).

Alternative site: cephalic or basilic veins of posterior hand (Fig. 14.34):

NOTE: If extravasation (infiltration) does occur, or if for some other reason the venipuncture must be terminated, withdraw the needle or catheter and apply light pressure on the site with gauze or a cotton ball. Follow department policy for maintenance of the extravasation site once bleeding from the IV insertion has been controlled. Always use a new needle for any subsequent punctures.

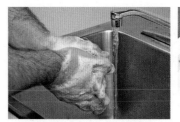
Fig. 14.28 Wash hands.

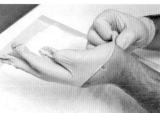
Fig. 14.29 Put on gloves.

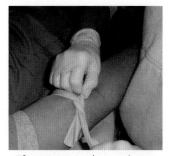
Fig. 14.30 Apply tourniquet.

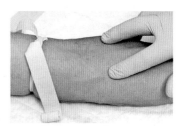
Fig. 14.31 Select vein.

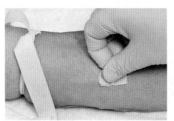
Fig. 14.32 Cleanse site.

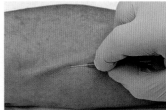
Fig. 14.33 Insert needle with bevel up, 20° to 45°, and advance slightly.

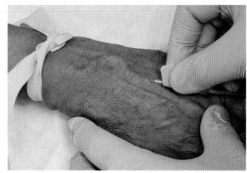
Fig. 14.34 With butterfly needle (posterior hand site), insert needle with bevel up, 20° to 25°, and advance slightly.

Step 4: Secure Access (Figs. 14.35 to 14.38)

A. **Butterfly needle:** Secure access by taping the needle in place. Tape should be placed over the hub of the butterfly across the flaps. Instructions should be given to the patient not to move or flex the arm. Observe the needle base for retrograde flow of blood. If no blood is seen, make slight adjustments to the needle position until blood "flashback" is seen in the tubing. Attach the IV tubing or a PRN adaptor to the extension tubing. Release the tourniquet.

B. **Over-the-needle catheter:** Once the needle is in the vein, firmly grasp the catheter with the thumb and index finger. Stabilize the needle and slowly advance the catheter into the vein. Apply pressure to the vein about 1 ½ inches (3.75 cm) above the insertion site. Deploy the needle retraction or covering device and properly dispose of the needle in a sharps container. Quickly attach the IV tubing or PRN adaptor to the hub of the catheter. Secure the catheter with tape and release the tourniquet.

Step 5: Proceed with Injection (Figs. 14.39 and 14.40)

A. It may be facility policy or technologist preference to quickly flush the IV catheter with 5 to 10 mL of normal saline in an effort to test the stability of the vein before it is attached to the contrast medium.

B. Ensure the contrast medium is administered at an appropriate rate, and watch the injection site for signs of extravasation.

C. After completion of injection, ensure patient comfort, remove gloves and wash hands.

D. The person who performs the venipuncture must write the following in the patient's chart:
   - Starting time of injection
   - Type and amount of contrast medium injected
   - Patient's tolerance to procedure
   - Further documentation of the procedure according to facility policy.

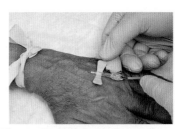

Fig. 14.35 With butterfly needle, observe backflow of blood.

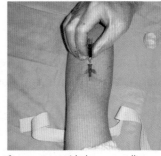

Fig. 14.36 Withdraw needle and release tourniquet.

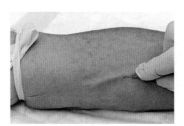

Fig. 14.37 Advance catheter into vein.

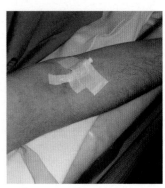

Fig. 14.38 Tape catheter in place.

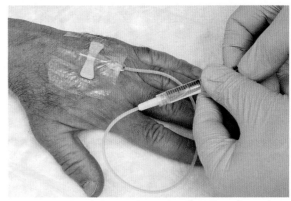

Fig. 14.39 Tape butterfly needle in place; ready to begin injection.

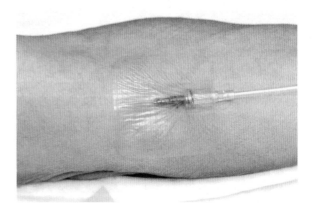

Fig. 14.40 Release tourniquet for over-the-needle catheter; ready for injection.

Step 6: Needle or Catheter Removal (Figs. 14.41 and 14.42)

For patient safety, maintain venous access during the entire examination or until the physician directs that the access be discontinued. **First, put on non-sterile gloves** to remove the securing device (e.g., tape, Tegaderm). Gently but quickly pull the IV catheter out of the vein and skin. Press firmly over the injection site using a 2 × 2-inch (5 × 5-cm) gauze or cotton ball. Direct pressure immediately over the puncture site and hold until the bleeding stops.

NOTE: If the patient is on blood thinning medication (e.g., heparin and Coumadin™), it will take longer to stop the bleeding.

Secure the gauze or cotton ball in place. Be sure to inform the patient that as long as the bleeding has stopped, the bandage may be removed after approximately 20 minutes.

SUMMARY OF SAFETY CONSIDERATIONS

1. Always wear non-sterile gloves during all aspects of the procedure.
2. Follow Occupational Safety and Health Administration (OSHA) Standard Precautions and properly dispose of all materials that contain blood or body fluids.
3. Place needles and syringes in a designated sharps container. Sharps containers should be replaced when half full.
4. If the initial puncture is unsuccessful, use a new butterfly or over-the-needle catheter for the second attempt. (The needle and/or catheter may have been damaged during the insertion.) Also select another puncture site. If the same vein is used, subsequent attempts for IV access must occur proximal to the site of the initial attempt.
5. If extravasation of contrast medium occurs, elevate the affected extremity and provide a cold compress over the site of injection for approximately 20 minutes followed by a warm compress. The cold compress will cause vasoconstriction to minimize bleeding and damage to the tissues and relieve pain. The warm compress then will increase circulation to encourage uptake of the extravasated contrast medium. This rotation of cold and warm compresses can continue for a length of time specified by the physician. A formal report of the extravasation may be required, depending on the amount extravasated and facility policy, and should be noted in the patient's chart.
6. Document the injection, including the injection site, time, amount, type of contrast agent injected, and any resultant complications.

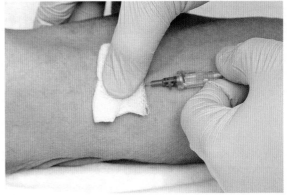

Fig. 14.41 Remove needle or catheter.

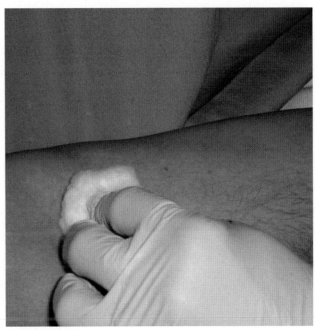

Fig. 14.42 Apply immediate pressure over injection site.

14

RADIOGRAPHIC PROCEDURES

Contrast Media and Urography

INTRODUCTION TO THE INTRAVENOUS UROGRAM

The plain abdominal radiographic image provides little information about the urinary system. The gross outline of the kidneys may be faintly demonstrated because of the fatty capsule surrounding the kidneys. However, in general, the urinary system blends in with the other soft tissue structures of the abdominal cavity, thus requiring contrast medium to radiographically demonstrate the internal, fluid-filled portion of the urinary system. This radiographic procedure in which contrast medium is injected intravenously is termed **intravenous urography (IVU)**. General radiographic examination of the urinary system is termed **urography** *(u″-rog′-rah-fe)*. *Uro-* is a prefix that denotes a relationship to urine or to the urinary tract.

IODINATED CONTRAST

Iodine is the **opacifying element** used in intravenous contrast media for urography. Its high atomic number (53) leads to increased attenuation and better visualization of the structures within the urinary system. The structure of all iodinated contrast agents is derived from a 6-sided benzene model, containing 3 iodine atoms, and referred to as a *tri-iodinated contrast agents*. Contrast agents can be **monomer** (Fig.14.43A), containing one tri-iodinated benzene ring or **dimer** (Fig.14.43B), containing two tri-iodinated benzene rings.

IONIC CONTRAST

Ionic iodinated contrast agents contain a positively charged side chain element called a **cation**. The cation is a salt, usually consisting of sodium, meglumine, or a combination of both. These salts increase the solubility of the contrast medium. The cation is combined with a negatively charged component called the **anion**. Diatrizoate, iothalamate, and metrizoate are common anions that help stabilize the contrast medium.

Once injected, the cation will disassociate (ionize) from the parent compound or anion, thus creating two separate particles in the blood. This action creates a hypertonic condition by increasing the blood plasma osmolality. **Osmolality** is the number of dissolved particles in a solution.

HIGH-OSMOLAR CONTRAST AGENTS (HOCA)

An ionic tri-iodinated monomer can greatly increase the osmolality of plasma and is considered a high-osmolar contrast agent (HOCA). In the 1950s HOCAs were the common agents used. This increase in osmolality can cause vein spasm, pain at the injection site, and fluid retention. More important, ionic contrast agents may increase the probability that a patient will experience a contrast medium reaction. Any disruption to the delicate balance of the body's physiologic functions may result in a reaction. This concept is the basis of the chemotoxic theory, which states that any disruption to the physiologic balance, called **homeostasis**, may lead to an adverse reaction.

NONIONIC CONTRAST

Nonionic contrasts contain the same tri-iodinated opacifying elements, but contain no positively charged cations. The ionizing carboxyl group is replaced with a non-dissociated group, such as amide or glucose. Therefore, when injected into the blood or other body cavities, the contrast medium remains intact. The term **nonionic** was coined to describe this type of contrast medium, based on its nonionizing characteristic (Fig. 14.44).

LOW-OSMOLAR CONTRAST AGENTS (LOCA)

In the 1980s a nonionic tri-iodinated monomer was developed. This agent slightly increases the osmolality of plasma, if at all, and is considered a low-osmolar contrast agent (LOCA). In the late 1980s to early 1990s dimer agents were introduced. A nonionic dimer will increase the number of iodine atoms to 6 and remain nearly isotonic. Once injected, the dimer remains as two particles but has twice the iodine concentration. Therefore, a smaller amount of contrast medium is needed to maintain opacification of the area of interest.

Research has indicated that patients are less likely to have contrast medium reactions when a LOCA is used. The cost for LOCAs used to be much higher than HOCAs. As patents expired in the mid 1990s the cost of LOCAs dropped. As a result, LOCAs are now the recommended contrast agent for use as intravenous contrast injections.[3] Table 14.1 presents a list of the iodine-based contrast agents.

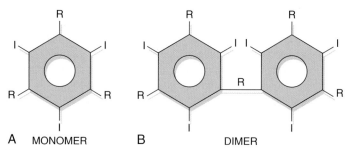

Fig. 14.43 A, Monomer. B, Dimer. (Case courtesy of Andrew Murphy, Radiopaedia.org, rID: 48581.)

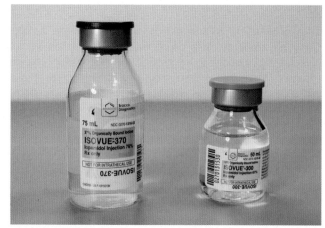

Fig. 14.44 Two examples of water-soluble nonionic contrast media.

TABLE 14.1	**CHARACTERISTICS OF IODINATED CONTRAST MEDIA**[4]		
NAME	**STRUCTURE**	**CHARGE**	**OSMOLALITY**
Renografin, Hypaque	Monomer	Ionic	High
Urografin	Monomer	Ionic	High
Conray	Monomer	Ionic	High
Telebrix	Monomer	Ionic	High
Hexabrix	Dimer	Ionic	Low
Isovue	Monomer	Nonionic	Low
Omnipaque	Monomer	Nonionic	Low
Imeron	Monomer	Nonionic	Low
Imagopaque	Monomer	Nonionic	Low
Oxilan	Monomer	Nonionic	Low
Optiray	Monomer	Nonionic	Low
Ultravist	Monomer	Nonionic	Low
Isovist	Dimer	Nonionic	Iso-osmolal
Visipaque	Dimer	Nonionic	Iso-osmolal

COMMON SIDE EFFECTS

Side effects occur in many patients as an expected outcome of injected iodinated contrast medium. They are brief and self-limiting.

Two common side effects that may occur after an IV injection of iodinated contrast medium are a **temporary hot flash** and a **metallic taste in the mouth.** Both the hot flash, particularly in the face, and the metallic taste in the mouth usually last only minutes. Discussion of these possible effects and careful explanation of the examination help reduce patient anxiety and prepare the patient psychologically.

PATIENT HISTORY

A careful patient history may serve to alert the medical team to a possible reaction (Fig. 14.45). Patients with a history of allergies are more likely to experience adverse reactions to contrast media than those who have no allergies. Questions to ask the patient include the following:

1. Are you allergic to anything?
2. Have you ever had hay fever, asthma, or hives?
3. Are you allergic to any drugs or medications?
4. Are you **allergic to iodine?**
5. Are you allergic to any foods?
6. Are you currently taking **metformin, Glucophage, Fortamet, Glumetza, Riomet, Glucovance, Metaglip, Jentadueto, ActoPlus Met, Prandimet, Avandamet, Kombiglyze XR, or Janumet[5]?**
7. Have you ever had an x-ray examination that required an injection into an artery or vein? If so, did you experience any difficulty with the injection of contrast media?

A positive response to any of these questions alerts the injection team to an increased probability of reaction.

BLOOD CHEMISTRY

The technologist must check the patient's chart to determine the **creatinine** and **blood urea nitrogen (BUN)** levels and/or the **estimated glomerular filtration rate (eGFR).** These laboratory tests should have been conducted and reported in the patient's chart before the urinary system study is undertaken. Creatinine and BUN levels are diagnostic indicators of kidney function. An elevated creatinine or BUN level may indicate acute or chronic renal failure, tumor, or other conditions of the urinary system. Patients with elevated blood levels have a greater chance of experiencing an adverse contrast medium reaction. **Normal creatinine levels** for the adult are **0.6 to 1.5 mg/dL.** The **BUN level** should range between **8 and 25 mg/100 mL.** The eGFR has shown to be a more sensitive predicter of kidney function. A **normal eGFR** for adults is **60 mL/min or greater.**

Metformin[5]

Metformin hydrochloride is a drug that is given for the management of non-insulin-dependent diabetes mellitus. Metformin decreases hepatic glucose and increases the body's response to insulin. Patients who are currently taking metformin can be given iodinated contrast media only if their kidney function levels are within normal limits. Because the combination of iodinated contrast medium and metformin may increase the risk for contrast medium–induced acute renal failure and/or lactic acidosis, the American College of Radiology recommends two categories for managing the risks:

Category I: If a patient has no evidence of acute kidney injury (AKI) and has an eGFR of 30 mL or greater, there is no need to discontinue metformin use prior to or following injection.

Category II: If a patient has an AKI or has an eGFR below 30 mL, Metformin should be withheld prior to injection and for 48 hours after the injection.

Individual site protocols may vary. The technologist must be aware of these policies prior to injecting contrast agents.[5]

The technologist must review the patient's chart and ask whether the patient is taking metformin. Trade names of medications that contain metformin include Glucophage, Glucophage XR, Fortamet, Glumetza, and Riomet. Combination products that contain metformin include Glucovance, Metaglip, Jentadueto, Actoplus Met, Actoplus Met XR, Prandimet, Avandamet, Janumet, Janumet XR, and Kombiglyze XR.[5]. If the patient says "yes," this should be brought to the immediate attention of the radiologist before injection.

SELECTION AND PREPARATION OF CONTRAST MEDIA

Selection and preparation of the correct contrast medium are important steps before injection (Fig. 14.46). Because labels on various containers are similar, one should **always read the label very carefully** several times. In addition, the **empty container should be shown to the radiologist or the person who is making the actual injection.** The empty contrast container should be kept in the examination room until the procedure is complete and the patient is dismissed, in the event a contrast reaction occurs. In some cases the lot number of the container must be documented as part of the patient file.

Whenever contrast medium is drawn into a syringe, the sterility of the medium, syringe, and needle must be maintained.

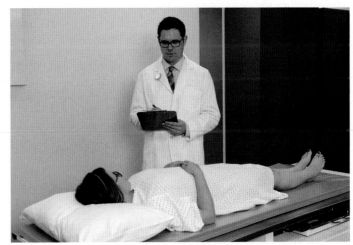

Fig. 14.45 Obtain patient history.

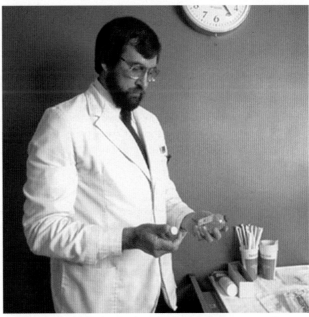

Fig. 14.46 Selection and preparation of contrast medium.

Reactions to Contrast Media

PREPARATION FOR POSSIBLE REACTION

Because a contrast medium reaction is possible and unpredictable, a fully stocked **emergency response cart** must be readily available whenever an IV injection is performed (Fig. 14.47). In addition to emergency drugs, the cart should contain cardiopulmonary resuscitation equipment, portable oxygen, suction and blood pressure apparatus, and possibly a defibrillator and monitor.

The technologist is responsible for ensuring that the emergency drug cart is stocked and available in the room. Masks and a cannula for oxygen support, suction tips, needles, and syringes must be readily available. The status of this equipment and the emergency drug cart should be verified before any contrast medium procedure is undertaken.

A common emergency drug is **epinephrine,** which should be available along with a syringe and needle ready for use (Fig. 14.48).

Premedication Procedure

To reduce the severity of contrast medium reactions, some patients may be premedicated before an iodinated contrast medium procedure is performed. The patient can be given a number of medications at different stages to reduce the risk of an allergic reaction to the contrast medium. One of the common premedication protocols includes a combination of an antihistamine and prednisone given over a period of 12 or more hours before the procedure. Patients who have a history of hay fever, asthma, or food allergy may be candidates for the premedication procedure. The technologist should ask patients whether they have received any premedication prior to the procedure and note their response in the appropriate chart.

Categories of Contrast Medium Reactions[5]

There are two categories of contrast media reactions, local and systemic. **Local reactions** are those that affect only the specific region of the body at which the contrast medium has been injected into the venous system. **Systemic reactions** are those that do not affect the site of injection, but rather the entire body or a specific organ system. Systemic reactions can range from mild to severe. Severe reactions can lead to significant complications following the reaction.

Local reactions Two local reactions to contrast medium injection can be found at or near the site of IV access. These include **extravasation** and **phlebitis.**

- **Extravasation:** Leakage of iodinated contrast medium outside the vessel and into surrounding soft tissues (sometimes also referred to as **infiltration**). This can occur when venous access is lost due to breakage of the accessed vein or when the needle is improperly placed within the surrounding tissue outside the intended vein. In either case, the contrast medium fills the soft tissue surrounding the access site. Extravasated contrast medium, particularly high-osmolality contrast agents, is known to be toxic to surrounding tissues. Acute, local inflammatory response to the skin peaks 24 to 48 hours following extravasation of the contrast medium. Ulceration and tissue necrosis may result within 6 hours following the event. Although consensus regarding treatment has not been reached, a common protocol for extravasation includes the following:
  - Notify department nurse and/or physician so that treatment can be administered quickly.
  - Elevate the affected extremity above the heart to decrease capillary pressure and promote resorption of extravasated contrast medium.
  - Use a cold compress followed by warm compresses first to relieve pain and then to improve resorption of contrast medium.
  - Document the incident.

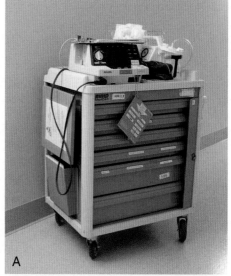

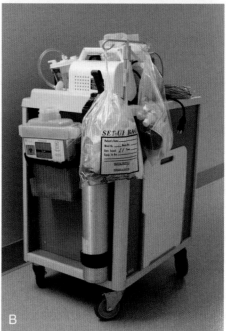

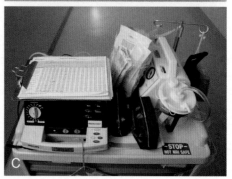

Fig. 14.47 Emergency response cart. (From Ehrlich RA, Coakes DM. *Patient care in radiography*, ed 10, St. Louis, 2021, Elsevier.)

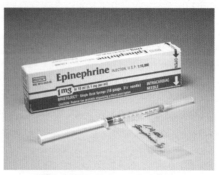

Fig. 14.48 Emergency drug.

URINARY SYSTEM AND VENIPUNCTURE **CHAPTER 14** **545**

Outpatients should be released only after the radiologist has confirmed the initial signs and symptoms have improved and no new signs and/or symptoms have developed. Outpatients should be instructed to follow up with their physician should signs and symptoms worsen.

- **Phlebitis:** Inflammation of a vein. This can be a complication of venous access related to the administration of IV contrast medium or simply venous access. Signs of phlebitis include pain, redness, and possibly swelling surrounding the venous access site.

 If signs of phlebitis are noted at the site a technologist intended to use for administration of the contrast medium, discontinue the venous access at this site and locate an alternative site above the affected area or on the opposite appendage. Phlebitis can escalate into a serious complication and should be documented in the patient's chart. The attending nurse and/or physician should also be notified so that the site can be appropriately treated, if necessary.

Systemic reactions Three general systemic categories of contrast media reactions have been identified: **mild, moderate,** and **severe.** These three reaction types are classified according to the degree of symptoms associated with the reaction.

Regardless of the type of contrast medium reaction that a patient may experience, it is important to document all symptoms in the patient's chart and notify the attending nurse and/or physician.

- **Mild reaction:** This **nonallergic reaction** typically does not require drug intervention or medical assistance (Fig. 14.49). Two of these symptoms are also considered side effects. This type of reaction may be based on anxiety and/or fear. Although this may not be a life-threatening situation, the technologist must be attentive to all needs of the patient. Symptoms of a mild reaction include the following (Table 14.2):
  - Anxiety
  - Lightheadedness
  - Nausea
  - Vomiting
  - Metallic taste (common side effect)
  - Mild erythema
  - Warm flushed sensation during injection (common side effect)
  - Itching
  - Mild scattered hives

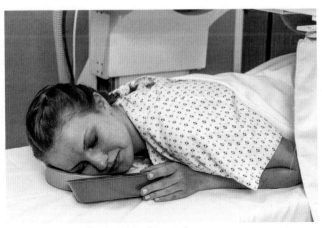

Fig. 14.49 Mild reaction—nausea.

TABLE 14.2 SUMMARY OF MILD REACTION TO CONTRAST MEDIUM

SYMPTOMS	TECHNOLOGIST RESPONSIBILITIES
All symptoms	Document all reactions to the contrast medium injection. Notify the attending nurse and/or physician of any unresolved reactions
Anxiety	Have patient take slow breaths and reassure patient. Continue to monitor patient.
Lightheadedness	Comfort and reassure patient.
Warm, flushed sensation, metallic taste	Comfort and reassure patient.
Nausea, vomiting	Have patient turn to side and provide emesis basin and cool washcloth (see Fig. 14.49).
Syncope (fainting)	Comfort and support patient and monitor vital signs.
Mild urticaria (scattered hives), itching	Inform nurse or physician. Continue to monitor patient.

TABLE 14.3 SUMMARY OF MODERATE REACTION TO CONTRAST MEDIUM

SYMPTOMS	TECHNOLOGIST RESPONSIBILITIES
All symptoms	Document all reactions to the contrast medium injection. Notify the attending nurse and/or physician
Moderate to severe urticaria (hives)	Call for medical assistance. Continue to monitor patient.
Laryngeal swelling (choking sensation from closure of larynx)	Call for medical assistance. Continue to monitor patient.
Angioedema (swelling of soft tissues)	Call for medical assistance. Continue to monitor patient.
Hypotension (low BP), moderate	Call for medical assistance. Continue to monitor patient.
Tachycardia (rapid heartbeat), moderate	Call for medical assistance. Continue to monitor patient.
Bradycardia (slow heartbeat), moderate	Call for medical assistance. Continue to monitor patient.

TABLE 14.4 SUMMARY OF SEVERE REACTION TO CONTRAST MEDIUM

SYMPTOMS	TECHNOLOGIST RESPONSIBILITIES
All symptoms	Document all reactions to the contrast medium injection. Immediately notify the attending nurse and/or physician.
Hypotension (systolic blood pressure < 80 mm Hg)	Declare medical emergency (code). Continue to monitor vital signs.
Bradycardia (heart rate < 50 beats/min)	Declare medical emergency (code). Continue to monitor vital signs.
No detectable pulse	Declare medical emergency (code). Continue to monitor vital signs.
Laryngeal swelling	Declare medical emergency (code). Continue to monitor vital signs.
Convulsions, loss of consciousness	Declare medical emergency (code). Continue to monitor vital signs.
Arrhythmias, cardiac arrest	Declare medical emergency (code). Continue to monitor vital signs.
Respiratory arrest	Declare medical emergency (code). Continue to monitor vital signs.
Diminished urine output	Notify physician.
Anuria (no urine output)	Notify physician.
No pulse	Notify physician.
Pulmonary edema (severe cough, shortness of breath)	Notify physician.
Vasculitis or limb pain	Notify physician.
Seizures	Notify physician.

Possible treatment for a mild reaction might include having the patient breathe slowly, providing a cool washcloth, and reassuring the patient. Continue to observe the patient to ensure that these symptoms do not advance into a more serious reaction.

- **Moderate reaction:** This second type of reaction is a **true allergic reaction (anaphylactic reaction)** that results from the introduction of iodinated contrast media. Symptoms of a moderate reaction include the following (Table 14.3):
  - Urticaria (moderate to severe hives)
  - Possible laryngeal swelling
  - Facial edema without dyspnea
  - Bronchospasm
  - Angioedema
  - Hypotension
  - Tachycardia (>100 beats/min) or bradycardia (<60 beats/min)

Because moderate reactions may lead to a life-threatening condition, medical assistance must be provided without delay. Treatment often involves drug intervention to counter the effects of the reaction.

- **Severe reaction:** This third type of reaction, also known as a **vasovagal reaction,** is a **life-threatening condition.** The introduction of iodinated contrast agents stimulates the vagus nerve, which may cause the heart rate to drop and the blood pressure to fall dangerously low. A fast response by the medical team is required. Symptoms of a severe reaction include the following (Table 14.4):
  - naphylactic shock (hypotension + tachycardia)
  - Cardiac arrhythmias
  - Laryngeal edema with stridor and/or hypoxia
  - Facial edema with dyspnea
  - Possible convulsions
  - Loss of consciousness
  - Cardiac arrest
  - Respiratory arrest
  - No detectable pulse

A medical emergency must be declared immediately. Ensure the emergency drug cart is nearby with oxygen and suction equipment available. Hospitalization for this patient is imminent.

A severe reaction may affect individual organ systems, leading to specific complications:
- Cardiac system: pulseless electrical activity
- Respiratory system: pulmonary edema
- Vascular system: venous thrombosis
- Nervous system: seizure induction
- Renal system: temporary failure or complete shutdown

A contrast medium reaction may start immediately following the contrast medium injection or may not be identifiable for up to 48 hours after the study has been completed. Treatment may include monitoring, possible hydration, administration of Lasix (a diuretic), interventional cardiac medications, antiseizure medications, and renal dialysis. Because a contrast medium reaction may occur several hours after a procedure has been completed, the patient should be instructed to alert the physician of any difficulty in producing urine or other unusual symptoms.

Excretory Urography—Intravenous Urography (IVU)

Excretory urography or **IVU,** is a radiographic examination of the urinary system. This examination often has been referred to as *intravenous pyelography,* or *IVP. Pyelo-,* however, refers only to the renal pelvises. Because the excretory urogram normally visualizes more anatomy than just the renal pelvis, the term *IVP* is not an accurate term for this procedure and should not be used.

IVU visualizes the minor and major calyces, renal pelvises, ureters, and urinary bladder after an intravenous injection of contrast medium. IVU is a **true functional test** because the contrast medium molecules are rapidly removed from the bloodstream and excreted completely by the normal kidney. (Today functional studies of the urinary system are conducted more frequently with computed tomography [CT].)

PURPOSE

The three purposes of IVU are as follows:
1. To visualize the collecting portion of the urinary system
2. To assess the functional ability of the kidneys
3. To evaluate the urinary system for pathology or anatomic anomalies

CONTRAINDICATIONS

Even though present-day contrast media are considered relatively safe, the technologist must take extra care in obtaining the patient history. Through the patient history, the technologist may become aware of certain conditions that prevent the patient from undergoing IVU. Major contraindications include the following:
1. Hypersensitivity to iodinated contrast media
2. Anuria, or absence of urine excretion
3. Multiple myeloma
4. Diabetes, especially diabetes mellitus
5. Severe hepatic or renal disease
6. Congestive heart failure
7. Pheochromocytoma *(fe-o-kro″-mo-si-to′-mah)*
8. Sickle cell anemia
9. Patients taking Metformin, Glucophage, Fortamet, Glumetza, Riomet, Glucovance, Metaglip, Jentadueto, ActoPlus Met, Prandimet, Avandamet, Kombiglyze XR, or Janumet[3]
10. Renal failure, acute or chronic (see the section Glossary of Urinary Pathologic Terms)

Certain conditions on this list, such as **multiple myeloma** and **pheochromocytoma,** warrant additional consideration. Multiple myeloma is a malignant condition of the plasma cells of the bone marrow, and a pheochromocytoma is a tumor of the adrenal gland. Research has indicated that these patients are at greater risk during IVU. Because **sickle cell anemia** can compromise the function of the kidney, these patients are also at higher risk. A patient with one of the listed contraindications may require evaluation with some other imaging modality. However, a patient with any of these high-risk conditions may still undergo IVU if the physician determines that the benefits of the procedure outweigh the risks.

Hydration therapy of a normal saline IV drip and diuretic before the procedure is begun may reduce the risk for patients with multiple myeloma, diabetes mellitus, and other conditions. These patients also may be candidates for the premedication protocol before the contrast medium study is performed.

GLOSSARY OF URINARY PATHOLOGIC TERMS

The following are common pathologic terms related to the urinary system that may be used to describe possible reactions to contrast media. These terms may be encountered in the patient's chart, examination requisition, or procedure results report.

Acute kidney injury (AKI) Formally known as acute renal failure (ARF); sudden kidney failure (see the term *renal failure*).

Angioedema *(an″-je-o-e-de′-ma)* Regions or areas of subcutaneous swelling (e.g., in the lips, other parts of the mouth, eyelids, hands and feet) caused by an allergic reaction to food or drugs.

Anuria *(an-ur′-e-a)* Complete cessation of urinary secretion by the kidneys; also called *anuresis.*

Bacteriuria *(bak-ter″-e-u′-re-a)* Presence of bacteria in the urine.

Bradycardia *(brad″-e-kar′-de-a)* Slowness of heartbeat, usually <60 beats/min.

Bronchospasm *(brong′-ko-spazm)* Contraction of the bronchi and bronchiolar muscles, producing restriction of air passages.

Diuretic *(di″-u-ret′-ik)* An agent that increases excretion of urine.

Fecaluria *(fe″-kal-u′-re-a)* Fecal matter in the urine.

Glucosuria *(gloo″-ko-su′-re-a)* Glucose in the urine.

Hematuria (he″-ma-tu′-re-a) Blood in the urine.

Hypotension (hi″-po-ten′-shun) Below normal arterial blood pressure.

Laryngospasm (la-ring′-go-spazm) Closure of the glottic aperture within the glottic opening of the larynx.

Lasix (la′-siks) Brand name for a diuretic.

Lithotripsy (lith″-o-trip′-se) A therapeutic technique that uses acoustic (sound) waves to shatter large kidney stones into small particles that can be passed.

Micturition (mik″-tu-ri′-shan) The act of voiding or urination.

Nephroptosis (nef″-rop-to′-sis) Excessive inferior displacement of the kidney when erect.

Oliguria (ol″-i-gu′-re-a) Excretion of a diminished amount of urine in relation to fluid intake, usually defined as less than 400 mL/24 hr; also called hypouresis and oligouresis.

Pneumouria (noo″-mo-u′-re-a) Presence of gas in the urine, usually as the result of a fistula between the bladder and the intestine.

Polyuria (pol″-e-u′-re-a) Passage of a large volume of urine in relation to fluid intake during a given period; a common symptom of diabetes.

Proteinuria (pro″-te-nu′-re-a) The presence of excessive serum protein levels in the urine; also termed albuminuria.

Renal agenesis (re′-nal a-jen′-a-sis) Absence of formation of a kidney.

Renal failure (acute or chronic) The inability of a kidney to excrete metabolites at normal plasma levels, or the inability to retain electrolytes under conditions of normal intake.

- **Acute renal failure:** Marked by uremia, oliguria, or anuria, with hyperkalemia and pulmonary edema; IVU demonstrates little or no contrast medium filtering through the kidney; possible exacerbation of patient's condition following use of iodinated contrast media; ultrasound considered a safe alternative for evaluation of signs of renal failure.
- **Chronic renal failure:** Results from a wide variety of conditions and may require hemodialysis or transplantation.

Retention The inability to void, which may be due to obstruction in the urethra or lack of sensation to urinate.

Syncope (sin′-ko-pe) Loss of consciousness caused by reduced cerebral blood flow; also known as **fainting.**

Tachycardia (tak-i-kar′-de-a) Rapid heartbeat, usually >100 beats/min.

Uremia (u-re′-me-a) An excess in the blood of urea, creatinine, and other nitrogenous end products of protein and amino acid metabolism; often present with chronic renal failure; also known as **azotemia.**

Urinary incontinence Involuntary passage of urine through the urethra; commonly caused by failure of voluntary control of the vesical and urethral sphincters.

Urinary reflux Backward or return flow of urine from the bladder into the ureter and kidney; also termed **vesicoureteral reflux,** a common cause of pyelonephritis, in which the backflow of urine may carry bacteria that can produce infection in the kidney.

Urinary tract infection (UTI) Infection that frequently occurs in adults and children caused by bacteria, viruses, fungi, or certain parasites; commonly caused by vesicoureteral reflux.

Urticaria (er″-ti-kar″-i-a) An eruption of wheals (hives) often caused by hypersensitivity to food or drugs.

Clinical Indications

The more common clinical indications for radiographic urinary system procedures include the following (Table 14.5).

Benign prostatic hyperplasia (BPH) is an enlargement of the prostate that generally begins in the fifth decade of life. Although it is a benign condition, it may cause urethral compression and obstruction. This obstruction often produces painful and frequent urination and possible vesicoureteral reflux.

The postvoid erect projection taken during IVU or cystography produces a defect along the base of the bladder indicative of BPH. The floor of the bladder may appear elevated and indented.

TABLE 14.5 SUMMARY OF CLINICAL INDICATIONS: URINARY SYSTEM

CONDITION OR DISEASE	MOST COMMON RADIOGRAPHIC EXAMINATION	POSSIBLE RADIOGRAPHIC APPEARANCE	EXPOSURE FACTOR ADJUSTMENT
Benign prostatic hyperplasia (BPH)	IVU—erect postvoid or recumbent bladder, cystography	Elevated or indented bladder floor	None
Bladder calculi	Cystography, sonography—CT (preferred)	Calcifications within bladder	None
Bladder carcinoma	Cystography, CT, and MRI (preferred)	Mucosal change within bladder	None
Congenital anomalies Duplication of ureter and renal pelvis Ectopic kidney Horseshoe kidney Malrotation	IVU, sonography—CT	Appearance dependent on nature of the anomaly	None
Cystitis	Cystography	Mucosal changes within bladder	None
Glomerulonephritis (Bright disease)	IVU, sonography—nuclear medicine	Acute—normal or enlarged kidneys with normal calyces; chronic—bilateral small kidneys, blunted calyces	None
Hydronephrosis	IVU (nephrography), sonography, retrograde urography	Enlarged renal pelvis and calyces and ureter proximal to obstruction; nephrogram becoming abnormally dense	None
Polycystic kidney disease (infantile, childhood, or adult)	IVU (nephrography), CT, MRI	Enlarged kidneys, elongated renal pelvis, radiolucency (cysts) throughout cortex	None
Prostate cancer	IVU (erect position) sonography, MRI	Elevated and distorted floor of contrast-filled bladder[a]	None
Pyelonephritis	IVU (nephrography), sonography	Chronic—patchy, blunting of calyces, with atrophy and thinning parenchyma	None
Renal calculi	IVU, CT (preferred), nuclear medicine	Signs of obstruction of urinary system	None
Renal cell carcinoma	IVU, sonography—CT (preferred)	Irregular appearance of parenchyma or collecting system	None
Renal hypertension	Hypertensive IVU series, sonography (preferred)	Small kidneys, with delayed excretion and overconcentration of contrast medium	None
Renal obstruction	IVU, CT (tumor, stones)	Signs of obstruction of the urinary system	None
Vesicorectal fistula (vesicocolonic)	Cystography—barium enema, CT (preferred)	Signs of inflammation or fluid collections	None

[a]Eisenberg RL, Johnson NM. Comprehensive radiographic pathology, ed 6, St. Louis, 2015, Mosby Elsevier.

14

Bladder calculi are stones that form in the urinary bladder. These stones are not as common as renal calculi, but they can grow large in the bladder (Fig. 14.50) and may be radiolucent or radiopaque. The radiolucent stones are most often uric acid stones. The presence of bladder stones can make urination difficult. These stones may be demonstrated during IVU or retrograde cystography. They also are seen clearly during a CT scan of the pelvis.

Bladder carcinoma is a tumor that is three times more common in males than in females.[6] This tumor usually is diagnosed after the age of 50 years. Symptoms of bladder carcinoma include hematuria and frequency in urination. The tumor is often a solid or papillary mass with mucosal involvement. Although the cystogram may be performed, CT and magnetic resonance imaging (MRI) are used to stage the tumor and determine the extent of tissue involvement.

Congenital anomalies are structural or chemical imperfections or alterations present at birth.

- **Duplication of the ureter and renal pelvis** involves two ureters and/or the renal pelvis originating from the same kidney. It is the most common type of congenital anomaly of the urinary system.[6] This anomaly usually does not cause a health concern for the patient. The IVU confirms this condition.
- **Ectopic kidney** describes a normal kidney that fails to ascend into the abdomen but remains in the pelvis. This type of kidney has a shorter than normal ureter. Although this condition does not pose a health concern for the patient, it may interfere with the birth process in females. Although IVU will confirm the location of the ectopic kidney, sonography and CT of the pelvis will also demonstrate this anomaly.
- **Horseshoe kidney** occurs as a fusion of the kidneys during development of the fetus (Fig. 14.51). Almost 95% of cases involve fusion of the lower poles of the kidneys.[6] This fusion usually does not affect the function of the kidney. Because of fusion of the lower poles, the kidneys do not ascend to their normal position in the abdomen and are typically situated in the lower abdomen–upper pelvis. CT and sonography of the abdomen demonstrate this congenital condition, as does IVU.
- **Malrotation** is an abnormal rotation of the kidney that is evident when the renal pelvis is turned from a medial to an anterior or a posterior direction. The UPJ may be seen lateral to the kidney. Usually, malrotation does not produce major complications for the patient.

Cystitis *(sis-ti'-tis)* describes an inflammation of the urinary bladder caused by a bacterial or fungal infection. It is seen most often in females because of the shorter urethra that more readily permits retrograde passage of bacteria into the bladder. Laboratory tests confirm the presence of infection. The cystogram may demonstrate signs of chronic cystitis in the form of mucosal edema.

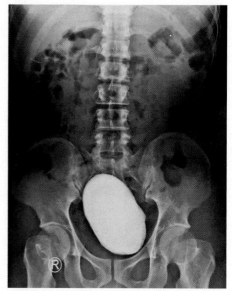

Fig. 14.50 Large stone in bladder. (From Nugroho EA et al. Giant bladder stone with history of recurrence urinary tract infections: A rare case. *Urology Case Reports* 26: 100945.)

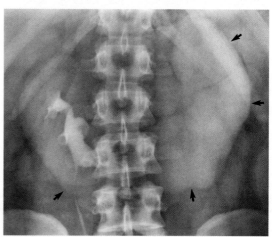

Fig. 14.51 A, Horseshoe kidney. (From Eisenberg RL, Johnson NM. *Comprehensive radiographic pathology*, ed 7, St. Louis, 2021, Elsevier.)

14

Glomerulonephritis (*glo-mer″-u-lo-na-fri′-tis*) (also known as *Bright disease*) is an inflammation of the capillary loops of the glomeruli of the kidneys. (*Nephritis* indicates inflammation of the nephron.)

- It occurs in acute, subacute, and chronic forms. With **acute glomerulonephritis,** the IVU may demonstrate an **enlarged kidney** with reduced concentrations of contrast medium in the collecting system. Sonography is the modality of choice and may show an enlarged, echolucent kidney with acute conditions.
- With the **chronic condition,** sonography demonstrates **small kidney size** caused by fibrosis and cortex destruction from long-standing inflammation. Thus, chronic forms of this disease result in **small kidneys with blunt, rounded calyces.** This condition is the most common cause of undeveloped kidneys in young adults.[7] It is characterized by hypertension and increased serum levels of BUN and creatinine. It may also result in increased levels of albumin in the urine.
- Nuclear medicine may be performed to demonstrate functional changes within the nephron caused by infection or restriction of blood flow through the capillary beds.

Hydronephrosis (*hi″-dro-na-fro′-sis*) is a distention of the renal pelvis and calyces of the kidneys that results from some obstruction of the ureters or renal pelvis. It may be present in both kidneys in a woman when the ureters are compressed by the fetus. Other, more common causes are calculi (stones) in the renal pelvis or ureter, tumors, and structural or congenital abnormalities (Figs. 14.52 and 14.53).

Polycystic kidney disease is a disorder marked by cysts scattered throughout one or both kidneys. This disease is the **most common cause of enlarged kidneys.**[7] Its cause may be genetic or congenital, depending on the type of polycystic disease. These cysts alter the appearance of the kidney and may alter renal function. In some cases, the liver may also have cysts.

The appearance of polycystic disease is described as a "bunch of grapes" scattered throughout the kidney.[6] Three major types of polycystic kidney disease include **infantile, childhood,** and **adult.** (See Chapter 16 for a description of infantile and childhood types.)

- **Adult:** This form of polycystic disease is hereditary. Although the condition is present at birth, symptoms are not seen until later in life.

  Symptoms include renal hypertension, proteinuria, and signs of chronic renal failure. If a cyst ruptures into a calyx, it may produce hematuria. The nephrogram or nephrotomogram taken during IVU may provide an indirect sign of cysts. High-resolution CT does an excellent job of demonstrating radiolucent regions characteristic of cysts, as does ultrasound and MRI.

Prostate carcinoma: The second most common malignancy in males over the age of 50 years. It is often a slow growing tumor and may not be detected for years. The most common metastases of prostate cancer is to bone[8] (Fig. 14.54).

IVU may demonstrate reduced excretion of contrast medium due to tumor involvement, but sonography and CT are the modalities of choice for demonstrating the extent of the tumor and its impact on surrounding tissues.

Pyelonephritis (*pi″-a-lo-na-fri′-tis*) describes an inflammation of the kidney and renal pelvis caused by pyogenic (pus-forming) bacteria. The inflammation process primarily affects the interstitial tissue between the tubules, whereas glomerulonephritis, described earlier, involves the glomeruli and tubules themselves.

With acute pyelonephritis, the intravenous urogram is frequently normal, but with chronic pyelonephritis, the hallmark urographic sign is patchy and blunted or rounded calyces with atrophy and thinning of renal parenchyma.

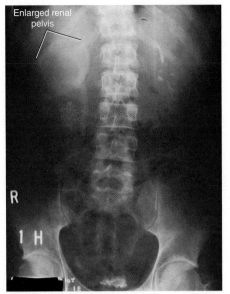

Fig. 14.52 IVU, delayed 1 hour; large hydronephrosis.

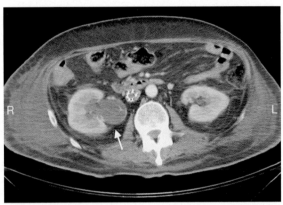

Fig. 14.53 Hydronephrosis CT. (From Kowalczyk N. *Radiographic pathology for technologists*, ed 6, St. Louis, 2014, Mosby Elsevier.)

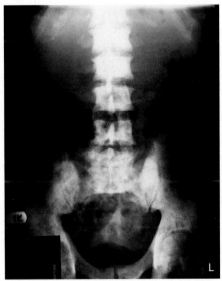

Fig. 14.54 Cancer of prostate with metastasis to pelvis and spine.

Renal calculi are calcifications that occur in the luminal aspect of the urinary tract (Figs. 14.55 and 14.56). These calcifications often lead to renal obstruction. Calcifications also occur in the renal parenchyma.

The causes of stone formation remain uncertain. Research indicates that patients with very acidic urine (pH 5 to 6) and elevated levels of calcium in the urine have a greater incidence of renal stones. Conditions that may produce elevated levels of calcium in the urine include hyperparathyroidism, bone metastasis, and multiple myeloma. Abnormal ingestion of calcium may increase the risk for renal calculi.

Although IVU demonstrates obstruction caused by renal calculi, CT of the urinary tract has become the gold standard for detecting stones.

- A **staghorn calculus** is a large stone that grows and fills the renal pelvis completely, blocking the flow of urine (Fig. 14.57). This type of stone most commonly is associated with chronic urinary tract infections (UTIs).

Renal cell carcinoma (hypernephroma) is the most frequent type of malignant tumor of the kidney.[6] It is three times more frequent in males than females. Symptoms include flank pain and hematuria. The tumor itself is typically a large irregular mass with internal areas of necrosis and hemorrhage.

Renal hypertension is increased blood pressure to the kidney through the renal artery due to atherosclerosis. This form of hypertension results from increased excretion of renin, which results in excessive vasoconstriction.

- **Severe hypertension** can result in localized necrosis of the renal parenchyma and **small kidneys,** with **delayed excretion** and overconcentration of contrast medium. Diabetes in conjunction with renal hypertension can accentuate the damage to the kidney.
- Renal hypertension often requires an alteration of the normal IVU routine. The filming sequence for the study allows for shorter spans of time between images. (The hypertensive IVU examination, which has largely been replaced by alternative modalities, is described more completely in a later section of this chapter.)

Renal obstruction may be caused by necrotic debris, calculus, thrombus, or trauma. Renal obstruction from any source may lead to renal damage. The longer the obstruction persists, the greater is the chance of functional injury.

- **Acute obstruction:** During IVU, the nephrogram demonstrates reduced perfusion of contrast medium through the kidney. Delayed opacification of the collecting system is another sign of acute obstruction. It may be hours after injection before the contrast medium is visible in the collecting system. This delay may require the technologist to take delayed films several hours after injection.
- **Chronic or partial obstruction:** During IVU, the collecting system may be opacified, but the calyces may show signs of enlargement and hydronephrosis.

Vesicorectal (vesicocolonic) fistula is a fistula (artificial opening) that forms between the urinary bladder and rectum or aspects of the colon. This condition may be due to trauma, tumor, or congenital defect.

Approximately 60% of fistulas result from diverticulosis (outpouching or herniation of an organ wall, usually in the small or large intestine). Another 20% are caused by an invading carcinoma, colitis, or trauma.[6] Pneumaturia and fecaluria are symptoms of a fistula.

Although a barium enema and cystography are performed to determine whether a fistula is present, they visualize only approximately 50% of the condition. CT is recommended to demonstrate signs of inflammation or air in the bladder, which may indicate a fistula.

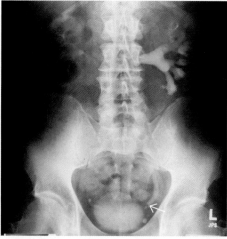

Fig. 14.55 Small triangular calculus in distal left ureter blocking flow of urine and contrast medium (*arrow*).

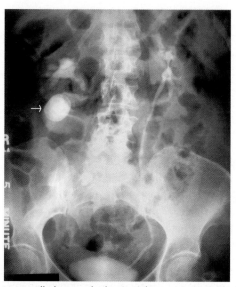

Fig. 14.56 Unusually large calculus in right ureter (*arrow*). (Courtesy Gateway Community College, Phoenix, Ariz.)

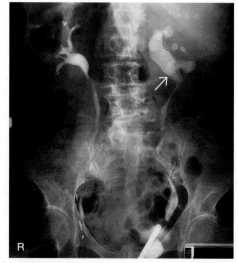

Fig. 14.57 Staghorn calculus in left kidney (*arrow*).

PATIENT PREPARATION

Patient preparation for IVU and the barium enema is similar. The intestinal tract should be free of gas and fecal material for both examinations. If they are to be performed on the same patient, they can be done on the same day. The IVU is done first, with the barium enema to follow.

General patient preparation for IVU includes the following:
1. Light evening meal before the procedure
2. Bowel-cleansing laxative
3. NPO after midnight (minimum of 8 hours)
4. Enema on the morning of the examination

Before the excretory urogram is performed, all clothing except shoes and socks should be removed and replaced with a short-sleeved hospital gown. The opening and ties should be in the back.

The patient should void just before the examination is performed for these two reasons:
1. A bladder that is too full could rupture, especially if compression is applied early in the examination.
2. Urine already present in the bladder dilutes the contrast medium that accumulates there.

Some department policies may require patients to urinate through a filter if the IVU study has been ordered to evaluate for renal stones.

PREGNANCY PRECAUTIONS

If the patient is a female, a menstrual history must be obtained. Irradiation of early pregnancy is one of the most hazardous situations in diagnostic radiography.

X-ray examinations, such as an IVU, that include the pelvis and uterus in the primary beam should be performed on pregnant females **only** when absolutely necessary and when the benefits exceed the risks. Abdominal radiography of a known pregnancy should be delayed until the third trimester if performed at all.

In certain cases IVU for a pregnant patient may be requested. Frequently it is ordered to rule out urinary obstruction. In these situations the technologist should communicate with the radiologist to determine whether the number of radiographs taken during the IVU can be reduced. A reduction in the number of projections taken may be the best way to reduce dose to the fetus. The use of a higher kV, with lower mAs exposure factors, also reduces patient exposure.

PREPARATION OF RADIOGRAPHIC EQUIPMENT AND SUPPLIES

Equipment and supplies needed for urography, in addition to a suitable radiography room, include the following (Fig. 14.58):
1. Correct type and amount of contrast medium drawn up in an appropriate syringe
2. The empty container of contrast medium to show the physician or assistant who is performing the injection
3. A selection of sterile needles, including 18-, 20-, and 22-gauge over-the-needle catheter and butterfly needles and tubing
4. Alcohol sponges or wipes

5. Clean procedure gloves
6. Tourniquet
7. Towel or sponge to support the elbow
8. Sharps container
9. Male gonadal shield
10. Emesis basin
11. Lead numbers, minute marker, and R and L markers
12. Emergency cart accessible
13. Epinephrine or Benadryl ready for emergency injection
14. Ureteric compression device (if used by department)
15. A cold towel for the forehead and/or injection site, and a warm towel if necessary
16. Operational and accessible oxygen and suction devices

These items should be assembled and ready before the patient is escorted to the radiography room.

URETERIC COMPRESSION

Ureteric compression is a method used to enhance filling of the pelvicalyceal system and proximal ureters. Furthermore, ureteric compression allows the renal collecting system to retain the contrast medium longer for a more complete study. A compression device is shown on the model in Fig. 14.59. It is a Velcro band that wraps around two inflatable pneumatic paddles. These paddles are held in place by a piece of Plexiglas and a sponge.

Before the contrast medium is injected, the device is placed on the patient, with the paddles deflated. The two paddles must be **placed over the outer pelvic brim** on each side to allow for compression of the ureters. The inner edges of the paddles should almost touch just lateral to the vertebral spine on each side. The greatest pressure is exerted in the center of the inflated paddles, which should be positioned over the point at which the ureters cross the psoas muscles. Without proper placement of the paddles, the contrast medium is excreted at its normal rate (see Fig. 14.59, inset).

Once the contrast medium has been introduced, the paddles are inflated and remain in place until the postcompression images are ready to be obtained.

Contraindications to Ureteric Compression

Certain conditions contraindicate the use of ureteric compression, including the following:
1. **Possible ureteric stones** (difficult to distinguish between the effects of compression versus the appearance caused by a stone)
2. **Abdominal mass** (may present the same radiographic appearance as ureteric compression)
3. **Abdominal aortic aneurysm** (compression device may lead to leakage or rupture of the aneurysm)
4. **Recent abdominal surgery**
5. **Severe abdominal pain**
6. **Acute abdominal trauma**

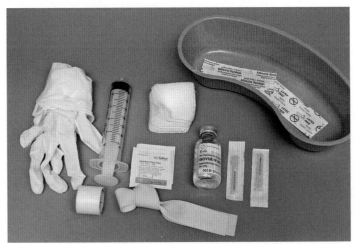

Fig. 14.58 Excretory urography supplies.

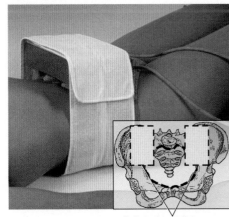

Inflated paddles over outer pelvic brim

Fig. 14.59 Ureteric compression. *Inset,* Inflated paddles over outer pelvic brim.

Alternative: Trendelenburg Position

The Trendelenburg position (wherein the head end of the table is lowered about 15°) provides some of the same results as the compression procedure without as much risk to the patient whose symptoms contraindicate ureteric compression (Fig. 14.60).

General Intravenous Urography Procedure

This section introduces a generic procedure for IVU; however, department routines vary. The department supervisor should be consulted for specific differences from the following description.

SCOUT IMAGE AND INJECTION

The patient's clinical history and other pertinent information are discussed with the radiologist before injection. The scout radiograph is taken for the following reasons: (1) to verify patient preparation; (2) to determine whether exposure factors are acceptable; (3) to verify positioning; and (4) to detect any abnormal calcifications. These scout radiographs should be shown to the radiologist before injection. If the patient has a urinary catheter in place, it should be clamped before injection.

When the injection is made, **the exact start time and duration of injection** should be noted. Timing for the entire series is based on the start of the injection, not the end of it. The injection usually takes 30 to 60 seconds and 1 minute to complete (Fig. 14.61). As the examination proceeds, the patient should be observed carefully for any signs or symptoms indicating a reaction to the contrast medium. Most contrast medium reactions will occur within the first 5 minutes following injection. Delayed reactions may also occur. The chart should note the amount and type of contrast medium given to the patient.

After the full injection of contrast medium, radiographs are taken at specific time intervals. Each image must be marked with a lead number that indicates the time interval when the radiograph was taken.

BASIC IMAGING ROUTINE (SAMPLE PROTOCOL)

A common routine for IVU is as follows (Box 14.1):
1. A **nephrogram** or **nephrotomogram** is taken immediately after completion of injection (or 1 minute after the start of injection) to capture the early stages of entry of the contrast medium into the collecting system (additional description on following page).
2. A **5-minute image** requires a full image of the kidneys, ureter, and bladder (KUB) to include the entire urinary system. The supine position (anteroposterior [AP]) is the preferred position.
3. A **10- to 15-minute image** requires a complete KUB to include the entire urinary system. Once again, the supine position (AP) is most commonly requested.
4. A **20-minute oblique** usually requires LPO and RPO positions to provide a different perspective of the kidneys and project the ureters away from the spine.
5. A **postvoid** radiograph is taken after the patient has voided. The positions of choice may include a prone (posteroanterior [PA]) or erect AP. The bladder should be included on this final radiograph.

NOTE: Prior to exposure, ensure that time markers are placed on the IR to record the time of exposure.

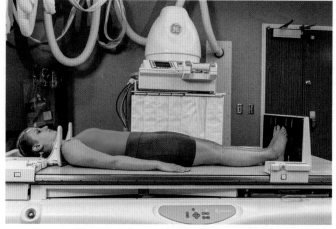

Fig. 14.60 IVU, Trendelenburg position.

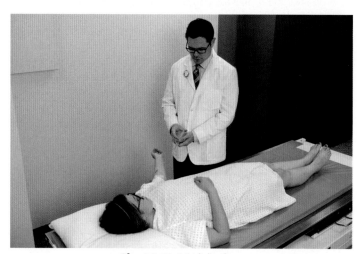

Fig. 14.61 IVU injection.

BOX 14.1 SUMMARY OF SAMPLE IVU PROTOCOL

1. Clinical history taken
2. Scout radiograph taken
3. Injection of contrast medium performed (Note start time of injection and type and amount of contrast medium injected.)
4. Basic imaging routine performed
   - 1-minute nephrogram or nephrotomogram
   - 5-minute AP supine
   - 10- to 15-minute AP supine
   - 20-minute posterior obliques
   - Postvoid (prone or erect)

ALTERNATIVES TO ROUTINE EXAMINATION

There are many variations or alternatives to the basic routine, and the radiologist may order specific positions at any time during the study. Three common variations include the following.

1. Postrelease or "spill" procedure with ureteric compression

   A full-size radiograph is taken after compression has been released. The procedure is explained to the patient and the air pressure is released, as illustrated in Fig. 14.62. The spill radiograph or any other delayed imaging usually is done with the patient in the supine position.

   To assess for asymmetric renal function, compression may be applied immediately after the 5-minute exposure (unless contraindicated) and then removed immediately before the 15-minute image.

2. Erect position for bladder

   If the patient has a history of prolapse of the bladder or an enlarged prostate gland, the erect bladder position taken **before voiding** may confirm these conditions.

3. Delayed radiographs

   Often, with urinary calculi, filling of the involved ureter is slow. The patient may be brought back to the department on a 1- or 2-hour basis. The radiology staff should be aware of when the next radiograph is due before leaving the department for the day.

   After completion of the usual IVU series, a postvoid radiograph is often obtained with the patient in the prone or upright position. Through emptying of the bladder, small abnormalities may be detected. The upright position also demonstrates any unusual movement of the kidneys.

   The radiologist should confirm that no additional images are required before releasing the patient from the department.

Nephrogram Versus Nephrotomogram

Radiographs taken very early in the series are termed **nephrograms** *(nef'-ro-grams)*. The renal parenchyma or functional portion of the kidney consists of many thousands of nephrons. Because individual nephrons are microscopic, the nephron phase is a blush of the entire renal parenchyma. This blush results from dispersion of contrast medium throughout the many nephrons, but not yet into the collecting tubules. The usual nephrogram is obtained with a radiograph at 1 minute after the start of injection. Ureteric compression, if used, tends to prolong the nephron phase to as long as 5 minutes in the normal kidney.

The most common imaging obtained during the nephron phase is a tomographic nephrogram, called a **nephrotomogram,** as opposed to a nontomographic nephrogram. Three separate focal levels are commonly taken with a nephrotomogram (Fig. 14.63) during this phase of the study. (See Chapter 19 for principles of conventional tomography.)

Because the primary interest in nephrography is the kidneys, centering and IR size should be confined to the kidneys. Centering should be halfway between the iliac crest and xiphoid process unless a better centering point is determined after the scout radiograph is viewed.

For determination of the initial fulcrum level, one method is to measure the thickness of the mid-abdomen using calipers. Once this number has been obtained, it is divided by 3. Therefore, with an abdomen that is 24 cm thick, one would first set the fulcrum at 8 cm. If the patient is lying on a thick pad or mattress, 1 cm is added to this calculation, which then results in an initial fulcrum setting of 9 cm.

Timing is critical on this radiograph, so the exposure must be made exactly 60 seconds after the start of the injection. The table, IR, and control panel must be set before the injection is initiated because the injection sometimes takes almost 60 seconds to complete.

Hypertensive Intravenous Urography
PURPOSE

A special type of IV urogram is the **hypertensive urogram.** This examination is performed on patients with high blood pressure (hypertension) to determine whether the kidneys are the cause of the hypertension. A much shorter time is allowed between projections for a hypertensive IV urogram compared with a standard IVU procedure.

PROCEDURE

During hypertensive urography, several early radiographs must be obtained. All image receptors must be available and marked with lead numbers to reflect the time sequence of each image. Once the procedure begins, radiographs must be taken at set intervals.

The hypertensive study includes at least **1-, 2-,** and **3-minute radiographs,** with the possibility of additional radiographs every 30 seconds. In most cases, timing begins at the start of injection.

After the initial radiographs, the imaging sequence may be similar to that of a standard IVU with imaging of the ureters and bladder.

NOTE: This procedure is not commonly performed today but may be done when alternative modalities are unavailable.

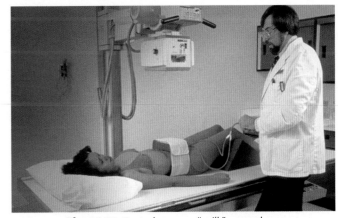

Fig. 14.62 Postrelease, or "spill," procedure.

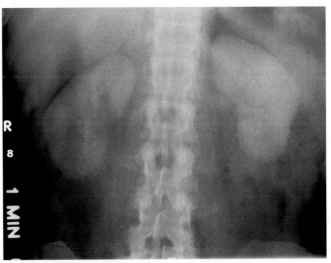

Fig. 14.63 Nephrotomogram, 1 minute.

Retrograde Urography

PURPOSE

Retrograde urography is a nonfunctional examination of the urinary system. Contrast medium is introduced directly retrograde (backward, against the flow) into the pelvicalyceal system via catheterization by a urologist during a minor surgical procedure. Retrograde urography is nonfunctional because the patient's normal physiologic processes are not involved in the procedure. This procedure is performed to determine the location of urinary calculi or other types of obstruction.

NOTE: This procedure is less frequently performed today because of the increased use of CT for locating urinary calculi or obstruction within the urinary system.

PROCEDURE

The patient is placed on the combination cystoscopy-radiography table, which is usually located in the surgery department. The patient is placed in the modified lithotomy position, which requires that the legs be placed in stirrups, as illustrated in Fig. 14.64. The patient is typically sedated or anesthetized for this examination. Additional details of this procedure are discussed in the section on surgical procedures in Chapter 15.

Retrograde Cystography

PURPOSE

Retrograde cystography *(sis-tog'ra-fe)* is a **nonfunctional** radiographic examination of the **urinary bladder** that is performed after instillation of an iodinated contrast medium via a urethral catheter. Cystography is a common procedure for ruling out trauma, calculi, tumor, and inflammatory disease of the urinary bladder.

PROCEDURE

No patient preparation is required for this examination, although the patient should empty the bladder prior to catheterization. After routine bladder catheterization is performed under aseptic conditions, the bladder is drained of any residual urine. The bladder then is filled with contrast medium, as illustrated in Fig. 14.65. The contrast material is allowed to flow in **by gravity only.** One should never hurry or attempt to introduce the contrast medium under pressure, which could result in rupture of the bladder.

After the bladder is filled, which may require 150 to 500 mL, fluoroscopic spot radiographs are taken by the radiologist, or various overhead positions may be exposed by the technologist.

Routine positioning for a cystogram includes an AP, with a **15° caudad angle** and **bilateral posterior oblique positions.**

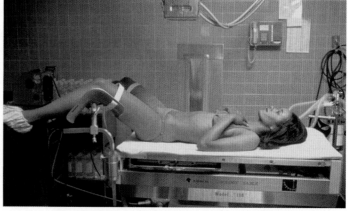

Fig. 14.64 Retrograde urogram (scout position).

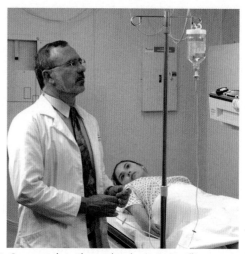

Fig. 14.65 Cystography. The technologist is instilling contrast medium through the catheter.

Voiding Cystourethrography
PURPOSE
Voiding radiographs may be taken after the routine cystography is complete. When images are combined in this manner, the examination is termed **cystourethrography** *(sist"-to-u"-re-throg'ra-fe)*, or **voiding cystourethrography (VCU).** This examination provides a study of the urethra and evaluates the patient's ability to urinate; therefore, it is a **functional study** of the bladder and urethra.

CLINICAL INDICATIONS
Trauma, posterior urethral valves, and **incontinence** are common clinical indications for a VCU examination. Posterior urethral valves are small leaflets of tissue that have a narrow, slitlike opening that partially impedes urine outflow.[9]

PROCEDURE
The voiding phase of the examination is best conducted using a fluoroscopy unit with image acquisition capability. The procedure is sometimes performed with the patient supine, although the upright position makes voiding easier. Before the catheter is removed from the bladder and urethra, all liquid must first be drained from the balloon portion of the catheter if this type of catheter is being used. Then the catheter is removed **very gently.** The urethra can be traumatized if care is not exercised.

The female is usually examined in the AP or slight oblique position, as shown on the radiograph in Fig. 14.66. The male is best examined in a 30° right posterior oblique position. An adequate receptacle or absorbent padding must be provided for the patient. Conventional or digital fluoroscopy may be used to capture specific phases of voiding.

After voiding is complete and adequate imaging is obtained, a postvoid AP may be requested.

Retrograde Urethrography
PURPOSE
Retrograde urethrography sometimes is performed on the **male patient** to demonstrate the full length of the urethra. Contrast medium is injected retrograde into the distal urethra until the entire urethra is filled (Fig. 14.67).

CLINICAL INDICATIONS
Trauma and **obstruction of the urethra** are clinical indications for this procedure.

PROCEDURE
Injection of contrast material sometimes is facilitated by a special device termed a **Brodney clamp** (Fig. 14.68), which is attached to the distal penis.

A **30° right posterior oblique** is the position of choice, with centering to the symphysis pubis. The special catheter is inserted into the distal urethra and the contrast medium is administered by injection. Ample contrast medium is used to fill the entire urethra, and exposures are made. An RPO retrograde urethrogram of a male patient is shown in Fig. 14.67. Ideally, the urethra is superimposed over the soft tissues of the right thigh. This position prevents superimposition of any bony structures except for the lower pelvis and proximal femur.

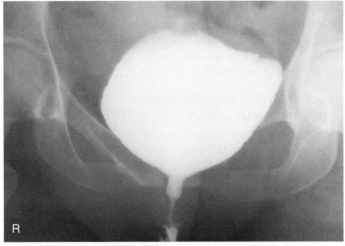
Fig. 14.66 Female voiding cystourethrogram.

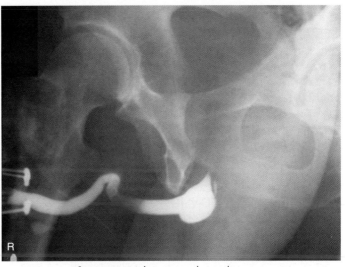
Fig. 14.67 Male retrograde urethrogram.

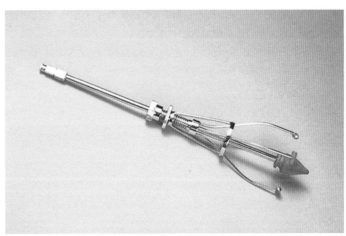
Fig. 14.68 Brodney clamp.

14

Summary of Urinary System Procedures

Urographic procedures may be categorized by the method of contrast medium administration used (Table 14.6). The contrast medium is introduced into the circulatory system or directly into the structure to be studied.

Special Patient Considerations
PEDIATRIC APPLICATIONS

The physiology of the pediatric patient is sensitive to changes in diet, fluid intake, and the presence of iodinated contrast media. Therefore, patient preparation for IVU of an infant or young child must be monitored carefully. Restricting fluids for a long time before the procedure is performed may cause severe dehydration, which can lead to added risk for a contrast medium reaction. Pediatric patients must be scheduled early in the day, so that they can return to a normal diet after the procedure. Furthermore, the technologist must carefully monitor the patient throughout the procedure.

The increased use of sonography for a variety of urinary conditions has provided a safer method (without radiation) of evaluating the pediatric patient.

GERIATRIC APPLICATIONS

Similar to pediatric patients, the older patient may be negatively affected by the change in diet and fluid intake before IVU. The technologist must monitor the older patient carefully during this procedure.

Because some older patients have a clinical history of diabetes, the technologist must ask whether they are taking the type 2 diabetes medications listed earlier. As noted, the use of iodinated contrast media may be contraindicated for patients who are taking these drugs.

BARIATRIC PATIENT CONSIDERATIONS

Technical factors may need to be increased for bariatric patients to penetrate excess adipose tissue. Bariatric patients may need additional assistance with moving between images. The panniculus (dense layer of fatty tissue growth, consisting of subcutaneous fat in the lower abdomen) may also need to be managed in an effort to visualize the bladder during postvoid or cone-down bladder images.

Digital Imaging Considerations

Digital imaging considerations for all urographic procedures, including IVU, are similar to those for other abdominal projections, as described in detail in Chapter 3 for the abdomen. These include (1) **close collimation;** (2) **accurate centering** of the central ray (CR) to the body part of interest and to the IR; and (3) **optimal exposure factors,** remembering the ALARA principle (exposure to patient *as low as reasonably achievable*), which is confirmed by the (4) **post-processing evaluation of exposure indicators.**

Alternative Modalities and Procedures
COMPUTED TOMOGRAPHY (CT)

The use of CT for renal studies has grown. It is an ideal modality for the evaluation of renal tumors and urinary obstructions. In many imaging departments, CT of the urinary system for renal calculi has replaced the IVU study. The patient does not require extensive bowel prep, and the location of the stone can be accurately pinpointed.

A high-speed, multi-detector CT scanner can be used to examine the entire urinary system quickly and efficiently. Contiguous, fine transverse slices from the kidneys through the urinary bladder can provide a noninvasive assessment for stones without the use of iodinated contrast media. This procedure, CT urography, also does not require any bowel prep, which often makes it the examination of choice.

CT departments are also performing what is referred to as a CT IVU (Fig. 14.69A). This procedure closely mimics protocols once regularly used in the diagnostic imaging department for IVU. The CT IVU typically requires the patient's bowel to be prepped with 32 oz of water at least 1 hour prior to the procedure. Once the patient has been prepped and centered on the CT table, an initial set of thin slice, contiguous, noncontrast images are taken from the top

TABLE 14.6 **SUMMARY OF UROGRAPHIC PROCEDURES**	
PROCEDURE	**CONTRAST MEDIUM DELIVERY**
IVU	IV injection: antegrade flow of contrast medium through superficial vein in arm
Retrograde urography	Retrograde injection through ureteral catheter by urologist as a surgical procedure
Retrograde cystography	Retrograde flow into bladder through urethral catheter driven by gravity
Voiding cystourethrography	Retrograde flow into bladder through urethral catheter, followed by withdrawal of catheter for imaging during voiding
Retrograde urethrography (male)	Retrograde injection through Brodney clamp or special catheter

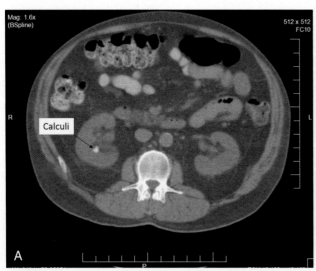

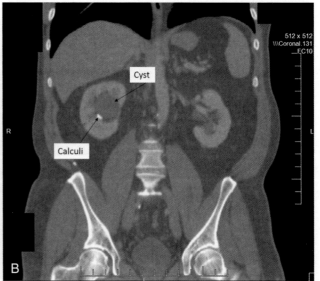

Fig. 14.69 A, Non-contrast CT of the abdomen showing renal calculi. B, Non-contrast CT of the abdomen with renal calculi and renal cyst.

of the kidneys through the bottom of the urinary bladder to evaluate for the presence and location of renal calculi. Noncontrast images are ideal because the attenuation factor of contrast and calculi are similar. Therefore, the use of contrast will preclude visualization of a calculi if present (Fig. 14.69B). Iodinated contrast medium then is introduced into the venous system using a power injector. A second set of contiguous images is taken at approximately 60 seconds from the start of the injection. This time, the images start just above the diaphragm through the pubic symphysis in an effort to evaluate the entire abdominal and pelvic cavities and the kidneys, ureters, and bladder post-contrast injection. Finally, a set of delayed images is again taken from just above the kidneys through the urinary bladder in an attempt to visualize the contrast-filled ureters. The time delay from the start of injection to initiation of the delayed image series can range from 5 to 10 minutes, depending on department protocol. Department protocol may also include three-dimensional reconstructions of the final delayed image series to demonstrate the entire contrast-filled urinary system.

CT has become the imaging modality commonly used for the evaluation and location of renal calculi because of the speed of the study and its ability to visualize the urinary system without superimposition of external structures. CT also provides physicians with the option to use iodinated contrast media or not, depending on the desire for a structural or structural and functional study.

CT DOSE REDUCTION MEASURES

The potential for high radiation exposure during CT is always on the mind of physicians and technologists. Many efforts have been made to improve the radiation safety measures used during CT series. Exposure factors can be adjusted to compensate for a decrease or increase in body size according to the patient's height and weight. Software applications can be initiated to decrease exposure as body part thickness decreases. Many facilities now also have the ability to conduct low-dose studies, which produce noisy images of lower diagnostic quality but may be appropriate for follow-up procedures and imaging of pregnant women. When the radiologist requires only a general overview, this option can save the patient and/or fetus exposure while still providing the necessary information.

Shielding during a CT procedure is always a possibility to decrease unnecessary patient exposure. It is important to remember that the radiation beam travels 360° around the patient, so lead shielding must follow this same pattern to be most effective. Special CT shields are now available to protect specific radiosensitive body parts such as the breasts, eyes, and thyroid during a procedure. These can even be placed over the breasts (Fig. 14.70) during chest CT or over the eyes during head CT. The materials used to create the shield do not interfere with image production like classic lead shielding. It is important to remember that these shields do not completely protect the tissues, but decrease their exposure. Other radiation exposure–reducing measures should still be used along with these shields.

SONOGRAPHY (ULTRASOUND)

Sonography provides a means to evaluate the kidney and bladder in a noninvasive manner. The filled bladder provides an acoustic window for demonstrating bladder calculi or masses in the bladder or organs that surround the bladder, such as the uterus. Ultrasound can also be used to evaluate the kidney to determine whether cysts or masses are present. It is the imaging modality of choice for evaluating the transplanted kidney. Sonography, along with nuclear medicine, can be used to measure parenchymal perfusion. Reduced blood flow or perfusion may be an indication of tissue rejection.

Endorectal ultrasound is highly effective for imaging of the prostate. It can be used to distinguish among solid, cystic, and mixed tissue masses in the prostate gland.

MAGNETIC RESONANCE IMAGING (MRI)

MRI is used to demonstrate subtle tissue changes in the urinary bladder and kidney. It can also be used to evaluate tumors, renal transplants, and patency of the renal artery and vein. On T1-weighted images, the kidney is well defined in contrast to the fat-laden perirenal space. Coronal, sagittal, and transverse perspectives of the urinary system provide a means of determining the spread of select tumors of the kidney to adjacent structures.

NUCLEAR MEDICINE (NM)

Specific NM procedures can measure renal function and excretion rates. NM studies provide a functional evaluation of the kidneys. They provide a less hazardous method of evaluating the kidneys for signs of chronic or acute renal failure without the use of iodinated contrast media. This is especially true in the evaluation of a transplanted kidney. Subtle signs of organ rejection can be seen in the degree of perfusion of radionuclides in the nephrons.

Radionuclides are also being used to determine whether a physical blockage exists in the ureter and to evaluate for vesicoureteral reflux. In the case of vesicoureteral reflux, the patient's bladder is filled with saline and a very small amount of radioactive material is instilled. During the act of voiding, any trace of reflux can be tracked and filmed.

In general, the role of NM in evaluating renal anatomy has been decreasing, but its use for confirming and analyzing renal function has increased.

Routine and Special Projections

Certain routine or special projections of the urinary system are demonstrated and described in this section. The radiologist and technologist must closely coordinate their efforts during examination of this anatomy.

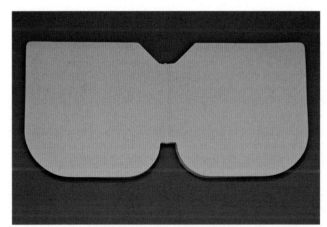

Fig. 14.70 CT breast shield.

14

AP PROJECTION (SCOUT AND SERIES): INTRAVENOUS (EXCRETORY) UROGRAPHY

Clinical Indications
- Scout demonstrates abnormal calcifications that may be urinary calculi.

  After injection, the AP projection may demonstrate signs of obstruction, hydronephrosis, tumor, or infection. See p. 552 for the IVU routine.

> **Intravenous (Excretory) Urography—IVU**
> ROUTINE
> - AP (scout and series)
> - Nephrotomogram
> - RPO and LPO (30°)
> - AP—postvoid erect or recumbent

Technical Factors
- Minimum SID—40 inches (100 cm)
- IR size—14 × 17 inches (35 × 43 cm), portrait; for nephrogram—10 × 12 inches (24 × 30 cm) landscape
- Grid
- kVp range—80–85
- Minute markers where applicable

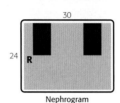

Nephrogram

Shielding Shield radiosensitive tissues outside the region of interest.

Patient Position Situate the patient supine, with a pillow for the head, arms at the sides, away from the body, and support under the knees to relieve back strain.

Part Position
- Align midsagittal plane to centerline of table and to CR.
- Ensure **no rotation** of trunk or pelvis.
- Include symphysis pubis on bottom of IR without cutting off upper kidneys (Fig. 14.71). (A second smaller IR for bladder area may be necessary on hypersthenic patients.)

CR
- CR is perpendicular to IR.
- Center CR and IR to level of iliac crest and to midsagittal plane.
- Nephrogram: Center CR midway between xiphoid process and iliac crest.

Recommended Collimation Collimate on all four sides to anatomy of interest.

Respiration Suspend respiration after expiration and expose.

NOTE: Have patient empty bladder immediately before beginning the examination so that contrast medium in the bladder is not diluted. Explain procedure and obtain a clinical history before injecting contrast medium. Be prepared for possible reaction to the contrast medium.

Evaluation Criteria
Anatomy Demonstrated: • Entire urinary system is visualized from upper renal shadows to distal urinary bladder (Figs. 14.72 and 14.73). The symphysis pubis should be included on lower margin of the IR. • After injection, only a portion of the urinary system may be opacified on a specific radiograph in the series.
Position: • No rotation as evidenced by symmetry of iliac wings and rib cage • Proper collimation applied.
Exposure: • No motion due to respiration or movement. • Appropriate technique with short-scale contrast demonstrating the urinary system.
Markers: • Minute markers and R or L markers visible on all series radiographs.

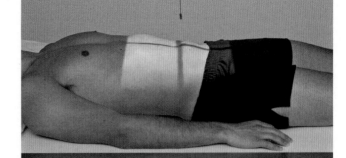
Fig. 14.71 IVU scout and series.

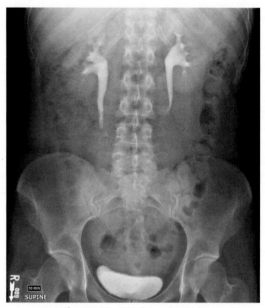
Fig. 14.72 IVU (10 minutes).

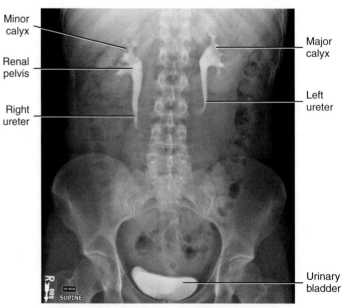

Minor calyx

Renal pelvis

Right ureter

Major calyx

Left ureter

Urinary bladder

Fig. 14.73 IVU; 10 minutes following injection.

NEPHROTOMOGRAPHY AND NEPHROGRAPHY: INTRAVENOUS (EXCRETORY) UROGRAPHY

Clinical Indications
- A nephrogram or nephrotomogram demonstrates conditions of and trauma to the renal parenchyma.

Renal cysts and/or adrenal masses may be demonstrated during this phase of IVU. A **nephrogram** involves a single AP radiograph of the kidney region taken within 60 seconds after injection.

Technical Factors
- Linear tomography
- Minimum SID—40 inches (100 cm) (or distance as required by specific tomographic equipment)
- IR size—10 × 12 inches (24 × 30 cm), landscape
- Grid
- kVp range—80–85
- Select correct exposure angle:
  - 10° angle or less, producing larger section of tissue in relative focus; the most common exposure angle performed during IVU
  - 40° exposure angle, producing thinner sections of tissue in relative focus; therefore, more tomographic exposures required to demonstrate the entire kidney

Shielding Shield radiosensitive tissues outside the region of interest.

Patient Position Position the patient supine, with a pillow for the head, arms at the sides, away from the body, and support under the knees to relieve back strain.

Part Position
- Align midsagittal plane to centerline of table or grid (Fig. 14.74).
- Ensure **no rotation** of trunk or pelvis.

CR
- Center CR midway between xiphoid process and iliac crest.

Recommended Collimation Collimate on four sides to anatomy of interest.

Respiration Suspend respiration after expiration and expose.

NOTE: Explain tomographic procedure to reduce anxiety for patient. Obtain a clinical history before injection of contrast medium. Remind the patient to remain immobile between exposures. Check scout image to verify focus level, optimal technique, and position of kidneys. Tomography procedures, including equipment setup and procedure, are described in Chapter 19.

Intravenous (Excretory) Urography—IVU

BASIC
- AP (scout and series)
- Nephrotomogram
- RPO and LPO (30°)
- AP—postvoid erect or recumbent

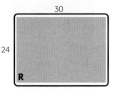

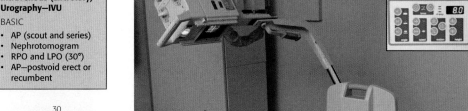

Fig. 14.74 Nephrotomogram (imaging system in starting position).

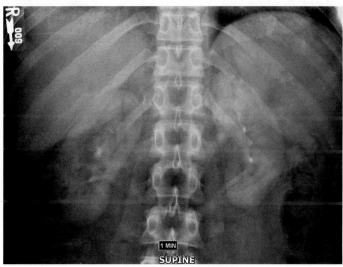

Fig. 14.75 Nephrogram taken at 1 minute following injection.

Evaluation Criteria
Anatomy Demonstrated: • Entire renal parenchyma is visualized, with some filling of collecting system with contrast medium (Fig. 14.75).
Position: • No motion due to respiration or movement is evident. • Proper collimation applied.
Exposure: • Appropriate technique is used to demonstrate renal parenchyma.
Markers: • Specific focus level markers should be visible on each radiograph, along with R or L and minute markers.

14

RPO AND LPO POSITIONS: INTRAVENOUS (EXCRETORY) UROGRAPHY

Clinical Indications
- Signs of infection, trauma, and obstruction of the elevated kidney are manifested.
- Trauma or obstruction of the downside ureter.

> **Intravenous (Excretory) Urography—IVU**
> BASIC
> - AP (scout and series)
> - Nephrotomogram
> - RPO and LPO (30°)
> - AP—postvoid erect or recumbent

Technical Factors
- Minimum SID—40 inches (100 cm).
- IR size—14 × 17 inches (35 × 43 cm), portrait, or 10 × 12 inches (24 × 30 cm), landscape (see NOTE)
- Grid
- kVp range—80–85
- Minute marker

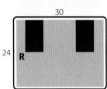

Shielding Shield radiosensitive tissues outside the region of interest.

Patient Position
The patient is supine and is partially rotated toward the right or left side.

Part Position
- Rotate body 30° for both R and L posterior oblique positions (Fig. 14.76).
- Flex elevated-side knee for support of lower body.
- Raise arm on elevated side and place across upper chest.
- Center vertebral column to midline of table or grid and to CR.

CR
- CR is perpendicular to IR.
- Center CR and IR to level of iliac crest and vertebral column.

Recommended Collimation
Collimate on four sides to anatomy of interest.

Respiration
Suspend respiration after expiration and expose.

NOTE: Some department routines include a smaller IR placed landscape to include the kidneys and proximal ureters, thus allowing gonadal shielding for males and females. Centering then would be midway between the xiphoid process and iliac crests.

Evaluation Criteria
Anatomy Demonstrated: • The kidney on elevated side is placed in profile or parallel to the IR and is best demonstrated with each oblique. • The downside ureter is projected away from the spine, providing an unobstructed view of this ureter (Figs. 14.77 and 14.78).

Position: • No excessive obliquity is evident. • The elevated kidney is parallel to the plane of IR and is not projected into the vertebral bodies of the lumbar spine. • Complete arch of symphysis pubis is visible on bottom margin of radiograph and the kidneys are included at the upper margin. • Proper collimation applied.

Exposure: • No motion due to respiration or movement is evident. • Appropriate technique with short-scale contrast is used to visualize the urinary system.

Markers: • Minute markers and R or L markers should be visible.

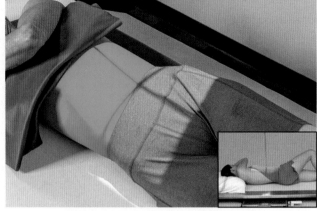

Fig. 14.76 RPO, 30°. *Inset,* 30° LPO.

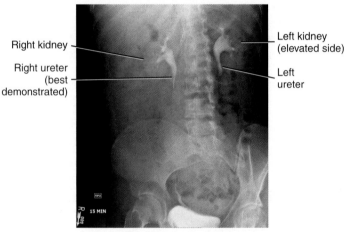

Right kidney
Right ureter (best demonstrated)
Left kidney (elevated side)
Left ureter

Fig. 14.77 RPO IVU.

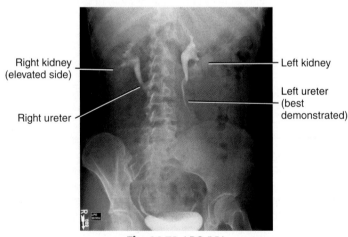

Right kidney (elevated side)
Right ureter
Left kidney
Left ureter (best demonstrated)

Fig. 14.78 LPO IVU.

AP PROJECTION: INTRAVENOUS (EXCRETORY) UROGRAPHY

POSTVOID

Clinical Indications
- Position may demonstrate enlarged prostate (possible BPH) or prolapse of the bladder. The erect position demonstrates nephroptosis (abnormal positional change of kidneys).

Intravenous (Excretory) Urography—IVU
ROUTINE
- AP (scout and series)
- Nephrotomogram
- RPO and LPO (30°)
- AP—postvoid erect or recumbent

Technical Factors
- Minimum SID—40 inches (100 cm).
- IR size—14 × 17 inches (35 × 43 cm), portrait
- Grid
- kVp range—80–85
- Erect and/or postvoid markers

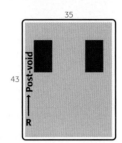

Shielding Shield radiosensitive tissues outside the region of interest.

Patient Position Patient is erect, with back against the table, or in prone position (Figs. 14.79 and 14.80).

Part Position
- Align midsagittal plane to center of table, grid, or IR, with no rotation.
- Position arms away from the body.
- Ensure that the symphysis pubis is included on bottom of the IR.
- Center low enough to include the prostate area, especially on older men.

CR
- Direct CR **perpendicular** to IR.
- Center to level of **iliac crest** and midsagittal plane or, for larger patients, 1 inch (2.5 cm) lower to ensure that the bladder area is included.

Recommended Collimation Collimate on four sides to anatomy of interest.

Respiration Suspend respiration after expiration and expose.
Alternative PA or AP Recumbent This image also may be taken as a PA or AP projection in the recumbent position, with centering similar to that described earlier.

Evaluation Criteria
Anatomy Demonstrated: · Entire urinary system is included, with only residual contrast medium visible (Fig. 14.81). • All of symphysis pubis (including prostate area on males) is included on radiograph.

Position: · No rotation is evident by symmetry of iliac wings. • Proper collimation applied.

Exposure: · No motion due to respiration or motion is evident. • Appropriate technique is used to demonstrate residual contrast medium in the urinary system.

Markers: · Erect and/or postvoid markers and R or L markers are visible.

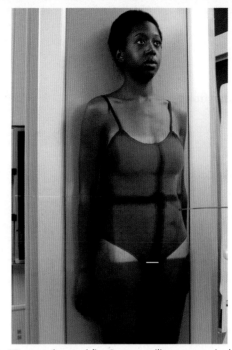

Fig. 14.79 AP erect (postvoid). Center at iliac crest to include the symphysis pubis.

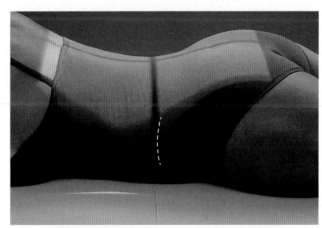

Fig. 14.80 Alternative—PA prone (postvoid).

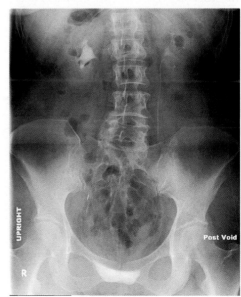

Fig. 14.81 AP erect (postvoid)—prolapse of bladder.

14

AP PROJECTION: INTRAVENOUS (EXCRETORY) UROGRAPHY

URETERIC COMPRESSION

WARNING: Compression should not be used for patients with a history of abdominal masses, obstructions (e.g., stones), abdominal aortic aneurysms, or recent surgery. (See the section Contraindications to Ureteric Compression. A Trendelenburg position with 15° tilt, which approximates the same effect, can be used for these patients.)

Clinical Indications
- Pyelonephritis and other conditions involving the collecting system of the kidney

Intravenous (Excretory) Urography—IVU
SPECIAL
• AP ureteric compression

Technical Factors
- Minimum SID—40 inches (100 cm).
- IR size—14 × 17 inches (35 × 43 cm) if available, landscape
- Grid
- kVp range—80–85

Shielding Shield radiosensitive tissues outside the region of interest.

Patient Position Position the patient supine, with the compression device in place (Figs. 14.82 and 14.83).

Part Position
- Align midsagittal plane to centerline of table or grid and to CR.
- Flex and support knees.
- Position arms away from body.
- Place upper edge of compression paddles at level of iliac crest. Inner edges of paddles should almost touch, just lateral to the vertebral spine on each side. (This places maximum pressure over the area of the ureters, which are just lateral to the lumbar spine and medial to the sacroiliac [SI] joints.)

CR
- CR is perpendicular to IR.
- Center to midway between xiphoid process and iliac crests.

Recommended Collimation Collimate on four sides to the anatomy of interest.

Respiration Suspend respiration after expiration and expose.

NOTE: Immediately after injection of contrast medium, the paddles are inflated and remain in place until the radiologist indicates that they should be released. The imaging sequence is to be determined by department protocol or by the radiologist.

Evaluation Criteria
Anatomy Demonstrated: • Entire urinary system is visualized, with enhanced pelvic calyceal filling (Fig. 14.84).
Position: • No rotation, as evident by symmetry of iliac wings and/or lumbar spine. • Proper collimation applied.
Exposure: • No motion due to respiration or movement is evident. • Appropriate technique is used, with short-scale contrast to visualize the urinary system.

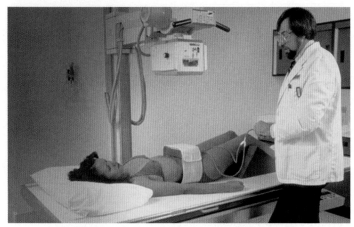

Fig. 14.82 AP—ureteric compression being applied.

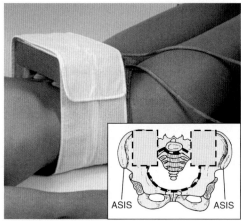

Fig. 14.83 Ureteric compression, with inflated paddles placed correctly. *Inset,* Paddles at medial to ASIS.

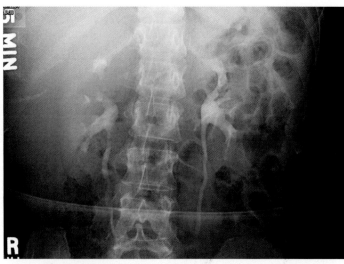

Fig. 14.84 AP, ureteric compression, 5-minute image.

AP PROJECTION: LPO AND RPO POSITIONS, LATERAL POSITION (OPTIONAL)—CYSTOGRAPHY

Clinical Indications

- Signs of cystitis, obstruction, vesicoureteral reflux, and bladder calculi are visualized.
- Lateral demonstrates possible fistulas between the bladder and uterus or rectum. See p. 554 for detailed procedure descriptions.

> **Cystography**
> ROUTINE
> - AP (10° to 15° caudad)
> - Both oblique positions (45° to 60°)
> SPECIAL
> - Lateral (optional)

Technical Factors

- Minimum SID—40 inches (100 cm).
- IR size—14 × 17 inches (35 × 43 cm) portrait
- Grid
- kVp range—80–90

Patient and Part Positions

AP

- Patient is supine, with legs extended and midsagittal plane to center of table (Fig. 14.85).

Posterior Oblique

- 45° to 60° body rotation (steep oblique positions are used to visualize posterolateral aspect of the bladder, especially UV junction) (Fig. 14.86).
- Partially flex downside leg for stabilization.

NOTE: Do not flex elevated-side leg more than necessary to prevent superimposition of the leg over the bladder.

Lateral This is optional because of the high gonadal radiation dose.
- Position patient in true lateral (no rotation) (Fig. 14.87).

CR

AP

- Center **2 inches** (5 cm) **superior to symphysis pubis,** with **10° to 15° caudad** tube angle (to project symphysis pubis inferior to bladder).
- To demonstrate urinary reflux, center higher at level of iliac crest.

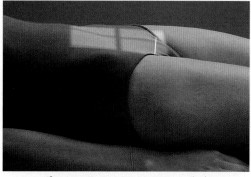

Fig. 14.85 AP, 10° to 15° caudad.

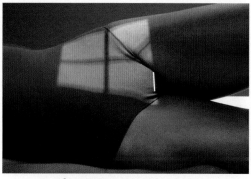

Fig. 14.86 RPO, 45° to 60°.

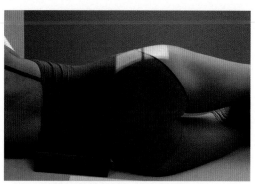

Fig. 14.87 Left lateral (optional).

14

Posterior Oblique
- For bladder projections only, CR perpendicular: Center 2 inches (5 cm) superior to symphysis pubis and 2 inches (5 cm) medial to anterior superior iliac spine (ASIS).
- To demonstrate urinary reflux, center at level of iliac crest.

Lateral (Optional)
- CR perpendicular: Center 2 inches (5 cm) superior and posterior to symphysis pubis.

Recommended Collimation Collimate on four sides to anatomy of interest.

Respiration Suspend respiration after expiration and expose.

NOTE: Unclamp and drain bladder before filling with contrast medium.

Contrast medium should **never** be injected under pressure but should be allowed to fill slowly by gravity in the presence of an attendant.

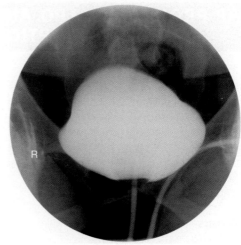

Fig. 14.88 AP (10° to 15° caudad).

Evaluation Criteria
Anatomy Demonstrated: • Distal ureters, urinary bladder, and proximal urethra on males should be included. • Appropriate technique is used to visualize the urinary bladder.
Position: • *AP:* Urinary bladder is not superimposed by pubic bones (Fig. 14.88). • *Posterior obliques:* Urinary bladder is not superimposed by partially flexed elevated side leg (Fig. 14.89). • *Lateral (optional):* Hips and femurs are superimposed. • Proper collimation applied.

Include the prostate area just distal to the pubis on older men.

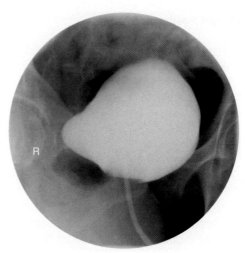

Fig. 14.89 45° posterior oblique.

RPO (30°) POSITION—MALE; AP PROJECTION—FEMALE: VOIDING CYSTOURETHROGRAPHY

Clinical Indications
- Possible vesicoureteral reflux
  A functional study of the urinary bladder and urethra determines the cause of urinary retention.

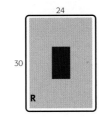

Voiding Cystourethrography
ROUTINE
- Male—RPO (30°)
- Female—AP

Technical Factors
- Minimum SID—40 inches (100 cm).
- IR size—10 × 12 inches (24 × 30 cm), portrait
- Grid
- kVp range—80–85

Shielding Shield radiosensitive tissues outside the region of interest.

Patient Position Take image with the patient **recumbent or erect.**

Part Position
Male
- Oblique body **30° into the RPO** position.
- Superimpose urethra over soft tissues of right thigh.

Female
- Position patient supine or erect into the AP position.
- Center midsagittal plane to table or film holder.
- Extend and slightly separate legs.

CR
- CR is perpendicular to IR.
- Center CR and IR to symphysis pubis.

Recommended Collimation Collimate on four sides to anatomy of interest.

Respiration Suspend respiration after expiration and expose.

NOTE: Fluoroscopy and spot imaging are best for this procedure. Catheter must be removed gently before voiding procedure. A radiolucent receptacle or absorbent padding should be provided for the patient. After voiding is complete, a postvoid AP projection may be requested.

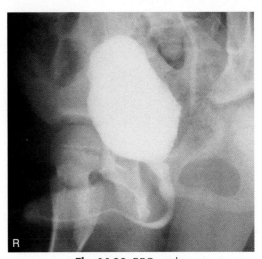

Fig. 14.90 RPO, male.

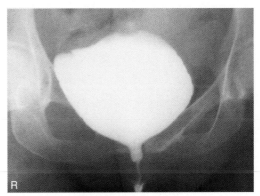

Fig. 14.91 AP, female.

Evaluation Criteria
Anatomy Demonstrated: • Contrast-filled urinary bladder and urethra are visualized.
Position: • *RPO:* Male urethra containing contrast medium is superimposed over soft tissues of right thigh (Fig. 14.90).
• *AP:* Female urethra containing contrast medium is demonstrated inferior to the symphysis pubis (Fig. 14.91).
• Proper collimation applied.
Exposure: • Appropriate technique is used to visualize the urinary bladder without overexposing the male prostate area and the contrast-filled urethra of the male or female.

14

CHAPTER 15

Trauma, Mobile, and Surgical Radiography

CONTRIBUTIONS BY **Bradley D. Johnson,** MED, RT(R)(ARRT)

RADIATION PROTECTION CONTRIBUTOR   W.R. Hedrick, PhD, FACR

CONTRIBUTOR TO PAST EDITIONS   Leslie E. Kendrick, MS, RT(R)(CT)(MR), Katrina Lynn Steinsultz, BS, RT(R)(M), Cindy Murphy, BHSc, RT(R), ACR

CONTENTS

TRAUMA AND MOBILE IMAGING

Introduction

This chapter is divided into two primary sections; the first section involves **trauma** and **mobile imaging,** and the second section discusses **surgical radiography.** Student radiographers may feel anxious and intimidated by these types of procedures because of the nature of the patient's condition, different equipment, unfamiliar surroundings, and working with personnel outside the radiology department. All of these factors can create a heightened perception of stress. To build confidence, reduce perceived stress, and perform these advanced exams with greater accuracy, it is important to view these experiences as an opportunity to build on knowledge previously acquired. There are multiple facets to these areas that could be discussed in great detail; however, the purpose of this chapter is to provide a basic foundation. Experience is truly the greatest resource in becoming prepared to face the challenges presented by these procedures. Maintaining an open mind, thinking critically, and accepting that learning is a product of effort and experience will allow for the development of the skills necessary to be proficient in trauma, mobile, and surgical radiography.

Skeletal Trauma and Fracture Terminology

The American Registry of Radiologic Technologists (ARRT) defines trauma as a serious injury or shock to the body, often requiring modifications that may include variations in positioning, minimal movement of the body part, and so on[1] (Fig. 15.1). This may mean that patients cannot be brought to the radiology department for routine radiographic procedures as described in other sections of this text. Instead, a mobile (portable) x-ray unit must be taken to the emergency department (ED) or to the patient's bedside (Fig. 15.2). Even if patients are brought to the radiology department, they may be immobilized in a number of ways. Some may present with one or more splints, indicating possible limb fractures or dislocations. Others may be strapped to a backboard with a cervical collar in place. In these cases, **a major adaptation of CR angles and image receptor placement is required.** Radiographers must use their knowledge of anatomy, technical factors, and positioning to acquire diagnostic images in difficult circumstances.

Skeletal trauma and surgical radiography require an understanding of terms that are unique to these situations, such as fracture-dislocation terminology. Knowing the terms used in patient histories or on examination requisitions allows the technologist to understand which type of injury or fracture is suspected and which projections are most important. It also is useful for knowing how to avoid positioning techniques or body positions that may result in additional pain or injury.

DISLOCATION

Dislocation refers to the displacement of a bone that is no longer in contact with its normal articulation.[2] Dislocations can frequently be clinically identified by the abnormal shape or alignment of the body parts. Any movement of these parts can be painful and must be avoided. As with fractures, dislocations should be imaged in two planes, 90° to each other, to demonstrate the degree of displacement. The most common dislocations encountered in trauma involve the shoulder (Fig. 15.3), fingers or thumb, patella, and hip.

If a bone has relocated itself following the injury, damage may still have occurred, and a minimum of two projections of the affected joint is required to assess for damage and/or possible avulsion fractures.

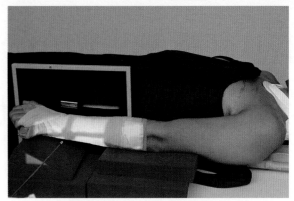

Fig. 15.1 Trauma radiography.

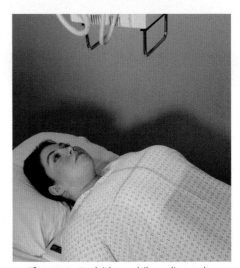

Fig. 15.2 Bedside mobile radiography.

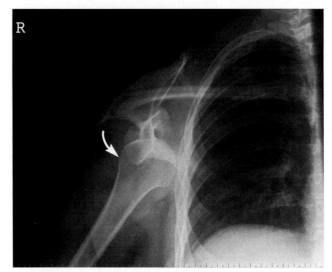

Fig. 15.3 Right shoulder dislocation (AP projection).

SUBLUXATION

A partial dislocation is illustrated in Fig. 15.4, in which a vertebra is displaced posteriorly. Another example is nursemaid elbow (so-called jerked elbow), which is a traumatic partial dislocation of the radial head of a child. This is caused by a hard pull on the hand and wrist of a child by an adult. It is frequently reduced when the forearm is supinated for an AP elbow projection.

SPRAIN

A sprain is a forced wrenching or twisting of a joint resulting in a partial rupture or tearing of supporting ligaments, without dislocation. A sprain may result in severe damage to associated blood vessels, tendons, ligaments, and/or nerves. Severe swelling and discoloration caused by hemorrhage of ruptured blood vessels frequently accompany a severe sprain. A severe sprain can be painful and must be handled with great care during the radiographic examination. Symptoms are similar to those of fractures; radiographs aid in differentiating a sprain from a fracture.

CONTUSION

This is a bruise type of injury with a possible avulsion fracture. An example is a hip pointer, a football injury involving contusion of bone at the iliac crest of the pelvis.

FRACTURE

A fracture (fx) is defined as a disruption of bone caused by mechanical forces applied either directly to the bone or transmitted along the shaft of the bone.[2] With any possible fracture, the technologist must use extreme caution in moving and positioning the patient so as not to cause further injury or displacement of fracture fragments. The technologist should **never force a limb or body part into position.** If the fracture is obvious, or if severe pain accompanies any movement, positioning should be adapted as needed.

FRACTURE ALIGNMENT TERMINOLOGY

Alignment refers to the associative relationship between long axes of the fracture fragments. A fracture is aligned if the long axes of the bone remain parallel to each other.

Apposition

Apposition describes how the fragmented ends of the bone make contact with each other. Three types of apposition are known:
1. **Anatomic apposition:** Anatomic alignment of ends of fractured bone fragments, wherein the ends of the fragments make end-to-end contact.
2. **Lack of apposition (distraction):** The ends of fragments are aligned but pulled apart and are not making contact with each other (e.g., as from excessive traction; Fig. 15.5).
3. **Bayonet apposition:** The fracture fragments overlap and the shafts make contact, but not at the fracture ends (Fig. 15.6).

Angulation

Angulation describes loss of alignment of the fracture; apex is the direction of the angulation and is opposite in relation to the distal part of the fracture fragments (Fig. 15.7). The following three terms can be used to describe the type or direction of angulation, which uses the apex or distal fragments as its reference point:
1. **Apex angulation:** Describes the direction or angle of the apex of the fracture, such as a medial or lateral apex, wherein the point or apex of the fracture points medially or laterally.
2. **Varus deformity:** The distal fragment ends are angled toward the midline of the body and the apex is pointed away from the midline.
3. **Valgus deformity:** The distal fragment ends are angled away from the midline and the apex is pointed toward the midline.

NOTE: The terms *varus* and *valgus* also are used as inversion and eversion stress movement terms (see Terminology, Chapter 1).

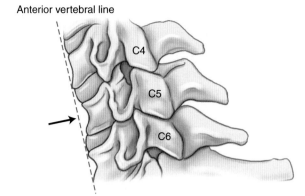

Fig. 15.4 Subluxation of cervical vertebra (C5 vertebra displaced posteriorly).

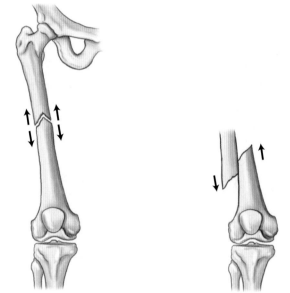

Fig. 15.5 Lack of apposition.   **Fig. 15.6** Bayonet apposition.

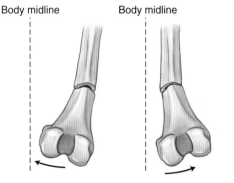

Fig. 15.7 Varus versus valgus deformity.

15

TYPES OF FRACTURES

Many terms are used in describing fractures. Terms that technologists are most likely to encounter are as follows.

Simple (Closed) Fracture

This is a fracture in which the bone does not break through the skin.

Compound (Open) Fracture

This is a fracture in which a portion of the bone (usually the fragmented end) protrudes through the skin (Fig. 15.8).

Incomplete (Partial) Fracture

This fracture does not traverse through the entire bone. (The bone is not broken into two pieces.) It is most common in children. Two major types of incomplete fractures are as follows:
1. **Torus fx (buckle fx):** This buckle of the cortex (outer portion of the bone) is characterized by localized expansion or torus of the cortex, possibly with little or no displacement, and no complete break in the cortex.
2. **Greenstick fx (hickory or willow stick fx):** Fracture is on one side only. The cortex on one side of the bone is broken and the other side is bent. When the bone straightens, a faint fracture line in the cortex may be seen on one side of the bone, and a slight bulging or wrinkle-like defect is seen on the opposite side (Fig. 15.9).

Complete Fracture

In this fracture, the break is complete and includes the cross-section of bone. The bone is broken into two pieces. There are three major types of complete fractures.
1. **Transverse fx:** Fracture is transverse at a near right angle to the long axis of the bone.
2. **Oblique fx:** The fracture passes through bone at an oblique angle.
3. **Spiral fx:** In this fracture, the bone has been twisted apart and the fracture spirals around the long axis (Fig. 15.10).

Comminuted Fracture

In this fracture, the bone is splintered or crushed at the site of impact, resulting in two or more fragments (Fig. 15.11). Three types of comminuted *(kom'-i-nu-ted)* fractures have specific implications for treatment and prognosis because of the possible substantial disruption of blood flow:
1. **Segmental fx:** A type of double fracture in which two fracture lines isolate a distinct segment of bone; the bone is broken into three pieces, with the middle fragment fractured at both ends.
2. **Butterfly fx:** A comminuted fracture with two fragments on each side of a main, wedge-shaped separate fragment; it has some resemblance to the wings of a butterfly.
3. **Splintered fx:** A comminuted fracture in which the bone is splintered into thin sharp fragments.

Impacted Fracture

In this fracture, one fragment is firmly driven into the other, such as the shaft of the bone being driven into the head or end segment. These most commonly occur at distal or proximal ends of the femur, humerus, or radius (Fig. 15.12).

SPECIFIC NAMED FRACTURES

Following are some examples and descriptions of named fractures, usually named by the type of injury or after the person who identified them.

Barton Fracture

This is an intra-articular **fracture** of the **distal radius** often associated with dislocation or subluxation of the **radiocarpal joint**.

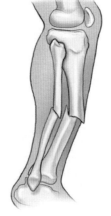
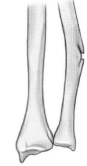

Fig. 15.8 Compound fx (tibia-fibula).

Fig. 15.9 Greenstick fx (ulna).

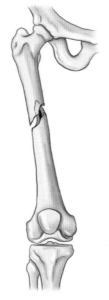
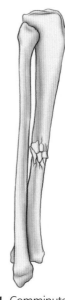

Fig. 15.10 Spiral fx (femur).

Fig. 15.11 Comminuted fx (tibia).

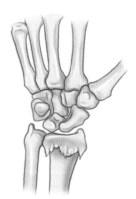

Fig. 15.12 Impacted fx (radius).

Baseball (Mallet) Fracture

This fracture of the distal phalanx is caused by a ball striking the end of an extended finger. The distal interphalangeal (DIP) joint is partially flexed, and an avulsion fracture is frequently present at the posterior base of the distal phalanx.

Bennett Fracture

This longitudinal fracture, which occurs at the base of the first metacarpal with the fracture line entering the carpometacarpal joint, generally includes a posterior dislocation or subluxation.

Boxer Fracture

This fracture usually involves the distal fifth metacarpal, with an apex posterior angulation best demonstrated on the lateral view. It results from punching someone or something.

Colles Fracture

This fracture of the wrist, in which the distal radius is fractured with the distal fragment displaced posteriorly, may result from a forward fall on an outstretched arm (Fig. 15.13).

Smith (Reverse Colles) Fracture

This is a fracture of the wrist with the distal fragment of the radius displaced anteriorly rather than posteriorly, as in a Colles fracture. It commonly results from a backward fall on an outstretched arm (Fig. 15.14).

Hangman Fracture

This fracture occurs through the pedicles of the axis (C2), with or without displacement of C2 or C3.

Hutchinson (Chauffeur) Fracture

This is an intra-articular fracture of the radial styloid process. (The name originates from the time when hand-cranked cars would backfire, with the crank striking the lateral side of the distal forearm.)

Monteggia (mon-tej´-ah) Fracture

This fracture of the proximal half of the ulna, along with dislocation of the radial head, may result from defending against blows with the raised forearm (Fig. 15.15).

Pott's Fracture

This term is used to describe a complete fracture of the distal fibula with major injury to the ankle joint, including ligament damage and frequent fracture of the distal tibia or medial malleolus (Fig. 15.16).

ADDITIONAL FRACTURE TYPES

Avulsion Fracture

This fracture results from severe stress to a tendon or ligament in a joint region. A fragment of bone is separated or pulled away by the attached tendon or ligament.

Blowout and/or Tripod Fracture

These fractures, which result from a direct blow to the orbit and/or maxilla and zygoma, create fractures to the orbital floor and lateral orbital margins.

Chip Fracture

This fracture involves an isolated bone fragment; however, this is not the same as an avulsion fracture because this fracture is not caused by tendon or ligament stress.

Compression Fracture

This vertebral fracture is caused by compression-type injury. The vertebral body collapses or is compressed. Generally, it is most evident radiographically by a decreased vertical dimension of the anterior vertebral body (Fig. 15.17).

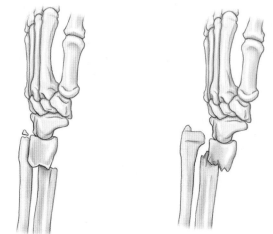

Fig. 15.13 Colles fx (radius).   **Fig. 15.14** Smith fx (reverse Colles fx).

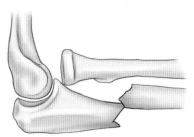

Fig. 15.15 Monteggia fx (ulna).

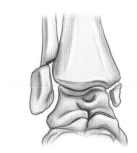

Fig. 15.16 Pott's fx (distal tibia-fibula).

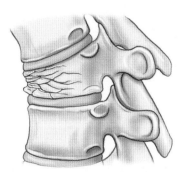

Fig. 15.17 Compression fx (body of vertebra).

15

Depressed Fracture (Sometimes Called a Ping-Pong Fracture)

In this fracture of the skull, a fragment is depressed. The appearance is similar to a Ping-Pong ball that has been pressed in by the finger, but if the indentation can be elevated again, it can assume its near-original position.

Epiphyseal Fracture

This is a fracture through the epiphyseal plate, the point of union of the epiphysis and shaft of a bone. It is one of the most easily fractured sites in long bones of children. Radiologists commonly use the Salter-Harris classification (Salter 1 to 5, with Salter 5 indicating the most complex) to describe the severity and reasonable indication of prognosis of these fractures.

Pathologic Fracture

These fractures are due to disease process within the bone, such as osteoporosis, neoplasia, or other bone diseases.

Stellate Fracture

In this fracture, the fracture lines radiate from a central point of injury with a starlike pattern. The most common example of this type of fracture occurs at the patella and is often caused by knees hitting the dashboard in a motor vehicle accident (Fig. 15.18).

Stress or Fatigue Fracture (Sometimes Called a "March" Fracture)

This type of fracture is nontraumatic in origin. It results from repeated stress on a bone, such as from marching or running. If caused by marching, these fractures usually occur in the midshafts of metatarsals; if caused by running, they are in the distal shaft of the tibia. Stress fractures are frequently difficult to demonstrate radiographically and may be visible only through subsequent callus formation at the fracture site or on a nuclear medicine bone scan.

Trimalleolar Fracture

This fracture of the ankle joint involves the medial and lateral malleoli as well as the posterior lip of the distal tibia.

Tuft or Burst Fracture

This comminuted fracture of the distal phalanx may be caused by a crushing blow to the distal finger or thumb (Fig. 15.19).

POSTFRACTURE REDUCTION

Closed Reduction

Fracture fragments are realigned by manipulation and are immobilized by a cast or splint. A closed reduction is a nonsurgical procedure; however, it may be done with the aid of fluoroscopy.

Open Reduction

For severe fractures with significant displacement or fragmentation, a surgical procedure is required. The fracture site is exposed and screws, plates, or rods are installed as needed to maintain alignment of the bony fragments until new bone growth can take place. This is called an open reduction with internal fixation (ORIF), as described later (see the section Surgical Radiography).

Mobile X-Ray Equipment

A study of trauma and mobile radiography requires an understanding of the functions and operations of the equipment being used. Trauma radiography may be performed with a conventional overhead tube in a dedicated trauma bay located in the ED or with **mobile (portable) units** that are brought to the ED, the patient's bedside, or the operating room (OR) for surgical procedures (Fig. 15.20). Radiographic examinations may also be performed in the

radiology department if the physician has deemed that the patient is stable. In this scenario, a nurse may accompany the patient to monitor the person's condition.

MOBILE X-RAY SYSTEMS

Major advances have been made in mobile radiographic and fluoroscopic equipment. Examples of general types commonly used are described and illustrated in this chapter.

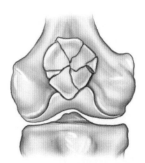

Fig. 15.18 Stellate fx (patella).

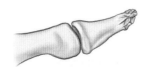

Fig. 15.19 Tuft fx (distal phalanx).

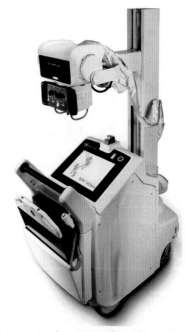

Fig. 15.20 GE Image Optima XR220amx. (Courtesy GE Healthcare.)

Battery-Driven, Battery-Operated, Mobile X-Ray Units

These systems are powered by 10 to 16 rechargeable, sealed, lead acid-type 12-volt batteries connected in series. The self-propelled systems of these units are also battery powered and have variable travel speeds up to an average walking speed of 2½ to 3 mph with a maximum incline of 7°. They have a driving range of up to 10 miles on a level surface after a full charge.

These units are driven and maneuvered by dual-drive motors that operate the two drive wheels. They also have a lower speed forward and reverse for maneuvering in close quarters. Parking brakes are automatically engaged when the control levers are not in use; this is known as dead man control. If the technologist releases the control levers, the mobile unit will come to an abrupt halt.

The unit can be plugged in for recharging when it is not being used and can be recharged at 110 or 220 V. The parking brakes are also used during charging. With 110-V, 5-amp outlets, the charging time is about 8 hours when fully discharged (Fig. 15.21).

Standard Power Source, Capacitor-Discharge, Non-Motor-Driven Units

A second type of mobile x-ray unit without battery power is now available. These models are much lighter in weight and usually are not motor driven. They operate with a 110-V, 15-amp power source or a 220-V, 10-amp power source. These units generally incorporate a capacitor discharge system, which stores electrical charges when plugged in and then discharges this electrical energy across the x-ray tube when exposure is initiated. This increases the electrical power (voltage) from the standard 110- or 220-V power source.

Other systems offer a dual power source with both battery power and plug-in electrical power for increased output. These generally also have a battery-assisted motor drive for easier transporting (Fig. 15.22).

The controls on these units may include some type of optional programmed memory system that is based on anatomic parts, or they may have operator-selected kVp and mAs technique controls.

NOTE: These are only two examples of available mobile systems. Other manufacturers offer various modifications, features, and options.

Digital Imaging Considerations

The widespread use of digital imaging in mobile systems is the most notable advancement in mobile equipment. As discussed in Chapter 1, digital imaging includes both computed radiography (CR) and digital radiography (DR). Digital imaging is especially well suited for trauma and mobile imaging in the ED, in the OR, and for bedside (mobile/portable) examinations. These procedures frequently are performed under difficult but urgent conditions in which opportunities for repeats are limited. The wide exposure latitude of digital images has improved the consistency of these images and has greatly reduced the need for repeat exposures due to positioning and technical variables.

Another advantage of digital imaging for trauma and mobile radiographic examinations is the ability to transfer these images electronically to more than one location simultaneously for interpretation or consulting. Radiologists can view the images and arrive at a diagnosis in a very short time and can communicate those findings to the ED physician, who then is able to create a plan of care for the trauma patient. In some instances, the images can be viewed directly on the mobile unit.

Following is a summary of guidelines that should be followed when digital imaging technology (computed radiography or digital radiography) is used for the lower limbs:

1. **Four-sided collimation:** Collimate to the area of interest with a minimum of two collimation parallel borders clearly demonstrated in the image. Four-sided collimation is always preferred if the study permits.

2. **Accurate centering:** It is important that the body part and the central ray be centered to the IR.

3. **Exposure factors:** With regard to exposure to the patient, it is important that the ALARA principle (as low as reasonably achievable) be followed and the lowest exposure factors required to obtain a diagnostic image be used. This includes the highest kVp and the lowest mAs that would result in desirable image quality. It may be necessary to increase kVp over that used for analog (film-screen) imaging for larger body parts, with 50 kVp as the minimum used on any procedure (exception is mammography).

4. **Post-processing evaluation of exposure indicator:** The exposure indicator value on the final processed image must be checked to verify that the exposure factors used were in the correct range to ensure optimal quality with the least radiation to the patient. If the index is outside of the acceptable range, the technologist must adjust kVp or mAs or both accordingly for any repeat exposures.

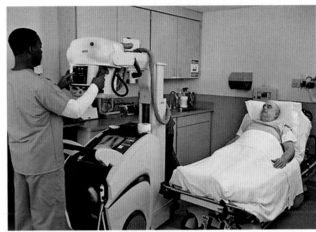

Fig. 15.21 Carestream DRX Revolution Mobile X-ray System. (Courtesy Carestream Health.)

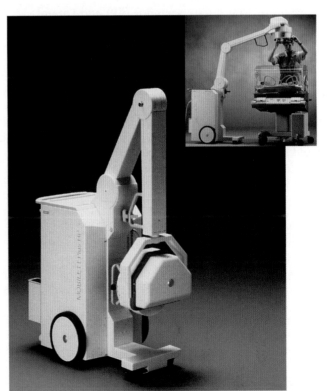

Fig. 15.22 Siemens Mobilett Plus—dual power source, battery and/or standard power, capacity discharge. (Courtesy Siemens Medical Solutions, Malvern, PA.)

Positioning Principles for Trauma and Mobile Radiography

Positioning principles for trauma and mobile radiography are similar to those applied for routine general radiography, as described in Chapter 1 of this text. The primary difference can be summarized by the word **adaptation**. Each trauma patient and situation is unique, and the technologist must evaluate the patient and adapt CR angles and IR placement as needed. However, all images must be as true to those of routine general radiography as possible.

The technologist must keep the following three principles in mind when performing trauma or mobile radiography:

1. Obtain two projections 90° to each other with true CR/part IR alignment
2. Include the entire structure or trauma area on the IR
3. Maintain the safety of the patient, health care workers, and the public

PRINCIPLE 1: TWO PROJECTIONS 90° TO EACH OTHER WITH TRUE CR/PART IR ALIGNMENT

Trauma radiography generally requires orthogonal views, **two projections taken at 90° (or right angles to each other)** while true CR/ part IR alignment is maintained. The preferences for the two projections are a true AP or PA and a true lateral achieved by turning the body part (standard positioning) or angling the CR and IR as needed (trauma adaptation positioning). In this way, the CR/part IR alignment can be maintained even if the patient cannot be turned or rotated. An example is shown in Figs. 15.23 and 15.24, in which true AP and lateral foot images are obtained without flexing or moving the lower limb. The AP projection is achieved by angling the CR and IR in relation to the foot, thus maintaining a true CR/part IR alignment.

When adaptations are made during the performance of any radiographic image, it is important to include as much information as possible as to how the image was achieved. This information includes CR angle, projection of the beam (AP, PA, lateral, oblique, horizontal beam lateral), and upright, semiupright, or supine position.

Exception to True Anteroposterior (AP) and Lateral Principle

Because of the patient's condition, occasionally it may not be possible to maintain this standard CR/part IR relationship for true anteroposterior (AP) and lateral projections. This may be due to unavoidable obstructions such as large splints, back supports, traction bars, or other apparatus. In this case, the technologist should still attempt two projections as near 90° to each other as possible, even if the anatomic part is partially rotated. **Only as a last resort should just one projection be taken.** When these exceptions are unavoidable, a note that explains the reason for this variance in routine should be left in the patient's record and/or examination requisition.

Exception to CR/Part IR Alignment

Generally, this principle involves placing the IR at right angles or perpendicular to the CR for minimal part distortion. However, in situations such as that shown in Fig. 15.25, the CR-part relationship can be maintained, but not the part-IR relationship. In this example, the AP axial oblique cervical spine is obtained with the patient supine and the IR flat on the table under the patient. This will result in some part distortion but, in trauma radiography, it may be an acceptable option.

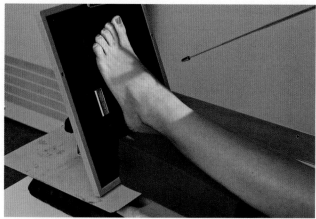

Fig. 15.23 AP foot (trauma adaptation positioning).

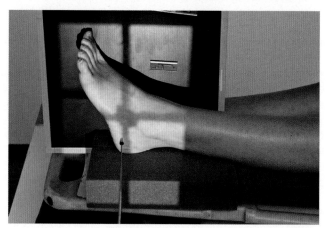

Fig. 15.24 Lateral foot.

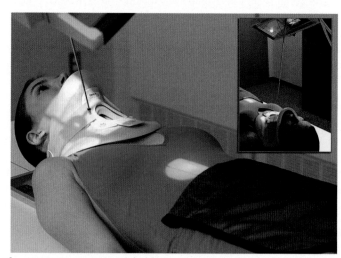

Fig. 15.25 Trauma AP axial oblique C-spine exception. The IR is not perpendicular to the CR.

PRINCIPLE 2: ENTIRE STRUCTURE OR TRAUMA AREA INCLUDED ON IMAGE RECEPTOR

Trauma radiography mandates that the **entire structure being examined should be included on the radiographic image** to ensure that no pathology is missed. This requires selection of sufficiently large IRs or the use of more than one IR if needed.

If an examination request on a trauma patient includes the long bones of the upper or lower limbs, **both joints should be included** for possible secondary fractures away from the primary injury. An example is a post-trauma examination request for a leg (tibia-fibula) with injury to the distal region. This may require a second, smaller IR of the knee to include the proximal tibia-fibula region if the patient's leg is too long to be included on a single image. Fractures of the distal tibia also may involve a secondary fracture of the proximal fibula. This principle of including both joints is true for AP and lateral projections.

For all upper and lower limb follow-up examinations, **always include a minimum of one joint nearest the site of injury.** Few if any exceptions to this rule exist, even if the obvious fracture shown on previous images is in the midshaft region. The joint nearest the fracture site should always be included (Figs. 15.26 and 15.27).

The principle of including the entire structure, or trauma region, also applies to these larger body areas. For example, the abdomen on a large patient may require two IRs placed landscape to include the entire abdomen. This may also be true for the chest or bony thorax.

Trauma patients often arrive in a supine position, and horizontal beam projections are commonly required for the lateral projections. Care must be taken to ensure that the divergent x-ray beam does not project the body part off the IR, especially when the IR is placed on edge directly beside the patient. This is true for the spine, skull, and other parts that rest directly on the tabletop. Examples of a horizontal beam, lateral skull projection, with and without a possible spine injury, are shown in Figs. 15.28 and 15.29. **With a questionable spinal injury, the head and neck cannot be moved or elevated.** Therefore, no support or pad can be placed between the head and tabletop. If the IR is placed on edge next to the patient's head, the divergent x-ray beam will project the posterior part of the skull off the IR.

To avoid cutoff of the posterior skull in this example, the patient can be moved to the edge of the table or cart and the IR placed below the level of the tabletop (see Fig. 15.29). This may result in an increase in the object–image receptor distance (OID), with resultant magnification. In these cases, this is an acceptable option. If cervical spine radiographs have ruled out cervical fracture or subluxation, the head may be raised and supported by a sponge to prevent posterior skull cutoff (see Fig. 15.28).

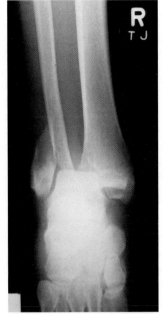
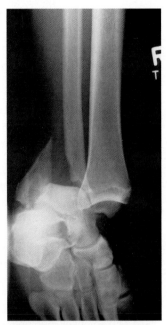

Fig. 15.26 AP distal lower leg and ankle.

Fig. 15.27 Lateral distal lower leg and ankle.

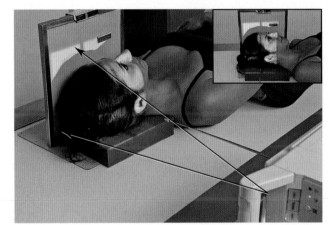

Fig. 15.28 Horizontal beam lateral skull without possible spine injury (head raised from tabletop).

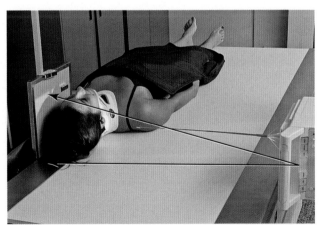

Fig. 15.29 With possible spine injury, head cannot be raised or moved (IR is placed below tabletop level to prevent posterior skull cutoff).

PRINCIPLE 3: MAINTAIN THE SAFETY OF THE PATIENT, HEALTH CARE WORKERS, AND THE PUBLIC

When trauma or mobile radiography is performed, it may be necessary to move room equipment and side rails to provide access to the patient. The technologist must take note of the equipment that is moved to make sure that it is not attached to the patient. Often, the technologist will be able to move equipment only a short distance because of space constraints. Side rails may have to be lowered to allow the technologist to place an IR under the patient. This must take place as quickly and as safely as possible. Never assume that a patient is unable to move. All side rails must be returned to the upright position, regardless of whether or not the patient already had the rails up. All equipment must be returned to its original location as well.

When performing mobile studies, **technologists are also responsible for ensuring the safety of the other health care workers in the immediate area**. In a trauma situation, time is of the essence. Although it is important that the technologist obtain trauma images while physicians, nurses, and other staff are attending to the patient, under no circumstances should an exposure take place with an unshielded person in the vicinity of the primary beam. The ALARA principle applies to other health care workers and the public, in addition to the patient.

Alternative Modalities

COMPUTED TOMOGRAPHY (CT)

The increased speed of computed tomography (CT) scanners has contributed to their increased use for emergency imaging. CT is commonly used for accurate diagnosis of a wide range of traumatic conditions that affect all body systems, thus replacing some of the traditionally ordered diagnostic examinations, such as spine and skull radiography. The three-dimensional reconstruction capability of CT is useful for fully assessing skeletal trauma.

SONOGRAPHY (MEDICAL ULTRASOUND)

Sonography (medical ultrasound) is indicated in the early assessment of certain trauma patients, such as those who have experienced blunt abdominal injury. It is a noninvasive technique used to detect free fluid or blood in the abdomen. Sonography is also the modality of choice for imaging emergency conditions of the female reproductive system (e.g., ectopic pregnancy). Sonography is used as required for specific emergency situations when other abdominal organs are imaged.

NUCLEAR MEDICINE (NM)

NM is useful for the evaluation of specific emergency conditions, such as pulmonary embolus, testicular torsion, and gastrointestinal (GI) bleeding. Blood flow to the areas under investigation is assessed through injection of the radionuclide.

ANGIOGRAPHY AND INTERVENTIONAL PROCEDURES

Angiography is indicated for studies of the aortic arch in the trauma patient, although the use of these procedures has declined because of the increased use of CT angiography. Interventional procedures performed on the trauma patient, as described in Chapter 17, include transcatheter embolization to occlude hemorrhaging vessels.

Routine and Special Projections

Certain routine and special projections for trauma, mobile, and surgical radiography are demonstrated and described on the following pages as suggested standard routine and special departmental routines or procedures.

TRAUMA AND MOBILE POSITIONING

AP CHEST

WARNING: With possible spinal injury or severe trauma, do not attempt to move the patient.

Clinical Indications
- According to the American College of Radiology (ACR), the AP chest radiograph is a standard part of the trauma workup at most level I trauma centers across the United States.[3]

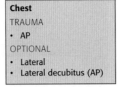

Chest
TRAUMA
• AP
OPTIONAL
• Lateral
• Lateral decubitus (AP)

- Approximately 25% of deaths from blunt trauma arise from chest injuries, although up to 50% of deaths are at least partially related to thoracic injuries.[2]
- Chest injuries include acute aortic injury, pulmonary injury, pneumothorax, hemothorax, extrapleural hematoma, large airway rupture, hemidiaphragmatic rupture, and musculoskeletal injury.[3]
- Ensure proper placement of lines and tubes.

Technical Factors
- Minimum SID—40 (100 cm). Use 72 inches (180 cm) if possible.
- IR size—14 × 17 inches (35 × 43 cm), **landscape,** for average to large patients (see NOTE 1)
- Grid (see NOTE 2)
- kVp range—90–125, depending on whether grid is required

Patient Position
AP Chest
- Patient is supine on cart; if patient's condition allows, the head end of the cart should be raised into an erect or semierect position.
- Rotate arms internally, if patient's condition allows, to move scapulae out of lung fields.

Part Position
AP Chest
- Enclose the IR in a plastic cover and place under or behind patient; place top of IR about 2 inches (4 to 5 cm) above the shoulders, aligning CR to IR. Ensure **no rotation** (coronal plane parallel to IR). (Place supports under parts of IR as needed.)

CR
AP Chest
- Direct CR 3 to 4 inches (8 to 10 cm) below jugular notch, **level of T7.**
- Angle CR 3° to 5° caudad, or raise head end of bed slightly, to place the CR perpendicular to long axis of sternum (unless grid prevents this). This simulates the PA projection and prevents the clavicles from obscuring the apices of the lungs (Fig. 15.30).
- If patient is able to attain only a semierect position, the CR must be angled to maintain the perpendicular relationship with the IR (Fig. 15.31).

Radiation Safety
- Exposure factor selection should be optimized in accordance with ALARA.
- Collimate on four sides to anatomy of interest.
- Shield radiosensitive tissues outside area of interest.

Respiration Expose at end of second full inspiration.

Optional lateral chest (not demonstrated here): A lateral image can be obtained with a horizontal beam CR if patient can raise arms at least 90° from body. Place IR parallel to midsagittal plane (MSP), with top of IR 2 inches (5 cm) above level of shoulders. Support patient on radiolucent pad to center chest to IR and center horizontal CR to level of T7.

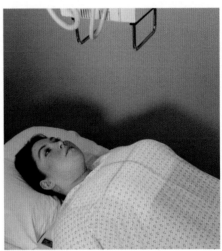

Fig. 15.30 AP supine chest, bedside (IR landscape), CR 3° to 5° caudad, perpendicular to sternum.

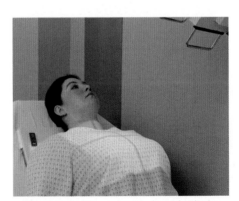

Fig. 15.31 AP semierect chest, bedside.

Lateral Decubitus AP Projection To determine air-fluid levels when the patient cannot be elevated sufficiently for an erect position, a lateral decubitus can be taken in bed with the IR placed behind the patient or on a stretcher in front of the IR holder, as shown in Fig. 15.32. Place radiolucent pads under the thorax and shoulders, and raise the arms above the head. CR/part IR alignment and centering are similar to that for supine AP, with necessary adaptations for the decubitus position.

NOTE 1: Costophrenic angle cutoff is a problem with recumbent chest positions taken with a shorter source–image receptor distance (SID) because of the divergence of the x-ray beam. Therefore, unless the patient is quite small, a **landscape IR placement is recommended.**

NOTE 2: Focused grids may be difficult to use for mobile chests because of the problems of grid cutoff.

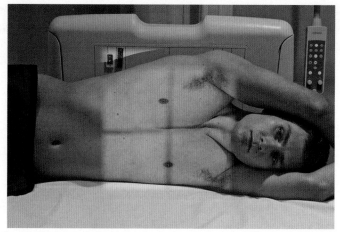

Fig. 15.32 Lateral decubitus (AP) chest, horizontal beam for detecting possible air-fluid levels.

AP SUPINE AND DECUBITUS: ABDOMEN

WARNING: With possible spinal injury or severe trauma, do not attempt to move the patient.

Clinical Indications

- Evaluate for fracture, free intraperitoneal air, abnormal fluid or gas.[4]
- Chest radiograph may be ordered along with an abdominal series.

Abdomen
TRAUMA
• AP supine
• Decubitus

Technical Factors

- Minimum SID—40 inches (100 cm)
- IR size—14 × 17 inches (35 × 43 cm), portrait (see NOTE 1)
- Grid
- kVp range—70–90
- Include decubitus and upside markers if applicable

Patient Position

AP Supine (Fig. 15.33)

- Place IR into plastic cover if taken at bedside.
- Align IR portrait to MSP.
- Arms placed at side, away from the body.

Left Lateral Decubitus AP (or PA) Projection (Fig. 15.34)

- This projection allows determination of air-fluid levels (see NOTE 2) and possible free intra-abdominal air when an upright image is not possible. The lateral decubitus can be taken in bed, on a stretcher in the ED, or on a stretcher in the radiography room in front of an upright wall bucky.
- Place supports or a positioning board under hips and thorax as needed to center abdomen to IR for lateral and dorsal decubitus projections, if performed bedside. This will create a flat surface, thus preventing the patient from sinking into the mattress and cutting off downside anatomy on the image.
- Raise arms up near head and partially flex the knees to stabilize patient.

Part Position 🔲

AP Supine

- Center IR to CR at level of iliac crest. Ensure that both sides of upper and lower abdomen are at equal distances from lateral IR margins.
- Place supports under parts of IR if needed to ensure that IR is level and perpendicular to CR (prevents patient rotation and grid cutoff on soft bed surfaces).

Left Lateral Decubitus AP (or PA) Projection

- Ensure that **diaphragm and upper abdomen are included.** Place center of IR 1 to 2 inches (2.5 to 5 cm) above level of iliac crests.
- Ensure no rotation and that the IR plane is perpendicular to CR.

CR

AP Supine

- Position CR perpendicular to **level of iliac crest** and to center of IR.

Left Lateral Decubitus AP (or PA) Projection

- Direct horizontal CR to center of IR, 2 inches (5 cm) above level of iliac crests.

Radiation Safety

- Exposure factor selection should be optimized in accordance with the ALARA.
- Collimate on four sides to anatomy of interest.
- Shield radiosensitive tissues outside area of interest.

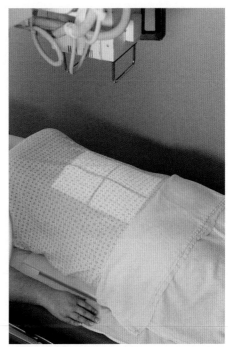

Fig. 15.33 Supine AP abdomen, bedside.

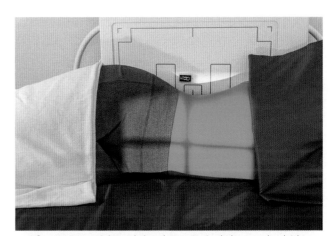

Fig. 15.34 Left lateral decubitus (AP) abdomen, bedside.

Respiration
AP Supine and Left Lateral Decubitus AP (or PA) Projection
- Make exposure at end of expiration.

NOTE 1: For patients with a large body habitus, two 14 × 17-inch (35 × 43-cm) IRs may be needed to ensure the entire anatomy is included. These IRs should be placed landscape, one for imaging the upper abdomen and diaphragm and the other for imaging the lower abdomen and symphysis pubis. Two separate exposures are necessary (see Chapter 3).

    NOTE 2: For lateral decubitus projections, have patients lie on the side for a minimum of **5 minutes** before taking exposure to allow air to rise to highest position within the abdomen.

Dorsal Decubitus, Lateral Position (Fig. 15.35)
- This is not a common bedside projection. The dorsal decubitus is a useful position for demonstrating a possible abdominal aortic aneurysm, or it may be used as an alternative to the lateral decubitus position if the patient cannot be moved.

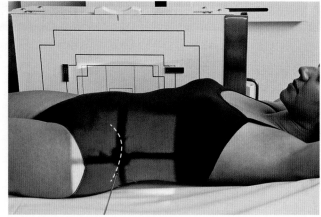

Fig. 15.35 Dorsal decubitus (lateral) abdomen, on stretcher in front of erect bucky.

UPPER LIMB

WARNING: With possible spinal injury or severe trauma, do not attempt to move the patient.

Clinical Indications
- Fractures, dislocations, and subluxations due to trauma.
- Hand and wrist fractures and dislocations are more common than those of any other part of the body.[5]
- Delayed diagnosis due to persistent clinical findings.

Upper Limb
TRAUMA
- AP or PA
- Lateral

OPTIONAL
- Oblique

Technical Factors
- Minimum SID—40 inches (100 cm)
- IR size—Smallest IR possible
- Grid—If part is thicker than 10 cm
- kVp range—50–70

Patient Position
- The patient will present in a multitude of positions. Some may be able to sit upright for their exam, whereas others may be supine on a back board. Because of the wide variance in patient positions, it is difficult to describe a specific protocol to follow in regard to patient positioning. The technologist must assess the patient's status and limitations to determine how to proceed in the best interest of the patient.

Part Position
- Obtain a minimum of two projections 90° to each other with true CR/part IR alignment (Figs. 15.36 and 15.37).
- Do not attempt to rotate a severely injured part.
- Do not remove splints or other immobilization devices.
- Be cautious working around foreign bodies that may be protruding from the area of interest.
- When placing the IR, minimally raise the affected limb while supporting both joints.

CR
- Include the entire structure or trauma area, including both joints for long bones.

Radiation Safety
- Exposure factor selection should be optimized in accordance with the ALARA.
- Collimate on four sides to anatomy of interest.
- Shield radiosensitive tissues outside area of interest.

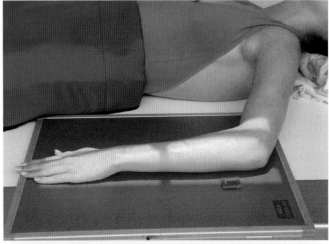

Fig. 15.36 PA forearm to include wrist and elbow.

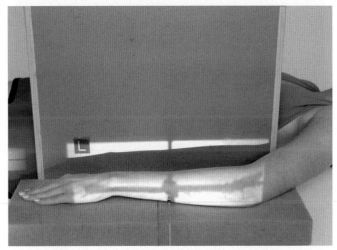

Fig. 15.37 Lateral forearm to include wrist and elbow.

15

Upper Limb Positioning Examples Figs. 15.38 to 15.50 provide examples of how radiographs can be produced when encountering a trauma situation involving the upper limb.

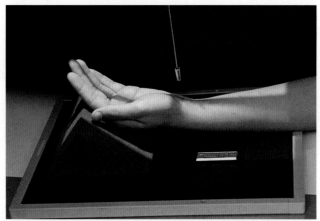

Fig. 15.38 AP proximal metacarpals and wrist.

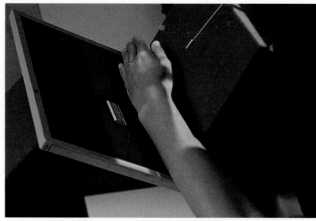

Fig. 15.42 Lateral wrist and hand.

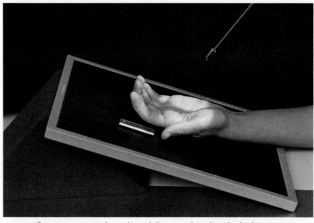

Fig. 15.39 AP hand and fingers for distal phalanges.

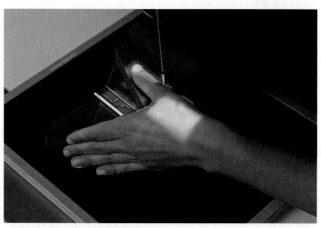

Fig. 15.43 PA thumb.

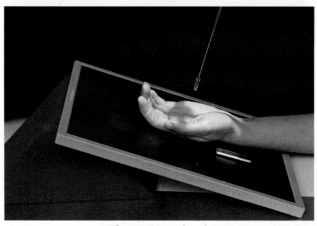

Fig. 15.40 AP hand.

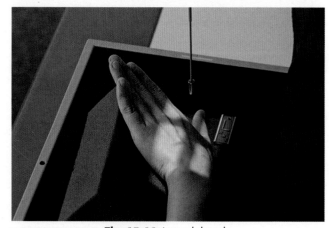

Fig. 15.44 Lateral thumb.

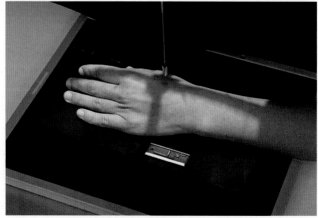

Fig. 15.41 Oblique—fingers, hand, and/or wrist.

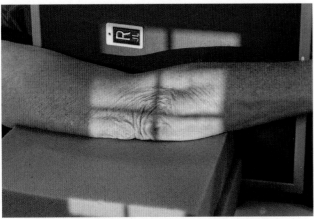

Fig. 15.45 PA horizontal beam elbow, CR perpendicular to interepicondylar plane.

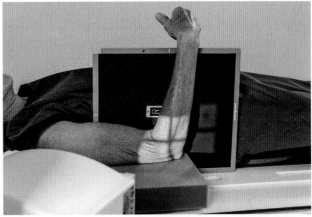

Fig. 15.48 Lateral for coronoid process, elbow flexed 80°, CR angled 45° distally (from shoulder).

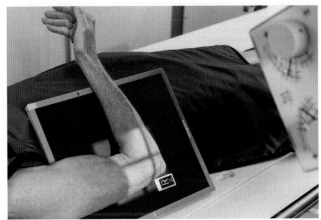

Fig. 15.46 Lateral elbow partially flexed, CR angled as needed to be parallel to interepicondylar plane.

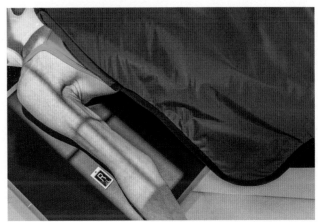

Fig. 15.49 AP humerus; should include both joints.

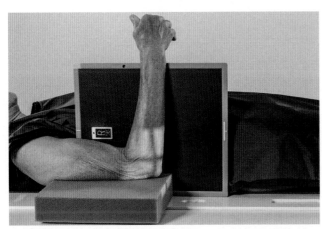

Fig. 15.47 Lateral for radial head, elbow flexed 90°, CR angled 45° proximally (toward shoulder).

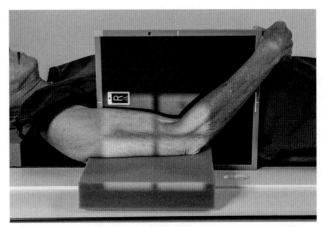

Fig. 15.50 Lateral, mid- and distal humerus to include elbow.

15

SHOULDER

WARNING: Do not attempt to rotate the arm if a fracture or dislocation is suspected; leave affected arm as presented.

NOTE: Local protocols for radiographic evaluation of the shoulder for trauma vary widely. However, the shoulder trauma protocol should have at least three views, two of which are orthogonal.[6]

> **Shoulder**
> TRAUMA
> • AP
> • Scapular Y lateral
> • Inferosuperior axial
> • Transthoracic lateral

Clinical Indications
• Fractures, dislocations, and subluxations due to trauma

Technical Factors
• Minimum SID—40 inches (100 cm)
• IR size—10 × 12 inches (24 × 30 cm) portrait
• Grid
• kVp range—70–85 with grid

Patient Position
AP Shoulder and Scapular Y Lateral—AP Oblique (Lateromedial Scapula) (Figs. 15.51 and 15.52)

• Patient will most likely be supine in the case of trauma; however, an erect position is usually more comfortable. Cervical spine and lower limb injuries must be ruled out before asking patient to stand or sit up.

Inferosuperior Axial (Fig. 15.53)

• Patient supine, with shoulder raised approximately 2 inches (5 cm) from the cart or tabletop.
• Place support under arm and shoulder to place area of interest near center of IR.

Transthoracic Lateral (Fig. 15.54)

• Patient will most likely be supine in case of trauma; however, an erect position is usually more comfortable.
• Place the affected shoulder closest to the IR.

Part Position
AP Shoulder
• Affected arm in neutral rotation, position at side.
• Center IR (grid IR under patient if on stretcher) to shoulder joint and to CR.

Scapular Y Lateral—AP Oblique (Lateromedial Scapula)
• Palpate borders of scapula by grasping medial and lateral borders of body of scapula with fingers and thumb. Carefully adjust body rotation as needed to bring the **plane of the scapular body perpendicular to the IR (approximately 25° to 30° away from IR).** Do not roll patient until the cervical spine has been cleared for fracture or subluxation.
• Center scapulohumeral joint to CR and center of IR.

Inferosuperior Axial
• Place IR as close to the neck as possible.
• Abduct affected arm 90° from body or as much as the patient can tolerate. Care should be taken when abducting the arm; support should be provided under arm. Do not abduct arm if fracture or dislocation is suspected.

Transthoracic Lateral
• Raise unaffected arm above head, elevating the unaffected shoulder.
• Center to level of surgical neck of affected arm to center of IR.

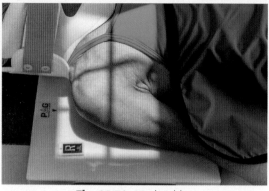

Fig. 15.51 AP shoulder.

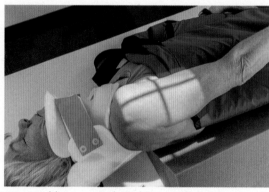

Fig. 15.52 AP oblique, scapular Y, lateromedial projection of scapula.

CR
AP Shoulder
- CR perpendicular to IR, directed to **midscapulohumeral joint.**

Scapular Y Lateral—AP Oblique (Lateromedial Scapula)
- Project CR perpendicular to IR, or if patient cannot be turned up sufficiently, angle CR as needed to be parallel to scapular blade (place grid horizontal to prevent grid cutoff) (see NOTE 1).
- Center CR to **scapulohumeral joint** (2 or 2½ inches [5 or 6 cm] below top of shoulder).

Inferosuperior Axial
- Direct CR **medially 15° to 30°** (less angle is required with less abduction of the arm).
- Center the CR **horizontally to axilla and humeral head.**

Transthoracic Lateral
- CR perpendicular to IR, directed through thorax **exiting at surgical neck** of affected arm (see NOTE 2).

Radiation Safety
- Exposure factor selection should be optimized in accordance with the ALARA.
- Collimate on four sides to anatomy of interest.
- Shield radiosensitive tissues outside area of interest.

Respiration
- Suspend respiration.
- A breathing technique may be preferred for the transthoracic lateral to blur out ribs and lung structures.

NOTE 1: Some distortion will occur with this medial CR angle if it is needed to achieve a lateral position of the scapula.

NOTE 2: A 10° to 15° cephalad angle may be required if superimposition of the shoulders occurs.

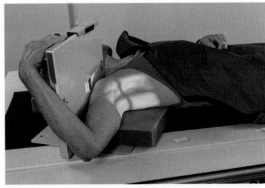

Fig. 15.53 Inferosuperior axial (transaxillary) shoulder.

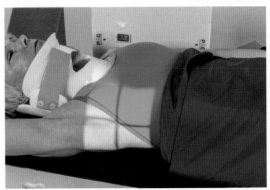

Fig. 15.54 Lateral, transthoracic proximal humerus.

LOWER LIMB

WARNING: With possible spinal injury or severe trauma, do not attempt to move the patient.

NOTE: Radiographs are the mainstay of initial medical imaging in the setting of acute foot trauma. Initial foot imaging typically consists of a three-view study with the possibility of additional views as indicated by the clinical setting.[7] An evaluation of the traumatized ankle should consist of AP, lateral, and mortise views of the ankle.[8] Several studies have found that the knee radiograph is commonly obtained after trauma but has the lowest yield for diagnosing clinically significant fractures.[9]

> **Lower Limb**
> TRAUMA
> • AP
> • Lateral
> OPTIONAL
> • Oblique

Clinical Indications
• Fractures, dislocations, and subluxations due to trauma

Technical Factors
• Minimum SID—40 inches (100 cm)
• IR size—Smallest IR possible
• Grid—If part is thicker than 10 cm
• kVp range—60–85

Patient Position
• The patient will present in a multitude of positions. Because of the wide variance in patient positions, it is difficult to describe a specific protocol to follow in regard to patient positioning. The technologist must assess the patient's status and limitations to determine how to proceed in the best interest of the patient.

Part Position
• Obtain a minimum of two projections 90° to each other with true CR/part IR alignment (Figs. 15.55 and 15.56).
• Do not attempt to rotate a severely injured part.
• Do not remove splints or other immobilization devices.
• Be cautious working around foreign bodies that may be protruding from the area of interest.
• When placing the IR, minimally raise the affected limb while supporting both joints.

CR
• Include the entire structure or trauma area, including both joints for long bones.

Radiation Safety
• Exposure factor selection should be optimized in accordance with the ALARA.
• Collimate on four sides to anatomy of interest.
• Shield radiosensitive tissues outside area of interest.

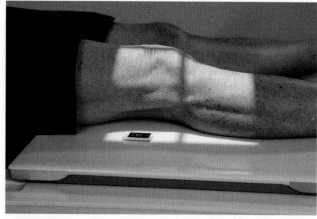

Fig. 15.55 AP knee, CR parallel to long axis of foot lateromedially. (No cephalic angle is required on average patients.)

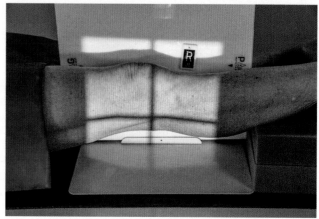

Fig. 15.56 Lateromedial knee, horizontal CR.

LOWER LIMB POSITIONING EXAMPLES

Figs. 15.57 to 15.67 provide examples of how radiographs can be produced when encountering a trauma situation involving the lower limb.

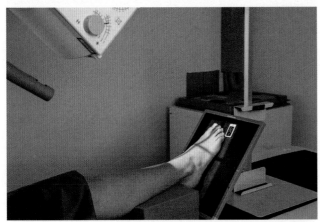

Fig. 15.57 AP foot and/or toes—CR perpendicular to IR.

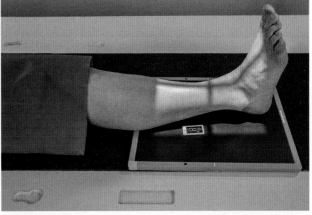

Fig. 15.60 Optional—AP ankle, CR perpendicular (parallel to long axis of foot).

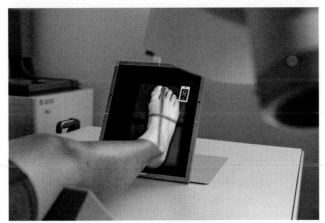

Fig. 15.58 Optional—oblique foot, CR cross-angled lateromedially 30° to 40°.

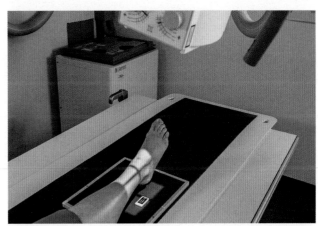

Fig. 15.61 AP mortise projection—CR 15° to 20° lateromedial angle, perpendicular to intermalleolar plane.

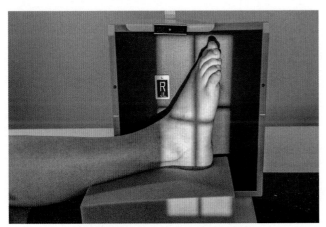

Fig. 15.59 Lateral foot or calcaneus.

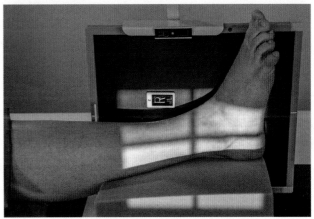

Fig. 15.62 Lateral ankle—CR horizontal.

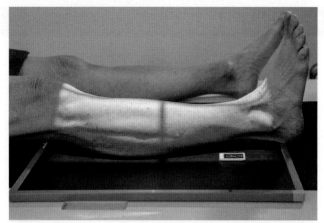

Fig. 15.63 AP lower leg—CR cross-angled lateromedially (parallel to long axis of foot).

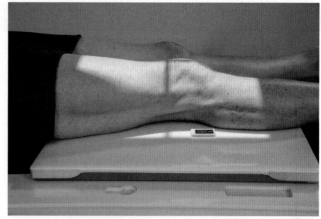

Fig. 15.66 AP mid- and distal femur.

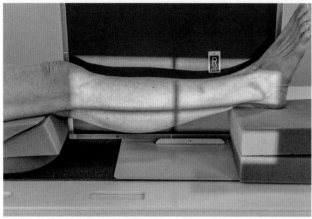

Fig. 15.64 Lateral lower leg.

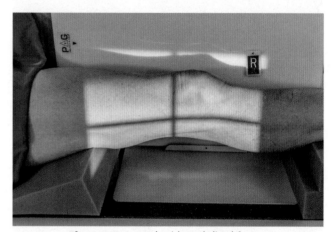

Fig. 15.67 Lateral mid- and distal femur.

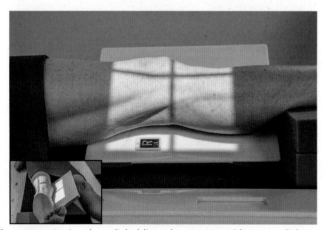

Fig. 15.65 Optional medial oblique knee—CR 45° lateromedial cross-angle, grid landscape (crosswise).

PELVIS

WARNING: Do not attempt to rotate leg internally if hip fracture is suspected.

NOTE: An AP pelvic radiograph is often combined with an AP chest and a lateral horizontal beam cervical spine radiograph to quickly assess the patient for emergent injuries and to triage patients.[3]

Pelvis
TRAUMA
• AP

Clinical Indications
• Fractures, dislocations, and subluxations due to trauma

Technical Factors
• Minimum SID—40 inches (100 cm)
• IR size—14 × 17 inches (35 × 43 cm), landscape
• Grid
• kVp range—75–90

Patient Position
AP Pelvis
• Patient supine, with arms removed from area of interest (Fig. 15.68).
• Direct CR perpendicular to center of IR and pelvis.

Part Position
AP Pelvis
• Place plastic cover over IR and slide under pelvis, **IR landscape**, centered to patient.
• Top of IR will be about 1 inch (2.5 cm) above iliac crest.
• Ensure **no rotation** and equal distances from anterior superior iliac spine (ASIS) to IR.
• Rotate feet internally 15° if possible (see previous WARNING).

CR
AP Pelvis
• CR is perpendicular to IR, directed **midway between level of ASIS and the symphysis pubis.** This is approximately 2 inches inferior to the level of ASIS.

Radiation Safety
• Exposure factor selection should be optimized in accordance with the ALARA.
• Collimate on four sides to anatomy of interest.
• Shield radiosensitive tissues outside area of interest.

Respiration Suspend respiration during exposure.

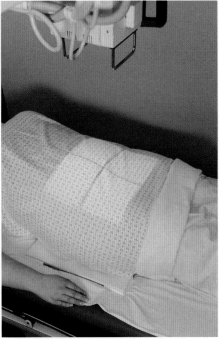

Fig. 15.68 AP pelvis—bedside mobile. (Right leg is not rotated internally in this example.)

HIP

WARNING: Do not attempt to rotate leg internally if hip fracture is suspected.

NOTE: Radiography is the established initial imaging study of choice for assessing the acutely painful hip. As with any trauma-related musculoskeletal radiographic studies, orthogonal projections (two or more views of the anatomy at right angles to each other) are considered standard.[10]

Hip
TRAUMA
• AP
• Lateral-axiolateral-inferosuperior hip— Danelius-Miller method

Clinical Indications
• Fractures, dislocations, and subluxations due to trauma

Technical Factors
• Minimum SID—40 inches (100 cm)
• IR size—14 × 17 inches (35 × 43 cm) or 10 × 12 inches (24 × 30 cm), portrait
• Grid
• kVp range—75–90

Patient Position
AP Hip and Axiolateral-Inferosuperior Hip—Danelius-Miller Method
• Patient supine, with arms removed from area of interest.

Part Position
AP Hip (Fig. 15.69)
• Place 14 × 17-inch (35 × 43-cm) portrait under hip with the top of the IR at the level of the iliac crest.
• Ensure no **rotation** and equal distances from anterior superior iliac spine (ASIS) to IR
• Rotate leg 15° internally, if possible (see previous WARNING).

Axiolateral-Inferosuperior Hip—Danelius-Miller Method (Fig. 15.70)
• Place IR against patient's side just above iliac crest and adjust so that it is **parallel to femoral neck.**
• Rotate leg 15° internally, if possible (see previous WARNING).
• Elevate opposite leg as much as possible.

CR
AP Hip
• CR is perpendicular to IR, directed 1 to 2 inches (2.5 to 5 cm) distal to midfemoral neck.

Axiolateral-Inferosuperior Hip—Danelius-Miller Method
• Direct horizontal CR perpendicular to femoral neck and to plane of IR.
• Ensure that CR is centered to the midline of the grid to prevent cutoff.

Radiation Safety
• Exposure factor selection should be optimized in accordance with the ALARA.
• Collimate on four sides to anatomy of interest.
• Shield radiosensitive tissues outside area of interest.

Respiration Suspend respiration during exposure.

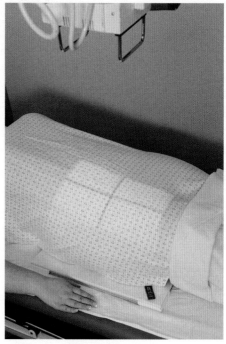
Fig. 15.69 AP hip.

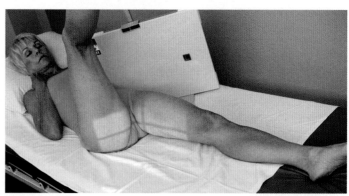
Fig. 15.70 Inferosuperior lateral—bedside mobile (Danelius-Miller method).

CERVICAL SPINE

WARNING: Do not remove cervical collar or move patient's head or neck until cervical fractures have been ruled out.

NOTE: A meta-analysis of seven studies that met strict inclusion criteria revealed that the pooled sensitivity of radiography for detecting cervical spine injuries (CSIs) was 52%, whereas the combined sensitivity of CT was 98%. Screening the cervical spine with multidetector CT (MDCT) is faster than performing radiography, with far fewer technical failures. The ACR panel concluded that thin-section MDCT, and not radiography, should be the primary screening study for suspected CSI. When motion artifacts are significant enough to prevent adequate evaluation of vertebral integrity, a single lateral view will suffice to show that there is normal alignment and no evidence of fracture.[11]

> **Cervical Spine**
> TRAUMA
> • Lateral, horizontal beam
> OPTIONAL
> • Cervicothoracic (swimmer) lateral

Clinical Indications
• Fractures, dislocations, and subluxations due to trauma

Technical Factors
• SID—60–72 inches (150–180 cm)
• IR size—10 × 12 inches (24 × 30 cm), portrait
• Grid or without grid (see **NOTE 1**)
• Specially designed compensating filter useful for obtaining uniform brightness on the swimmer lateral (see Chapter 1).
• kVp range—70–85; lateral, horizontal beam; 75–95; cervicothoracic (swimmer) lateral

Patient Position
Lateral, Horizontal Beam and Cervicothoracic (Swimmer) Lateral

• Patient supine with potential spinal injury

Part Position
Lateral, Horizontal Beam (Fig. 15.71)
• Vertical IR against shoulder, parallel to MSP, with **top of IR 1 to 2 inches (2.5 to 5 cm) above level of EAM.** Ensure that C7–T1 region is included.
• Have patient relax and depress shoulders as much as possible (see **NOTE 2**).

Cervicothoracic (Swimmer) Lateral (Fig. 15.72)
• Vertical IR placement is similar to lateral, horizontal beam placement.
• Elevate arm and shoulder closest to IR and depress opposite shoulder as much as possible (see **NOTE 3**).

CR
Lateral, Horizontal Beam
• Direct CR **horizontal to C4** (upper thyroid cartilage) and to center of grid to prevent grid cutoff, or turn grid with centerline vertical to prevent grid cutoff if necessary.

Cervicothoracic (Swimmer) Lateral
• Direct CR horizontal, **centered to C7–T1** (approximately 1 inch [2.5 cm] above level of jugular notch). Center the center of grid to CR to prevent grid cutoff (grid lines vertical).

Radiation Safety
• Exposure factor selection should be optimized in accordance with the ALARA.
• Collimate on four sides to anatomy of interest.
• Shield radiosensitive tissues outside area of interest.

Respiration Suspend respiration on full expiration.

NOTE 1: It is estimated that, for a small body part (4 inches [10 cm], a 10-inch (25-cm) air gap will clean up scatter as well as a 15:1 grid. The cleanup is not as efficient for a larger body part (8 inches [20 cm]).[12]

NOTE 2: Traction on the arms will help depress the shoulders but should be done only by a qualified assistant and/or with the consent or assistance of a physician. If the C7–T1 junction cannot be visualized on the initial horizontal beam lateral C-spine image, a horizontal beam swimmer's lateral should be performed.

NOTE 3: A 5° CR caudal angle may be required if patient cannot depress shoulder opposite IR.

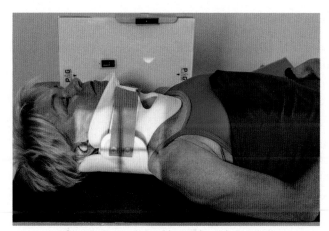

Fig. 15.71 Horizontal beam lateral, C spine.

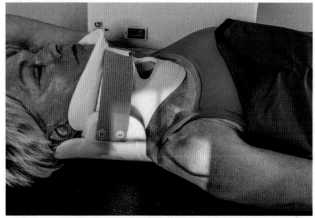

Fig. 15.72 Swimmer's lateral—C–T1.

THORACIC AND LUMBAR SPINE

WARNING: With possible spinal injury or severe trauma, do not attempt to move the patient.

Lateral projections are typically reviewed by a physician prior to obtaining additional spine images as described in Chapters 8 and 9.

NOTE: Currently MDCT is the imaging procedure of choice for evaluating trauma patients with possible spinal fractures or injuries.[11]

> **Thoracic and Lumbar Spine**
> TRAUMA
> • Lateral, horizontal beam
> OPTIONAL
> • Cervicothoracic (swimmer) lateral (previous page)

Clinical Indications
• Fractures, dislocations, and subluxations due to trauma

Technical Factors
• Minimum SID—40 inches (100 cm)
• IR size—14 × 17 inches (35 × 43 cm), portrait
• Grid (see NOTE 1)
• kVp range—80–95 lateral thoracic spine; 90–95 lateral lumbar spine

Patient Position

Lateral Thoracic Spine, Horizontal Beam and Lateral Lumbar Spine, Horizontal Beam

• Patient supine, raise arms sufficiently so as to not obscure anatomy of interest.

Part Position
Lateral Thoracic Spine, Horizontal Beam and Lateral Lumbar Spine, Horizontal Beam
• Build up patient with backboard (see Fig. 15.73) or move patient to edge of table and place vertical IR below level of tabletop. Use IR holder or tape and/or sandbags to support IR (see NOTE 2).

CR
Lateral Thoracic Spine, Horizontal Beam
• Center horizontal CR to vertebral column (**midway between midcoronal plane and posterior aspect of thorax**); near centerline of grid at **level of T7**, 3 to 4 inches (8 to 10 cm) inferior to jugular notch (see Fig. 15.73).

Lateral Lumbar Spine, Horizontal Beam
• Center horizontal CR centered to vertebral column (**midcoronal plane**); near centerline of grid at **level of L4** or the iliac crest (see Fig. 15.74).

Radiation Safety
• Exposure factor selection should be optimized in accordance with the ALARA.
• Collimate on four sides to anatomy of interest.
• Shield radiosensitive tissues outside area of interest.

Respiration Suspend respiration on full expiration.

NOTE 1: A decubitus-type grid with lead strips aligned horizontally can be used to prevent grid cutoff. The grid then may be placed landscape to patient, for better centering of the CR to the near centerline of the grid. This applies to both horizontal beam thoracic and lumbar spine projections.

NOTE 2: Both lateral thoracic and lumbar examinations can be performed with the patient remaining on the gurney. The stretcher can be moved to an upright bucky and the CR aligned with the patient positioned appropriately.

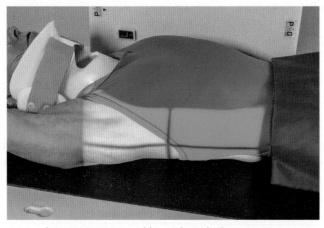

Fig. 15.73 Horizontal beam lateral—thoracic spine.

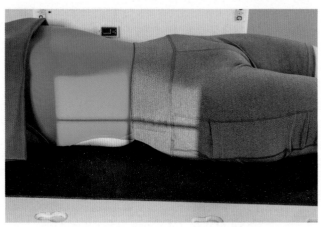

Fig. 15.74 Horizontal beam lateral—lumbar spine.

CRANIUM—LATERAL, HORIZONTAL BEAM

WARNING: Cervical spine fractures and subluxations or dislocations must be ruled out before attempts are made to move or manipulate the patient's head or neck.

NOTE: Rapid CT scanning is readily available in most hospitals that treat patients with head injuries; thus the routine use of CT has been advocated as a screening tool to triage patients with minor or mild head injuries who require hospital admission or surgical intervention from those who can be safely discharged without hospital admission.[13]

> **Cranium**
> TRAUMA
> • Lateral, horizontal beam
> • AP
> • AP axial

Clinical Indications
• Calvarial fractures, penetrating injuries, and radiopaque foreign bodies

Technical Factors
• Minimum SID—40 inches (100 cm)
• IR size—10 × 12 inches (24 × 30 cm), landscape (aligned to the anterior to posterior dimension of the skull).
• Grid
• kVp range—70–85

Patient Position
• Patient supine; remove all metal, plastic, or other removable objects from head. Do not remove cervical collar unless approved by attending physician

Part Position
AP Lateral, Horizontal Beam
• If patient's head can be manipulated (see previous WARNING), carefully elevate skull on a radiolucent sponge (Fig. 15.75). If you cannot manipulate head, move patient to edge of table and then place grid IR at least 1 inch (2.5 cm) below tabletop and occipital bone, as shown in Fig. 15.76. The divergent beam then will not project the posterior skull off the IR. Place the side of interest closest to the IR.
• Place head in true lateral position by ensuring that the MSP is parallel to the IR, the image plate (IP) is perpendicular to the IR, and the infraorbitomeatal line (IOML) is perpendicular to the tabletop (see previous WARNING).
• Adjust IR to ensure that the entire skull will be included on image and center of grid is centered to CR.
• Make sure not to cut off the top of the skull. If required, use a larger IR to include the entire skull.

CR
AP Lateral, Horizontal Beam
• A **horizontal beam** (essential for visualization of intracranial air-fluid levels) is directed perpendicular to IR.
• Center to a point **2 inches (5 cm) superior to the EAM.**

Radiation Safety
• Exposure factor selection should be optimized in accordance with the ALARA.
• Collimate on four sides to anatomy of interest.
• Shield radiosensitive tissues outside area of interest.

Respiration
• Suspend respiration during exposure.
REMINDER: On a patient with a cervical spine injury, do not attempt to raise and place support under the head or to move any portion of the head or neck, as shown in Fig. 15.75, until cervical pathology has been ruled out with a horizontal beam lateral cervical.

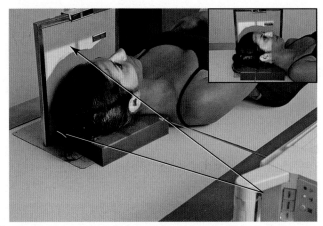

Fig. 15.75 Trauma lateral after cervical injury has been ruled out. Support is placed under elevated head.

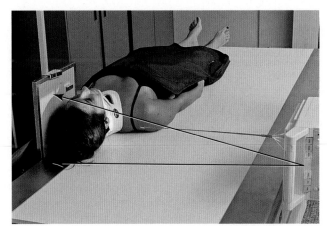

Fig. 15.76 Trauma lateral without head manipulation.

CRANIUM—AP, AP AXIAL 15° (REVERSE CALDWELL METHOD)

WARNING: Cervical spine fractures and subluxations or dislocations must be ruled out before attempts are made to move or manipulate the patient's head or neck.

NOTE: Rapid CT scanning is readily available in most hospitals that treat patients with head injuries; thus the routine use of CT has been advocated as a screening tool to triage patients with minor or mild head injuries who require hospital admission or surgical intervention from those who can be safely discharged without hospital admission.[13]

> **Cranium**
> TRAUMA
> • Lateral, horizontal beam
> • AP
> • AP axial

Clinical Indications
• Calvarial fractures, penetrating injuries, and radiopaque foreign bodies

Technical Factors
• Minimum SID—40 inches (100 cm)
• IR size—10 × 12 inches (24 × 30 cm), portrait
• Grid
• kVp range—75–90

Patient Position
• Patient supine; remove all metal, plastic, and other removable objects from head. Do not remove cervical collar unless approved by attending physician.

Part Position
AP and AP Axial 15°
• Align MSP perpendicular to midline of grid or table (see previous WARNING)
• Center IR to CR

CR
AP to Orbitomeatal Line Projection (Fig. 15.77)

• Angle **CR parallel to orbitomeatal line (OML)**: With patient in a cervical collar, this often occurs approximately 10° to 15° caudad, but each patient and situation will be different.
• Center CR **to glabella**; then center IR to projected CR.

AP Axial 15° Reverse Caldwell Method Projection (Fig. 15.78)

• Angle **CR 15° cephalad to OML:** To accomplish this, first find the OML on the patient; this varies in patients in cervical collars with the neck extended. Then, angle the CR 15° cephalic to the patient's OML.
• Center CR **to nasion**; then center IR to projected CR.

Radiation Safety
• Exposure factor selection should be optimized in accordance with the ALARA.
• Collimate on four sides to anatomy of interest.
• Shield radiosensitive tissues outside area of interest.

Respiration Suspend respiration during exposure.

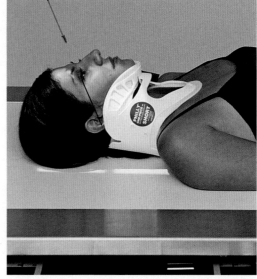

Fig. 15.77 AP CR parallel to OML, centered to glabella.

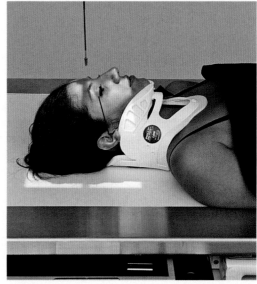

Fig. 15.78 AP axial 15° reverse Caldwell method—CR 15° cephalad to OML, centered to nasion.

CRANIUM—AP 30° AXIAL (TOWNE METHOD)

WARNING: Cervical spine fractures and subluxations or dislocations must be ruled out before attempts are made to move or manipulate the patient's head or neck.

NOTE: Rapid CT scanning is readily available in most hospitals that treat patients with head injuries; thus the routine use of CT has been advocated as a screening tool to triage patients with minor or mild head injuries who require hospital admission or surgical intervention from those who can be safely discharged without hospital admission.[13]

Cranium
TRAUMA
• Lateral, horizontal beam
• AP
• AP axial

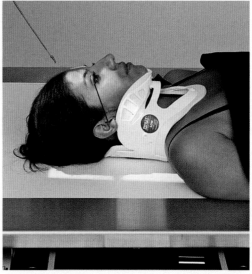

Fig. 15.79 AP axial Towne—CR 30° caudad to OML, centered to midpoint between EAMs.

Clinical Indications
- Calvarial fractures, penetrating injuries, and radiopaque foreign bodies

Technical Factors
- Minimum SID—40 inches (100 cm)
- IR size—10 × 12 inches (24 × 30 cm), portrait
- Grid
- kVp range—75–90

Patient Position
- Patient supine; remove all metal, plastic, and other removable objects from head. Do not remove cervical collar unless approved by attending physician.

Part Position
AP Axial (Towne Method) Projection
- Align MSP perpendicular to midline of grid or table (see previous WARNING)
- Center IR to CR

CR
AP Axial (Towne Method) Projection (Fig. 15.79)

- Angle **CR 30° caudad to OML, or 37° caudad to the IOML.** (Once again, note that a patient in a cervical collar with the neck extended will have OMLs and IOMLs that vary from the conventional parallel and perpendicular relationships formed through routine positioning; see NOTE).
- Center CR to pass **midway between EAMs** and exiting the foramen magnum. This centers CR to midsagittal plane 2¼ inches (6 cm) above superciliary arch; then center IR to projected CR.

NOTE: The CR for the AP axial should not exceed 45°, or excessive distortion will hinder the visualization of essential anatomy. If the CR cannot be angled 30° to the OML (before the maximum angle of 45° is reached), the dorsum sella and posterior clinoid processes will be visualized **superior** to the foramen magnum.

Radiation Safety
- Exposure factor selection should be optimized in accordance with the ALARA.
- Collimate on four sides to anatomy of interest.
- Shield radiosensitive tissues outside area of interest.

Respiration Suspend respiration during exposure.

FACIAL BONES—LATERAL, HORIZONTAL BEAM

WARNING: Cervical spine fractures and subluxations or dislocations must be ruled out before attempts are made to move or manipulate the patient's head or neck.

NOTE: Rapid CT scanning is readily available in most hospitals that treat patients with head injuries; thus the routine use of CT has been advocated as a screening tool to triage patients with minor or mild head injuries who require hospital admission or surgical intervention from those who can be safely discharged without hospital admission.[13]

Facial Bones
TRAUMA
• Lateral, horizontal beam
• Acanthioparietal (reverse Waters method)
• AP (see previous pages)
OPTIONAL
• Modified acanthioparietal (modified reverse Waters method)

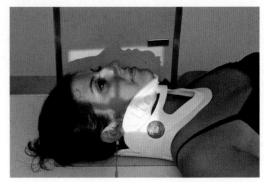
Fig. 15.80 Trauma horizontal beam lateral—facial bone projection.

Clinical Indications
• Fractures, penetrating injuries, and radiopaque foreign bodies

Technical Factors
• Minimum SID—40 inches (100 cm)
• IR size—10 × 12 inches (24 × 30 cm), portrait
• Grid
• kVp range—75–85

Patient Position
AP Lateral, Horizontal Beam
• Patient supine; remove all metal, plastic, or other removable objects from head. Do not remove cervical collar unless approved by attending physician.

Part Position
AP Lateral, Horizontal Beam (Fig. 15.80)
• Place head in true lateral position by ensuring that the MSP is parallel to the IR, the image plate (IP) is perpendicular to the IR, and the infraorbitomeatal line (IOML) is perpendicular to the tabletop (see previous WARNING).

CR
• A **horizontal beam** (essential for visualization of intracranial air-fluid levels) is directed perpendicular to IR.
• Center CR **to the zygoma,** midway between the outer canthus and EAM.

Radiation Safety
• Exposure factor selection should be optimized in accordance with the ALARA.
• Collimate on four sides to anatomy of interest.
• Shield radiosensitive tissues outside area of interest.

Respiration Suspend respiration during exposure.

FACIAL BONES—ACANTHIOPARIETAL (REVERSE WATERS METHOD) AND MODIFIED ACANTHIOPARIETAL (MODIFIED REVERSE WATERS)

WARNING: Cervical spine fractures and subluxations or dislocations must be ruled out before attempts are made to move or manipulate the patient's head or neck.

NOTE: Rapid CT scanning is readily available in most hospitals that treat patients with head injuries; thus the routine use of CT has been advocated as a screening tool to triage patients with minor or mild head injuries who require hospital admission or surgical intervention from those who can be safely discharged without hospital admission.[13]

Facial Bones
TRAUMA
• Lateral, horizontal beam
• Acanthioparietal (reverse Waters method)
• AP (see previous pages)
OPTIONAL
• Modified acanthioparietal (modified reverse Waters method)

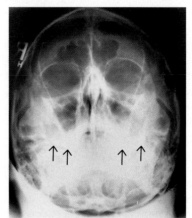

Fig. 15.81 Acanthioparietal (reverse Waters method)—CR parallel to MML, centered to acanthion.

Clinical Indications
• Fractures, penetrating injuries, and radiopaque foreign bodies

Technical Factors
• Minimum SID—40 inches (100 cm)
• IR size—10 × 12 inches (24 × 30 cm), portrait
• Grid
• kVp range—70–85

Patient Position
Acanthioparietal (Reverse Waters Method)
• Patient supine; remove all metal, plastic, or other removable objects from head. Do not remove cervical collar unless approved by attending physician.

Part Position
Acanthioparietal (Reverse Waters Method) (Fig. 15.81)
• Position MSP perpendicular to midline of grid or table (see previous WARNING).

Fig. 15.82 Acanthioparietal (reverse Waters method).

CR
Acanthioparietal (Reverse Waters Method)
• Angle CR cephalad as needed to align CR parallel to MML.

NOTE: This projection best visualizes facial bone structures and the maxillary region by projecting the maxilla and maxillary sinuses above the petrous ridges (see arrows in Fig. 15.82).

• Center **to acanthion**; then center IR to projected CR.

Part Position
Modified Acanthioparietal (Modified Reverse Waters Method) (Fig. 15.83)
• Position MSP perpendicular to midline of grid or table (see previous WARNING).

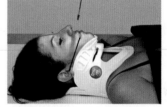

Fig. 15.83 Modified acanthioparietal (modified reverse Waters method)—CR parallel to LML, centered to acanthion.

CR
• Angle CR cephalad as needed to align CR parallel to LML.

NOTE: This projection best demonstrates the floor of the orbits and provides a view of the entire orbital rims. Petrous ridges are visualized in midmaxillary sinus region (Fig. 15.84).

• Center **to acanthion**; then center IR to projected CR.

Radiation Safety
• Exposure factor selection should be optimized in accordance with the ALARA.
• Collimate on four sides to anatomy of interest.
• Shield radiosensitive tissues outside area of interest.

Respiration Suspend respiration during exposure.

Fig. 15.84 Modified acanthioparietal (modified reverse Waters method).

15

SURGICAL RADIOGRAPHY

Radiography in surgery is one of the most demanding challenges encountered by a radiologic technologist. The technologist will be called on to perform procedures quickly and accurately in a sterile environment, with a minimum number of repeat exposures (Fig. 15.85). For most surgical procedures, the patient is under general anesthesia and time is of the essence, because the less time a patient spends under general anesthesia, the less likely it is that complications will occur. Therefore, the surgeon expects the technologist to perform any requested procedure without error or delay. These added pressures may create uncertainty and anxiety for the radiography student or recent graduate. However, with a solid knowledge of the surgical procedure and operation of the imaging equipment, the technologist can function effectively in the surgical suite.

Through supervised observations with an experienced surgical technologist, the student can become comfortable and confident in the surgical environment. It is essential that the student technologist be kept under the direct supervision of an experienced technologist in the OR until he or she has achieved competency for a specific procedure.

This section of the chapter identifies essential skills and commonly used equipment, and previews the surgical environment to provide the student radiographer with a baseline knowledge. More commonly performed procedures are discussed at the end of this chapter; however, it is important for student radiographers to understand that they will participate in a variety of surgical procedures based on their clinical setting. Rather than focus on specific surgical procedures, student radiographers should focus their efforts on developing the essential skills and transfer their newly acquired skills from one procedure to the next.

Essential Attributes of the Radiologic Technologist in Surgical Radiography

Although confidence and knowledge of procedures are needed in all aspects of radiography, certain personal attributes, skills, and insight are the trademark of a competent radiologic technologist in the surgical setting.

CONFIDENCE

Although no one can teach a technologist confidence, it is the first attribute that the other members of the surgical team expect to see in the technologist. **Confidence is judged by the technologist's level of comfort and ease in the OR suite, including the skilled use of imaging equipment, ability to problem-solve situations, and respect for the sterile field.** The surgical team expects the technologist to be confident in his or her abilities to perform the procedure quickly and accurately, with a minimum of repeat exposures. However, confidence comes only with experience and knowledge of all aspects of radiography. As the technologist gains experience and success in the OR, confidence will grow.

COMMUNICATION

It is essential that the technologist be an excellent communicator. He or she must communicate with other members of the surgical team regarding any concerns that arise during the procedure. **Clear communication between the technologist, surgeon, and anesthesiologist is paramount for most radiographic procedures.** For example, during operative cholangiography, the technologist must coordinate the exposure with the surgeon who is injecting the contrast medium and with the anesthesiologist who is suspending respiration. Without this team approach, motion may result and the quality of the exposure may be compromised.

The technologist must communicate radiation safety concerns with the surgical team, including failure to wear aprons, overuse of C-arm real-time imaging, and placement of hands into the radiation field. In these situations during surgery, the technologist is the radiation safety expert and must minimize exposure for the surgical team.

PROBLEM-SOLVING SKILLS

Even when the technologist has used the best knowledge and preparation, unexpected problems can occur during surgery. C-arms can cease to work, reliable exposure factors may fail to produce a diagnostic image, or the sterile field may be violated. Although it is difficult to predict every situation that might occur in the OR, the radiologic technologist **must be able to find solutions** to these problems quickly. Perhaps the most important skill of the technologist is the ability to problem-solve unforeseen situations immediately.

MASTERY

Mastery of all aspects of radiography, including use of the C-arm and mobile radiographic equipment, is essential. The technologist must be able to operate and troubleshoot conventional and digital equipment. The technologist must also know reliable exposure factors for patients of different sizes and for various procedures.

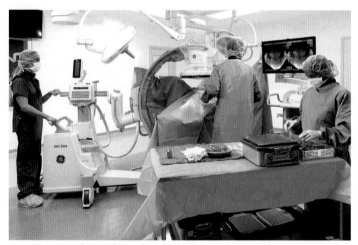

Fig. 15.85 Radiography in the surgical suite. (Courtesy GE Healthcare.)

Surgical Team

The composition of the surgical team will vary, depending on the surgeon, institutional policy, type of procedure, and other factors. A typical surgical team consists of the following members (Fig. 15.86).

SURGEON

The surgeon is a physician licensed and trained in general surgery or a specialty such as cardiovascular or orthopedic procedures. She or he has the primary responsibility for the entire surgical procedure and for the well-being of the patient prior to, during, and immediately following surgery.

ANESTHESIOLOGIST

A physician anesthesiologist or a certified nurse anesthetist specializes in administering anesthetic drugs to induce and maintain anesthesia in the patient during surgery. This person has the responsibility of ensuring the safety of the patient and monitoring physiologic functions and fluid levels of the patient during surgery.

SURGICAL ASSISTANT

A physician, physician assistant, certified surgical technologist (CST), or registered nurse (RN) assists the surgeon. This person's range of responsibilities may include suctioning, tying and clamping blood vessels, and assisting in cutting and suturing tissue.

CERTIFIED SURGICAL TECHNOLOGIST

A CST is a health professional who prepares the OR by supplying it with the appropriate supplies and instruments. Other CST responsibilities include preparing the patient for surgery and helping connect surgical equipment and monitoring devices. During surgery, CSTs have the primary responsibility for maintaining the sterile field.

CIRCULATOR

A circulator is a nonsterile CST or RN who assists in the OR by responding to the needs of scrubbed members in the sterile field before, during, and after the surgical procedure. Duties may include recording of pertinent information, retrieval of additionally needed items, and connecting nonsterile surgical equipment.

SCRUB

A scrub is a CST or RN who prepares the sterile field scrubs, gowns the members of the surgical team, and prepares and sterilizes the instruments before the surgical procedure is begun (Fig. 15.87).

NOTE: During OR cases, the radiologic technologist receives instructions from a physician (surgeon, anesthesiologist).

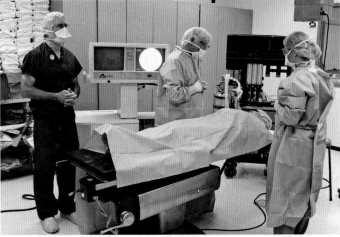

Fig. 15.86 Surgical team—surgeon, certified surgical technologist (CST), and radiologic technologist discussing procedure with patient.

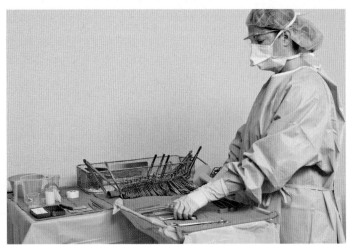

Fig. 15.87 Scrub preparing and maintaining sterile surgical field.

Surgical Radiography Imaging Equipment

The technologist must be familiar with the location of power outlets to be used for a procedure. Ideally, all imaging equipment should be in place and checked for correct operation before the procedure is begun. Although most surgical equipment remains in the surgical area, it must be cleaned and checked frequently for correct operation. Once the procedure has begun, there is no time to troubleshoot equipment or fix problems.

Daily, weekly, and monthly quality control protocols should be followed for all surgical radiographic equipment. Even a small problem, such as a frayed electrical cord, must be addressed before it results in an equipment failure.

CLEANING

Mobile (portable) units and C-arm equipment should be cleaned before and after use in the surgical area. An approved antiseptic cleaner should be used to wipe down the equipment. A liquid-type cleaner rather than an aerosol is recommended to prevent the introduction of airborne contaminants into the surgical area. The technologist must wear gloves when cleaning equipment, especially if blood or other body fluids are present.

Equipment permanently stored in the surgical area must be cleaned weekly or as needed. IRs and grids must be inspected for contamination and cleaned weekly.

OPERATIONAL CHECK

Before imaging equipment is used, an operational check should be performed. A log of any problems and failures should be maintained and monitored.

PROPER EQUIPMENT LOCATION

The technologist must be familiar with the location of power outlets (and data ports for uploading images to a picture archiving and communications system [PACS]) to be used for a procedure. Ideally, all imaging equipment should be in place and checked for correct operation before the procedure.

If C-arm fluoroscopy units are being used, place monitors in clear vision of the surgeon. Make sure that placement of the C-arm or portable unit is not interfering with normal foot traffic.

MOBILE C-ARM DIGITAL FLUOROSCOPY SYSTEMS

Another type of mobile imaging equipment is the C-arm mobile fluoroscopy system. The term *C-arm* describes a basic design of a mobile fluoroscopy unit, which forms a large C shape with the x-ray tube located at one end of the C-arm and the image intensifier tower at the other (Fig. 15.88).

Familiarity with the C-arm, monitor, and image controls is essential for the technologist who is performing ED or procedures, during which these systems are most commonly used. One also must become familiar with the various types of special beds or carts used with the C-arm. For example, a surgical bed may not accommodate the C-arm x-ray tube under the table in the abdominal area because of the base supports unless the patient's head is placed at the correct end of the bed or cart (Fig. 15.89).

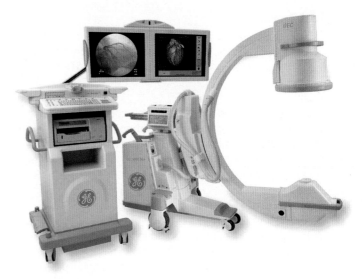

Fig. 15.88 OEC 9900 Elite. (Courtesy GE Healthcare.)

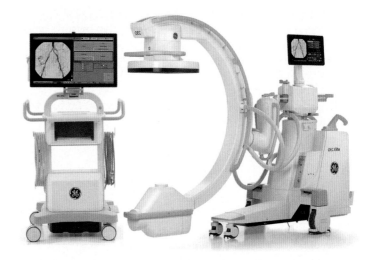

Fig. 15.89 OEC 9900 Elite. (Courtesy GE Healthcare.)

Maneuverability

The equipment is designed to be very maneuverable. The C-arm itself is attached to a beam located on the base of the C-arm that can be raised, lowered, or extended as needed. The base of the C-arm and the supporting beam provide a much-needed counterbalance to the C-arm portion. This counterbalance stabilizes the machine during any needed rotation, tilt (cephalic or caudal angles), or horizontal-beam, projection (Fig. 15.90). The C-arm can also be rotated 180° to place the tube on top and the intensifier on the bottom. However, this is not recommended because of the increase in OID, which decreases image resolution and increases scatter radiation. The tube-on-top position also results in a significant increase in exposure to the eyes, head, and neck areas of the surgeon or radiologist because of the exposure pattern of the C-arm in this orientation (see Fig. 15.97).

Overall, the unit is flexible to use. The technologist must be familiar with a variety of built-in joints, extensions, and adjustments. With its three-wheel base, steerable rear wheels, and a swiveling nose wheel, the operator can easily maneuver the unit into almost any possible configuration, with reasonable space.

Display Monitors and Control Cart

Two monitors are generally used, so the active image can be displayed on one monitor while the second monitor can be used to hold an image for reference purposes. Generally, the active monitor is on the technologist's left and the hold monitor is on the right. Images also can be rotated or flipped as needed for preferred viewing by the surgeon and/or radiologist.

Uses of C-Arm

The technologist will use the C-arm unit with various types of procedures in which mobile fluoroscopy and/or still frame imaging is needed. Common surgical procedures may include cholangiography, open or closed reductions of fractures, and hip pinnings.

Images can be stored temporarily by video memory or on hard disks. With the advancement and popularity of the PACS, images can be directly uploaded to a PACS with the appropriate data connection. Optional hard copy printers are also available for printouts. Cine loop capability, wherein images are recorded in rapid succession while contrast medium is injected and then displayed as a moving (or cine) image, is possible.

As with other types of digital imaging, image enhancement and manipulation are possible, including overall brightness and contrast controls, magnification, edge enhancement, masking, and digital subtraction studies. These manipulations can be made during fluoroscopy or for postimage processing, depending on the manufacturer.

Controls and Operation Modes

The digital C-arm fluoroscopy systems include a variety of operating mode control options with which the technologist must be familiar. These control panels may be located on the display monitor control cart, on the C-arm unit itself (Fig. 15.91), or on an attached or detached remote control.

The magnification mode is the ability of a system to magnify the image for better visualization of structures because surgeons frequently need to view the image at a specified distance from the monitor.

The pulse mode is used to create an x-ray beam that pulsates at timed increments to reduce exposure.

The snapshot or digital spot mode activates a digital spot, which results in a higher quality computer-enhanced image as compared with a held fluoroscopic image.

Auto/manual exposure control allows for exposure by the operator if desired, or the use of automatic exposure control (AEC).

Additional optional modes available on some equipment that allow more complicated procedures include subtraction (digital subtraction) and roadmapping. Subtraction is a technique in which an initial image is recorded during continuous fluoroscopy. The initial image then is used as a filter for the next fluoroscopic images. Essentially, the C-arm subtracts the initial image from all the other images produced. All stationary structures are removed (subtracted) from the image, and only moving (or new/different) structures are imaged. When fluoroscopy ends, the C-arm resets back to normal mode. For example, subtraction is sometimes used for operative cholangiography. Use of subtraction will eliminate the stationary ribs, spine, and surrounding soft tissues, leaving only the moving injected contrast medium to be imaged. Therefore, the final images show the contrast-filled biliary system free from superimposition of the surrounding structures.

Roadmapping is a method of image display wherein a specific fluoroscopic image is held on the screen in combination with continuous fluoroscopy. It is similar to subtraction in that it removes stationary structures from the viewing screen. This is especially useful in interventional procedures that require the placement of catheters.

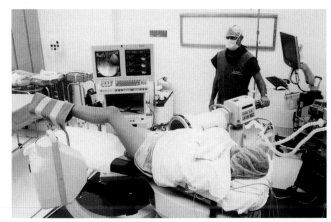

Fig. 15.90 Horizontal setup for lateral hip.

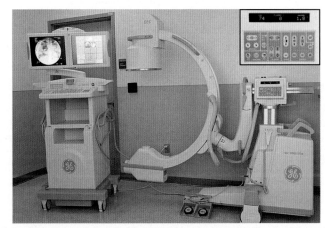

Fig. 15.91 Control panels of OEC 9600 ELITE series C-arm. (Courtesy GE OEC Medical Systems, Salt Lake City, UT.)

15

Foot Pedal

The foot pedal allows the physician or other operator to have hands-free operation of the C-arm. A fully equipped foot pedal has multiple controls for various functions, as shown in Fig. 15.92.

Image Orientation

The flexibility of the C-arm for imaging a variety of anatomic structures at almost any conceivable angle from any side or direction requires correct image orientation each time it is set up for use. This should be completed during setup time before the initial image is obtained to avoid needless exposure to the patient and personnel.

Because of the variety of policies and procedures reported in various hospitals and medical centers, technologists must develop their own methods of achieving correct image orientation before the patient is imaged. One method is to bring the C-arm into the room in the same position and orientation that will be used for the procedure. Place an R lead marker on the flat surface of the x-ray tube collimator, oriented in the same way the patient will be oriented. The top of the letter R should be to the head end, indicating the patient's right side, to appear anatomically correct on the monitor to the viewer's left. (This is the same orientation as for viewing radiographs; that is, the patient's right to the viewer's left.) At this point, the image can be flipped or rotated as needed to produce the correct orientation necessary for the procedure. An exposure can be provided during this setup with an apron or other shielding covering the C-arm to shield other personnel in the room. Correctly viewing and orienting the test image of the R on the monitor is an important preparation for the procedure.

O-ARM

The O-arm is a new type of surgical imaging equipment that a radiologic technologist may operate during select procedures (Fig. 15.93). The O-arm imaging system is a mobile x-ray system designed for 2D fluoroscopic and 3D imaging and is intended to be used where a physician benefits from 2D and 3D information of anatomic structures and objects with high x-ray attenuation such as bony anatomy and metallic objects. The O-arm imaging system is compatible with certain image-guided surgery systems.[14]

The O-arm is an example of new technology that can be operated in the surgical setting by a radiologic technologist; however, the C-arm continues to be the primary imaging equipment with fluoroscopic capabilities used, and therefore, the C-arm is the focus of this section.

Radiation Protection in Surgical Radiography

Conscientious radiation protection practices are especially important in mobile radiography and surgery suites in which fixed protective barriers do not provide a shielded place to stand during exposures. This is true with all mobile x-ray examinations, but even more so with C-arm mobile fluoroscopy, which potentially results in considerably more scatter radiation to the immediate area over a longer time. The technologist must continually be aware of the three important cardinal rules of radiation protection—time, distance, and shielding.

STAFF RADIATION EXPOSURE

The primary source of radiation exposure to the fluoroscopy staff is from scattered radiation from the patient. Scattered x-rays originate from the volume of tissue irradiated by the x-ray beam (structures within the field of view). Nearby radiation levels depend on C-arm orientation, technique factors, and patient size, but decrease rapidly with distance from the patient.

The operator and all who remain in the room during the exposure should always wear a lead apron. A 0.5-mm lead equivalent apron, which reduces the exposure by a factor of 50% or more over the diagnostic x-ray energy range, is recommended.[15] A wrap-around apron is necessary if the person's back is repeatedly turned toward the patient. In addition, staff members should always move away from the patient during x-ray beam activation if their immediate presence is not required. Extra care must be taken to ensure that all personnel are conscientious about the location of the C-arm and each adjusts their position appropriately so that the lead shield remains between themselves and the C-arm. In addition, the operator, even if wearing a lead apron, should always stand a minimum of 6 feet (2 m) from the x-ray tube during all exposures.

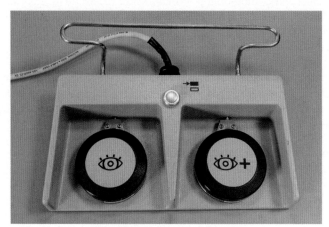

Fig. 15.92 Foot pedal controls.

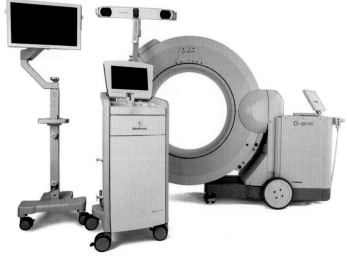

Fig. 15.93 O-arm imaging system. (Reprinted with the permission of Medtronic, Inc. © 2017.)

C-ARM ORIENTATION AND EXPOSURE PATTERNS
Vertical Posteroanterior Projection CR

If it is assumed that the patient is supine, keeping the C-arm posteroanterior (PA; the fluoroscopy tube is located below the patient, and the image intensifier is located above the patient) and directly perpendicular to the floor minimizes exposure to the neck and facial region (Fig. 15.94). If the C-arm is tilted as much as 30°, as shown in Fig. 15.95, the configuration of the exposure fields changes to increase exposure significantly to the upper body and facial region not shielded by the lead apron. **Studies have shown that even a 30° C-arm tilt will increase the dose to the face and neck region of an operator of average height who stands next to the C-arm by a factor of 4.**

Horizontal Projection CR

The configuration of the exposure fields with a horizontal beam is demonstrated in Fig. 15.96. Note that the **exposure region on the x-ray tube side of the patient is significantly larger** than that in the region near the intensifier tower. This should be an important consideration for the surgeon or other operator who may need to stay near the patient.

Vertical AP Projection CR

Occasionally, the technologist may be asked to reverse the C-arm, tube on top and image intensifier on bottom. This may provide the surgeon more room for manipulation; however, **this is not recommended due to a significant increase in exposure to the operator**, as shown in Fig. 15.97 (up to 100 times higher dose to the eyes of the operator).

Patient Dose

Modern fluoroscopic units produce images with an image intensifier (or flat panel detector) that captures the x-rays exiting the patient. The detector converts the time sequence of incident x-rays to a series of images displayed on the monitor. With manual technique, the image quality and brightness are adversely affected when the operator pans across tissues of different thickness and composition. For this reason, fluoroscopy is almost exclusively performed using automatic brightness control (ABC). Technical factors (e.g., kVp, mA, filtration, and/or pulse length) are then adjusted automatically to maintain image brightness at a constant, proper level.

The exposure rate depends on operational mode, field size, patient size, tissue composition, and ABC design. Attenuation of x-rays along the beam path influences the number of x-rays reaching the detector. The ABC compensates brightness loss caused by lower transmission of x-rays through the patient by generating more x-rays and/or producing more penetrating x-rays (reducing image contrast). The maximum exposure rate at 1 foot (30 cm) from the image receptor (IR) cannot exceed an air kerma rate of 88 mGy/min, which equals an exposure rate of 10 R/min. In high-level fluoroscopy (HLF) mode, the maximum exposure rate at the same reference point cannot exceed 20 R/min, corresponding to an air kerma rate of 176 mGy/min. Generally, the entrance exposure rate to the patient is 1 to 3 R/min, but the ABC can boost the exposure rate to maximum for large patients.

Digital spot film acquires a single, static radiographic image of the structures of interest with a low radiation dose. This is an excellent dose reduction method to evaluate static spatial relationships or document the proper location of a device.

Gonadal shielding should be applied when the x-ray beam is directed toward the abdomen and pelvis if the presence of such shielding does not interfere with the examination.

Summary of Radiation Protection in Surgical Radiography

Sound radiation protection practices are important for protection of all personnel during mobile imaging, as already described. A summary of what this includes in the surgical setting follows.

TIME
Use of Intermittent Fluoroscopy

- Single-exposure capacity can greatly reduce fluoroscopy time.
- The image hold feature allows the last image to remain on the monitor.

Minimize Boost Exposures

The boost feature on most C-arms provides an improved and brighter image for the patient with a large body habitus, or thick anatomy. However, this feature increases radiation, primarily mA, which also increases exposure to the patient and surrounding surgical team by a factor of three to four times compared with standard fluoroscopy. Use the boost feature only when no other alternative or adjustment will improve the image.

DISTANCE
Vertical Alignment

Place the vertical alignment of the C-arm so the x-ray tube is away from the operator's head and neck region. This is achieved by placing the x-ray tube beneath the OR table, thus reducing the dose to the head and neck region of the surgical team. (See p. 604 for details of C-arm orientation and exposure patterns.)

Minimize Distance between Anatomy and Image Receptor

Reducing the distance between the anatomy and the image intensifier creates a brighter, sharper, and less magnified image, with a reduction in radiation to the immediate area.

SURGICAL TEAM RADIATION PROTECTION SHIELDING
Protective Lead Aprons

- Provide aprons for all personnel.
- Wear a thyroid collar.
- Secure aprons tightly to prevent them from touching the sterile field or sterile personnel.
- Clean aprons weekly or as needed with a liquid-type cleaner.
- Intermittently check aprons for cracks in the lead lining.

COMMUNICATION
Coordination of Exposure with Surgical Team

Coordinate exposures among the anesthesiologist, surgeon, and surgical team. For studies such as operative cholangiography, injection of contrast media, and suspension of patient breathing, x-ray exposure must be closely coordinated among team members.

The technologist should clearly announce "x-ray" or "x-ray on" before initiating an exposure to enable nonessential staff to leave the area or get behind lead shields. Announcing "x-ray off" communicates to nonessential staff that it is safe to return to the area.

Monitor Personal Dosimetry Report

Technologists who frequently perform C-arm procedures should closely monitor their personal dosimetry. Personnel dosimeters must be worn at collar level outside of protective apron. If they discover excessively high levels, they may have to modify their work habits and discuss strategies to reduce dose levels with the department radiation safety officer.

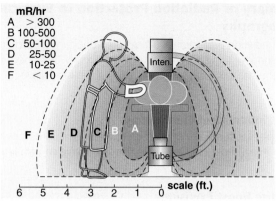

Fig. 15.94 Exposure levels—CR vertical, PA projection, intensifier on top (least exposure to operator).

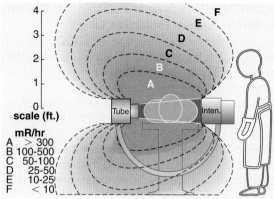

Fig. 15.96 Exposure patterns and levels—CR horizontal (least exposure at intensifier side). (Adapted from Technical reference, Salt Lake City, Utah, 1996, OEC Medical Systems; and Geise RA, Hunter DW: Personnel exposure during fluoroscopy procedures, *Postgrad Radiol* 8:162–173, 1988.)

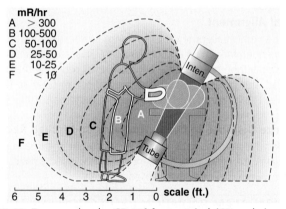

Fig. 15.95 Exposure levels—CR 30° from vertical (CR angle increases exposure to operator). (Adapted from Technical reference, Salt Lake City, Utah, 1996, OEC Medical Systems; and Geise RA, Hunter DW: Personnel exposure during fluoroscopy procedures, *Postgrad Radiol* 8:162–173, 1988.)

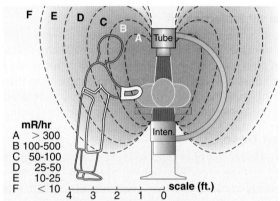

Fig. 15.97 Exposure levels, AP projection (tube on top) (not recommended). (Adapted from Technical reference, Salt Lake City, Utah, 1996, OEC Medical Systems; and Geise RA, Hunter DW: Personnel exposure during fluoroscopy procedures, *Postgrad Radiol* 8:162–173, 1988.)

Surgical Asepsis Principles

Unfortunately, it is impossible to remove all infectious organisms from the OR. Surgical asepsis consists of the practice and procedures used to **minimize the levels of infectious agents present in the surgical environment.** Through the use of safe practices, wearing proper surgical attire, and ensuring that care is taken around the surgical incision, the patient's exposure to these infectious agents is greatly minimized. This requires a clear separation of sterile items and areas from nonsterile areas in the surgical suite (Fig. 15.98).

To reduce the risk for infection of the patient during surgery, the following principles of surgical asepsis must be followed:

1. Only sterile items are allowed within the sterile field.
2. If the sterility of an object is in doubt, it must be considered nonsterile.
3. If a sterile drape or cover is touched by a nonsterile object or person, it must be considered contaminated.
4. Nonsterile personnel must not come into contact with a sterile barrier, drape, surgical instrument, or sterile personnel.
5. Any contaminated sterile drape or cover must be reported and replaced by sterile personnel.
6. Sterile gowns are considered sterile from the shoulder to the level of the sterile field, and at the sleeve from the cuff to just above the elbow.
7. OR tables are considered sterile only at the level of the tabletop.
8. Only sterile personnel can touch sterile items.

Surgical Suite Environment

The typical surgical suite has two general regions known as **sterile** and **nonsterile** areas.

The **sterile** area includes the patient, surgical field, surgeon and surgical assistants, surgical equipment, tables, and carts. (In some facilities, the sterile area includes the area surrounding the sterile field, up to 1 foot wide.) Often, most of the sterile area is located to one side of the room, leaving the other side of the room available for necessary nonsterile personnel. **The technologist and the imaging equipment must not violate the sterile area.** Student technologists new to the OR must have a clear understanding of the differences between sterile and nonsterile areas. When in doubt, ask the radiologic technologist, CST, or circulator for clarification. If the sterile area is violated, which may contaminate the instruments used for the procedure, the technologist must report this event immediately. Because the violation may have not been noticed by the surgical team, the technologist has a critical responsibility to report it. In most cases, additional sterile drapes or a new set of sterile instruments can be used to create a safe and sterile environment again.

The **nonsterile** area is where the technologist and other nonsterile surgical personnel, such as the anesthesiologist and the circulator, is located. The technologist can safely stand and operate imaging equipment within this area. For select procedures, a plastic drape or shower curtain may be erected to indicate the dividing point between sterile and nonsterile areas.

IMAGING EQUIPMENT/PERSONNEL AND STERILE FIELDS

C-Arm

C-arm use in surgical settings requires special attention in maintaining sterile fields. Vertical alignment with the intensifier on top often causes it to be placed over open incisions. Three basic approaches are commonly used to maintain a sterile field.

The first (and most commonly used) method involves draping the image intensifier, x-ray tube, and C-arm with a sterile cloth and/or bags, with a tension band or adhesive tape holding the cloth or

plastic cover in place (Fig. 15.99). Another type of image intensifier cover, called a snap cover, has a band that makes a snapping sound when it is released into position (Fig. 15.100). These types of covers also make it possible for the technologist (with guidance from the surgeon) to position the image intensifier precisely as needed over the sterile surgical site for correct centering.

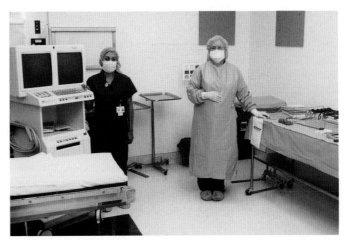

Fig. 15.98 Surgical asepsis—separation of sterile and nonsterile areas.

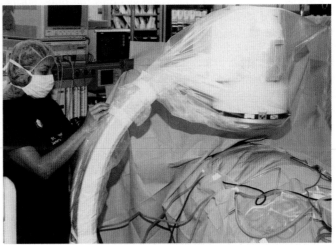

Fig. 15.99 Draping the C-arm with sterile plastic C-arm cover.

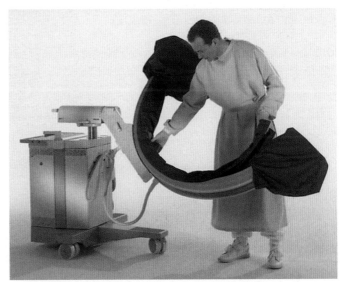

Fig. 15.100 Draping the C-arm and intensifier with snap cover. (Courtesy Philips Healthcare, Andover, MA.)

A second approach is to drape the patient (or surgery site) temporarily with an additional sterile cloth before the undraped C-arm is positioned over the anatomy. Once a satisfactory image has been obtained and the C-arm removed, the sterile cloth (or drape) is then removed from the patient and discarded. This process is repeated with a new (unused) sterile cloth if it becomes necessary to use the C-arm again. This approach is used in cases in which the physician does not need to interact with the surgical site during fluoroscopy or when snap covers are not available.

The third method of maintaining a sterile area uses a shower curtain. Hip pinnings or femoral roddings require frequent manipulation of the C-arm between PA and lateral projections to the surgical incision, making these procedures ideal for the shower curtain. A long horizontal metal bar attached to two vertical suspending rods is placed along the lateral longitudinal axis of the affected side (Fig. 15.101). A large, sterile, clear plastic sheet (called a shower curtain) is suspended from the horizontal bar, which is positioned about 3 feet (1 m) above the patient. A special opening in the middle of the plastic is attached with a second adhesive strip to the lateral aspect of the hip–proximal femur and is used for access to the incision. The curtain forms a sterile barrier between the physician and patient as the C-arm is positioned for a standard PA and horizontal beam lateral hip from the nonaffected side of the patient.

IMAGE RECEPTORS

When an IR must be used within the sterile field, it must be placed in a sterile plastic cover. Keep in mind that **only the outer surface of the cover is sterile.** The inner surface of the cover is nonsterile and comes in contact with the IR. The procedure for placing and removing an IR in a sterile cover is as follows:

1. Sterile surgical personnel hold the plastic cover open, with the top cover folded over to maintain sterility of the outer surface and their gloved hands.
2. The technologist carefully slips the IR into the cover, ensuring that the IR touches only the inner surface of the plastic cover (Fig. 15.102).
3. Surgical personnel wrap the top of the cover over and secure it.
4. The surgical staff, with verbal directions from the radiologic technologist, places the covered IR in the necessary location and the exposure is taken.
5. Once the exposure has been taken, the surgical staff removes the covered IR and hands it to the radiologic technologist.
6. The technologist removes the IR from the plastic cover by sliding the IR onto a nonsterile table or surface, with care taken not to transfer any possible body fluids from the outer cover of the plastic bag, to dispose of the IR cover in the appropriate receptacle, and to remove gloves (Fig. 15.103).
7. The image is processed.

NOTE: The technologist must wear nonsterile gloves when handling the cover because of possible blood or other body fluid exposure.

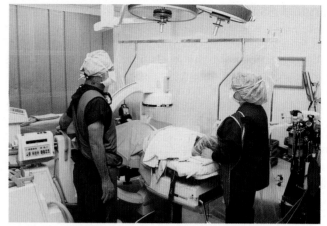

Fig. 15.101 Shower curtain, view from the technologist's (nonsterile) perspective

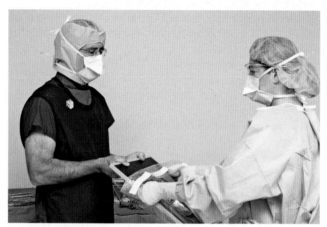

Fig. 15.102 Procedure for placing IR into sterile cover.

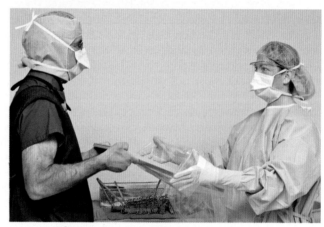

Fig. 15.103 Removing IR from sterile cover.

Surgical Attire

The technologist must change from normal work dress into the appropriate surgical attire before entering the OR. Because the technologist's typical uniform may pose a health concern for the operative patient, proper surgical attire must be worn in all restricted and nonrestricted areas in surgery (Fig. 15.104). Proper surgical attire includes the following items.

SCRUBS

Even if surgical scrubs are normally worn in the general radiology department, the radiologic technologist must change into approved surgical scrubs. Surgical scrubs should be made of a low lint-producing material, which minimizes bacterial shedding. Two-piece scrubs should fit properly, with the top tucked in at the waist. The pant legs of the scrub bottoms must not drag on the floor. In some facilities, scrub jackets are also available. Surgical scrubs must be changed following the procedure and laundered by the hospital. If soiled with blood, perspiration, or food, scrubs must be changed before the wearer reenters the surgical suite.

SCRUB COVER

Scrub covers are button-up or snapped covers worn by the technologist between procedures. They are designed to prevent soiling or cross-contamination of the scrubs while the technologist is outside the surgical suite. Scrub covers must be removed before the technologist enters the surgical suite.

HEAD COVER

A proper-fitting head cover must be worn before entry into a surgical area. The bouffant and hood types of covers are preferred because they cover the head best. All hair must be tucked inside the head covers. The hood type of cover must be worn by the technologist with a beard or other facial hair. Head covers must be discarded immediately after use and changed for each procedure.

SHOE COVERS

Shoe covers are designed to keep the shoes clean and decrease the quantity of soil and bacteria tracked into the surgical suite. They must be changed if they become soiled or torn. They should be worn even in the presurgical and recovery areas.

SHOES

Because of the volume of fluid and presence of sharps in the OR, soft cloth shoes should not be worn. A durable shoe with plenty of support and closed hard toe and heel will minimize injuries caused by falling objects, needles, and image receptors.

MASKS

A surgical mask must be worn to reduce the dispersal of microbial droplets from the technologist during surgery. Masks also will reduce the risk that pathogenic organisms present in the surgical suite may be inhaled by the technologist. A single high-filtration mask is recommended for most procedures. This mask has a pliable nose stripe and two sets of ties to secure it. The nose stripe provides a contoured fit for the wearer and helps prevent fogging for eyeglass wearers. **Masks must be changed between procedures or when moisture is detected on the outside of the mask.**

PROTECTIVE EYEWEAR

If the technologist is present during a procedure in which blood, body fluids, or tissue debris may strike the eye region, Occupational Safety and Health Administration (OSHA)–approved protective eyewear must be worn. However, this equipment will not be necessary for most of the radiographic procedures performed in surgery. In the angiography suite, specialized lead eyewear is sometimes worn to protect the eyes of the wearer from long-term exposure to the x-ray field.

NONSTERILE GLOVES

When handling contaminated IRs or soiled IR covers, or when cleaning equipment after procedures have been performed, the technologist must wear nonsterile gloves. Once the gloves are removed, the hands must be washed.

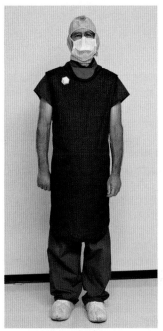

Fig. 15.104 Surgical attire—scrubs, mask, shoe covers, head cover, nonsterile gloves, and protective apron.

SURGICAL RADIOGRAPHIC PROCEDURES

Biliary Tract Procedures

OPERATIVE (IMMEDIATE) CHOLANGIOGRAPHY

Overview of Procedure

First performed in 1932, the operative or immediate cholangiography is performed during surgery to demonstrate anatomy of the biliary ductal system, drainage into the duodenum, and any residual stones in the biliary ducts. In many cases, the patient has a previous history of gallstones and the surgeon may be concerned about residual stones remaining undetected in one of the biliary ducts.

The operative cholangiography may be performed before or following surgical removal of the gallbladder. The surgeon places a small catheter into the biliary ducts and injects iodinated contrast media into the ducts. Once respiration has been suspended, the technologist initiates exposure and produces images using mobile radiographic or C-arm equipment.

Equipment Used and Setup

C-arm Digital Fluoroscopic Cholangiography The C-arm should be set up and correctly oriented prior to the beginning of the procedure, with the monitors set up in clear view of the surgeon. The C-arm will be positioned in vertical alignment, with the x-ray tube beneath the table. A sterile drape or cover must be placed over the image intensifier, as shown in Fig. 15.105. Make sure that the C-arm is moved away from the surgical field until needed, and then place the image intensifier over the anatomy to be imaged. Coordinate all exposures with the surgeon and anesthesiologist.

Mobile Radiographic Cholangiography A conventional mobile radiographic unit also can be used for this procedure and should be brought into the surgical suite and positioned carefully near the surgical field. Once the surgical incision has been draped by the surgeon, the x-ray tube is brought in and centered over the anatomy. Often, the surgeon will indicate the centering point with a twist or mark on the sterile towel (Fig. 15.106). The IR is placed in the IR holder ("pizza pan") and is placed into a special slot under the surgical table that allows the IR and IR holder to slide under the surgical table until the appropriate location is reached. The IR and holder are placed into the table near the end of the table closest to the anesthesiologist. With the use of a handle, the IR is advanced until it is centered over the right upper quadrant of the abdomen. With an IR of 14 × 17 inches (35 × 43 cm), the top of the image receptor is just below the right axilla.

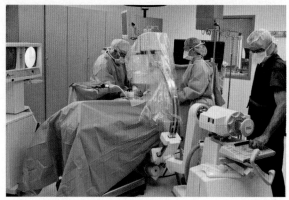

Fig. 15.105 C-arm–guided operative cholangiography.

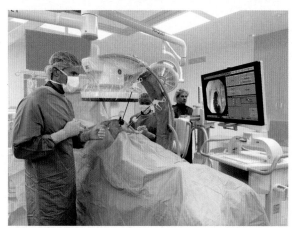

Fig. 15.106 Conventional mobile x-ray unit positioned for AP projection (centering point indicated by surgeon). (Courtesy GE Healthcare.)

LAPAROSCOPIC CHOLECYSTECTOMY

Laparoscopic cholecystectomy provides a less invasive approach for the removal of diseased gallbladders. The surgeon makes a small opening in the umbilicus and passes an endoscope into the abdominal cavity. This type of procedure has long been used for visual assessment of the abdomen to detect signs of pathology or trauma. It is referred to as a laparoscopic *(lap″-ah-ro-skop′-ik)* procedure. This technique has been modified so that cholecystectomy and cholangiography can be performed with a minimal amount of surgical trauma to the patient.

Advantages of Laparoscopy

There are three advantages of laparoscopy:
1. It can be performed as an outpatient procedure.
2. It is a minimally invasive procedure. Previous surgical techniques required the creation of a large opening to remove the gallbladder. This degree of invasive surgery required the patient to remain in the hospital for at least 2 days.
3. It involves a shorter hospital stay than other procedures, with reduced cost. Many patients who undergo the laparoscopic technique can return home the same day and, in some cases, can return to work in 2 to 3 days.

The laparoscopic cholecystectomy, however, is not suited for every patient. More complex disease processes or involved procedures may require the more traditional surgical approach.

Summary of Procedures for Operative and Laparoscopic Cholangiography

1. The technologist changes into surgical attire and ensures that the portable unit or C-arm is functional and clean. The C-arm should be set to the cine loop function, if available.
2. If a portable unit is used, a scout image is taken before the patient is surgically prepped. The distance that the IR is advanced from the head of the table is noted. A special ruler and tray setup may be used in positioning the IR.
3. The scout image is processed and exposure factors adjusted with the IR positioned correctly.
4. Once the surgeon places the catheter into the biliary ducts, the portable unit is again readied for another image or the C-arm is placed over the desired anatomy. Once the radiologic technologist is prepared to obtain images, and surgeon injects contrast media.
5. Images are obtained with the cooperation and synchronization of the surgeon, anesthesiologist, and technologist. The anesthesiologist controls the breathing of the patient. Some surgeons prefer to inject all the contrast and image after injection; others prefer to view the contrast filling the biliary ducts, moving to the hepatopancreatic sphincter, and spilling into the duodenum.
6. If the OR table is tilted for the oblique positions and a mobile unit is being used, the grid and IR are placed landscape (crosswise) to avoid objectionable grid cutoff.
7. Images are processed and may have to be reviewed by a radiologist. The technologist may convey a written report from the radiologist to the surgeon.

Images Obtained

At least two and preferably three radiographic images are obtained in slightly different positions. Each exposure is preceded by a fractional injection of contrast medium. Positions may include an **AP,** a **slight right posterior oblique (RPO),** and a **slight LPO.** The RPO is helpful in projecting the biliary ducts away from the spine, especially with a hyposthenic patient.

The C-arm may have to be tilted to project the biliary ducts away from the spine.

Anatomy Demonstrated

Contrast-enhanced biliary ducts, including the common bile duct, hepatic ducts, and cystic ducts, are shown (Fig. 15.107). If the cholangiography is performed before the gallbladder is removed, the gallbladder also will be enhanced. If stones or biliary duct stenosis is present, the opacity of the biliary ducts will be restricted.

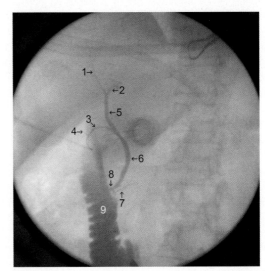

Fig. 15.107 Normal intraoperative cholangiogram. (1) Right hepatic duct; (2) left hepatic duct; (3) cystic duct; (4) two surgical clips holding the cholangio catheter in the cystic duct; (5) common hepatic duct; (6) common bile duct; (7) pancreatic duct; (8) ampulla of Vater; (9) duodenum. (From Massarweh NN, Flum DR. Role of intraoperative cholangiography in avoiding bile duct injury. *Journal of the American College of Surgeons* 204(4):656–664.)

Urinary Tract Procedures

RETROGRADE UROGRAPHY

Overview of Procedure

Retrograde urography is a nonfunctional examination of the urinary system during which contrast medium is introduced directly retrograde (backward, against the flow) into the pelvicalyceal system via catheterization by the urologist during a minor surgical procedure. Retrograde urography is nonfunctional because the patient's normal physiologic processes are not involved in the procedure. This procedure is frequently performed to determine the location of undetected calculi or other types of obstruction in the urinary system. The procedure may also be performed to study the renal pelvis and calyces for signs of infection or structural defect.

Equipment Used and Setup

The procedure usually is done as outpatient surgery in a dedicated urography room. The urography room generally contains a combination cystoscopic-radiographic table, which includes a dedicated x-ray tube (which may also house fluoroscopic capabilities), with a bucky tray built into the table. If such a table is not available, a mobile radiographic unit or C-arm may be used to image the urinary system. The patient is usually sedated or anesthetized for this examination. If the unit does not have fluoroscopy, conventional film-screen or digital imaging receptors are used for creating radiographs.

Summary of Procedure

1. The technologist changes into surgical attire and ensures that the unit (or portable unit or C-arm) is functional and clean.
2. The patient is placed in the modified lithotomy position, with the legs placed in stirrups, as illustrated in Fig. 15.108.
3. The urologist inserts a cystoscope through the urethra into the bladder. After examining the inside of the bladder, the urologist inserts ureteral catheters into one or both ureters. Ideally, the tip of each ureteral catheter is placed at the level of the renal pelvis.
4. After catheterization, a scout radiograph is exposed. The scout radiograph allows the technologist to check technique and positioning and the urologist to check catheter placement. Center to the level of the iliac crest when using a 14 × 17-inch (35 × 43-cm) IR, portrait alignment.
5. The second radiograph in a common retrograde urographic series is a **pyelogram.** The urologist injects 3 to 5 mL of contrast media directly through the catheter into the renal pelvis of one or both kidneys. Respiration is suspended immediately after injection, and the exposure is made.
6. The third and final radiograph in a common series is a **ureterogram.** The head end of the table may be elevated for this radiograph. The urologist withdraws the catheters and simultaneously injects contrast material into one or both ureters. The urologist indicates when the exposure should be made.

This examination is used to visualize the internal structures of one or both kidneys and ureters directly.

Anatomy Demonstrated

A retrograde **urogram** (Fig. 15.109) on the right side, with catheter in place, best demonstrates the renal pelvis and contrast-filled major and minor calyces. The left side shows the left ureter after the left catheter has been withdrawn; therefore, this is called a **ureterogram.**

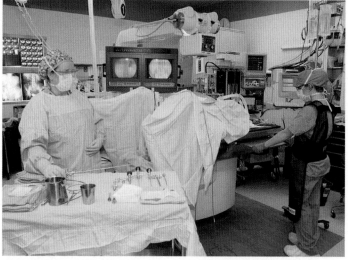

Fig. 15.108 Modified lithotomy position for retrograde urography. (From Long BW, Rollins J, Smith B. *Merrill's atlas of radiographic positioning and procedures,* ed 14, St. Louis, 2019, Elsevier.)

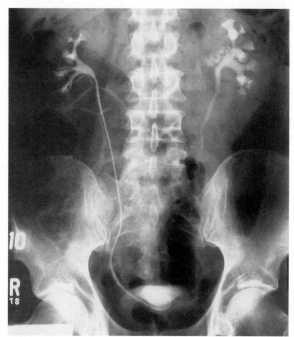

Fig. 15.109 Retrograde urogram—catheter in right ureter, left catheter withdrawn.

Orthopedic Procedures

Orthopedic procedures performed in surgery are intended to reestablish the length, shape, and alignment of fractured bones and joints or to restore function and range of motion of joints affected by trauma or disease. Radiography is required for many orthopedic surgical procedures to provide guidance to the surgeon while reducing fractures, inserting various orthopedic devices, or inserting stabilizing rods in long bones.

Technologists have an important role and responsibility during these procedures. They operate the technology that provides the surgeon with "eyes" or vision during the procedure. C-arm or mobile radiographic units are used extensively during most orthopedic procedures.

ORTHOPEDIC SURGICAL TERMINOLOGY AND CONCEPTS

The following terms, procedures, and concepts are common in orthopedic surgery. Knowledge of these terms is essential because they will be used frequently to describe various orthopedic surgical procedures.

Closed Reduction

Fracture fragments are realigned by manipulation and are immobilized by a cast or splint. A closed reduction is a nonsurgical procedure. The fracture site of the patient is not cut open during the procedure; however, small pins are sometimes placed through the skin of the patient into the proper location and are left in place or later removed.

Open Reduction

For severe fractures with significant displacement or fragmentation, a surgical procedure is required. The fracture site is exposed, and a variety of screws, plates, or rods are inserted as needed to maintain alignment of the bony fragments until new bone growth can take place. This surgical procedure is called an **ORIF.** Images obtained from a C-arm unit or from a mobile radiographic unit are frequently used to guide the orthopedic surgeon during these surgical procedures.

Internal Fixation

During open reduction of fractures, a variety of compression plates, screws, pins, intramedullary rods, nails, or wires are applied to reduce or realign the fracture (Fig. 15.110). Based on the age and condition of the patient, the type of procedure performed, and the extent of the fracture, these devices are left in place and the skin is closed around the devices. In some minor surgeries, these fixation devices may be removed later.

External Fixation

The use of an external fracture-stabilizing device permits bone healing without the immediate requirement for internal fixation. External fixators can also be used in conjunction with internal fixation procedures. Indications for external fixation include severe open fractures, comminuted closed fractures, arthrodesis, infected joints, and major alignment and length deficits. As with internal fixators, several varieties of external fixators are available to aid the surgeon. The Ilizarov device (Fig. 15.111) is a prime example of an external fixator used to correct a length deficit. Through a process of tension stress and distraction, bone length can increase over time through new bone formation. A second external fixation device used for alignment stabilization of the pelvis is shown in Fig. 15.112.

Intramedullary Fixation

Intramedullary rods and nails are inserted within the shaft of long bones to stabilize fractures (Fig. 15.113). This technique is popular for reducing shaft fractures of the humerus, tibia, and femur. In some cases, the intramedullary rods are a better option than the use of compression plates and screws for reducing midshaft fractures. Intramedullary fixation devices minimize the amount of tissue exposed during surgery, decrease surgical and healing time, and reduce opportunities for postsurgical infection.

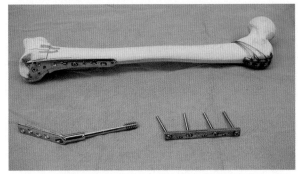

Fig. 15.110 Internal fixation devices.

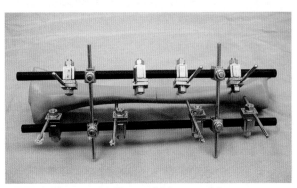

Fig. 15.111 Ilizarov tibial external fixator.

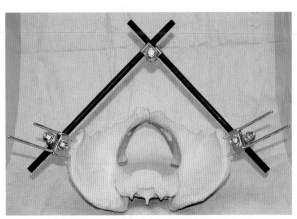

Fig. 15.112 Pelvic external fixator.

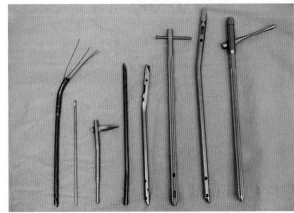

Fig. 15.113 Examples of intramedullary fixators—intramedullary rods and nails.

15

HIP FRACTURES (PINNING, OPEN REDUCTION WITH INTERNAL FIXATION)

Proximal femur (hip) fractures are classified according to their anatomic location. Common hip fractures include **femoral neck** fractures, **intertrochanteric** fractures, and **subtrochanteric** fractures. Each of these fractures can be subclassified (Fig. 15.114). These fractures require an ORIF procedure. Sometimes these ORIF procedures are distinguished by the types of internal fixators used. For a hip pinning, the procedure generally involves the use of long screws for nondisplaced femoral neck fractures (Fig. 15.115).

In a hip ORIF, a longer fixator is placed on the lateral side of the fractured hip and secured by inserting screws through the fixator into the neck and head of the femur, followed by smaller screws below the trochanters that traverse the shaft of the femur. The goals of these surgeries are to reduce and stabilize the fracture and restore use of the lower limb with minimal loss of blood. Internal fixation devices for hip fractures require the use of cannulated screws, compression screws, lag screw and plate combinations, and pins. During the operative procedure, the patient is placed on a special fracture (orthopedic) table that permits traction of the involved limb and fluoroscopy during the procedure (Fig. 15.116).

Based on the type of fracture and fixation device to be used, the fracture first is reduced through traction and manipulation. An incision then is made at the level of the greater trochanter, and the guide pins are inserted through the fracture, thus stabilizing it. For femoral neck fractures, once the guide pins are aligned, large cannulated screws or some other type of internal fixation pin-type device is inserted through the fracture (see Fig. 15.115A to F).

Fluoroscopy is used throughout the procedure to verify the position and location of guide pins and the internal fixator. In some cases, the physician may order a postoperative image of the hip and prosthetic device to verify final alignment of the fracture.

Imaging Equipment Used and Setup

With the fracture table in place, an isolation drape or shower curtain is erected that essentially divides the room into sterile and nonsterile sections and allows easy access and movement of the C-arm outside the sterile field (Fig. 15.117). The C-arm must be free to move easily from a PA to a horizontal beam lateral position. Although the C-arm is located outside the sterile field, a nonsterile bag should cover the x-ray tube (remember that the x-ray tube is located beneath the patient) to prevent blood and povidone-iodine (Betadine) from leaking onto it. The C-arm monitors must be set to allow easy viewing by the surgeon. This generally requires placing the monitors to one side of the surgeon, just behind the shower curtain, where the images can be viewed by the surgeon and technologist without contamination of the sterile area.

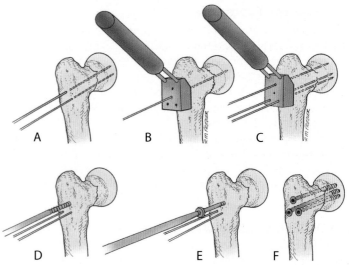

Fig. 15.115 Internal fixation of fractured hip with cannulated screws inserted over guidewires—cannulated screw fixation for nondisplaced femoral neck fractures. (From Rothrock JC. *Alexander's care of the patient in surgery*, ed 16, St. Louis, 2019, Elsevier.)

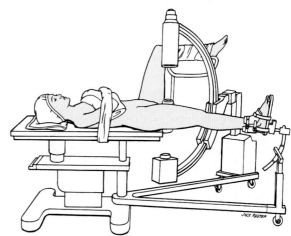

Fig. 15.116 Fracture orthopedic table with C-arm in position. (Adapted from Rothrock JC. *Alexander's care of the patient in surgery*, ed 16, St. Louis, 2019, Elsevier.)

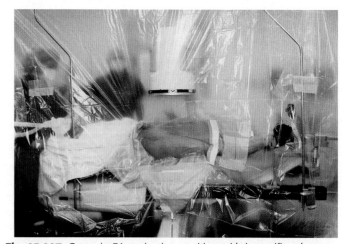

Fig. 15.117 C-arm in PA projection position with intensifier above and tube below, and shower curtain in position separating sterile from nonsterile areas.

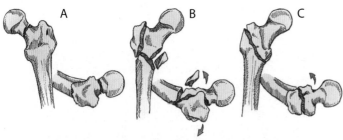

Fig. 15.114 Proximal femur fractures. A, Femoral neck. B, Comminuted subtrochanteric. C, Intertrochanteric. (From Rothrock JC. *Alexander's care of the patient in surgery*, ed 16, St. Louis, 2019, Elsevier.)

Lateral Hip C-Arm Projection

The surgeon will ask the technologist to move the C-arm from its PA position into a lateral hip C-arm projection. This can be accomplished in two ways. One is by sliding the C-arm underneath the affected leg until the x-ray tube is located superiorly and the image intensifier inferiorly (Fig. 15.118). This is not the most desirable manner of placing the C-arm because it increases radiation exposure to the head and neck of the surgeon; however, it may be requested because it is the easiest and quickest way to obtain a lateral hip projection during the surgical case. All images in this projection should have short exposure times, according to the ALARA principle.

The recommended alignment of the C-arm during a lateral projection hip pinning is to place the x-ray tube inferiorly and the image intensifier superiorly and exteriorly above the hip (Fig. 15.119). This alignment will produce the clearest image of the hip while reducing exposure to the head and neck of the surgeon and surgical personnel (see p. 604 in this draft for radiation exposure patterns for the C-arm).

Summary of Procedure

1. The technologist changes into surgical attire and ensures that the mobile unit is functional and clean.
2. After the patient has been sedated and placed on the fracture table, the fracture is reduced and the lower limb is placed in traction to maintain proper alignment of the fracture.
3. Fluoroscopy is used to verify alignment in both PA and lateral perspectives.
4. An incision is made just below the greater trochanter.
5. Guide pins are inserted through the fracture site. The location and position of guide pins are verified with fluoroscopy as needed by the surgeon.
6. A bone reamer is used to provide a channel for a screw or other internal fixator device.
7. A cannulated, lag, or compression screw assembly is inserted over the guide pins. The position of the screws is verified with fluoroscopy in the PA and lateral perspectives.
8. Guide pins are removed and traction is released.
9. The surgical wound is closed.
10. If postoperative radiographs are requested, include the entire orthopedic prosthesis for all projections (Figs. 15.120 and 15.121). This may require an adaptation of positioning principles to ensure that the entire orthopedic prosthesis is included on a single image.

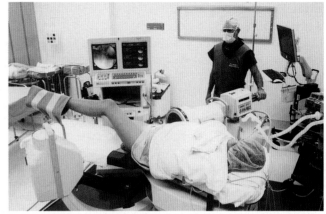

Fig. 15.119 Recommended C-arm alignment for lateral right hip imaging.

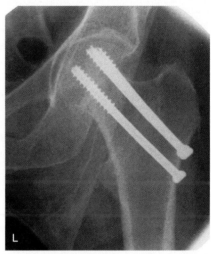

Fig. 15.120 Postoperative radiographic images of hip pinning showing internal fixation devices in place—AP projection. (From Frank E, Long B, Smith B. *Merrill's atlas of radiographic positioning and procedures*, ed 12, St. Louis, 2012, Mosby.)

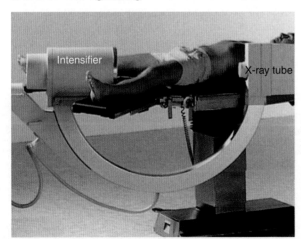

Fig. 15.118 Alternative C-arm alignment if requested by surgeon; not recommended because of increased radiation exposure pattern at tube end. (Courtesy Philips Healthcare, Andover, MA.))

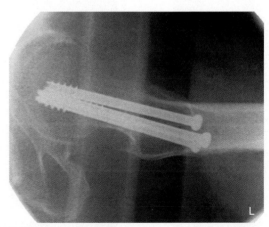

Fig. 15.121 Postoperative radiographic images of hip pinning showing internal fixation devices in place—lateral projection. (From Frank E, Long B, Smith B. *Merrill's atlas of radiographic positioning and procedures*, ed 12, St. Louis, 2012, Mosby.)

Spinal Procedures
LAMINECTOMY

Laminectomy is a surgical procedure performed to alleviate pain caused by neural impingement. This surgery is designed to remove a small portion of the bone or herniated disk material impinging on the nerve root. The surgery is intended to give the nerve root more space by removing the source of impingement or irritation. Based on the number of vertebrae on which the surgeon operates during the laminectomy, an additional procedure called a **spinal fusion,** which uses rods, plates, and screws to stabilize the surgically altered vertebrae, may be necessary (Figs. 15.122 and 15.123).

Interbody fusion devices, or cages, are another alternative to traditional spinal fusion or the use of pedicle screws to stabilize the vertebrae. **Interbody fusion cages** are titanium cages filled with bone that are inserted between the vertebral bodies to maintain disk space height and fuse the joint, thereby eliminating abnormal movement (Fig. 15.124).

A laminectomy is also effective in decreasing pain and improving function for patients with lumbar spinal stenosis. **Spinal stenosis** is a condition that primarily afflicts older patients; it is caused by degenerative changes that result in enlargement of the facet joints. The enlarged joints then place pressure on the nerves, which may be effectively relieved with a lumbar laminectomy.

A laminectomy can be performed on the cervical or lumbar region. Cervical laminectomy is performed to remove bony obstructions such as bone spurs (osteophytes) and herniated disk materials that cause pain by impinging on the spinal cord or spinal nerves in the cervical region. Lumbar laminectomy is performed for a myriad of reasons, including bony obstructions, stenosis, and spinal cord impingement.

Equipment Used and Setup

The laminectomy may require the use of C-arm or mobile radiographic units. The roles of radiography are to confirm the correct level (or vertebrae) for the laminectomy and provide fluoroscopic guidance if orthopedic plates and/or screws are used during surgery. The C-arm must be free to move easily from an AP or PA to a horizontal beam lateral position (Figs. 15.125 and 15.126). A sterile drape is placed over the image intensifier; a nonsterile bag should cover the x-ray tube to prevent blood and Betadine from leaking onto it. When the x-ray tube is moved to the horizontal beam lateral position, it may be covered by a sterile drape because this generally places the x-ray tube near the sterile field. C-arm monitors must be set to allow easy viewing by the surgeon.

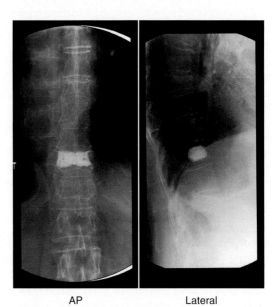
AP   Lateral
Fig. 15.124 Interbody fusion device—AP and lateral projections.

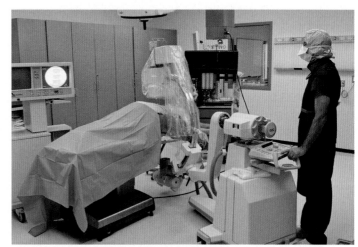
Fig. 15.125 AP projection (patient prone, tube below) for lumbar laminectomy.

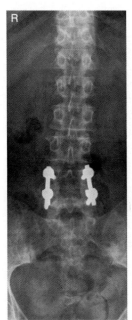
Fig. 15.122 Lumbar laminectomy-fusion—AP projection.

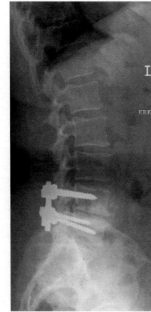
Fig. 15.123 Lumbar laminectomy-fusion—lateral projection.

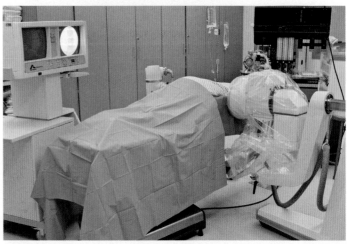
Fig. 15.126 Lateral projection in position for lumbar laminectomy.

Summary of Procedure

Cervical procedure (anterior approach) The patient is placed in a supine position with the arms drawn down by the sides of the body. The arms may be placed in traction to ensure visibility of the lower cervical vertebrae.

1. The technologist changes into surgical attire and ensures the portable unit or the C-arm is functional and clean.
2. A needle is placed at the level of the laminectomy. The correct vertebral level is verified by C-arm fluoroscopy in both AP and lateral perspectives. A mobile radiographic unit may also be used to confirm correct needle placement by obtaining a horizontal beam lateral projection of the cervical spine. Visualization of the entire spine is necessary for the surgeon to count the number of vertebrae correctly and determine the correct level (vertebral) at which the procedure should be performed.
3. The C-arm must be parallel to the vertebrae to avoid distortion of visible structures.
4. Cervical plates and screws may be used during the procedure to stabilize the vertebrae. C-arm fluoroscopy may be used as needed to guide placement of the orthopedic appliances.

Lumbar procedure (posterior approach) The patient is prone with a bolster under the abdomen to flex the spine. The arms usually are above the head on arm boards.

1. The technologist changes into surgical attire and ensures that the portable unit or C-arm is functional and clean.
2. A needle is placed at the level of the laminectomy. The correct vertebral level is verified by C-arm fluoroscopy in both AP and lateral perspectives. A mobile radiographic unit may also be used to confirm correct needle placement by obtaining a horizontal beam lateral projection of the lumbar spine. Visualization of the entire spine is necessary for the surgeon to correctly count the number of vertebrae and determine the correct level (vertebral) at which the procedure should be performed.
3. The C-arm must be parallel to the vertebrae to avoid distortion of visible structures.
4. Pedicle screws, interbody fusion cages, rods, and other appliances may be used during the procedure. C-arm fluoroscopy may be used as needed to assist with the placement of orthopedic appliances.

Anatomy demonstrated The spine in the PA-AP and lateral perspectives at the desired level within the entire vertebral (cervical or lumbar) column is seen. The total vertebrae, including the spinous processes, must be demonstrated.

Thoracic Procedures
PACEMAKER INSERTION

More than 500,000 Americans have an implantable permanent **pacemaker** device. A pacemaker implantation is performed under local or general anesthesia in a hospital by a surgeon assisted by a cardiologist. An insulated wire called a *lead* is inserted into an incision below the clavicle and is guided through a large vein into the chambers of the heart. These electrodes stimulate the heart muscle, causing it to beat at a predetermined rate. This process is referred to as *pacing* of the heart.

Electrodes often are inserted through a vein in the arm or chest and are advanced into the right ventricle under fluoroscopic guidance. The pulse generator or battery that provides the electrical sensation to control the heartbeat may be external (temporary) or may be inserted into the superficial tissues of the thoracic wall.

Equipment Used and Setup

A pacemaker or other line insertion procedure can be performed in the surgical suite, outpatient surgery suite, or radiology department. The use of fluoroscopy is essential during the insertion of electrodes into the right ventricle of the heart.

C-arm mobile fluoroscopy is used in the surgical suite (Fig. 15.127). The C-arm must be free to move easily from a PA to a horizontal beam lateral position. A sterile drape is placed over the image intensifier. C-arm monitors must be set to allow easy viewing by the cardiologist or surgeon.

Summary of Procedure—Transvenous Approach

1. The technologist changes into surgical attire and ensures that the C-arm is functional and clean.
2. Venotomy is performed (vein is accessed).
3. Under fluoroscopic guidance, the electrode is advanced through the vein into the right atrium, through the tricuspid valve, and into the right **ventricle.** The tip of the electrode is advanced until it reaches the right ventricular apex.
4. A pulse generator is inserted into the chest wall.

Once the procedure is complete, the patient's vital signs are monitored.

A postoperative AP or PA chest x-ray is taken to ensure that the pacemaker and leads are properly positioned. In this example, the patient must be positioned as upright as possible to confirm proper positioning of the lead wires (Figs. 15.128 and 15.129).

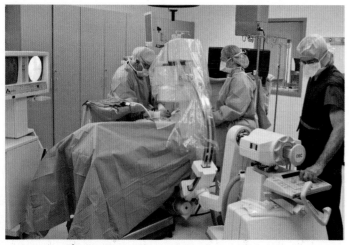

Fig. 15.127 Radiography in the surgical suite.

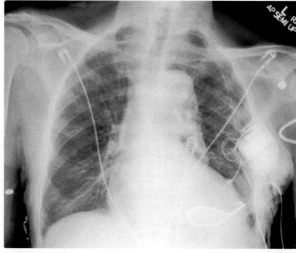

Fig. 15.128 PA chest with pacemaker in place. (From Jaroszewski DE et. al. Nontraditional surgical approaches for implantation of pacemaker and cardioverter defibrillator systems in patients with limited venous access. *The Annals of Thoracic Surgery* 88(1):112–116.)

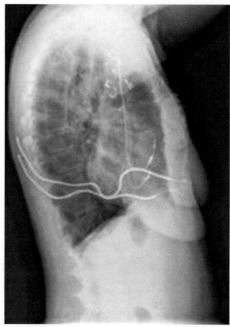

Fig. 15.129 Lateral chest with pacemaker in place. (From Jaroszewski DE et. al. Nontraditional surgical approaches for implantation of pacemaker and cardioverter defibrillator systems in patients with limited venous access. *The Annals of Thoracic Surgery* 88(1):112–116.)

Glossary of Surgical Abbreviations, Terminology, and Procedures

ACL Anterior cruciate ligament

Arthrodesis *(ar-thro-de'-sis)* Stiffening of a joint by operative means

Arthropathy *(ar"-throp'-a-the)* Any disease that affects a joint

Arthroplasty *(ar'-thro-plas-te)* Creation of an artificial joint to correct ankylosis

Asepsis *(a-sep'-sis)* A state of sterility; condition in which living pathogens are absent

Cancellous screw Orthopedic screw designed to enter and fix porous and spongy bone

Cannulated screw Large screw used for internal fixation of non-displaced fractures of proximal femur

Cardiac pacemaker An artificial regulator for cardiac rate and rhythm

Cerclage wire Orthopedic wire that tightens around fracture site to reduce shortening of limb

Cesium *(se'-ze-um)* **implants** The use of radioactive cesium in the treatment of certain malignancies, including prostate cancer

Cholecystectomy *(ko"-le-sis-tek'-to-me)* Surgical removal of gallbladder

Closed reduction Procedure in which bone fragments are reduced manually without surgical intervention

Cortical screw Narrow orthopedic screw designed to enter and fix cortical bone

CR Closed reduction (cast or traction)

Cystoscope *(sis'-to-skop)* Lighted tubular endoscope used for examination of the urinary bladder

DHS Dynamic hip screw

Dynamic compression plate Screw and plate combination used to apply forces through the fracture site; used commonly for long bone shaft fractures in which stress may be great

ESWL (extracorporeal shock wave lithotripsy) Electrohydraulic shock waves used to break apart calcifications in the urinary system

EX-FIX External fixation

Fracture (orthopedic) table A special OR table used for hip pinnings and other orthopedic procedures to provide traction to the involved limb and allow fluoroscopy to be performed during the procedure

Hip pinning Surgical procedure designed to reduce proximal femoral fractures through the use of various internal fixation devices

HTO High tibial osteotomy

Ilizarov technique Procedure in which a special external fixator is used to lengthen long bones as treatment for severe fracture or congenital deformity

IM nail Intramedullary nail

Interbody bone fusion device Titanium or other alloy cage filled with bone and inserted between the vertebral bodies to maintain disk space height and permit fusion of the intervertebral joint

Intramedullary rod A flexible or rigid device placed within the medullary cavity to reduce a fracture or stabilize a diseased long bone

Kirschner *(kirsh'-ner)* **wire (K-wire)** Unthreaded (smooth) or threaded metallic wire used to reduce fractures of the wrist (carpals) and individual bones of the hands and feet; also may be used for skeletal traction

Laminectomy *(lam"-i-nek'-to-me)* A surgical procedure performed to alleviate pain caused by neural impingement by removing an aspect of the lamina in the vertebral arch

Laminotomy *(lam"-i-not'-o-me)* Surgical opening into one or more laminae of the vertebral arch

Laparoscopic *(lap"-ah-ro-skop'-ik)* **cholecystectomy** Use of a special endoscopic device to visualize and assist with surgical removal of the gallbladder

Lithotripsy *(lith'-o-trip-se)* Crushing of calcification in the renal pelvis, ureter, or urinary bladder by mechanical force or sound waves

Microdiskectomy *(mi"-kro-dis-kek'-to-me)* Microsurgical procedure performed on the spine to remove bony fragments or disk material that may be causing neural impingement

Neural impingement A condition in which bony changes or a herniated disk produces impingement of the spinal nerves that pass through the vertebral arch of the vertebra

Open reduction of fracture fragments through surgical intervention

Operative (immediate) cholangiography Radiographic procedure performed during surgery to visualize and locate undetected stones or obstructions within the biliary ducts

ORIF Open reduction with internal fixation

PCL Posterior cruciate ligament

Prosthesis *(pros-the'-sis)* Fabricated (artificial) substitute for a diseased or missing anatomic part

Reduce To align two bone fragments in the correct position as treatment for a fracture, as applied in orthopedic medicine

Retrograde urography A nonfunctional examination of the urinary system during which contrast medium is introduced directly retrograde (backward, against the flow) into the pelvicalyceal system via catheterization by a urologist during a minor surgical procedure

Semitubular plate Flexible and thin orthopedic plate used to fix and connect fractures

Shower curtain An isolation drape that separates the sterile field from the nonsterile environment; often used to permit the use of C-arm fluoroscopy during a hip pinning procedure

Spinal fusion Surgical fusion of one vertebra to another, which stabilizes them following laminectomy or as treatment for a degenerative condition or fracture

Spinal stenosis Condition caused by degenerative changes that result in enlargement of the facet joints, which often leads to impingement of the spinal nerves that pass by them

Strike-through Soaking of moisture through a sterile or nonsterile drape, cover, or protective barrier, permitting bacteria to reach sterile areas

THR, THA Total hip replacement, total hip appliance

TKR, TKA Total knee replacement, total knee appliance

Total joint arthroplasty The use of artificial joint implants to restore motion and function of a joint—for example, total hip replacement is common orthopedic procedure performed on patients with degenerative joint disease (e.g., avascular necrosis [AVN] of proximal femur)

Traction The process of putting a limb, bone, or group of muscles under tension with the use of weights and pulleys to align or immobilize the part

CHAPTER 16

Pediatric Radiography

CONTRIBUTIONS BY **Chad Hensley,** PhD, RT(R)(MR)

CONTRIBUTORS TO PAST EDITIONS   Bette Schans, PhD, RT(R), Claudia Calandrino, MPA, RT(R), Jessie R. Harris, RT(R), Cecilie Godderidge, BS, RT(R), Linda Wright, MHSA, RT(R)

CONTENTS

INTRODUCTION AND PRINCIPLES

Introduction

Successfully completing pediatric radiographic studies starts with **room preparation** and the **technologist's attitude toward children**. Properly preparing the room for a pediatric patient can reduce the amount of time the child is in the exam room and create a better workflow for the technologist. This includes organizing the room to remove potential hazards, setting the technical components, and having immobilization devices available.

Working with pediatric patients can be challenging at times because of their inability to follow instructions. It is important to remember that the pediatric patient might be scared, confused, hurting, or a combination of all three. The pediatric technologist must view children as special persons to be handled with care and understanding. This approach requires patience and taking the necessary time to talk to and build a rapport with the child. Explaining instructions to children in a way they can understand is extremely important in developing trust and cooperation.

AGE OF UNDERSTANDING AND COOPERATION

All children do not reach a sense of understanding at the same predictable age. This ability varies from child to child, and the pediatric technologist must not assume a child will comprehend what is occurring. However, by age **2 or 3 years,** most children can be talked through a diagnostic radiographic study without immobilization or parental aid. Most important is a sense of trust, which begins at the first meeting between the patient and the technologist; the first impression the child has of the technologist is everlasting and forges the bond of a successful relationship.

PRE-EXAMINATION INTRODUCTION AND CHILD AND PARENT EVALUATION

Introduction of Technologist

At the first meeting, most children are accompanied by at least one parent or caregiver. The following steps are important:
- Introduce yourself as the technologist who will be working with the child (Fig. 16.1).
- Find out what information the attending physician has given to the parent and patient.
- Explain what you are going to do and what your needs will be (Fig. 16.2).

Tears, fear, and combative resistance are common reactions for a young child. The technologist must take the time to communicate to the parent and the child, in language they can understand, exactly what he or she is going to do. The technologist must try to build an atmosphere of trust in the waiting room before the patient is taken into the radiography room; this includes discussing the necessity of immobilization as a last resort if the child cannot cooperate.

Evaluation of Parent's Role

The first meeting is also the time to evaluate the role of the parent or caregiver. Three possibilities are as follows:
1. Parent is in room as an observer, lending support and comfort by his or her presence.
2. Parent actively participates, assisting with immobilization.
3. Parent is asked to remain in the waiting area and not accompany the child into the radiography room.

Sometimes a child who acts fearful and combative in the waiting room with a parent present is more cooperative without his or her presence. This is the time when the technologist's communication skills are tested.

The assessment of the parent's role is important and requires an objective evaluation by the technologist. If it is determined that the parent's anxiety would interfere with the child's cooperation, option 3 should be chosen. However, parents generally do wish to assist in immobilizing the child. If this option is chosen (assuming the parent is not pregnant and is properly shielded), the technologist should carefully explain the procedure to both the parent and the patient. This explanation includes instructions to the parent on correct immobilization techniques. Parental cooperation and effectiveness in assisting tend to increase when the parent understands how proper but firm immobilization improves the diagnostic quality of the image and reduces radiation exposure to the patient by reducing the potential of repeats. If the parent is unable or unwilling to assist with immobilization, soliciting help from another technologist or using immobilization devices is the next best option.

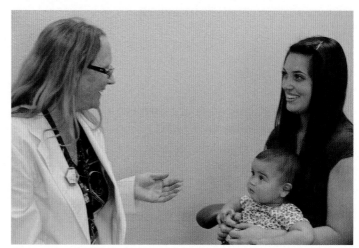

Fig. 16.1 Technologist introducing herself to the patient and developing trust.

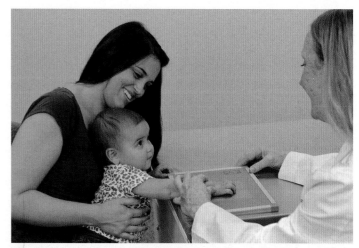

Fig. 16.2 Technologist explaining the procedure to the patient and parent.

Immobilization

Pediatric patients generally include infants through children up to age 12 years. Older children may be treated more like adults, except that special care must be taken with gonadal shielding and reducing exposure factors because of their smaller size. This chapter describes and illustrates radiography primarily of infants (birth to 1 year old) and toddlers (1 to 3 years old) who require special attention to prevent motion during the exposure.

In general, pediatric radiography should **always use mAs with short exposure times** to minimize image blurring that may result from patient motion. However, even with short exposure times, preventing motion during exposures is a constant challenge in pediatric radiography, and effective methods of immobilization are essential.

Before using a pediatric immobilizer, good communication with the parent or guardian is important. The more cooperation there is from the parent, the better chances there are for a successful examination. Unless there are extenuating circumstances, the parent is responsible for the care of the pediatric patient; therefore, consent from the parent is required prior to using an immobilization device. If a parent or guardian refuses to allow an immobilization device, the technologist should seek advice from a radiologist or referring physician. There are a variety of pediatric immobilization devices available depending on the need. Before an immobilization device is used, it is crucial the technologist have a full understanding of its proper usage to ensure the safety of the child.

UPRIGHT

Devices such as the Pigg-O-Stat (Fig. 16.3A) or the Pediatric Restraining Chair (Fig. 16.3B) may be used for upright images such as the chest or abdomen. The child can be safely restrained in these devices in such a way that the arms are elevated, allowing for proper positioning.

RECUMBENT

Devices used for recumbent positioning in routine radiography and fluoroscopy include the Tam-em board (Fig. 16.4A), Papoose Board (Fig. 16.4B), or Octostop (Fig. 16.4C). These instruments allow the infant or child to lie on a radiolucent board with Velcro straps placed across the head, torso, and legs to restrict movement.

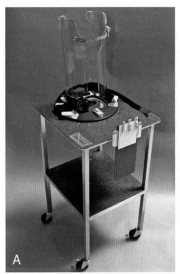
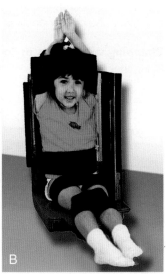

Fig. 16.3 Upright immobilizers. A, Pigg-O-Stat (with IR holder). B, EC Pediatric Restraining Chair. (**B** Courtesy Edwin Cabansag.)

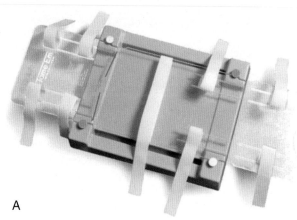
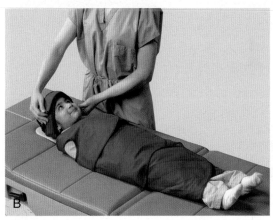
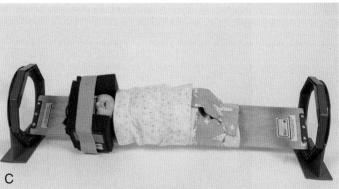

Fig. 16.4 A, Tam-em Board. B, Papoose Board. C, Octostop. (**A** Courtesy Cone Instruments; **B** Courtesy Natus Medical. All rights reserved; **C** From http://octostop.com/en/product/universal-octopaque/.)

16

OTHER FORMS OF IMMOBILIZATION

Extremity immobilization devices, such as a radiolucent paddle (Fig.16.5A), are available. Radiolucent paddles apply pressure to the area being imaged to restrict motion. Care must be taken, and pressure should not be applied when there is a possible fracture. Radiolucent sponge blocks (Fig. 16.5B) are effective tools, but will require assistance. Radiolucent sponges allow for the child to be held firmly without superimposition of the holders' hands. Proper shielding should be given to the holder, who will be in close proximity to the primary beam. Other methods such as sandbags, tape or compression bands may also be used. Care must be taken if tape is used. Tape can cause damage if applied directly to the skin. Skin-sensitive tape should be used if possible. If regular adhesive tape is used, twist the tape to ensure the adhesive surface is not directly on the skin, or apply gauze as a barrier.

Wrapping with Sheets or Towels ("Mummifying")

Using sheets or towels in "mummifying" or wrapping may be necessary to immobilize infants and some children up to 3 years old for certain radiographic procedures. Wrapping is very effective for immobilization if performed correctly. A four-step method is shown in Figs. 16.6 to 16.9. The room should be set up and prepared before the patient is brought into it.

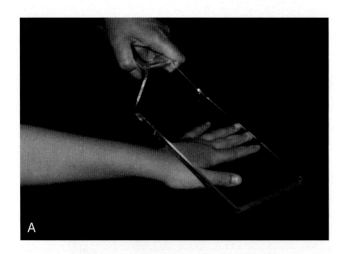

A

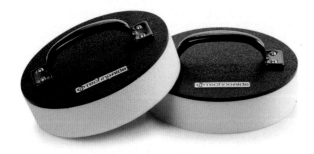

B

Fig. 16.5 A, Hand immobilizer. B, Head paddle. (**A** from https://www.chamcousa.com/store/p11/pediatrichandimmobilizer .html#/. **B** courtesy of Techno-Aide, Inc. All rights reserved.)

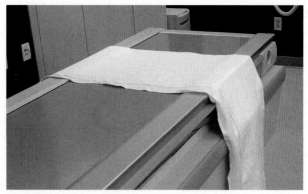

Fig. 16.6 Step 1. Place the sheet on the table folded in half or in thirds lengthwise, depending on the size of the patient.

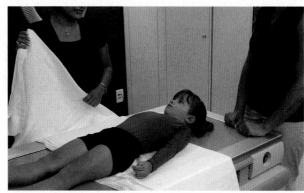

Fig. 16.7 Step 2. Place the patient in the middle of the sheet; place the patient's right arm beside his or her body. Take the end of the sheet closest to the technologist and pull the sheet across the patient's body tightly, keeping the arm next to the patient's body.

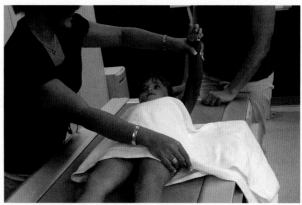

Fig. 16.8 Step 3. Place the patient's left arm beside his or her body on top of the top sheet. Bring the free sheet over the left arm to the right side of the patient's body and around under the body as needed.

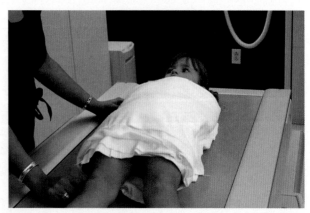

Fig. 16.9 Step 4. Complete the wrapping process by pulling the sheet tightly enough so that the patient cannot free the arms.

Bone Age Study

The bones of infants and small children go through various growth changes from birth through adolescence. The pelvis is an example of ossification changes that are apparent in children. As shown in Fig. 16.10, the divisions of the hip bone between the ilium, the ischium, and the pubis are evident. They appear as individual bones separated by a joint space, which is the cartilaginous growth region in the area of the acetabulum. Pediatric long bone anatomy can be seen in Fig. 16.11. It includes the diaphysis (shaft or body) (D), the primary center of ossification; the epiphysis (E), the secondary center of ossification; the metaphysis (M), the area where bone grows in length; and the epiphyseal plate (EP), the cartilaginous area between the epiphysis and metaphysis.

PURPOSE

A bone age study is a radiologic examination to determine skeletal maturity. Bone age studies may be done for a variety of reasons including forensic and pathologic purposes and to determine future growth potential. Pathologic conditions may result in a delay of normal bone growth. Examples of pathologic conditions that may delay bone aging include malnutrition, endocrine disorders (e.g., hypothyroidism), and nonendocrine disorders (e.g., cystic fibrosis).[1]

PROCEDURE

The most common image evaluated is a single PA of the left hand and wrist. However, the knee, foot and ankle, fibula, or hemiskeleton (radiographs of half the skeleton) have also been used.[2] Protocols may differ based on the radiologist's or pediatrician's preference, and technologists should be familiar with the routines specific to their facility.

OSSIFICATION PATTERNS (TABLE 16.1)

The bones in the hand and wrist of a healthy child will mature at a fairly consistent rate. Although there are slight variations between genders (females mature more quickly than do males), some assumptions can be made about the anatomy seen on a radiograph. At birth, the metacarpals, phalanges, radius and ulna can be radiographically demonstrated (Fig. 16.12). Around 3 to 14 months of age, the capitate and hamate begin to ossify and are then radiographically visible (Fig. 16.13). Between 14 months and 3 years the epiphyses of the phalanges, metacarpals, and distal radius are radiographically visible (Fig. 16.14). Between the ages of 3 and 9 years, the epiphyses widen to the width of their associated metaphysis and the triquetrum, lunate, trapezium, trapezoid, and scaphoid become radiographically visible (Fig. 16.15). Between the ages of 9 and 14 years, the epiphyses extend to cover the metaphysis, and the pisiform and sesamoid bone of the first digit become radiographically visible (Fig. 16.16). After 14 years of age the epiphyses will narrow as it continues to fuse to their associated metaphysis[3] (Fig. 16.17).

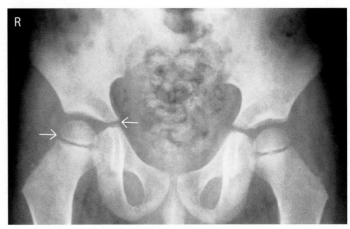

Fig. 16.10 Normal 3-year-old pelvis.

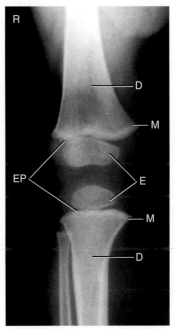

Fig. 16.11 Normal 1-year-old lower limb.

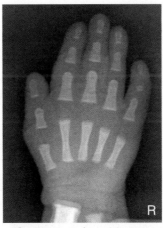

Fig. 16.12 0 days. (Courtesy Bonepit.com)

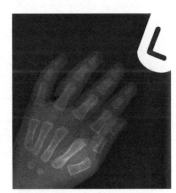

Fig. 16.13 5 months. (Case courtesy Dr Aneta Kecler-Pietrzyk, Radiopaedia.org, rID: 53220.)

TABLE 16.1 OSSIFICATION PATTERNS OF THE HAND/WRIST	
AGE	**RADIOGRAPHIC ANATOMY**
Birth – 3 month	Metacarpals, phalanges, radius, ulna
3 month – 14 months	Capitate, hamate
14 month – 3 years	Epiphyses of metacarpals, phalanges, distal radius
3 years – 9 years	Epiphyseal widening, triquetrum, lunate, trapezium, trapezoid, scaphoid
9 years – 14 years	Epiphyseal overlap on metaphysis, pisiform, sesamoid
14 years+	Epiphyseal fusion to metaphysis

Data from Gilsanz V, Ratib O. *Hand bone age*, Berlin, 2005, Springer.

MEASUREMENTS

More specific age calculations are completed by using either the Greulich-Pyle (GP) or Tanner-Whitehouse (TW) method. The GP method is the most common technique used by radiologists for estimating bone age.[2] The GP method compares the overall radiographic appearance of the hand/wrist to the standards found in the *Radiographic Atlas of Skeletal Development of the Hand and Wrist*, originally published in 1959.[4] Although there may be variances due to enthicity at older ages, the GP method is a reliable technique to estimate a child's age.[5,6]

The TW method[7] assigns a numeric value to specific areas of the hand and produces an overall score which is then calculated to determine age. Specifically, this method calculates the characteristics of the radius, ulna, and carpals, including the size and shape of the bones and epiphyses. Although this method has been shown to be more accurate in estimating age, it takes considerably longer and therefore is not the predominant method used by radiologists.[1]

Digital methods are now available in a variety of computer software programs. These methods combine GP and TW techniques to estimate bone age, and they are proving to be reliable and to produce results faster than the GP or TW method.[8]

Child Abuse

A radiographer is likely to be exposed to nonaccidental trauma of children, more commonly referred to as child abuse. According to the U.S. Department of Health and Human Services Administration for Children and Families, most reported abuse occurs in children younger than 3 years old, with the highest victimization rates in those younger than 1 year old. Radiology is an important tool in the diagnosis of child abuse cases.

Technologists should have an understanding of the laws surrounding the reporting of child abuse in their specific location. Although the technologist may not initiate the reporting process, he or she is an important component. The technologist's primary role is to obtain quality images and communicate effectively with the radiologist. Part of this communication involves obtaining a thorough history from the parents or guardians. It should be noted that most abuse is committed by one or both parents; therefore, the history given may not be accurate in cases of abuse.[9] If the mechanism of the pathology seen does not correlate with the history given, a stronger case for child abuse can be made.

CLASSIFICATION

Child abuse can be classified into types (listed in order of frequency):
1. Neglect (includes medical neglect)
2. Physical abuse
3. Sexual abuse
4. Other/unknown
5. Psychological or emotional maltreatment[9]

Medical imaging can play an important role in the diagnosing of child abuse; specifically, radiography has a dominant role in detecting physical abuse.

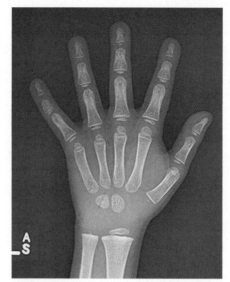

Fig. 16.14 3 years. (Case courtesy Dr Jeremy Jones, Radiopaedia.org, rID: 23244.)

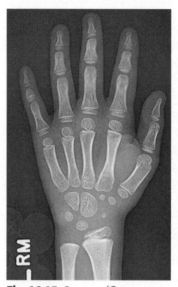

Fig. 16.15 8 years. (Case courtesy Dr Jeremy Jones, Radiopaedia.org, rID: 23244.)

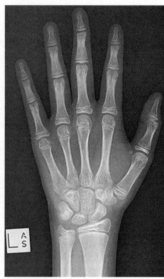

Fig.16. 16 13 years (Case courtesy Dr Jeremy Jones, Radiopaedia.org, rID: 23244.)

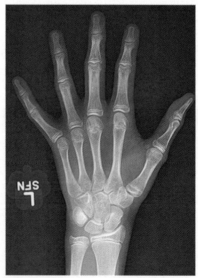

Fig. 16.17 15 years (Case courtesy Dr Jeremy Jones, Radiopaedia.org, rID: 23244.)

RADIOGRAPHIC INDICATIONS

Classic Metaphyseal Lesion

Specific fractures have a high indication of child abuse, and the classic metaphyseal lesion (CML) is one such fracture. The CML is a fracture along the metaphysis that results in a tearing or avulsion of the metaphysis. Other names for the CML include *corner fracture* (Fig. 16.18A) and *bucket-handle fracture* (Fig. 16.18B), based on the fracture's appearance and location. The CML will appear radiographically as a crescent-shaped osseous density adjacent to the avulsion fragment (arrows). The CML is caused by forces exerted on the metaphysis, such as pulling on an extremity, or by holding a child around the thorax and shaking violently, as seen in *shaken baby syndrome.*

Rib Fractures

Rib fractures, especially multiple and posterior, are a strong indicator of child abuse. The common mechanism for this is shaken baby syndrome. When a child is held under the axillae and shaken, the amount of force exerted on the anterior to posterior thorax is enough to fracture multiple ribs. This squeezing of the thorax promotes fractures at the costovertebral and costotransverse articulations. Additional indicators of child abuse may be fractures of the scapula and spinous process posteriorly and the sternum anteriorly resulting from squeezing.

Healing Fractures

The presence of multiple fractures in various stages of healing can also raise suspicion for child abuse. However, a thorough history may reveal these fractures to be pathologic in nature, such as fractures seen in osteogenesis imperfecta.

RADIOGRAPHIC IMAGING

The accepted method in imaging a child for suspected child abuse is with the skeletal survey. The skeletal survey[10] consists of the following:

- AP skull
- Lateral skull (to include C-spine)
- AP chest
- Lateral chest
- Right and left oblique thorax to include sternum, ribs, thoracic and upper lumbar spine
- AP abdomen to include pelvis
- Lateral lumbar spine
- AP humeri
- AP forearms
- PA hands
- AP femurs
- AP lower legs
- AP feet

The skeletal survey can assist in determining normal variants or disease versus child abuse. The technologist should obtain the best images possible while maintaining the ALARA principle (as low as reasonably achievable) owing to the number of exposures required. A method that is *not* acceptable is a technique known as the "babygram," in which a child is placed on the image receptor (IR) and the collimators are opened to image as much as possible.

ALTERNATIVE IMAGING MODALITIES

Computed Tomography (CT)

Computed tomography (CT) is very useful in the diagnosis of child abuse. The advantages of CT include the visualization of visceral damage, especially within the abdomen and head, and skeletal fractures. CT is a valuable tool in the diagnosis of brain injuries associated with child abuse, specifically injuries resulting from shaken baby syndrome. Because of the violent anterior and posterior shaking and lack of head support, the brain can strike the cranium both anteriorly and posteriorly, which can cause contusions (concussion) or hemorrhaging such as subdural hematomas. Care must be taken to reduce the radiation dose, and pediatric-specific CT protocols must always be used.

Magnetic Resonance Imaging (MRI)

MRI can assist in assessing soft tissue and central nervous system damage. However, because of the length of time required and the necessity for a child to remain motionless, MRI is not generally the modality of choice on the initial assessment.

Sonography

Sonography is beneficial in imaging visceral damage such as hemorrhage and certain skeletal damage. A benefit of sonography is that ionizing radiation is not needed to obtain the images.

Nuclear Medicine (NM)

NM is useful in assessing the healing bone. In cases of multiple fractures, some may be radiographically occult. NM can visualize the bone in its various stages of healing. NM is often used in conjunction with the skeletal survey if multiple fractures are found.

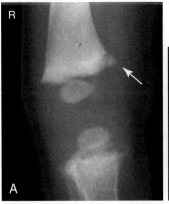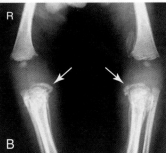

Fig. 16.18 A, Corner fracture of femur. B, Bucket-handle fracture. (Courtesy Dr. Loren Yamamoto. In Boychuk R.B.: Bucket handle and corner fractures. *Radiology Cases in Pediatric Emergency Medicine,* Vol. 4, Case 2, http://www.hawaii.edu/medicine/pediatrics/pemxray/v4c02.html.)

Radiation Protection and Image Gently®

With the advent of digital imaging, a heightened concern for increased radiation dose to pediatric patients has emerged. In 2007, the Society for Pediatric Radiology collaborated with the American College of Radiology, the American Society of Radiologic Technologists, and the American Association of Physicists in Medicine to begin a campaign to raise awareness of an increased pediatric dose rate among imaging professionals and with the public. From that first meeting, the Image Gently® campaign was launched.

The campaign examined dose rate in radiographic, fluoroscopic, and interventional imaging, in addition to CT, and protocols were written to reduce exposure during examinations. In radiography, the dose rate for more radiosensitive pediatric patients can be reduced by (1) eliminating the use of a grid if the part of interest is less than 4 inches (10 cm) thick; (2) collimating to the field size of the part of interest; (3) increasing the kVp to reduce mAs (exposure); and (4) taking into account the relationship of the thickness of the part of interest, the technique, and the exposure value. There is a wealth of information on pediatric imaging dose and suggestions for reducing exposure on the Image Gently® website[11] (www.imagegently.org).

MINIMIZING EXPOSURE DOSE

Reduction of repeat exposures and avoiding "dose creep" are critical in pediatric imaging.
- Proper immobilization and mAs with short exposure time techniques reduce the incidence of motion artifact (blurriness).
- Accurate manual technique charts with patient body weights should be available.
- Radiographic grids should be used only when the body part examined is more than 4 inches (10 cm) in thickness.

Each radiology department should keep a list of specific routines for pediatric imaging examinations, including specialized views and limited examination series, to ensure appropriate projections are obtained and no unnecessary exposures are made.

GONADAL PROTECTION

Gonads of a child can be shielded with contact-type shields, unless it is not recommended by site protocols or such shields obscure the essential anatomy of the lower abdomen or pelvic area. Various shapes, sizes, and gender-specific types of contact shields are shown in Figs. 16.19 and 16.20.

Other safeguards for radiation protection should also be used such as **close collimation, low-dosage techniques,** and a **minimum number of exposures.** To relieve parents' fears, the technologist should explain in simple language the practice of radiation protection and the rationale behind it.

PARENT PROTECTION

If parents are to be in the room, they must be supplied with **lead aprons.** If they are immobilizing the child and their hands are in or near the primary beam, they should also be given **lead gloves** (Fig. 16.21).

If the mother or other female guardian is of childbearing age and wishes to assist in the procedure, the technologist must **ask whether she is pregnant** before allowing her to remain in the room during the radiographic exposure. If she is pregnant, she should not be allowed in the room and must stay in the waiting area.

Pre-Examination Preparation

The following preparations should be completed before the patient is brought into the room:
- The necessary immobilization and shielding paraphernalia should be in place. IRs and markers should be in place, and techniques should be set.

- Specific projections should have been determined, which may require consultation with the radiologist.
- If two technologists are working together, the responsibilities of each technologist during the procedure should be clarified. The assisting technologist can set techniques, make exposures, and process the images. The primary technologist can position the patient; instruct the parents (if assisting); and position the tube, collimation, and required shielding.

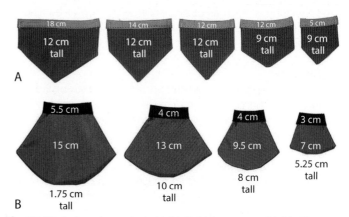

Fig. 16.19 A, Female contact shield. B, Male contact shield. (Courtesy Techno-Aide, Inc. All rights reserved)

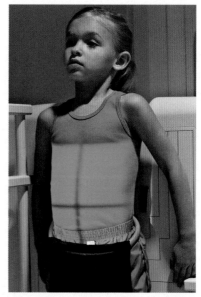

Fig. 16.20 Lead waist apron in place for erect abdomen.

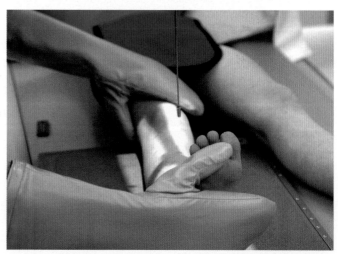

Fig. 16.21 Lead aprons and gloves for parents.

CHILD PREPARATION

After the child is brought into the room and the procedure is explained to the child's and parent's satisfaction, the parent or technologist must remove any clothing, bandages, or diapers from the body parts to be radiographed. Removal of these items is necessary to prevent the items from casting shadows and creating artifacts on the radiographic image because of the low exposure factors used for the patient's small size.

Digital Imaging Considerations

Guidelines listed here should be followed when digital imaging systems (computed radiography or digital radiography) are used for imaging infants and young children (these are described in greater detail in Chapter 1 and in preceding chapters for adult patients).

1. **Collimation:** Four-sided collimation is important to ensure that the final image after processing is of optimal quality. Collimation also is required for accurate reading of the imaging plate or exposed field size.
2. **Accurate centering:** Because of the way the image plate reader scans the exposed imaging plate in computed radiography, it is important that the body part and the central ray (CR) be accurately centered to the IR.
3. **Exposure factors:** The ALARA principle must be followed, and the lowest exposure factors required to obtain a diagnostic image must be used. For children, this also means that kVp ranges recommended for the age and size of the patient should be used, along with mAs using short exposure times to minimize the chance of motion artifact (blurriness). Lower mAs values can produce quantum mottle when a higher kVp is set.
4. **Post-processing evaluation of exposure indicator:** After the image is processed and ready for viewing, it must be checked for an acceptable relative exposure indicator, to verify the exposure factors used were in the correct range and to ensure an image of optimal quality with the least possible radiation dose to the patient.
5. **Grid use:** If direct digital imaging (digital radiography) receptors are used, the grid should be removed for body parts smaller than 4 inches (10 cm). Chest and abdomen images on smaller patients can be visualized appropriately without a grid; this reduces the exposure considerably.
6. **SID:** The minimum source to image receptor distance (SID) for many examinations has traditionally been 40 inches (100 cm). However, increasing the SID to 50 inches (130 cm) without a change in technique has been shown to reduce patient exposure without a loss of image detail.[12]

Alternative Modalities
COMPUTED TOMOGRAPHY (CT)

CT is used to produce cross-sectional images of body parts when slight differences in soft tissue densities must be demonstrated. Examples include CT scans of the head, which can visualize various soft tissue pathologies such as blood clots, cerebral edema, and neoplastic processes.

Chest pathology such as parenchymal lung disease can be demonstrated with high-resolution CT and the use of thin sections.

Renal CT scans have largely replaced intravenous urography studies in diagnostic radiography.

Reducing Pediatric Dose during CT

Although the benefits of properly performed CT examinations almost always outweigh the risks for an individual child, unnecessary exposure is associated with unnecessary risk. Minimizing radiation exposure from pediatric CT, whenever possible, is always desirable. Image Gently® provides examples of CT protocols that can be used to reduce the pediatric dose; these are available at http://imagegently.org/Procedures/ComputedTomography.aspx.

It is important the CT technologist remember the following in regard to pediatric scanning:

1. **Perform only necessary CT examinations:** When appropriate, use other modalities such as ultrasound or magnetic resonance imaging.
2. **Adjust exposure parameters for pediatric CT** based on:
   - **Child size:** Guidelines based on individual size/weight parameters should be used.
   - **Region scanned:** The region of the body scanned should be limited to the smallest necessary area.
   - **Organ system scanned:** Lower mA and/or kVp should be considered for skeletal or lung imaging and some CT angiographic and follow-up examinations.
3. **Scan resolution:** The highest quality images (i.e., those that require the most radiation) are not always required to make diagnoses.[13]

SONOGRAPHY (MEDICAL ULTRASOUND)

A major advantage of medical ultrasound for pediatric patients is the lack of ionizing radiation exposure; this is especially important for children and pregnant women. The role of ultrasound in pediatric radiology includes assisting in neurosurgical procedures, such as shunt tube placement in infants with open fontanels; visualization of intracranial structures; skeletal examinations, such as for congenital hip dysplasia; and gastrointestinal examinations for pyloric stenosis.

MAGNETIC RESONANCE IMAGING (MRI)

The advantages of MRI include the lack of ionizing radiation and improved imaging detail. Longer examination times compared with CT are a major disadvantage of MRI in pediatric use, and sedation is commonly recommended. However, MRI is an effective tool for neurologic, musculoskeletal, renal, liver, and vascular examinations.

Functional MRI is used along with clinical evaluation to study and diagnose functional brain diseases and disorders. In children, these include disorders that affect how young children can function at home or in school, such as attention-deficit/hyperactivity disorder, Tourette syndrome (multiple motor tics), and autism (compulsive and ritualistic behavior). See Chapter 20 for more information on MRI and functional MRI.

NUCLEAR MEDICINE (NM)

NM procedures can be used for various organ function studies. In addition, NM can be used to identify radiographically occult fractures and fractures in various stages of healing.

Clinical Indications

Technologists should be familiar with certain pathologies that are unique to newborns (neonates) and young children. Pediatric patients cannot describe their symptoms, and optimal procedures or projections should be performed correctly the first time without repeats. Being familiar with pathologic indications, as noted on patient records, provides the technologist with information that can suggest how the patient should be handled and what precautions should be taken. This information is also important for deciding what technique adjustments are needed for images of optimum quality and for ensuring that the correct procedures or projections are performed (Tables 16.2 to 16.4).

PEDIATRIC CHEST

Aspiration (mechanical obstruction) is most common in small children when foreign objects are swallowed or aspirated into the air passages of the bronchial tree. The obstruction is most likely to be found in the right bronchus because of bronchus size and the angle of divergence. Obstruction can cause other disease processes such as atelectasis and bronchiectasis (see Chapter 2).

Asthma is most common in children and generally is caused by anxiety or allergies. Airways are narrowed by stimuli that do not affect the airways in normal lungs. Breathing is labored, and increased mucus in the lungs may result in some increase in the radiodensity of lung fields; however, chest radiographs frequently appear normal.

Croup (primarily seen in children 1 to 3 years old) is caused by a viral infection. It is evidenced by labored breathing and a harsh dry cough that frequently (but not always) is accompanied by fever. It is treated most commonly with antibiotics. AP and lateral radiographs of the neck and upper airway may be requested to look for the characteristic smooth but tapered narrowing of the upper airway ("steeple sign"), which is most obvious on the AP projection.

Cystic fibrosis is an inherited disease in which secretions of heavy mucus cause progressive "clogging" of bronchi and bronchioles, which may be demonstrated on chest radiographs as increased radiodensities in specific lung regions. Hyperinflation of the lung results from blocked airways. Symptoms in the lungs generally are not obvious at birth but may develop later.

Epiglottitis (supraglottitis) is a bacterial infection of the epiglottis that is most common in children 2 to 5 years old but that may also affect adults. Epiglottitis is a **serious condition that can rapidly become fatal** (within hours of onset); it results from blockage of the airway caused by swelling. Examination usually must be performed in an emergency department by a specialist using a laryngoscope; the airway can be reopened by inserting an endotracheal tube or by performing a tracheostomy (opening through the front of the neck). A physician or other attendant should accompany the patient during any radiographic procedure to ensure that the airway remains open.

Hyaline membrane disease is now called **respiratory distress syndrome,** although this condition still is commonly known as hyaline membrane disease in infants. This is one of the most common indications for chest radiographs in newborns, especially premature infants. In this emergency condition, the alveoli and capillaries of the lung are injured or infected, resulting in leakage of fluid and blood into the spaces between alveoli or into the alveoli themselves. The normally air-filled spaces are filled with fluid, which can be detected radiographically as increased density throughout the lungs in a granular pattern.

Meconium aspiration syndrome During the birth process, the fetus under stress may pass some meconium stools into the amniotic fluid, which can be inhaled into the lungs. Meconium aspiration may result in blockage of the airway, causing the air sacs to collapse, which may cause a lung to rupture, creating a pneumothorax or atelectasis.

Table 16.2 presents a summary of the clinical indications for pediatric chest radiography.

TABLE 16.2 **SUMMARY OF CLINICAL INDICATIONS: PEDIATRIC CHEST**	
CONDITION OR DISEASE	**RADIOGRAPHIC EXAMINATION**
Aspiration (mechanical obstruction)	AP and lateral chest or AP and lateral upper airway for obstruction
Asthma	PA and lateral chest
Croup (viral infection)	PA and lateral chest and AP and lateral upper airway
Cystic fibrosis (may develop meconium ileus)	PA and lateral chest
Epiglottitis (acute respiratory obstruction)	AP and lateral chest and lateral upper airway
Hyaline membrane disease or respiratory distress syndrome (primarily in premature infants)	PA and lateral chest
Meconium aspiration syndrome (newborns)	AP and lateral chest (possible pneumothorax)

PEDIATRIC SKELETAL SYSTEM

Craniostenosis (craniosynostosis) refers to a deformity of the skull caused by premature closure of skull sutures. The type of deformity depends on which sutures are involved. The most common type involves the sagittal suture and results in AP (front to back) elongation of the skull.

Developmental dysplasia of the hip In developmental dysplasia of the hip, the femoral head is separated by the acetabulum in the newborn. The cause of this defect is unknown; it is more common in girls, in infants born in breech (buttocks first), and in infants who have close relatives with this disorder. Ultrasound is commonly used to confirm dysplasia in newborns. Frequent hip radiographs may be required later; gonadal shielding is important when x-rays are performed.

Idiopathic juvenile osteoporosis (in which bone becomes less dense and more fragile) occurs in children and young adults.

Osteochondrodysplasia refers to a group of hereditary disorders in which the bones grow abnormally, most often causing dwarfism or short stature.

- **Achondroplasia** is the most common form of short-limbed dwarfism. Because this condition results in decreased bone formation in the growth plates of long bones, the upper and lower limbs usually are short with a near-normal torso length.

Osteochondrosis primarily affects the epiphyseal or growth plates of long bones, resulting in pain, deformity, and abnormal bone growth.

- **Kohler bone disease** causes inflammation of bone and cartilage of the navicular bone of the foot. It is more common in boys, beginning at age 3 to 5 years, and rarely lasts more than 2 years.
- **Legg-Calvé-Perthes disease** leads to abnormal bone growth at the hip (head and neck of femur). It affects children 5 to 10 years old; the femoral head first appears flattened and then later appears fragmented. It usually affects only one hip and is more common in boys.
- **Osgood-Schlatter disease** causes inflammation at the tibial tuberosity (tendon attachment). It is more common in 5- to 10-year-old boys and usually affects only one leg.
- **Scheuermann disease** is a relatively common condition in which bone development changes in the vertebrae result in kyphosis (humpback). Scheuermann disease is more common in boys, beginning in early adolescence.

Osteogenesis imperfecta is a hereditary disorder in which the bones are abnormally soft and fragile. Infants with this condition may be born with many fractures, which can result in deformity or dwarfism or both. Sutures of the skull are unusually wide, containing many small wormian bones.

Infantile osteomalacia (rickets) is a condition in which developing bones do not harden or calcify, causing skeletal deformities. The most common sign is bowed legs, with bowing of the bones of the distal femur and the tibia and fibula, as seen on radiographs of the entire lower limbs.

Salter-Harris fractures involve the epiphyseal plates. They can be classified based on the location of the fracture and the involvement of surrounding anatomy. There are nine classifications; however, the most common are types I through V (Fig. 16.22):

- Type I: Transverse fracture along the epiphyseal plate; this may involve slipping of the epiphyses such as seen with slipped capital femoral epiphyses (SCFE)
- Type II: Fracture through the metaphysis and epiphyseal plate
- Type III: Fracture through the epiphyseal plate and epiphysis
- Type IV: Fracture through the metaphysis, epiphyseal plate, and epiphysis
- Type V: Compression fracture of the epiphyseal plate

Spina bifida In spina bifida, the posterior aspects of the vertebrae fail to develop, exposing part of the spinal cord. Spina bifida can be discovered before birth by ultrasound or by clinical tests of the amniotic fluid. Various degrees of severity exist.

- **Meningocele** is a more common and severe form of spina bifida that involves the protrusion of the meninges through the undeveloped opening of the vertebrae. The cerebrospinal fluid–filled bulge under the skin is called a *meningocele*.
- **Myelomeningocele** In myelomeningocele, the most severe type of spina bifida, the meninges and spinal cord protrude through the opening. This condition is most serious when it occurs in the cervical region and causes major physical handicaps, deterioration of kidney function, and frequently an associated hydrocephalus (water on the brain).
- **Spina bifida occulta** is a mild form of spina bifida that is characterized by some defect or splitting of the posterior arch of the L5–S1 vertebrae without protrusion of the spinal cord or meninges (membranes covering the spinal cord and brain).

Talipes Equinovarus (clubfoot) is a congenital deformity of the foot that can be diagnosed prenatally with the use of real-time ultrasound. It also is commonly evaluated radiographically in an infant with frontal and lateral projections of each foot. (The Kite method is described on p. 638.)

Table 16.3 presents a summary of the clinical indications for the pediatric skeletal system.

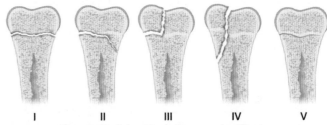

| I | II | III | IV | V |

Fig. 16.22 Salter-Harris fracture classification.

TABLE 16.3 **SUMMARY OF CLINICAL INDICATIONS: PEDIATRIC SKELETAL SYSTEM**	
CONDITION OR DISEASE	**RADIOGRAPHIC EXAMINATION AND (+) OR (−) EXPOSURE ADJUSTMENTS[a]**
Craniostenosis (craniosynostosis)	AP and lateral skull
Developmental dysplasia of hip or congenital dislocation of hip	Sonography, AP hip
Idiopathic juvenile osteoporosis	Bone survey study or AP of bilateral upper or lower limbs (−) slight decrease
Osteochondrodysplasia Achondroplasia	Bone survey study of long bones
Osteochondrosis	AP (possible oblique) and lateral projections of:
Kohler	Affected limbs
Legg-Calvé-Perthes	Navicular (foot)
Osgood-Schlatter	Hip
Scheuermann	Tibia (proximal)
	Spine (kyphosis)
Osteogenesis imperfecta	Bone survey, including AP and lateral skull (−), significant decrease, up to 50%
Infantile osteomalacia (rickets)	AP lower limbs (−) moderate decrease, depending on severity and age
Salter-Harris fractures	AP (possible oblique) and lateral projections of affected limbs
Spina bifida	Prenatal sonography, PA and lateral spine, and CT or MRI of affected region
Meningocele Myelomeningocele Spina bifida occulta	
Talipes Equinavarus (clubfoot)	AP and lateral foot (Kite method)

[a]Exposure adjustments depend on severity or stage of condition for manual exposure settings.

16

PEDIATRIC ABDOMEN

Atresias (or clausura) is a congenital condition that requires surgery because an opening to an organ is absent. One example is an anal atresia (imperforate anus), in which the anal opening is absent at birth. Other examples are biliary, esophageal, duodenal, mitral, and tricuspid atresias.

Hematuria Blood in the urine, or hematuria, may be caused by various conditions, such as cancer of the kidneys or bladder (intermittent bleeding), kidney stones, kidney cysts, or sickle cell disease (an inherited blood disease in which the red blood cells are crescent shaped or sickle shaped and deficient in oxygen).

Hirschsprung disease (congenital megacolon) is a congenital condition of the large intestine in which nerves that control rhythmic contractions are missing. This serious condition results in severe constipation or vomiting. It usually is corrected surgically by connecting the distal portion of the normal part of the large intestine to an opening in the abdominal wall (colostomy).

Intestinal obstruction In adults, intestinal obstruction is caused most frequently by fibrous adhesions from previous surgery. In newborns and infants, it is caused most often by birth defects such as intussusception, volvulus, or meconium ileus.

- **Ileus**, which also is called *paralytic ileus* or *adynamic ileus,* is an intestinal obstruction that is **not a mechanical obstruction** (e.g., a volvulus or an intussusception), but rather an obstruction caused by lack of contractile movement of the intestinal wall.
- **Intussusception** is a mechanical obstruction that is caused by the telescoping of a loop of intestine into another loop. It is most common in the region of the distal small bowel (ileus).
- **Meconium ileus** is a mechanical obstruction whereby the intestinal contents (meconium) become hardened, creating a blockage. This can be found in conjunction with cystic fibrosis.
- **Volvulus** is a mechanical obstruction that is caused by twisting of the intestine itself.

Necrotizing enterocolitis is inflammation of the inner lining of the intestine that is caused by injury or inflammation. It occurs most often in premature newborns and may lead to tissue death (necrosis) of a portion of the intestine. This condition may be confirmed with plain radiographs of the abdomen that show gas produced by bacteria inside the intestinal wall.

Polycystic kidney disease (infantile or childhood) is an inherited renal condition in which many cysts form in the kidney, causing enlarged kidneys in infants and children. Generally, this disease is fatal without dialysis or kidney transplantation if it affects both kidneys.

Pyelonephritis is a bacterial infection of the kidneys that is most commonly associated with or is caused by vesicoureteral reflux of urine from the bladder back into the kidneys.

Hypertrophic pyloric stenosis is an overgrowth in the muscles of the pylorus, causing narrowing or blockage at the pylorus or stomach outlet. It occurs in infants and frequently results in repeated, forceful vomiting.

TABLE 16.4 SUMMARY OF CLINICAL INDICATIONS: PEDIATRIC ABDOMEN

CONDITION OR DISEASE	RADIOGRAPHIC EXAMINATION
Atresias (clausura)	AP abdomen or GI series, or both
Hematuria	Sonography
Hirschsprung disease (congenital megacolon)	AP abdomen or GI series (frequently requires a colostomy), or both

Intestinal obstruction
  Ileus
  Intussusception
  Meconium ileus
  Volvulus
	Acute abdomen series and small bowel series or barium enema

Necrotizing enterocolitis	Acute abdomen series
Polycystic kidney disease	Sonography, CT, or MRI
Pyelonephritis	Sonography
Hypertrophic pyloric stenosis	Upper GI series or ultrasound, or both

Tumors
  Neuroblastoma
  Wilms tumor
	Radiographic studies of affected body part, CT, sonography

Urinary tract infection	Voiding cystourethrogram (VCUG)
Vesicoureteral reflux	VCUG or nuclear medicine

Tumors (neoplasms) Malignant tumors (cancer) occur less frequently in children than in adults and are more curable in children.

- **Neuroblastomas** are associated with childhood cancer (generally children younger than 5 years of age). They occur in parts of the nervous system, most frequently the adrenal glands. This cancer is the second most common type in children.
- **Wilms tumor** is a cancer of the kidneys of embryonal origin. It usually occurs in children younger than 5 years old. Wilms tumor is the most common abdominal cancer in infants or children, and it typically involves only one kidney.

Urinary tract infection frequently occurs in adults and children and is caused by bacteria, viruses, fungi, or some type of parasite. Bacterial infections in newborns involving the bladder and urethra are most common in boys, but after age 1, they are more common in girls. A common cause of urinary tract infection in children is vesicoureteral reflux.

Vesicoureteral reflux causes a backward flow of urine from the bladder into the ureters and kidneys, increasing the chance of spreading infection from the urethra and bladder into the kidneys.

Table 16.4 presents a summary of the clinical indications for pediatric abdominal radiography.

Routine and Special Projections

Certain routine and special projections for pediatric radiography are demonstrated and described on the following pages as suggested standard routine and special departmental routines or procedures.

AP AND PA CHEST PROJECTION: CHEST

Clinical Indications
- Pathology involving lung fields, diaphragm, bony thorax, and mediastinum, including the heart and major vessels

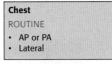

NOTE: Patient should be **erect if possible to demonstrate air/fluid levels.** Generally, pediatric patients, if old enough, should be examined in an erect position with the use of a Pigg-O-Stat or similar erect immobilization device (see Fig. 16.24). Exceptions are infants in an isolette and infants too young to support their heads.

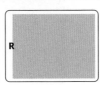

Technical Factors
- Minimum SID—50 to 60 inches (125 to 150 cm); x-ray tube raised as high as possible (if supine)
- IR size and placement—determined by size of patient (if supine, place cassette under patient)
- Grid not required
- Shortest exposure time possible
- kVp range—75–85

Shielding Shield radiosensitive tissues outside region of interest.

Patient Position—Patient Supine
- Immobilization techniques should be used when necessary (Fig. 16.23).
- Patient is supine, arms extended to remove scapula from the lung fields. Legs are extended to prevent rotation of the pelvis.
- With parental assistance (if parent is not pregnant), do the following:
  1. Have parent remove child's chest clothing.
  2. Provide parent with lead apron and gloves or shield.
  3. Place child on IR.
  4. Parent should extend child's arms over head with one hand while keeping head tilted back to prevent superimposing upper lungs. With other hand, parent holds child's legs at level of the knees, applying pressure as necessary to prevent movement.
  5. Place parent in a position that does not obstruct technologist's view of patient while exposure is made.
  6. Place lead gloves or lead shield over the top of parent's hands if parent is not wearing the gloves. (It may be easier to hold on to the patient if not wearing the lead gloves.)

Part Position
- Place patient in the middle of IR with shoulders 2 inches (5 cm) below top of IR.
- Ensure that thorax is **not rotated.**

CR
- CR **perpendicular** to IR, centered to the midsagittal plane at the **level of midthorax,** which is approximately at the **mammillary (nipple) line**

Recommended Collimation Closely collimate on four sides to outer chest margins.

Respiration Make exposure on second full inspiration. If child is crying, watch respiration and make exposure immediately after the child fully inhales.

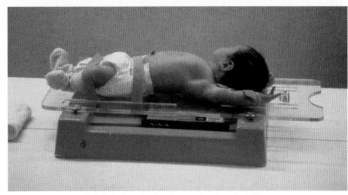

Fig. 16.23 Supine AP using immobilizer.

AP AND PA CHEST PROJECTION: CHEST

ERECT PA CHEST WITH PIGG-O-STAT

Patient Position—Patient Erect
- Patient is placed on seat with legs down through center opening. Adjust seat to correct height so that top of IR is about 1 inch (2.5 cm) above shoulders.
- Arms are raised and side body clamps are placed firmly against patient and are secured by base adjustment and adjustable strap.
- Lead shield is raised to a level about 1 inch (2.5 cm) above iliac crest.
- Correct R and L markers and "insp" (inspiration) marker are set to be exposed on lower image (Fig. 16.24).
- Ensure **no rotation.**

CR
- CR perpendicular to IR at level of midlung fields (at mammary line)
- Minimum SID—72 inches (180 cm)

Recommended Collimation Collimate closely on four sides to outer chest margins.

Respiration If child is crying, watch respiration and make exposure as child fully inhales and holds breath. (Children can frequently hold their breath on inspiration after a practice session.)

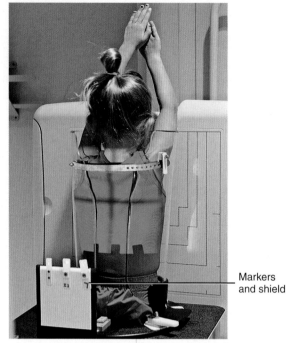

Markers and shield

Fig. 16.24 Immobilized by Pigg-O-Stat.

Evaluation Criteria
Anatomy Demonstrated: • Entire lungs should be included from apices (C7–T12 level) to costophrenic angles. • Air-filled trachea from T1 down is demonstrated, in addition to hilum region markings, thymus, heart, and bony thorax (Fig. 16.25).
Position: • Chin is sufficiently elevated to prevent superimposition of apices. • **No rotation** exists, as evidenced by equal distance from lateral rib margins on each side to the spine and distance from both sternoclavicular (SC) joints to the spine. • **Full inspiration** visualizes 9 (occasionally 10) posterior ribs above diaphragm on most patients. • Collimation to area of interest.
Exposure: • Lung contrast is sufficient to visualize fine lung markings within lungs. • Faint outlines of ribs and vertebrae are visible through heart and mediastinal structures. • **No motion** is present, as evidenced by sharp outlines of rib margins, diaphragm, and heart shadows.

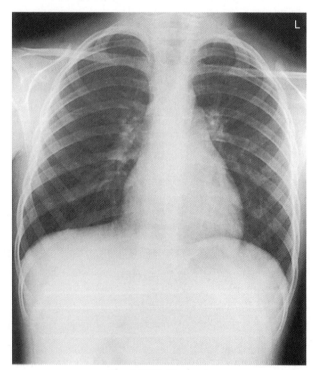

Fig. 16.25 PA chest.

LATERAL CHEST POSITION: CHEST

Clinical Indications
- Pathology involving lung fields, trachea, diaphragm, heart, and bony thorax
- Hemothorax or pulmonary edema; horizontal beam projection is needed to visualize air-fluid levels

Chest
ROUTINE
• AP or PA
• Lateral

Technical Factors
- Minimum SID—50 to 60 inches (130 to 155 cm)
- IR size—determined by size of patient
- IR portrait under patient (unless horizontal beam is taken on immobilizer)
- Grid not required
- Shortest exposure time possible
- kVp range—80–85

Shielding Shield radiosensitive tissues outside region of interest.

Patient Position—Patient Recumbent
- Immobilization techniques should be used when necessary.
- Patient is lying on side in true lateral (generally left lateral) position (Fig. 16.26) with arms extended above head to remove arms from lung field. Bend arms at the elbows for patient comfort and stability with head placed between arms. If immobilizer is used, patient position does not change from AP projection. Turn x-ray tube into horizontal beam projection. Place immobilized child adjacent to imaging device or cassette (Fig. 16.27).
- If parental assistance is required, perform the following steps:
  1. Place patient on IR in left lateral position (unless right lateral is indicated).
  2. Bring arms above the head and hold with one hand. Place the other hand across patient's lateral hips to prevent child from rotating or twisting.
  3. Place parent in a position that does not obstruct technologist's view of patient while exposure is made.
  4. Place lead gloves or shield over top of parent's hands if parent is not wearing the gloves.

Part Position
- Place the patient in the middle of IR with the shoulders about 2 inches (5 cm) below top of IR.
- **No rotation** should exist; ensure a true lateral position.
- CR
- CR **perpendicular** to IR **centered to the midcoronal plane** at the level of the mammillary (nipple) line

Recommended Collimation Closely collimate on four sides to outer chest margins.

Respiration Make exposure on second full inspiration. If child is crying, watch respiration and make exposure when the child fully inhales.

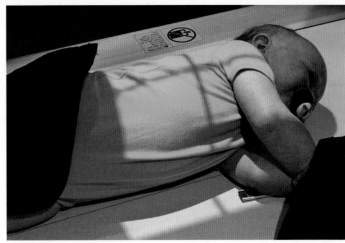

Fig. 16.26 Recumbent lateral chest (with immobilization aids).

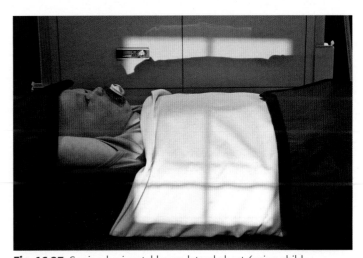

Fig. 16.27 Supine horizontal beam lateral chest (using child immobilizer).

LATERAL CHEST PROJECTION: CHEST

ERECT LATERAL CHEST WITH PIGG-O-STAT

This position can be used with young children up to approximately age 4 years (patient in Fig. 16.28 is 4 years old).

Patient Position—Patient Erect
- Patient is placed on seat and adjusted to correct height so that top of IR holder is about 1 inch (2.5 cm) above the shoulders.
- Arms are raised and side body clamps are placed firmly against patient and secured by base adjustment and by adjustable strap.
- Lead shield is raised to a level about 1 inch (2.5 cm) above iliac crest.
- Correct R and L markers and inspiration marker are set to be exposed on image.
- Ensure that **no rotation** exists.

Procedure if Lateral Follows PA Projection If patient is already in position from the PA projection, patient and swivel base are turned 90° to lateral position. Lead shield remains in position, and lead marker is changed to indicate correct lateral. IR is placed in film holder mount.

CR
- CR perpendicular to IR at level of midthorax (mammillary line)
- Minimum SID of 72 inches (180 cm)

Recommended Collimation Collimate closely on four sides to outer chest margins.

Respiration If child is crying, watch respiration and make exposure as child fully inhales and holds breath.

> **Evaluation Criteria**
> **Anatomy Demonstrated:** • Entire lungs from apices to costophrenic angles and from sternum anteriorly to posterior ribs are demonstrated (Fig. 16.29).
> **Position:** • Chin and arms are elevated sufficiently to prevent excessive soft tissues from superimposing apices. • **No rotation** exists; bilateral posterior ribs and costophrenic angles are superimposed. • Collimation to area of interest.
> **Exposure:** • **No motion** is evidenced by sharp outline of diaphragm, rib borders, and lung markings. • Exposure is sufficient to visualize faintly rib outlines and lung markings through the heart shadow and upper lung region without overexposing other regions of the lungs.

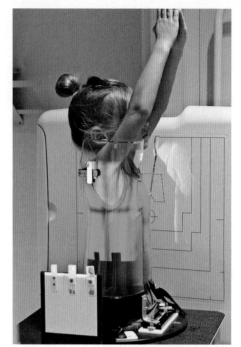

Fig. 16.28 Pigg-O-Stat: left lateral.

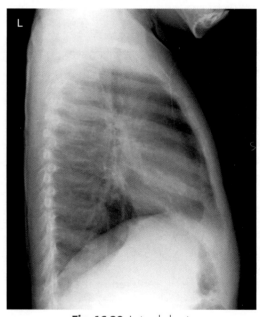

Fig. 16.29 Lateral chest.

AP AND LATERAL: UPPER LIMBS

NOTE 1: Department routines and protocols should be followed in regard to specific positioning routines for the upper limbs at various ages and for specific diagnostic indicators. The entire upper limb may be included on infants and young children, as shown in Fig. 16.30. For older children with more bone growth in the joint regions (except for general survey examinations), individual joints such as the elbow or wrist are radiographed separately, with the CR centered to the joint of interest. For older children, if the area of interest is the hand, generally a PA, oblique, and lateral hand should be taken, as for an adult.

Upper Limbs
ROUTINE
• AP
• Lateral

Clinical Indications

- Fractures, dislocations, and congenital anomalies
- Pathologies involving the upper limbs

Technical Factors

- Minimum SID—40 inches (100 cm)
- IR size and placement—determined by size of patient
- Grid not used for infants and small children
- Shortest exposure time possible
- kVp range—50–60

Shielding Shield radiosensitive tissues outside region of interest.

Patient Position

- Immobilization techniques should be used when necessary.
- Place patient in supine position.
- When radiographing a long bone, place IR under limb to be radiographed, including proximal and distal joints.
- When radiographing a joint, place IR under joint to be radiographed, including a minimum of 1 to 2 inches (2.5 to 5 cm) of proximal and distal long bones.

Part Position

- Align the part to be radiographed to the long axis of the IR, or cross-cornered if necessary, to include entire upper limb and both joints (see Fig. 16.30).

AP

- Supinate hand and forearm into the AP position (with hand and fingers extended) (Fig. 16.31).

Lateral

- If patient is in supine or erect position, adduct the arm and turn the forearm and wrist into a lateral position (Fig. 16.32).

CR

- CR perpendicular to IR directed to midpoint of part to be radiographed

Recommended Collimation Collimate closely on four sides to area of interest.

NOTE 2: A positioning angle sponge was not used with oblique hand (see Fig. 16.38); therefore, digits are not parallel to IR, resulting in obscured interphalangeal joints.

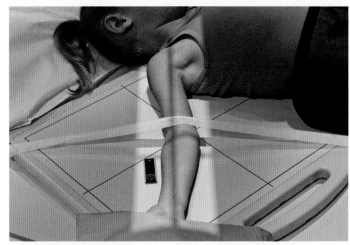

Fig. 16.30 AP upper limb (secured with tape and sandbag) using cassette-less detector.

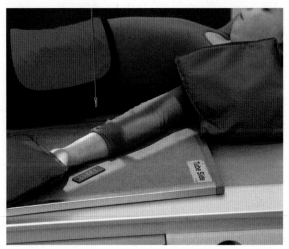

Fig. 16.31 AP forearm: 7-year-old (secured with sandbags).

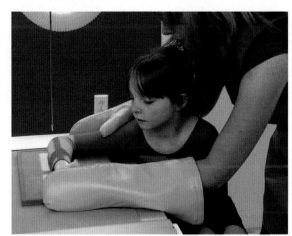

Fig. 16.32 Lateral forearm (parent immobilizing).

16

Evaluation Criteria
Anatomy Demonstrated: • See NOTE 1 regarding departmental routines and protocols on how much of the upper limb to include.
Position: • Generally two views 90° from each other are obtained. • An exception is the hand requiring a PA and an oblique. • Collimate to area of interest (Figs. 16.33 to 16.38).
Exposure: • **No motion** is evidenced by sharp trabecular markings and bone margins. • Optimal exposure demonstrates soft tissue and joint space regions without underexposing the more dense shaft regions of long bones.

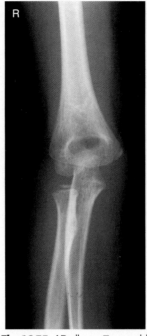 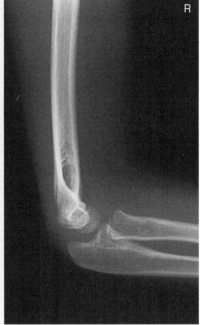

Fig. 16.35 AP elbow: 7-year-old. **Fig. 16.36** Lateral elbow: 7-year-old.

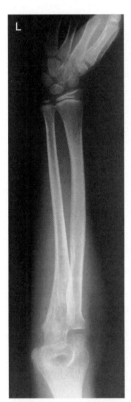 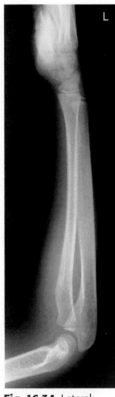

Fig. 16.33 AP forearm: 7-year-old.   **Fig. 16.34** Lateral forearm: 7-year-old.

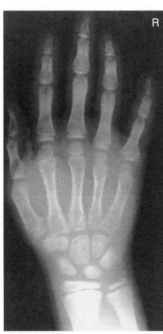 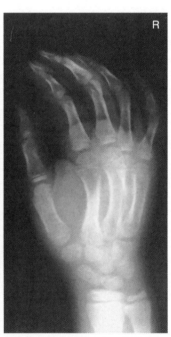

Fig. 16.37 PA hand: 9-year-old.   **Fig. 16.38** Oblique hand: 9-year-old.

AP AND LATERAL: LOWER LIMBS

Clinical Indications
- Fractures, dislocations, and congenital or other anomalies
- Diseases such as Osgood-Schlatter disease or osteomalacia

Lower Limbs
Routine
• AP
• Lateral

Technical Factors
- Minimum SID—40 inches (100 cm)
- IR size and placement—determined by size of body part to be radiographed, portrait frequently
- Grid not necessary for infants and small children
- Shortest exposure time possible
- kVp range—50–60

Shielding Shield radiosensitive tissues outside region of interest.

Patient Position and CR
AP and Lateral
- Immobilization techniques should be used when necessary.
- Patient is supine with IR under patient centered to affected limb (Figs. 16.39 and 16.40) or placed diagonally for bilateral limbs if needed to include entire limbs from hips to feet.
- For bilateral limbs, abduct both limbs into frog-leg position. CR is perpendicular to mid area of limbs.

NOTE: For infants or young children, bilateral examinations may be requested on one IR for a bone survey or for comparison purposes (Figs. 16.41 and 16.42).

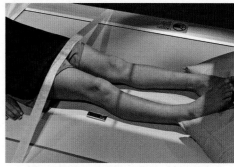

Fig. 16.41 AP (bilateral) lower limbs.

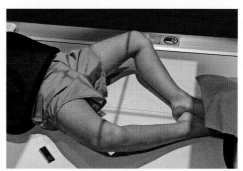

Fig. 16.42 Lateral (bilateral) lower limbs—frog-leg.

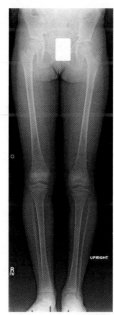

Fig. 16.43 AP (bilateral) lower limbs.

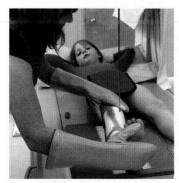

Fig. 16.39 AP lower leg.

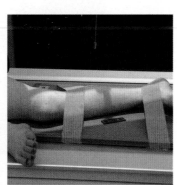

Fig. 16.40 Lateral lower leg.

Evaluation Criteria
Evaluation criteria are similar to upper limb criteria except for specific positioning criteria for lower limbs as follows.
AP: • Lateral and medial epicondyles of distal femur appear symmetric and in profile. • Tibia and fibula appear alongside each other with minimal overlap (Fig. 16.43).
Lateral: • Medial and lateral condyles and epicondyles of distal femur are superimposed. • Tibia and fibula appear mostly superimposed (Fig. 16.44).

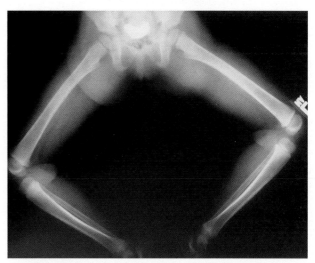

Fig. 16.44 Lateral (bilateral) frog-leg for lower limbs.

AP AND LATERAL: LOWER LEG AP AND LATERAL FOOT

KITE METHOD

16

NOTE: Department routines and protocols should be followed in regard to specific positioning routines for the lower limbs at various ages and for specific diagnostic indicators. If the specific area of interest is the **knee, ankle, or foot region,** separate images should be obtained, with the CR centered to the joint of interest (see Figs. 16.47 and 16.48.)

Lower Leg and Foot
LOWER LEG
Routine
• AP
• Lateral
FOOT
Routine
• AP
• Lateral

Clinical Indications

• Fractures, dislocations, congenital deformities, or other anomalies of lower limbs

Technical Factors

• Minimum SID—40 inches (100 cm)
• IR size and placement—determined by size of body part to be radiographed
• Grid not necessary for infants and small children
• Shortest exposure time possible
• kVp range—50–60 for lower leg; 40–50 for foot

Shielding Shield radiosensitive tissues outside region of interest.

Patient Position and CR

AP Lower Leg

• Immobilization techniques should be used when necessary.
• With patient supine, immobilize the arms and the leg that is not being radiographed, if needed.
• If parent is helping with immobilization, have the parent hold the leg in this position with one hand firmly on the pelvis and the other holding the feet.
• Place IR under limb being radiographed; include knee and ankle.
• Place leg as for a true AP projection, rotating knee internally slightly until the interepicondylar line is parallel to plane of IR. The feet and ankles should be in a true anatomic position (Fig. 16.45).
• CR is perpendicular to midleg.

Lateral Lower Leg

• Rotate patient toward affected side with leg in a frog-lateral position (Fig. 16.46) while bending knee at an approximate 45° angle.
• Immobilize body parts not being radiographed.
• If parent is helping with immobilization, have parent hold the feet and hips in position.
• CR is perpendicular to midleg.

Recommended Collimation Collimate closely on four sides to area of leg, including knee and ankle.

AP and Lateral Foot

AP Foot

• Immobilization techniques should be used when needed.
• Seat child on elevated support with knee flexed and foot placed on IR. CR is perpendicular to midfoot (Fig. 16.47).

Lateral Foot

• With patient lying or seated on table, rotate leg externally to place foot into lateral position. Use appropriate immobilizer when necessary (Fig. 16.48).
• CR is perpendicular to midfoot.

Recommended Collimation Collimate closely on four sides to area of the foot.

Talipes Equinovarus (Congenital Clubfoot)—Kite Method The foot is positioned for AP and lateral views as demonstrated, with **no attempt made to straighten the foot when placing it on the IR.** Because of shape distortion, it may be difficult to obtain a true AP and lateral, but two projections 90° from each other should be obtained. The two feet generally are imaged separately for comparison purposes.

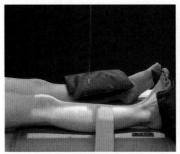
Fig. 16.45 AP lower leg.

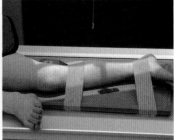
Fig. 16.46 Lateral lower leg.

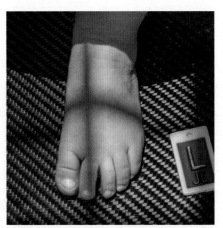
Fig. 16.47 AP foot using cassette-less detector.

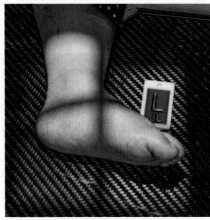
Fig. 16.48 Lateral foot.

AP AND LATERAL: PELVIS AND HIPS

WARNING: Do not attempt the frog-leg hip position on trauma patients until fractures have been ruled out from the AP pelvis projection.

Clinical Indications
- Fractures, dislocations, and congenital anomalies
- Pathologies involving the pelvis and hips, such as Legg-Calvé-Perthes disease and hip dysplasia.

> **Pelvis and Hips**
> ROUTINE
> - AP
> - Lateral (bilateral frog-leg)
>
> R

Technical Factors
- Minimum SID—40 inches (100 cm)
- IR size—determined by size of body part to be radiographed, IR landscape
- Grid if larger than 4 inches (10 cm)
- Shortest exposure time possible
- kVp range—50–60

Shielding Before exposing the patient, discuss the examination with the radiologist. The patient's history may require that a gonad shield not be used if it obscures an area of interest.
- **Girls:** Carefully shield the gonadal area. Place the female pediatric shield under the umbilicus and above the pubis; this avoids covering the hip joints (Figs. 16.49 to 16.51).
- **Boys:** Carefully place the upper border of the male pediatric shield at the level of the symphysis pubis.

Patient and Part Position
- Immobilization techniques should be used when necessary to ensure pelvis is not rotated.
- Align patient to center of table and IR.

AP
- With patient in supine position, position hips for AP projection by rotating knees and feet internally so that the anterior feet cross each other.

Lateral
- Abduct the legs by placing the soles of the feet together, knees bent and abducted. Bind soles of feet together, if needed.

CR
- CR perpendicular to IR, centered at the level of the hips

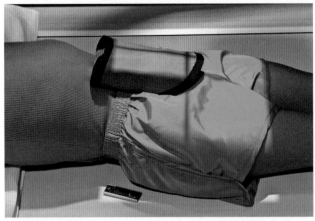

Fig. 16.49 AP pelvis (female gonadal shield in place).

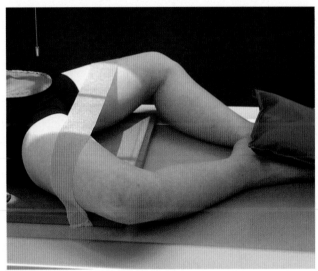

Fig. 16.50 Lateral hips and proximal femora (shielding female gonadal shielding in place).

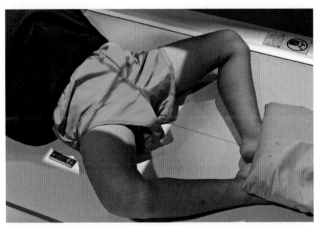

Fig. 16.51 AP pelvis with lateral hips (shielding above iliac crest).

Recommended Collimation Collimate to area of interest.

Respiration
- With infants and small children, watch their breathing pattern. When the abdomen is still, make the exposure.
- If the patient is crying, watch for the abdomen to be in full extension.

NOTE: Correctly placed gonadal shielding should be evident on both male and female patients without obscuring the hip joints (unless contraindicated by radiologist). See shield placement errors in Figs. 16.52 and 16.53.

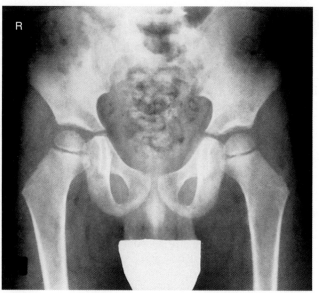

Fig. 16.52 AP hips and proximal femora. (Shielding error: Shield should have been placed higher with the top of the shield at the lower margins of the symphysis pubis, unless pubic bones are an area of interest.)

> **Evaluation Criteria**
> **Anatomy Demonstrated:** • Sufficiently large IR should be used to include all of pelvis and proximal femora.
> **Position:** • No rotation of pelvis is evidenced by symmetric alae or wings of ilium and by bilateral obturator foramina.
> **AP:** • Correct internal rotation of both legs is evidenced by femoral neck and greater trochanter region seen in profile. • Lesser trochanters are not visible.
> **Lateral:** • Proper lateral position of proximal femur regions is evident by superimposition of greater trochanter and neck with lesser trochanters in profile inferiorly. • Collimation to area of interest.
> **Exposure:** • Sharp trabecular markings and bone margins indicate **no motion.** • Optimal exposure visualizes soft tissue and bony detail. • Outline of femur heads should be visible through a portion of the acetabulum and ischium.

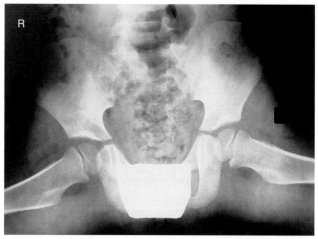

Fig. 16.53 Lateral hips (boy). (Shielding error: Shield is placed too high and covers symphysis pubis, does not adequately cover genitals.)

AP, AP REVERSE CALDWELL, AND AP TOWNE: SKULL

Clinical Indications
- Fractures, congenital anomalies of the cranium, including sutures or fontanels, head size, shunt check, bony tumors
- Other pathologies of the skull

Skull (Head)
ROUTINE
• AP
• AP reverse Caldwell
• AP Towne
• Lateral

Technical Factors
- Minimum SID—40 inches (100 cm)
- IR size—determined by size of body part to be radiographed, portrait
- Grid if larger than 4 inches (10 cm)
- Shortest exposure time possible
- kVp range—70–80

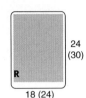

24
(30)

R

18 (24)

Shielding Shield radiosensitive tissues outside region of interest.

Patient Position
- Immobilization techniques should be used when necessary.
- Patient is supine, aligned to midline of table or grid.

Part Position
- Position head with **no rotation.**
- Adjust chin so that **orbitomeatal line (OML) is perpendicular to IR** (Fig. 16.54).

CR
- CR centered to glabella
  AP skull: CR parallel to OML
  AP reverse Caldwell: CR 15° cephalad to OML
  AP Towne: CR 30° caudad to OML
- IR centered to CR

Recommended Collimation Collimate closely on four sides to outer margins of skull.

NOTE: Generally, holding by parent is *not* needed for examinations of the head if immobilization devices are used.

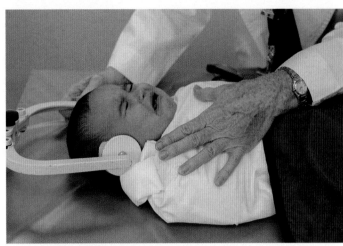

Fig. 16.54 Patient mummified; head clamps in use.

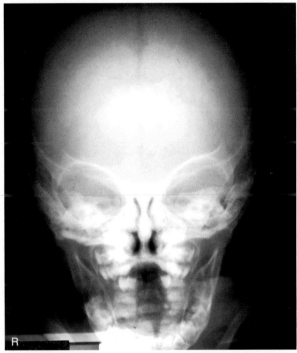

Fig. 16.55 AP skull (CR <10° cephalad to OML).

Evaluation Criteria
Anatomy Demonstrated: • Entire skull, including cranial and facial bones, is demonstrated.
Position: • No rotation occurs, as evidenced by symmetric orbits at equal distances from outer skull margins. • *AP 0°:* Petrous ridges superimpose superior orbital margins. • *AP with 15° cephalad angle:* Petrous pyramids and internal auditory canals are projected into lower one-half to one-third of orbits (Fig. 16.55). • *AP Towne with 30° caudal angle:* Petrous pyramids are projected below the inferior orbital rim, allowing visualization of the entire orbital margin (see Chapter 11). • Dorsum sellae and posterior clinoids are projected into foramen magnum. • Collimation to area of interest.
Exposure: • No motion is present, as evidenced by sharp margins of bony structures. • Penetration and exposure are sufficient to visualize frontal bone and petrous pyramids through the orbits.

LATERAL PROJECTION: SKULL (HEAD)

Clinical Indications
- Clinical indications are the same as shown for AP projection on preceding page

Skull (Head)
ROUTINE
• AP
• AP Caldwell
• AP Towne
• Lateral

Technical Factors
- Minimum SID—40 inches (100 cm)
- IR size and placement—determined by size of body part to be radiographed
- Grid if larger than 4 inches (10 cm)
- Shortest exposure time possible
- kVp range—70–80

Shielding Shield radiosensitive tissues outside region of interest.

24 (30)
18 (24) R

Patient Position
- Immobilization techniques should be used when necessary.
- Patient is in semiprone position, centered to midline of table.

Part Position
- Rotate head into true lateral position, and maintain position by placing a sponge or folded towel under mandible (Figs. 16.56 and 16.57).

CR
- CR perpendicular to IR, centered midway between glabella and occipital protuberance or inion, 2 inches (5 cm) above external acoustic meatus
- IR centered to CR

Recommended Collimation Collimate closely on four sides to outer margins of skull.

Evaluation Criteria
Anatomy Demonstrated: • Entire cranium is demonstrated (Fig. 16.58).
Position: • No rotation is evidenced by superimposed rami of mandible, orbital roofs, and greater and lesser wings of sphenoid. • Sella turcica and clivus are demonstrated in profile without rotation. • Collimation to area of interest.
Exposure: • No motion, as evidenced by sharp margins of bony structures. • Penetration and exposure are sufficient to visualize parietal region and lateral view outline of sella turcica without overexposing perimeter margins of skull.

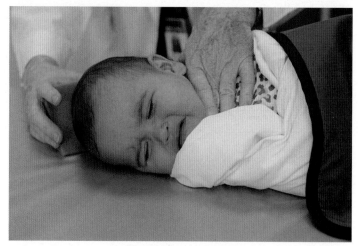
Fig. 16.56 Lateral skull.

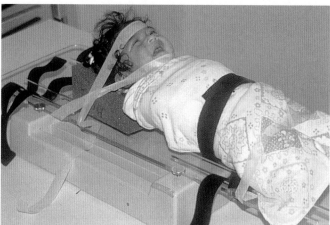
Fig. 16.57 Horizontal beam lateral with Tam-em board.

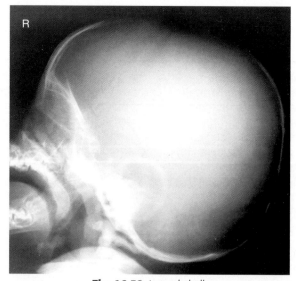
Fig. 16.58 Lateral skull.

RADIOGRAPHIC PROCEDURES OF PEDIATRIC ABDOMEN

Differences Between Children and Adults

Differences between children and adults are seen not only in size but also in the many developmental changes that occur from birth to puberty. The chest and abdomen are almost equal in circumference in a newborn. The pelvis is small and is composed more of cartilage than bone. The abdomen is more prominent and the abdominal organs are higher in infants than in older children. Accurate centering may be difficult for technologists who are more used to radiographing adults and using the iliac crest and the anterior superior iliac spine as positioning landmarks, which for all practical purposes are nonexistent in a young child. As a child grows, bone and musculature develop, the body outline and characteristics become distinctive, and familiar landmarks are located more easily.

It is difficult to distinguish on a radiograph between small and large bowels in infants and toddlers because the haustra of the large bowel are not as apparent as in older children and adults. Also, little intrinsic body fat exists, so an outline of the kidneys is not as well seen as in adults. Even so, visualization of the soft tissues is important in children, and a good plain radiograph of the abdomen provides valuable diagnostic information. Radiologists commonly say that the gas in the GI tract may be the best contrast medium in evaluating the pediatric abdomen.

Precise collimation is important, and the diaphragm, symphysis pubis, and outer edges of the abdomen all should be included in a plain supine radiograph in a child. Radiographs of young children tend to look "flat," and less contrast is seen than in radiographs of adults. This appearance is to be expected because bones are less dense, there is less fat, muscles are undeveloped, and the range of soft tissues is softer and less defined.

Patient Preparation for Contrast Media Procedures

Patient history is important in evaluating pediatric patients because this assists the radiologist in deciding the order and type of radiographic procedures to be performed. When it is necessary to withhold feeding for an upper GI study, the examination should be scheduled early in the morning. Children become irritable when hungry, and technologists need to be understanding of the difficulties in having a young child fast and must be supportive of both parent and child before and during fluoroscopic examinations of the GI tract. Having the infant's stomach empty is important not only because this ensures a good diagnostic upper GI study but also because infants, when hungry, are more likely to drink the barium.

UPPER GI TRACT

Infants and young children require minimal preparation for upper GI studies. Length of fasting is determined by age; the older the child, the slower the gastric emptying. **Neonates and young infants** should have nothing to eat or drink from 3 hours before the examination. Infants can have an early morning feed at 6:00 am and be scheduled for a barium swallow and upper GI study at 10:00 am (Table 16.5).

Written instructions should be given to the parent, and the reason for "absolutely nothing by mouth" should be explained and emphasized.

LOWER GI TRACT

Patient history determines the preparation for a lower GI examination. This examination is usually a single-contrast barium enema in children. Double-contrast enemas are performed less frequently than in adults

CONTRAINDICATIONS

Patients with the following clinical symptoms or conditions should not be given laxatives or enemas: Hirschsprung disease, extensive diarrhea, appendicitis, obstruction, and conditions in which the patient cannot withstand fluid loss.

PATIENT PREP

Similar to adults, pre-exam preparations may be needed to properly visualize the anatomic structures of the GI. Careful review of site specific prep-protocols are needed which are created with consultations from the radiologist. Newborn to 2 years old typically do not require any preparations. Children older than 2 may require diet restrictions such as a low-residual meal the evening before the exam and NPO until after the exam. A pediatric laxative and enema may also be required based on the advice of a physician.[14]

INTRAVENOUS UROGRAM

The preparation of children for intravenous urogram (IVU) is simple. No solid foods are given for 4 hours before the examination to diminish the risk for aspiration from vomiting. The patient should be encouraged to drink plenty of clear liquids until 1 hour before the examination.

TABLE 16.5 SAMPLE NPO PROTOCOL: AGE SUMMARY

Neonates and young infants	NPO 3 hours before procedure
Older infants and children	NPO 4 hours before procedure
Adolescents	NPO 6 hours before procedure

ACR–SPR Practice Parameters for the Performance of Contrast Esophagrams and Upper Gastrointestinal Examinations in Infants and Children. https://www.acr.org/-/media/ACR/Files/Practice-Parameters/UpperGI-Infants.pdf.

16

AP PROJECTION (KUB): ABDOMEN

Clinical Indications
- Pathology of the abdomen—evaluate gas patterns, soft tissue, and possible calcifications
- Other anomalies or diseases of abdomen

Abdomen
ROUTINE
• AP (KUB)
SPECIAL
• AP erect
• Lateral and dorsal decubitus

Technical Factors
- Minimum SID—40 inches (100 cm)
- IR size—determined by size of patient, portrait
- Grid if 4 inches (10 cm) or larger
- Shortest exposure time possible
- kVp range—60–75

R

Shielding Shield radiosensitive tissues outside region of interest.

Patient and Part Position
- Patient is supine, aligned to midline of table or IR (Fig. 16.59).
- Apply immobilization if necessary.

Newborns and Young Infants
- Infants are usually calm if they feel snug and warm, unless they are in pain. If an infant is crying, a pacifier may help and would not interfere with the examination.

Infants and Toddlers Apply immobilization if necessary. If parents are providing assistance, do the following:
- Provide parent with lead apron and gloves.
- Position tube and IR and set exposure factors before positioning.
- Position parent so that technologist's view is not obstructed.
- Usually it is only necessary to have a parent hold the child's arms.

CR
- Infants and small children – CR and cassette centered **1 inch (2.5 cm) above umbilicus**
- Older children and adolescents – CR centered at **level of iliac crest**

Respiration
- With **infants and young children,** watch the breathing pattern. When abdomen is still, make the exposure. If the patient is crying, make the exposure as the patient takes a breath to let out a cry.
- Children older than 5 years of age usually can hold their breath after a practice session.

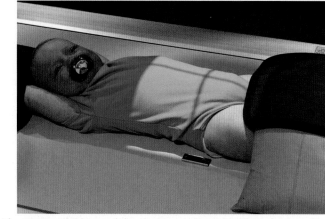

Fig. 16.59 Child immobilized with sandbags for AP abdomen. (Note sandbags under and over lower limbs.)

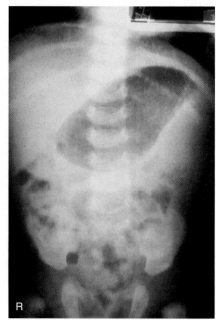

Fig. 16.60 AP abdomen, supine (demonstrates distended air-filled stomach).

Evaluation Criteria
Anatomy Demonstrated: • Soft tissue border outlines and gas-filled structures such as the stomach and intestines, calcifications (if present), and faint bony skeletal structures are shown (Fig. 16.60).
Position: • Vertebral column is aligned to center of radiograph. • **No rotation** exists; pelvis, hips, and lower rib cage are symmetric. • **Collimation** to area of interest.
Exposure: • **No motion** is evident, and diaphragm and gas patterns appear sharp. • Optimal contrast and exposure visualize bony structure outlines such as ribs and vertebrae through abdominal contents without overexposing gas-filled structures.

AP ERECT PROJECTION: ABDOMEN

Clinical Indications
- Pathology of the abdomen, including possible intestinal obstruction by demonstration of air-fluid levels or free intra-abdominal air.

Generally, this projection is part of a three-way or acute abdomen series (supine, erect, and decubitus).

Abdomen
ROUTINE
• AP (KUB)
SPECIAL
• AP erect
• Lateral and dorsal decubitus

Technical Factors
- Minimum SID—40 inches (100 cm)
- IR size—determined by size of patient, portrait
- Grid if 4 inches (10 cm) or larger
- Shortest exposure time possible
- kVp range—60–75

Shielding Shield radiosensitive tissues outside region of interest.

Patient and Part Position
- Have patient sit or stand with back against upright IR.
- Seat younger child on large foam block with legs slightly apart. Immobilize legs if necessary. Ask parent to hold arms away from side or over the child's head (Fig. 16.61). Hold infant's head between arms.
- Small children may be placed in a Pigg-O-Stat as an immobilization device and to improve positioning accuracy (Fig. 16.62).
- Children 4 years old or older (unless too ill) can stand with assistance.
- With parental assistance (if parent is not pregnant):
  - Provide parent with lead apron and gloves.
  - Position tube and cassette and set exposure factors before positioning.
  - Position parent so that technologist's view is not obstructed.

CR
- With infants and small children, center CR and IR 1 inch (2.5 cm) above umbilicus.
- With older children and adolescents, center CR at approximately 1 inch (2.5 cm) to 2 inches (5 cm) (depending on the height of the child) above the level of the iliac crest, which should place top collimation border and top of film at level of the axilla to include the diaphragm on IR.

Respiration
- With infants and children, watch the breathing pattern. When the abdomen is still, make the exposure. If the patient is crying, make the exposure as the patient takes a breath in to let out a cry.
- Children older than 5 years usually can hold their breath after a practice session.

Evaluation Criteria
Anatomy Demonstrated: • Entire contents of abdomen are shown, including gas patterns and air-fluid levels and soft tissue if not obscured by excessive fluid in distended abdomen, as shown in Fig. 16.63.
Position: • Vertebral column is aligned to center of radiograph. • **No rotation** exists; pelvis and hips should be symmetric. • Collimation to area of interest.
Exposure: • **No motion** is evident, and diaphragm and gas pattern borders appear sharp. • Bony pelvis and vertebral body outlines are evident through abdominal contents without overexposing air-filled structures.

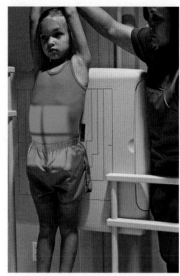

Fig. 16.61 Erect AP abdomen. (Parent holding child should be wearing lead apron and gloves.)

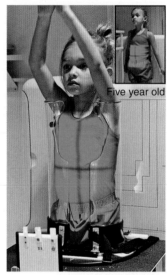

Five year old

Fig. 16.62 Erect AP abdomen with Pigg-O-Stat. Note top of cassette at axilla to include diaphragm. *Inset,* A 5-year-old child in front of the IR.

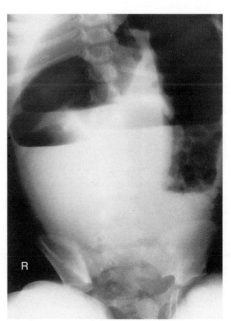

Fig. 16.63 Erect AP abdomen (demonstrates fluid levels and distended air-filled large bowel).

LATERAL DECUBITUS AND DORSAL DECUBITUS: ABDOMEN

16

NOTE: When clinically indicated, a dorsal decubitus abdomen may be performed instead of a right or left lateral decubitus.

Abdomen
ROUTINE
• AP (KUB)
SPECIAL
• AP erect
• Lateral and dorsal decubitus

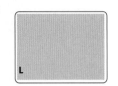

Clinical Indications
• Air-fluid levels and free air in abdomen
• Possible calcifications, masses, or other anomalies; dorsal decubitus demonstrates prevertebral region of abdomen

Technical Factors
• Minimum SID—40 inches (100 cm)
• IR size—determined by the size of patient, portrait to anatomy
• Grid if 4 inches (10 cm) or larger
• Shortest exposure time possible
• kVp range—60–75

Shielding Shield radiosensitive tissues outside region of interest.

Patient and Part Position
Lateral Decubitus
• Patient on side on a radiolucent foam block with back against IR (Fig. 16.64)
• Horizontal CR directed to 1 inch (2.5 cm) superior to umbilicus

Dorsal and Ventral Decubitus
• Patient is supine on a rectangular radiolucent foam block for dorsal decubitus (Fig. 16.65).
• Patient is prone on a rectangular radiolucent foam block for ventral decubitus.
• Gently pull arms above head and ask parent to hold arms and head with newborn or small infant. Immobilize as necessary.
• Place IR portrait, parallel to the midsagittal plane against side of patient (support with cassette holder device or with sandbags).

CR
• CR **horizontal**, centered to midcoronal plane for dorsal and ventral decubitus:
  • Infants and small children – CR and IR centered 1 inch (2.5 cm) superior to level of umbilicus
  • Older children and adolescents – CR centered at level of 1 to 2 inches (2.5 to 5 cm) superior to iliac crest

Evaluation Criteria (Dorsal and Ventral Decubitus)
Anatomy Demonstrated: • Abdominal structures in the prevertebral region and air-fluid levels within abdomen are demonstrated; diaphragm is included superiorly, and pelvis and hips are included inferiorly (Fig. 16.66). • Ventral decubitus demonstrates rectosigmoid area.
Position: • No rotation exists; posterior ribs are superimposed.
Collimation and CR: • At least minimal collimation borders should be visible on four sides, with CR to midcoronal plane, midway between diaphragm and symphysis pubis.
Exposure: • No motion is evident, and diaphragm and gas patterns appear sharp. • Abdominal soft tissue detail is visible without overexposing gas-filled structures. • Faint rib outlines are visible through abdominal contents.

Respiration
• With **infants and small children,** watch the breathing pattern. When the abdomen is still, make the exposure. If the patient is crying, make the exposure after the patient takes a breath to let out a cry.
• Children older than 5 years usually can hold their breath after a practice session.

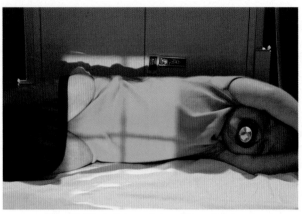

Fig. 16.64 Left lateral decubitus abdomen.

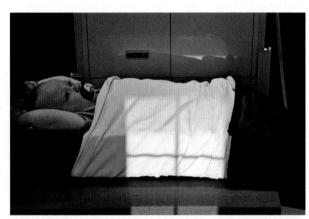

Fig. 16.65 Dorsal decubitus abdomen—left lateral position.

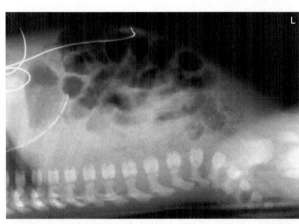

Fig. 16.66 Dorsal decubitus abdomen (demonstrates necrotizing enterocolitis in infant).

UPPER GI TRACT STUDY

BARIUM SWALLOW, UPPER GI, AND SMALL BOWEL COMBINATION STUDY

Clinical Indications

• Diseases or conditions involving the GI tract (see summary of clinical indications for the pediatric abdomen, Table 16.4, p. 630)

Room Preparation The fluoroscopic procedure room should be prepared before the child is brought into the room. The table is placed in the horizontal position, and the fluoroscopic controls are set (Fig. 16.67). A cotton or disposable sheet should be placed over the table. Depending on the examination, the appropriate barium or contrast media, feeding bottle, nipple, straw, feeding catheter, and syringe should be ready for use. Suction and oxygen also should be readily available in the event of an emergency.

Shielding A section of 1-mm lead vinyl may be placed under the child's buttocks to shield the gonads from scatter radiation if the fluoroscopy tube is under the tabletop.

Barium Preparation Liquid barium may be used according to a particular manufacturer's instructions. The barium may have to be diluted for younger children and infants. Dilution is usually necessary when a feeding bottle is used, and it is helpful to widen the hole in the nipple with a sterile needle or scalpel so that the infant can feed more easily.

The amount of barium for an upper GI study varies with the age of the child. Typical volumes range from 30 to 75 mL (1 to 2.5 oz) in infants to 480 mL (16 oz) in older adolescents. This can be adjusted based the discretion of the radiologist.[4]

Patient and Parent Preparation The parent should accompany the child into the procedure room before the study is started. A few minutes spent explaining the examination and how the equipment works is beneficial to both parent and child (Fig. 16.68). The large equipment and strange noises that seem so normal to the technologist are terrifying to many young children. An explanation and demonstration of how the image intensifier is brought down over the chest and abdomen lessen fears that the child might have of being crushed. On the monitor, children can be shown how they can watch the "milk shake" going down into the stomach.

Barium procedures on children are usually performed with the patient lying down. Parents (if not pregnant) may be given a lead apron and gloves so that they can remain in the room during the fluoroscopic procedure. Holding the child's hand and assisting the technologist in feeding the child reduces anxiety and helps in providing a supportive environment for both parent and child. Continual words of encouragement help the child with ingestion of the barium.

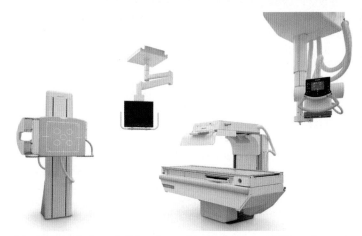

Fig. 16.67 Modern digital radiographic/fluoroscopy (R/F) equipment for GI study. (Courtesy of Royal Philips.)

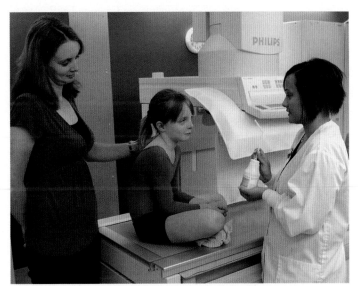

Fig. 16.68 Providing clear explanations to the parent and child is beneficial.

Procedure

Drinking Barium An infant drinks from a feeding bottle. An older child usually drinks through a straw, which prevents spillage (Fig. 16.69).

In some cases, a child may insist on drinking directly from a cup. This entails sitting the child up to drink and then laying the child down for fluoroscopy. If the esophagus must be outlined, barium paste can be spooned onto the palate or tongue. Another tactic is to squirt barium into the child's mouth with a 10-mL syringe while gently holding the nose. If a child refuses to swallow the barium, it may be necessary for the radiologist to pass a nasogastric tube into the stomach.

Fluoroscopy Positioning Sequence Radiologists follow a particular sequence of positions for a upper GI study starting with the **patient supine.** This generally is followed by a **left lateral, left posterior oblique (LPO), right anterior oblique (RAO),** and **right lateral** with the patient turned onto the right side; in this position, the stomach empties quickly (Fig. 16.70). It is important to check the location of the duodenojejunal junction to rule out malrotation before the jejunum fills. The final position is **prone.** This is a standard procedure even in patients who do not have symptoms of malrotation.

Permanent images are recorded during fluoroscopy. These digital images can be displayed on monitors and manipulated later as needed before sending to the picture archiving and communication system (PACS).

Small Bowel Follow-Through An AP or PA abdomen is taken at **20- to 30-minute intervals,** either supine or prone, depending on the age and condition of the patient. Transit time is quite rapid in young children; the barium may reach the ileocecal region in **1 hour** (Fig. 16.71).

Postprocedure Instructions After the examination is complete and the radiographs have been checked, the patient may eat and drink normally if diet permits. The child should be encouraged to drink plenty of water and fruit juices if diet permits. The technologist should ensure that the digital images are processed and saved to PACS. The number of images recorded and fluoroscopic time should be noted on the requisition and in the radiology information system.

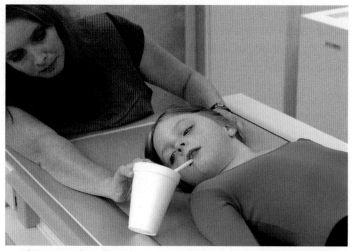

Fig. 16.69 "Drinking" barium just before beginning fluoroscopy.

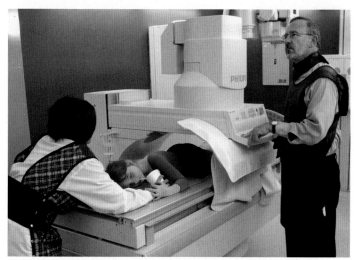

Fig. 16.70 Patient being placed in an oblique position in preparation for upper GI fluoroscopy. (Parent will step back before fluoroscopy begins.)

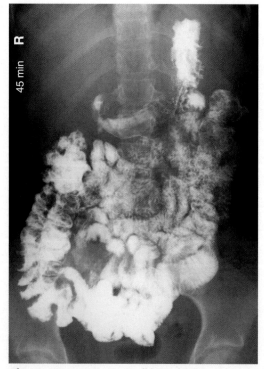

Fig. 16.71 45-minute small bowel follow-through.

LOWER GI TRACT STUDY: BARIUM ENEMA

SINGLE-CONTRAST, DOUBLE-CONTRAST, OR AIR ENEMA

Clinical Indications See summary of clinical indications for pediatric abdomen in Table 16.4, p. 630.

Contrast Medium and Materials – Barium Enema, Single Contrast

Children Older Than 1 Year

- A disposable enema bag is used with barium sulfate, tubing, and clamp. Add tepid (not cold) water according to manufacturer's instructions (Fig. 16.72).
- **Pediatric flexible enema tip:** Some of these catheters are designed so that they cannot be inserted beyond the rectum. Taping the tube in place prevents leakage.

WARNING: Latex tips must *not* be used because of the potential for a life-threatening allergic response to latex. Inflatable balloon-type retention tips also must *not* be used because they may perforate the rectum.

Neonates (Newborn to 1 Year)

- 10F flexible silicone catheter and 60-mL syringe; barium injected manually and slowly

All Patients

- Water-soluble lubricating jelly
- Hypoallergenic (and skin sensitive) tape
- Gloves
- Washcloths and towels for cleanup

Contrast Media and Materials – Barium Enema, Double Contrast

- High-density barium and air contrast enema kit or enema bag with double-line tip, including tube through which air is introduced
- Air insufflation device
- Remainder of materials same as for a single-contrast barium enema

Air Enema An air enema is performed under fluoroscopy for the pneumatic reduction of an intussusception. This condition occurs when one portion of the large bowel telescopes into an adjacent portion (Figs. 16.73 and 16.74). The pneumatic reduction most often is performed as an emergency because the patient is in severe abdominal pain. It is a specialized procedure that must be done carefully to avoid perforation of the bowel. When the procedure is successful, the child's pain dissipates quickly, and in many cases, the reduction helps to prevent an operative procedure. An intussusception also may be reduced by barium enema, depending on the preference of the radiologist.

Materials

- Air insufflation device
- Aneroid air pressure gauge
- Disposable tubing with three-way stopcock
- Flexible enema tip
- Hypoallergenic tape
- Gloves
- Washcloths and towels for cleanup

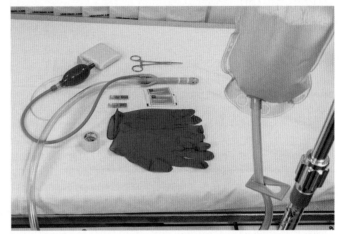

Fig. 16.72 Barium enema room setup with disposable enema bag, tubing, enema tip (use pediatric flexible-type enema tip), and other supplies.

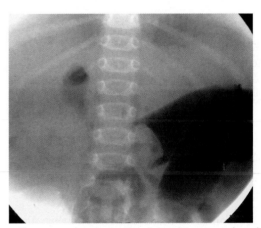

Fig. 16.73 Air enema demonstrating air in transverse colon, the most common site of intussusception. (From Godderidge C: *Pediatric imaging,* Philadelphia, 1995, Saunders.)

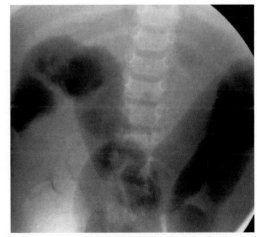

Fig. 16.74 Air enema spot image following the image shown in Fig. 16.73, showing the air having pushed out the telescoped bowel. (From Godderidge C: *Pediatric imaging,* Philadelphia, 1995, Saunders.)

Room Preparation The room should be prepared as for a upper GI with the table horizontal, covered with a disposable or cotton sheet, and the fluoroscopic controls set. The enema bag with barium, tubing, stand, clamp, and tip should be assembled and ready for use. The barium is administered slowly, by gravity, from **24 inches (61 cm)** above the tabletop unless otherwise directed by the radiologist.

Shielding The gonads cannot be shielded during a fluoroscopic examination of the large bowel.

Patient and Parent Preparation The patient and the parent should be brought into the room, and the procedure should be explained clearly and simply. It is particularly important to explain why the tube is being inserted into the rectum and how the barium enhances the bowel on the television screen. Appropriate technology and language should be used in the explanation, depending on the age of the child. A young child is likely to be frightened by having someone touch the buttocks and genital area.

Technologists should be reassuring and supportive and should explain to parent and child that the examination does not hurt, although the child may feel a desire to go to the bathroom while the barium is passing into the bowel (Fig. 16.75).

A parent should stay with the child throughout the examination. Talking and giving words of encouragement help the examination go smoothly.

Procedure

Fluoroscopy and spot imaging
- Digital imaging during fluoroscopy; image size depending on age of child and equipment
- Supine or prone abdomen at completion of fluoroscopy
- Right and left lateral decubitus images of the abdomen for double contrast
- AP supine abdomen after evacuation of barium

NOTE: In contrast to the follow-up images taken for adults, fewer radiographs (sometimes none) are taken at the completion of fluoroscopy.

After Reduction of Intussusception Following Air or Barium Enema
- AP supine abdomen to document that air or barium, depending on the contrast medium used, has passed through the ileocecal region into the ileum, proving that the intussusception has been reduced (Fig. 16.76).

Postprocedure Tasks
- After the examination is complete and the radiographs have been checked, encourage the patient to drink plenty of water and fruit juices, if diet permits.
- Ensure that digital images are labeled and sent to PACS. Record the number or images taken and the fluoroscopic time on the requisition and in the radiology information system.

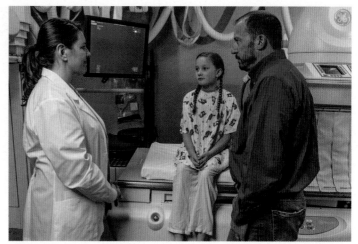

Fig. 16.75 The technologist providing clear explanations to the child and parent.

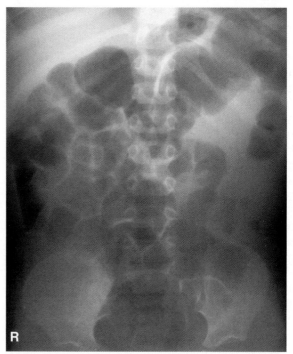

Fig. 16.76 Postreduction of intussusception demonstrating air in terminal ileum. (From Godderidge C: *Pediatric imaging,* Philadelphia, 1995, Saunders.)

GENITOURINARY SYSTEM STUDY: VOIDING CYSTOURETHROGRAM (VCUG)

Clinical Indications See summary of diagnostic indications for the pediatric abdomen in Table 16.4, p. 630.

VCUG may be performed before IVU or an ultrasound scan of the kidneys. **Urinary tract infection** is a very common condition in young children, and this study may be performed to check or evaluate **vesicoureteral reflux,** a common cause of urinary tract infection.

Technical Factors
- Minimum SID—40 inches (100 cm)
- IR size—determined by the size of patient, IR portrait to anatomy
- Grid if 4 inches (10 cm) or larger
- Shortest exposure time possible
- kVp range—70–80

Shielding
- Gonadal shielding can be used on boys for plain images of the abdomen and for excretory urography except for voiding images. Shielding is not used during voiding cystourethrogram (VCUG).
- Gonadal shielding cannot be used on girls except when the kidney area only is radiographed because the ovaries of younger children are higher in the abdomen and their location is variable. The lower abdomen may be shielded for the initial contrast image of the kidneys taken during IVU unless shielding obscures the area of diagnostic interest.

Preparation VCUG requires no special preparation. If the procedure is to be followed by IVU, the child should be prepared for IVU. This procedure should be described to the patient beforehand, and depending on the age of the child, the timing of the procedure should be left to the parent (Fig. 16.77). Simple written instructions given to the parent assist in the explanation.

Contrast Media and Materials
- Iodinated contrast media for cystography
- Intravenous stand, tubing, and clamp
- Sterile tray with small bowls, sterile gauze, and gloves
- Urine specimen container
- 8F feeding tube (inflatable balloon-retaining catheters should not be used for children)
- Lidocaine lubricating jelly
- Skin cleanser-antiseptic, washcloths, and towels
- 10-mL syringe and fistula tip for boys
- Urine receptacle

Room Preparation The table should be in a horizontal position, covered with a disposable or cotton sheet, and the fluoroscopic controls should be set. The bottle of contrast medium should be warmed slightly and hung from an intravenous stand with tubing and clamp attached. Warmed antiseptic skin cleanser is poured into a small sterile bowl ready for use, and the tray is covered until the patient is on the table.

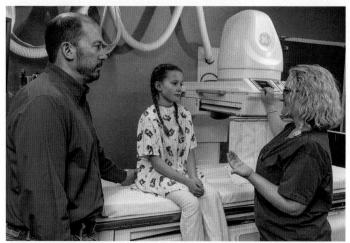

Fig. 16.77 It is important to talk to the child and parent.

Patient and Parent Preparation The patient and the parent should be brought into the room and the procedure explained again simply and clearly. The child should be shown the equipment and how it works and should be reassured that the image intensifier will not hurt him or her. The explanation of the procedure should be given in language appropriate for the age of the child. "Void" or "voiding" is frequently used by technologists or radiologists, but words such as "tinkle" or "pee" are more likely to be understood by young children, enabling them to follow instructions. Because so many terms are used for urination, ask the parent what word is used at home.

VCUG is just as embarrassing and difficult for a young child as it is for an adult. A child who has just been toilet trained has difficulty understanding why urinating lying down on a table is acceptable. As much privacy as possible is recommended; only staff members who are participating in the examination should be allowed in the room. If possible, a technologist or radiology nurse who is the same sex as the patient should perform the catheterization.

Procedure An older child should be asked to empty the bladder before entering the room. An infant's bladder is drained at catheterization. After the perineum is cleaned, the catheter is inserted into the bladder, and a urine specimen is taken. After the contrast medium is run to clear air from the tubing, the catheter is attached to the tubing and bottle of contrast medium, and the bladder is slowly filled.

Images are taken when the patient's bladder is full and when voiding because this is when reflux is most likely to occur (Fig. 16.78). AP and oblique positions often are performed during the voiding phase of the study. A postvoid image of the bladder and kidneys is taken. If reflux occurs, a late image of the abdomen may be taken to check whether the kidneys have emptied (Fig. 16.79). If a patient is being followed for reflux or postoperatively, a radionuclide VCUG may be performed at a reduced radiation dose instead of a fluoroscopic procedure.

Postprocedure Tasks The parent and child should be told that when the child first urinates after the procedure, a slight burning sensation may occur and the urine might be pink. Drinking plenty of clear fluids quickly helps to alleviate this problem.

Images should be properly processed and sent to PACS. The amount and type of contrast material, the number of images, and fluoroscopic times should be recorded. A urine specimen should be sent for culture.

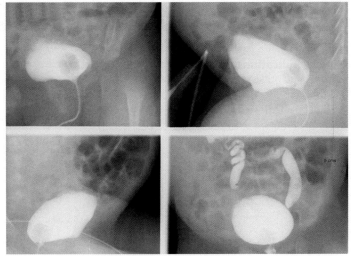

Fig. 16.78 Voiding cystourethrogram: AP and oblique projections demonstrate reflux of both kidneys (16-day-old boy).

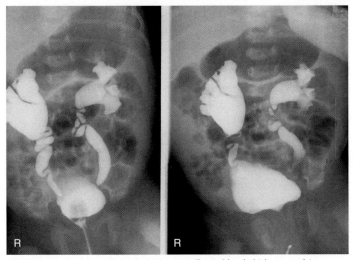

Fig. 16.79 VCUG: various positions, reflux of both kidneys. This pediatric patient is demonstrating vesicoureteral reflux (reflux is most likely to occur during the voiding phase of VCUG; see right image).

CHAPTER 17

Angiography and Interventional Procedures

CONTRIBUTIONS BY **Nicolle M. Hightower,** MEd, RT(R)(VI)

CONTRIBUTORS TO PAST EDITIONS   Cindy Murphy, BHSc, RT(R), ACR, Marianne Tortorici, EdD, RT(R), Patrick Apfel, MEd, RT(R), Barry T. Anthony, RT(R)

CONTENTS

RADIOGRAPHIC ANATOMY

Introduction

DEFINITION

Angiography refers to the radiographic examination of vessels after injection of contrast media. Because of the relative densities of the soft tissues of the body, contrast media must be added to visualize the circulatory system. For example, the routine lateral skull radiograph in Fig. 17.1 demonstrates none of the vessels of the cranial circulatory system, whereas the lateral cerebral carotid arteriogram in Fig. 17.2 clearly demonstrates the blood vessels by subtracting out the bony anatomy. This is also true for the circulatory systems of other body regions, such as the thorax, abdomen, and upper and lower limbs (peripheral). A good understanding of the vascular anatomy, as covered in the first part of this chapter, is essential for performing angiography.

DIVISIONS OR COMPONENTS OF THE CIRCULATORY SYSTEM

The circulatory system consists of the cardiovascular and lymphatic components. The cardiovascular portion includes the heart, blood, and vessels that transport the blood.

The **lymphatic component** of the circulatory system is composed of a clear, watery fluid called **lymph, lymphatic vessels,** and **lymphatic nodes.** The cardiovascular and lymphatic components differ in their function and method of transporting their respective fluids within the vessels. This chapter focuses solely on the cardiovascular portion of the circulatory system.

The **cardiovascular,** or blood circulatory, division may be divided further into the **cardio** (circulation within the heart) and **vascular** (blood vessel) components. The vascular, or vessel, component is divided into the **pulmonary** (heart to lungs and back) and general, or **systemic,** (throughout the body) components (Box 17.1).

CARDIOVASCULAR SYSTEM

The **heart** is the major organ of the cardiovascular system; it functions as a pump to maintain circulation of blood throughout the body. The **vascular component** comprises a network of blood vessels that carry blood from the heart to body tissues and back to the heart again.

Functions

Functions of the cardiovascular system include the following:
1. Transportation of oxygen, nutrients, hormones, and chemicals necessary for normal body activity
2. Removal of waste products through the kidneys and lungs
3. Maintenance of body temperature and water and electrolyte balance.

These functions are performed by the blood components: red blood cells, white blood cells, and platelets suspended in plasma.

Blood Components

Red blood cells, or **erythrocytes,** are produced in the red marrow of certain bones and transport oxygen by the protein hemoglobin to body tissues.

White blood cells, or **leukocytes,** are formed in bone marrow and lymph tissue and defend the body against infection and disease. **Platelets,** also originating from bone marrow, repair tears in blood vessel walls and promote blood clotting.

Plasma, the liquid portion of the blood, consists of 92% water and about 7% plasma protein and salts, nutrients, and oxygen.

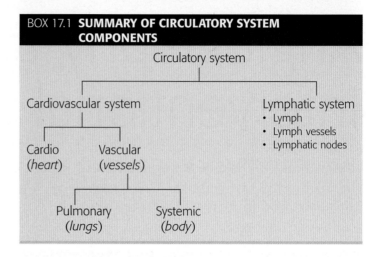

BOX 17.1 **SUMMARY OF CIRCULATORY SYSTEM COMPONENTS**

SYSTEMIC CIRCULATION

Arteries

Vessels that transport oxygenated blood from the heart to tissues are called **arteries.** Arteries that originate directly from the heart are large, but they subdivide and decrease in size as they extend from the heart to various parts of the body. The smaller arteries are termed **arterioles.** As blood travels through the arterioles, it enters the tissues through the smallest subdivision of these vessels, known as **capillaries** (Fig. 17.3).

Veins

The deoxygenated blood returns to the heart through the venous system. The venous system extends from venous capillaries to **venules** to **veins,** increasing in size as it nears the heart.

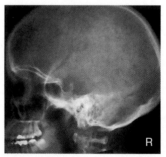
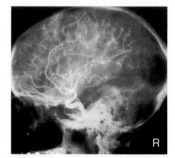

Fig. 17.1 Lateral skull radiograph. **Fig. 17.2** Lateral cerebral carotid arteriogram demonstrates the blood vessels through the use of contrast media.

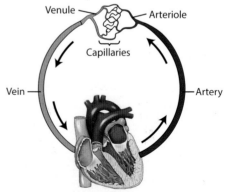

Fig. 17.3 General cardiovascular circulation.

Pulmonary Circulation

The elements of the blood vessel circuit (veins, venules, capillaries, arterioles, and arteries) that supply blood to the lungs and back make up the **pulmonary circulation** component of the cardiovascular system.

As previously noted, arteries generally carry oxygenated blood away from the heart to the capillaries. Exceptions are the **pulmonary arteries,** which carry **deoxygenated blood** to the lungs that has been returned to the heart through the superior and inferior venae cavae. The **superior** and **inferior venae cavae** (singular, *vena cava*) empty the returning deoxygenated blood into the **right atrium** of the heart.

The heart pumps this deoxygenated blood from the **right ventricle** through the pulmonary arteries to the lungs, where oxygen and carbon dioxide (CO_2) are exchanged through the small air sacs or alveoli of the lungs. The **oxygenated blood** returns through the **pulmonary veins** to the **left atrium** of the heart (Fig. 17.4).

General Systemic Circulation

HEART

The heart is a muscular organ that pumps blood throughout the body. Anatomically, the heart lies within the mediastinum and rests on the **diaphragm** (Fig. 17.5). Cardiac tissue differs from other muscle tissues of the body in its construction and is termed **myocardium.** The left side of the heart is responsible for the extensive systemic circulation; the left muscle wall is about three times as thick as the right side.

The heart is divided into four chambers: the **right** and **left atria** and the **right** and **left ventricles.** Each chamber functions to receive or pump blood. The blood circulation is a closed system by which unoxygenated blood enters the **right atrium** from all parts of the body, is reoxygenated in the lungs, and is returned to the body by the **left ventricle.**

Blood returning to the heart enters the right atrium through the **superior** and **inferior venae cavae** (Fig. 17.6). Blood in the superior vena cava originates from the head, chest, and upper limbs. The inferior vena cava (IVC) delivers blood into the right atrium from the abdomen and lower limbs.

From the **right atrium,** blood is pumped through the **tricuspid (right atrioventricular) valve** to the **right ventricle.** The right ventricle contracts, moving the blood through the **pulmonary (pulmonary semilunar) valve** to the **pulmonary arteries** and on to the lungs. While in the lungs, the blood is oxygenated and then is returned to the left atrium of the heart by the **pulmonary veins.** As the left atrium contracts, blood is transported through the **mitral (left atrioventricular or bicuspid) valve** to the left ventricle.

When the left ventricle contracts, the oxygenated blood exits the chamber by the **aortic (aortic semilunar) valve,** flows through the aorta, and is delivered to various body tissues (Box 17.2).

BOX 17.2 SUMMARY OF GENERAL SYSTEMIC CIRCULATION

Venae cavae	Aorta
↓	↑ (Aortic valve)
Right atrium	Left ventricle
↓ (Tricuspid valve)	↑ (Bicuspid valve)
Right ventricle	Left atrium
↓ (Pulmonary valve)	↑ (Pulmonary valves)
Pulmonary arteries → Lungs → Pulmonary veins	
(Unoxygenated blood)	(Oxygenated blood)

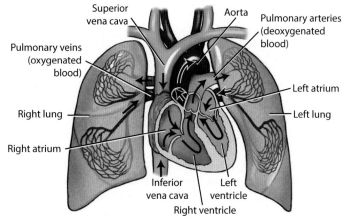

Fig. 17.4 Pulmonary circulation.

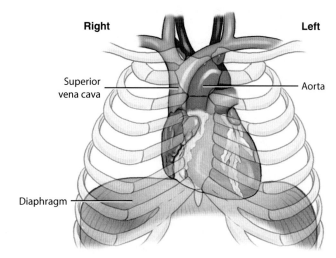

Fig. 17.5 Heart and mediastinal structures.

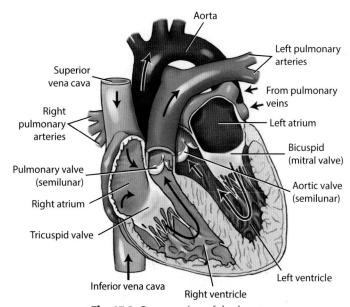

Fig. 17.6 Cross section of the heart.

CORONARY ARTERIES

The **two coronary arteries** are the vessels that deliver blood to the heart muscle. These arteries are called the **right coronary artery** and the **left coronary artery.** Both originate from the **aortic bulb (root).**

The right coronary artery arises from the right (anterior) sinuses of the aortic bulb, and the left coronary artery originates from the left (posterior) aortic bulb sinus. The **right coronary artery** supplies much of the **right atrium** and the **right ventricle** of the heart (Fig. 17.7).

The **left coronary artery** supplies blood to **both ventricles** and the **left atrium** of the heart. Many interconnections or anastomoses exist between the left and right coronary arteries. Blood returns to the right atrium of the heart via the coronary veins.

CORONARY VEINS

The coronary sinus system returns blood to the right atrium for recirculation. The **coronary sinus** is a large vein on the posterior side of the heart between the atria and ventricles. The coronary sinus has three major branches: the **great, middle,** and **small cardiac veins.**

The **great cardiac vein** receives blood from both ventricles and the left atrium. The **middle cardiac vein** drains blood from the right ventricle, right atrium, and part of the left ventricle. The **small cardiac vein** returns blood from the right ventricle. The coronary sinus drains most of the blood from the heart. Some small veins drain directly into both atria (Fig. 17.8).

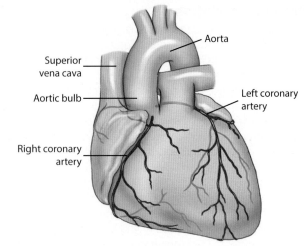

Fig. 17.7 Arteries of the heart (anterior view).

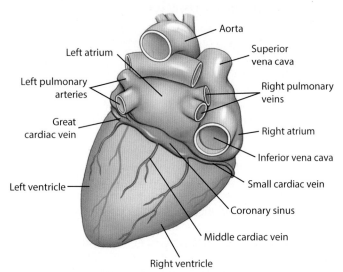

Fig. 17.8 Veins of the heart (posterior view).

Cerebral Arteries

BLOOD SUPPLY TO BRAIN

The brain is supplied with blood by major arteries of the systemic circulation. The four major arteries that supply the brain are as follows (Fig. 17.9):

1. Right common carotid artery
2. Left common carotid artery
3. Right vertebral artery
4. Left vertebral artery

Major branches of the two common carotid arteries supply the anterior circulation of the brain, and the two vertebral arteries supply the posterior circulation. Radiographic examination of the neck vessels and the entire brain circulation is referred to as a **four-vessel angiogram** because these four vessels are collectively and selectively injected with contrast media. Another common series is the **three-vessel angiogram,** in which the two carotids and only one vertebral artery are studied.

BRANCHES OF AORTIC ARCH

The aorta is the major artery leaving the left ventricle of the heart. Three major branches arise from the **arch** of the **aorta** as follows (Fig. 17.10):

1. Brachiocephalic artery
2. Left common carotid artery
3. Left subclavian artery

The brachiocephalic trunk is a short vessel that bifurcates into the **right common carotid artery** and the **right subclavian artery.** This bifurcation occurs directly posterior to the right sternoclavicular joint. The right and left vertebral arteries are branches of the subclavian arteries on each side as described earlier (see Fig. 17.9). Because the left common carotid artery rises directly from the arch of the aorta, it is slightly longer than the right common carotid artery.

In the cervical region, the two common carotid arteries resemble one another. Each common carotid artery passes cephalad from its origin along either side of the trachea and larynx to the level of the upper border of the **thyroid cartilage.** Each common carotid artery divides here into **external** and **internal carotid arteries.** The site of bifurcation for each common carotid artery is at the approximate level of the **fourth cervical vertebra.**

NECK AND HEAD ARTERIES

The major arteries supplying the head, as seen from the right side of the neck, are shown in Fig. 17.11A (only right-side vessels are identified on this drawing). The **brachiocephalic trunk artery bifurcates** into the **right common carotid artery** and the **right subclavian artery.**

The right common carotid artery ascends to the level of the fourth cervical vertebra to branch into the **external carotid artery** and **internal carotid artery,** also described earlier. Each external carotid artery primarily supplies the anterior neck, the face, and the greater part of the scalp and meninges (brain coverings). Each internal carotid artery supplies the cerebral hemispheres, the pituitary gland, the orbital structures, the external nose, and the anterior portion of the brain.

The **right vertebral artery** arises from the right subclavian artery to pass through the transverse foramina of C6 through C1. Each vertebral artery passes posteriorly along the superior border of C1 before angling upward through the foramen magnum to enter the cranium.

A common carotid arteriogram is shown on the right visualizing the right internal carotid artery (A), right external carotid artery (B), and right common carotid artery (C) (Fig. 17.11B).

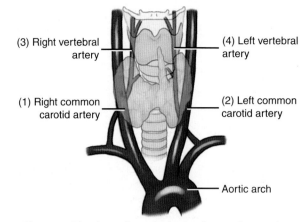

Fig. 17.9 Blood supply to the brain—four major arteries.

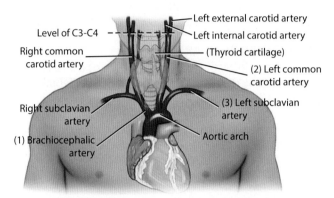

Fig. 17.10 Three branches of the aortic arch.

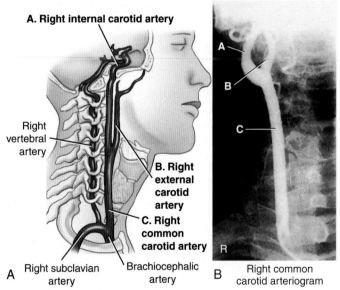

Fig. 17.11 Neck and head arteries.

EXTERNAL CAROTID ARTERY BRANCHES

The four major branches of the external carotid artery include the following:

1. Facial artery
2. Maxillary artery
3. Superficial temporal artery
4. Occipital artery

INTERNAL CAROTID ARTERY

Each **internal carotid artery** ascends to enter the carotid canal in the petrous portion of the temporal bone. Within the petrous pyramid, the artery curves forward and medially. Before supplying the cerebral hemispheres, each internal carotid artery passes through a collection of venous channels around the sella turcica. Each internal carotid artery passes through the dura mater, medial to each anterior clinoid process, to bifurcate into the cerebral branches.

The S-shaped portion of each internal carotid artery is termed the **carotid siphon** and is studied carefully by the radiologist.

ANTERIOR CEREBRAL ARTERY

The two end branches of each **internal carotid artery** are the **anterior cerebral** (Fig. 17.12) and the **middle cerebral arteries** (Fig. 17.13). Each anterior cerebral artery and branches supply much of the forebrain near the midline. The anterior cerebral arteries curve around the corpus callosum, giving off several branches to the midportions of the cerebral hemisphere. Each anterior cerebral artery connects to the opposite one and to the posterior brain circulation.

MIDDLE CEREBRAL ARTERY

The middle cerebral artery is the largest branch of each internal carotid artery. This artery supplies the **lateral aspects of the anterior cerebral circulation** (see Fig. 17.13). As the middle cerebral artery courses toward the periphery of the brain, branches extend upward along the lateral portion of the insula or central lobe of the brain. These small branches supply brain tissue deep within the brain.

INTERNAL CAROTID ARTERIOGRAM

When one internal carotid artery is injected with contrast media, both the anterior cerebral artery and the middle cerebral artery fill. The arterial phase of a cerebral carotid angiogram is similar to the drawings in Fig. 17.14.

In the frontal view or posteroanterior (PA) projection, little superimposition of the two vessels occurs because the anterior cerebral artery courses toward the midline, and the middle cerebral artery extends laterally.

Some superimposition exists in the lateral position. The internal carotid artery supplies primarily the anterior portion of the brain.

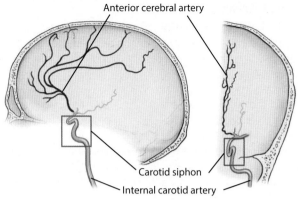

Fig. 17.12 Internal carotid and anterior cerebral artery.

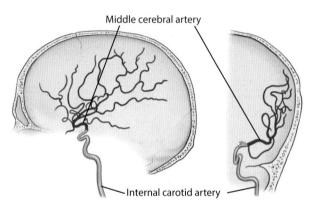

Fig. 17.13 Middle cerebral artery.

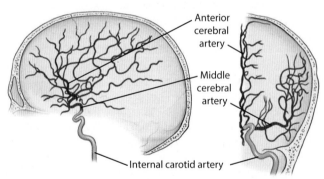

Fig. 17.14 Internal carotid arteriogram; both anterior and middle cerebral arteries are visualized.

VERTEBROBASILAR ARTERIES

The two vertebral arteries enter the cranium through the foramen magnum and unite to form the single basilar artery. The vertebral arteries and the basilar artery and their branches form the vertebrobasilar system. Omitting much of the occipital bone in Fig. 17.15 allows these arteries to be shown along the base of the skull. Several arteries arise from each vertebral artery before their point of convergence to form the basilar artery. These branches supply the spinal cord and the hindbrain. The basilar artery rests on the clivus, a portion of the sphenoid bone, and the base of the occipital bone anterior to the foramen magnum and posterior to the dorsum sellae.

ARTERIAL CIRCLE (CIRCLE OF WILLIS)

The blood to the brain is supplied by the internal carotid and vertebral arteries. The posterior brain circulation communicates with the anterior circulation along the base of the brain in the **arterial circle** or **circle of Willis** (Fig. 17.16). The five arteries or branches that make up the arterial circle are (1) the **anterior communicating artery,** (2) the **anterior cerebral arteries,** (3) branches of the **internal carotid arteries,** (4) the **posterior communicating artery,** and (5) the **posterior cerebral arteries.**

Not only are the anterior and posterior circulations connected, but also both sides connect across the midline. An elaborate anastomosis interconnects the entire arterial supply to the brain. As the basilar artery courses forward toward the arterial circle, it gives off several branches to the hindbrain and posterior cerebrum. The posterior cerebral arteries are two of the larger branches.

Certain aneurysms may occur in these vessels that make up the arterial circle; they need to be well demonstrated on cerebral angiographic studies (Fig. 17.17).

The important "master" gland, the **hypophysis** (pituitary gland), and its surrounding bony structure, the **sella turcica,** are located within the arterial circle. See Fig. 17.15 for the location of the **basilar artery** resting on the **clivus** and the relationship of these structures to the **dorsum sellae.**

VERTEBROBASILAR ARTERIOGRAM

A standard vertebrobasilar arteriogram appears similar to the simplified drawing in Fig. 17.18. The **vertebral arteries, basilar artery,** and **posterior cerebral arteries** can be seen. Several branches to the cerebellum have not been labeled on this drawing.

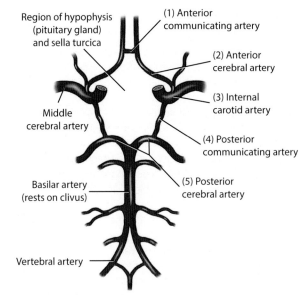

Fig. 17.16 Arterial circle (circle of Willis)—five arteries or branches.

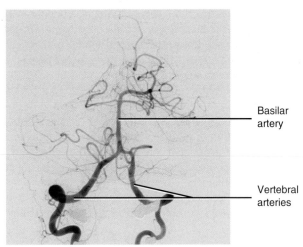

Fig. 17.17 Vertebrobasilar arteriogram. (From Nadgir R, Yousem DM: *Neuroradiology: The requisites,* ed 4, Philadelphia, 2017, Elsevier.)

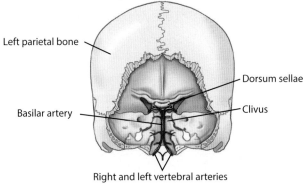

Fig. 17.15 Vertebrobasilar arteries.

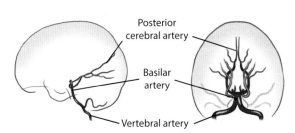

Fig. 17.18 Vertebrobasilar arteriogram.

Cerebral Veins
GREAT VEINS OF NECK

The **three pairs** of major veins that drain the head, face, and neck region (Fig. 17.19) include the following:
1. Right and left internal jugular veins
2. Right and left external jugular veins
3. Right and left vertebral veins

Each **internal jugular vein** drains the meninges and brain. In addition, many smaller veins join each internal jugular vein as it passes caudad eventually to become the **brachiocephalic vein** on each side. The right and left brachiocephalic veins join to form the superior vena cava, which returns blood to the right atrium of the heart.

The two **external jugular veins** are more superficial trunks that drain the scalp and much of the face and neck. Each external jugular vein joins the respective **subclavian vein.**

The right and left **vertebral veins** form outside the cranium and drain the upper neck and occipital region. Each vertebral vein enters the transverse foramen of C1, descends to C6, and enters the subclavian vein.

DURAL VENOUS SINUSES

The dural sinuses are venous channels that drain blood from the brain (Fig. 17.20). These sinuses are situated between the two layers of the dura mater, as described in Chapter 18, which discusses brain coverings and meningeal spaces.

A space between the two layers of the dura, along the superior portion of the longitudinal fissure, contains the **superior sagittal sinus.** The **inferior sagittal sinus** flows posteriorly to drain into the **straight sinus.** The straight sinus and the superior sagittal sinus empty into opposite transverse sinuses.

Each **transverse sinus** curves medially to occupy a groove along the mastoid portion of the temporal bone. The sinus in this region is termed the **sigmoid sinus.** Each sigmoid sinus curves caudad to continue as the **internal jugular vein** at the jugular foramen.

The **occipital sinus** courses posteriorly from the foramen magnum to join the superior sagittal sinus, straight sinus, and transverse sinuses at their confluence. The **confluence of sinuses** is located near the internal occipital protuberance. Other major dura mater sinuses drain the area on either side of the sphenoid bone and sella turcica.

CRANIAL VENOUS SYSTEM

The major veins of the entire cranial venous system are labeled in Fig. 17.21. Only the most prominent veins are identified. One group not individually named is the *external cerebral veins,* which, along with certain dural sinuses, drain the outer surfaces of the cerebral hemispheres. Similar to all veins of the brain, the external cerebral veins possess no valves and are extremely thin because they have no muscle tissue.

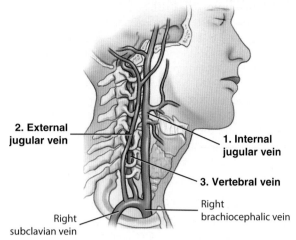

Fig. 17.19 Great veins of the neck.

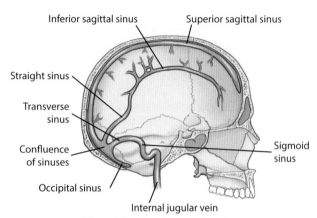

Fig. 17.20 Dura mater sinuses.

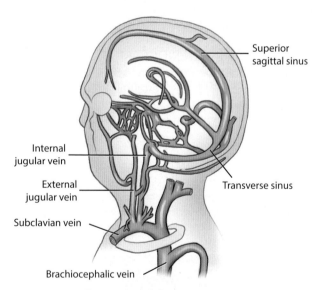

Fig. 17.21 Dural venous system.

Thoracic Circulatory System

THORACIC ARTERIES

The **aorta** and **pulmonary arteries** are the major arteries located within the chest. The pulmonary arteries supply the lungs with deoxygenated blood (as shown earlier in Fig. 17.4, p. 655).

The aorta extends from the heart to about the fourth lumbar vertebra and is divided into thoracic and abdominal sections. The **thoracic section** is subdivided into the following **four segments** (Fig. 17.22):

1. Aortic bulb (root)
2. Ascending aorta
3. Aortic arch
4. Descending aorta

The **bulb**, or root portion, is at the proximal end of the aorta and is the area from which the coronary arteries originate. Extending from the bulb is the **ascending portion** of the aorta, which terminates at approximately the second sternocostal joint and becomes the **arch.** The arch is unique from the other segments of the thoracic aorta because three arterial branches arise from it: the brachiocephalic artery, left common carotid artery, and left subclavian artery. (This is also shown in Fig. 17.10, p. 657.)

Many variations of the aortic arch exist. Three more common variations sometimes seen in angiography include the following (Fig. 17.23):

A. **Left circumflex aorta** (normal arch with the descending aorta downward and arched to the left)
B. **Inverse aorta** (arch is arched to the right)
C. **Pseudocoarctation** (arched descending aorta)

At its distal end, the arch becomes the **descending aorta** (see Fig. 17.22). The descending aorta extends from the isthmus to the level of the twelfth dorsal vertebra. Numerous intercostal, bronchial, esophageal, and superior phrenic arterial branches arise from the descending aorta (not shown in Fig. 17.22). These arteries transport blood to the organs for which they are named.

THORACIC VEINS

The major veins within the chest are the **superior vena cava, azygos,** and **pulmonary arteries.** The superior vena cava returns the blood transported from the thorax to the right atrium. The **azygos vein** is the major tributary that returns blood from the posterior thoracic wall to the superior vena cava (Fig. 17.24). The azygos vein enters the superior vena cava posteriorly. Blood from the chest enters the azygos vein from the intercostal, bronchial, esophageal, and phrenic veins. A section of the vena cava has been removed on this drawing to visualize the azygos and intercostal veins better. Blood from the right ventricle of the heart is carried to lungs by **pulmonary arteries.**

The **superior** and **inferior pulmonary veins** return oxygenated blood from the lungs to the left atrium, as previously shown. The **IVC** returns blood from the abdomen and lower limbs to the right atrium (see Figs. 17.4 and 17.6, p. 655).

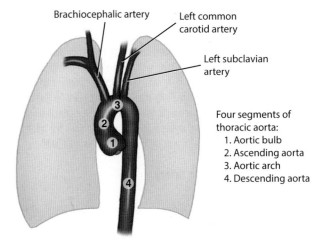

Brachiocephalic artery
Left common carotid artery
Left subclavian artery

Four segments of thoracic aorta:
1. Aortic bulb
2. Ascending aorta
3. Aortic arch
4. Descending aorta

Fig. 17.22 Thoracic aorta.

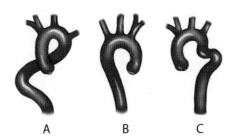

A B C

Fig. 17.23 Variations of the arch.

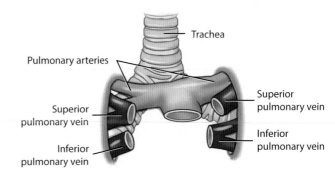

Trachea
Pulmonary arteries
Superior pulmonary vein
Superior pulmonary vein
Inferior pulmonary vein
Inferior pulmonary vein

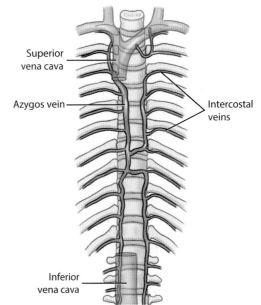

Superior vena cava
Azygos vein
Intercostal veins
Inferior vena cava

Fig. 17.24 Thoracic veins.

Abdominal Circulatory System

ABDOMINAL ARTERIES

The abdominal aorta is the continuation of the thoracic aorta. The abdominal aorta is anterior to the vertebrae and extends from the diaphragm to approximately L4, where it bifurcates into the right and left common iliac arteries. **Five major branches** of the abdominal aorta exist that are of greatest interest in angiography. Any one of these branches may be selectively catheterized for study of a specific organ. These are shown in Fig. 17.25 as follows:

1. Celiac artery
2. Superior mesenteric artery
3. Left renal artery
4. Right renal artery
5. Inferior mesenteric artery

The **trunk** of the **celiac artery** arises from the anterior aspect of the aorta just below the diaphragm and about ½ inch (1.5 cm) above the origin of the superior mesenteric artery. Organs supplied with blood by the three large branches of the celiac trunk are the **liver, spleen,** and **stomach.**

The **superior mesenteric artery** supplies blood to the pancreas, most of the small intestine, and portions of the right side of the large intestine (cecum, ascending colon, and about one half of the transverse colon). It originates from the anterior surface of the aorta at the level of the first lumbar vertebra about ½ inch (1.5 cm) below the celiac artery.

The **inferior mesenteric artery** originates from the aorta at about the third lumbar vertebra approximately 1¼ to 1½ inches (3 to 4 cm) above the level of the bifurcation of the common iliac arteries). Blood is supplied to portions of the large intestine (left half of the transverse colon, descending colon, sigmoid colon, and most of the rectum) by the inferior mesenteric artery.

The **right** and **left renal arteries** supplying blood to the kidneys originate on each side of the aorta just below the superior mesenteric artery at the level of the disk between the first and second lumbar vertebrae.

The distal portion of the abdominal aorta bifurcates at the level of the fourth lumbar vertebra into the **right** and **left common iliac arteries.** Each common iliac artery divides into the **internal** and **external iliac arteries.** The internal iliac arteries supply the pelvic organs (urinary bladder, rectum, reproductive organs, and pelvic muscles) with blood.

The lower limbs receive blood from the **external iliac arteries.** The **external iliac artery** is significant in angiography and is used to **study each lower limb.**

ABDOMINAL VEINS

Blood is returned from structures below the diaphragm (the trunk and lower limbs) to the right atrium of the heart by the **IVC.** Several radiographically important tributaries to the IVC exist. These veins include the right and left **common iliacs, internal iliacs, external iliacs, renal veins** (Fig. 17.26), and **hepatic portal system.** The iliac veins drain the pelvic area and lower limbs, and the renal veins return blood from the kidneys.

The **superior** and **inferior mesenteric veins** return blood from the small and large intestine through the **hepatic portal vein** and the **hepatic veins** and into the **IVC.** This is best shown in Fig. 17.27.

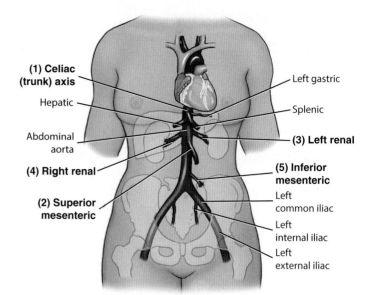

Fig. 17.25 Abdominal arteries.

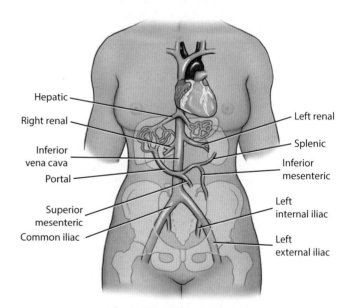

Fig. 17.26 Abdominal veins.

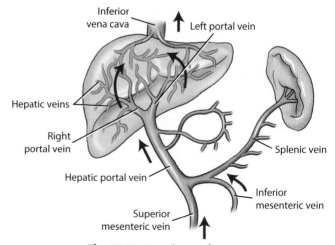

Fig. 17.27 Hepatic portal system.

HEPATIC PORTAL SYSTEM (HEPATOPORTAL SYSTEM)

The hepatic portal system includes all veins that drain blood from the abdominal digestive tract and from the spleen, colon, and small intestine. From these organs, this blood is conveyed to the liver through the **hepatic portal vein.** While in the liver, this blood is "filtered" and is returned to the IVC by the hepatic veins. Several major tributaries to the **hepatic veins** exist. The **splenic vein** is a large vein with its own tributaries, which return blood from the spleen.

The **inferior mesenteric vein,** which returns blood from the rectum and from parts of the large intestine, usually opens into the splenic vein, but in about 10% of cases, it ends at the angle of union of the splenic and superior mesenteric veins. The **superior mesenteric vein** returns blood from the small intestine and parts of the large intestine. It unites with the splenic vein to form the portal vein.

Peripheral Circulatory System

UPPER LIMB ARTERIES

The arterial circulation of the upper limb is generally considered to begin at the **subclavian artery** (Fig. 17.28). The origin of the subclavian artery differs from the right side to the left side. On the right side, the subclavian arises from the **brachiocephalic artery,** whereas the left subclavian originates directly from the aortic arch.

The subclavian continues to become the **axillary artery,** which gives rise to the **brachial artery.** The brachial artery bifurcates into the **ulnar** and **radial arteries** at approximately the level of the neck of the radius. The radial and ulnar arteries continue to branch until they join together to form **two palmar arches** (deep and superficial). Branches of these arches supply the hand and fingers with blood.

UPPER LIMB VEINS

The venous system of the upper limb may be divided into two sets: **deep** and **superficial veins** (Fig. 17.29). They communicate with each other at frequent sites and form two parallel drainage channels from any single region. The **cephalic** and **basilic veins** are the primary tributaries of the superficial venous system. Both veins originate in the arch of the hand. Anterior to the elbow joint is the **median cubital vein** (the vein most commonly used to draw blood), which connects the superficial drainage systems of the forearm. The upper basilic vein empties into the large **axillary vein,** which flows into the **subclavian** and eventually the **superior vena cava.** The lower basilic vein joins the median cubital vein, continuing to the upper basilic vein.

The deep veins include the **two brachial veins** that drain the **radial vein, ulnar vein,** and **palmar arches.** The deep brachial veins join the superficial basilic vein to form the axillary vein, which empties into the subclavian and finally into the **superior vena cava.**

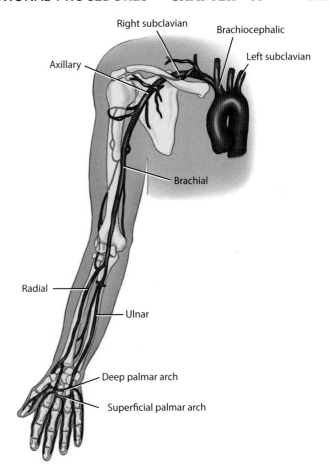

Fig. 17.28 Upper limb arteries.

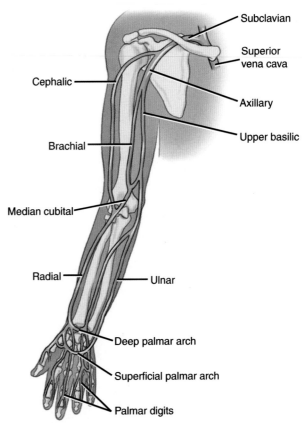

Fig. 17.29 Upper limb veins.

LOWER LIMB ARTERIES

The arterial circulation of the lower limb begins at the **external iliac artery** and ends at the arteries of the foot (Fig. 17.30). The first artery to enter the lower limb is the **common femoral artery**. The common femoral artery divides into the **femoral** and **deep femoral arteries**. The femoral artery extends down the leg and becomes the **popliteal artery** at the level of the knee. Major branches of the popliteal artery are the **anterior tibial and posterior tibial arteries**.

The **anterior tibial artery** continues as the **dorsalis pedis artery,** with branches to the ankle and foot. The **posterior tibial artery** supplies the calf and plantar surface of the foot.

LOWER LIMB VEINS

The veins of the lower limb are similar to those of the upper limb in that both have a **superficial** and a **deep venous system**. The superficial venous system contains the **great (long)** and **small (short) saphenous veins** and their tributaries and the superficial veins of the foot.

The **great saphenous vein** is the longest vein in the body; it extends from the foot, along the medial aspect of the leg, to the thigh, where it opens into the **femoral vein**. The **small saphenous vein** originates in the foot and extends posteriorly along the leg, terminating at the knee, where it empties into the **popliteal vein**.

The **major deep veins** are the **posterior tibial, anterior tibial, popliteal,** and **femoral**. The posterior tibial and anterior tibial veins join up with the dorsal venous arch (dorsalis pedis) to drain the foot and lower leg. The posterior tibial vein extends upward and unites with the **anterior tibial vein** to become the **popliteal vein** at the level of the knee. The popliteal vein continues upward to become the **femoral vein** before becoming the **external iliac vein** (Fig. 17.31).

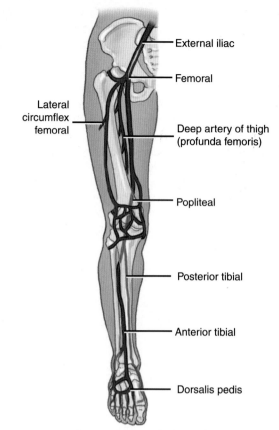

Fig. 17.30 Lower limb arteries.

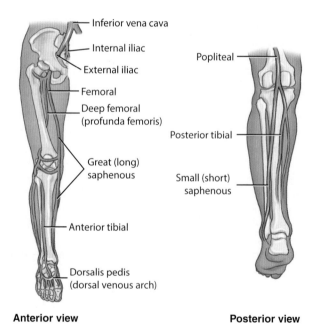

Anterior view   Posterior view

Fig. 17.31 Lower limb veins.

ANGIOGRAPHIC PROCEDURES

Overview

As defined at the beginning of this chapter, **angiography** refers to **radiologic imaging of blood vessels after injection of contrast media.** To visualize these low-contrast structures, a contrast medium is injected by a catheter that is placed in the vessel of interest. Positive contrast media are more commonly used, but there are instances when use of negative contrast media is indicated. Highly specialized imaging equipment is required for these procedures.

Angiography can be more specifically described as follows:

- **Arteriography:** Imaging of the arteries
- **Venography:** Imaging of the veins
- **Angiocardiography:** Imaging of the heart and associated structures

NOTE: This chapter is designed to be an introduction to angiography and interventional procedures and is not inclusive of the variety of techniques, information, and procedures available.

ANGIOGRAPHY TEAM

Angiography is performed by a team of health professionals, including (1) a **radiologist** (or other qualified angiographer), (2) a **"scrub" nurse or technologist who assists with sterile and catheterization procedures,** and (3) a **radiologic technologist.** Depending on the departmental protocol and the specific situation, an additional physician, nurse, technologist, or hemodynamic technologist may be available to assist with the procedure (Fig. 17.32).

Angiography is often an area of specialty practice for technologists and other health professionals. A competent, efficient team is crucial to the success of the procedure (Fig. 17.33).

CONSENT AND PATIENT CARE BEFORE PROCEDURE

A **medical history** should be obtained before the procedure is begun. This history should include questions intended to assess the patient's ability to tolerate the contrast media injection (e.g., allergy history, cardiopulmonary status, renal function). The patient also is interviewed regarding medication history and symptoms. Medication history is important because some medications are anticoagulants and cause excessive bleeding during and after the procedure. Knowing the medication history is also important when one is selecting the premedication. Previous laboratory reports and other pertinent data also are reviewed.

A detailed explanation of the procedure is given to the patient, which is important to ensure full understanding and cooperation. The explanation includes possible risks and complications of the procedure so that the patient is fully informed before signing the consent.

Solid food is withheld for approximately 8 hours before the procedure to reduce the risk for aspiration. However, ensuring that the patient is well hydrated is important to reduce the risk for contrast media–induced renal damage.

Premedication is usually given to patients to help them relax before the procedure. The patient may be made more comfortable on the table by placing a sponge under the knees to reduce strain on the back; however, in many procedures this is not an option. Vital signs are obtained and recorded; pulses in the distal extremities should be checked. The puncture site is subsequently shaved, cleaned, and draped using sterile technique (Fig. 17.34).

Continuous communication and monitoring of the patient by the technologist, nurse, and the rest of the angiography team greatly alleviates patient discomfort and fear.

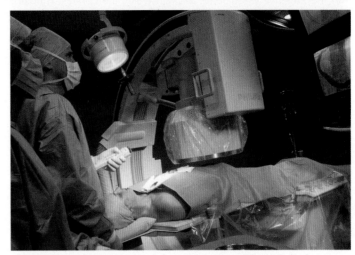

Fig. 17.32 Angiographic procedure. (Courtesy Philips Medical Systems.)

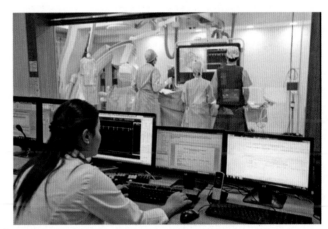

Fig. 17.33 Angiography team. (Courtesy Medipol Health Group. All rights reserved. Available at https://www.medipol.com.tr/en/technology/biplane-digital-flat-detector-angiography-system)

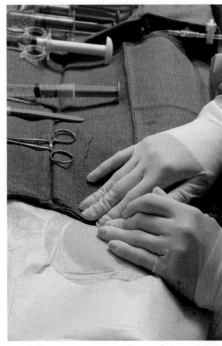

Fig. 17.34 Pulse assessment at femoral artery injection site.

VESSEL ACCESS FOR CONTRAST MEDIA INJECTION

To visualize the vessel of interest, a catheter must be introduced into the patient's vasculature, through which the contrast medium is injected. Often with the use of ultrasound guidance, the Seldinger technique is used for catheterization (Fig. 17.35). This commonly used method of vessel access was developed by Seldinger in the 1950s and remains popular today. It is a percutaneous (through the skin) technique that can be used for arterial or venous access, in addition to access to other structures.

Four vessels are typically considered for catheterization: (1) femoral, (2) axillary, (3) brachial, and (4) radial. The angiographer, who consults with the performing physician, makes the selection based on the presence of a strong pulse and the absence of vessel disease. The **femoral artery is the preferred site** for an arterial puncture because of its size and easily accessible location. It is punctured just inferior to the inguinal ligament. If a femoral artery puncture is contraindicated because of previous surgical grafts, the presence of an aneurysm, or occlusive vascular disease, the axillary, brachial, or radial artery may be selected. The **femoral vein** would be the vessel of choice for venous access; however, this is also dependent on physician preference and the procedure itself.

A step-by-step description of the Seldinger technique follows.

SELDINGER TECHNIQUE (FIG. 17.36)

Step 1. Insertion of Compound (Seldinger) Needle The compound needle with an inner cannula (see Fig. 17.36) is placed in a small incision and advanced so that it punctures both walls of the vessel. Newer needles have a single cannula for both vessel puncture and catheterization.

Step 2. Placement of Needle in Lumen of Vessel Placement of the needle in the lumen of the vessel is achieved by removing the inner cannula and slowly withdrawing the needle until a steady blood flow returns through the needle.

Step 3. Insertion of Guidewire When the desired blood flow is returned through the needle, the flexible end of a guidewire (Fig. 17.37) is inserted through the needle and is advanced about 4 inches (10 cm) into the vessel.

Step 4. Removal of Needle After the guidewire is in position, the needle is removed by withdrawing it over the portion of the guidewire that remains outside the patient.

Step 5. Threading of Catheter to Area of Interest The catheter is threaded over the guidewire and is advanced to the area of interest under fluoroscopic control. This "catheter" placement may involve dilation of the tract and placement of an introducer sheath that protects vessel access and contains a one-way valve to prevent leakage (Fig. 17.38).

Step 6. Removal of Guidewire When the catheter is located in the desired area, the guidewire is removed from inside the catheter. The catheter or introducer sheath remains in place as a connection between the exterior of the body and the area of interest.

If the vessel cannot be accessed through the Seldinger technique, a cutdown may be performed. A cutdown requires a minor surgical procedure to expose the vessel to be catheterized; this is rarely performed outside of surgery.

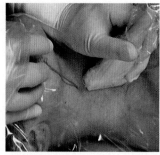

Fig. 17.35 Ultrasound-guided venous access. (With permission from Dr. Brian Pollard.From Ultrasound Guidance for Vascular Access and Regional Anesthesia.)

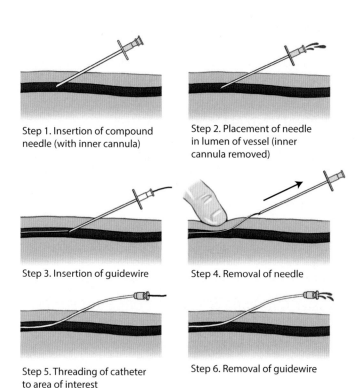

Step 1. Insertion of compound needle (with inner cannula)

Step 2. Placement of needle in lumen of vessel (inner cannula removed)

Step 3. Insertion of guidewire

Step 4. Removal of needle

Step 5. Threading of catheter to area of interest

Step 6. Removal of guidewire

Fig. 17.36 Six steps of Seldinger technique.

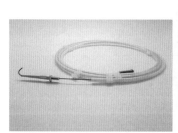

Fig. 17.37 Sample of guidewire as used with Seldinger technique. (Shutterstock.com/panpilaipaipa.)

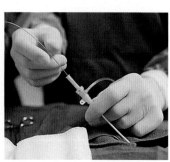

Fig. 17.38 Introducer sheath placement. (Shutterstock.com/ Monkey Business Images.)

Fig. 17.39 shows sterile items that have been placed and are ready for arterial puncture by the radiologist. In addition to the syringes and supplies shown, a manifold (or three-way stopcock) may be connected to one or more lengths of tubing to (1) a transducer for vessel pressure readings, (2) a heparinized saline drip under pressure, or (3) an appropriate contrast media. This setup also allows the physician to inject contrast media or medications by hand and to connect to an angiographic catheter.

Angiographic catheters have different shapes at the distal end to permit easy access to the vessel of interest. It is important for the technologist to be familiar with the types, radiopacity, sizes, construction, and tip design of the catheters and guidewires in use. Many types of angiographic catheters are available (Fig. 17.40).

The catheter should be flushed frequently during the procedure to prevent the formation of blood clots that may become emboli.

ANGIOGRAPHIC TRAY

A sterile tray contains the basic equipment necessary for a Seldinger catheterization of a femoral artery. Basic sterile items include the following:

1. Hemostats
2. Preparation sponges and antiseptic solution (Fig. 17.41)
3. Scalpel blade
4. Syringe and needle for local anesthetic
5. Basins and medicine cup
6. Sterile drapes and towels
7. Band-Aids
8. Sterile image intensifier cover (not shown)

CONTRAST MEDIA

The contrast medium of choice is a water-soluble, nonionic, iodinated substance because of its low osmolality and reduced risk for allergic reaction. The amount required depends on the vessel being examined. As for all procedures that use contrast media, emergency equipment should be readily available, and the technologist must be familiar with the protocol in case of an allergic reaction by the patient. Patients who have known sensitivities may require premedication to minimize the risk. Chapter 14 provides an overview of contrast media and levels of reactions.

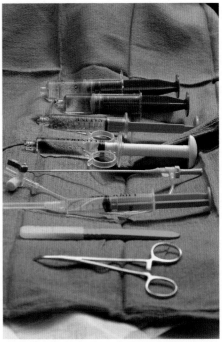

Fig. 17.39 Sterile items ready for arterial puncture and catheterization.

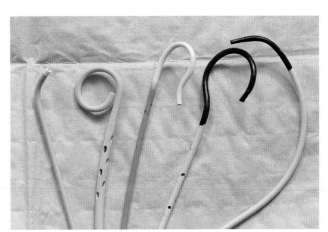

Fig. 17.40 Angiographic catheters.

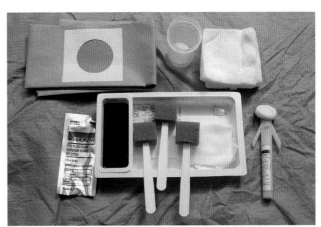

Fig. 17.41 Skin prep tray.

17

RISKS AND COMPLICATIONS

Angiographic procedures always involve some level of risk for the patient. Common risks and complications include the following:

- **Bleeding at the puncture site:** Bleeding usually can be controlled by applying compression.
- **Thrombus formation:** A blood clot may form in a vessel and disrupt the flow to distal parts.
- **Embolus formation:** A piece of plaque may be dislodged from a vessel wall by the catheter. A stroke or other vessel occlusion may result.
- **Dissection of a vessel:** The catheter may tear the intima of a vessel.
- **Infection of puncture site:** Infection is caused by contamination of the sterile field.
- **Contrast media reaction:** The reaction may be mild, moderate, or severe (see Chapter 14).

If the axillary, brachial, or radial artery is used for catheterization, an additional risk may be damage to nearby nerves and arterial spasm.

Rarely, a portion of the guidewire or catheter may break off inside a vessel. The fragment becomes an embolus; this causes great risk to the patient and is treated immediately. This fragment may be retrieved with the use of a special type of retrieval catheter (see Figs. 17.87 and 17.88).

POSTPROCEDURAL CARE

After the angiographic procedure has been completed, the catheter is removed, and either compression is applied to the puncture site or a closure device is used to seal the artery. The patient remains on bed rest for a minimum of 4 hours, but the head of the bed or stretcher may be elevated approximately 30°. (This may depend on physician preference or department protocol.) During this time, the patient is monitored closely; vital signs and peripheral pulses distal to the puncture site continue to be checked. The affected extremity is also checked for warmth, color, and numbness to ensure that circulation has not been disrupted. Oral fluids are given, and analgesics are provided if required.

Patients should be instructed on what to do if the puncture site spontaneously begins to bleed: **apply pressure** and **call for help.**

More recent advances include the development of devices used to close the puncture site percutaneously. Percutaneous closure of the puncture site reduces the risk for hemorrhage. In addition, the angiographer is usually not required to compress the puncture site with the use of these closure devices. This technique is often effective for patients who are taking anticoagulants, another added benefit.

Special Patient Considerations

PEDIATRIC APPLICATIONS

Pediatric patients who require angiography generally are heavily sedated or under general anesthesia for these procedures, depending on the patient's age and condition. Neonates from special care nurseries are covered with warming blankets during the procedure to maintain their body temperature.

Parents and guardians usually are not permitted in the angiography unit. However, they should be given a thorough explanation of the procedure before signing the consent.

Pediatric patients may have pathologies similar to those of adult patients. However, angiographic procedures, especially cardiac catheterization, often are indicated to investigate congenital defects.

GERIATRIC APPLICATIONS

Sensory loss (e.g., eyesight, hearing) associated with aging may result in the need for additional patience, assistance, and monitoring throughout the procedure. It is not unusual for geriatric patients to feel anxious before their procedure; they may fear falling from the narrow examination table. Reassurance and additional care from the technologist throughout the procedure enable patients to feel secure and comfortable.

A radiolucent mattress of additional padding on the examination table provides comfort to geriatric patients. Extra blankets should be made available after the procedure to keep them warm.

Older patients may have tremors or difficulty holding steady; use of high mA results in shorter exposure times, which helps to reduce the risk for motion on the images.

TABLE 17.1 SKIN DOSE FOR COMMON PROCEDURE	
PROCEDURE	**APPROXIMATE SKIN DOSE**
TIPS	2168 mGy
Nephrostomy	258 mGy
Neuroembolization—head	1977 mGy
Neuroembolization—spine	3739 mGy
IVC filter placement	193 mGy
Biliary drainage	781 mGy
Hepatic embolization	1959 mGy
PCI	2 Gy
PTCA and CA	1407 mGy

CA, Coronary artery; *IVC,* intravenous catheter; *PCI,* percutaneous coronary intervention; *PTCA,* percutaneous transluminal coronary angioplasty; *TIPS,* transjugular intrahepatic portosystemic shunt.
Reproduced with permission from Rothrock J: Alexander's care of the patient in surgery, ed 15, St. Louis, 2015, Mosby; modified from Conference of Radiation Control Program Directors, Inc: *Monitoring and tracking fluoroscopic dose,* 2010, available at www.crcpd.org/Pubs/Handout-MonitoringAndTrackingFluoroDosePubE-10-8.pdf.

RADIATION PROTECTION

A potential risk exists for increased radiation dose to the health professionals who are members of the angiography team because of the use of fluoroscopy and their proximity to the patient and equipment during the procedure. Conscientious use of **radiation protection devices,** such as wrap-around lead aprons, thyroid shields, and lead glasses, is required, as is dose monitoring of staff. Ensuring that **fluoroscopy time is absolutely minimized** is also vital to reducing dose.

Lead shields may be suspended from the ceiling as an additional means of protecting the angiographer's face and eyes. Angiography units may have specialized beam filtration and pulsed fluoroscopic capabilities to help ensure that the dose is kept to a minimum. Fig. 17.42 demonstrates the importance of the positioning of team members during fluoroscopy exposure. Because scatter radiation largely contributes to staff dose, maximizing the distance between the staff member, the x-ray source, and the scattering object (the patient) is crucial.

Precise collimation, beam limitation, is important for reducing the dose to the patient and the angiography team. The limitation of the beam decreases the amount of secondary radiation produced and improves overall image quality. Fig. 17.43 demonstrates several important points regarding reducing patient dose. The distance between the image intensifier and the patient should be minimized, whereas the distance between the x-ray source and the patient should be maximized. In addition, using tools such as last image hold or the review of previously stored images may also assist in reducing dose to all. Table 17.1 gives examples of patient skin dose received during common procedures performed in angiography.

CONTRAINDICATIONS

Contraindications to angiography include contrast media allergy, impaired renal function, blood-clotting disorders, anticoagulant medication, and unstable cardiopulmonary or neurologic status.

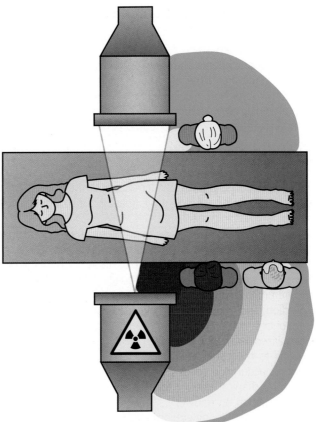

Fig. 17.42 Effect of scatter radiation on team members. (From Rothrock JC: *Alexander's care of the patient in surgery,* ed 16, St. Louis, 2019, Elsevier.)

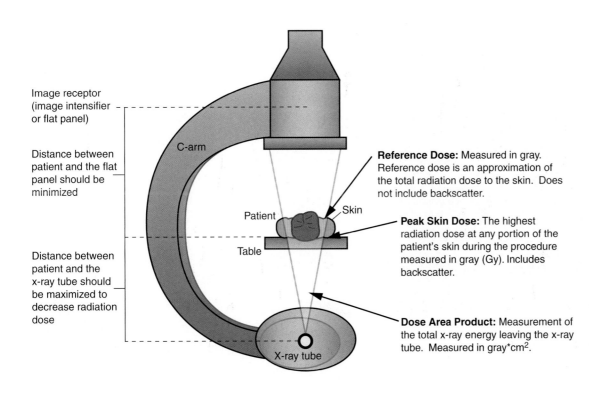

Image receptor (image intensifier or flat panel)

Distance between patient and the flat panel should be minimized

C-arm

Distance between patient and the x-ray tube should be maximized to decrease radiation dose

Patient

Skin

Table

X-ray tube

Reference Dose: Measured in gray. Reference dose is an approximation of the total radiation dose to the skin. Does not include backscatter.

Peak Skin Dose: The highest radiation dose at any portion of the patient's skin during the procedure measured in gray (Gy). Includes backscatter.

Dose Area Product: Measurement of the total x-ray energy leaving the x-ray tube. Measured in gray*cm².

Fig. 17.43 Minimizing patient dose. (From Rothrock JC: *Alexander's care of the patient in surgery,* ed 16, St. Louis, 2019, Elsevier.)

Angiographic Imaging Equipment

ANGIOGRAPHY ROOM

An angiography room is equipped for all types of angiographic and interventional procedures and has a wide variety of needles, catheters, and guidewires close at hand. It is larger than conventional radiography rooms and usually includes a sink and scrub area and a patient holding area. The room must have outlets for oxygen and suction, and emergency medical equipment must be kept nearby.

EQUIPMENT REQUIREMENTS

An angiography unit generally requires the following:

- An island-type table that provides access to the patient from all sides; it should have four-way floating capability, adjustable height, and a tilting mechanism
- An analog-to-digital conversion fluoroscopy imaging system with intensifier or the newer flat detector digital fluoroscopy acquisition type; both of these systems are available in C-arm configurations single or biplane, as shown in Figs. 17.44 and 17.45
- Programmable digital image acquisition system that allows selection and acquisition of the imaging rate, in addition to sequencing and processing of the images
- Specialized x-ray tube with high heat load capacity and rapid cooling to meet the need for high mA, high frame rates, and multiple acquisition series
- Electromechanical injector for delivery of contrast media (see full description on p. 671)
- Physiologic monitoring equipment that allows monitoring of the patient's venous and arterial pressures, oxygen levels, and electrocardiogram (especially important for angioplasty and cardiac catheterization)
- Image archiving method linked to a picture archiving and communications system (PACS) from Chapter 1.

DIGITAL ACQUISITION

As described earlier, two types of technology are available for digital fluoroscopy and image acquisition: (1) analog-to-digital conversion type (less commonly seen) and (2) flat detectors (direct digital conversion).

Digital acquisition allows images to be archived directly to a PACS with all the inherent advantages (e.g., ease of access to images by specialists, elimination of lost images, simultaneous viewing of images).

Digital Subtraction Angiography

One advantage of digital technology is the ability to perform **digital subtraction angiography (DSA)** in real time. With digital technology, a highly sophisticated computer "subtracts" or removes overlying anatomic structures so that the resultant image shows only the vessel or vessels of interest that contain contrast media (Fig. 17.46). The subtracted image appears as a reversed image and may demonstrate diagnostic information not apparent on a conventional nonsubtracted image (Fig. 17.47).

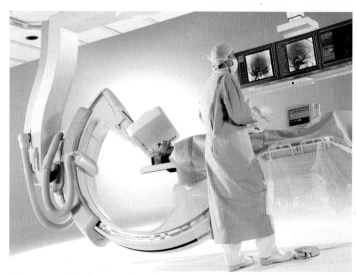

Fig. 17.45 Flat detector digital angiographic system, single plane. (Courtesy Philips Medical Systems.)

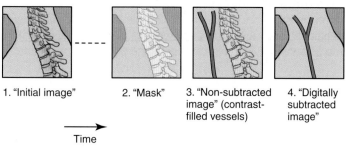

1. "Initial image" 2. "Mask" 3. "Non-subtracted image" (contrast-filled vessels) 4. "Digitally subtracted image"

Time

Fig. 17.46 Steps for DSA.

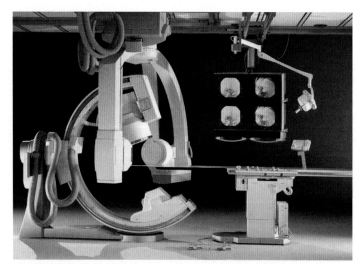

Fig. 17.44 Biplane digital angiographic system. (Courtesy Philips Medical Systems.)

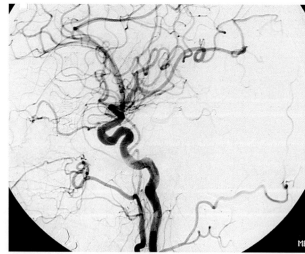

Fig. 17.47 Carotid DSA, lateral view.

Post-Processing Images

Because the images are digital and are stored electronically, several **post-processing options** are available to improve or modify the image. Examples of post-processing functions include **pixel shifting** or **remasking,** which allows the technologist to improve the quality of the subtracted image. The image may be **magnified, or "zoomed,"** to reveal specific structures; images also may be **quantitatively analyzed** to measure distances and calculate stenosis.

Road mapping is a technique that allows accurate positioning of a catheter, guidewire, or other interventional device during the procedure. An image of a structure that contains contrast media is overlaid on a live fluoroscopic image. The resultant image shows the structure as if it were completely filled with contrast media. This is termed the "road map" image. Subsequent fluoroscopy shows the progress of the procedure over this reference image.

See Chapter 1 for additional information on post-processing of digital images.

AUTOMATIC ELECTROMECHANICAL CONTRAST MEDIA INJECTOR

As the contrast medium is injected into the circulatory system, it is diluted by blood. The contrast medium must be injected with sufficient pressure to overcome the patient's systemic arterial pressure and to maintain a bolus to minimize dilution with blood. To maintain the flow rates necessary for angiography, an automatic electromechanical injector is used. The flow rate is affected by many variables, such as the viscosity of the contrast medium, the length and diameter of the catheter, and the injection pressure. Depending on these variables and the vessel to be injected, the desired flow rate can be selected before injection.

After the vessel of interest is catheterized under fluoroscopic guidance, a small hand injection of contrast medium is administered to ensure that the catheter is in an accurate position (i.e., it is in the vessel lumen and is not lodged against the wall). For the imaging series, the electromechanical injector is set to deliver a preset amount of contrast medium. The rate of image acquisition is rapid, often in the range of several frames per second. The series is reviewed to determine what, if any, additional series are needed.

A typical contrast media injector is shown in Fig. 17.48. Every injector is equipped with syringes, a heating device, a high-pressure mechanism, and a control panel. The syringes in common use are disposable. Reusable syringes must be disassembled for sterilization. The heating device warms and maintains the contrast medium at body temperature, reducing the viscosity of the medium. The high-pressure mechanism is usually an electromechanical device that consists of a motor drive that moves a piston into or out of the syringe.

In addition to safety, convenience, ease of use, and reliability of flow-rate settings, other features of an automatic mechanical injector include (1) ready light when armed and set for injection, (2) a slow or manual injector control to remove air bubbles from the syringe, and (3) controls to prevent inadvertent injection or excessive pressure or volume injection.

Alternative Modalities and Procedures

In addition to the specific angiographic procedures described on subsequent pages, alternative modalities and procedures are available in clinical imaging centers for imaging the vascular system.

COMPUTED TOMOGRAPHY (CT)

Volume acquisition, multislice technology, subsequent reconstruction of images, and sophisticated software have made computed tomography (CT) a valuable tool in vessel assessment. CT is used to study a wide variety of intracranial, thoracic, abdominal, and peripheral vascular pathologies, such as aortic aneurysms. If equipment specifications permit, CT is also useful in diagnosis of pulmonary embolism.

CT angiography provides images of the vascular structures in cross-section, which, depending on the capability of the scanner and software, can be reconstructed into a three-dimensional (3D) image. Multislice technology has allowed the acquisition of thinner slices, enhancing the resolution of CT angiography images. CT angiography provides the advantage of intravenous administration of contrast media, eliminating the need for an arterial puncture and catheter insertion.

NUCLEAR MEDICINE (NM)

NM is often used in conjunction with angiography in the investigation of cardiovascular pathologies, including pulmonary embolus, gastrointestinal bleed, renovascular hypertension, and coronary artery disease. NM complements other imaging modalities because it provides primarily physiologic information but little anatomic detail.

SONOGRAPHY (ULTRASOUND)

The role of ultrasound (sonography) in cardiovascular imaging has increased. Sonography may be used to image the patency of vessels and to demonstrate thrombus formation, plaque, or stenosis. Color duplex (color flow Doppler) is also used in sonography to demonstrate the presence or absence of flow within a vessel, the direction of flow, and, with more sophisticated equipment, the velocity of flow. Echocardiography provides detailed images of the heart for investigation of numerous cardiac conditions, including valve disease, aneurysm, cardiomyopathy, myocardial infarction, and congenital defects.

MAGNETIC RESONANCE ANGIOGRAPHY (MRA)

MRA provides highly detailed images of the patient's vasculature. This modality is advantageous because a contrast medium is not always required and vessel puncture is avoided.

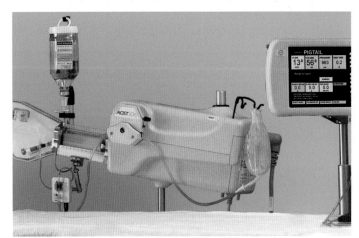

Fig. 17.48 ACIST CVi contrast delivery system. (Courtesy ACIST Medical Systems.)

ROTATIONAL ANGIOGRAPHY

During contrast media injection and while the images are acquired, the C-arm configuration on an angiography unit is rotated up to 180° around the patient. The vascular structure and the system are visualized from a wide variety of angles with a single injection. Resultant images (usually a cerebral, abdominal, or coronary angiogram) may be played back digitally in a **cine loop** mode to provide a dynamic image presentation. Rotational imaging can provide information regarding which vessels require additional investigation or the optimal equipment angle that should be used in future studies.

3D ROTATIONAL ANGIOGRAPHY

A 3D image may be produced from the image data acquired during a rotational acquisition. These data are processed by a sophisticated computer system through the use of digital reconstruction techniques similar to the techniques used in CT.

3D imaging reconstruction systems are valuable for visualizing complex intracranial vascular pathologies (e.g., arteriovenous malformations, aneurysms with unusual locations or characteristics) (Fig. 17.49A). Information from 3D images is often used when an interventional approach to these pathologies is planned (Fig. 17.49B).

ALTERNATIVE CONTRAST MEDIA: CO_2 AND GADOLINIUM

Alternatives to iodine-based contrast media may be required for patients with cardiopulmonary disease, diabetes mellitus, renal insufficiency, or iodinated contrast media allergy.

CO_2 is used at some centers for selected procedures when iodinated contrast agents are contraindicated. Specialized CO_2 injectors have been developed to provide accurate, well-timed delivery of gas into the vessels being examined. Some angiographic equipment includes specialized digital imaging software to optimize the use of CO_2. The primary limitation of the use of CO_2 as an intravascular contrast agent is the risk for neurotoxicity. Experimental findings have indicated that CO_2 may cause ischemic infarction as a result of gas embolism of cerebral vessels. It has been suggested by early proponents of this technique that CO_2 should not be used in vessels above the diaphragm.

The limitations of CO_2 as a contrast agent have prompted angiographers to seek alternative agents for patients who cannot tolerate iodinated contrast media. **Gadolinium,** a popular injectable agent used in magnetic resonance imaging (MRI), has been used more recently in angiography and has shown promise for various vessels. Images obtained are diagnostic, and adverse effects have not been observed. However, gadolinium is contraindicated in patients with renal disease.

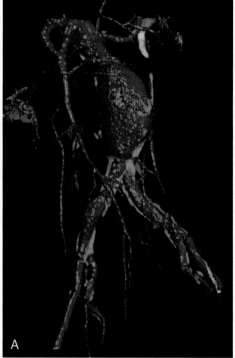

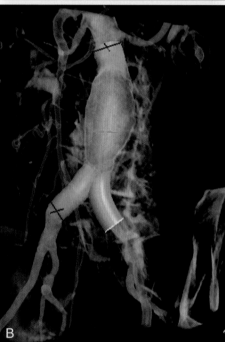

Fig. 17.49 A, 3D rotational angiography image of abdominal aortic aneurysm. B, Same patient with virtual stent for abdominal aortic aneurysm. (Courtesy Philips Medical Systems.)

Specific Angiographic Procedures

Five additional common angiographic procedures that are performed in a typical clinical imaging center are introduced and briefly described in this section. (The specific routines for each of these procedures are determined by radiologist preferences or department protocol.) The following procedures are described:

1. Cerebral angiography
2. Thoracic angiography
3. Angiocardiography
4. Abdominal angiography
5. Peripheral angiography

CEREBRAL ANGIOGRAPHY

Purpose

Cerebral angiography is a **radiologic study of the blood vessels of the brain.** The primary purpose of cerebral angiography is to provide a vascular road map that enables physicians to localize and diagnose pathology or other anomalies of the brain and neck regions.

Clinical Indications

Clinical indications for cerebral angiography include the following:

- Vascular stenosis and occlusions
- Aneurysms
- Trauma
- Arteriovenous malformations
- Neoplastic disease

Catheterization

The femoral approach is preferred for catheter insertion. The catheter is advanced to the aortic arch, and the vessel to be imaged is selected. Vessels commonly selected for cerebral angiography include the **common carotid arteries, internal carotid arteries, external carotid arteries,** and **vertebral arteries.**

Contrast Media

The amount of contrast media required depends on which vessel is being examined, but it usually ranges from 5 to 10 mL.

Imaging

Digital C-arm equipment and/or flat detector digital fluoroscopy is preferred for cerebral angiography (Fig. 17.50). The imaging sequence selected must include all phases of the circulation—arterial, capillary, and venous. The projections required depend on the vessels being examined. Examples follow.

Common Carotid Arteriography Carotid arteriograms are among the most frequently performed cerebral angiography studies. Occasionally, cervical carotid arteries are injected before catheterization of the cerebral branches (Figs. 17.51 and 17.52). The right common carotid artery is demonstrated in the PA (fluoroscopy tube under table) projection and the lateral position for examination of this artery and its bifurcation into internal and external carotid arteries. The area of bifurcation is studied carefully for occlusive disease (see arrows). The left common carotid artery is studied in a similar manner during the examination.

Internal Carotid Arteriography A second cerebral arteriogram demonstrates the internal carotid arteries. Representative subtracted images of the arterial phase of a left internal carotid angiogram are shown in the radiographs in Figs. 17.53 and 17.54. PA and lateral images allow visualization of the bifurcation of the internal carotid artery into the anterior and middle cerebral arteries.

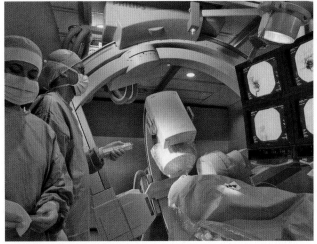

Fig. 17.50 Patient in position for cerebral angiogram. (Courtesy Philips Medical Systems.)

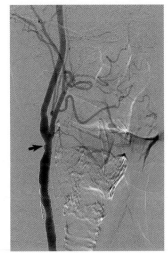

Fig. 17.51 PA projection of right common carotid arteriogram—subtracted image. (Courtesy Philips Medical Systems.)

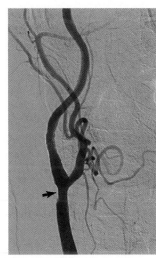

Fig. 17.52 Lateral projection of common carotid artery with stenosis—subtracted image. (Courtesy Philips Medical Systems.)

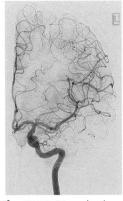

Fig. 17.53 PA projection—left internal carotid arteriogram. (Courtesy Philips Medical Systems.)

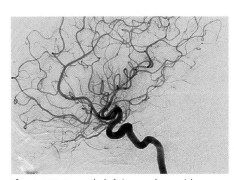

Fig. 17.54 Lateral—left internal carotid arteriogram. (Courtesy Philips Medical Systems.)

17

THORACIC ANGIOGRAPHY

Purpose

Thoracic angiography demonstrates the contour and integrity of the thoracic vasculature. Thoracic aortography is an angiographic study of the **ascending aorta**, the **arch**, the **descending portion of the thoracic aorta**, and the **major branches.**

Pulmonary arteriography is an angiographic study of the pulmonary vessels that usually is performed to investigate for pulmonary embolus. As mentioned earlier, pulmonary angiography is performed infrequently because of the availability of alternative modalities.

Clinical Indications

Clinical indications for thoracic and pulmonary angiography include the following:

- Aneurysms
- Congenital abnormalities
- Vessel stenosis
- Embolus
- Trauma

Catheterization

The preferred puncture site for a thoracic aortogram is the femoral artery. The catheter is advanced to the desired location in the thoracic aorta. Selective procedures may be performed with the use of specially designed catheters to access the vessel of interest.

Because of the location of the pulmonary artery, the femoral vein is the preferred site for catheter insertion. The catheter is advanced along the venous structures, into the IVC, through the right atrium of the heart into the right ventricle, and into the pulmonary artery. Typically, both pulmonary arteries are examined.

Contrast Media

The amount of contrast media injected varies according to the procedure; however, an average amount for thoracic angiography is 30 to 50 mL. For selective pulmonary angiography, the average amount is 25 to 35 mL.

Imaging

Serial images for thoracic angiography are acquired over several seconds. The imaging rate and sequence depend on many factors, including vessel size, patient history, and physician preference. Respiration is suspended during image acquisition.

Thoracic Aortogram Because of the structure of the proximal aorta, an oblique is required to visualize the aortic arch. A 45° left anterior oblique (LAO) is preferred to prevent superimposing the structures and to visualize any anomalies (Figs. 17.55 and 17.56). This projection is achieved by manipulating the C-arm, rather than the patient, into the desired obliquity.

Pulmonary Arteriogram Fig. 17.57 demonstrates the arterial phase of a pulmonary angiogram (DSA). The imaging sequence usually is extended when the pulmonary artery is imaged, to visualize the venous phase of circulation.

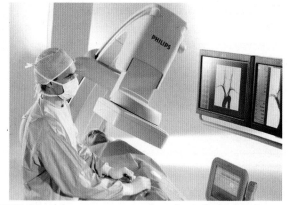

Fig. 17.55 Thoracic aortogram—aortic arch. Catheter is advanced through femoral artery to selected portion of thoracic aorta. (Courtesy Philips Medical Systems.)

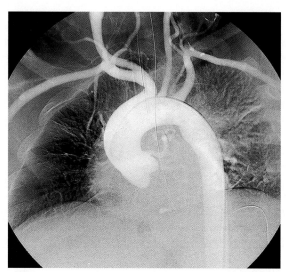

Fig. 17.56 Thoracic aortogram—aortic arch, 45° LAO.

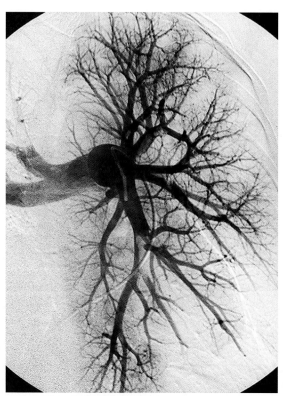

Fig. 17.57 Pulmonary arteriogram—DSA.

ANGIOCARDIOGRAPHY

Purpose

Angiocardiography refers specifically to radiologic imaging of the **heart** and **associated structures. Coronary arteriography** typically is performed at the same time to visualize the **coronary arteries.**

Cardiac catheterization is a more general term that is used to describe placing a catheter in the heart; it includes studies in addition to radiologic imaging, such as obtaining blood samples to measure oxygen saturation (oximetry) and measuring hemodynamic pressures and gradients. Specialized physiologic monitoring equipment is required for these sensitive measurements. For the purposes of this text, the focus is on the imaging aspect of cardiac catheterization.

Clinical Indications

Clinical indications for angiocardiography and coronary arteriography include the following:

- Coronary artery disease and angina
- Myocardial infarct
- Valvular disease
- Atypical chest pain
- Congenital heart anomaly
- Other heart and aorta pathology

Catheterization

In addition to the femoral artery, the radial artery may also be a preferred site for catheterization (Fig. 17.58). The catheter is advanced to the aorta and along its length into the left ventricle for the **left ventriculogram.** A pigtail catheter is used because a large volume of contrast media is injected. For the coronary arteriogram, the catheter is changed, and the coronary artery is selected; both right and left coronary arteries are routinely examined. Specially shaped catheters are designed to fit each of the coronary arteries.

After injection of contrast media into the coronary arteries, the catheter is immediately removed to prevent occlusion of the vessel.

Access to the right side of the heart is obtained by catheterizing the femoral vein and advancing the catheter through the venous structures until the right side of the heart is reached.

Contrast Media

Approximately 30 to 40 mL of a nonionic, low-osmolar, water-soluble iodinated contrast medium is injected for the ventriculogram. The coronary arteries typically require 7 to 10 mL of contrast media per injection.

Imaging

The imaging rate for angiocardiography is very rapid, in the range of 15 to 30 frames per second, and even higher for pediatric patients.

If biplane equipment is available for left ventriculography, right anterior oblique (RAO) and LAO images are obtained. If equipment is single plane, a 30° RAO is obtained routinely (Fig. 17.59). With the use of the ventriculogram, the **ejection fraction** can be calculated. The ejection fraction is expressed as a percentage and provides an indication of the pumping efficiency of the **left ventricle** (Fig. 17.60).

A series of oblique images is obtained to visualize the coronary arteries fully. Routinely, six views of the left coronary artery and two views of the right coronary artery are obtained (more views of the left coronary artery are obtained in most people because it and its branches supply blood to most of the heart) (Figs. 17.61 and 17.62). If it is available, biplane imaging equipment is advantageous in that it reduces the amount of contrast media required because two oblique projections can be obtained simultaneously. Respiration is suspended for the image acquisition.

The images are archived into a PACS. When played back, the images are viewed in cine mode. Once cardiac catheterization examinations are archived to a PACS, a system that has been specifically designed for cardiology applications should be used for reviewing.

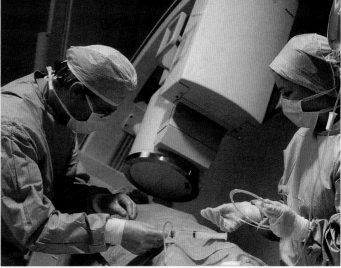

Fig. 17.58 Cardiac catheterization—advancing catheter through femoral artery and aorta to left ventricle. (Courtesy Philips Medical Systems.)

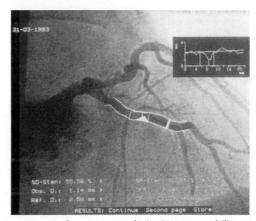

Fig. 17.59 Automated coronary analysis. (Courtesy Philips Medical Systems.)

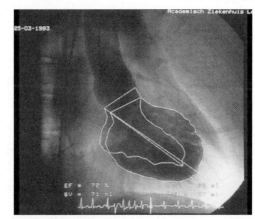

Fig. 17.60 Left ventricle analysis. (Courtesy Philips Medical Systems.)

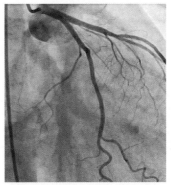 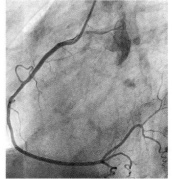

Fig. 17.61 Left coronary artery. (Courtesy Philips Medical Systems.)   **Fig. 17.62** Right coronary artery. (Courtesy Philips Medical Systems.)

ABDOMINAL ANGIOGRAPHY

Purpose

Abdominal angiography demonstrates the contour and integrity of the **abdominal vasculature.** The placement or displacement of abdominal vessels being studied and possible obstructions or vessel tears (e.g., aneurysm ballooning) are demonstrated. Any displacement of vessels may indicate a space-occupying lesion.

Aortography refers to an angiographic study of the aorta, and selective studies refer to the catheterization of a specific vessel. **Venacavography** demonstrates the superior and inferior venae cavae.

Clinical Indications

Clinical indications for abdominal angiography include the following:

- Aneurysm
- Congenital abnormality
- Gastrointestinal bleed
- Stenosis or occlusion
- Trauma

Catheterization

For an aortogram, the aorta typically is accessed by the femoral artery, Fig. 17.63. The type and size of catheter required depend on the structure, but a pigtail catheter usually is used because a larger amount of contrast media, as is needed for an abdominal aortogram, is delivered.

Selective angiographic studies require the use of specially shaped catheters to access the vessel of interest. Common selective studies performed include the celiac artery, the renal arteries (Fig. 17.64), and the superior and inferior mesenteric arteries, which are selected when a gastrointestinal bleed is investigated. A superselective study involves selecting a branch of a vessel. A common example is selection of the hepatic or splenic artery; these are two of the branches of the celiac artery.

Catheterization for **venacavography** is obtained by a femoral vein puncture. The catheter is advanced to the level for inferior vena cava filter placement (see p. 682).

Contrast Media

The amount of contrast media needed for selective studies varies depending on the vessel under examination. As for other angiographic procedures, the contrast medium of choice is nonionic, water-soluble, and iodinated with low osmolality.

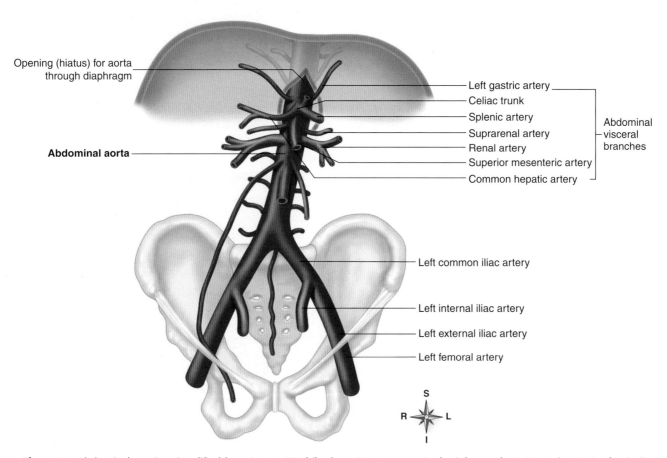

Fig. 17.63 Abdominal arteries. (Modified from Patton KT, Thibodeau GA: *Anatomy & physiology*, ed 10, St. Louis, 2019, Elsevier.)

Imaging

Imaging is done with the patient in the supine position; any obliquity required is obtained by manipulating the C-arm. Serial images are acquired, typically over several seconds. The imaging sequence and rate depend on many factors, including vessel size, patient history, and physician preference.

Before any arterial abdominal selective studies are performed, an abdominal aortogram generally is obtained, preferably including the area from the diaphragm to the aortic bifurcation. Associated branches of the aorta, such as the right and left renal arteries and the superior and inferior mesenteric arteries, are visualized, as is shown in the images in Fig. 17.65.

The imaging sequences for the selective studies usually are extended to visualize the venous phase. Respiration is suspended for the image acquisition.

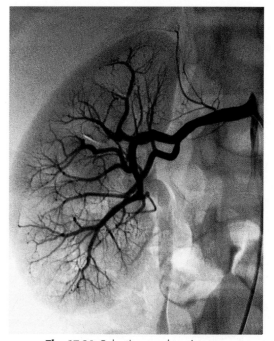

Fig. 17.64 Selective renal angiogram.

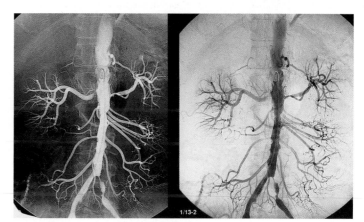

Fig. 17.65 Lower abdomen angiogram, with DSA image on the right.

PERIPHERAL ANGIOGRAPHY

Purpose

Peripheral angiography is a radiologic examination of the **peripheral vasculature** after the injection of contrast media. Peripheral angiography may be an **arteriogram** (Fig. 17.66), in which case the injection is administered by a catheter in an artery, or a **venogram,** in which the injection is placed into a distal vein of the extremity being examined. Extremity venograms may have been replaced, in part, with sonography (color duplex).

Clinical Indications

Clinical indications for peripheral angiography include the following:

- Atherosclerotic disease
- Vessel occlusion and stenosis
- Trauma
- Neoplasm
- Embolus and thrombus

Catheterization

The Seldinger technique is used to access the femoral artery or an alternative injection site for a peripheral arteriogram. For lower limb arteriograms, the side of access may vary depending on whether the study is unilateral or bilateral. Unilateral studies usually require access from the contralateral side of interest. For bilateral studies, either femoral artery may be accessed; the catheter is advanced just superior to the aortic bifurcation.

For an upper limb arteriogram, the catheter is advanced along the abdominal and thoracic aorta. For a study of the left upper limb, the left subclavian artery is selected; for a study of the right upper limb, the right subclavian artery is selected from the brachiocephalic trunk.

Contrast Media

The average amount of contrast media required for an upper limb arteriogram is much less than for a lower limb arteriogram because of the difference in part size and the fact that the upper limb examination is unilateral, whereas the lower limb examination may be a bilateral study.

Imaging

Lower Limb Because variance in blood flow through the two lower limbs exists as a result of vessel patency and occlusion, the time of circulation must be determined to ensure that contrast is visible in the vessels during imaging. Different methods can be used to time the imaging. It can be done manually by controlling the speed of table movement during acquisition, or it can be programmed into the computer.

With current technology, when the timing of blood flow has been established, the table moves at a predetermined rate, and images are acquired in the PA projection. These images can be reconstructed to provide visualization of the entire lower limb (Figs. 17.67 and 17.68), or they can be viewed by region. In addition, the placement of filters next to and in between the lower extremities before image acquisition provides filtration and uniform density while improving image quality.

Respiration is suspended for the image acquisition.

Upper Limb Upper limb imaging also requires timing of the blood flow; a technique similar to the one described previously may be used. The primary difference between upper and lower limb imaging is that imaging is unilateral for the upper limb and may be either unilateral or bilateral for the lower limb depending on the area of interest.

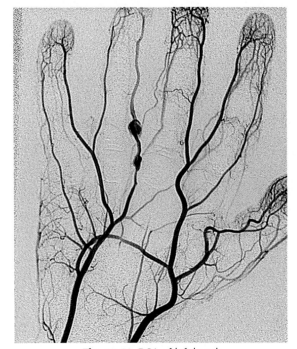

Fig. 17.66 DSA of left hand.

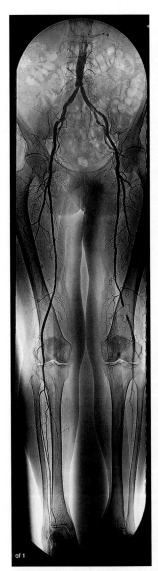
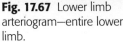

Fig. 17.67 Lower limb arteriogram—entire lower limb.

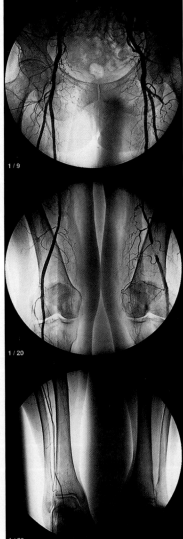

Fig. 17.68 Lower limb arteriogram—spot images.

INTERVENTIONAL IMAGING PROCEDURES

Definition and Purpose

Interventional imaging procedures are radiologic procedures that intervene in a disease process, providing a therapeutic outcome. Simply stated, interventional procedures use angiographic techniques for the treatment of disease, in addition to providing certain diagnostic information. This is a continuously growing specialty in medical imaging, because interventional procedures have become an important tool in the management of an ever-growing list of pathologies.

The purpose of these procedures and the benefits to the patient and health care system include the following:

- Techniques that are minimally invasive with lower risk compared with traditional surgical procedures
- Procedures that are less expensive than traditional medical and surgical procedures
- Shorter hospital stays for the patient
- Shorter recovery time because of a safer, less invasive procedure
- Alternatives for patients who are not candidates for surgery

These procedures typically are performed in an angiographic suite under the direction of an interventional radiologist. Fluoroscopic guidance is crucial to follow the path of the required needles and catheters.

The increase in complexity of the type of interventional procedures performed has resulted in upgrading of many angiography units to meet operating room specifications. This reduces the risk for infection and allows rapid surgical management in case of complications.

Interventional procedures may be categorized as **vascular** or **nonvascular** procedures.

Vascular Interventional Angiography

EMBOLIZATION

Transcatheter **embolization** is a procedure that uses an angiographic approach to **create an embolus in a vessel,** restricting blood flow. Numerous clinical indications for this procedure exist, including the following:

- Stop blood flow to a site of pathology
- Reduce blood flow to a highly vascular structure and tumor before surgery
- Stop active bleeding at a specific site
- Deliver a chemotherapeutic agent

The following sections provide examples of specific embolization procedures.

Uterine Fibroid Embolization

Uterine fibroid embolization (UFE) is a procedure used to treat symptomatic fibroids. Small microspheres or beads are injected into the uterine artery cutting off blood supply to the fibroid. Embolization of the uterine artery can shrink fibroids and eliminate associated pain and bleeding, replacing a hysterectomy (Figs. 17.69 and 17.70).

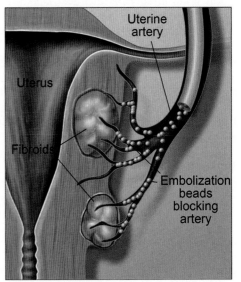

Fig. 17.69 Uterine fibroid embolization. (Courtesy of Fresenius Vascular Care.)

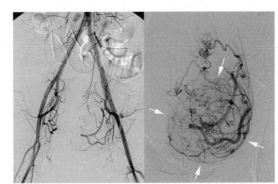

Fig. 17.70 Aortogram following uterine fibroid embolization. (Courtesy UCSF Department of Radiology & Biomedical Imaging.)

17

Chemoembolization

Chemoembolization is used most commonly for hepatic malignancies. The chemotherapy agent is injected into the tumor vasculature. The survival rate with this procedure is comparable to survival after treatment by a more invasive surgical resection (Figs. 17.71 and 17.72). Investigation is underway regarding the use of this technique for other locally advanced cancers (e.g., lung, breast, brain).

Intracranial Endovascular Coil Embolization

Intracranial endovascular coil embolization provides an alternative to patients with **brain aneurysms** that are inoperable or of high surgical risk. With the use of specially designed microcatheters, this procedure uses **detachable coils** to **occlude the aneurysmal sac and neck completely.**

Special catheters are used to place the embolic agent, which may be temporary (e.g., absorbable gelatin sponge [Gelfoam]) or permanent (e.g., stainless steel coils), depending on the clinical application of the procedure. Embolization procedures can also be performed for trauma-related accidents to stop active bleeding at a specific site, as mentioned earlier.

Risks and Complications

The complications of embolization procedures are similar to complications of other angiographic procedures, including vessel perforation, stroke, and hemorrhage. For these procedures, the added risk of occluding the inappropriate vessel exists; great care is taken to prevent this.

Examples

An example of an embolization procedure used successfully to occlude an aneurysm of the anterior communicating artery is shown in Figs. 17.73 and 17.74. It demonstrates the site of the aneurysm (see arrow) to be completely occluded after microcatheterization was performed and nine detachable coils were placed into the aneurysm.

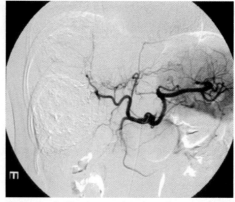

Fig. 17.72 Chemoembolization angiogram. (From Jarnagin WR: *Blumgart's surgery of the liver, biliary tract and pancreas,* ed 6, Philadelphia, 2017, Elsevier.)

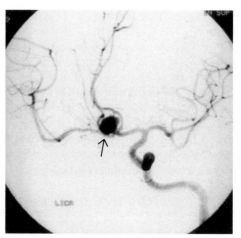

Fig. 17.73 Angiogram (DSA) before embolization procedure. (Courtesy Philips Medical Systems.)

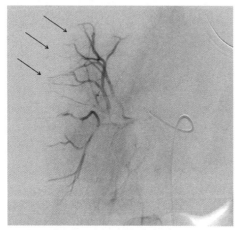

Fig. 17.71 Selective right hepatic arteriography after embolization with Gelfoam slurry. Successful hemostasis was achieved *(arrows).* (From Gutovich JM, Van Allan RJ. Hepatic artery embolization for hepatic rupture in HELLP syndrome. *Journal of Vascular and Interventional Radiology* 27(12): 1931-1933.)

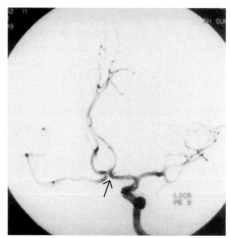

Fig. 17.74 Angiogram (DSA) after embolization procedure (aneurysm occluded). (Courtesy Philips Medical Systems.)

PERCUTANEOUS TRANSLUMINAL ANGIOPLASTY AND STENT PLACEMENT

Angioplasty

Percutaneous transluminal angioplasty uses an angiographic approach and specialized catheters to dilate a stenosed vessel. This procedure is a long-standing interventional technique that has applications for a wide variety of vessel types and sizes (e.g., coronary, iliac, renal arteries).

A catheter with a deflated balloon is advanced to the vessel of interest (Fig. 17.75). Hemodynamic pressures proximal and distal to the stenosis are obtained, and an angiogram is performed before angioplasty. The balloon portion of the catheter is placed at the vessel stenosis, and the balloon is inflated. The pressure of the inflation is monitored by a pressure gauge to prevent vessel rupture; more than one inflation may be required. The duration of the inflations is carefully timed to eliminate damage to distal tissue because the blood supply is temporarily occluded.

Final steps of the procedure include obtaining arterial pressures proximal and distal to the dilated portion of the vessel and performing an angiogram after angioplasty. This angiogram allows assessment of the effectiveness of the procedure.

Stent Placement

To assist in maintaining patency of the vessel, a stent is inserted across the treated area during the angioplasty. A stent is a cage-like metal device that is placed in the lumen of a vessel to provide support (Fig. 17.76). The stent may be a self-expanding type or a balloon-expandable type. The self-expanding type automatically expands when the stent cover is removed from the vessel. The balloon-expandable type (the compressed stent covers the balloon on the catheter) is positioned during the balloon inflation phase of the angioplasty (Fig. 17.77). Many of the stents currently in use are impregnated with a pharmacologic agent that inhibits the regrowth of vascular tissue within the artery and interferes with the process of restenosis.

Risks and Complications

Risks of transluminal angioplasty include vessel rupture and perforation, embolus, stent thrombosis, vessel occlusion, and dissection.

STENT-GRAFT PLACEMENT

Stent-grafts are a combination of interventional stents and surgical grafts. The primary clinical indications for stent-graft placement include aortic aneurysms and traumatic vascular injuries. This procedure offers an option for patients who are not candidates for surgical procedures and offers a lower-risk procedure option for patients who are candidates for surgical procedures. These procedures often involve both the interventional radiology team and the vascular surgical team.

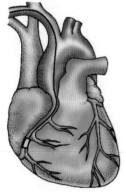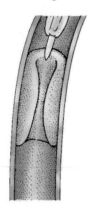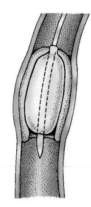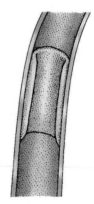

1. The balloon-tipped catheter is positioned in the artery.

2. The uninflated balloon is centered in the obstruction.

3. The balloon is inflated, which flattens plaque against the artery wall.

4. The balloon is removed, and the artery is left unoccluded.

Fig. 17.75 Transluminal angioplasty—balloon catheter. (From Ignatavicius DD, Workman ML: *Medical-surgical nursing: critical thinking for collaborative care*, ed 7, St. Louis, 2010, Mosby.)

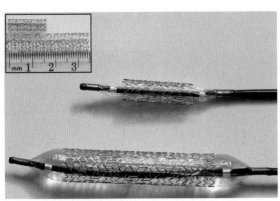

Fig. 17.76 Balloon-expanding stent.

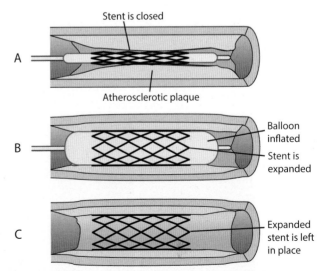

Fig. 17.77 A, Balloon-expanding stent—closed. B, Balloon stent—deployed. C, Expanded stent in vessel. (From Lovaasen K, Schwerdtfeger J: *2012 ICD-09-CM coding theory and practice with ICD-10*, St. Louis, 2012, Saunders.)

Through an angiographic cutdown or percutaneous approach, fluoroscopy is used to follow the progress of a catheter. The stent-graft self-expands after delivery through the catheter; the attached struts anchor it to the vessel wall (Fig. 17.78).

Risks and Complications

Complications of this procedure include leakage around the stent-graft and migration of the device. Rupture of the vessel is also a risk.

IVC FILTER

An **IVC filter** is indicated for patients who have recurrent pulmonary emboli or who are at high risk for developing them (e.g., patients with pelvic and lower extremity fractures after trauma). A filter is placed in the IVC to trap potentially fatal emboli that originate in the lower limbs. A variety of filter designs are available for this procedure (Fig. 17.79).

A femoral or jugular vein puncture is used to gain access to the IVC; the approach depends on physician preference or the presence of deep vein thrombosis. An angiographic technique is used to deploy the filter through a catheter. The filter has struts that anchor it to the walls of the vessel. The filter must be placed inferior to the renal veins to prevent renal vein thrombosis (Fig. 17.80).

Risks and Complications

In addition to the usual angiographic complications (e.g., infection, bleeding), an added risk is that the filter may migrate into the heart and lungs. The filter also may become occluded over the long term.

INSERTION OF VENOUS ACCESS DEVICES

The placement of venous access devices has become a common procedure in vascular and interventional units because the insertion of a catheter may be followed under fluoroscopy. Ultrasound is used frequently to identify the location of vessels such as the internal jugular vein for line placement (Fig. 17.81A). These venous catheters are used for administering chemotherapy, large amounts of antibiotics, frequent blood tests, hemodialysis, or total parenteral nutrition. The catheters may remain in place for several months; this depends on the type of catheter used and the clinical indication. In addition, many central venous lines and devices are designed for CT power injections (of radiographic contrast media). The three most common devices inserted include the following:

- **Peripherally inserted central catheters** (PICC lines) may remain in place for 6 months if good care is taken of the line. The proximal catheter tip is positioned near the right atrium, and the distal end remains exposed (usually on the patient's upper extremity) and must be kept covered and dry to prevent infection.

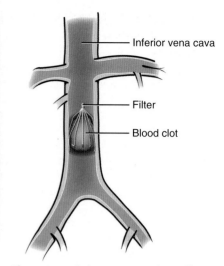

Fig. 17.78 Stent-graft placed for abdominal aortic aneurysm. (Courtesy Cook Canada, Inc.)

Fig. 17.79 Inferior vena cava (IVC) filter diagram. (Copyright Memorial Sloan Kettering Cancer Center.)

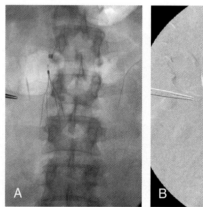

Fig. 17.80 A, IVC filter—initial scout, unsubtracted. B, Determining location of renal vein—subtracted and final IVC filter placement. (From Joseph N Jr: *Imaging pulmonary embolism. CEEssentials*, January 22, 2017, https://www.ceessentials.net/article12.html)

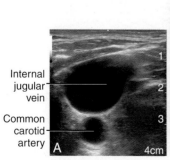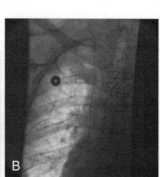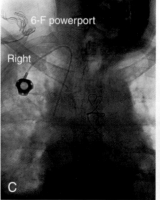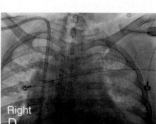

Fig. 17.81 A, Ultrasound image for insertion. B, Central venous cathether. C, Powerport. D, Hemodialysis catheter.

- **Central lines,** which may be tunneled under the chest wall (see Fig. 17.81B), come in many brands and types. Although some of these central lines may be used for hemodialysis (Fig. 17.81D), other central lines are used for general venous access, as listed previously, and may be CT injectable. **Many central lines are now designed for CT injections.** These come in the form of portacaths, PICC lines, or other central venous catheters (see Fig. 17.81C). The catheter tips are also positioned near the right atrium.
- **Subcutaneous ports** are the most permanent and generally the most expensive devices. The catheter tip is placed near the right atrium; the injection port for chemotherapy rests just beneath the chest wall (see Fig. 17.81C).

All central lines must be inserted under the strictest aseptic conditions; this is crucial because most of these patients are immunocompromised. Access to the venous system usually occurs through the cephalic vein or the jugular vein and requires the use of ultrasound-guided access.

Risks and Complications

Complications include infection, bleeding, thrombosis, and pneumothorax.

TRANSJUGULAR INTRAHEPATIC PORTOSYSTEMIC SHUNT

A transjugular intrahepatic portosystemic shunt (TIPS) is a vascular interventional procedure developed to treat variceal bleeding (caused by portal hypertension), refractory ascites, and cirrhosis. TIPS is useful in managing various patients, ranging from patients with end-stage liver disease to patients awaiting liver transplantation. This procedure creates an artificial passageway to allow portal venous circulation to bypass the normal route through the liver (Fig. 17.82).

The hepatic portal system is accessed through the right jugular vein. A sheath is inserted to protect vessels from needle and catheter manipulations. With the use of fluoroscopic guidance and a transjugular needle, the needle is advanced following the venous structures until it reaches the **hepatic vein.** The needle is advanced **through an intrahepatic vein, through the liver, and into the portal vein.** A guidewire is advanced through the needle and is removed so that a balloon (angioplasty) catheter may be advanced. The balloon on the catheter is inflated to create a tract through the liver. A metallic stent is placed across the tract that has been formed to maintain its patency.

Risks and Complications

Primary complications of the procedure include hemorrhage and thrombus formation. Later, there is risk for stenosis or occlusion of the TIPS; patient progress is monitored closely. After this procedure, the incidence of hepatic encephalopathy is increased. Because much of the blood is bypassing the liver, the blood contains a higher than normal level of toxins. This affects the brain and may cause confusion, disorientation, and, in extreme cases, coma. In severe cases of hepatic encephalopathy, the TIPS may have to be occluded.

Research is ongoing to find methods to increase the long-term effectiveness of TIPS. Possible adjuncts to the procedure include anticoagulation therapy and development of a stent-graft.

THROMBOLYSIS AND THROMBECTOMY

If diagnostic angiographic studies indicate that a vessel is blocked by a thrombus (clot), a **thrombolysis or thrombectomy** procedure, or a combination of the two, may be indicated; blood-clotting coagulation laboratory studies must support this procedure. During thrombolysis, the clot or thrombus is lysed (disintegrated) by passage of a guidewire and catheter through the clot or as far into the clot as possible (Fig. 17.83). A dissolving agent is injected through the catheter into the region of the thrombus. Various types of

catheters, such as a pulse spray type or an infusion type, may be used for this injection (Fig. 17.84). The pulse spray method involves hand injections with a syringe, whereas the infusion method generally involves an injection process with a pump to infuse the dissolving agent slowly over hours or several days. The catheter may be advanced during this time as the thrombus is being dissolved.

Thrombectomy machines, such as the Angiojet shown in Fig. 17.85, uses a thrombectomy device designed to mechanically remove clots from vessels large or small, providing a restoration of blood flow.

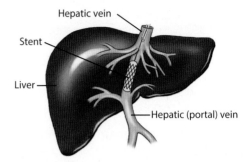

Fig. 17.82 Intrahepatic stent placement in TIPS procedure.

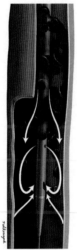

Fig. 17.83 Thrombolysis. (From Kaproth-Joslin K, et al: *Interventional ultrasound. Ultrasound Clinics* 8(2), April 2013, Elsevier.)

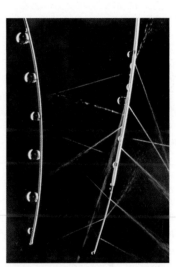

Fig. 17.84 Thrombolysis pulse spray and infusion catheters. (Courtesy Medi-tech/ Boston Scientific Corporation.)

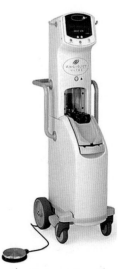

Fig. 17.85 Angiojet thrombectomy system. (Image provided courtesy of Boston Scientific. © 2017 Boston Scientific Corporation or its affiliates. All rights reserved.)

Risks and Complications

Possible complications with this procedure include bleeding and partially dissolved clots that may move on to block other smaller vessels.

INFUSION THERAPY

The infusion of therapeutic drugs may occur through a systemic or a superselective approach. Treatment duration ranges from a few days to several weeks. The type of approach and the duration of infusion therapy are determined by the pathology present, the area to be treated, the patient's condition, and the results of previous therapeutic methods. Vasoconstrictors, vasodilators, chemotherapeutic drugs, and radioactive materials may be used for infusion therapy. Although vasoconstrictors are used to help control bleeding, vasodilators are useful in the treatment of vascular spasm or constriction. Other drugs may be infused for chemotherapy in patients with advanced nonresectable malignancies.

EXTRACTION OF NONVASCULAR AND VASCULAR FOREIGN BODIES

Most foreign bodies found in the vascular system are limited to fragments of vascular catheters or guidewires, pacemaker electrodes, or shunts. Stone retrieval baskets (Fig. 17.86) are used frequently in the urinary system for nonvascular procedures. Instruments used to retrieve foreign bodies in the vascular system include those demonstrated in Figs. 17.87 and 17.88. For removal of foreign bodies with a snare wire loop, the catheter is inserted beyond the foreign body, collapsed onto the object, then withdrawn to catch the foreign body (Fig. 17.87). Retrieval instruments can also be used to capture and extract foreign bodies (Fig. 17.88).

Risks and Complications

Care should be taken to avoid tearing the vascular intima lining when foreign bodies that are adhered to the vessel are removed; these must be removed surgically.

Nonvascular Interventional Procedures

PERCUTANEOUS VERTEBROPLASTY AND KYPHOPLASTY

Vertebroplasty

Percutaneous vertebroplasty is used to treat patients who have vertebral pain and instability caused by osteoporosis, spinal metastases, compression fractures, or vertebral angiomas. Percutaneous injection of acrylic cement into the vertebral body under fluoroscopic guidance contributes to stabilization of the spine and long-term pain relief.

This procedure is performed in the operating room or in the interventional suite. The surgeon or interventional radiologist places a small hollow needle through the patient's back until it reaches the affected area of the vertebra. When the needle is in place and this has been verified by C-arm fluoroscopy (Fig. 17.89), the physician injects an orthopedic cement mixture that also may include a contrast medium (for better visibility on the monitor). The physician usually asks for continuous fluoroscopy while the cement mixture is being injected. At this point, the physician checks to ensure that the cement has filled the entire affected vertebral area and then withdraws the needle. The orthopedic cement hardens quickly and stabilizes the fractured vertebra, which often results in pain relief.

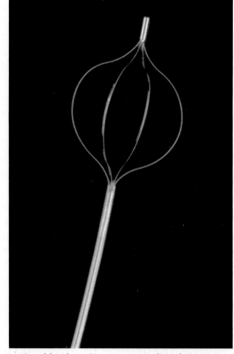

Fig. 17.86 Retrieval basket. (Courtesy Medi-tech/Boston Scientific Corporation.)

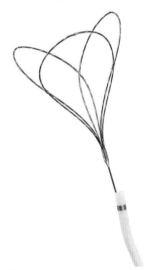

Fig. 17.87 Loop snare catheter. (Courtesy Merit Medical.)

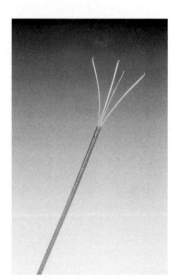

Fig. 17.88 Retrieval instruments—grasping forceps. (Courtesy Meditech/Boston Scientific Corporation.)

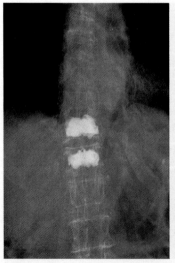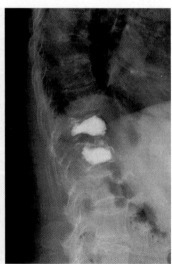

Fig. 17.89 PA and lateral views of fractured vertebra with the insertion of cement. (From Liu H et al. Reperfusion revision surgery for augmented vertebral nonunion with movable cement. *World Neurosurgery* 132: 429–433.e1.)

Kyphoplasty

The vertebroplasty technique has been modified more recently, resulting in a procedure known as *kyphoplasty*. Through small incisions in the patient's back, a kyphoplasty balloon is inserted into a collapsed vertebral body. The balloon is inflated for the purpose of restoring the collapsed portion of the vertebra (Fig. 17.90). Acrylic cement is injected to stabilize the vertebra in a procedure similar to vertebroplasty.

Risks and Complications

Complications of vertebroplasty include leakage of the cement into adjacent structures, which may result in the need for emergency surgery. A less common complication is pulmonary embolus, which causes migration of the cement into perivertebral veins.

Fewer complications are associated with kyphoplasty than with vertebroplasty because less cement is required, and it is injected in a more controlled fashion.

NEPHROSTOMY

Nephrostomy tubes may be placed for diagnostic or therapeutic reasons; they are also useful in treating several types of kidney pathologies or disorders. Placement of a nephrostomy tube is useful as a diagnostic tool for renal function assessment, urine culture, brush biopsy, determining the cause of urinary tract dilation, nephroscopy, and failed attempts at retrograde pyelography. Therapeutic reasons for performing nephrostomy include ureteral obstruction secondary to stones or other obstructive pathology, chemolysis, and abscess drainage.

In this procedure, a catheter is introduced through the skin and kidney parenchyma to the renal pelvis or other target area (Figs. 17.91 and 17.92). After correct catheter placement, a specific intervention, such as drainage or stone removal, is performed. A ureteral stent may be inserted to keep the ureter open.

PERCUTANEOUS BILIARY DRAINAGE

Percutaneous biliary drainage (PBD) can be used for many reasons, such as internal or external drainage, stone removal, dilation of an obstructed bile duct, and biopsy. The most common use of PBD is as a palliative procedure for unresectable malignant disease. Less common uses include the treatment of biliary obstruction, suppurative cholangitis, postoperative or post-traumatic biliary leakage, and stone removal.

Patients who undergo PBD may have infected bile. To avoid the spread of infection, antibiotics should be administered at least 1 hour before the procedure.

A common use of PBD is internal or external drainage. External treatment usually involves placement of the catheter in the duodenum, whereas internal drainage uses a stent or catheter. An external drain may be in place for a couple of days, then capped, ultimately resulting in internal drainage.

PERCUTANEOUS ABDOMINAL ABSCESS DRAINAGE

Percutaneous abdominal drainage has a success rate of greater than 80%. It is indicated when an abdominal or pelvic abscess cannot be readily treated by simple incision and when the abscess is located in a safe place for needle entry. If present, foreign bodies should be removed because they serve as foci of infection. If no improvement is seen in 24 to 48 hours, another treatment method may be considered.

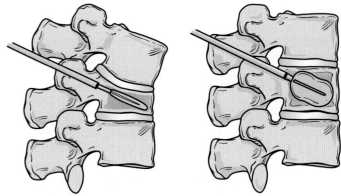

Fig. 17.90 Kyphoplasty drawings illustrate vertebrae before and after balloon is inflated.

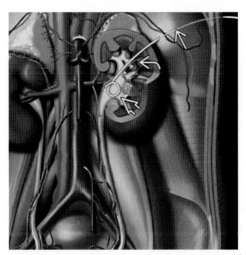

Fig. 17.91 Percutaneous nephrostomy diagram. (From Wible BC: *Diagnostic imaging: Interventional procedures*, ed 2, Philadelphia, 2018, Elsevier.)

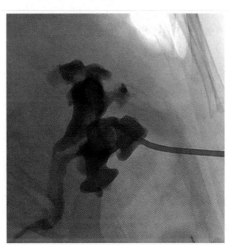

Fig. 17.92 Percutaneous nephrostomy with contrast injection. (From Krohmer S et al. Image-guided nephrostomy interventions: How to recognize, avoid, or get out of trouble. *Techniques in Vascular and Interventional Radiology* 21(4): 261–266.)

17

Needle Aspiration

Needle placement may be performed under CT (Fig. 17.93) or with ultrasound guidance. Sonography is preferred for superficial abscesses, abscesses in solid material, and abscesses not surrounded by bowel. The advantage of sonography is that it allows continuous monitoring. The procedure requires positioning of a needle in the abscess; fluid is withdrawn and sent for laboratory tests. If the fluid is purulent, the drainage procedure continues. If the material is sterile, the fluid is withdrawn, and the needle is removed. The fluid is removed with the use of gravity or a special suction pump. The gravity method is preferred because suction may erode the abscess wall or may cause the wall to adhere to the catheter.

Catheter Drainage

With catheter drainage, the Seldinger over-the-wire technique may be used for inserting the catheter. One example is the Van Sonnenberg sump drain-type catheter illustrated in Fig. 17.94. If a sump pump type of arrangement is used, a double-lumen type of catheter is required, by which room air can flow into the abscess region while the suction is being applied. This simultaneous drainage and venting prevents suction, which causes the abscess material to cling to the walls of the catheter, blocking the drainage holes. The "pigtail" type of design at the end of the catheter aids in retention and prevents accidental withdrawal.

The catheter is removed when no more symptoms exist or signs of infection disappear (normal white blood cell count), when no more drainage occurs, or when a postprocedural CT or sonography scan is normal (Fig. 17.95).

PERCUTANEOUS NEEDLE BIOPSY

Percutaneous needle biopsy is performed when primary or metastatic malignancy is suspected. A biopsy is useful in providing information about the stage and extent of disease, confirming tumor recurrence, and diagnosing infection.

In performing a biopsy, site and depth of pathology are determined. Correct positioning of the needle may be achieved by monitoring needle introduction with sonography, CT, or fluoroscopy. Sonography is the modality of choice for lesions in organs that differ significantly in echogenicity from adjacent structures—as long as the lesion is not surrounded by gas, fat, or calcified structures, such as liver, kidney, and pelvic organs. CT is ideal for small, deep lesions, especially lesions surrounded by large vessels or bowel. Fluoroscopy may be used for lesions that differ significantly in radiopacity from surrounding tissue, such as pulmonary pleurae, osseous lesions, and lymph nodes filled with contrast media.

A tissue sample is obtained by advancing the needle to the target, alternately moving and rotating it vertically about ½ to ¾ inch (1 to 2 cm). The needle is removed, and the sample is prepared for immediate examination. At least four samples generally are taken to include the center and peripheral areas.

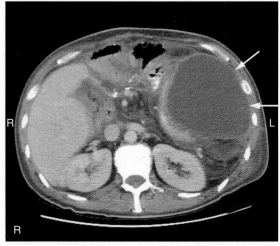

Fig. 17.93 CT-guided drainage: Before drainage of abdominal abscess (arrows point to large dark area).

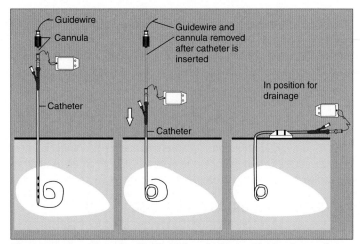

Fig. 17.94 Over-the-wire (Seldinger) technique with Van Sonnenberg sump drain catheter. (Courtesy Medi-tech/Boston Scientific Corporation.)

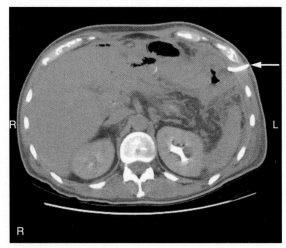

Fig. 17.95 CT-guided drainage: After drainage of abscess (arrow points to drainage tube).

PERCUTANEOUS GASTROSTOMY

Percutaneous gastrostomy is performed for extended feeding (>4 weeks) of patients unable to eat, for gastric decompression, or for dilation of the upper gastrointestinal tract when the oral approach fails. Individuals who may be candidates for gastrostomy include patients with impaired swallowing; this may be due to neurologic disease or obstructive oropharyngeal or esophageal pathology. Gastrostomy tubes may also be helpful for patients with burn injuries, trauma, or types of cancer.

In this procedure, examinations are performed beforehand to ensure that no organ is located over the puncture site; this is important to avoid puncturing these organs. A nasogastric tube is placed in the stomach to inflate the stomach with 500 to 1000 mL of air. The puncture site is located in the upper or middle area of the stomach. A tube is placed and secured in the stomach. When the tube is in position, the patient is suctioned for 24 hours, and feeding may begin.

RADIOFREQUENCY ABLATION

Radiofrequency ablation (RFA) is a minimally invasive procedure that is used to treat patients with neoplastic disease, especially certain liver, kidney, bone, lung, and soft tissue tumors. Under imaging guidance, a special needle electrode is placed in the tumor. A radiofrequency current is passed through the electrode to heat the tumor tissue near the needle tip and "ablate" it. The application of current agitates ions in the tissues that surround the electrode, causing them to generate frictional heat, which destroys the tissue. Dead tumor cells are gradually replaced by scar tissue that shrinks over time. The procedure may be performed with the patient sedated or under general anesthesia. If the patient is awake, he or she typically feels little or no pain during the procedure and often can go home the same day or the next day. Vital signs are monitored throughout RFA to ensure patient safety.

Patients whose disease is unsuitable for surgical resection are candidates for RFA. Tumors treated with RFA ideally should measure about 1¼ inches (3 cm) or less; larger tumors (if treatable) often require more than one procedure.

Risks associated with RFA depend on the site that was treated. Patients may experience localized inflammation or thermal damage to tissue. Hemorrhage is also a risk in this procedure, although the heat from radiofrequency energy cauterizes small blood vessels, reducing the risk.

17

CHAPTER 18

Computed Tomography

CONTRIBUTIONS BY **Andrew Woodward,** MA, RT(R)(CT)(QM)

CONTRIBUTORS TO PAST EDITIONS   Cindy Murphy, BHSC, RT(R), ACR, Barry T. Anthony, RT(R), James D. Lipcamon, RT(R)

ANATOMY CONTRIBUTOR TO PAST EDITION   Timothy C. Chapman, RT(R)(CT)

CONTENTS

RADIOGRAPHIC ANATOMY

This chapter describes the anatomy of the central nervous system, including the brain and spinal cord.

Gross Anatomy of the CNS–Brain and Spinal Cord

The anatomy related to **cranial or head computed tomography (CT)** includes the bony anatomy of the skull and facial bones, as described in Chapter 11. The anatomy of the **central nervous system (CNS),** as seen on head and spine CT images, includes the **brain** and **spinal cord.**

NEURONS

Neurons, or nerve cells, are the specialized cells of the nervous system that conduct electrical impulses. Each neuron is composed of an **axon,** a **cell body,** and one or more **dendrites.**

Dendrites are processes that conduct impulses **toward** the neuron cell body. An axon is a process that **leads away from** the cell body.

A **multipolar motoneuron** is shown in Fig. 18.1. This type of neuron is typical of the neurons that conduct impulses from the spinal cord to muscle tissue. A multipolar neuron is one **with several dendrites and a single axon.**

The **dendrites** and **cell bodies** make up the **gray matter** of the brain and spinal cord, and the large myelinated **axons** make up the **white matter,** as is seen in later drawings and CT scans.

DIVISIONS OF CNS

One must know the general gross anatomy of the brain and CNS before learning sectional anatomy as seen on tomographic sections or slices.

The CNS has two main divisions: (1) the **brain,** which occupies the cavity of the cranium, and (2) the solid **spinal cord,** which extends inferiorly from the brain and is protected by the bony vertebral column. The solid spinal cord terminates at the lower border of **L1,** with a tapered area called the **conus medullaris.** Nerve root extensions of the spinal cord continue down to the first coccyx segment. The subarachnoid space continues down to the second segment of the sacrum (S2).

SUMMARY OF SPINAL CORD ANATOMY

The drawing in Fig. 18.2 demonstrates three anatomic factors of the brain and spinal cord that are important radiographically, as follows:

1. The **conus medullaris** is the distal tapered ending of the spinal cord at the **lower level of L1.**
2. The **subarachnoid space,** which contains cerebrospinal fluid (CSF), a clear, colorless watery liquid, surrounds both the spinal cord and the brain and continues down to the lower **S2.**
3. A common **lumbar puncture site,** as required for a spinal tap or for removal of CSF and the injection of contrast media for a myelogram, is **between L3 and L4.** The needle can enter the subarachnoid space without danger of striking the spinal cord, which ends at the lower level of the L1 vertebra.

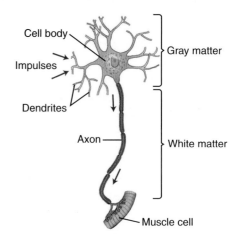

Fig. 18.1 Multipolar motoneuron (several dendrites, one axon).

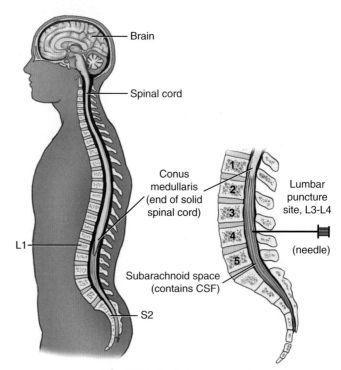

Fig. 18.2 Central nervous system.

Brain and Spinal Cord Coverings—Meninges

Both the brain and the spinal cord are enclosed by **three** protective coverings or membranes termed **meninges** (Fig. 18.3). Starting externally, these are the (1) **dura mater**, (2) **arachnoid**, and (3) **pia mater.**

DURA MATER

The outermost membrane is the **dura mater,** which means "hard" or "tough mother." This strong, fibrous brain covering has an **inner layer** and an **outer layer.** The outer layer of the dura mater is tightly fused to the inner layer, except for spaces that are provided for large venous blood channels called **venous sinuses** or **dura mater sinuses.** The outer layer adheres closely to the inner table of the **cranium,** or skull. The inner layers of dura mater below these sinuses join to form the **falx cerebri,** as seen on CT scans extending down into the longitudinal fissure between the two cerebral hemispheres (see Fig. 18.7).

ARACHNOID

Between the pia mater and the dura mater is a delicate avascular membrane called the **arachnoid** mater. Delicate, threadlike trabeculae attach the arachnoid membrane to the pia mater; hence its name, meaning "spider mother."

PIA MATER

The innermost of these membranes is the pia mater, literally meaning "tender mother." This membrane is very thin and highly vascular and lies next to the brain and spinal cord. It encloses the entire surface of the brain, dipping into each of the fissures and sulci.

MENINGEAL SPACES

Immediately exterior to each meningeal layer is a space or potential space (see Fig. 18.3). There are three of these spaces, or potential spaces: (1) **epidural space,** (2) **subdural space,** and (3) **subarachnoid space.**

Epidural Space

Exterior to the dura mater, between the dura and the inner table of the skull, is a potential space termed the *epidural space.*

Subdural Space

Beneath the dura mater, between the dura and the arachnoid, is a narrow space called the *subdural space,* which contains a thin film of fluid and various blood vessels. Both the epidural space and the subdural space are potential sites for hemorrhage after trauma to the head.

Subarachnoid Space

Beneath the arachnoid membrane, between the arachnoid and the pia mater, is a comparatively wide space termed the *subarachnoid space.* The subarachnoid spaces of the brain and spinal cord normally are filled with **CSF.**

Three Divisions of Brain

The brain can be divided into three general areas: (1) **forebrain,** (2) **midbrain,** and (3) **hindbrain.** These three divisions of the brain are divided further into specific areas and structures, as shown on the midsagittal sectional drawing in Fig. 18.4 and in the summary (Fig. 18.5) of brain divisions on the right. Each of these divisions is described in greater detail later in this chapter.

BRAINSTEM

The brainstem is comprised of the **midbrain, pons,** and **medulla (oblongata)** which passes through the large opening at the base of the skull, the foramen magnum, to become the **spinal cord.** The medulla is the final portion of the brainstem, located at the level of the foramen magnum, the opening at the base of the skull.

Secondary terms for these brain divisions are included as indicated in parentheses in the summary chart on the right.

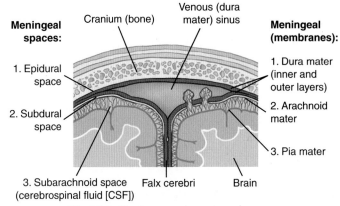

Fig. 18.3 Meninges and meningeal spaces.

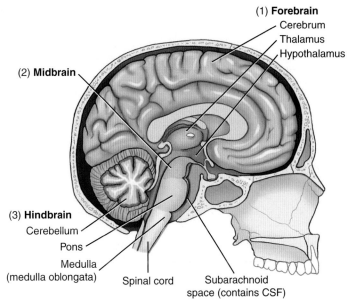

Fig. 18.4 Brain (midsagittal section).

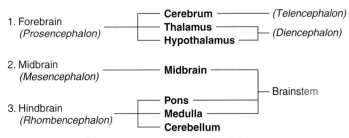

Fig. 18.5 Summary of brain divisions.

FOREBRAIN

The first part of the forebrain to be studied is the large **cerebrum.**

Cerebrum

A sagittal section through the head and neck leaving the brain and upper spinal cord intact is demonstrated in Fig. 18.4, which shows the relative sizes of various structures. The surface layer of the entire cerebrum (about 2 to 4 mm in thickness) directly under the bony skullcap is called the **cerebral cortex.** As can be seen, the total cerebrum occupies most of the cranial cavity.

Five Lobes of Each Cerebral Hemisphere Each side of the cerebrum is termed a *cerebral hemisphere* and is divided into five lobes. The four lobes seen in Figs. 18.6 lie beneath the cranial bones of the same name. The **frontal lobe** lies under the frontal bone, with the **parietal lobe** under the parietal bone. Similarly, the **occipital lobe** and the **temporal lobe** lie under their respective cranial bones. The fifth lobe, termed the **insula,** or **central lobe,** is more centrally located and cannot be seen on these views.

Cerebral Hemispheres The top of the brain is shown in Fig. 18.7. The cerebrum is partially separated by a deep **longitudinal fissure** in the midsagittal plane. This fissure divides the cerebrum into right and left cerebral hemispheres. Parts of the **frontal, parietal,** and **occipital lobes** are visualized on this top-view drawing.

The surface of each cerebral hemisphere is marked by numerous grooves and convolutions, which are formed during the rapid embryonic growth of this portion of the brain. Each convolution or raised area is termed a **gyrus.** Two such gyri that can be identified on CT sectional radiographs are an **anterior central (precentral) gyrus** and a **posterior central (postcentral) gyrus,** as shown on each side of the **central sulcus.** A sulcus is a shallow groove, and the central sulcus, which divides the frontal and parietal lobes of the cerebrum, is a landmark used to identify specific sensory areas of the cortex.

A deeper groove is called a **fissure,** such as the deep **longitudinal fissure** that separates the two hemispheres.

The **corpus callosum,** located deep within the longitudinal fissure and not visible on this drawing, consists of an arched mass of transverse fibers (white matter) connecting the two cerebral hemispheres.

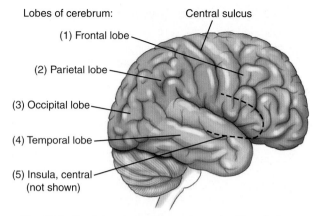

Fig. 18.6 Five lobes located in each cerebral hemisphere.

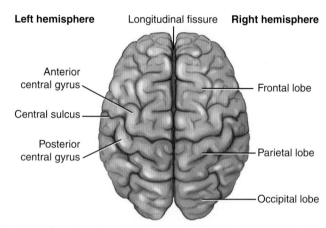

Fig. 18.7 Top view of cerebral hemispheres, showing frontal, parietal, and occipital lobes and the relative differences among gyrus, sulcus, and fissure.

18

Cerebral Ventricles A thorough understanding of the cerebral **ventricles** is important for cranial CT because they are readily identified on sectional CT radiographs. The ventricular system of the brain is connected to the subarachnoid space. There are **four cavities** in the ventricular system. These four cavities are filled with CSF and interconnect through small tubes.

The **right** and **left lateral ventricles** are located in the right and left cerebral hemispheres. The **third ventricle** is a single ventricle that is located centrally and inferior to the lateral ventricles. The **fourth ventricle** is also a single ventricle located centrally, just inferior to the third ventricle (Fig. 18.8).

CSF is formed in the lateral ventricles in specialized capillary beds called **choroid plexus,** which filter the blood to form CSF. According to *Gray's Anatomy,* although 500 mL of CSF is formed daily, only about 140 mL of CSF is present within and around the entire CNS, with the balance being reabsorbed into the venous circulatory system. CSF is believed to serve some nutrient role during development, but in the adult, it serves a protective role for the CNS.

Lateral Ventricles Each lateral ventricle comprises four parts. The superior and lateral views in Fig. 18.9 demonstrate that each of the lateral ventricles has a centrally located **body** and three projections, or horns, extending from the body. The **anterior,** or **frontal, horn** is toward the front. The **posterior,** or **occipital, horn** is toward the back, and the **inferior,** or **temporal, horn** extends inferiorly.

The two lateral ventricles are located on each side of the midsagittal plane within the cerebral hemispheres and are mirror images of each other. Certain pathologic processes, such as a space-occupying lesion or a "mass lesion," alter the symmetric appearance of the ventricular system, as seen on CT images.

Third Ventricle Each of the lateral ventricles connects to the third ventricle through an **interventricular foramen.** The **third ventricle** is located in the midline and is roughly four sided. It lies just below the level of the bodies of the two lateral ventricles (Figs. 18.10 and 18.11). The **pineal gland** is attached to the roof of the posterior part of the third ventricle directly above the cerebral aqueduct, which causes a recess in the posterior part of this ventricle. (The pineal gland also is shown in Fig. 18.16 in relationship to the thalamus portion of the forebrain.)

Fourth Ventricle The cavity of the third ventricle connects posteroinferiorly with the **fourth ventricle** through a passage known as the **cerebral aqueduct.** The diamond-shaped fourth ventricle connects with a wide portion of the subarachnoid space called the **cisterna cerebellomedullaris** (see Figs. 18.10 and 18.12).

On each side of the fourth ventricle is a lateral extension termed the **lateral recess,** which also connects with the subarachnoid space through an opening or foramen.

Superior View of Ventricles A superior view of the ventricles is shown in Fig. 18.11. This view shows the relationship of the **third and fourth ventricles** to the two **lateral ventricles.** The third ventricle is seen on this view only as a narrow, slitlike structure lying in the midline between and below the bodies of the lateral ventricles.

The **cerebral aqueduct** is clearly shown connecting the third ventricle to the fourth ventricle.

The **lateral recess** is shown on each side of the fourth ventricle, providing a communication with the subarachnoid space.

The **body, inferior horn,** and **anterior** and **posterior horns** of each of the lateral ventricles again are well demonstrated on this top view.

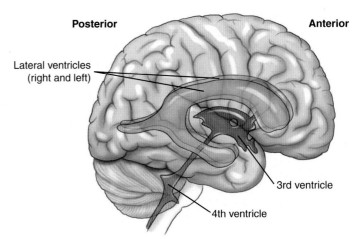

Fig. 18.8 Cerebral ventricles.

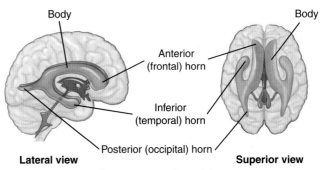

Fig. 18.9 Lateral ventricles.

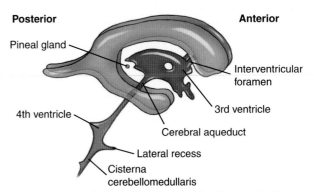

Fig. 18.10 Third and fourth ventricles (lateral view).

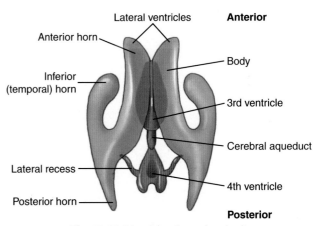

Fig. 18.11 Ventricles (superior view).

18

Anterior View of Ventricles An anterior view of the ventricles within the brain is shown in Fig. 18.13. The **interventricular foramina** connect the body of each lateral ventricle to the third ventricle. This view emphasizes the fact that the **third** and **fourth ventricles** are midline structures. The **anterior horn, body,** and **inferior horn** of each lateral ventricle are shown on this drawing as they would appear on a frontal projection. The region of the **lateral recess** that connects the fourth ventricle to the subarachnoid space is also shown.

Subarachnoid Cisterns As already noted, CSF normally is manufactured within each lateral ventricle. It passes through the third ventricle into the fourth ventricle. After CSF leaves the **fourth ventricle,** it completely surrounds the brain and spinal cord by filling the **subarachnoid space,** as shown in Fig. 18.12. Any blockage along the pathway leading from the ventricles to the subarachnoid space may cause excessive accumulation of CSF within the ventricles, a condition known as *hydrocephalus.*

Various larger areas within the subarachnoid space or system are called **cisterns,** the largest being the **cistern cerebellomedullaris** (cisterna magna), located inferiorly to the fourth ventricle and the cerebellum.

Cisternal Puncture The cistern cerebellomedullaris is the site for a **cisternal puncture,** in which a needle inserted into this cistern between C1 and the occipital bone to introduce an anesthetic into the subarachnoid space. This location is a secondary puncture site; the L3–L4 space is a primary lumbar puncture site, as shown in Fig. 18.13).

The **cisterna pontis** is located just inferior and anterior to the **pons.** Each of the larger black "dots" in these drawings indicates specific cisterns that usually are named according to their locations. The **chiasmatic cistern,** shown in the top-view drawing of the brain in Fig. 18.14, is so called because of its relationship to the optic chiasma, the site of crossings of optic nerves, which is identified in later drawings.

Various other cisterns lie along the base of the brain and brainstem. Because the midbrain is totally surrounded by fluid-filled cisterns, this area can be well seen on a CT scan.

The CSF-filled subarachnoid space and the ventricular system are important in CT because these areas can be differentiated from tissue structures.

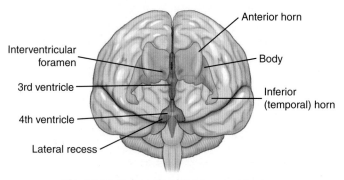

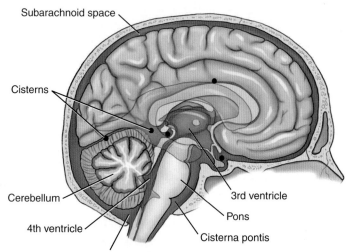

Fig. 18.12 Subarachnoid cisterns—side view.

Fig. 18.13 Ventricles (anterior view).

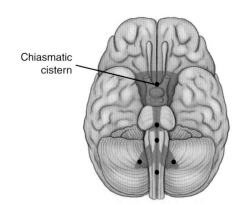

Fig. 18.14 Subarachnoid cisterns—top view.

Thalamus

Following the large cerebrum, the second part of the forebrain is the **thalamus** (Figs. 18.15 and 18.16). The thalamus is a small oval structure (about 1 inch [2.5 cm] in length) that is located just above the midbrain and under the corpus callosum. It consists of two oval masses of primarily gray matter or nuclei that **form part of the walls of the third ventricle,** just superior to the midbrain.

These groups of nuclei (gray matter) of the thalamus serve as relay stations for most of the sensory impulses as they pass from the spinal cord and midbrain structures into the cerebral cortex. The thalamus serves as an **interpretation center** for certain sensory impulses, such as **pain, temperature,** and **touch,** and for **certain emotions** and **memory.**

The thalamus and the hypothalamus together make up the diencephalon portion of the forebrain, as described previously.

Hypothalamus

The third and final division of the forebrain is the **hypothalamus** (see Figs. 18.15 and 18.16). *Hypo-* means "under"—hence its location **under the thalamus.** The hypothalamus forms the **floor and lower walls of the third ventricle.** Three significant structures associated with the hypothalamus are the **infundibulum** *(in″-fun-dib′-u-lum),* **posterior pituitary gland,** and **optic chiasma** *(ki-as′-mah).*

The infundibulum is a conical process that projects downward and ends in the posterior lobe of the pituitary gland. The infundibulum plus the posterior pituitary are known as the **neurohypophysis.**

The **optic chiasma** (see Fig. 18.15) is so named because it resembles the Greek letter χ (chi). The crossing of the optic nerves at the chiasma creates this appearance. It is located superior to the pituitary gland and anterior to the third ventricle.

The hypothalamus is small, but it **controls important body activities** through a link with the endocrine system. Most of these activities are related to **homeostasis,** the tendency or ability of the body to stabilize its normal body states.

MIDBRAIN AND HINDBRAIN

The **midbrain** is seen as a short, constricted portion of the upper brainstem that connects the forebrain to the hindbrain.

The **hindbrain** consists of the **cerebellum, pons,** and **medulla.** As seen in the drawing in Fig. 18.16, the cerebellum is the largest portion of the hindbrain and the second largest portion of the entire brain. The hindbrain is described in detail on the following page.

Pituitary and Pineal Glands

Two important midline structures are the pituitary and pineal glands. The **pineal gland** was shown in its relationship to the third ventricle in Fig. 18.10. This small gland (approximately ¼ inch [5 mm] in length) is an **endocrine gland,** which secretes hormones that aid in regulation of certain secretory activities.

The important **pituitary gland,** also called the **hypophysis,** is referred to as the **"master" gland** because it regulates so many body activities. It is located in and protected by the **sella turcica** of the sphenoid bone and is attached to the hypothalamus of the brain by the **infundibulum** (shown in Figs. 18.15 and 18.16). This gland, which is also relatively small, about ½ inch (1.3 cm) in diameter, is divided into anterior and posterior lobes. The hormones secreted by this master gland control a wide range of body functions, including growth and reproductive functions.

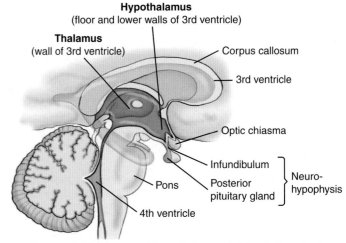

Fig. 18.15 Thalamus and hypothalamus (midsagittal section).

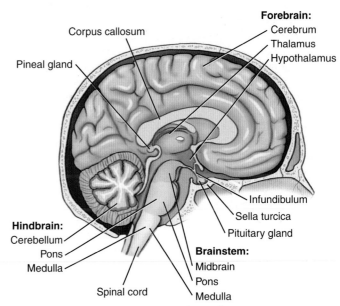

Fig. 18.16 Brain (midsagittal section).

18

Cerebellum

The last part of the brain to be described, the **cerebellum** (Fig. 18.17), occupies the major portion of the inferior and posterior cranial fossae. In the adult, the size proportion between the cerebrum and the cerebellum is about 8:1.

The cerebellum is shaped like a butterfly and consists of **right** and **left hemispheres** united by a narrow median strip, the **vermis.** Toward the superior end of the anterior surface is the wide, shallow **anterior cerebellar notch.** The fourth ventricle is located within the anterior cerebellar notch, separating the pons and the medulla from the cerebellum.

Inferiorly, along the posterior surface, the cerebellar hemispheres are separated by the **posterior cerebellar notch.** An extension of the dura mater, termed the **falx cerebelli,** is located within the posterior cerebellar notch.

The cerebellum primarily coordinates the important motor functions of the body, such as coordination, posture, and balance.

Gray Matter and White Matter

The CNS can be divided by appearance into white matter and gray matter. **White matter** in the brain and spinal cord is composed of **tracts,** which consist of bundles of **myelinated axons.** Myelinated axons are axons wrapped in a myelin sheath, a fatty substance having a creamy white color. The white matter comprises mostly axons.

The **gray matter** is composed mainly of **neuron dendrites** and **cell bodies.** A section of brain tissue through the cerebral hemispheres is shown in Fig. 18.18. At this level of the brain, gray matter forms the **outer cerebral cortex,** whereas the brain tissue under the cortex is white matter. This underlying mass of white substance is termed the **centrum semiovale.** Deep within the cerebrum, inferior to this level, is more gray matter termed the **cerebral nuclei,** or **basal ganglia.**

Because a cranial CT scan can differentiate between white matter and gray matter, a section through the cerebral nuclei provides a wealth of diagnostic information. The horizontal or axial section of the right cerebral hemisphere in Fig. 18.19 shows the areas that usually can be visualized. Areas of white matter include the **corpus callosum** and the **centrum semiovale.** Gray matter areas include the **cerebral nuclei, thalamus,** and **cerebral cortex.**

SUMMARY: WHITE MATTER VERSUS GRAY MATTER

White Matter

White matter consists of **myelinated axons** that are commonly identified on CT brain sections as light-appearing or white-appearing tissue. It is most commonly seen on sectional scans of the cerebral hemispheres as subcortical white masses of **centrum semiovale,** which are fibers that connect the gray matter of the cerebral cortex with the deep, more caudal parts of the midbrain and spinal cord.

The second major white matter structure is the **corpus callosum,** a band of fibers that connect the right and left cerebral hemispheres deep within the longitudinal fissure.

Gray Matter

The gray matter comprises the thin outer layer of the folds of the **cerebral cortex** and is composed of dendrites and cell bodies.

Other gray matter of the brain includes more central brain structures, such as the **cerebral nuclei** or **basal ganglia,** located deep within the cerebral hemispheres, and the groups of **nuclei** that make up the **thalamus.**

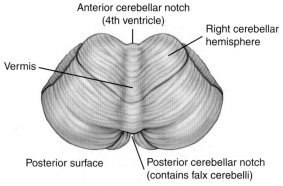

Fig. 18.17 Cerebellum.

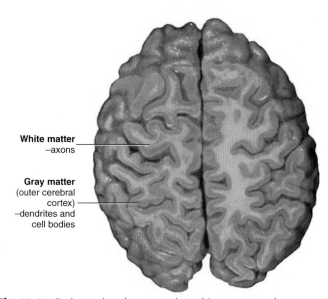

Fig. 18.18 Brain section demonstrating white matter and gray matter.

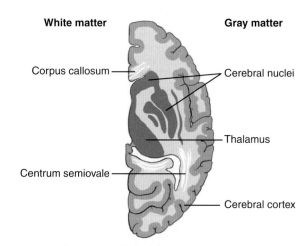

Fig. 18.19 White matter and gray matter.

CEREBRAL NUCLEI (BASAL GANGLIA)

The **cerebral nuclei,** or basal ganglia, are paired collections of gray matter deep within each cerebral hemisphere (Fig. 18.20). There are four specific areas or groupings of these cerebral nuclei; three of them are shown in this cutaway drawing: the **caudate nucleus;** the **lentiform nucleus,** comprising the putamen and globus pallidus; and the **amygdaloid nucleus,** or body. (The **claustrum** is not visible in this drawing.)

The relationships of the **brainstem** and the **cerebellum** to three of the cerebral nuclei and to the **thalamus** are shown in Fig. 18.20. The cerebral nuclei are bilaterally symmetric collections of gray matter located on **both sides of the third ventricle.**

Brain—Inferior Surface

Fig. 18. 21 shows a drawing of the inferior surface of the brain, demonstrating the **infundibulum, pituitary gland,** and **optic chiasma,** which are anterior to the **pons** and **midbrain.** Extending forward from the optic chiasma are the large **optic nerves,** and extending posterolaterally are the **optic tracts.** A portion of the **corpus callosum** is shown to be located deep within the longitudinal fissure.

Cranial Nerves

The 12 pairs of cranial nerves are attached to the base of the brain and leave the skull through various foramina. Identifying all of these cranial nerves on radiographs or drawings is generally beyond the scope of anatomy required of technologists.

Technologists should know all the names and general functions described subsequently (summarized in Table 18.1). The nerves are numbered in order from anterior to posterior with Roman numerals. The **smallest** of the cranial nerves are **IV,** the **trochlear nerves,** and the **largest** are **V,** the **trigeminal nerves.**

The mnemonic **On Old Olympus' Towering Tops, A Finn And German Viewed Some Hops** gives the first letter of each of the 12 pairs of cranial nerves, as shown in Table 18.1.

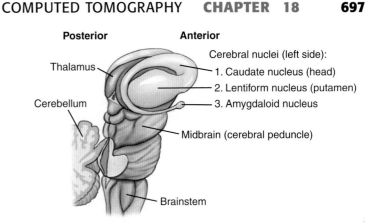

Fig. 18.20 Midsagittal view of cerebral nuclei (basal ganglia) deep within cerebrum.

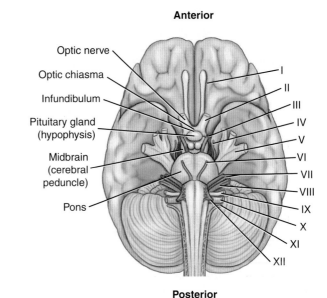

Fig. 18.21 Brain (inferior surface).

TABLE 18.1 **SUMMARY OF CRANIAL NERVES**		
I	Olfactory nerve (smell)	On
II	Optic nerve (vision)	Old
III	Oculomotor nerve (eye movement)	Olympus'
IV	Trochlear nerve (eye movement)	Towering
V	Trigeminal nerve (mixed sensory and motor with three branches)	Tops
VI	Abducens nerve (eye movement)	A
VII	Facial nerve (sensory and motor)	Finn
VIII	Vestibulocochlear (acoustic) nerve (hearing)	And
IX	Glossopharyngeal nerve (taste and swallowing)	German
X	Vagus nerve (sensory and motor)	Viewed
XI	Accessory (spinal accessory) nerve (swallowing)	A (Some)
XII	Hypoglossal nerve (tongue, speech, and swallowing)	Hop(s)

Orbital Cavity

The orbital cavities are often filmed as a routine part of a cranial CT scan. The orbital cavity as dissected from the front includes the **bulb** of the eye and numerous associated structures, as illustrated in Fig. 18.22. Orbital contents include the **ocular muscles, nerves** (including the large optic nerve), **blood vessels, orbital fat, lacrimal gland,** and **lacrimal sac and duct.**

ORBITAL CAVITIES (SUPERIOR VIEW)

The orbital cavities are exposed from above, as shown in Fig. 18.23, by removal of the orbital plate of the frontal bone. The right orbit illustrates the normal fullness of the orbital cavity. The **lacrimal gland** in the upper outer quadrant, **orbital fat,** and **ocular muscles** help fill the entire cavity. The **internal carotid artery** is seen entering the base of the skull. At this point, the internal carotid artery has already given off an artery that supplies the orbital contents.

The left orbital cavity, with fat and some muscles removed, illustrates the course of the larger **optic nerve** as it emerges from the bulb to course medially to the **optic chiasma.** Orbital tumors and foreign bodies can be readily detected through CT scan of the orbits.

VISUAL PATHWAY

Axons leaving each eyeball travel via the **optic nerves** to the **optic chiasma.** Within the optic chiasma, some fibers cross to the opposite side, and some remain on the same side, as shown in Fig. 18.24. After passing through the optic chiasma, the fibers form an **optic tract.** Each optic tract enters the brain and terminates in the **thalamus.**

In the thalamus, fibers synapse with other neurons, axons of which form the **optic radiations,** which pass to the **visual centers** in the cortex of the occipital lobes of the cerebrum. Because of the partial crossing of fibers, sight can be affected in various ways, depending on the location of a lesion in the visual pathway. An example is **hemianopia,** which causes blindness or defective vision in only half the visual field of each eye.

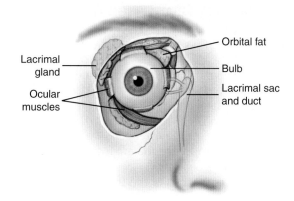

Fig. 18.22 Orbital cavity.

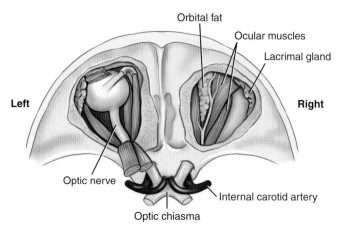

Fig. 18.23 Orbital cavities (superior view).

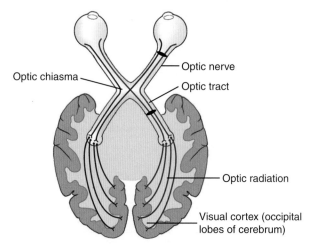

Fig. 18.24 Visual pathway.

BASIC PRINCIPLES

Basic Principles of CT

The radiographic term **tomography** is derived from the Greek words *tomos,* meaning "slice," and *graphein,* meaning "to write." CT uses a complex computer and mechanical imaging system to provide sectional anatomic images in the **axial, sagittal, and coronal planes.** The concept of CT may be simplified by comparing a procedure with imaging a loaf of bread; conventional radiography captures images of the loaf as a whole, whereas CT takes the loaf and images it in individual *slices* (also called sections, or cuts), which are viewed independently. Fig. 18.25 illustrates this example; the anteroposterior (AP) abdomen is the "loaf," and the CT image on the right is the "slice."

A CT unit uses an x-ray tube and a detector array to gather anatomic data from a patient. These data are reconstructed into an image. This chapter provides an introduction to CT equipment, imaging principles, and clinical applications; additional study on the topic is required for competence in performing CT procedures.

CT TERMINOLOGY

As CT technology has evolved, so have the terms used to describe it. Initially, *computer-assisted tomography* and *computerized axial tomography (CAT)* were used, but as the technology advanced, the accepted term became *computed tomography (CT)*. Although the term *CAT scan* may still be heard, it is not accurate because CT images are routinely reconstructed in the sagittal and coronal planes as well as in oblique planes.

EVOLUTION OF CT

Since the introduction of clinical CT scanning in the early 1970s, systems have evolved through multiple generations. The difference between generations is related primarily to the design and construction of *detectors,* the devices that measure the attenuation of the transmitted x-ray beam. Additional differences include dual energy imaging, shorter scan times and the ability to obtain volumetric data sets with the latest generation of CT scanner. Dual energy imaging uses two different kVp levels for image data sets that allow for improved tissue differentiation, in addition to material analysis. The shorter scan times allow for the elimination of motion, and volumetric data sets allow for the generation of three-dimensional volume rendered images.

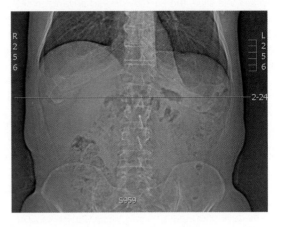

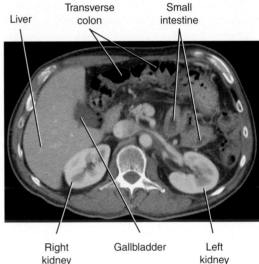

Fig. 18.25 CT scan of the abdomen at level of kidneys, L2.

MULTIDETECTOR CT SCANNERS (MDCT)

X-ray tube movement in early CT scanners was restricted by high-tension cables. The x-ray tube first would rotate 360° in one direction to obtain one slice, the CT table would advance a set distance, and the x-ray tube would rotate 360° in the opposite direction to obtain the next slice. The development of slip-ring technology in the early 1990s allowed CT technology to move beyond single-slice acquisition.

Slip rings replaced the high-tension cables and now allow for **continuous rotation of the x-ray tube.** This, combined with simultaneous continuous table movement through the gantry, permits data acquisition in a helical or spiral fashion (Fig. 18.26). The general term used to describe this acquisition of a volume of data is *volume scanning.* The terms *helical* and *spiral scanning* are sometimes also used to refer to this scanning technique, but these are vendor-specific terms. Volume CT scanners are also capable of single-slice acquisition.

Scanners developed before 1992 were single-slice scanners that were capable of imaging only one slice at a time. By late 1998, CT manufacturers announced new **multislice technology scanners** capable of imaging **four slices simultaneously** per x-ray tube rotation. The drawing in Fig. 18.27 shows the usual single-detector bank scanner on the left with the four-multidetector array bank type on the right.

Multislice CT (Fig. 18.28) has continued to progress rapidly, largely because of advances in computer technology. Currently, multislice scanners are available that can image 320 slices per x-ray tube rotation. Although it is important that radiologic technologists have an understanding of this technology, specific information on the physics and instrumentation of this technology is beyond the scope of this chapter.

Advantages

Multislice CT offers several advantages over single-slice or volume CT, as follows:

- **Shorter scan time:** A 64-slice system with a 360° tube rotation time of 1 second would be able to acquire 64 images per second versus a 1-slice-per-second scanner. This faster imaging is advantageous for procedures that require a single breath hold or in cases in which patient motion is a problem. It also makes possible procedures that require shorter exposure times (e.g., cardiac CT).
- **Decreased amount of contrast medium:** A decreased amount of intravenous contrast medium can be used because of the increased acquisition speed of multislice scanners.
- **Improved spatial resolution:** Submillimeter slice thickness is possible as a result of multislice technology. This is especially advantageous for examinations of the inner ear and other complex structures. Also, a decreased amount of contrast medium is required because of the increased speed of image acquisition.
- **Improved temporal resolution:** Temporal resolution is the ability to image fast moving objects and relates to the speed (time) at which data may be captured. The faster the data can be captured translates into increased temporal resolution. Temporal resolution is especially important in cardiac imaging, in which the beating heart motion needs to be stopped for optimal image quality.
- **Improved image quality:** Image quality for CT angiography and 3D multiplanar reconstruction is improved as a result of the acquisition of thinner slices.
- **Multiplanar reconstruction (MPR):** Volumetric data allow more accurate reconstruction of patient data into alternative planes (coronal, sagittal, oblique, and three-dimensional [3D]); hence the term *multiplanar reconstruction.*
- **Artifacts reduced:** Artifacts caused by patient motion are reduced.

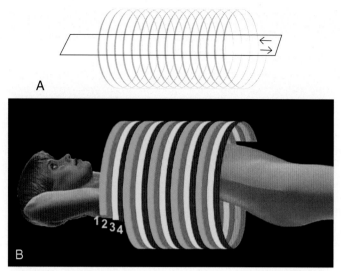

Fig. 18.26 A and B, Volume (spiral) multislice scan; 360° continuous rotation of tube and detectors while patient moves in or out. (**A** courtesy GE Medical Systems; **B** courtesy Philips Medical Systems.)

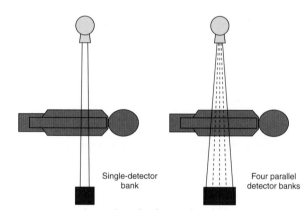

Fig. 18.27 Comparison of single-slice and multislice scanner concepts.

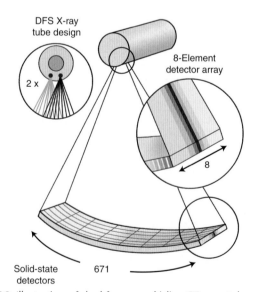

Fig. 18.28 Illustration of dual-focus, multislice CT x-ray tube with an 8-element detector array, resulting in 16 slices per rotation.

CT SYSTEM COMPONENTS

CT systems are typically fixed installations. Mobile CT scanners are available but are not commonly used (Fig. 18.29). Mobile CT scanners are used in trauma and intensive care units and in intraoperative imaging; they also serve as an auxiliary or backup system within an imaging department. They are useful in military field hospitals and for imaging patients in strict isolation.

CT systems consist of three major components: **gantry, computer,** and **operator console.** These systems include highly complex computing and imaging devices. The following sections provide a broad introduction to a very technical topic.

Gantry

The gantry consists of the **x-ray tube, detector array,** and **collimators.** Depending on the technical specifications of the unit, the gantry typically can be angled 30° in each direction, as required for CT scanning of the head or spine. The central opening in the gantry is the **aperture.** The CT **table** (sometimes called the **patient couch**) is electronically linked to the gantry for controlled movement during the scan (Fig. 18.30). The patient anatomy within the aperture is the area being scanned at that time.

X-ray Tube The x-ray tube is similar to a general radiographic tube in construction and operation; however, design modifications often are required to ensure the tube is able to withstand additional heat capacity because of increased exposure times.

Detector Array Detectors are solid state and are composed of photodiodes coupled with scintillation crystal materials (cadmium tungstate or rare earth oxide ceramic crystals). Solid-state detectors convert transmitted x-ray energy into light, which is converted into electrical energy and then into a digital signal. The detector array affects patient dose and the efficiency of the CT unit.

Collimator Assembly Collimation in CT is important because it reduces patient dose and improves image quality. Current-generation CT scanners generally use **one collimator-prepatient** (at the x-ray tube), which shapes and limits the beam. The slice thickness on modern multidetector CT units is determined by the size of the detector row used.

Computer

The CT computer requires **two types** of highly sophisticated software: one for the **operating system** and one for **applications.** The operating system manages the hardware, whereas the applications software manages preprocessing, image reconstruction, and a wide variety of post-processing operations.

The CT computer must possess staggering speed and memory capacity. For instance, consider that for one CT slice (image) with a 512 × 512 matrix, the computer must simultaneously perform 262,144 mathematical calculations per slice.

Operator Console

The components of the operator console include a keyboard, a mouse, and single or dual monitors, depending on the system (Fig. 18.31). The operator console allows the technologist to control the parameters of the examination, called the *protocol,* and view or manipulate the images generated. The protocol, which is predetermined for each procedure, includes factors such as kilovoltage, milliamperage, pitch, field of view, slice thickness, table indexing, reconstruction algorithms, and display windows. These parameters may be modified by the technologist, if required, based on patient presentation or clinical history.

Networking and Archiving

Networking of computer workstations, a setup in which workstations are situated in other locations for use by the radiologist or technologist, is common. These workstations may be within the imaging department or located in remote areas with electronic transmission of data.

Image archiving for most CT systems involves the use of digital media that are housed in the *picture archiving and communications system* (PACS) archive. Images not stored in a PACS may use a combination of optical disks and hard disk drives for high-capacity permanent storage of data. Laser printers may also be used to print a hard-copy image for storage. Interpretation of the examination findings generally is performed by the radiologist on a high-resolution workstation.

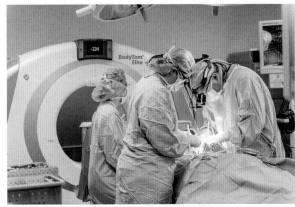

Fig. 18.29 Mobile CT unit. (Courtesy NeuroLogica, A Subsidiary of Samsung Electronics Co., Ltd. All rights reserved.)

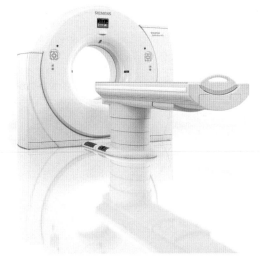

Fig. 18.30 CT scanning unit—patient table (couch) and gantry. (Courtesy of Siemens Medical Solutions USA, Inc.)

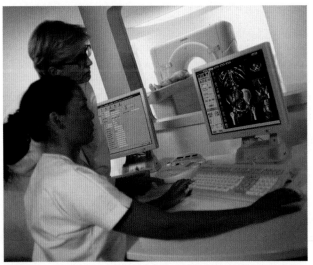

Fig. 18.31 Operator at control console. (Courtesy Philips Medical Systems.)

Image Reconstruction

As in conventional radiography, CT images display various shades of gray. The incident radiation is differentially attenuated by the patient, and the remnant radiation is measured by the detectors. Low-density structures (lungs and air-filled structures) attenuate very little of the x-ray beam, whereas higher density structures (bones and contrast media) attenuate all or nearly all of the x-ray beam. The attenuation information exits the detectors in analog form and is converted to a digital signal by an analog-to-digital converter. The digital values are used in the next step, which consists of reconstruction of the image based on a series of reconstruction algorithms.

VOLUME ELEMENT (VOXEL)

The display matrix of the digital image is composed of rows and columns of tiny blocks called *pixels* (picture elements). Each of the pixels is a two-dimensional (2D) representation of the 3D volume of tissue in the CT slice (Fig. 18.32). These 3D tissue volumes are called **volume elements,** or *voxels.* Voxels have height, width, and depth. The depth of a voxel is determined by the slice thickness, as selected by the technologist. Each voxel is represented by a pixel in the 2D reconstructed image (Fig. 18.33).

As stated previously, multislice CT allows submillimeter slice thicknesses, whereby voxels have equal dimensions in all three axes (height, width, and depth, or *x, y,* and *z* planes). Data sets from these voxels are said to be *isotropic.* Isotropic data sets allow optimal MPR and 3D images with equal spatial resolution in all planes. Isotropic imaging is especially useful when high-resolution MPR images are required, such as in CT angiography, inner ear imaging, and skeletal imaging.

Any CT image, such as in Fig. 18.34, is composed of a large number of pixels that represent various degrees of attenuation, depending on the anatomic density of the tissue in the voxel that is being represented.

ATTENUATION (DIFFERENTIAL ABSORPTION) OF EACH VOXEL

Each voxel in the tissue slice is assigned a number by the computer that is proportional to the degree of x-ray attenuation of that tissue volume. In CT, data from differential absorption of tissues in each voxel are collected and processed by the processing unit of the computer.

CONVERTING 3D VOXELS TO 2D PIXELS

When the degree of attenuation of each voxel is determined, the 3D tissue slice is displayed on the computer monitor as a **2D image.** Each voxel of tissue is represented on the computer display as a pixel. The number of pixels capable of being displayed is determined by the manufacturer.

Fig. 18.34 shows an example of a 2D display of a slice of brain tissue created by the attenuation or differential absorption of these tissues. CSF within the ventricles results in less attenuation of the voxels of these tissues than is seen in the voxels of the dense bony regions of the cranium or the calcified pineal gland seen midline to the brain that appears white. The choroid plexuses (capillaries within the ventricle) are also calcified.

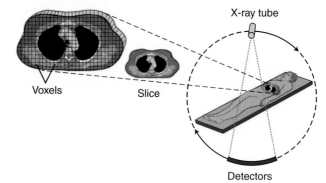

Fig. 18.32 CT image reconstruction—voxels (3D display) to pixels (2D display).

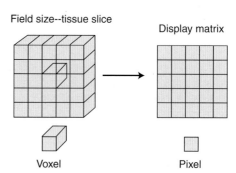

Fig. 18.33 CT image—voxels and pixels.

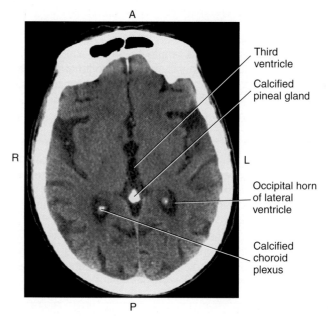

Fig. 18.34 Cranial CT (axial slice).

COMPUTED GRAY SCALE AND CT NUMBERS

After the CT computer (through thousands of mathematic calculations) determines the degree of attenuation (called the *linear attenuation coefficient*) for each voxel, these values are converted to another numeric scale called **CT numbers,** which are used in the display matrix. Originally, CT numbers were called *Hounsfield units,* after Hounsfield, an English scientist who in 1970 produced the first head CT scan. (Hounsfield and Cormack won the Nobel prize in medicine in 1979 for their work on CT.)

Shades of gray are assigned to the CT numbers. The baseline for CT numbers is **water,** which is assigned the CT number value of **0.** Scanners are calibrated so that water is always valued as 0. Dense cortical bone has a value of +1000, or up to +3000, and air (which produces the least amount of attenuation) has a value of −1000. Between these two extremes are tissues and substances that possess various CT numbers according to their attenuation. Different shades of gray are assigned specific CT numbers to create the displayed image. Table 18.2 lists common tissue types and structures, along with their associated CT numbers and appearances.

As can be seen on the chest CT scan in Fig. 18.35, bone, soft tissue, muscle, and fat all appear differently on a CT image because of their attenuation and the resultant CT number. Dense tissues, such as **bone,** appear white. **Contrast medium–filled structures** also appear white (Fig. 18.36). **Air,** which is not dense compared with tissues, appears black. **Fat, muscle,** and **organs,** which fall between the densities of bone and air, appear as varying shades of gray.

WINDOW WIDTH AND WINDOW LEVEL (WINDOWING)

Window width (WW) refers to the range of CT numbers that are displayed as shades of gray. Wide window width indicates more CT numbers as a group (long scale or low contrast). **WW controls the displayed image contrast** (wide window width, low contrast as in chest imaging; narrow window width, high contrast as in cranial imaging).

Window level (WL) controls image brightness or determines the CT number that is the center of the window width. WL usually is determined by the tissue density that occurs most frequently within an anatomic structure.

PITCH WITH VOLUME SCANNERS

The x-ray tube and detector array, in addition to the patient, are in continuous motion during a volume acquisition. The amount of anatomy covered during a particular scan is determined by the *pitch.* Pitch is a ratio that reflects the relationship between table speed and slice thickness. The formula for pitch is as follows:

$$Pitch = \frac{Couch\ movement\ (mm/sec)\ per\ 360°\ rotation\ of\ tube}{Collimation}$$

A **1:1 pitch** indicates that table speed and slice thickness are equal. A 1.5:1 pitch would be created if table speed equaled 15 mm/sec with a slice thickness of 10 mm. A 2:1 pitch increases the risk that pathology may be missed as a result of **undersampling** of the anatomy. A 0.5:1 ratio would increase patient dose because of **oversampling** of the anatomy. Pitch is determined by the radiologist or technologist according to the nature of the study or the pathologic indications.

IMAGE RECONSTRUCTION SUMMARY

During a CT procedure, the tube and the detector array rotate around the patient. Thousands of measurements are taken to determine the radiation attenuation value (linear attenuation coefficient) for each tissue volume element (voxel). When the linear attenuation coefficient has been determined, the data are converted into CT numbers for display purposes. On the monitor, a 2D image is displayed as a matrix of picture elements (pixels), with each pixel representing the CT number of a specific volume element (voxel) in the CT slice. The window width and level may be adjusted to alter the image appearance.

TABLE 18.2 TISSUE TYPE AND CT NUMBERS

TISSUE TYPE	CT NUMBERS	APPEARANCE
Cortical bone	+1000	White
Muscle	+50	Gray
White matter	+45	Light gray
Gray matter	+40	Gray
Blood	+20	Gray[a]
CSF	+15	Gray
Water	0 (baseline)	
Fat	−100	Dark gray to black
Lung	−200	Dark gray to black
Air	−1000	Black

[a]White if iodinated contrast medium is present.

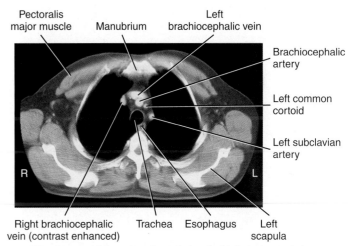

Fig. 18.35 Axial section through level of inferior manubrium.

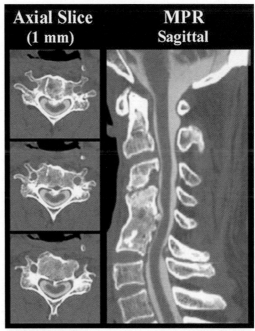

Fig. 18.36 MPR (multislice) volume scan of cervical spine in axial and sagittal slices; demonstrates superior contrast resolution compared with conventional radiography.

CLINICAL APPLICATION OF CT

CT Versus Conventional Radiography

CT is widely used today. It has several advantages compared with conventional radiography, as follows:

- **Anatomic structures are visualized with no superimposition.** 3D anatomic information is presented as a series of thin slices of the internal structure of the part in question (Fig. 18.37).
- **CT images have increased contrast resolution.** The CT system is more sensitive in tissue-type differentiation compared with conventional radiography; thus differences in tissue types can be delineated more clearly and studied. Conventional radiography can display tissues that have at least a 10% difference in density, whereas CT can detect tissue density differences of 1% or less. This detection aids in differential diagnosis of

pathologies; a solid mass can be distinguished from a cyst, or (in some cases) a benign neoplasm may be distinguished from a malignant neoplasm. Fig. 18.38 demonstrates a subdural hematoma on the left side of the brain.

- **MPR:** Acquired data may be reconstructed and viewed in alternative planes with no additional radiation exposure to the patient (Fig. 18.39).
- **Manipulation of attenuation data:** Tissue attenuation data collected by the detectors may be manipulated and measured by the computer. Lesions visualized on the image may be measured, and the recorded numeric value (CT number) of the lesion may be viewed to assess its composition (e.g., fat, calcium, water) (Fig. 18.40).

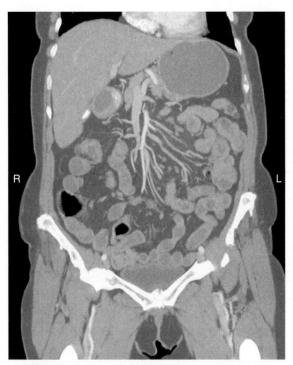

Fig. 18.37 Coronal abdomen CT–reconstruction.

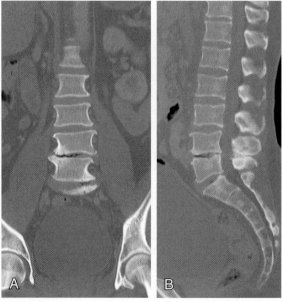

Fig. 18.39 A and B, Lumbar spine reconstructed in coronal and sagittal planes.

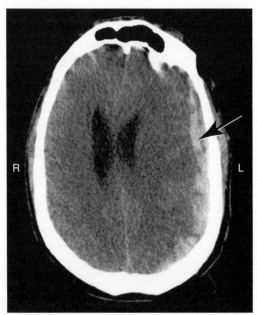

Fig. 18.38 Left subdural hematoma.

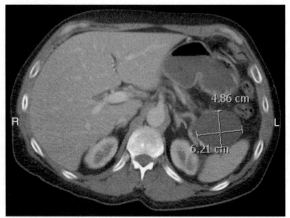

Fig. 18.40 Measurement of tumor in abdomen.

Patient Communication and Consent

The CT procedure must be fully explained to the patient (Fig. 18.41). The explanation should include the nature of the examination and what the patient can expect, how long it will take, the need to remain still, and reassurance that the technologist will be monitoring the patient throughout the procedure. Breathing instructions should be given, and breathing can be rehearsed if required. If a clinical history has not already been provided by the referring physician, the technologist should take one.

The equipment can appear intimidating to a patient, and a thorough explanation by the technologist can alleviate fears and ensure a successful diagnostic procedure.

Procedure

Following the explanation of the procedure, the patient is positioned on the CT table. This position (supine versus prone; head first versus feet first) depends on the examination being performed. A preliminary image of the area being examined is obtained. This preliminary image is called a **scanogram** (Fig. 18.42), scout, or topogram, depending on the brand of CT equipment used; the term *scanogram* is used in this chapter. The technologist uses the scanogram to select the range of the CT scan. Additional parameters important to the examination are contained in the selected protocol and include kilovoltage, milliamperage, pitch, field of view, slice thickness, table indexing, reconstruction algorithms, and display windows.

VIEWING CT IMAGES

When CT images are viewed, the patient's right is placed to the viewer's left, as in conventional radiography. Axial scans are viewed as though the viewer were facing the patient and looking at the scan from the foot end of the patient.

INTRAVENOUS CONTRAST MEDIA

An intravenous injection of iodinated contrast medium is frequently required to distinguish between normal tissue and pathology. An electromechanical injector is necessary because of the short scan time in multislice CT. Careful selection of the volume of the injection and the rate of flow peak ensures optimal vascular and organ enhancement levels.

It has become common practice in CT to follow the contrast medium injection with a saline bolus injection (saline flush). Injecting a saline bolus at this time allows for increased duration of contrast enhancement as the pooled contrast material is flushed from the veins and the contrast medium bolus is propelled forward. It also may allow for a reduction in the amount of contrast medium used. Double-barreled electromechanical injectors are available for this technique. The injector automatically switches to a saline syringe after the contrast medium has been injected.

Refer to Chapter 14 for information regarding venipuncture, contrast medium contraindications, and reactions.

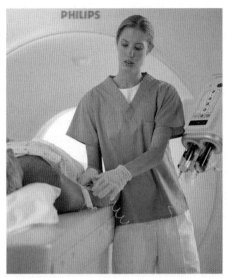

Fig. 18.41 Patient being prepared for CT examination. (Courtesy Philips Medical Systems.)

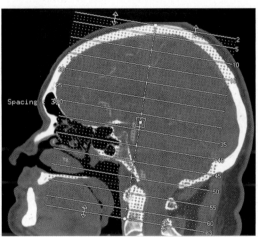

Fig. 18.42 Scanogram slice plan.

18

Contrast Media and Blood-Brain Barrier

It is estimated that 50% to 90% of all head CT scans require an intravenous injection of contrast medium. Contrast media used are similar to media used for intravenous urography. These iodinated contrast media usually are administered as bolus injections but may be introduced slowly via an intravenous infusion.

The brain is well supplied with blood vessels that carry oxygen and nutrients. Oxygen must be in constant supply because total oxygen deprivation for 4 minutes can lead to permanent brain cell damage. Similarly, glucose must be continually available because carbohydrate storage in the brain is limited. Glucose, oxygen, and certain ions pass readily from the circulatory blood into extracellular fluid and then into brain cells. Other substances found in the blood normally enter brain cells quite slowly. Still others, such as proteins, most antibiotics, and contrast media, do not pass at all from the normal cranial capillary system into brain cells.

Brain tissue differs from other tissues in that it possesses a natural barrier to the passage of certain substances. This natural phenomenon is termed the **blood-brain barrier.** Figs. 18.43 and 18.44 demonstrate contrast media outside of normal vasculature due to an intraparenchymal and subarachnoid hemorrhage.

RADIATION DOSE

As for all radiologic examinations, CT procedures should be performed only if there is a clinical indication. Additionally, when these procedures are performed, adherence to the ALARA principle (as low as reasonably achievable) is required to reduce dose to patients and personnel.

Patient Dose

Radiation dose for CT procedures is higher than the dose of a conventional radiographic examination of the same part. Patient dose is related to pitch: a lower pitch results in a higher dose (slice overlap). Thinner slices also result in a higher dose. To compensate for the potential increased dose with CT (especially multislice CT), some manufacturers have incorporated technology called *dose modulation*. This technique allows the minimum dose required per slice to be determined by the scanogram; each slice then is obtained with the use of optimal mAs. Dose to radiosensitive organs (eyes, breasts, pelvis, and thyroid) also can be reduced by applying bismuth shields to the patient. Image quality is not compromised through these techniques.

In 2007 the Alliance for Radiation Safety in Pediatric Imaging, in a joint effort with the Society for Pediatric Radiology, American College of Radiology, American Society for Radiologic Technologists, and American Association of Physicists in Medicine, implemented the Image Gently® campaign. This campaign asks that every member of the health care team take the following pledge:

- To make the Image Gently® message a priority in staff communications this year
- To review the protocol recommendations and, where necessary, implement adjustments to our processes
- To respect and listen to suggestions from every member of the imaging team on ways to ensure changes are made
- To communicate openly with parents[1]

In October 2010 the American College of Radiology, Radiological Society of North America, American Society of Radiologic Technologists, and American Association of Physicists in Medicine jointly developed the Image Wisely© campaign to promote the reduction of radiation exposure to adult patients. The Image Wisely© campaign uses the following pledge:

1. To put my patient's safety, health, and welfare first by optimizing imaging examinations to use only the radiation necessary to produce diagnostic quality images
2. To convey the principles of the Image Wisely© program to the imaging team in order to ensure that my facility optimizes its use of radiation when imaging patients

3. To communicate optimal patient imaging strategies to referring physicians, and to be available for consultation
4. To routinely review imaging protocols to ensure that the least radiation necessary to acquire a diagnostic quality image is used for each examination[2]

Pediatric CT Scans

Protocols have been established to minimize exposure to pediatric patients during CT scans. Ideal exposure factors, slice thickness, and critical organ dose-sparing measures must be used. The CT technologist must be trained in pediatric procedures to ensure the best procedure is produced with a minimal amount of exposure to the patient.

Technologist and Personnel Exposure

Anyone who must remain in the CT examination room during an examination must wear protective lead apparel. The highest radiation exposure occurs nearest the patient because of the scatter produced in the patient; if possible, it is desirable to maintain maximum distance from the source.

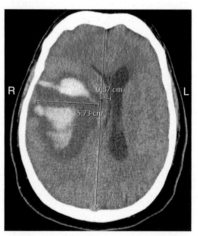

Fig. 18.43 Intraparenchymal hemorrhage with midline shift.

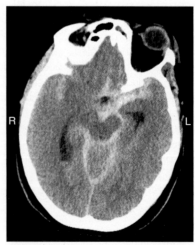

Fig. 18.44 CT scan demonstrating subarachnoid hemorrhage.

Cranial CT—Head CT

Injury and pathology of the head often involve the brain and associated soft tissues; however, plain radiographic images provide a 2D view of the bony skull only. CT is a vital tool in evaluation of the patient because it can allow for differentiation of acute hemorrhage, fluid collections, calcifications, white matter and gray matter, CSF, cerebral edema, and neoplasms.

The term *head CT* refers to CT imaging of the brain. Specific CT procedures are also available for investigation of pathology of orbits, sella turcica, sinuses, temporal bones, and temporomandibular joints. This section focuses on CT imaging of the brain.

PATHOLOGIC INDICATIONS

Any suspected disease process involving the brain is an indication for a head CT scan. Common indications include the following:

- **Tumors**—metastatic lesions, meningioma, glioma
- **Headache**
- **Circulatory pathology**—cerebrovascular accident, aneurysm, arteriovenous malformation
- **Inflammatory** or **infectious conditions**—meningitis, abscess
- **Degenerative disorders**—brain atrophy
- **Trauma**—epidural and subdural hematoma, fracture
- **Congenital abnormalities**
- **Hydrocephalus**

HEAD CT PROCEDURE

The basic principles of skull positioning in conventional radiography also apply to CT; however, specific positioning for head CT scan varies, depending on radiologist preferences and departmental protocols.

Metallic items (e.g., earrings, hair pins) and dentures must be removed. The patient is placed supine on the CT table and is positioned so there is no rotation (Figs. 18.45 and 18.46) or tilt (Fig. 18.47) of the midsagittal plane. Rotation is corrected by aligning the midsagittal plane perpendicular to the floor of the room. Evaluation for tilt is achieved by assessing the symmetry of bony structures. Two anatomic structures frequently compared are the external auditory canals and zygomatic arches for symmetry. Ensuring the proper positioning of the head allows for a more accurate assessment of anatomy and pathology without the influence of positional asymmetry.

After being properly positioned, the head is immobilized. Movement of the head and neck for correction of tilt and rotation should not be performed in a patient with a suspected cervical spine injury.

A scanogram must be obtained before the procedure is begun to allow the technologist to determine the range of the scan. A routine head CT scan includes the region from the base to the vertex of the skull in 5- to 8-mm slices. Gantry and beam angulation also can be determined from the scanogram. Typically, the x-ray beam is aligned parallel to the infraorbitomeatal line.

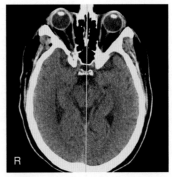

Fig. 18.45 Axial CT head scan—no rotation.

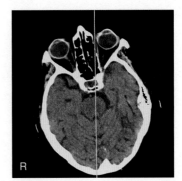

Fig. 18.46 Axial CT head scan—rotation.

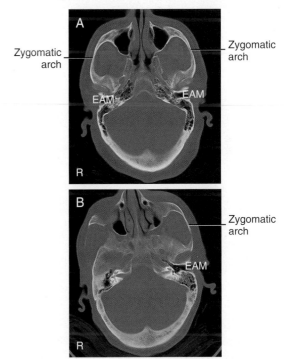

Fig. 18.47 A, Axial CT head scan—no tilt. B, Axial CT head scan—tilt.

Head CT images are viewed with **two window settings or window widths.** A narrow WW allows optimal **visualization of soft tissue and brain** (Fig. 18.48), and a wide WW displays optimal **bony detail** (Fig. 18.49). In addition to the window setting for soft tissue and bone, there are other special processing **algorithms** (mathematical calculations and processes applied during image reconstruction) for demonstration of specific anatomy. Figs. 18.50 and 18.51 are axial and coronal images, respectively, of the temporal bone for middle and internal ear anatomy, in which a bony algorithm is applied during reconstruction.

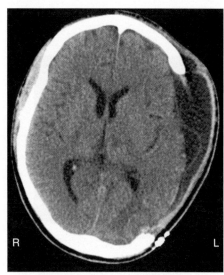

Fig. 18.48 Subdural hematoma post craniotomy—subdural fluid collection.

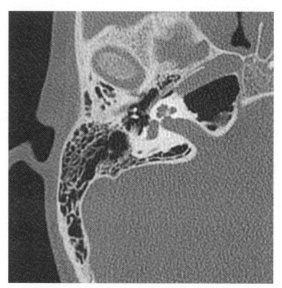

Fig. 18.50 Axial CT image of temporal bone.

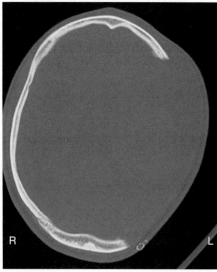

Fig. 18.49 Subdural hematoma post craniotomy—bone window.

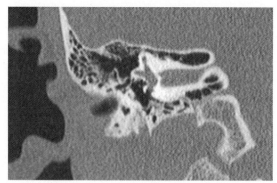

Fig. 18.51 Coronal CT image of temporal bone.

Sectional Anatomy

AXIAL SECTIONS OF BRAIN

Figs. 18.52 through 18.57 are axial CT images demonstrating specific structures the technologist should be able to recognize when comparing these images with unlabeled axial CT images. Included with the axial images is the corresponding lateral skull radiograph showing the slice level.

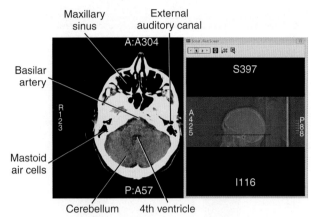

Fig. 18.52 Axial CT scan—level of fourth ventricle and cerebellum.

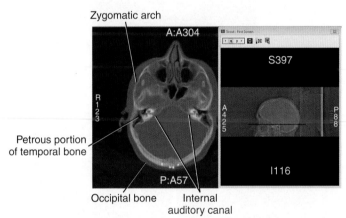

Fig. 18.53 Axial CT scan—level of internal auditory canals.

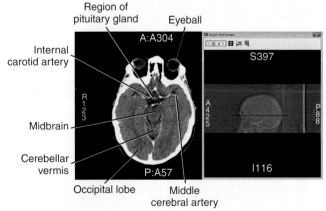

Fig. 18.54 Axial CT scan—level of pons.

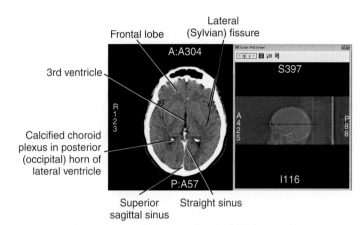

Fig. 18.55 Axial CT scan—level of third ventricle.

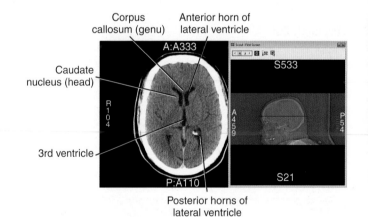

Fig. 18.56 Axial CT scan—level of lateral (anterior and posterior horns) ventricles.

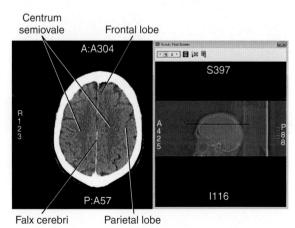

Fig. 18.57 Axial CT scan—level of upper cerebrum.

18

EXAMPLES OF PATHOLOGY
Metastatic Lesion
An example of a positive CT scan is shown in Fig. 18.58. The patient has a history of cancer that has metastasized to the brain, as demonstrated by the three separate lesions. Contrast medium enhancement is necessary for most suspected neoplasia because of possible breakdown of the normal blood-brain barrier, as described in the discussion of contrast media and the blood-brain barrier. Fig. 18.59 demonstrates contrast enhancement of a nonmetastatic brain tumor.

Subdural Hematoma
Figs. 18.60 and 18.61 demonstrate a subdural hematoma. A subdural hematoma is a blood clot that forms between the dura mater and the surface of the brain as a result of damage to cerebral venous circulation.

Subarachnoid Hemorrhage
Fig. 18.44 (see page 706) demonstrates a subarachnoid hemorrhage. A subarachnoid hemorrhage may be traumatic or nontraumatic and represents bleeding into the subarachnoid space.

Cerebrovascular Accident (Stroke)
A cerebrovascular accident may be caused by a rupture or occlusion of an artery in the brain. The rupture of an artery in the brain leads to a hemorrhagic stroke as demonstrated in Fig. 18.62. The occlusion of an artery in the brain can result in an ischemic stroke as seen in Fig. 18.63.

Hydrocephalus
Hydrocephalus refers to an increase in the volume of CSF within the brain. The increase in the volume of CSF leads to the enlargement of the ventricles and subsequent compression of surrounding brain structures. Fig. 18.64 demonstrates the enlargement of the ventricular system as a result of hydrocephalus. Fig. 18.64B shows a shunt that has been placed into the lateral ventricle to eliminate excess CSF.

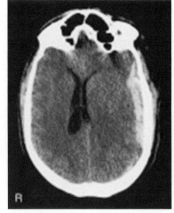 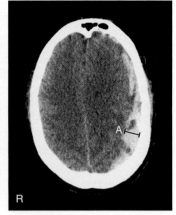
Fig. 18.60 Subdural hematoma.   **Fig. 18.61** Subdural hematoma.

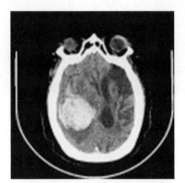
Fig. 18.62 Cerebrovascular accident.

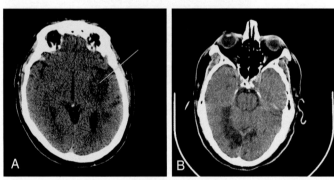
Fig. 18.63 A, Middle cerebral artery infarction. B, Occipital lobe infarction.

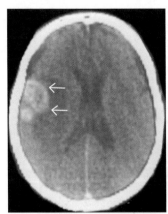 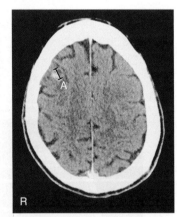
Fig. 18.58 Metastatic lesion—level of cerebrum.   **Fig. 18.59** CT image demonstrating nonmetastatic brain tumor.

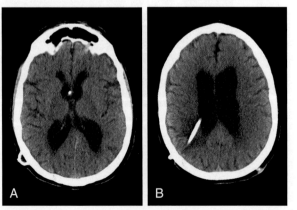
Fig. 18.64 A, Hydrocephalus. B, Hydrocephalus with ventricular shunt.

Additional CT Procedures

NECK CT

Neck CT allows visualization of complex low-contrast anatomy. Common pathologic indications include the following:

- Congenital abnormalities
- Trauma
- Infection or abscess
- Tumors of the nasopharynx, oropharynx, parotid gland, and larynx

Before the procedure begins, metallic objects must be removed, and the patient is positioned supine on the table. A scanogram, or scout image, is obtained to determine the range of the examination, usually from the skull base to the thoracic inlet, with the use of 2- to 3-mm slices. The patient should be instructed to refrain from swallowing and from causing any form of upper airway movement (e.g., talking, gum chewing, and breathing). To help distinguish the esophagus from surrounding soft tissue, the patient may be asked to swallow low-density radiopaque esophageal paste. Intravenous contrast medium is frequently indicated in a neck CT scan to determine the extent of soft tissue tumors and to visualize vascular structures. The Valsalva maneuver may be required. MPR is often used for a CT scan of the neck, and images are viewed with soft tissue and bone windows.

MUSCULOSKELETAL CT

Musculoskeletal CT demonstrates bone destruction and soft tissue. Upper and lower limbs and extremities, shoulders, and hips may be examined (the hip examination is similar to a pelvic CT scan). When extremities are imaged, it is desirable to image both extremities for comparison purposes.

Common **pathologic indications** include the following:

- Trauma
- Tumor

The protocol is determined by the clinical history, with the patient's plain radiographs used as a reference. A scanogram, or scout image, is required to establish the parameters of the scan. When the CT images are reviewed, both **soft tissue window settings** and **bone window settings** should be used. Images may be reconstructed into alternative planes or 3D images if required. Intravenous contrast media may be helpful in assessing tumors, and an intra-articular injection of contrast medium (negative or positive) may be required to study the joints.

SPINE CT

Common **pathologic indications** for spine CT include the following:

- Disk herniation
- Tumor
- Infection
- Trauma or fracture
- Spinal stenosis

A scanogram, or scout image, is required to establish the parameters of the scan. Slice thickness is generally 3 mm or less.

Fig. 18.65 demonstrates a lumbar vertebra fracture in the axial, coronal, and sagittal planes. Fig. 18.66 demonstrates a cervical vertebra fracture in the axial, coronal, and sagittal planes.

Specialized CT Procedures

Advances in CT technology and the development of specialized software have led to a variety of new CT procedures and applications.

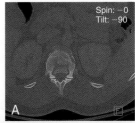
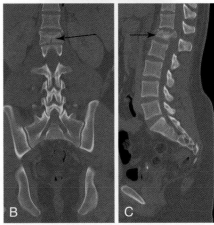

Fig. 18.65 Lumbar vertebra fracture. A, Axial plane. B, Coronal plane. C, Sagittal plane.

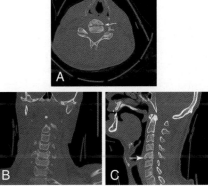

Fig. 18.66 Cervical vertebra fracture. A, Axial plane. B, Coronal plane. C, Sagittal plane.

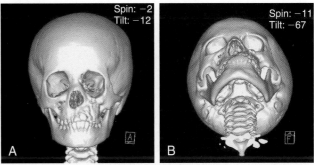

Fig. 18.67 A and B, Skull 3D reconstructions.

3D RECONSTRUCTION

A data set obtained in a volume acquisition may be reconstructed into a 3D image if the required software and hardware are available. Clinical applications include assessment of trauma to the face, spine, pelvis, shoulder, and knee and evaluation of congenital abnormalities and trauma. Fig. 18.67 demonstrates examples of 3D CT images of the skull used for planning reconstructive surgery.

CT (VIRTUAL) ENDOSCOPY

One application of 3D imaging is **virtual endoscopy.** 3D reconstruction software is used to simulate endoscopic views, typically bronchoscopy, laryngoscopy, and colonoscopy. This technique requires high contrast between the lumen and surrounding tissues so that the internal surfaces of the structure of interest can be identified for image formatting. Most endoscopic applications rely on air as the contrast medium of choice; however, depending on the procedure, there may be an indication for another contrast medium. Anatomic structures can be visualized in various formats.

CT colonography, sometimes referred to as virtual colonoscopy, is the most widely used CT endoscopic application at the present time. It is useful in the investigation of colon pathology, including polyps, tumors, diverticula, and other defects and strictures within the large intestine.

Before the procedure is begun, the patient must undergo bowel preparation to ensure that no fecal debris in the large intestine may obscure anatomy or pathology.

To provide the required contrast, air or carbon dioxide is instilled into the large intestine through a small tube inserted into the rectum. This gas serves to distend the large intestine to demonstrate the intestinal wall completely. Oral contrast solutions may be given to identify fecal artifacts.[3]

The patient is scanned in both supine and prone positions to allow visualization of all bowel structures. The scan data obtained are processed through special software to create 3D images and virtual "fly-through" of the anatomy (Fig. 18.68). Because no sedation is (typically) required, the patient is able to leave and resume normal diet and activities after the procedure.

Risks for the procedure are related to bowel preparation, rectal tube insertion, and colon insufflation. Feedback from patients typically indicates that they find the virtual endoscopy procedure less uncomfortable and painful than conventional colonoscopy. See Chapter 13 for further information on the advantages and disadvantages of CT colonography.

CT ENTEROCLYSIS

In a CT examination of the abdomen, the small bowel is visualized with the ingested contrast medium. However, if the small bowel is the focus of the examination, a procedure called *CT enteroclysis* may be performed. Clinical indications for CT enteroclysis include investigation of Crohn disease, small bowel tumors, and cause or degree of low-grade small bowel strictures.

Before the procedure is performed, solid food should be withheld from the patient for 8 to 12 hours, but the patient should be well hydrated.

Under fluoroscopic guidance, an intestinal catheter is inserted nasally and is advanced distal to the duodenojejunal flexure. Although uncomfortable for the patient, this nasal approach usually is better tolerated than the oral approach. The patient is taken to the CT unit and is positioned for the scan; up to 2000 mL of contrast medium is instilled through the tube into the small bowel. Use of an electromechanical injector and a high injection rate are necessary to ensure rapid and equal small bowel distention. Antiperistaltic drugs (e.g., glucagon) often are administered to assist with small bowel distention and to enhance patient comfort. An intravenous injection of iodinated contrast medium often is given during this procedure to gain additional clinical information. A volumetric acquisition (slice thickness ≤1.25 mm) is obtained, and multiplanar reformatting is often done (Fig. 18.69).

Contrast media used for CT enteroclysis depend on the patient's clinical history. Two commonly used substances include a dilute barium sulfate solution and a methylcellulose preparation. If there is risk of perforation or leakage, the barium sulfate solution is contraindicated.

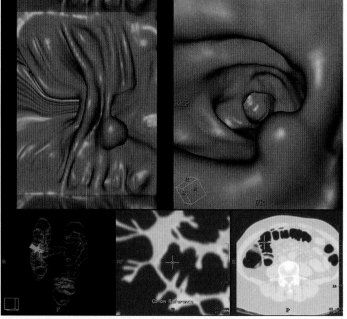

Fig. 18.68 CT colonography. Note polyp localized on intestinal wall. (Courtesy Philips Medical Systems.)

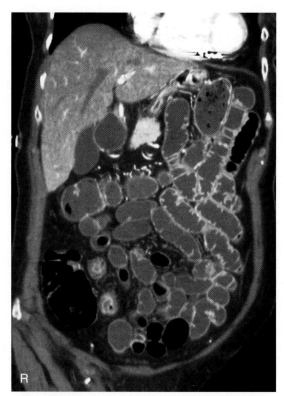

Fig. 18.69 CT enteroclysis—coronal reconstruction.

CT ANGIOGRAPHY

CT angiography is a general term for a CT examination that provides 3D images of vascular structures in the axial, coronal, and sagittal planes. Although conventional angiography is an invasive procedure in that it requires an arterial puncture, CT angiography provides the advantage of administering contrast medium intravenously. Contraindications for CT angiography are related to risks associated with contrast medium injection (e.g., renal function, contrast medium sensitivity).

Images in CT angiography often are viewed through a technique called maximum intensity projection (MIP). With information from the data set from the volumetric acquisition, an image is created from the brightest voxels. In CT angiography, the brightest voxels are the ones that contain the contrast medium; the resultant MIP image shows the vascular structures extracted from the data sets. The image is best viewed in animated format because this shows surface information best, although depth and occlusion information is lost.

Clinical indications for CT angiography, which depend on the vessel or structure that is being examined, are the same as those in conventional angiography. Studies frequently are done to investigate aneurysms and vessel dissections.

Fig. 18.70 demonstrates CT angiography images of the arterial circle (circle of Willis) within the brain with only the vessels shown. Fig. 18.71 is a 3D CT angiography scan within the skull demonstrating the cerebral arterial circle (circle of Willis).

Fig. 18.72 is a CT angiography scan of the upper extremity. Fig. 18.73 shows images before and after intra-arterial treatment of an abdominal aortic aneurysm. Fig. 18.73B also shows the presence of the endovascular repair device.

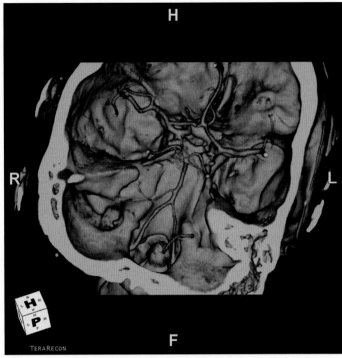

Fig. 18.71 CT angiography of arterial circle (circle of Willis) with sphenoid bone.

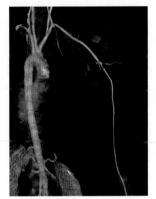

Fig. 18.72 CT angiography of upper extremity.

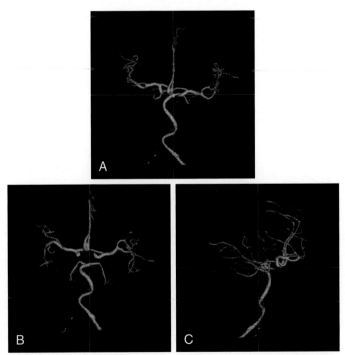

Fig. 18.70 A to C, CT angiography of the arterial circle (circle of Willis).

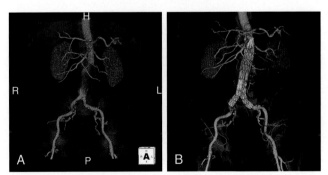

Fig. 18.73 Abdominal aortic aneurysm. A, Before procedure. B, After procedure with endovascular repair device.

CARDIAC CT AND CORONARY CT ANGIOGRAPHY

Multislice technology and specialized software have led to the development of cardiac CT procedures that previously were not possible.

Clinical indications for cardiac CT and coronary CT angiography include congenital heart disease, cardiomyopathy, cardiac aneurysms, ischemic heart disease, cardiac tumors, pericardial disease, postoperative or postinterventional procedure follow-up, and trauma.

Because cardiac motion is rapid and causes CT image artifacts, subsecond rotation times and use of electrocardiogram (ECG) gating techniques provide the required temporal and spatial resolution. Two types of ECG gating techniques are used:

- **Prospective ECG gating:** The heart is scanned only during times of least motion in the cardiac cycle (cardiac motion is least during diastole).
- **Retrospective ECG gating:** The heart is imaged continuously, but the images are generated retrospectively from data at certain ECG points. The dose is higher with retrospective ECG gating because oversampling is required (a high pitch).

Patients may be medicated during cardiac CT to stabilize or lower the heart rate to reduce motion artifacts further. An injection of iodinated contrast medium during cardiac CT allows assessment of cardiac morphology, coronary artery calcium scoring, and integrity of the coronary arteries. It is recommended that cardiac scanning be done with a single breath hold.

Although traditional coronary angiography is the gold standard for evaluation of the coronary arteries, cardiac CT provides diagnostic information noninvasively. Cardiac CT demonstrates the degree of coronary vessel stenosis, and it is able to visualize atherosclerotic plaque (fatty and fibrous) in the vessel wall. Calcified plaque, which occurs in chronic coronary artery disease, also may be visualized. Fig. 18.74 demonstrates a 3D CT of the coronary artery.

CT FLUOROSCOPY

Dynamic images may be obtained in CT fluoroscopy, as they are in conventional fluoroscopy. The patient table or couch is stationary, with the body section that is being imaged positioned in the gantry. In CT fluoroscopy, the same kVp is used as in conventional scanning; however, a lower mA is used. Partially reconstructed images can be obtained and displayed at the rate of 8 to 12 images per second. Technical advances have provided improved image quality and speed and will continue to do so.

CT fluoroscopy has an application for biopsies and CT interventional procedures, such as abscess drainage, in which the availability of real-time images facilitates accurate placement of needles. It is important for the operator to adhere to radiation safety guidelines; lead aprons, thyroid shields, and lead goggles must be worn, and special needle holders must be used to keep the operator's hands out of the beam because the skin dose to the hands can be high. Special filters are used to reduce the patient's skin dose.

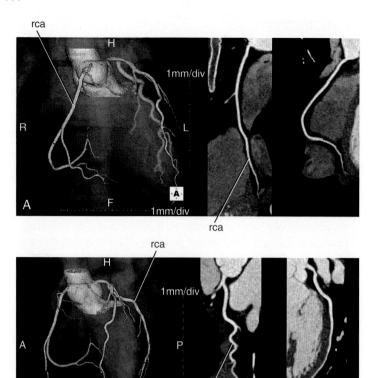

Circumflex branch of the left coronary artery

Fig. 18.74 A and B, Coronary CT angiography (stent in place).

INTERVENTIONAL CT

The two most common interventional CT procedures are percutaneous biopsy and abscess drainage (Fig. 18.75).

Percutaneous Biopsy

Core biopsy and aspiration biopsy performed under CT guidance are less invasive than a surgical biopsy procedure and have a high accuracy rate. Depending on the site for biopsy, the patient may be positioned supine, prone, or lateral. The patient is scanned to localize the tumor, the area is prepared and anesthetized, and the needle is placed. The area is scanned again, to ensure the needle is correctly placed (CT fluoroscopy is helpful here); the needle tip can be accurately visualized within a tumor (Fig. 18.76). The specimen is obtained and sent to the laboratory.

Possible complications associated with the procedure include infection, hemorrhage, pneumothorax (from a transpleural puncture for a lung lesions), and pancreatitis (if a pancreatic biopsy is performed).

Percutaneous Abscess Drainage

Abscesses are potentially life-threatening for the patient and must be treated. CT allows accurate localization of the abscess and placement of a needle into the abscess (Fig. 18.77).

For percutaneous abscess drainage, the patient is scanned to localize the abscess, the area is prepared and a Rich: Does this still apply? **Multiplanar reconstruction** maximum intensity projection nesthetized, and the needle is placed. The area is scanned again to ensure that the needle is correctly placed (CT fluoroscopy is helpful here). When the needle is in optimal position, a guidewire is placed, followed by a catheter. The catheter is sutured into place, and the abscess drains for approximately 24 to 48 hours. The success rate of CT percutaneous abscess drainage is 85%.

Terminology

Algorithm: Set of mathematical calculations and processes applied in image reconstruction.

Artifact: Undesirable feature or density in an image not representative of anatomy.

Computed tomography (CT): Radiographic examination that displays sectional anatomic images in axial, sagittal, or coronal planes.

CT number: Number that represents the attenuation value for each pixel, relative to water.

Gantry: Component of a CT system that houses the x-ray tube, detectors, and collimators.

Isotropic: Having the same value of a property in all directions; used to describe voxels that have the same value (size) in all directions (cubic).

Linear attenuation coefficient: Numeric expression of the decrease in radiation intensity that follows transmission through matter.

Matrix: Series of rows and columns (of pixels) that give form to the digital image.

Maximum intensity projection (MIP): Technique used to view vessels as demonstrated in CT angiography.

Multiplanar reconstruction (MPR): Method by which images acquired in the axial plane may be reconstructed in the coronal or sagittal plane.

Networking: Hardware and software that allow computers to be connected for the purpose of sharing resources and interacting.

Pixel: Picture element; an individual matrix box; each pixel is assigned a CT number.

Protocol: Predetermined procedure; in CT, *protocol* refers to the parameters of an examination.

Scanogram: Preliminary image of a CT examination that is used to plan the range of the scan; depending on the vendor, it may be called a *topogram* or a *scout.*

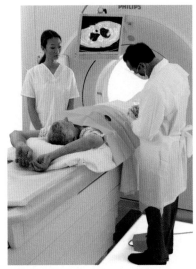

Fig. 18.75 Interventional CT procedures, as for biopsy or abscess drainage. (Courtesy Philips Medical Systems.)

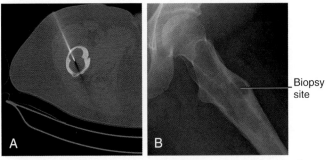

Biopsy site

Fig. 18.76 A, Bone biopsy under CT guidance. B, Radiograph of biopsy site.

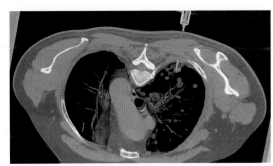

Fig. 18.77 Percutaneous abscess drainage under CT guidance. (Courtesy of Siemens Medical Solutions USA, Inc.)

Slice: Section of the object that is being scanned.

Slip rings: Devices that transmit electrical energy and allow continuous rotation of the x-ray tube for volumetric acquisition.

Volume scanning: Refers to acquisition of a volume of CT data; the patient moves through the gantry with uninterrupted rotation and output of the x-ray tube; also may be referred to as *helical* or *spiral scanning.*

Voxel: Volume element; corresponds to a three-dimensional tissue volume, having height, width, and depth; each pixel represents a voxel when an image is viewed.

Window level: Controls the brightness of an image within a certain range.

Window width: Controls the gray level of an image (the contrast).

Windowing: Adjustment of the window level and window width (brightness and image contrast) by the user.

Workstation: Computer that serves as a digital post-processing station or an image review station.

CHAPTER 19

Special Radiographic Procedures

CONTRIBUTIONS BY **Bradley D. Johnson,** MEd, RT(R)(ARRT)

CONTRIBUTORS TO PAST EDITIONS   Brenda K. Hoopingarner, MS, RT(R)(CT), Marianne Tortorici, EdD, RT(R), Patrick Apfel, MEd, RT(R)

CONTENTS

INTRODUCTION

This chapter discusses special radiographic procedures that may be performed in the general imaging department. As a result of the development and use of advanced imaging techniques in magnetic resonance imaging (MRI), computed tomography (CT), and sonography, these examinations are performed far less frequently by entry-level technologists. The use of other imaging modalities often provides a level of detail that can exceed fluoroscopic or conventional imaging. However, the special procedures discussed in this chapter are still being performed in medical centers and clinics, and technologists should have a basic understanding of them.

When these procedures are performed in the general imaging department, it is important for the technologist to follow Image Gently and Image Wisely guidelines or principles (see Chapter 1). Advances in imaging technology provide a way for physicians and technologists to reduce medical radiation exposure greatly. The use of other imaging modalities, such as MRI and sonography, coupled with these special procedures reduces radiation dose to the patient. The physician ultimately determines the modality of choice, but the technologist always plays a role in keeping the exposure as low as reasonably achievable (ALARA principle).

ARTHROGRAPHY

Introduction

Arthrography *(ar-throg'-rah-fee)* is a study of synovial joints and related soft tissue structures that uses contrast media. Joints studied include the hip, knee, ankle, shoulder, elbow, wrist, and temporomandibular joints (TMJs).

Some physicians prefer arthrography for examination of these joints; others prefer MRI or CT in place of, or in addition to, arthrography, especially for the knee (Figs. 19.1 and 19.2) and shoulder (see Figs. 19.15 and 19.16).

NOTE: Arthrography of the TMJs has become a rare procedure. Most physicians prefer MRI to evaluate the TMJs.

Arthrograms of the shoulder and knee, the most common arthrography procedures performed today, are described and illustrated in this chapter.

Knee Arthrography
PURPOSE

Knee arthrography is performed to demonstrate and assess the knee joint and associated soft tissue structures for pathologic

processes. Structures of major interest include the joint capsule; menisci; and collateral, cruciate, and other minor ligaments (Figs. 19.3 and 19.4). These structures are visualized through the introduction of a contrast agent into the joint capsule with conventional or digital fluoroscopy.

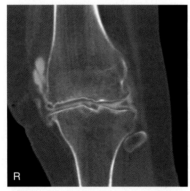

Fig. 19.1 CT knee arthrogram—coronal view.

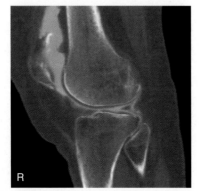

Fig. 19.2 CT knee arthrogram—sagittal view.

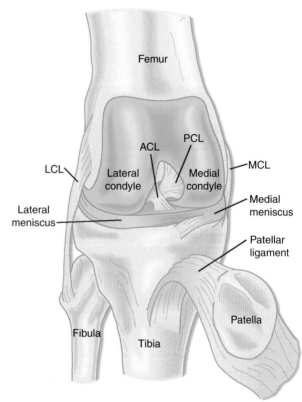

Fig. 19.3 Knee joint and cruciate ligaments. *ACL,* Anterior cruciate ligament; *LCL,* lateral collateral ligament; *MCL,* medial collateral ligament; *PCL,* posterior cruciate ligament.

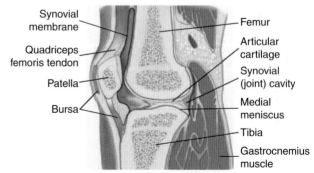

Fig. 19.4 Knee joint—cross section.

CLINICAL INDICATIONS

Knee arthrography is indicated when tears of the joint capsule, menisci, or ligaments are suspected. The knee is subject to considerable stress, especially during sports activities, and many of the pathologic processes that occur in the knee are due to trauma.

An example of a **nontraumatic pathologic process** for which arthrography is indicated is **Baker cyst,** which communicates with the joint capsule in the popliteal area.

CONTRAINDICATIONS

Arthrography of any joint is generally contraindicated when the patient is known to be allergic to an iodine-based contrast medium or to local anesthetics.

PATIENT PREPARATION

Any arthrographic procedure should be thoroughly explained to the patient before the examination to preclude patient anxiety. The patient should be advised of any complications and must sign an informed consent form.

IMAGING EQUIPMENT

The imaging equipment used for knee arthrography varies. Typically, image acquisition is obtained during fluoroscopy. A table-mounted patient-restraining device arranged as a sling around the knee area should be available (Fig. 19.5, inset). The sling is used to provide lateral or medial stress to "open up" the appropriate area of the joint to visualize the meniscus better during fluoroscopy. Specific positioning criteria are discussed later in this section.

ACCESSORY EQUIPMENT

Except for items needed for contrast injection and preparation of the injection site, accessory equipment for examination of the knee varies according to the method of imaging. The items for contrast injection and preparation of the injection site are basically the same for any sterile arthrogram tray (Fig. 19.6). The technologist should be aware of any specific accessory equipment needs a particular physician may have to ensure that the procedure is efficiently performed.

CONTRAST MEDIA

Knee arthrography can be accomplished through the use of a radiolucent (negative) agent; a radiopaque (positive) iodinated, water-soluble agent; or a combination of the two media (double-contrast). The double-contrast study is most common.

NEEDLE PLACEMENT AND INJECTION PROCESS

A retropatellar, lateral, anterior, or medial approach may be used during needle placement. The actual site of injection is the site preferred by the physician.

With the site prepared, draped, and anesthetized, the physician introduces the needle through the skin and underlying tissues into the joint space. Joint fluid is aspirated. If the fluid is normal in appearance (i.e., clear and tinged yellow), it may be discarded. If the fluid appears abnormal (cloudy), it should be sent to the laboratory for assessment.

When all the fluid has been aspirated, the contrast agent or agents are injected into the joint. With the contrast agent injected, the knee is gently flexed, which produces a thin, even coating of the soft tissue structures with the positive medium.

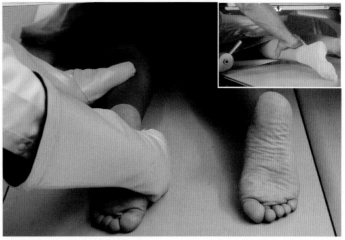

Fig. 19.5 Knee arthrogram (stressed during fluoroscopy). *Inset,* Compression band used to restrain distal femur.

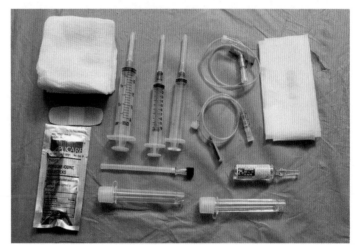

Fig. 19.6 Arthrogram tray.

POSITIONING ROUTINES
Radiographic Routines
The routine positioning and procedure for knee arthrography vary with the method of examination used, such as fluoroscopy, conventional radiography, or a combination of the two.

Conventional or Digital Fluoroscopic Imaging
During fluoroscopy, the radiologist usually takes a series of closely collimated views of **each meniscus,** rotating the leg approximately **20° between exposures** (Fig. 19.7). The result is nine spot images of each meniscus, which demonstrates the meniscus in profile throughout its diameter (Fig. 19.8). The images are stored in a picture archiving and communications system (PACS) for final viewing or archiving or are printed to hard copy.

Evaluation Criteria
- Each meniscus should be visualized clearly in various profiles on each of the nine exposed areas of the image receptor (IR). Additional exposures may be necessary to demonstrate pathologic processes.
- The meniscus that is being visualized should be in the center of the collimated field.
- Correct exposure and adequate penetration should be evident to visualize the meniscus and contrast media.
- The meniscus under examination should be appropriately marked as M (medial) or L (lateral) with small anatomic side markers.
- The R or L marker should be visualized without superimposition of the anatomy.

Conventional Radiographic Projections
In addition to digital fluoroscopy imaging, routine anteroposterior (AP) and lateral radiographs of the entire knee, obtained with use of the radiographic tube, usually are included (Figs. 19.9 and 19.10).

Evaluation Criteria
- AP and lateral images should demonstrate the entire articular capsule as outlined by the combination of negative and positive contrast media.
- Positioning criteria should be similar to criteria used for conventional AP and lateral knee views, as described in Chapter 6.
- The R or L marker should be visualized without superimposing anatomy.

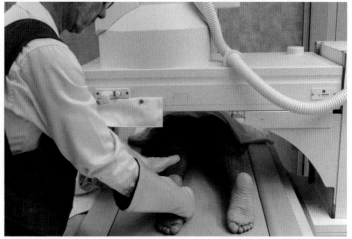

Fig. 19.7 Fluoroscopic spot imaging (left knee).

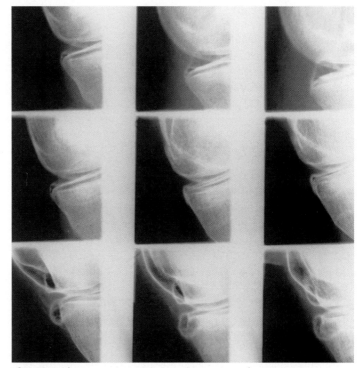

Fig. 19.8 Fluoroscopic spot image (approximately 20° rotation between exposures).

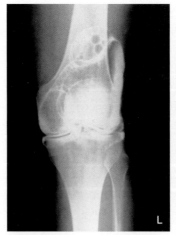
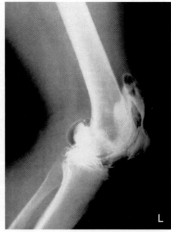

Fig. 19.9 AP knee post injection.   **Fig. 19.10** Lateral knee post injection.

19

Shoulder Arthrography

PURPOSE

Arthrography of the shoulder uses single-contrast or double-contrast injection to **demonstrate the joint capsule, rotator cuff** (formed by conjoined tendons of four major shoulder muscles), **long tendon of the biceps muscle, and articular cartilage** (Fig. 19.11).

CLINICAL INDICATIONS

Shoulder arthrography is indicated when a patient presents with chronic pain or generalized weakness and when tears in the rotator cuff are suspected.

IMAGING EQUIPMENT

A radiography/fluoroscopy room is needed for the procedure. Contrast injection is monitored under fluoroscopic control, and conventional imaging is done with the overhead x-ray tube.

ACCESSORY EQUIPMENT

Accessory equipment for examination of the shoulder includes a standard sterile arthrogram tray and a spinal needle. As with the knee arthrogram, the technologist should be aware of any specific accessory equipment needs a particular physician may have to ensure that the procedure is efficiently performed.

CONTRAST MEDIA

Arthrography of the shoulder can be accomplished with a positive contrast agent (single contrast) or a combination of positive and negative contrast agents (double contrast). A double-contrast study demonstrates specific areas better, such as the inferior portion of the rotator cuff, when images are obtained with the patient upright.

NEEDLE PLACEMENT AND INJECTION PROCESS

The injection site, directly over the joint, is prepared as in any arthrographic procedure (Fig. 19.12). After the area has been anesthetized, the physician uses fluoroscopy to guide the needle into the joint space. Because the joint is quite deep, a spinal needle (2¾ to 3½ inches) must be used. A small amount of contrast medium is injected so that the physician can determine whether the bursa has been penetrated. When the contrast medium has been fully instilled, imaging begins.

POSITIONING AND IMAGING SEQUENCE

Radiography of the shoulder joint varies, and imaging can be accomplished with the patient upright or supine. It is becoming common practice for physicians to manipulate the patient under fluoroscopy, taking spot images as needed to demonstrate the area of interest (Figs. 19.13 and 19.14), thus eliminating the need for conventional radiographic images. A suggested imaging sequence can include **scout AP projections,** with **internal and external rotation** as standard, and a **glenoid fossa, transaxillary, or intertubercular (bicipital) groove projection** (per departmental routine).

After the contrast agent has been injected, the images are repeated. If the radiographs appear normal, the patient is directed to exercise the shoulder, and the radiographs are repeated.

CT and MRI Arthrography

The conventional arthrogram routine has been largely replaced by CT and MRI; however, conventional or fluoroscopic imaging may be used in conjunction with these imaging modalities. Under fluoroscopic guidance, the physician places a needle at the preferred site and injects the contrast agent (typically an iodinated water-soluble contrast agent for CT and gadolinium for MRI). The physician manipulates the joint and takes fluoroscopic spot images as the area of interest is demonstrated by the contrast agent. After the physician has evaluated the joint adequately under fluoroscopy, the patient is transferred to CT or MRI for further imaging, as seen in Figs. 19.15 and 19.16. The exact protocol and procedure for CT or MRI arthrography depends on the area of interest being examined and the protocol of the facility or physician. Conventional radiographic imaging is not typically performed in these instances.

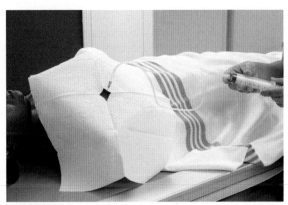

Fig. 19.12 Shoulder arthrogram needle placement.

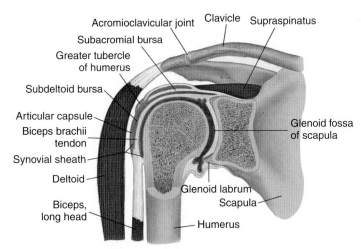

Fig. 19.11 Shoulder joint—cross section. (From Monahan F, Sands J, Neighbors M, et al: *Phipps' medical-surgical nursing,* ed 8, St. Louis, 2006, Mosby.)

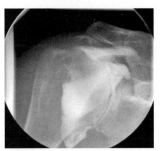

Fig. 19.13 External rotation. Shoulder arthrogram fluoroscopic spot image.

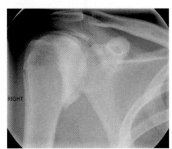

Fig. 19.14 Shoulder arthrogram fluoroscopic spot image.

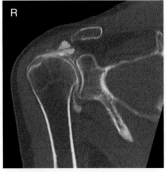

Fig. 19.15 CT arthrogram of the shoulder—coronal view.

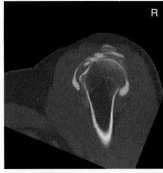

Fig. 19.16 CT arthrogram of the shoulder—coronal oblique view.

BILIARY DUCT PROCEDURES

Postoperative (T-Tube or Delayed) Cholangiography

PURPOSE

Postoperative cholangiography, also termed *T-tube* or *delayed cholangiography*, usually is performed in the radiology department after a cholecystectomy. The surgeon may be concerned about residual stones in the biliary ducts (Fig. 19.17) that went undetected during surgery. If these concerns exist, the surgeon places a special T-tube–shaped catheter into the common bile duct during the cholecystectomy. The catheter extends to the outside of the body and is clamped off.

Clinical Indications

Residual Calculi Undetected stones may remain in the biliary ducts after the operative cholangiogram. The T-tube cholangiogram enables the radiologist to determine the location of stones and remove them, if possible, through a specialized catheter.

Strictures A region of the biliary ducts may have been narrowed as demonstrated during the operative cholangiogram; this may warrant further investigation.

CONTRAINDICATIONS

Primary contraindications to T-tube cholangiography include hypersensitivity to iodinated contrast media, acute infection of the biliary system, and elevated creatinine or blood urea nitrogen (BUN) levels.

PATIENT PREPARATION

Patient preparation for the T-tube cholangiogram varies based on department protocol. The procedure should be clearly explained to the patient, and a careful clinical history should be taken. The patient should be placed in a hospital gown and should be kept NPO (nothing by mouth) for at least 8 hours before the procedure.

IMAGING EQUIPMENT

Fluoroscopy is required during injection of a contrast medium. Radiographic images may be taken after the fluoroscopic procedure.

ACCESSORY EQUIPMENT

Syringes of various sizes, syringe adapters, emesis basins, gloves, and sterile drapes are needed.

CONTRAST MEDIA

T-tube cholangiography can be accomplished through the use of an iodinated, water-soluble contrast medium (possibly a diluted concentration to prevent obscuring of small calculi).

INJECTION PROCESS

Because the T-tube catheter has been clamped off, drainage of excess bile is performed at the beginning of the procedure. An emesis basin should be provided for this task. **Follow standard precautions when handling bile. Wear gloves throughout the procedure.**

After duct drainage and under fluoroscopic control, the iodinated contrast agent is injected fractionally, and fluoroscopic spot images are obtained (Fig. 19.18). It is important not to introduce any air bubbles while injecting contrast medium because these bubbles may be mistaken for radiolucent stones.

If residual stones are detected, the radiologist may elect to remove them. A basket catheter may be passed over a guidewire, and the stones may be removed.

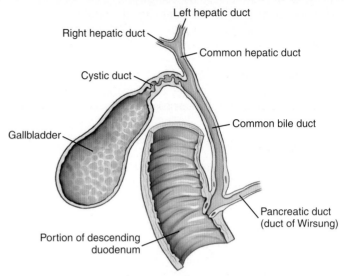

Fig. 19.17 Anatomy of biliary ducts.

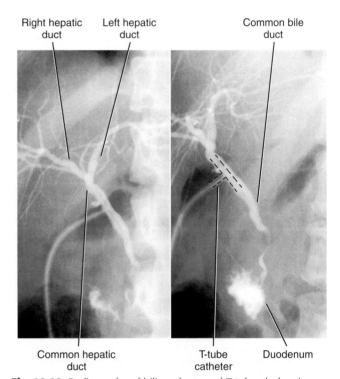

Fig. 19.18 Radiographs of biliary ducts and T-tube cholangiogram.

Endoscopic Retrograde Cholangiographic Pancreatography

ENDOSCOPY

Endoscopy (en-dos'-ko-pee) refers to inspection of any cavity of the body using an endoscope, an instrument that allows illumination of the internal lining of an organ. Various fiberoptic endoscopes are available for use in examining the interior lining of the stomach, duodenum, and colon. Older types of endoscopes allow for individual viewing only through an eyepiece, but newer videoendoscopes project the image onto video monitors for viewing by multiple persons. Also, a special type of fiberoptic endoscope, called a *duodenoscope,* is commonly used for performing endoscopic retrograde cholangiopancreatography (ERCP). When a duodenoscope is inserted into the duodenum through the mouth, esophagus, and stomach, it provides a wide-angle side view that is useful for locating and inserting a catheter or cannula into the small opening of the hepatopancreatic sphincter, leading from the duodenum into the common bile duct and the main pancreatic ducts (Fig. 19.19).

PURPOSE

ERCP is performed frequently for examination of the biliary and main pancreatic ducts. ERCP can be a diagnostic or a therapeutic procedure. Therapeutically, ERCP can be performed to relieve certain pathologic conditions through the removal of choleliths or small lesions or for other purposes, such as to repair a stenosis (narrowing or blockage of a duct or canal) of the hepatopancreatic sphincter or associated ducts.[1]

For diagnostic purposes, the ERCP procedure generally includes endoscopic insertion of the catheter or injection cannula into the common bile duct or main pancreatic duct under fluoroscopic control, followed by retrograde injection (backward or reverse direction) of contrast media into the biliary ducts. The procedure usually is performed by a gastroenterologist, who is assisted by a team that comprises the technologist, one or more nurses, and perhaps a radiologist.

CLINICAL INDICATIONS

Residual Calculi

Stones may be located in one or more branches of the biliary ducts (Fig. 19.20); during the ERCP procedure, the gastroenterologist may be able to remove them with a specialized catheter.

Strictures

A region of the biliary ducts may have been narrowed; this warrants further investigation.

CONTRAINDICATIONS

Primary contraindications to ERCP include hypersensitivity to iodinated contrast medium, acute infection of the biliary system, possible pseudocyst of the pancreas, and elevated creatinine or BUN levels.

PATIENT PREPARATION

Patient preparation for ERCP varies based on departmental protocol. The procedure should be clearly explained to the patient, and a careful clinical history should be taken. The clinical history should be reviewed to determine whether the patient has pancreatitis or a pseudocyst of the pancreas. Injecting contrast medium into a pseudocyst may lead to rupture of the pseudocyst and produce infection of the pancreas and surrounding tissues.

The patient should be placed in a hospital gown and should be kept NPO for at least 8 hours before the procedure. In addition, because the patient's throat is anesthetized during the procedure, the patient should remain NPO for at least 1 hour (or more) after the procedure to prevent aspiration of food or liquid into the lungs.

IMAGING EQUIPMENT

Fluoroscopy is required during placement of a catheter into the biliary ducts and injection of a contrast medium. Radiographic images may be taken after the fluoroscopic procedure.

ACCESSORY EQUIPMENT

Syringes of various sizes, syringe adapters, emesis basins, gloves, and sterile drapes are required.

CONTRAST MEDIA

ERCP can be accomplished through the use of an iodinated, water-soluble contrast medium (possibly a diluted concentration to prevent obscuring of small calculi).

INJECTION PROCESS

The physician introduces the endoscope through the mouth, esophagus, stomach, and duodenum until the hepatopancreatic ampulla (ampulla of Vater) is located. A catheter is inserted into the common bile duct; the physician may use fluoroscopy to verify placement before injection of the contrast agent. When the physician is satisfied with placement of the catheter, the contrast agent is injected into the common bile duct. Fluoroscopy and spot images are used to evaluate the common bile duct and surrounding structures. Rotation of the equipment or patient may be necessary to evaluate the biliary tract fully.

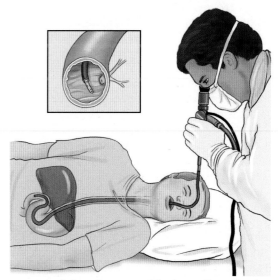

Fig. 19.19 Cannulation of common bile duct using a duodenoscope.

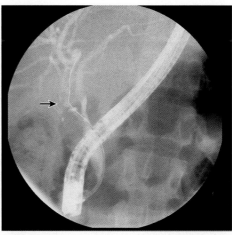

Fig. 19.20 ERCP showing large biliary calculi within the right hepatic duct.

HYSTEROSALPINGOGRAPHY

Introduction

The **hysterosalpingogram** *(his"-tar-o-sal"-pin'-go-gram)* primarily demonstrates the **uterus** and **uterine** (fallopian) **tubes** of the female reproductive system. The female pelvic organs and their relationship to the abdominal peritoneal cavity are described in Chapter 14. Technologists should have an understanding of the detailed anatomy demonstrated during **hysterosalpingography (HSG)**, as described in the following section.

Anatomy

Anatomic considerations for HSG include the principal organs of the **female reproductive system**—the **vagina, uterus, uterine tubes,** and **ovaries.** Emphasis is placed on the uterus and uterine tubes. Additional anatomic considerations include the subdivisions, layers, and supporting structures of the female organs. The female reproductive organs are located within the **true pelvis.** Differentiation between the true pelvis and the false pelvis is defined by a plane through the brim or inlet plane of the pelvis, as described in Chapter 7.

UTERUS

The **uterus** is the central organ of the female pelvis. It is a pear-shaped, hollow, muscular organ that is bordered posteriorly by the rectosigmoid colon and anteriorly by the urinary bladder (Fig. 19.21). The size and shape of the uterus vary, depending on the patient's age and reproductive history. The uterus is positioned most commonly in the midline of the pelvis in an anteflexed position supported chiefly by the various ligaments. The position may vary with bladder or rectosigmoid distention, age, and posture.

The uterus is subdivided as follows: (1) **fundus,** (2) **corpus** (body), (3) **isthmus,** and (4) **cervix** (neck) (Fig. 19.22). The **fundus** is the rounded, superior portion of the uterus. The **corpus** (body) is the larger central component of the uterine tissue. The narrow, constricted segment, often described as the lower uterine segment that joins the cervix at the **internal os,** is the **isthmus.** The **cervix** is the distal cylindrical portion that projects into the **vagina,** ending as the **external os.**

The uterus is composed of inner, middle, and outer layers. The inner lining is the **endometrium,** which lines the **uterine cavity** and undergoes cyclic changes in correspondence to the woman's menstrual cycle. The middle layer, the **myometrium,** consists of smooth muscle and constitutes most of the uterine tissue. The outer surface of the uterus, the **serosa,** is lined with peritoneum and forms a capsule around the uterus.

UTERINE TUBES

The **uterine** (fallopian) **tubes** communicate with the uterine cavity from a superior lateral aspect between the body and the fundus. This region of the uterus is referred to as the **cornu.** The uterine tubes are approximately 4 to 4¾ inches (10 to 12 cm) in length and 1 to 4 mm in diameter. They are subdivided into four segments: (1) The proximal portion of the tube, the **interstitial** segment, communicates with the uterine cavity. (2) The **isthmus** is the constricted portion of the tube, where it widens into the central segment termed the **ampulla,** which arches over the bilateral **ovaries.** (3) The most distal end, the **infundibulum,** contains fingerlike extensions termed **fimbriae,** one of which is attached to each ovary. (4) The ovum passes through this **ovarian fimbria** into the uterine tube, where—if it is fertilized—it then passes into the uterus for implantation and development.

The distal infundibulum portion of the uterine tubes containing the fimbriae **opens into the peritoneal cavity.**

Purpose

HSG is the **radiographic demonstration of the female reproductive tract with a contrast agent.** The radiographic procedure best demonstrates the **uterine cavity** and the **patency** (degree of openness) **of the uterine tubes.** The uterine cavity is outlined by injection of contrast medium through the cervix. The shape and contour of the uterine cavity are assessed to detect any uterine pathologic process. As the contrast agent fills the uterine cavity, the patency of the uterine tubes can be demonstrated as the contrast material flows through the tubes and spills into the peritoneal cavity.

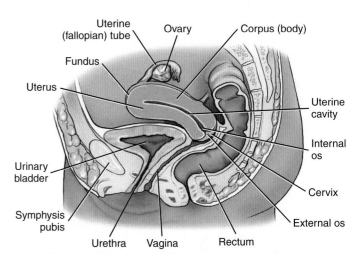

Fig. 19.21 Female reproductive organs—sagittal section.

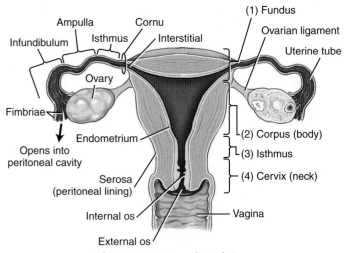

Fig. 19.22 Uterus—frontal view.

Clinical Indications

INFERTILITY ASSESSMENT

One of the most common indications for HSG is **assessment of female infertility.** The procedure is performed to diagnose any **functional** or **structural defects.** A blockage of one or both uterine tubes may inhibit fertilization. In some cases, HSG can be a **therapeutic tool.** Injection of contrast medium may dilate or straighten a narrowed, tortuous, or occluded uterine tube.

DEMONSTRATION OF INTRAUTERINE PATHOLOGY

Although ultrasound is generally the modality of choice, an HSG may also be performed when patient symptoms indicate the presence of **intrauterine pathologic processes.** Abnormal uterine bleeding, pelvic pain, and pelvic fullness are typical symptoms exhibited by patients. **Lesions** that are demonstrated include endometrial polyps, uterine fibroids, and intrauterine adhesions. HSG also is used to diagnose pelvic masses, fistulas, habitual spontaneous abortions, and congenital defects.

A third indication is evaluation of the uterine tube after tubal ligation or reconstructive surgery.

Contraindications

Pregnancy is a contraindication to HSG. To avoid the possibility the patient may be pregnant, the examination typically is performed 7 to 10 days after the onset of menstruation.

Other contraindications include acute pelvic inflammatory disease and active uterine bleeding.

Patient Preparation

Departmental protocol should determine the requirements for patient preparation. These procedures may include proper bowel preparations to ensure adequate visualization of the reproductive tract unobstructed by bowel gas or feces. Preparation may include a mild laxative, suppositories, or a cleansing enema, or some combination of these, before the procedure. In addition, the patient may be instructed to take a mild pain reliever before the examination to alleviate some of the discomfort associated with cramping.

To prevent displacement of the uterus and uterine tubes, the patient should be instructed to empty her bladder immediately before the examination.

The procedure and possible complications should be explained to the patient, and informed consent must be obtained. In some instances, the physician also may perform a manual pelvic examination before the radiographic procedure is begun.

Imaging Equipment

The major equipment required for HSG is conventional or digital fluoroscopy (Fig. 19.23). Ideally, the table should have the capability to tilt the patient to a Trendelenburg position if needed. If available, gynecologic stirrups should be attached to the table to assist the patient in the lithotomy position.

Accessory and Optional Equipment

Routinely, a sterile, disposable HSG tray is used (Fig. 19.24). The tray contains the equipment and ancillary materials required for the procedure.

An additional instrument that may be requested by the physician is a **tenaculum** (an instrument with a hooked clamp for gathering and holding tissues and structures in place).

Contrast Media

Radiopaque (positive) iodinated contrast media is used for an HSG. **Water-soluble iodinated** contrast medium is preferred. It is absorbed easily by the patient, does not leave a residue within the reproductive tract, and provides adequate visualization. However, this medium causes pain when injected within the uterine cavity, and the pain may persist for several hours after the procedure.

The amount of contrast medium to be introduced into the reproductive tract varies depending on physician preference. Fractional injections may be performed during the study.

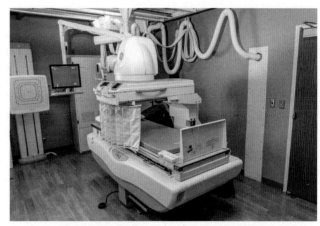

Fig. 19.23 Radiography/fluoroscopy room.

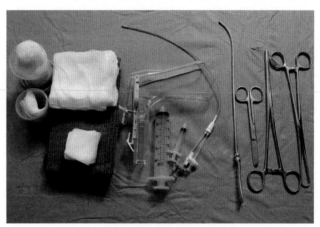

Fig. 19.24 HSG tray.

19

Cannula or Catheter Placement and Injection Process

At the beginning of the procedure, the patient lies supine on the table in the lithotomy position. If gynecologic stirrups are unavailable, the patient bends her knees and places her feet at the end of the table. The patient is draped with sterile towels; with sterile technique, a vaginal speculum is inserted into the vagina. The vaginal walls and cervix are cleansed with an antiseptic solution. A cannula or balloon catheter is inserted into the cervical canal. Dilation with a balloon catheter helps to occlude the cervix, preventing contrast medium from flowing out of the uterine cavity during the injection phase. A tenaculum may be necessary to aid in insertion and fixation of the cannula or catheter.

When cervical placement of the cannula or catheter has been obtained, the physician may remove the speculum and place the patient in a slight Trendelenburg position. This position facilitates the flow of contrast medium into the uterine cavity. A syringe filled with contrast medium is attached to the cannula or balloon catheter. Using fluoroscopy, the physician slowly injects contrast medium into the uterine cavity. If the uterine tubes are patent (open), contrast medium flows from the distal ends of the tubes into the peritoneal cavity.

Positioning

RADIOGRAPHIC ROUTINE

Routine positioning for HSG varies with the method of examination. Fluoroscopy, conventional or digital radiography, or a combination of both may be used.

DIGITAL FLUOROSCOPY OR CONVENTIONAL IMAGING

Imaging of the reproductive tract is most commonly acquired with the use of spot cassette fluoroscopy or, more recently, digital fluoroscopy. Typically, a collimated scout image is obtained with fluoroscopy. During injection of the contrast medium, a series of collimated images may be obtained while the uterine cavity and uterine tubes are filling (Figs. 19.25 and 19.26). After injection of the contrast medium, an additional image may be taken to document spillage of the contrast medium into the peritoneum (Fig. 19.27). The patient most commonly remains in the supine position during imaging, but additional images may be obtained with the patient in a left posterior oblique (LPO) or right posterior oblique (RPO) position to visualize pertinent anatomy adequately.

RADIOGRAPHY

A radiographic AP scout image may be obtained on a 10 × 12-inch (24 × 30-cm) IR. The central ray (CR) and IR are centered to a point 2 inches (5 cm) superior to the symphysis pubis. If fluoroscopy is unavailable, fractional injection of contrast medium is implemented, with a radiograph performed after each fraction to document filling of the uterine cavity and uterine tubes and contrast medium within the peritoneum. Additional images as determined by the radiologist may include LPO or RPO positions.

EVALUATION CRITERIA

- The pelvic ring as seen on an AP projection should be centered within the collimation field.
- The cannula or balloon catheter should be seen within the cervix.
- An opacified uterine cavity and uterine tubes are seen centered to the IR (see Fig. 19.27).
- Contrast medium is seen within the peritoneum if one or both uterine tubes are patent.
- Appropriate brightness (density—analog) and contrast demonstrate anatomy and contrast medium.
- R or L marker should be visualized without superimposition of anatomy.

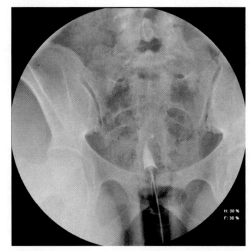

Fig. 19.25 Hysterosalpingogram. Initiation of contrast injection.

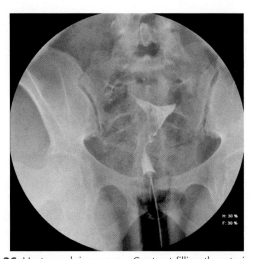

Fig. 19.26 Hysterosalpingogram. Contrast filling the uterine cavity.

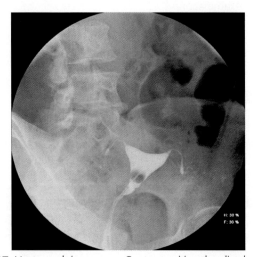

Fig. 19.27 Hysterosalpingogram. Contrast exiting the distal uterine tubes into the peritoneal cavity.

MYELOGRAPHY

NOTE: The myelogram procedure has largely been replaced by MRI or CT procedures, but technologists should still be proficient in performing it when requested.

Purpose

A myelogram *(mi'-e-lo-gram)* is a radiographic study of the spinal cord and its nerve root branches that uses a contrast medium.

The spinal cord and nerve roots are outlined by injection of a contrast agent into the subarachnoid space of the spinal canal. The shape and contour of the contrast agent are assessed to detect possible pathologic processes. Because most conditions demonstrated by this procedure occur in the lumbar and cervical areas, myelography of these areas of the spine is most common.

Clinical Indications

Myelography is performed when patient symptoms indicate the presence of a **lesion that may be present within the spinal canal or may protrude into the canal.** If the pathologic process impinges on the spinal cord, patient symptoms may include pain and numbness, often in the upper or lower limbs. The lesions most commonly demonstrated by myelography include **herniated nucleus pulposus, which is the most common clinical indication for myelography; cancerous or benign tumors; cysts;** and (in the case of trauma) **possible bone fragments.** If a lesion is present, myelography identifies the extent, size, and level of the pathologic process.

Another important feature of myelography is the identification of **multiple lesions.**

Contraindications

The following are contraindications to myelography:
- **Blood in the cerebrospinal fluid (CSF):** The presence of blood in the CSF indicates probable irritation within the spinal canal, which can be aggravated by the contrast medium.
- **Arachnoiditis** (inflammation of the arachnoid membrane): Myelography is contraindicated in the case of arachnoiditis because the contrast medium may increase the severity of the inflammation.
- **Increased intracranial pressure:** In cases of elevated intracranial pressure, tapping of the subarachnoid space with needle insertion may cause severe complications to the patient as the pressure equalizes between the areas of brain and spinal cord.
- **Recent lumbar puncture** (within 2 weeks of the current procedure): Performing myelography on a patient who has had a recent lumbar puncture may result in extravasation of the contrast medium outside the subarachnoid space through the hole left by the previous puncture.

Patient Preparation

Patients scheduled for myelography may be apprehensive about the procedure. To reduce anxiety and relax the patient, an injectable sedative or muscle relaxant usually is administered 1 hour before the examination. The type and amount of premedication used are determined by the radiologist who performs the procedure.

Before the examination, the physician should explain the procedure and possible complications to the patient, and an informed consent must be signed by the patient.

Imaging Equipment

Equipment for myelography includes a radiography/fluoroscopy room with a 90°/45° (or 90°/90°) tilting table, shoulder braces, and a foot rest with myelography ankle restraints (Fig. 19.28). Shoulder braces and a foot rest are used to secure the patient during the procedure, which may require tilting of the table in the Trendelenburg position (head lower than feet). Use of shoulder rests and ankle restraints together rather than separately is advised. The foot rest is used to support the patient when the table is moved to the upright position.

Accessory and Optional Equipment

Accessory equipment for myelography includes grid cassettes with holders for horizontal beam radiography, a myelography tray, sterile gloves, an antiseptic solution, appropriate laboratory requisitions, and a large position sponge or pillow. The number and sizes of grid cassettes used depend on the level of the spinal canal that is being examined.

The myelography tray is generally a commercial prepackaged, sterilized, disposable unit (Fig. 19.29).

Contrast Media

The ideal contrast medium for myelography is one that is miscible (mixes well) with CSF, easily absorbed, nontoxic, and inert (nonreactive) and has good radiopacity. None of the currently available commercial contrast media meet all these criteria. In the past, air or gas (radiolucent) and oil-based iodinated (radiopaque) media were used for myelography. However, **nonionic, water-soluble, iodine-based media** are primarily used at the present time because of their relatively low osmolality (see Chapter 14).

Water-soluble contrast media provide excellent radiographic visualization of the nerve roots, are easily absorbed into the vascular system, and are excreted by the kidneys. Absorption begins approximately 30 minutes after injection, with good radiopacity evident up to about 1 hour after injection. After 4 to 5 hours, the contrast medium has a hazy radiographic effect, and it is radiographically undetectable after 24 hours.

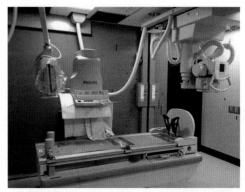

Fig. 19.28 Myelography-equipped room. (Courtesy Sutter Health.)

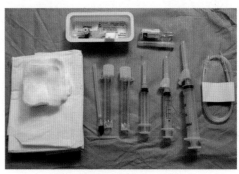

Fig. 19.29 Myelogram tray.

19

DOSAGES

The dosage for myelographic contrast media is recommended by the manufacturer and varies with the concentration of the medium used and the area of the spine under examination. Generally, a range of approximately **9 to 15 mL** is used.

Care should be taken to prevent contrast medium from entering the brain. For example, during examination of the cervical region with the patient prone or in Trendelenburg position, the chin is hyperextended to prevent the medium from flowing into the cranial region of the subarachnoid space.

Needle Placement and Injection Process

Introduction of contrast media for myelography is accomplished via puncture of the subarachnoid space. Generally, two locations are used as puncture sites: the **lumbar** (L3–L4) and **cervical** (C1–C2) areas (Fig. 19.30). Of these two locations, the lumbar area is safer and easier on the patient and is used most often for the procedure. Cervical puncture is indicated if the lumbar area is contraindicated, or if a pathologic condition indicates complete blockage of the vertebral canal above the lumbar area, obstructing the flow of contrast medium to the upper spinal region.

Two body positions generally are used for a **lumbar puncture.** The patient may be **prone,** with a firm pillow or large positioning block placed under the abdomen to flex the spine (Fig. 19.31), or may lie in a **left lateral position** with the spine flexed. Flexion of the spine widens the interspinous space, which facilitates introduction of the spinal needle.

For a **cisternal puncture,** the patient may be seated in an **erect position** (Fig. 19.32) or **prone,** with the head flexed to open the interspinous space.

The radiologist may use fluoroscopy to facilitate needle placement after the puncture site has been selected. With the area anesthetized, the spinal needle is introduced through the skin and underlying tissues into the subarachnoid space. The location of the needle in the subarachnoid space is verified by an unobstructed backflow of CSF, which generally is allowed to flow through the needle. Allowing free flow of the CSF rather than drawing it out with a syringe reduces the risk for spinal cord trauma at the distal end of the needle within the canal. A sample of CSF is first collected and sent to the laboratory for analysis.

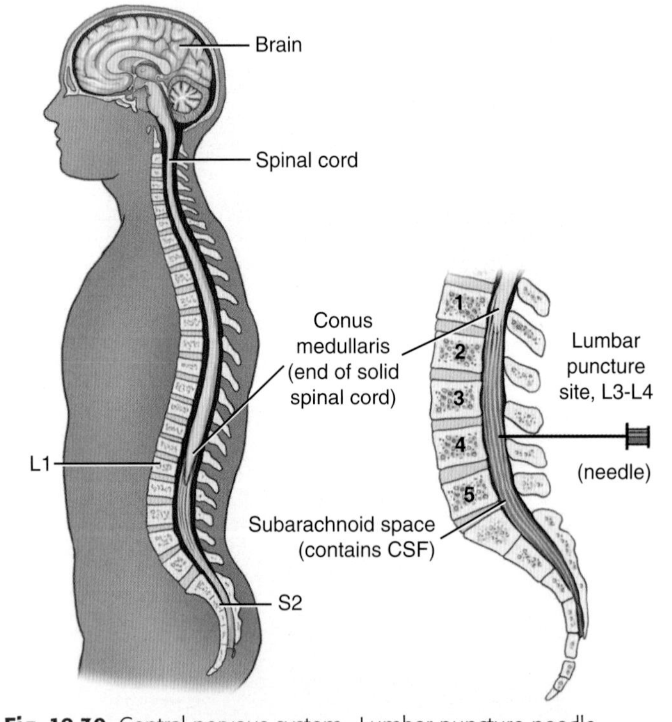

The amount of CSF collected is dictated by the amount needed for the laboratory tests ordered. After the CSF has been collected, the spinal needle is left in place for the contrast agent injection.

The contrast agent is injected through the spinal needle into the subarachnoid space. When the injection has been completed, the needle is removed, and images are acquired.

Positioning

FLUOROSCOPY OR SPOT IMAGING OR DIGITAL FLUOROSCOPY OR IMAGING

During fluoroscopy, the table (and patient) is tilted from erect through Trendelenburg positions. This movement facilitates the flow of contrast medium to the area under examination.

Under fluoroscopic control, once the contrast agent has reached the desired area, the radiologist may image the patient in various positions from prone to supine and in anterior or posterior oblique positions (Figs. 19.33 and 19.34). Images may be obtained with the use of conventional or digital technology, depending on available equipment. After fluoroscopy, the technologist takes conventional radiographs that are appropriate for the area under examination, as requested by the radiologist.

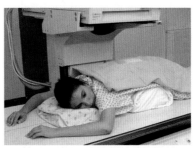
Fig. 19.31 Prone position for lumbar puncture.

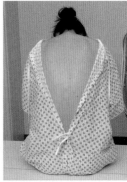
Fig. 19.32 Erect position for cisternal (C1–C2) puncture.

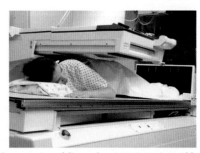
Fig. 19.33 Left posterior oblique for spot imaging of lumbar myelogram. (X-ray tube is under table, making this a posterior oblique projection.)

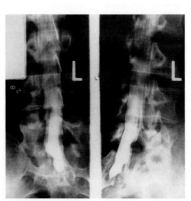
Fig. 19.34 Spot images of lumbar myelogram (RPO and LPO).

Fig. 19.30 Central nervous system. Lumbar puncture needle placement.

RADIOGRAPHIC MYELOGRAPHY POSITIONING (AFTER FLUOROSCOPY)

Although departmental radiographic routines for myelography may vary significantly, the following positions and projections represent suggested **basic** routines for different levels of the spinal column. Additional positions and projections that may be considered routine or special are included.

Before routine radiography begins, the radiologist adjusts the table tilt as needed to concentrate the contrast medium to the level of the spinal cord that is being radiographed.

CERVICAL REGION
Horizontal Beam Lateral (Figs. 19.35 and 19.36)
- The patient is positioned prone, with the arms extended along the sides of the body and the shoulders depressed.
- The chin is extended and is resting on a small positioning sponge or folded linen.
- The CR is directed to the level of C4–C5.
- The field should be collimated to reduce scatter radiation.
- Respiration is suspended during the exposure.

Cervicothoracic (Swimmer) Lateral Horizontal Beam (Figs. 19.37 and 19.38)
- The patient is positioned prone, with the chin extended.
- For a right lateral, the right arm is extended along the right side of the body, with that shoulder depressed. The left arm is flexed (i.e., stretched superior to the head).
- The CR is directed to the level of C7.
- The field is collimated to reduce scatter radiation.
- Respiration is suspended during the exposure.

NOTE: Additional positions may include anterior oblique projections.

THORACIC REGION
Right Lateral Decubitus Position—AP or PA Projection with Horizontal Beam (Fig. 19.39)
- The patient is positioned in a true right lateral, with the right arm flexed, superior to the head. The left arm is extended and rests along the left side of the body.
- To maintain the alignment of the spine parallel to the tabletop, the patient may rest the head on the arm. If needed, a small positioning sponge or folded linen may be placed between the head and the arm to maintain alignment.

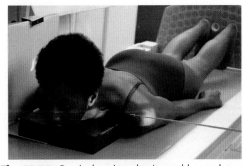
Fig. 19.35 Cervical region—horizontal beam lateral.

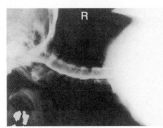
Fig. 19.36 Transcervical (horizontal beam) lateral.

- The CR is directed to the level of T7.
- The field is collimated to reduce scatter radiation.
- Respiration is suspended during the exposure.

Left Lateral Decubitus Position—AP or PA Projection with Horizontal Beam (Fig. 19.40)
- The patient is positioned in a true left lateral position, with the left arm raised and flexed above the head. The right arm is extended down and rests on the right side of the body as shown.
- The spine remains parallel to the tabletop.
- The CR is directed to T7.
- The field is collimated to reduce scatter radiation.
- Respiration is suspended during the exposure.

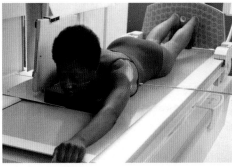
Fig. 19.37 Cervical region (C7 to T1 region)—swimmer (horizontal beam) lateral.

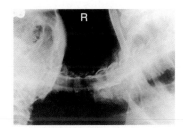
Fig. 19.38 Cervicothoracic (swimmer) (horizontal beam) lateral.

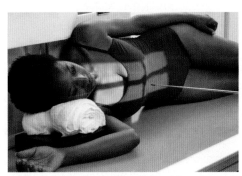
Fig. 19.39 Thoracic region—right lateral decubitus (AP horizontal beam projection).

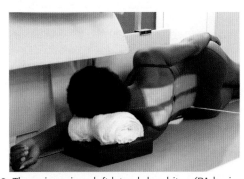
Fig. 19.40 Thoracic region—left lateral decubitus (PA horizontal beam projection).

Right or Left Lateral—Vertical Beam (Fig. 19.41)
- The patient is positioned in a true lateral, with the knees flexed. Both arms are semiflexed.
- The alignment of the spine should be maintained parallel to the tabletop. The patient may rest the head on the hands, or a small positioning sponge or folded linen may be placed between the hands and the head to maintain alignment of the spine.
- The CR is directed to the level of T7.
- The field is collimated to reduce scatter radiation.
- Respiration is suspended during the exposure.
  Additional positions may include a supine (AP projection) and a lateral with a horizontal beam.

NOTE: A supine AP and a horizontal beam lateral generally are not recommended; in the supine position, pooling of contrast medium occurs in the midthoracic region as a result of the usual thoracic curvature. This pooling is more prominent in some patients. To demonstrate best the entire spinal canal of the thoracic region, **AP and PA projections** should be taken in both **right and left lateral decubitus positions,** in addition to the **vertical beam lateral position** as described and illustrated.

LUMBAR REGION
Semierect Lateral—Horizontal Beam (Figs. 19.42 and 19.43)
- Position the patient prone, with the arms flexed superior to the head.
- The table and the patient are semierect. The radiologist, under fluoroscopic control, adjusts the angulation of the table to concentrate the contrast medium in the lumbar area.
- The CR is directed to L3.
- The field is collimated to reduce scatter radiation.
- Respiration is suspended during the exposure.
  Additional positions may include oblique projections with a vertical or horizontal beam and a supine AP projection.

Radiographs
EVALUATION CRITERIA (FOR ALL LEVELS OF SPINAL COLUMN)
- The appropriate level of the spinal column, with contrast medium present, should be demonstrated.
- Correct exposure factors and adequate penetration help to demonstrate anatomy and contrast medium.
- Patient identification markers and anatomic markers (right or left) should be clearly visualized without superimposing anatomy.
- Collimation should be evident.

CT Myelography
The conventional myelogram routine has been largely replaced by the imaging modalities of CT and MRI; however, conventional or fluoroscopic imaging may be used in conjunction with CT. Under fluoroscopic guidance, the physician places a needle into the subarachnoid space and injects the contrast agent (typically, iodinated water-soluble contrast is used for CT). The physician manipulates the table and obtains fluoroscopic spot images as the area of interest is demonstrated by the contrast agent. The physician may also request one or two post–contrast injection radiographs (Fig. 19.44). Then, after the spinal cord has been evaluated adequately under fluoroscopy, the patient is transferred to CT for further imaging (Fig. 19.45).

The exact procedure for CT myelography depends on the area of interest being examined and the protocol of the facility or physician. Conventional radiographic imaging is not typically performed in these instances.

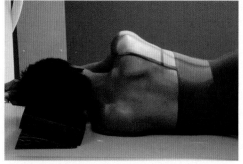
Fig. 19.41 Thoracic region—left vertical beam lateral.

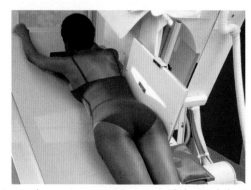
Fig. 19.42 Lumbar region—semierect transabdominal (horizontal beam right lateral).

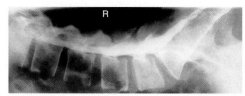
Fig. 19.43 Lumbar—transabdominal (horizontal beam) lateral.

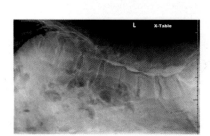
Fig. 19.44 Myelogram. Horizontal beam lateral lumbar spine.

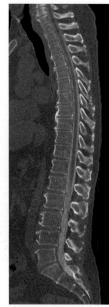
Fig. 19.45 CT myelogram of thoracic/lumbar region—sagittal view.

HIP-TO-ANKLE LONG BONE MEASUREMENT

The hip-to-ankle study is being more commonly performed in radiology departments as a way for orthopedic physicians to assess the lower extremities bilaterally (Fig. 19.46). This image allows the physician to determine limb length discrepancies and lower extremity alignment. Measurements can also be made to determine hardware requirements when surgery has been indicated. Some surgical appliance manufacturers have developed software with the capability to overlay the prosthesis or other appliance on the image receptor itself to facilitate surgical planning.

TECHNICAL FACTORS
- SID—120 inches (300 cm)
- IR size—14 × 52 inches (35 × 132 cm), portrait
- kVp range—80–95
- Magnification marker placed on medial aspect of knee
- Wedge filter may be used; anode-heel effect should be applied

POSITIONING AND CR
- Remove patient's shoes and position patient standing; separate the legs approximately 8 inches (20 cm) apart
- Ensure knees are in true AP position
- Make sure CR is perpendicular to knee joint
- Suspended respiration

EVALUATION CRITERIA
- Image demonstrates bilateral lower extremity to include iliac crest superiorly and level of calcaneus inferiorly, including the pelvis, femur, tibia, fibula, and talar domes (see Fig. 19.46).
- Femorotibial joint space is open.

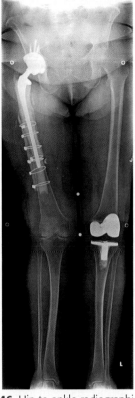

Fig. 19.46 Hip-to-ankle radiographic image.

RADIOGRAPHIC SKELETAL SURVEY (BONE SURVEY)

A radiographic skeletal survey is a series of radiographic images that encompass the entire skeleton or those anatomic regions appropriate for the clinical indications.[2] The specific imaging protocol will depend on the clinical situation. The goal of the skeletal survey is to accurately identify the focal and diffuse abnormalities of the skeleton, including acute or healing fractures, bone lesions, evidence of metabolic bone disease or characteristics of skeletal dysplasia, and to differentiate them from developmental changes and other anatomic variants[2] (Box 19.1).

There are several imaging and interventional techniques for the initial detection and follow-up of metastatic bone disease: radiography, radionuclide bone scanning, CT, MRI, fine-needle aspiration, and core-needle biopsy[3] (Fig 19.47). In some instances, a radiographic skeletal survey may be performed as the initial imaging procedure. Based upon the findings, or lack thereof, a physician may follow up by ordering additional imaging in another modality. Conversely, if a radionuclide bone scan detects an abnormality, it should be x-rayed to make sure it does not represent a benign process.[3]

Further information related to the radiographer's role in radiographic skeletal surveys performed due to known or suspected abuse involving pediatric patients can be found in Chapter 16.

BOX 19.1 COMPLETE SKELETAL SURVEY[2]

APPENDICULAR SKELETON

Humeri (AP)
Forearms (AP)
Hands (PA)
Femurs (AP)
Lower legs (AP)
Feet (AP)

AXIAL SKELETON

Thorax (AP, lateral, right and left obliques), to include sternum, ribs, thoracic and upper lumbar spine
Abdomen, to include the pelvis (AP)
Lumbosacral spine (lateral)
Skull (frontal and lateral), to include cervical spine (if not completely visualized on lateral skull)

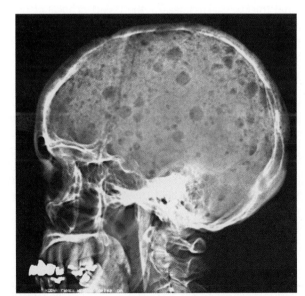

Fig. 19.47 Multiple myeloma. (From Tepper JE: *Gunderson and Tepper's clinical radiation oncology*, ed 5, Philadelphia, 2021, Elsevier.)

CONVENTIONAL TOMOGRAPHY

NOTE: The following section provides a brief overview of the basic principles and setup required to perform linear tomography because most conventional procedures have been replaced with advanced imaging modalities such as digital tomosynthesis, CT and MRI. However, conventional linear tomograms are still obtained for certain procedures such as intravenous urography (see Chapter 14). Previous editions of this textbook and physics and imaging-related textbooks provide an in-depth description of tomography.

Purpose

Tomography is a special type of imaging that is used to **obtain a diagnostic image of a specific layer of tissue or an object that is superimposed by other tissues or objects.** This image is accomplished with the use of accessory equipment that allows the x-ray tube and IR to move about a fulcrum point during the exposure. The resulting radiograph, called a **tomogram,** demonstrates a clear image of an object lying in a specific plane, with blurring of the structures located above and below the specific plane. The specific plane of interest in Fig. 19.48 is set at 8 cm from the radiographic tabletop. This is a frequent tomographic level taken during nephrotomography.

Terminology

Because the tomogram represents a section of the body, this type of imaging sometimes is termed **body section radiography.** In 1962, the International Commission on Radiological Units and Measures (ICRU) established the term *tomography* to describe all forms of body section radiography.

Because terminology may differ, following is a list of terms and their definitions as used in this textbook:

Blur: Area of distortion of objects outside the object plane.

Exposure angle (or exposure amplitude): Total distance the x-ray tube travels during the actual exposure. There is an inverse relationship between the exposure angle and section thickness.

Fulcrum: Pivot point between the movement of the x-ray tube and IR. The level or height of the fulcrum is measured in centimeters or inches from the tabletop.

Object plane (focal plane): Plane in which the target anatomy is clear and in relative focus. It is controlled by the level of the fulcrum.

Sectional thickness: Thickness of the object or focal plane (variable, controlled by exposure angle).

Tomographic angle (or tomographic amplitude): Total distance the x-ray tube travels.

Basic Principles

FULCRUM

The fulcrum is the **pivot point through which the x-ray tube and IR move** (Fig. 19.49). This pivot point is important because all structures located at this level are included in the object plane. The structures within the object plane remain in the same position on the IR during the exposure, remaining relatively clear and in focus. Conversely, all structures located outside the object plane, either above or below, are projected from one point on the IR to another, resulting in movement or blurring (Fig. 19.50).

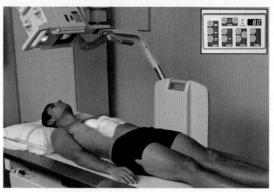

Fig. 19.48 Linear tomographic unit.

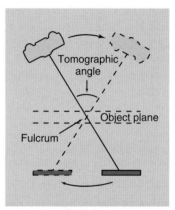

Fig. 19.49 Fulcrum.

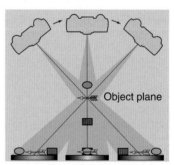

Fig. 19.50 Object plane.

Determining Fulcrum Level and Centering

With a general knowledge of the relative locations of organs or structures of interest, the technologist can approximate the area of specific interest and center to this area. The initial scout tomogram is obtained with the fulcrum set at the estimated level or plane of the specific area of interest. For example, on a nephrotomogram, centering is to the area of the kidneys, and the fulcrum level for the initial scout image would be set to the level of the kidneys (Figs. 19.51 and 19.52). This centering and fulcrum level setting is described for a nephrotomogram procedure in Chapter 14.

DETERMINING SECTIONAL THICKNESS (OBJECT PLANE THICKNESS)

It is advantageous to adjust the thickness of the object plane to correspond to the structure or structures being imaged. Large structures, such as the lung, are best imaged with the use of a thick object plane created by using a reduced exposure angle (10°), often referred to as a *thick cut* (see Fig. 19.51A). Small structures are best imaged with the use of a thin object plane created by using a greater exposure angle (40°), often referred to as a *thin cut* (see Fig. 19.51B).

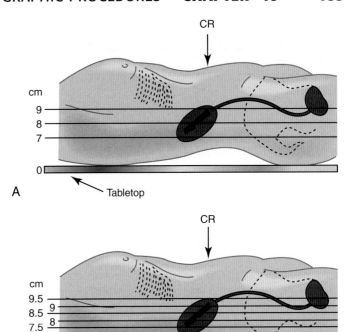

Fig. 19.51 A and B, Effect of exposure amplitude on section thickness.

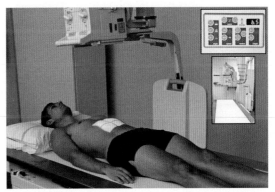

Fig. 19.52 Patient positioned for nephrotomography.

DIGITAL TOMOSYNTHESIS

Tomography is not a new concept in radiography; however, new applications of the concept have been made possible due to advancements in imaging technology. With the advent of digital radiography and flat-panel detectors, development of digital tomosynthesis (DTS) became technically feasible and practical.[4] DTS has been applied to angiographic, dental, orthopedic, breast, and chest imaging, with the latter two currently generating the most research interest.[5] These high-resolution images can often be produced with a much lower radiation dose than in CT and at a lower cost.[6]

With DTS, multiple very low-dose x-ray projection images are acquired from different angles during a single linear sweep of the x-ray tube across a stationary detector[5] (Fig 19.53). Depending on the manufacturer, this tube angle can have a range of 10° to 60°. Unlike conventional tomography, which delivers continuous exposure, the DTS detector receives pulsed x-ray exposures at different tube angles.[4] This allows the system to acquire as many as 60 images in a single linear sweep. An arbitrary number of images can be reconstructed at multiple depths from a single set of projection images that encompass the entire thickness of the patient in a single sweep.[4] This was not possible with conventional tomography.

The fundamental principle behind DTS takes advantage of parallax from the projected images obtained at varying angles.[7] Parallax is the effect whereby the position or direction of an object appears to differ when viewed from different positions. An easy way to understand parallax is to place your thumb out in front of your eyes, and notice how its position changes relative to the eye from which you are viewing it.

The data acquired during the DTS imaging process is automatically reconstructed to form tomographic sections through the imaged object, with each section parallel to the detector imaging plane.[5] Planes are synthesized by aligning all the projection images so that structures in the plane of interest all align precisely (Fig. 19.54).[7]

Essentially, DTS addressed the limitations of a standard x-ray, which are superimposition or overlapping structures. DTS removes overlapping/overlying structures, allowing the physician to see injuries or abnormalities that are otherwise obscured in standard x-rays, thereby enhancing the conspicuity of anatomy in the different slices (Fig. 19.55). The structures in each plane are more clearly visible without the interference of tissue in front or in back of the plane of interest.[7]

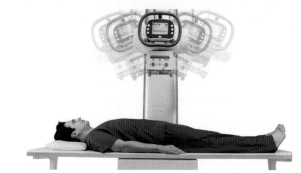

Fig 19.53 GE VolumeRAD digital tomosynthesis. (Courtesy GE Healthcare.)

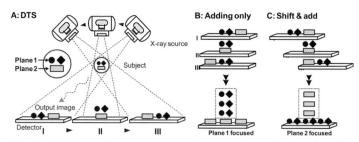

Fig. 19.54 Schematic representation of the principle of shift and add tomosynthesis method. (From Woong K et al. Digital tomosynthesis (DTS) for quantitative assessment of trabecular microstructure in human vertebral bone. *Medical Engineering & Physics* 37(1): 109-120.)

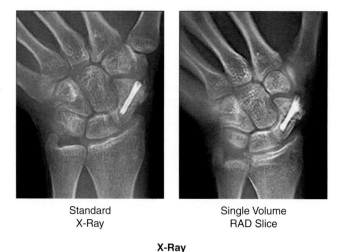

Standard X-Ray

Single Volume RAD Slice

X-Ray

Fig. 19.55 DTS of carpal region. (Courtesy GE Healthcare.)

CHAPTER 20

Diagnostic and Therapeutic Modalities

CONTRIBUTOR TO NUCLEAR MEDICINE **Jeanne Dial,** MEd, CNMT, RSO

CONTRIBUTOR TO POSITRON EMISSION TOMOGRAPHY (PET) **Derek Lee,** BS, CNMT, PET

CONTRIBUTOR TO RADIATION ONCOLOGY THERAPY **Shaun T. Caldwell,** MS, RT(R)(T)

CONTRIBUTOR TO SONOGRAPHY **Joie Burns,** MS, RT(R)(S), RDMS, RVT

CONTRIBUTOR TO MAMMOGRAPHY **Michelle A Wilt,** M.H.A., RT(R)(M)(ARRT)

CONTRIBUTOR TO BONE DENSITOMETRY **Sharon R. Wartenbee,** RTR, BD, CBDT, FASRT

CONTRIBUTOR TO MAGNETIC RESONANCE IMAGING (MRI) **Kathryn A. Wissink,** RT(R)(MR)

CONTRIBUTORS TO PAST EDITIONS Molly E. Lampignano, CNMT, PET, Kathleen Murphy, MBA, RDMS, RT(R), Kristi Blackhurst, BS, RT(R)(MR), Daniel J. Bandy, MS, CNMT, Nancy L. Dickerson, RT(R)(M), Eugene D. Frank, MA, RT(R), FASRT, FAERS, Brenda K. Hoopingarner, MS, RT(R)(CT), Manjusha Namjoshi, BS, RDMS, RT(R), Sandra J. Nauman, RT(R)(M), Charles R. Wilson, PhD, FAAPM, FACR, Cheryl DuBose, Ed.D, RT(R) (MR), (CT) (QM)

CONTENTS

PART ONE ▪ NUCLEAR MEDICINE (NM)

Contributor: **Jeanne Dial,** MEd, CNMT, RSO

Definition and Introduction

Nuclear Medicine (NM) is the modality of diagnostic medical imaging that uses radiopharmaceuticals to create an image that demonstrates the physiology or function or an organ at the molecular level. The examination is accomplished by introducing a radiopharmaceutical into the body, most commonly by intravenous injection; however, a radiopharmaceutical can also be introduced into the body by inhalation (i.e., ventilation lung scan), ingestion (i.e., gastric emptying study), or instillation (i.e., nuclear medicine cystogram). Nuclear medicine techniques differ from other imaging modalities because they evaluate changes in organ function or physiology rather that changes in anatomy.

Radiopharmaceuticals are defined as radioactive drugs used in the diagnosis and treatment of disease. They are created by tagging, or attaching a radionuclide to a pharmaceutical. The radiopharmaceutical is formulated to go to a specific organ. Before they are introduced into a patient, the pharmaceutical and radionuclide are chelated, or attached together. Once administered to the patient, the pharmaceutical, by virtue of its chemical makeup, will go to a specific organ or body part intended to be examined. The radionuclide emits a gamma ray as it decays. The gamma rays create an image that is digitally displayed. Areas of abnormal accumulation (either increased or decreased concentrations of the radiopharmaceutical) are called "hot spots" or "cold spots," which indicate a physiologic change within the organ. These images provide an anatomic view of the organ structure and provide diagnostic insights regarding the function of the organ.

The nuclide most commonly used in NM is technetium 99m (Tc 99m). Tc 99m has an energy of **140 keV** and a physical half-life of 6 hours. **Half-life** is the time it takes for radiation to decay by one-half of its original activity. The short half-life of Tc 99m provides adequate time for imaging yet allows the target organ to decay background radiation levels within 2 days. Typical doses for most diagnostic nuclear medicine procedures range from 200 microcuries (μCi) to 30 millicuries (mCi).

Nuclear Imaging Equipment

Gamma cameras have evolved tremendously as a result of the development of hybrid imaging systems. The simplest type of nuclear imaging is **planar or static imaging,** in which the image looks like a single "snapshot" of the target anatomy. **Dynamic imaging** provides a series of images that demonstrate blood flow in the body and within specific organs. A gamma camera can acquire three-dimensional (3D) images in a technique called **single photon emission computed tomography (SPECT).**

SPECT images also can be acquired on a hybrid system, which combines two types of imaging equipment into one camera system (Fig. 20.1). A common example of a hybrid system combines the SPECT gamma camera with computed tomography (CT). This form of imaging is capable of demonstrating the physiology of the organ being examined through nuclear medicine and the target anatomy during the CT scan. This information is reconstructed by a computer into various sectional perspectives with the anatomy overlaid with the physiologic activity.

Another example of hybrid imaging includes positron emission tomography (PET) nuclear medicine imaging. This technqiue examines metabolic function combined with magnetic resonance imaging (MRI) or CT images that examine anatomy in one hybrid imaging system. These forms of hybrid imaging are termed PET/MRI and PET/CT.

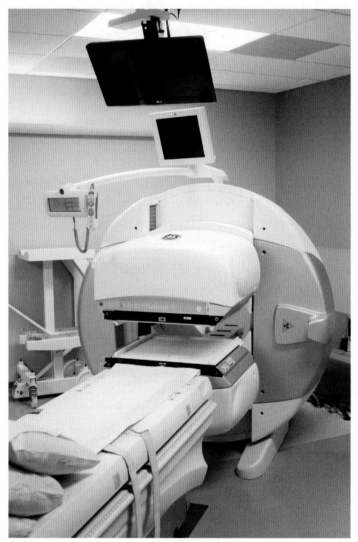

Fig. 20.1 Fusion imaging system (CT and SPECT). (Courtesy Scottsdale Medical Imaging, Scottsdale, Arizona.)

Clinical Applications

BONE SCAN

Bone scans image the skeletal system to detect abnormalities such as metastasis, a stress fracture, or a loose prosthesis (orthopedic device implanted in the body). A bone scan can detect a fracture 2 years after an injury. Technologists may have to perform closely collimated radiographs of skeletal hot spots as determined by bone scans.

GENITOURINARY STUDIES

Both anatomic and functional evaluations of the kidneys are obtained with nuclear genitourinary studies. This modality is excellent for assessment of a kidney transplant.

GASTROINTESTINAL STUDIES

The gastrointestinal studies performed most commonly in the nuclear medicine department are gastric emptying and hepatobiliary scans. A gastric emptying study can evaluate the motility of solids and liquids through the gastrointestinal tract. Hepatobiliary scans evaluate gallbladder function and can identify a bile leak after removal of a patient's gallbladder. Other gastrointestinal scans include gastroesophageal reflux and spleen scans, a cystogram, and a gastrointestinal bleeding scan, which identifies the location of bleeding in the stomach, small intestine, or large intestine.

HEART (CARDIAC) STUDIES

Cardiac perfusion imaging, also called *stress/rest cardiac imaging*, accounts for approximately half of all imaging performed in nuclear medicine. Freestanding clinics and mobile units can be found in most communities that perform only cardiac examinations. The patient is given a cardiac radiopharmaceutical intravenously. The radiopharmaceutical is extracted from the blood pool into the heart muscle within 2 minutes; SPECT images are then acquired. The patient returns in approximately 3 hours and receives a second injection of the radiopharmaceutical during the stress phase of the test. During the second visit, stressing of the heart is accomplished by having the patient run on a treadmill or by administering one of a variety of pharmacologic stressing agents. These stressing agents are given through an intravenous line, followed by the imaging agent. Delivery of the radiopharmaceutical injection is intended to coincide with maximum cardiac stress, as determined by an electrocardiogram (ECG) obtained under the direction of a physician, nurse practitioner, or physician assistant trained in these examinations. SPECT images are acquired after each phase of the test and are compared with each other during interpretation to determine the presence of ischemia or infarction (Fig. 20.2).

LUNG SCAN (VENTILATION AND PERFUSION STUDIES)

Lung scans examine both ventilation (the movement of air into the lungs) and perfusion (blood flow in the pulmonary vessels). They are most commonly performed to identify a pulmonary embolism. The ventilation scan is usually performed first, followed by the perfusion scan. Both sets of images use radiopharmaceuticals tagged to Tc 99m; this requires the number of counts from the perfusion images to be tripled to overshadow the counts from the ventilation images.

THYROID UPTAKE STUDY

Thyroid uptake measurements are obtained to evaluate the function of the thyroid gland (Fig. 20.3). The radiopharmaceutical sodium iodide ^{123}I (iodine-123) is taken orally, and images are obtained 6 hours after ingestion. The amount of radioactive iodine uptake by the thyroid is evaluated at 6- hour and 24-hour intervals. **Hyperthyroidism** (overactive thyroid) results in a higher uptake reading, which may indicate Graves disease (diffuse toxic goiter) (Fig. 20.4),

Plummer disease (toxic multinodular goiter), or thyroid adenomas. Thyroid therapy with ^{131}I (iodine-131), with its high energy, can be given to reduce the function of the thyroid. A lower thyroid reading indicates hypothyroidism (thyroid with reduced activity).

Nuclear Medicine Team

Nuclear medicine procedures are performed by a team of professionals consisting of the following individuals:

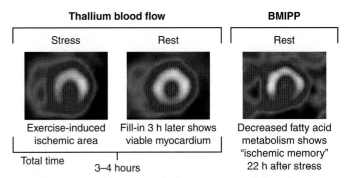

Fig. 20.2 Cardiac perfusion study demonstrates a defect during stress phase of study. (Dilsizian V, Bateman TM, Bergmann SR, et al. Metabolic imaging with beta-methyl-p-[123I]-iodophenyl-pentadecanoic acid identifies ischemic memory after demand ischemia. Circulation. 2005;112:2169–2174, March, 2008.)

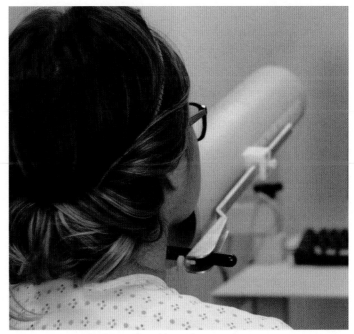

Fig. 20.3 Thyroid uptake measurement.

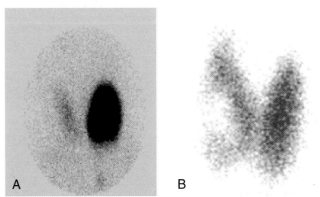

Fig. 20.4 I-131 scans showing (A) a hot nodule and (B) a cold nodule. (From Shah JP, et. al.: *Jatin Shah's head and neck surgery and oncology*, ed 5, Philadelphia, 2020, Elsevier.)

Nuclear medicine technologist: The technologist has a strong background in radiation physics, anatomy and physiology, radiation safety, computers, and imaging procedures. Patient safety and accurate documentation are key responsibilities of the nuclear medicine technologist. After images have been acquired, the nuclear medicine technologist must perform statistical analysis of the data and must digitally process the images.

Nuclear medicine physician: A nuclear medicine physician is a radiologist who has received additional training in the performance and interpretation of nuclear medicine procedures. The nuclear medicine physician is licensed to acquire and use radioactive materials.

Radiation safety officer (RSO): The nuclear medicine physician often serves as the RSO. Duties include reviewing the imaging protocols used in the nuclear medicine department and reviewing all dosimetry records for the facility. RSOs also serve on the radiation safety committee.

Health physicist: This individual has received advanced training in nuclear physics, computers, and radiation safety. Responsibilities of the health physicist include calibrating and maintaining imaging equipment and running audits on the record keeping of the nuclear medicine department.

Glossary of Nuclear Medicine Terms[1]

Alpha particle: Helium nucleus that consists of two protons and two neutrons.

Attenuation: Process by which radiation is reduced in intensity when it passes through some material.

Becquerel (Bq): Unit of radioactivity in SI (International System of Units).

Beta emission: Release of high-energy beta particles through disintegration of certain radioactive nuclides.

Beta particle: Ionizing radiation with characteristics of an electron emitted from the nucleus of a radioactive atom.[2]

Biologic half-life: Time required for an organism to eliminate half of an administered dose of any substance through normal processes.

Collimator: Device used to confine the elements of a beam within an assigned solid angle.

Contamination (radioactive): Deposition of radioactive material in any place where its presence is not desired.

Count: External indication of a device designed to enumerate ionizing events.

Curie (Ci): Traditional or standard unit of radioactivity. It has been replaced by the SI unit, the becquerel.

Cyclotron: Device for accelerating charged particles in a spiral fashion to high energies via an alternating electrical field.

Daughter: Synonym for a product of decay.

Decay: Spontaneous transmutation of a radionuclide that results in a decrease in the number of radioactive events in a sample.

Disintegration (nuclear): Spontaneous nuclear transmutation characterized by emission of energy or mass or both from the nucleus.

Dose: Amount of radiopharmaceutical given to a patient.

Electron capture: Method of radioactive decay that involves the capture of an orbital electron by its nucleus.

Equilibrium: Stage in a reaction in which the concentration of the reactive species is no longer changing.

Fusion imaging: Use of software or hybrid cameras to superimpose nuclear medicine scans on images from modalities such as CT or MRI. Also referred to as *image fusion* or *coregistration.*

Gamma rays: High-energy, short-wavelength electromagnetic radiation emanating from the nucleus of a nuclide.

Half-life: Time required for disintegration of half of the original activity of a radioactive nuclide.

Hybrid imaging[3]: Combination of two (or more) imaging modalities to form a new technique.

In vitro: Outside of the patient; occurring or being in an artificial environment, such as a test tube or a culture plate.

In vivo: Inside of the patient; describes a process or reaction that occurs within the patient.

Infarction: Development and formation of a localized area of necrosis within a tissue.

Ion: Atom or chemical radical that bears an electrical charge that is either positive or negative.

Isotope: Nuclides of the same element that have different atomic mass (neutrons) but the same atomic number (protons).

Microcurie (μCi): Unit of radioactivity equal to one-millionth of a curie.

Millicurie (mCi): Unit of radioactivity equal to one-thousandth of a curie.

Parent: Radionuclide that yields another nuclide during disintegration.

Pharmaceutical: Any chemical substance intended for use in the medical diagnosis, cure, treatment, or prevention of disease.

Radioactivity: Spontaneous disintegration of an unstable atomic nucleus, resulting in the emission of ionizing radiation.

Radionuclide: Type of atom whose nucleus disintegrates spontaneously.

Radiopharmaceutical: Group of radioactive drugs used in the diagnosis and treatment of disease.

Scintillation: Emission of light flashes from certain materials as a result of interaction with ionizing radiation.

Single photon emission computed tomography (SPECT): Imaging system that uses one to three gamma detectors to produce tomographic images of an organ or structure.

Technetium 99m (Tc 99m): Common radionuclide of technetium used for 90% of nuclear medicine procedures.

PART TWO ▪ POSITRON EMISSION TOMOGRAPHY(PET)

Contributor: **Derek Lee,** BS, CNMT, PET

Definition and Description

PET is a branch of nuclear medicine in the category of functional imaging. PET is distinguished from nuclear medicine by the physics of positron decay. PET scanners use the phenomenon of positron decay to detect and place biochemical functions in 3D space (Fig. 20.5). Because of this, PET is often used to aid in the diagnosis of disease processes; it can detect functional changes long before they manifest themselves physically or symptomatically.

PET also has the unique ability to quantify the activity of a lesion by means of the standard uptake value (SUV). The SUV is a ratio derived from the radioactivity concentration of a region of interest (ROI) to the whole-body concentration of injected radioactivity. The SUV is typically reported as a unitless measurement. This measurement becomes particularly important in oncology applications for assessing the efficacy of treatment and in research applications for evaluating new therapies.

COMPARISON WITH NUCLEAR MEDICINE

PET is similar to nuclear medicine in that it uses an external source of radiation, the radiopharmaceutical inside the patient, to produce an image. Both modalities collect photon energy and use algorithms to position the events in space. PET is inherently a 3D modality; nuclear medicine imaging is inherently two dimensional (2D) but can be imaged in three dimensions with SPECT. The physics of positron decay enable PET to obtain a higher level of resolution than SPECT.

USE OF POSITRON EMITTERS

Unlike conventional nuclear medicine radioisotopes, PET uses positron emitters. These isotopes undergo radioactive decay by positron emission. As these isotopes decay, a positron is emitted from the nucleus of the atom. When the positron comes to rest, approximately 2 mm from the origin, it creates two 511-keV annihilation photons exactly 180° apart. It should be noted that there is a degree of uncertainty associated with the point of origin. Positron-emitting nuclides travel different distances prior to annihilation, depending on the initial energy of the positron. For example, ^{18}F (fluorine-18) can travel up to 2.4 mm before annihilation, whereas ^{82}Rb (rubidium-82) travels up to 14.1 mm. This lends a sphere of uncertainty to the origin of the event and subsequently degrades the resolution of PET relative to modalities such as CT and MRI. These annihilation photons are detected by a ring of detectors surrounding the patient. The detectors consist of a photomultiplier tube (PMT) attached to a crystal made of bismuth germanate (BGO) or lutetium oxyorthosilicate (LSO).This crystal material is another key differentiator from SPECT. These materials are key to stopping the high-energy photons. Newer systems are now moving to digital detection technologies, such as silicon photomultipliers (SiPMs) and avalanche photodiodes (APDs). These photon pairs are filtered, collected, and sorted by their time signature, allowing the point of origin to be determined (Fig. 20.6).

POSITRON-EMITTING ELEMENTS

There are several known positron-emitting elements. The most commonly used elements in PET include oxygen, carbon, nitrogen, rubidium, gallium, and fluorine. On the horizon are iodine and copper. Oxygen, carbon, and nitrogen are among the building blocks of life. This makes the positron-emitting isotopes more readily substitutable in many compounds without compromising the biologic behavior of these compounds. Some of the common imaging radiopharmaceuticals are ^{15}O water, ^{11}C methionine, ^{13}N ammonia, ^{82}Rb chloride, ^{68}Ga DOTATATE, and ^{18}F-fluorodeoxyglucose (^{18}F-FDG).

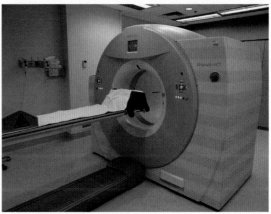

Fig. 20.5 PET/CT imaging system. (Courtesy Derek S. Lee, BS, CNMT.)

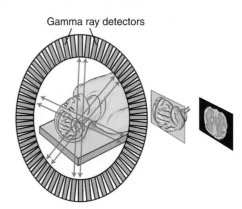

Fig. 20.6 Positron emission and detector array.

Cyclotron

A PET scanner is of no use without a positron-emitting source. The source, a PET radiopharmaceutical, must be compounded with a positron-emitting isotope. Most positron emitters (^{11}C, ^{13}N, ^{15}O, and ^{18}F) are created by a cyclotron (Fig. 20.7). Some are derived from a generator (^{82}Rb and ^{68}Ga).

Most PET tracers have very short half-lives (120 seconds to 110 minutes), necessitating proximity to a production facility. Currently, ^{18}F-FDG is the most common tracer, with a 110-minute half-life that allows more location flexibility in relation to the production radiopharmacy. Shorter-lived tracers require an on-site cyclotron to be viable in daily use. These are typically found at teaching and research centers.

ANATOMIC AND FUNCTIONAL IMAGE COREGISTRATION

Virtually all new PET scanners sold are hybrid PET/CT scanners that combine the functional information of the PET scan with the attenuation correction and anatomic localization of the CT scan. The CT portion of the system is housed in the front portion of the gantry, and the PET ring of detectors and its associated electronics are housed in the rear portion of the gantry. These systems allow imaging of the biochemical functions to be fused/coregistered with the higher-resolution anatomic images of the CT scan acquired in a single, sequential imaging session. The CT scan is acquired first and defines the area of the body to be covered by the PET scan. The CT is completed in less than a minute, followed by the longer PET scan. These two data sets can be overlaid, allowing for more precise localization of a pathologic condition discovered on the PET scan.

On these hybrid PET/CT systems, the CT also allows for attenuation correction of the PET images (Fig. 20.8). Attenuation correction is needed in PET imaging to correct for the different tissue densities of the human body. In nonhybrid systems, attenuation correction requires the use of separate sealed radioactive sources housed within the scanner. This sealed source method also requires a significantly longer acquisition time to create an attenuation correction map for the PET scan.

The latest addition to the hybrid scanner family is the PET/MRI (Fig. 20.9). In a similar fashion to the PET/CT, the PET/MRI combines a PET scanner with an MRI scanner. In these systems, the MRI is used for attenuation correction and anatomic localization. The MRI offers superior soft tissue resolution, in addition to other functional imaging aspects to be combined with the PET data. In these hybrid systems, the PET detector ring is located in the isocenter of the gantry, and the PET and the MRI sequences are acquired simultaneously. This does help mitigate the overall longer imaging times necessitated by the MRI. These systems are just gaining traction worldwide, with only a handful of units currently installed in the United States.

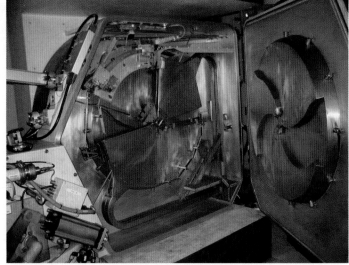

Fig. 20.7 PET medical cyclotron with radiation shields retracted to show internal components. (Courtesy Biotech Cyclotron LLC.)

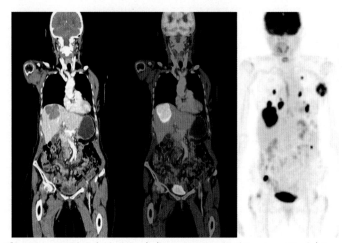

Fig. 20.8 PET/CT fusion study liver metastasis. (Courtesy Daniel J. Bandy, MS, CNMT.)

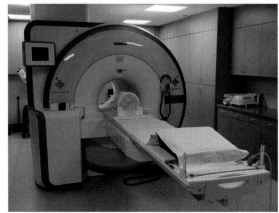

Fig. 20.9 PET/MRI imaging system. (Courtesy Derek S. Lee, BS, CNMT.)

Clinical Applications

ONCOLOGY (STUDY OF TUMORS)

PET is a valuable tool for assessing the metabolism of tumors. Generally, malignant cells have an accelerated glucose metabolism because of their unregulated growth; they readily use sugar as an energy source. The glucose analog fluorodeoxyglucose or 2-deoxy-2-[^{18}F]fluoro-D-glucose either term is acceptable (FDG) also is taken up readily by active tumors. PET scans for this application generally are done to determine the initial sites of cancers and to see whether cancer has spread to other areas of the body (Fig. 20.10). An increase in glycolysis (increased use of sugar by the cells) in a specific organ or region of the body is an indicator of malignancy. PET may be used for the initial diagnosis, for staging of a malignancy, and as a follow-up technique for determining response to treatment. Oncology staging studies are further aided by the use of the SUV calculation available in PET.

Newer, non-glucose-based PET radiopharmaceuticals are allowing targeted visualization of certain neuroendocrine tumors (^{68}Ga DOTATATE) and prostate-specific malignancies (^{18}F fluciclovine) that were not visualized with FDG. These new radiopharmaceuticals are changing the way physicians manage these disease processes. Imaging for neuroendocrine tumors previously relied on whole-body and SPECT imaging over the course of 3 days; it now is completed within 2 hours, with a much greater degree of accuracy. Evaluating for biochemically recurrent prostate cancer is now possible; PET imaging allows us to see processes that were invisible prior to their use. These newer agents are part of a group of radiopharmaceuticals that has been dubbed **theranostic agents.** Theranostic agents are given to diagnose a specific disease process, and they then can be used to eradicate the disease process by using a different radioisotope attached to the theranostic agent. This provide a more targeted approach to delivering a radiation dose to the offending tissue.

CARDIOLOGY

Coronary Artery Disease

The leading cause of heart failure is coronary artery disease (CAD). Coronary artery disease begins when blood flow to the heart is obstructed. Chest pain, heart attack, and death may occur as a result of this disease. PET can be used to assess how coronary artery disease affects the normal functioning of the heart. A PET perfusion tracer (e.g., ^{13}N ammonia or ^{82}Rb chloride) is used to investigate whether certain areas of the heart are receiving insufficient blood flow (Fig. 20.11). PET perfusion imaging has the ability to quantify myocardial blood flow (MBF) and myocardial flow reserve (MFR) in absolute terms to facilitate diagnosis of multivessel CAD. Newer PET/CT scanners can be equipped with multislice CT units, which can permit CT angiography or calcium scoring to be performed in conjunction with PET perfusion scanning. CT can provide anatomic

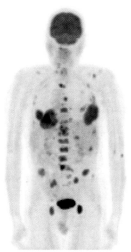

Fig. 20.10 Coronal view of a whole-body PET scan. Darker areas indicate increased uptake of ^{18}F-FDG. It is normal to see activity in the brain because this organ naturally consumes a great deal of glucose. It is also normal to see activity in the collecting system of the kidneys or in the bladder as the tracer is excreted into the urinary system. The two focal areas in the liver are indicative of metastatic spread of breast cancer.

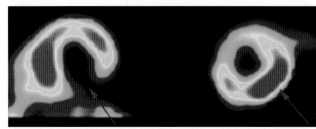

Fig. 20.11 Short-axis images of the heart with the use of ^{13}N-ammonia *(left)* and ^{18}F-FDG *(right)* to assess perfusion and glucose metabolism. Perfusion images reveal a defect in the inferior-lateral area of the heart, as evidenced by decreased function *(arrows)*. FDG images have increased glucose metabolism in this same region. This mismatched pattern is indicative of viable myocardium. (Courtesy Daniel J. Bandy, MS, CNMT.)

information regarding the location of an atherosclerotic lesion, and PET can demonstrate its functional impact on perfusion. Additional studies using the FDG sugar tracer can tell clinicians whether these same areas of decreased blood flow are still viable and would be able to resume normal function if blood flow is restored. Using these images, clinicians can obtain a more complete picture of the scope of disease and can help identify patients who may or may not benefit from other procedures that reroute blood to areas of the heart that are in need.

NEUROLOGY

Epilepsy

PET can be used to investigate the location of seizure sites in patients with epilepsy who are unresponsive to drug therapy; this is accomplished by measuring changes in how the brain uses the sugar tracer (FDG) in the affected areas. PET can detect seizure sites within the brain, regardless of whether a patient is experiencing a seizure at the time of scanning. During a seizure, the image that is created shows an increase in sugar use at the seizure site (Fig. 20.12). If the patient is seizure free at the time of scanning, the image shows a decrease in sugar use in the area of the seizure site. With results of these types of PET scans, the surgeon can identify the affected seizure site for the purpose of removing it. Electroencephalography often is performed immediately after FDG is injected to determine whether any epileptic activity is present.

Brain Mapping

Lesions are described as abnormalities involving tissues or organs that result from disease or injury. When lesions are found in areas of the brain that are vital to the performance of behaviors involved in language, memory, vision, and movement, neurosurgery is associated with the risk of permanent disability. PET brain mapping techniques are able to minimize the risk of injury to a key motor or sensory region of the brain by allowing evaluation of the patient before surgery so the locations of these vital areas can be mapped (Fig. 20.13).

Central Nervous System Tumor Imaging

PET can be used to characterize central nervous system tumors in the same way that it is used for imaging tumors elsewhere in the body. Actively growing brain tumors concentrate FDG. In addition to FDG, another tracer, ^{11}C methionine, can be used to assess amino acid metabolism. This agent is much more sensitive to the presence of even low-grade tumors (Fig. 20.14). By combining ^{11}C methionine scanning with FDG, it is possible to detect the presence of a tumor and to determine how aggressive it is.

Evaluation of Dementia

PET scanning is capable of evaluating and characterizing various types of dementias, such as Alzheimer disease. Using FDG, PET can measure glucose metabolism in the brain. During the normal aging process, glucose metabolism naturally decreases uniformly throughout the brain. In patients with Alzheimer disease, glucose metabolism is dramatically decreased in several key areas of the brain (Fig. 20.15). PET can help confirm the diagnosis of Alzheimer disease and monitor the effects of treatment. PET scanning with FDG and/or beta-amyloid protein imaging agents can assist in the evaluation and characterization of various types of dementia. Using amyloid agents, PET can detect abnormally high levels of a specific beta-amyloid plaque in the brain, which can be indicative of Alzheimer disease.

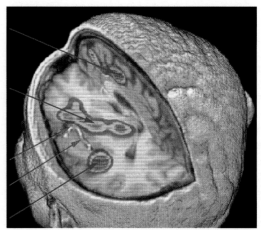

Fig. 20.13 Increases in cerebral blood flow during a language activation examination *(blue arrows)* relative to an arteriovenous malformation *(red arrows)*. (Courtesy Daniel J. Bandy, MS, CNMT.)

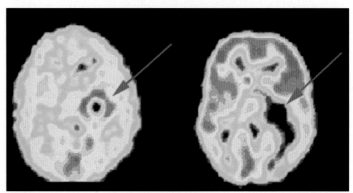

Fig. 20.14 Tumor imaging with the use of ^{11}C-methionine *(left)* and ^{18}F-FDG *(right)* in a patient being evaluated for a newly discovered brain tumor. ^{11}C-Methionine demonstrates a rim of hyperactivity with a cold cystic center *(arrow, left image)*. ^{18}F-FDG shows little or no uptake in the same region *(arrow, right image)*. This pattern is indicative of a low-grade tumor. ^{11}C-Methionine is used to determine the presence or extent of tumor, whereas ^{18}F-FDG is used to determine the grade of the tumor. (Courtesy Daniel J. Bandy, MS, CNMT.)

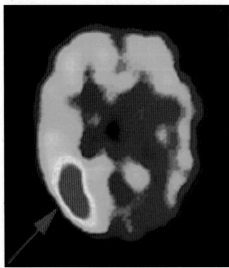

Fig. 20.12 FDG PET scan of a 6-month-old boy with infantile spasms. PET scan shows increased glucose (FDG) uptake *(arrow)* relative to surrounding brain areas. This is indicative of an active seizure focus. (Courtesy Daniel J. Bandy, MS, CNMT.)

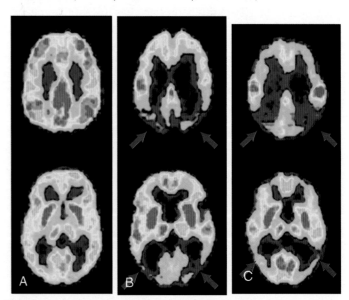

Fig. 20.15 A, B, and C represent FDG brain studies of three individuals: a normal person (A), a patient with mild dementia (B), and a patient with severe dementia (C). Within each column, the top image and the bottom image represent superior and midbrain slices of an FDG brain study. Note the characteristic decreases in glucose metabolism *(blue shade)* in the posterior parietal regions indicated by arrows. (Courtesy Daniel J. Bandy, MS, CNMT.)

PART THREE ▪ RADIATION ONCOLOGY THERAPY

Contributor: **Shaun T. Caldwell,** MS, RT(R)(T)

Introduction

Medical science is finding new ways to treat, cure, and prevent cancer. Death rates from cancer continue to decline in the United States. It is not uncommon for cancer patients to have surgery, chemotherapy, and radiation therapy treatments to eradicate, control, or manage the symptoms of this life-threatening disease.

Radiation oncology is a field of medicine that uses ionizing radiation (radiation therapy treatments), computers, and a team of health care professionals to treat cancer. According to the American Cancer Society (ACS), cancer is the second leading cause of death in the United States. The ACS estimated that in 2020, 1.8 million people in the United States would be diagnosed with some type of cancer. However, it was also noted that 5-year survival rates in general have improved since the 1960's from 27%–39% to 64%–70% depending on type of cancer, treatments, and ethnicity.[4] Approximately 66% of these patients have received or will receive radiation therapy for cure or for palliation.[5] Palliative radiation therapy treatments are not given to cure the patient of the cancer, but to relieve the symptoms associated with the disease, such as pain, bleeding, or obstruction. Patients who receive radiation therapy treatments for palliation may experience an improved quality of life, allowing them to live with and manage their cancer.

Radiation therapy uses x-rays, gamma rays, and particulate radiation (electrons and protons) to destroy cancer cells. A prescribed dose of radiation is delivered in a variety of ways, depending on the type and location of the cancer. Two primary mechanisms used to deliver therapeutic or palliative radiation are **external beam irradiation (also known as** *teletherapy* **or** *long-distance therapy***)** and **brachytherapy (short-distance therapy).**

External Beam Irradiation

The use of megavoltage irradiation for cancer treatments was developed for widespread clinical use in the 1950s. These units, known as cobalt-60 units, used a radioactive ^{60}Co source. The 1.25-MeV gamma rays emitted by the ^{60}Co source were used to deliver the radiation therapy treatments. Beginning in the 1970s, the cobalt-60 units were gradually replaced by **linear accelerators.**

A medical linear accelerator (Fig. 20.16) produces a photon beam by using microwave technology to accelerate electrons fired from an electron gun. These electrons interact and transmit through a tungsten target, creating the high-energy x-ray beam used for treatment. If the tungsten target is removed, a type of particulate irradiation known as an *electron beam* is created. Medical linear accelerators used today are able to produce photon and electron treatment beams at varying energies. The ability to treat with photons or electrons at different energies has led to the development of cancer treatment protocols that are based on the type, size, and location of the malignancy. These protocols are always designed to give a maximum dose of radiation to the tumor and a minimum dose to the surrounding normal tissue.

Radiation therapy has been able to capitalize on the development of 3D and four-dimensional (4D) imaging by integrating this technology into treatment planning and delivery. 4D Imaging depicts the tumor in the *X, Y,* and *Z* planes and in the fourth dimension of time. The fourth dimension of time takes into account movement of the tumor caused by breathing and other body functions. CT, MRI, and PET scanning are used singularly or in combination for 3D or 4D definition of the tumor. With these images a treatment plan (Fig. 20.17) is developed through the use of sophisticated computers and treatment-planning software. This advanced technology allows ablative **(destruction of tissue)** doses of radiation to be directed at the tumor while significantly limiting the dose to the surrounding normal tissue.

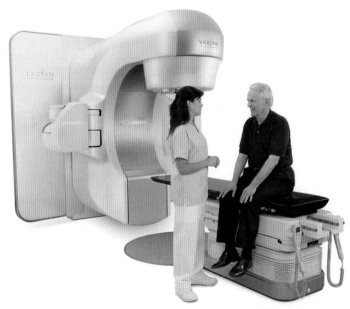

Fig. 20.16 Medical linear accelerator—high-energy x-rays or low-energy electron beam. (Courtesy Varian Medical Systems, Inc. All rights reserved.)

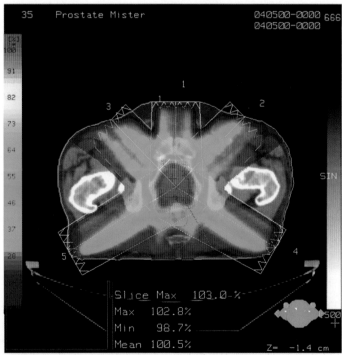

Fig. 20.17 Treatment plan for prostate cancer. (Courtesy Varian Medical Systems, Inc. All rights reserved.)

Other types of external beam irradiation include intraoperative radiation therapy, stereotactic radiosurgery (SRS), and stereotactic body radiation therapy (SBRT). With intraoperative radiation therapy, a dose of radiation is given directly to an organ or area at the time of surgery. This technique is generally used when the likelihood of tumor recurrence postoperatively is high. With SRS and SBRT, multiple beams of radiation are used to target a tumor. With these techniques, ablative radiation is delivered to a small area, usually in one to five treatments. Two types of units are available for SRS and SBRT: cobalt-60–sourced units, also known as Gamma *Knife surgery* (Fig. 20.18), and a specialized or modified linear accelerator–based unit. **Gamma Knife surgery** is a bloodless procedure for neurologic diseases. The surgery does not require the skull to be incised during the procedure. A gamma radiation source is directed to a tumor or lesion with pinpoint accuracy. The treatment is conducted in one procedure and often on an outpatient basis.[6]

Brachytherapy

Brachytherapy (short-distance therapy) uses sealed radioactive isotopes or a miniaturized high-dose-rate x-ray source. Sealed radioactive isotopes may be placed in tissue (interstitial irradiation), and sealed sources or a miniaturized high-dose-rate x-ray source may be placed within a body cavity (intracavitary irradiation) or on a body surface. This method allows for high doses of radiation to be given to the affected tissue without significant irradiation of the surrounding normal tissue.

Proton Therapy

Proton therapy for cancer treatments uses protons (positively charged nuclear particles) to deliver a high dose of radiation to the tumor with almost no radiation dose to the surrounding normal tissue. This exciting advancement in the treatment of cancer and some other diseases means being able to eradicate a cancerous tumor with surgical precision, dramatically lowering a patient's risk for treatment side effects (Fig. 20.19).

Radiation Oncology Team

Radiation oncology is a unique field that combines technology with direct patient care. The field requires the collaboration of dedicated professionals to ensure that the prescribed doses of radiation are given accurately and safely. Patients who receive radiation therapy must be monitored physically and on a psychosocial level for their response to treatment. Members of this team include the following:

Radiation oncologist is the physician responsible for determining the treatment volume and dose of radiation that should be given to a patient. In addition, the radiation oncologist medically manages the patient's response to treatment.

Medical physicists and dosimetrists are charged with planning the treatment as prescribed by the radiation oncologist. The medical physicist also maintains and directs the quality control and quality assurance activities associated with the use of ionizing radiation.

Radiation oncology nurses assist in the monitoring, care, and education of patients who are treated with radiation therapy. The radiation oncology nurse also serves as a conduit for patient referrals to social services, nutritional counseling, and other support groups.

Radiation therapists are responsible for the accurate delivery and documentation of daily radiation treatments. The radiation therapist also provides daily patient assessment, monitoring, and education.

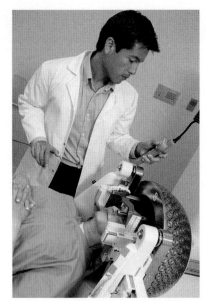

Fig. 20.18 Gamma Knife procedure. (© Getty Images.)

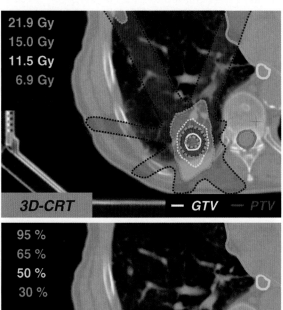
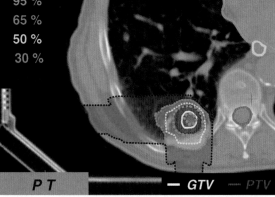

Fig. 20.19 Dose reduction with proton therapy for lung lesion. (From Dietmar G, Hillbrand, M et al. Can protons improve SBRT for lung lesions? Dosimetric considerations. *Radiotherapy and Oncology* 88(3):2008.)

PART FOUR ▪ SONOGRAPHY

Contributor: **Joie Burns,** MS, RT(R)(S), RDMS, RVT

Definition and Introduction

Diagnostic medical sonography (also called *sonography, ultrasound, ultrasonography,* and *echosonography*) is the use of high-frequency sound waves to produce medical images of soft tissue structures. In diagnostic imaging, *sonography* and *ultrasound* are the preferred terms for this modality. Ultrasound refers to sound that is above the range of human hearing. Commonly used diagnostic ultrasound frequencies range from 2 to 20 MHz and higher, depending on the application.

Sonographic equipment creates waves of energy when an electrical voltage is applied to the hundreds of elements housed inside the transducer. Sound waves are transmitted into the body, and echoes are reflected back from each organ the wave encounters. The transducer then acts as a receiver that processes the echoes returning from inside the body. These received echoes create a composite image that is displayed in real time on a monitor and can be viewed, manipulated, and stored. The sonographer maneuvers the transducer into specific planes and angles to obtain images based on the examination ordered by the patient's health care provider (Fig. 20.20).

Transducers come in a variety of sizes, shapes, and frequencies for specific applications (Fig. 20.21). Lower-frequency transducers permit greater penetration for imaging large organs such as the liver. Higher-frequency transducers permit less penetration but provide a higher-resolution image for superficial structures such as breast tissue.

Diagnostic sonography has three major imaging specialty areas: general imaging, echocardiography, and vascular imaging. Within these specialty areas are subsets of abdominal and superficial parts, obstetrics and gynecology, fetal/pediatric/adult cardiac, breast, musculoskeletal, vascular, pediatric, and miscellaneous applications. Sonography is the preferred modality for imaging the male and female reproductive system and for obstetrics and pediatrics. It does not use ionizing radiation and can be performed both quickly and effectively to obtain a diagnosis.

History and Physical Principles of Ultrasound

The technique of echo location is not new in nature. For example, bats locate their prey by listening for insects far away and are successful despite very poor vision. Medical applications for imaging emerged, as many inventions do, from the military. During World War I, detection of submarines underwater using high-frequency sound was developed and termed *sound navigation and ranging* (SONAR). Echo location was perfected and became a very effective tool for detecting submarines during World War II.

The medical use of ultrasound became more prevalent after World War II, when peaceful uses for sonar were explored by medical pioneers who imaged a variety of anatomic structures inside the body. For the first time images of soft tissues and organs such as the brain, liver, uterus, and fetus were created, and ultrasound became a diagnostic tool for clinicians. The evolution of diagnostic medical sonography is closely aligned with improvements in computer capabilities, speed, miniaturization, and sophistication (Fig. 20.22; also see Fig. 20.25).

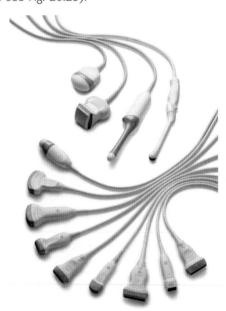

Fig. 20.21 Transducers and probes—LOGIQ E9 suite of transducers. (Courtesy GE Healthcare.)

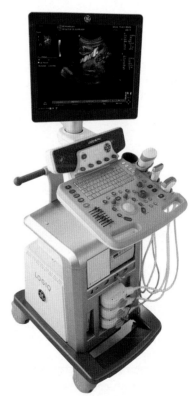

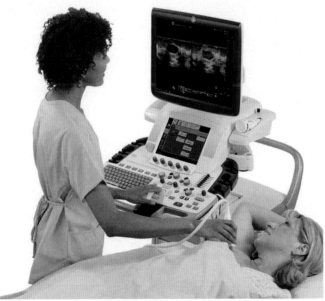

Fig. 20.20 Sonographer scanning on LOGIQ 9. (Courtesy GE Healthcare.)

Fig. 20.22 Ultrasound system. (Courtesy GE Healthcare.)

A-MODE

The first ultrasound unit was built in the early 1950s. Amplitude mode (A-mode) was used to display echoes produced at each organ border. Each echo appeared as a spike on an oscilloscope. The strength of an echo was correlated to the height of the spike – hence the term *amplitude*. The higher the spike, the stronger the echo. Although this display was very primitive, it allowed physicians to begin to assess anatomic structures deep within the body.

B-MODE

The growth and evolution of ultrasound continued in the 1960s. With increasing computer complexity and capacity, the ultrasound display changed to create a 2D image, or frame, made up of a series of dots. This display was called *brightness mode* (B-mode). Each dot represented varying shades of gray, or "gray scale." The strength of an echo was correlated to the whiteness of the dot – the whiter the dot, the stronger the echo. This more intuitive display allowed the examiner to determine the characteristics of each organ, and it provided information about whether a structure was solid (e.g., the liver) or fluid filled (e.g., the bladder).

M-MODE

Motion mode (M-mode) is a way to display movement of a structure on a scale (Fig. 20.23). This mode is commonly used in echocardiography to demonstrate movement of the heart valves and walls. It is also used to demonstrate early fetal heart activity, the motion of a nonadherent clot within a vein, or an intimal flap associated with an arterial dissection.

REAL-TIME IMAGING

In the 1970s, as computer technology improved, B-mode imaging moved to a new era as images in two dimensions, or frames, were recorded fast enough to be displayed in "real time." The increased speed of image display allowed the sonographer to observe anatomic movement for the first time. The fetus moving inside the uterus and the fetal heartbeat, using M-mode, could be recorded instantly. At this time, the equipment was gaining widespread acceptance as part of routine care in areas such as obstetrics.

DOPPLER

Explosive growth for diagnostic sonography occurred in the 1980s and 1990s as computer technology continued to advance. Applications to detect blood flow and direction with spectral, color, and power/energy Doppler allowed organs and vascular structures to be accurately mapped, measured, and imaged and blood flow velocities to be assessed. More transducers with a wider range of applications and sophistication were introduced, and image quality improved with each technologic update or upgrade to the imaging platforms.

DIGITAL SYSTEMS

As in other areas of electronics, digital imaging allowed miniaturization, stabilization, faster image processing and manipulation, viewing, and storage to expand the limits of sonography. Images could be created in one location and sent to the reading physician across the world or down the street for instant viewing. Saving images on other types of media, such as film, has become obsolete, because digital imaging allows electronic storage and web-based access.

Diagnostic medical sonography units are generally small enough to be portable, and the equipment becomes more versatile with each new generation. Newer applications include 3D imaging to allow the display of an object in three dimensions (Fig. 20.24). 4D Imaging allows real-time display of 3D images. Fusion technology allows ultrasound images to be merged and aligned with a prior study from another modality such as MRI or CT. Elastography, a technique that assesses the compressibility of soft tissue, is being used to detect fibrotic change in the liver associated with cirrhosis and tissue changes in the breast, thyroid, and prostate associated with cancer.

The explosion of digital imaging and miniaturization has created laptop, handheld, and smart phone diagnostic sonography units. Sonography can be performed literally anywhere in the health care setting, such as the emergency department, physician offices, operating room, bedside, acute care setting, and patient transport vehicles (Fig. 20.25).

A negative outcome of digital imaging has been higher rates of job-related musculoskeletal injury for sonographers. Proposed reasons for injury include increased reporting of injuries, shortages of skilled sonographers, examination speed and productivity, increasing patient obesity, and other factors related to scheduling or reimbursement issues. Proper ergonomic scanning technique and equipment, rest, and adequate time between patients are important factors in maintaining the health of sonographers so they are not scanning in pain (Fig. 20.26).

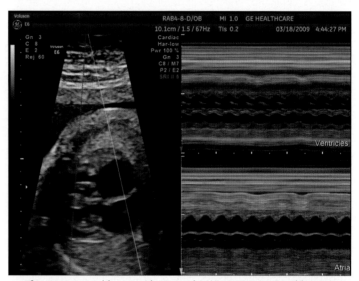

Fig. 20.23 Fetal heart with M mode. (Courtesy GE Healthcare.)

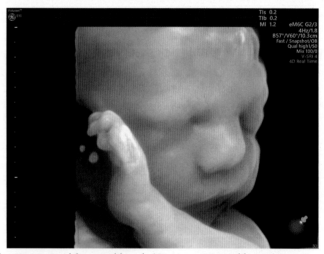

Fig. 20.24 Fetal face and hand. (Courtesy GE Healthcare.)

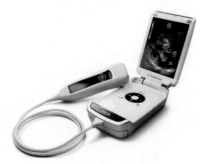

Fig. 20.25 V scan—pocket sized. (Courtesy GE Healthcare.)

Limitations and Advantages of Sonography in Medical Imaging

Sound wave energy at ultrasound frequencies has been proven in epidemiologic studies to create changes in tissue known as *bioeffects,* or biologic effects. The bioeffects that occur in tissue fall into two categories, thermal and mechanical (nonthermal) effects. Thermal changes are associated with the friction created as the wave disturbs cells from their resting position. Mechanical effects are associated with changes that occur as the waves interact with microscopic gas bodies within tissues. Indices have been created to be displayed on the ultrasound system's monitor to increase the sonographer's awareness of the potential for adverse biologic effects to occur. These indices are the thermal index (TI), which is related to heating, and the mechanical index (MI), which is related to mechanical or nonthermal effects on tissue. TI and MI values measure the potential for thermal and mechanical bioeffects to occur and are displayed on each image acquired during the scan. Sound wave energy is an important safety issue for the patient, especially for the developing embryo and fetus. The sonographer keeps the ALARA principle (as low as reasonably achievable) in mind to ensure that a diagnostic scan is performed in the least amount of time, with the lowest power applied to the patient.

The Statement on Prudent Use and Safety, issued by the American Institute of Ultrasound in Medicine (2019), states[7]:

No independently confirmed adverse effects caused by exposure from present diagnostic ultrasound instruments have been reported in human patients in the absence of microbubble contrast agents. Biological effects...have been reported in mammalian systems at diagnostically relevant exposures but the clinical significance of such effects is not yet known. Ultrasound should be used by qualified health professionals to provide medical benefit to the patient.

Air reflects nearly 100% of the sound between the face of the transducer and the patient's skin. Sound waves travel very efficiently through water and most other liquids, so a water-based coupling medium or gel is generously applied between the patient and the transducer to perform any ultrasound study. Sonography is well suited for imaging anatomy such as the liver, kidneys, gallbladder, uterus, thyroid, testicles, and blood vessels because there is little interference from bone or air. Air in the gastrointestinal (GI) tract reduces ultrasound's use in this area. However, inflammatory changes, such as appendicitis, intussusception, and Crohn disease, in addition to hypertrophic changes associated with pyloric stenosis, are well demonstrated. Additionally, water may be used to fill portions of the GI tract to allow ultrasound evaluation of a specific area such as the stomach, duodenum, or colon. Because of its density, bone also is not a ready medium for diagnostic ultrasound. However, bones seen in growing fetuses and young infants are not as well calcified as adult bones. This makes ultrasound examination of the infant for hip dysplasia and fetal assessment of skeletal growth and development possible.

Advances in Sonography

Promising applications continue, because sonography shows great portability in the health care setting. Ultrasound examinations can be performed at any point-of-care location. Lung ultrasound is an increasingly common diagnostic tool used at the bedside to assess lung consolidation, pleural effusion, and pneumonia. Some experts in the field indicate that lung ultrasound may replace the routine chest x-ray for pediatric patients with pneumonia.

Automated breast volume scanning (ABVS) is a technique that acquires a series of consecutive B-mode pictures and reconstructs 3D data sets of the entire breast volume. The ability to visualize breast cancers in the coronal plane has improved diagnosis of the disease. The automated acquisition also reduces the musculoskeletal stress on the sonographer.

The extended focused assessment with sonography for trauma (EFAST) scan in emergency medicine has enhanced the demand for sonography in trauma settings to identify fluid and blood collections in the thorax and abdomen and pneumothorax. Early identification of these abnormalities may mean the difference between life and death for a patient.

Sonographic contrast agents consist of microbubbles of gas encased in a lipid coat. These bubbles are tiny enough to pass through the entire circulatory system without rupturing. Just as iodinated contrast is used to demonstrate the vascular characteristics of anatomy and lesions during an intravenous urogram (IVU) or a contrast-enhanced CT, an ultrasound microbubble contrast medium demonstrates the vascular characteristics of a lesion under ultrasound. Contrast-enhanced ultrasound (CEUS) is performed with great success in many countries around the world on a variety of organs and body systems. The U.S. Food and Drug Administration (FDA) has approved the use in the United States of an intravenous microbubble contrast medium for liver and echocardiographic examinations.

Elastography is a scanning technique that assesses the relative stiffness of tissue or a lesion. Manual compression or strain elastography has been used in breast imaging for several years to differentiate stiff, fibrotic changes associated with breast cancer from soft, benign masses. This method of elastography creates a B-mode image superimposed with colors that represent the tissue's relative hardness (H) or softness (S) as indicated on the adjacent scale (Fig. 20.27). This qualitative imaging technique is not useful in patients with fibrocystic dysplasia of the breast. A quantifiable form of elastography to assess fibrotic change in patients with chronic liver disease has recently become widely accepted. Instead of manually compressing the tissue, the ultrasound system measures shear waves that are generated by the tissue. Multiple ROIs are measured throughout the anatomy during an exam (Fig. 20.28). This imaging method is well suited to comparison over time. It is anticipated that this noninvasive scanning technique may replace the current practice of a biopsy to assess changes. Thick adipose tissue and other disease may reduce this technique's reliability. Assessment of the masses with elastography is in the investigational stage but shows promise.

Clinical Applications
ABDOMEN

Abdominal sonography is performed to assess all of the abdominal organs, gastrointestinal tract, bile ducts, and vessels of the abdomen and their branches (Fig. 20.29). This area of practice presents a

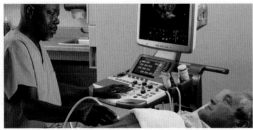

Fig. 20.26 Sonographer scanning a patient. (Courtesy GE Healthcare.)

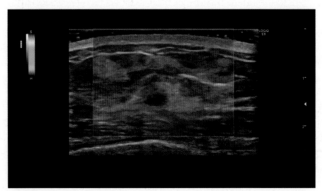

Fig. 20.27 Breast elastogram. Scale indicates S (soft) to H (hard). (Courtesy GE Healthcare.)

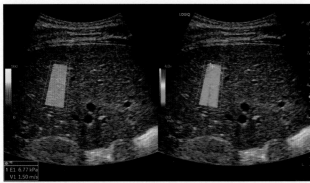

Fig. 20.28 2D Shear Wave elastography–liver. (Courtesy GE Healthcare.)

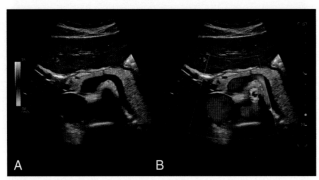

Fig. 20.29 Transverse epigastrium. A, Normal pancreas in B-mode. B, Normal vasculature surrounding pancreas in color Doppler. (Courtesy GE Healthcare.)

significant challenge for the sonographer, because the patient's age may range from infancy to old age, with a variety of pathologic conditions associated with each stage of life.

OBSTETRICS AND GYNECOLOGY

Real-time images of the gravid uterus are used to detect the initial pregnancy implantation site, in addition to the growth and well-being of the embryo and fetus throughout pregnancy. The 3D image in Fig. 20.30 depicts an early pregnancy in the first trimester.

Gynecologic imaging is used to assess the nongravid female pelvis in patients with complaints of pelvic pain, pelvic mass, menstrual irregularities, and postmenopausal bleeding. In Fig. 20.31, the uterus and endometrium are seen in three planes: axial, longitudinal, and coronal.

CARDIAC EVALUATIONS

Sonography for cardiac applications may be performed on adults, children, and the fetus during pregnancy. Echocardiography may be performed two ways, by transthoracic or transesophageal means. Transthoracic cardiac imaging is performed through the chest wall. Transesophageal echocardiography (TEE) requires patient sedation because the transducer is introduced into the esophagus immediately adjacent to the heart. The TEE approach allows high-resolution imaging of the posterior heart and aorta. A microbubble contrast medium may be used to assess cardiac chamber function and size. Fig. 20.32 demonstrates a B-mode (gray scale) and M-mode scan of a fetal heart. With early diagnosis of fetal heart abnormalities, the parents and the health care provider can plan a course of treatment before delivery.

SUPERFICIAL PARTS

Patients undergoing mammography often have a sonographic examination of the breast when a mass is identified. Sonography is used to examine the corresponding breast tissue identified on the mammogram and determine if the mass is cystic or solid (Fig. 20.33). Breast sonography may also be performed in lactating and adolescent patients whose breasts are considered dense, which reduces the effectiveness of a mammogram.

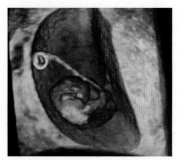

Fig. 20.30 Obstetric scan—first trimester. (Courtesy GE Healthcare.)

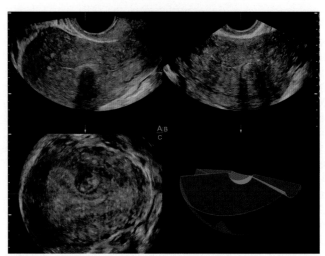

Fig. 20.31 Uterus and endometrium in three dimensions. (Courtesy GE Healthcare.)

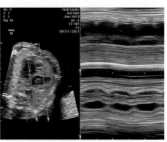

Fig. 20.32 Fetal heart with atrioventricular block imaged in gray scale and M mode. (Courtesy GE Healthcare.)

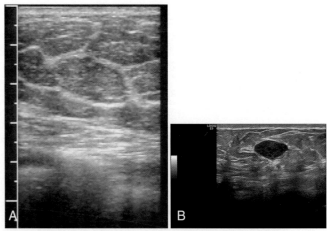

Fig. 20.33 A, Normal breast. B, Complex solid breast mass. (**A** courtesy Robert Kuo; **B** courtesy GE Healthcare.)

Thyroid and parathyroid sonography is performed to assess and characterize lesions in these endocrine glands. Ultrasound may be used to guide the biopsy or fine needle aspiration, ensuring accurate tissue sampling of suspicious tissue.

Patients with complaints of scrotal pain, swelling, or a palpable mass are referred for a scrotal ultrasound. Common pathologic conditions include inflammatory processes (e.g., epididymitis and orchitis) or vascular concerns (e.g., testicular torsion and trauma), in addition to testicular cancers.

Sonography is often used to assess and monitor brain hemorrhage and ventricular enlargement in the neonatal intensive care unit (NICU). Images are obtained by directing the ultrasound beam through the infant's fontanels.

VASCULAR IMAGING

Sonography of the vascular system is used to diagnose and assess vascular patency, in addition to blood flow adequacy and direction. Arteries are examined for atherosclerotic changes, aneurysm, and dissection. Veins are assessed for thrombus and valvular sufficiency. Commonly examined vessels include those in the upper and lower extremities, the abdominal and pelvic vasculature, and the carotid and subclavian arteries. Ultrasound is also frequently used to assess vascular grafts, stents, and fistulas for patency and changes associated with failure. Additionally, ultrasound may be used to guide the placement of central lines for patients requiring chemotherapy or long-term intravenous (IV) medications. The sonographic vascular examination uses color and spectral Doppler, in addition to grayscale imaging, to provide both anatomic and physiologic information to assist in making a diagnosis (Fig. 20.34).

MUSCULOSKELETAL IMAGING

Ultrasound is well suited to assess the musculoskeletal system because it can assess skin lesions in addition to connective tissues and deeper muscles. Ultrasound is especially useful for imaging joints throughout their range of motion and for assessing muscles and tendons for masses, ruptures, and tears. Additionally, inflamed bursae, effusions, and other fluid collections may be identified for treatment. Commonly examined areas include the shoulder for rotator cuff tear and impingement, the elbow and ankle in athletes, and the wrist for carpal tunnel complaints. The Achilles tendon is assessed in this image to determine if there is normal insertion, a tear, or some other type of injury (in Fig. 20.35 the arrow points to the Achilles tendon).

SONOGRAPHY TEAM MEMBERS

Sonographers are professionals whose education and certification enable them to use high-frequency sound waves and other diagnostic techniques for medical diagnosis. Sonographers are highly skilled and competent individuals who must be able to produce and evaluate ultrasound images, correlate related data that are used by physicians to render a medical diagnosis, and provide quality patient care. Sonographers must have the following skill sets: a patient-centered perspective with extensive patient care competencies, outstanding written and spoken communication abilities, knowledge of normal and pathologic conditions, a thorough knowledge of sectional anatomy and anatomic variants, visual acuity and attention to subtle details, the ability to create diagnostic images consistently, and excellent critical thinking skills.[7]

Sonologists are physicians, often radiologists, who are qualified by training to interpret the imaging studies performed by the sonographer. Sonologists work closely with sonographers, formulate the diagnosis, and create the final report that is sent to the ordering health care provider.

Students in sonography programs must complete significant hours of clinical practice, laboratories, and courses designed to prepare them to become competent entry-level sonographers. According to the Society of Diagnostic Medical Sonography, at the time of this publication only four states (New Hampshire, New Mexico, North Dakota, and Oregon) required certification and licensing of sonographers. However, most employers require the graduate to pass a certification examination to gain employment.[8]

The **American Registry for Diagnostic Medical Sonography (ARDMS)** offers certification in specialty areas, depending on the candidate's qualifications, such as abdominal/superficial parts, OB/GYN, breast, adult/pediatric/fetal cardiac, pediatric, musculoskeletal, and vascular. All ARDMS candidates first must pass the Sonography Principles and Instrumentation examination, and then a specialty examination, to gain certification as registered sonographers. The **American Registry of Radiologic Technologists (ARRT)** also offers a sonography pathway leading to certification in sonography (abdominal, OB/GYN, and superficial parts), vascular, or breast imaging. Evidence of continuing education and recertification every 10 years is required to maintain certification with both the ARDMS and the ARRT (https://www.ardms.org and https://www.arrt.org).

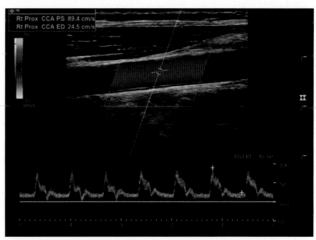

Fig. 20.34 Common carotid artery with color and spectral Doppler. (Courtesy GE Healthcare.)

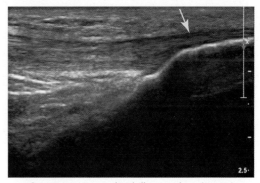

Fig. 20.35 Normal Achilles tendon (arrow).

SONOGRAPHY TERMINOLOGY

ALARA: As low as reasonably achievable; this is the goal, to keep thermal and mechanical effects of ultrasound as low as possible and still obtain a diagnostic imaging examination for the patient.

Bioeffects: Ultrasound has the potential to cause thermal and mechanical changes in tissue. Thermal changes occur when the intensity of the sound waves heat tissue. Mechanical changes occur when gas bubbles in the cells become deformed. To date, diagnostic ultrasound has not been shown to be harmful to humans.

B-mode: Abbreviation for brightness modulation mode; basis for all gray-scale ultrasound images; echoes converted to bright dots that vary in intensity according to the strength of the echo.

Color-flow Doppler: Ultrasound technique that measures the average velocity and direction of blood within a vessel; changes in velocity and direction are seen as different shades of color or color variance.

Doppler effect: Alteration in frequency or wavelength of sound waves reflected from moving structure or medium.

Doppler ultrasound: Application of the Doppler effect to ultrasound to detect frequency and velocity shifts of a moving structure or medium; used for blood flow studies of the body.

Echo: Measurements of the intensity of acoustic energy reflected and received from anatomic structures.

EFAST scans: Extended focused assessment with sonography for trauma; this scan application in trauma is seen in the emergency department and may include the chest, abdomen, and pelvis.

Elastography: Techniques that use sonography to compare the mechanical properties of tissues and their relative stiffness to distinguish benign from malignant lesions.

Element: Manufactured crystal that has a voltage applied to it, causing it to deform, creating the piezo or pressure electric effect that results in the creation of wavelets.

Fusion imaging: Combination of two imaging modalities (e.g., MRI or CT and sonography) to create a single study demonstrating anatomy and function together.

Gray scale: Display of various levels of echo brightness or intensity represented in shades of gray.

M-mode: The ultrasound demonstration of a structure's movement with time. M-mode is frequently used to measure the fetal heart rate in early pregnancy, in addition to valve and heart wall motion during an echocardiographic exam.

Power/energy Doppler: Ultrasound technique that displays and measures the average velocity of blood within a vessel; changes in velocity are seen as different shades of one color. This technique is not capable of demonstrating changes in direction.

Real-time imaging: Ultrasound images that demonstrate dynamic motion or changes within a structure in real time.

Reflection: Acoustic energy that is reflected from a structure back toward the transducer.

Sonar: Acronym for "sound navigation and ranging"; a naval instrument used to detect objects underwater.

Spectral Doppler: Ultrasound technique that measures and displays the velocities and direction of blood within a vessel; changes in velocity and direction are seen as dots on a scale on which velocity is indicated on the vertical (x-axis) and time is represented along the horizontal (y-axis).

Sonography: Process of generating images with ultrasound.

Three-dimensional and four-dimensional ultrasound (3DUS/4DUS): Volume imaging using 2D images to create a volume rendering of specific tissue or organs for greater diagnostic clarification in three planes of section acquired in real time.

Transducer: Device that contains specific types of crystals that undergo mechanical stress to produce an ultrasound wave; serves as a sender and receiver of the ultrasound signal.

Wave: Acoustic energy that travels through a medium.

PART FIVE: MAMMOGRAPHY

Contributor: **Michelle A Wilt,** MHA, RT(R)(M)(ARRT)

Breast Cancer

Breast cancer is the second most common cancer among women (the most common is skin cancer). Until recently, breast cancer was the leading cause of death from cancer among women; lung cancer is now the leader.

Breast cancer accounts for 15.2% of all new cancers detected in U.S. women and 6.9% of all cancer deaths.[9] The American Cancer Society (ACS) estimates that 1 in 8 American women will develop a breast cancer at some time in her life. In the United States, approximately 268,600 cases were diagnosed in 2019. Of those, 62,930 were carcinoma in situ. Nationwide, approximately 41,760 women and 500 men died from breast cancer in 2019.[10]

Worldwide, breast cancer is still the most common cancer in women, with 2 million new cases documented in 2018.[11] This is down from 2.7 million reported in 2008. Female breast cancer incidence rates have increased slightly, by approximately 0.4%, in recent years. In 2019 there were more than 3.1 million breast cancer survivors in the United States.[10] These statistics indicate that cancers are being found earlier and treatments have improved; however, the chance that breast cancer will be responsible for a woman's death is about 1 in 38.[10]

Men also can develop breast cancer, but their risk is between 1% and 2% of a woman's risk. Breast cancer accounts for less than 0.1% of all cancers found in men; however, there has been a 26% increase in incidence over the past three decades. Because breast cancer is uncommon among men, the symptoms may not be recognized as early, and often the disease progresses to an advanced stage before it is diagnosed.[12]

The first step in prevention of any disease is to understand the risk factors for that disease. Over time, certain risk factors have been identified for breast cancer, yet specific causes of most breast cancers are still unknown. The current best defense against this disease continues to be women having regular mammograms so that early detection is possible. The ACS sets guidelines for early detection practices for all common types of cancer. Breast cancer guidelines vary, depending on a woman's age. These guidelines include mammography and clinical breast examination, and MRI has been added for women who have a high-risk profile.

Regular mammography can be the key to survival with breast cancer because many breast lesions may be detected before they become symptomatic or metastasize. Mammograms can detect a lesion 2 mm in size; such lesions may take 2 to 4 years to be palpable on breast self-examination or clinical breast examination. It is reported that once a breast tumor has reached about ¾ inch (2 cm) in size, it often has already metastasized or spread to other regions. The average survival time for a patient with metastatic breast cancer is only 2 years.[13] It is recommended (if supported by their health care provider) that at-risk women and men undergo annual mammograms in an effort to detect breast lesions prior to metastasis. The earlier a lesion is detected, the more treatment options the patient has, and the better the prognosis.

Mammography has evolved into one of the most critical and demanding radiologic examinations that can be performed. Mammographic procedures are highly dependent on the knowledge and skills of the mammographer. A mammographer is a radiologic technologist who has received additional training in mammography. Accurate and careful positioning of the breast during mammography is imperative in diagnosing breast cancer. The maximum amount of breast tissue must be clearly demonstrated on each projection. Mammographic images are characterized by optimal contrast and high resolution, and they must contain no artifacts that may potentially obscure a pathologic condition. Technologists become qualified through didactic coursework, professional training, and hands-on experience, and they are required to pass an additional certification examination. The mammographer is required to continue education in mammography on a yearly basis to maintain certification.

Current recommendations from the ACS, the American College of Radiology (ACR), and other health organizations are that all women who are 40 years old should be able to choose to undergo a screening mammogram and regular mammograms thereafter. High-risk patients with a family history of breast cancer may be advised to begin screening mammograms at an earlier age. As previously stated, although the number of new breast cancer cases is increasing, the mortality rate has decreased in recent years, as reported by the National Cancer Institute.[9] This increase in detection is not alarming because more women and men are getting tested, and the overall life expectancy has risen. The decreased mortality rate supports the fact that clinicians are finding the disease at an earlier, more treatable stage. There is no given age at which a woman should discontinue the screening mammogram regimen. According to the ACS, as long as a woman is in good health, would be a good candidate for breast cancer treatment, and has a life expectancy of 10 years or more, she should continue to have a screening mammogram to increase the chances of early detection[13] (although it should be noted that the National Cancer Risk Assessment tool does not include women over the age of 85). Despite the many technologic advances made in breast imaging, screening mammography remains one of the best diagnostic tools that can be used to detect early breast cancers, before metastasis.

Mammography Quality Standards Act

In 1992 the U.S. federal government enacted the **Mammography Quality Standards Act (MQSA).** The MQSA came about as a result of a high-visibility public relations campaign by the ACS, which recommended that all women older than age 40 should undergo screening mammography. Additionally, the recommendation included that federal legislation should provide reimbursement for screening mammography in women who are eligible for Medicare. The MQSA was written as a result of lobbying by the ACR because of great concern about the poor quality of mammography that was being performed. The act, which went into effect **October 1, 1994,** requires all facilities (except Veterans Administration facilities) that provide mammography services to meet quality standards and become certified for operation by the secretary of the U.S. Department of Health and Human Services (DHHS). Enactment of the MQSA marks the first time the use of an x-ray machine and a specific examination were regulated by the federal government. All pertinent facilities are required to (1) be accredited by an approved body, (2) be certified by the DHHS, and (3) receive an on-site inspection by a state agency acting on behalf of the DHHS (or by DHHS inspectors). All mammography facilities were to have met these regulations by April 28, 1999. The final rules of the MQSA are known as Public Law 105-248. In Canada, mammography guidelines are set by the Canadian Association of Radiologists.

The technical aspects of mammography are tightly controlled, and mammography must be performed on a dedicated mammography unit. The mammography unit must be state of the art and must be monitored regularly through an intensive quality assurance program. Although film-based systems are considered the gold standard in breast imaging, digital mammography (discussed later in this section) is becoming more and more common.

Anatomy of the Breast

Each of the mammary glands or breasts in a woman is a conic or hemispheric eminence that is located on the anterior and lateral chest walls. Breast size varies from one individual to another and often even during a woman's life span, depending on her age and the interplay of various hormones. These hormones are very influential in tissue development, growth, and eventually milk production in the woman. Until puberty, breast tissue is identical in males and females, comprised of fatty tissue and ducts. Breast shape undergoes numerous changes throughout a woman's lifetime. In younger women, breast skin stretches and expands as the breast grows, producing a rounder appearance. Breast tissue in a young woman tends to be slightly denser and more glandular than breast tissue in an older woman. The average breast extends from the anterior portion of the **second rib** down to the **sixth** or **seventh rib** (midsternum) and from the lateral border of the sternum into the axilla. Each breast comprises 15 to 20 lobes, which are covered by adipose tissue that primarily accounts for the breast's size and shape.

SURFACE ANATOMY

The surface anatomy (Fig. 20.36) includes the **nipple,** a small projection that contains a collection of 15 to 20 duct openings from secretory glands within the breast tissue. The circular, darker pigmented area surrounding the nipple is termed the **areola.** The **Montgomery glands** are small oil glands whose purpose is to keep the nipple lubricated and protected, especially while the woman is nursing an infant. The junction of the inferior part of the breast with the anterior chest wall is called the **inframammary fold** (IMF). The **axillary tail** (AT) is a band of tissue that wraps around the pectoral muscle laterally.

On most women the width of the breast, called the **mediolateral diameter,** is greater than the vertical measurement (from top to bottom). The vertical measurement, which may be described as the **craniocaudad diameter,** averages 4¾ to 6 inches (12 to 15 cm) at the chest wall. In positioning, the mammographer realizes that more breast tissue is present beyond the obvious tissue that extends from the chest wall. Breast tissue overlies the costocartilage area near the sternum and extends well up into the axilla. This breast tissue extending into the axilla is called the **tail of the breast** or the **axillary prolongation** of the breast and is the most common site for breast cancer to occur.

SAGITTAL SECTION ANATOMY

A sagittal section through a mature breast is illustrated in Fig. 20.37, which shows the relationship of the mammary gland to the underlying structures of the chest wall. In this illustration, the **IMF** is at the level of the sixth rib, but a great deal of variation can exist among individuals.

The large **muscle,** known as the *pectoralis major,* is seen overlying the bony thorax. A layer of fibrous tissue encompasses the breast because of its location below the skin surface and covering the pectoralis major muscle. The area where these tissues meet superiorly to inferiorly is termed the **retromammary space.** This retromammary space must be demonstrated on **at least one projection** during the radiographic study of the mammary gland as an indication that all breast tissue has been visualized. This is possible because the connections within the retromammary space are loose, and the area of the IMF is the most mobile within the normal breast.

The relative position of glandular tissue versus adipose (fatty) tissue is illustrated in Fig. 20.38. The central portion of the breast is primarily **glandular tissue.** Varying amounts of **adipose,** or **fatty, tissue** surround the glandular tissue. The ratio of glandular to adipose tissue varies from individual to individual, primarily secondary to genetics and age.

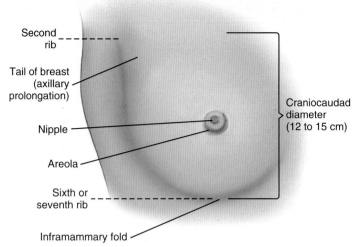
Fig. 20.36 Surface anatomy.

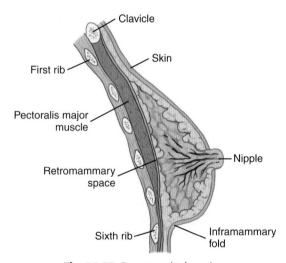
Fig. 20.37 Breast sagittal section.

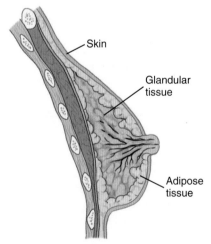
Fig. 20.38 Breast tissue sagittal section.

The primary function of the mammary gland is the secretion of milk, or lactation. The size of the female breast or amount of glandular and fatty tissue has no bearing on the functional ability of the gland.

The skin that covers the breast is seen to be uniform in thickness except in the area of the areola and nipple, where the skin is thicker.

METHODS OF LOCALIZATION

Two methods are commonly used to subdivide the breast into smaller areas for localization purposes. These methods, the **quadrant system** and the **clock system,** are shown in Figs. 20.39 and 20.40, respectively. Of the two, the quadrant system is easier to use for generalized lesion localization. Four quadrants can be described by using the nipple as the center. These quadrants are the **UOQ** (upper outer quadrant), the **UIQ** (upper inner quadrant), the **LOQ** (lower outer quadrant), and the **LIQ** (lower inner quadrant).

The **clock system** (see Fig. 20.40) compares the surface of the breast with the face of a clock. Although this method provides a more accurate description of a lesion, what is described at 3 o'clock in the right breast must be described at 9 o'clock in the left breast.

These methods of lesion localization are very similar to methods used for breast self-examination and clinical examination with respect to examining the breast by quadrant or a circular clock method. If the referring physician or the patient has felt a mass of any suspicious area in either breast, one of these methods is used to describe the area of special interest to radiology personnel.

ANTERIOR VIEW ANATOMY

The glandular tissue of the breast is divided into **15** or **20 lobes** that are arranged similarly to the spokes of a wheel surrounding the nipple (Fig. 20.41). The glandular lobes, which include several individual **lobules,** are not clearly separated but are grouped in a radial arrangement, as shown in the figure.

Distally, the smallest lobules consist of clusters of rounded **alveoli.** On glandular stimulation, peripheral cells of the alveoli form oil globules in their interior, which, when ejected into the lumen of the alveoli, constitute milk globules. The clusters of alveoli that make up the lobules are interconnected and drain through individual **ducts.** Each duct enlarges into a small **ampulla** that serves as a reservoir for milk just before terminating in a tiny opening on the surface of the **nipple.**

Various subdivisions of these ducts and associated ampullae are activated during pregnancy to prepare for lactation and after birth to produce milk for the newborn.

A layer of adipose tissue just under the skin surrounds and covers the glandular tissue. Lobular mammary fatty tissue, **subcutaneous fat,** is interspersed between the glandular elements. **Interlobular connective** or fibrous tissues surround and support the lobes and other glandular structures. Bandlike extensions of this fibrous tissue, known as **Cooper (suspensory) ligaments** of the breast, provide support for the mammary glands.

Each breast is abundantly supplied by blood vessels, nerves, and lymphatic vessels. The veins of the mammary gland usually are larger than the arteries and are located more peripherally. Some larger veins usually can be seen distinctly on a mammogram. The term **trabeculae** is used by radiologists to describe various small structures seen on the finished radiograph, such as small blood vessels, fibrous connective tissues, ducts, and other small structures that cannot be differentiated.

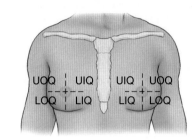

Fig. 20.39 Breast localization—quadrant method.

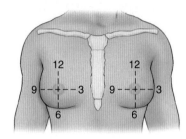

Fig. 20.40 Breast localization—clock system.

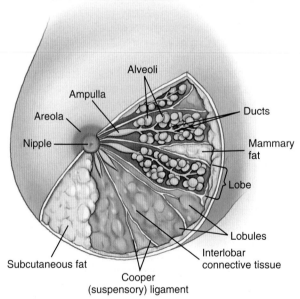

Fig. 20.41 Breast—anterior view (glandular tissue).

BREAST TISSUE TYPES

A major challenge associated with imaging the breast radiographically is that the various tissues have low inherent subject contrast or breast tissue "makeup." Breast tissue can be divided into three main types: (1) **glandular,** (2) **fibrous** or **connective,** and (3) **adipose** (Fig. 20.42). Because the breast is a soft tissue structure, no high-density or air-filled tissue is present to provide contrast. The fibrous and glandular tissues are of almost heterogeneous density, which means that radiation is absorbed by these tissue types in a similar fashion.

The major difference among breast tissues is that adipose or fatty tissue is less dense than either fibrous or glandular tissue. This difference in density between the fatty tissue and the remaining tissues accounts for the contrast differences apparent on the final image.

SUMMARY

Three types of breast tissue exist:
1. Glandular
2. Fibrous or connective – similar higher density (appears lighter)
3. Adipose – less density (appears darker)

The analog (film-screen) mammogram image (Fig. 20.43A) shows the differences in tissue density. These differences provide the basis for the radiographic image of the breast. The more dense glandular and fibrous or connective tissues appear as "light" structures or regions. The less dense adipose or fatty tissues appear as various shades of gray, depending on the thickness of these tissues. Fig. 20.43B demonstrates digital mammography. Note how image contrast is enhanced compared to the analog image.

Breast Classifications

Technical exposure factors for any one part of the anatomy are determined primarily by the thickness of that particular part. For example, a large elbow requires greater exposure factors than a small elbow. This is also true in mammography; however, the mammographer has some control in this relationship. In mammography, two determinants contribute to the exposure factors used: **compressed breast thickness** and **tissue density.** The breast size or thickness is easy to determine, but breast density is less obvious and requires additional information unless previous mammograms are available for review.

The relative density of the breast is affected primarily by the patient's inherent breast characteristics (genetics), hormone status, age, and number of pregnancies. The mammary gland undergoes cyclic changes associated with the increase and decrease of hormonal secretions during the menstrual cycle, changes during pregnancy and lactation, and gradual changes that occur throughout a woman's lifetime (Box 20.1).

Generally, breasts can be classified into **three broad categories,** depending on the relative amounts of fibroglandular tissue versus fatty tissue. These categories are the fibroglandular breast, the fibrofatty breast and the fatty breast.

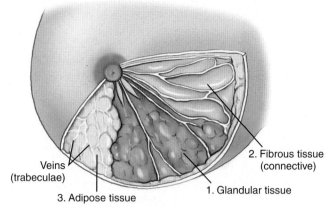

Fig. 20.42 Breast—anterior view (three tissue types).

Veins (trabeculae)
3. Adipose tissue
1. Glandular tissue
2. Fibrous tissue (connective)

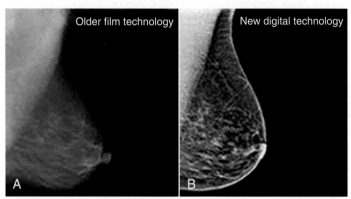

Older film technology | New digital technology

Fig. 20.43 Analog (film-screen) (A) versus digital mammography (B). (Courtesy Hologic, Inc., Bedford, MA.)

BOX 20.1 SUMMARY OF BREAST CLASSIFICATIONS

FIBROGLANDULAR BREAST
- Common age group: 15 to 30 years (and childless women >30 years old)
- Pregnant or lactating women
- Radiographically dense
- Very little fat

FIBROFATTY BREAST
- Common age group: 30 to 50 years
- Young women with three or more pregnancies
- Average radiographic density
- 50% fat and 50% fibroglandular

FATTY BREAST
- Common age group: ≥50 years
- Postmenopausal
- Minimal radiographic density
- Breasts of children and men

FIBROGLANDULAR BREAST

The first category is the fibroglandular breast. The breast of a young woman normally is quite dense because it contains relatively little fatty tissue. The common age group for the fibroglandular category is post puberty to about 30 years old. However, women older than age 30 who have never been pregnant or given birth to a live infant usually fit into this category. Pregnant, prepregnancy, and lactating women of any age also may be placed in this category because their breast tissue is very dense during this time (Fig. 20.44). In addition, genetics can play a part in this tissue type. A technologist may find fibroglandular tissue in a patient beyond menopause, so age is not the sole determining factor. Technologists need to understand that this type of breast tissue, because of its glandular nature, can make breast compression very uncomfortable for the patient.

FIBROFATTY BREAST

The second general category is the fibrofatty breast. As a woman ages and changes in breast tissue continue to occur, the low amount of fatty tissue gradually shifts to a more equal distribution of fat and fibroglandular tissue. In women 30 to 50 years old, the breast is usually not quite as dense as in younger women.

Radiographically, the breast tissue of women in this age group is of average density and requires less exposure than fibroglandular breast tissue. Because of the more equal distribution of fatty tissue and glandular tissue ("50-50" breast), fibrofatty breast tissue produces better radiographic contrast than either very glandular breast tissue or fatty breast tissue.

Several pregnancies early in a woman's reproductive life accelerate the conversion of her breast tissue to this fibrofatty category (Fig. 20.45).

FATTY BREAST

The third category is the fatty breast, which generally occurs after menopause, commonly in women 50 years of age or older. After a woman's ability to reproduce has ended, most glandular breast tissue is converted to fatty tissue in a process called *involution*. This type of breast tissue is compressed easily, requiring less exposure (Fig. 20.46).

The breast tissue of children and most men contains mostly fat in small proportions and falls into the fatty breast category. Although most mammograms are performed on women, 1% to 2% of all breast cancers are found in men. Mammograms are occasionally performed on men for diagnostic purposes. A notable difference when the male breast is imaged is that male breast tissue does not have the same mobility as female breast tissue. Please note that compression can be just as uncomfortable for a male patient as for a female patient.

SUMMARY

In addition to breast size or thickness on compression, the density of breast tissue determines exposure factors. The densest breast tissue is the **fibroglandular** type. The least dense breast tissue is the **fatty** type. A breast with more or less equal amounts of fatty and fibroglandular tissue is termed **fibrofatty.**

Breast density is one of the strongest risk factors associated with breast cancer, and it also makes cancer diagnosis the most challenging. Although there is no national standard for disclosing breast density to women undergoing mammography, in 2019 the FDA proposed an amendment to the MQSA, moving the notification movement in the right direction. The movement began in 2009 in Connecticut, where the first density reporting law was enacted. Since then 38 states have followed suit by enacting density-reporting legislature. Federal advocacy groups are currently involved in these educational efforts. In February, 2015, bills were reintroduced into Congress as the Breast Density and Mammography

Reporting Act of 2015. The most recent recommendation will help address varied reporting disparities among states, requiring consistent reporting from mammography facilities. Patients across the nation will be provided with a report informing them of their personal breast density assessment.[14]

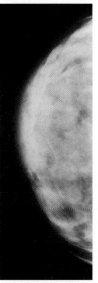

Fig. 20.44 Fibroglandular breast (younger or prepregnancy).

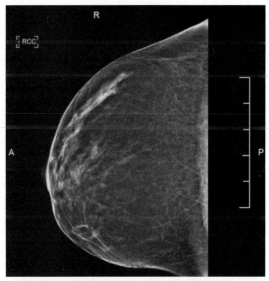

Fig. 20.45 Fibrofatty breast.

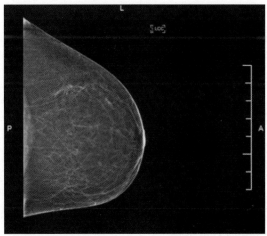

Fig. 20.46 Fatty breast (68-year-old woman).

RADIOGRAPHIC POSITIONING

Positioning And Technical Considerations
PATIENT PREPARATION

Before the mammography examination begins, the technologist asks the patient to put on a gown (preferably one designed for mammography), which allows exposure of only the breast that is being examined. The patient is instructed to remove any jewelry, talcum powder, or deodorant/antiperspirant that may cause artifacts on the radiographic image. Certain lotions, especially lotions with sparkles or glitter, can also cause artifacts on the image.

The technologist explains the procedure and documents any relevant patient history per departmental protocol. Generally, the patient history includes the following:

- Number of pregnancies and live births
- Family history of cancer, including breast cancer (relationship of relative)
- Medications (e.g., hormone therapy) currently taken
- Previous breast surgery
- Previous mammograms, when and where performed, possibly other prior breast imaging studies
- Reason for current visit, such as screening mammogram, lumps, pain, or discharge

The mammographer also should note the location of any scars, palpable masses, moles, warts, and tattoos.

BREAST POSITIONING

In mammography, the patient's tissue type, the shape and contour of the breast, and the patient's individual tolerance for the examination can pose challenges to the mammographer who is striving to produce the highest quality diagnostic images for interpretation.

The **base** of the breast is the portion near the chest wall, and the area near the nipple is termed the **apex**. In either the craniocaudal (CC) or the mediolateral (ML) projection, the base of the breast is much thicker and contains denser tissues than are found at the apex. To overcome this normal anatomic difference found in the breast, a compression device is used in combination with a specially designed tube so that the more intense central ray (CR) of the x-ray beam penetrates the thicker base of the breast.

X-RAY TUBE

The most distinctive aspect of the mammography machine is the unique design of the x-ray tube, which has a **molybdenum target** with small focal spots of **0.3 and 0.1 mm. Rhodium** also has been introduced as an optional anode material. The focal spots must be of this smaller size because of the microscopic size of cancer calcifications, which typically measure less than 1 mm.

The anode configuration produces a **prominent heel effect**, which results from the short source to image receptor distance (SID) and the use of a narrow reference target angle. Mammography units are manufactured so the x-ray tube is aligned with the cathode placed over the base of the breast (at the chest wall) and the anode outward toward the apex (nipple area); in this way, the heel effect can be used to maximum advantage (Fig. 20.47). The cathode side of the x-ray beam has a significantly greater intensity of x-rays compared with the anode side; this assists in the creation of a breast image with more uniform density because the more intense x-rays arrive at the base, where tissue thickness is greater.

Most mammographic units use grids, automatic exposure control (AEC), and the important breast compression device.

AEC chamber selection

The AEC chambers on most mammographic systems are adjustable in up to 10 positions from the chest wall to the nipple region.

Generally, for a blind examination (prior images are unavailable for preview), to ensure adequate exposure of the more dense or thick tissues, the **chamber under the chest wall** or the **denser tissue area** should be selected. Exceptions include special projections, such as magnification and spot compression views, for which the chamber would be placed directly under the region of interest.

Generally, selection of the AEC chamber position depends on tissue density or the region of interest. For example, in Fig. 20.48 the breast tissue is denser toward the nipple, and in this case, the detector would be positioned posterior to the nipple rather than the chest wall to ensure adequate exposure.

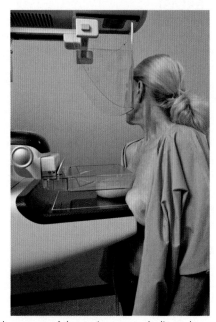

Fig. 20.47 Placement of the patient on a dedicated mammography unit for CC projection. *Note:* Vertical CR is placed directly over the chest wall structures, which allows the posterosuperior breast structures to be imaged.

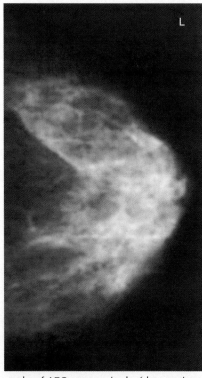

Fig. 20.48 Example of AEC nearer nipple (denser tissue area). (Courtesy Hologic, Inc., Bedford, MA.)

Compression[15]

All mammographic systems contain a compression device that is used to even out the thickness of the breast tissue. Improvements in breast compression technology in recent years have greatly enhanced the visibility of detail in breast images. The compression device is made of plastic, which allows transmission of low-energy x-rays. The device should have a straight edge that allows the compression to grasp the breast tissues close to the chest wall. Compression is controlled by the technologist and typically is applied at **15 to 30 pounds of pressure, although up to 40 pounds of pressure is allowable.** Slow, steady application allows the patient time to adjust to the sensation and generally allows application of adequate compression. It is important to keep visual contact with the patient during application of compression so that assessment of her or his comfort level is possible. Gentle, verbal encouragement from the technologist usually leads to the desired results.

In addition to the standard compression device, a smaller "spot" compression paddle may be used to better visualize a possible lesion or region of superimposition of tissue that might be obscuring a pathologic condition. All compression devices should be checked regularly to ensure they are working properly and applying the correct amount of pressure. This is part of the MQSA regimen.

Appropriately applied compression is a critical component of the production of a high-quality mammogram. **Six reasons for the use of compression** are as follows:

1. To decrease the thickness of the breast and make it more uniform
2. To bring the breast structures as close to the image receptor (IR) as possible
3. To decrease the dose needed and the amount of scattered radiation
4. To decrease motion and increase geometric sharpness
5. To increase contrast by allowing a decrease in exposure factors and dose
6. To separate breast structures that may be superimposed

These six factors allow improved image quality or resolution by reducing scatter and by reducing magnification of breast structures. The drawings in Fig. 20.49 compare uncompressed and compressed tissue states. Note the location of the microcalcifications and the lesion surrounded by dense breast tissue illustrated in Fig. 20.49A, and how compression brings them closer to the IR and in a parallel plane with the IR (Fig. 20.49B). Overall breast thickness has also been greatly reduced, which reduces the ratio of scatter to primary radiation by 50%. Geometric sharpness has been preserved in that the CR now is perpendicular to the breast structures. In addition, had there been any superimposed structures, the compression would have brought them into a more side-by-side alignment.

MAGNIFICATION

Magnification mammography (Fig. 20.50) is used to enlarge specific areas of interest, such as small lesions or microcalcifications. An x-ray tube with a **0.1-mm focal spot** is required to maintain image resolution. Magnification of up to ×2 can be attained by inserting a specially constructed magnification platform between the IR and the breast, magnifying the part through an **increased object to image receptor distance (OID).** A well-trained, skilled mammographer can use this magnification technique with all mammographic projections to visualize better or rule out potential breast pathologic changes.

PATIENT DOSE

Mammography is soft tissue imaging for an inherently low-contrast anatomic structure. It is the objective of every mammographer to produce a high-quality image that best demonstrates breast anatomy and any signs of existing disease without any unnecessary radiation. The dose to the breast of an individual patient is determined by a combination of three factors: (1) the characteristics of the equipment being used, (2) the technique factors selected for the examination, and (3) the size and density of the patient's breasts. The dose unit most referenced in mammographic imaging is that of **mean glandular dose (MGD),** which would be the average dose to the patient's glandular tissue, considered to be the most sensitive to the effects of radiation.

Digital imaging is replacing analog imaging in mammography. Some advantages of digital over film-screen mammography are:
- Information is quickly available on the screen for making a diagnosis.
- Information can be transmitted electronically to others and images can be printed on films as necessary.
- Digital units provide the ability to localize small lesions and guide the radiologist during biopsy.
- Image storage is easier and less bulky, and access is much quicker.
- Digital imaging also has the potential to reduce patient doses because there may be fewer repeat images and higher kVp levels may be used (reducing MGD) without affecting the quality of the image.
- Chemical processing is not required to produce the images, and this reduces the environmental impact because there are no waste chemicals.[16]

The principal way in which patient dose is controlled in mammography is by careful and accurate positioning, which minimizes the need for repeat exposures. The ACR recommends a repeat rate of **less than 5%** for mammography. The only shielding possible is a waist apron that is used to shield the gonadal region. Although generally thought to be unnecessary, a thyroid shield could also be used to protect the thyroid region, but the technologist must be very careful in its placement to ensure it does not accidentally obscure any chest wall anatomy, causing a repeat projection to be necessary.

ANALOG (FILM-SCREEN) MAMMOGRAPHY

Film-screen mammography continues to be the standard in current breast imaging. The greatest benefit of the film-screen system,

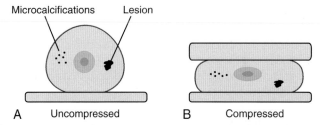

Fig. 20.49 Effects of breast compression. A, Decreased tissue thickness (less scatter, better resolution). B, breast structures closer to IR.

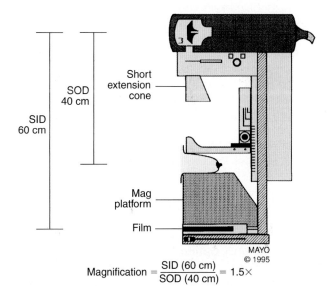

$$\text{Magnification} = \frac{\text{SID (60 cm)}}{\text{SOD (40 cm)}} = 1.5\times$$

Fig. 20.50 Magnification—breast in position on a raised platform to produce a 1.5× magnification image. *SOD,* source to object distance. (Courtesy Mayo Foundation.)

excellent image quality with a low radiation dose, allows women to undergo this examination as needed with less worry. The ability to see fine detail, edge sharpness, and soft tissue is a hallmark of a good film-screen mammogram. However, digital mammography (computed radiography or digital radiography [DR]) is developing rapidly and, as in all digital imaging, has certain distinct advantages over film-screen mammography, as previously mentioned.

Digital Mammography

One challenge of mammography comes from the similarity in the x-ray attenuation of normal breast tissue and cancerous breast tissue. To maximize contrast in film-screen mammography, a low kVp is commonly used, which increases the patient dose. In digital mammography, the film-screen system is replaced by a detector, which produces an electronic signal and uses reconstruction algorithms. Digital mammography can use a higher kVp level, thus reducing the absorbing dose to the patient.[17]

DIGITAL VERSUS ANALOG (FILM-SCREEN) MAMMOGRAPHY

Although contrast resolution is outstanding with a digital system, the overall spatial resolution of the digital image currently may still fall slightly short of the analog system. As a result, radiologists may not be as confident about detecting microcalcifications and tissue changes in the breast when examining a digital breast image. However, improvements in detector technology and monitor design have made this concern almost negligible. In addition, post-processing features, such as magnification (all or part of the image), edge enhancement, image reversal (reversal of black to white), and adjustment of image contrast and brightness, can be applied to enhance specific mammographic images and improve their diagnostic quality.

COMPUTED RADIOGRAPHY MAMMOGRAPHY

Computed radiography can be used for mammography in much the same way as it is used in general radiography with its image plate and image processor, as described in Chapter 1. Computed radiography cassettes containing imaging plates can be used in most existing mammographic systems. Advantages of computed radiography mammography include operating costs, telemammography, archiving and picture archiving and communication system (PACS) options, and image manipulation.

Operating Costs

Computed radiography imaging plates can be exposed many times before they have to be replaced. Given the cost of film and expenses associated with chemical (wet) processing, the use of computed radiography is more economical.

Telemammography

In communities where expertise in breast imaging interpretation is lacking, the ability to send images to another location where such expertise exists is very beneficial. In another scenario, a patient may have moved since her previous study was taken and does not have images from her previous study at the time of her present examination. Digital mammography provides the ideal solution to this problem. As a result of the Digital Imaging and Communications in Medicine (DICOM) standard (see Chapter 1), which includes a specialized module for digital mammography, it is convenient today to transmit images from a digital mammography system to a remote diagnostic workstation for interpretation.

Archiving and PACS Options

After images have been interpreted, they can be stored electronically at any desired location using PACS (see Chapter 1). The necessity of physical storage space for hard-copy films is eliminated because mammographic images are incorporated into existing PACS. Depending on the specifications of the PACS in use, outside referring health care providers may have access to these images from their offices. This is convenient for both the patient and the health care provider because the images are readily available and do not require duplication, transport, or the possibility of permanent loss or damage.

Image Manipulation

Computed radiography mammography and digital mammography allow for post-processing image manipulation. Image manipulation can reduce the number of repeat images taken, provided that correct exposure factors and positioning techniques were used. Fewer repeats lead to lower radiation dose and less discomfort for the patient.

MAMMOGRAPHY WORKSTATION

A digital mammography unit workstation is a second form of digital imaging that continues to be refined and developed and is now commonly used in mammography, especially in metropolitan areas. These mammographic systems contain a flat panel detector that is permanently mounted on the x-ray unit (Fig. 20.51). Comparison studies have shown that newer digital mammographic systems have improved contrast resolution while providing reductions in patient dose compared with film-screen imaging. The flat panel detector captures the remnant x-rays and produces a digital image. The digital image is projected onto a monitor at the technologist's workstation for direct viewing and post-processing as needed (Fig. 20.52). As in all digital imaging, the incorporation of algorithms in digital mammography allows the technologist to use a higher kVp technique without compromising the image contrast. The increased kVp level also reduces the overall dose to the patient and allows exceptional imaging of the dense breast compared with film-screen.

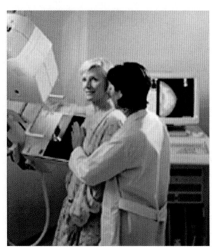

Fig. 20.51 Digital mammography unit. (Courtesy GE Medical Systems.)

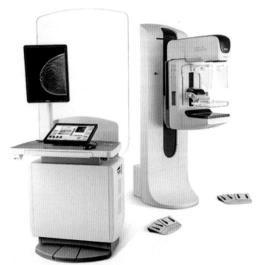

Fig. 20.52 Digital mammography unit workstation for direct viewing and post-processing options. (Courtesy Hologic Inc., Bedford, MA.)

CONTRAST MAMMOGRAPHY[18]

The clinical benefit of mammography lies in the ability to identify cancers through their differing absorption of x-rays with respect to the surrounding tissue. In mammography, the majority of cancers appear white, which is also the appearance of normal glandular tissue. Herein lies the challenge and the dilemma, and even more so in the dense breast.

In other radiographic procedures, the use of a contrast agent often enhances the ability to make an accurate diagnosis of a pathologic condition. It is anticipated that contrast media will be used in breast imaging.

Contrast mammography is the imaging of the breast using an iodinated contrast agent (Fig. 20.53). It is referred to as contrast-enhanced (CE) imaging and uses the same contrast agents as those for CT studies.

Tumors need a blood supply and cell multiplication (capillary growth) to deliver the blood to the needed area. Contrast in mammography has been shown to be useful because a contrast medium will accumulate in lesions that are metabolically active. Therefore, it complements the morphologic image acquired during imaging. In addition, the contrast agent is unaffected by dense breast tissue, so its use is extremely beneficial in patients with dense breast tissue, particularly when an area of possible malignancy is visualized.

Contrast-enhanced breast imaging is complicated and requires dual-energy imaging because only a very small dose of iodine is intravenously administered. The low energy level (28 to 33 kVp) is for the breast tissue imaging, and the higher energy level (45 to 49 kVp) is for the contrast agent. The final image is a subtraction of the two images, which removes the breast parenchyma and adipose tissue and leaves an image that demonstrates the distribution of the iodine within the breast.

Contrast-enhanced mammography is used as an alternative imaging option once a possible lesion has been identified on mammography or sonography. The criteria are similar to those for MRI breast imaging:

- Evaluate a breast difficult to diagnose with standard mammography
- Identify potential undetected malignancies
- Image patients who have contraindications to MRI breast imaging
- Monitor the effectiveness of treatments
- Evaluate the extent of disease identified

COMPUTER-AIDED DETECTION SYSTEMS

The computer continues to be used as one of the "second readers" in mammographic interpretation. Computer-aided detection (CAD) technology has had a dramatic impact on the diagnosis of breast cancer. CAD systems use computerized detection algorithms to analyze digital or digitized images for possible lesions, abnormal calcifications, and parenchymal distortions. Certain studies have shown that using a second reader to interpret screening mammographic images improves the cancer detection rate by 5% to 15%. However, CAD does not detect all cancers, and it should not be used as a primary evaluator of screening mammograms.[19]

CAD devices are advantageous in that they do not get fatigued or distracted, and they do not demonstrate intraobserver variation. Clusters of microcalcifications are a good example of objects appropriate for CAD viewing because they differ from normal anatomic structures in density, shape, and size. Detection and classification of microcalcifications and borders of lesions are possible with CAD systems. Some studies show improvement in microcalcification detection rates. The use of CAD systems is increasing because many insurance plans cover this extra expense, but they are not expected to replace the radiologist. The CAD report alerts the radiologist to a region of interest in which a possible lesion may be present. The radiologist decides whether the area is worrisome or requires follow up.[20]

Alternative Modalities and Procedures
SONOGRAPHY (ULTRASOUND)

Sonography has been used to image the breast since the mid-1970s. Along with the film-screen mammogram and physical examination, a sonogram provides valuable adjunct information for the radiologist. Sonography is an integral part of the breast imaging department. Its major value is its ability to **distinguish between a cyst and a solid lesion** (Fig. 20.54). It also is used extensively to reveal fluid, abscess, hematoma, and silicone gel. Ultrasound has the ability to find cancers in women with dense breasts in whom lesions may be hidden radiographically. Through the American Society of Radiologic Technologists (ASRT), mammographers now find breast ultrasound within their scope of practice once proper educational and hands-on training has been attained. Image quality depends heavily on sonographer expertise.

Conventional Scanner and Handheld Transducer

When a high-resolution conventional scanner (Fig. 20.55) is used, the patient is positioned supine or is rolled slightly onto one side. The handheld transducer is placed on a palpable mass or on an area noted on a mammographic image.

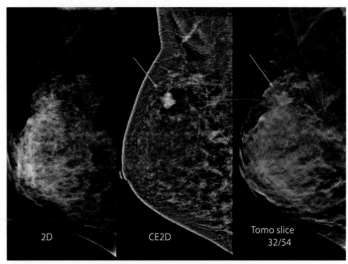

Fig. 20.53 Contrast-enhanced mammography. *Left,* 2D image MLO. *Center,* Contrast-enhanced 2D image MLO. *Right,* 3D image MLO. (Courtesy Hologic, Inc., Bedford, MA.)

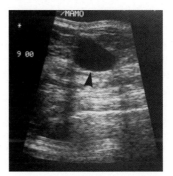

Fig. 20.54 Breast sonogram obtained with conventional scanner showing a cyst *(arrowhead).*

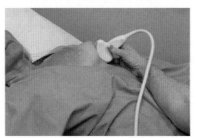

Fig. 20.55 Conventional ultrasound scanner with handheld transducer.

NUCLEAR MEDICINE (NM)

Nuclear medicine also plays a role in breast disease diagnosis and may be a valuable adjunct examination to the mammogram. Nuclear breast imaging refers to functional imaging of the breast using radiopharmaceuticals. According to a 2010 article by Ferrara in the ASRT journal *Radiologic Technology,* "the radiopharmaceuticals do not change normal physiological processes, but rather allow the clinicians to visualize them."[21] Functional imaging can demonstrate alterations in cell metabolism that occur as a result of malignancies and can often identify a disease process earlier than anatomic imaging.

Nuclear medicine procedures used for imaging breast pathologic conditions include the following:

- **Scintimammography (sestamibi)** may be helpful in confirming a breast cancer diagnosis. ^{99m}Tc sestamibi, a radionuclide, is injected as a tracer into the arm opposite the affected breast; breast imaging begins 10 minutes later. This procedure has fallen slightly out of favor because of the high number of false-positive results. The distance from the detector to the breast being imaged has also made this modality unreliable for any lesion smaller than ½ inch (1 cm).
- **Sentinel node studies** are useful for patients with melanoma, and they are becoming increasingly useful for detection of breast cancer. This procedure involves injecting sulfur colloid around the lesion subcutaneously. (Patients must have undergone a localization procedure previously.) The flow is followed through the lymph vessels to localize the sentinel node. In surgery, once identified, the sentinel node is removed and sent to the laboratory for assessment of the possibility of metastasis. Results determine the treatment path to be taken.

POSITRON EMISSION TOMOGRAPHY (PET) MAMMOGRAPHY

PET mammography is a very specific modification of positron emission tomography. Although it is a new breast imaging modality, it is approved by the FDA for imaging patients who have a known history of breast cancer. In contrast to scintimammography, PET mammography places the detectors very near the breast. This imaging procedure uses the tracer ^{18}F-FDG, approximately 10 mCi, and a scan time of about 10 minutes per projection; the same projections taken for a routine mammogram are obtained. Because PET mammography uses a compression device, it can detect lesions as small as 1.5 mm, which is far smaller than lesions detectable by conventional PET scans. The PET mammography compression device is solely for reducing the likelihood of motion from the patient and providing a more accurate reading. In contrast to mammographic compression, it is not used to thin the breast tissue.

PET has proven to be a very important tool in monitoring the treatment response of patients undergoing cancer treatments and is still considered unequaled in whole-body staging of breast cancer.

Tumor cells have an increased metabolic rate. This increased metabolism uses sugar, and the ^{18}F-FDG tracer molecules are taken up by the tumor at a greater rate compared with normal breast tissue, making the location of the cancer visible with PET mammography and PET. PET also is used after surgery or treatment for breast cancer to determine whether recurrent disease is present in the breast or in other parts of the body. PET can quantify the metabolic activity of the tumor site to assist in assessing the effectiveness of therapy both during and after treatment, allowing for rapid alterations of treatment when needed.

Two disadvantages of using PET for breast imaging are **higher cost** and **radiation exposure.** Although PET has certain valuable applications for early detection of breast disease (and restaging of breast cancer), the cost of the equipment required and the use of radioactive tracers with a short half-life make the use of PET impractical as a screening tool. Radiation exposure from the ^{18}F-FDG tracer is approximately six times greater than the exposure from a ^{99m}Tc sestamibi study as used in nuclear medicine.

BREAST-SPECIFIC GAMMA IMAGING

Breast-specific gamma imaging (BSGI) is a new technology that is often referred to as "molecular breast imaging" (MBI) and is considered the newer version of scintimammography. Similar to scintimammography, BSGI uses sestamibi as its imaging agent. The biggest difference is that compared to scintimammography, the gamma camera for BSGI is much smaller and much closer to the patient's breast and the source of radiation.

BSGI imaging uses a small single or dual-headed gamma camera. Units have a compression plate, and the breast is placed between the detector and the plate for imaging. BSGI is considered a functional study because the images capture the activity of breast tissue and cells. BSGI is complementary to traditional mammography, not a substitute.

Studies of these new modalities continue, with the focus being the specificity and sensitivity of each modality in finding breast cancer at its earliest stage. If trials validate the new advances in functional imaging of the breast, nuclear breast imaging will play a much larger role in the diagnosis of breast cancer.

MAGNETIC RESONANCE IMAGING (MRI)

MRI has proven to be an important adjunct screening tool for breast imaging (Fig. 20.56). The number of breast MRI scans performed in the United States is increasing annually. Although its cost makes it prohibitive for general clinical use, MRI has been clinically proven to be effective for certain special applications such as the following:

- Palpable masses not seen with mammography or ultrasound
- Assessment of lesions in extremely dense, glandular breast tissue
- Possible screening of a young woman at very high risk for breast cancer because of familial history or women who carry the *BRCA1* and *BRCA2* genes (the *BRCA1* and *BRCA2* genes were identified by geneticists in 1994 and are associated with a greater risk of developing breast, *ovar*ian, *and t*esticular *cancers*)
- Staging of breast cancer (locating additional areas of malignancy not imaged initially)
- Assessment of leakage from silicone breast implants (Figs. 20.57 and 20.58)

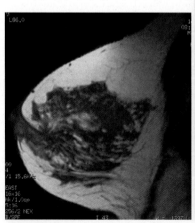
Fig. 20.56 T1-weighted MRI image of dense breast.

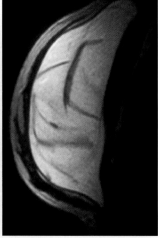
Fig. 20.57 MRI image—normal silicone implant.

Advantages of MRI

One advantage of MRI is that it can **show the whole breast maximally** with greater comfort for the patient. Also, more recent work with contrast agents indicates that MRI can show evidence of **vascularization of lesions.** It provides better sensitivity and specificity than ultrasound and x-ray mammography.

MRI allows the diagnostician to view all body structures, including soft tissue, which proves valuable in the early discovery of cancers and in the staging of existing disease such as breast cancer. The 3D capabilities of MRI yield valuable information about the cancer itself, especially in the dynamic contrast-enhanced image.

Breast Implants

More than 300,000 breast augmentations (surgical implants) are performed each year in the United States. Silicone and saline implants are radiopaque and, depending on their placement within the breast, can obscure the breast tissue and any existing disease. Mammograms can be performed on patients with implants. In order to obtain mammogram images, the mammographer obtains implant displaced (ID) views (via the Eklund method).These views are *in addition* to routine mammogram images. Although rupture or damage to the implant is highly unlikely, compression for patients with implants requires careful assessment and application by the mammographer.

The compression used for views with the implant in place should be firm enough to control movement of the implant so that the integrity of the implant can be adequately visualized but without the amount of compression applied to the displaced implant tissue. These nondisplaced views are *not* used for breast tissue evaluation. AEC cannot be used with augmented breast (nondisplaced) views. Implants come in all sizes, therefore the mammographer must be knowledgeable about manual techniques related to breast thickness to avoid repeating an image. These factors make imaging of breast tissue with implants a challenge.

MRI has been clinically proven to be most effective in diagnosing problems related to breast implant imaging. With MRI, it is possible to evaluate potential intracapsular and extracapsular rupture, including the area posterior to the implant, which can be very problematic with mammographic or sonographic studies. The MRI images in Figs. 20.58 and 20.59 clearly demonstrate intracapsular and extracapsular rupture of silicone implants.

In addition to detecting implant rupture, it is important to demonstrate the breast tissue surrounding and posterior to the implants for possible malignant growth. Physical examination is more difficult with implants, which also increases the risk for cancer growth without detection. In contrast to mammography or sonography, MRI is not hindered by the presence of an implant.

Clinical testing is being done with a new kind of radiolucent implant that would allow more effective use of film-screen mammography, including the use of AECs. However, the more than 2 million women with radiopaque implants, many of whom are nearing the life expectancy limits of their implants, will require continued evaluation of their breast implants for possible rupture or other related problems. This increases the potential role of MRI in breast implant imaging.

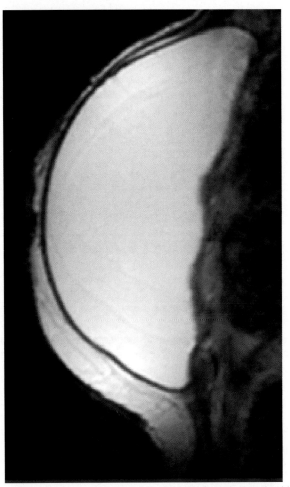

Fig. 20.58 MRI image—intracapsular rupture (silicone contained by fibrous capsule).

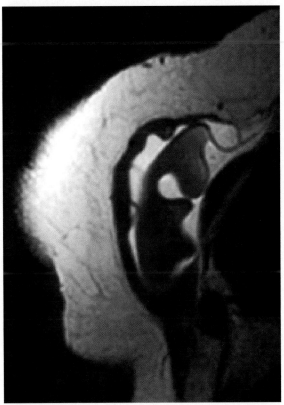

Fig. 20.59 MRI image—saline component inside, silicone outside.

Disadvantages of MRI

The primary disadvantages of MRI are its **high false-positive rate, high costs,** and **length of the examination itself,** all of which limit its use as a breast screening procedure. However, research and clinical use continue as MRI is beginning to play a larger role in the diagnostic workup for breast lesions. Additionally, not all patients are candidates for an MRI. Patients must undergo a strict screening process to determine if they are MRI eligible.

DIGITAL BREAST TOMOSYNTHESIS

Digital breast tomosynthesis (DBT) (Fig. 20.60), also known as 3D mammography imaging, represents the marriage of traditional 2D mammography and the latest technology in full-field digital mammography (FFDM). Digital breast tomosynthesis is a screening and diagnostic modality that acquires images of a breast at multiple angles during a short scan (Fig. 20.61). The individual images are then reconstructed into a series of thin, high-resolution slices typically 1-mm thick, which can be displayed individually or in a dynamic ciné mode.

A tomosynthesis data set virtually eliminates detection challenges associated with overlapping structures in the breast, which is the primary drawback of conventional 2D analog and digital mammography (Fig. 20.62). In addition, breast tomosynthesis offers other potential benefits, including increased lesion and margin visibility, help in localizing structures in the breast, a reduction in recall rates, and increased cancer detection.

Developers of this technology believe eventually it may replace both analog (film-screen) mammography and FFDM. However, DBT and FFDM can be cost prohibitive for screening purposes, with costs of approximately $400,000 per unit for FFDM and $700,000 per system for DBT.

Pathologic Indications

Screening mammography is important for the early detection of pathologic changes in the breast. These changes can be either benign (noncancerous) or malignant (cancerous). The ACR Breast Imaging Reporting and Data Systems (BI-RADS) defines a breast mass as a 3D space-occupying lesion seen on at least two mammographic images. Benign masses do not invade the surrounding tissue. Malignant masses extend through the basement membrane and invade the surrounding glandular tissue. These determinations are based on their imaging characteristics and histology. The most common benign and malignant pathologic findings in the breast are discussed in the following sections.

BREAST CARCINOMA (CANCER)

Carcinoma of the breast is divided into two categories, **noninvasive** and **invasive.** Noninvasive carcinoma is a distinct lesion of the breast that has the potential to become invasive cancer. These lesions are restricted to the glandular lumen and do not have access to the lymphatic system or blood vessels. Noninvasive cancer also may be termed **in situ. Ductal carcinoma in situ** is isolated within the breast duct and has not spread to other areas of the breast. **Lobular carcinoma in situ** consists of abnormal cells that have been detected in one or more lobes of the breast. Noninvasive cancers (ductal carcinoma in situ and lobular carcinoma in situ) account for approximately 15% to 20% of all breast cancer diagnoses.

The most common form of breast cancer is invasive or infiltrating ductal carcinoma. This type accounts for approximately 80% of all breast cancer diagnoses. Invasive cancer is believed to arise in the terminal duct lobular unit. This form of cancer is found in both the female and the male breast (Fig. 20.63). Most of these cancers cannot be specified without histologic evaluation. Invasive cancer of the breast carries the worst overall prognosis of the invasive cancers.

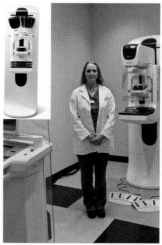

Fig. 20.60 Hologic 3D breast tomosynthesis system. (Courtesy SimonMed Imaging, Scottsdale, AZ. courtesy Hologic, Inc., Bedford, MA.)

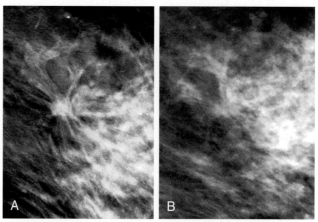

Fig. 20.61 A, DBT image. B, Same region of breast without the use of DBT. (Courtesy Mary Carrillo.Obtained through Aunt Minnie.)

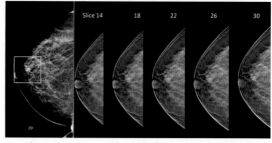

Fig. 20.62 The 2D image on the left shows a potential lesion in the subareolar region of the breast. However, the 3D breast tomosynthesis image on the right shows that in fact there is no lesion present. Individual structures can be picked out on the separate slices, which summate to form the potential lesion seen on the 2D projection image. (Courtesy Hologic Inc. Bedford, MA.)

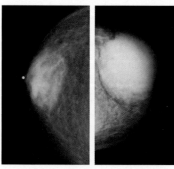

Fig. 20.63 Invasive ductal cancer in a male patient. (Modified from Ikeda DM: *Breast imaging*, St. Louis, 2005, Mosby.)

CYSTS

Cysts are **fluid-filled sacs** that are **benign** and appear as well-circumscribed masses. Their density is usually that of the surrounding tissue; however, they may appear denser. In some cases, high concentrations of calcium particles may be suspended within the cyst fluid. This condition is known as *milk of calcium*.[22] A 90° lateral projection of the breast assists in determining milk of calcium versus other, more worrisome calcium formations because milk of calcium particles layer out in the 90° lateral projection. For positive diagnosis of a cyst, ultrasonography and needle biopsies are required.

FIBROADENOMA

Fibroadenomas are the most common **benign,** solid lumps or tumors composed of fibrous and glandular tissue. They are well-circumscribed lesions with clearly defined edges that may be felt during palpation. They typically have the same density as the surrounding tissue. The mass is an overgrowth of fibrous tissue of the breast lobule.[23]

FIBROCYSTIC CHANGES

Fibrocystic changes constitute a common, benign condition that is usually bilateral and occurs in premenopausal women. It includes a variety of conditions; the most obvious are fibrosis and cystic dilation of ducts. Multiple cysts with increased fibrous tissue commonly are distributed throughout the breasts.

GYNECOMASTIA

The term *gynecomastia* is derived from a Greek term meaning "woman-like breasts." In this benign condition of the male breast, a benign glandular enlargement of the breast occurs. Gynecomastia may be unilateral or bilateral but seems to be more pronounced in one breast. It typically manifests as a palpable mass near the nipple (Fig. 20.64).

INTRADUCTAL PAPILLOMA

An intraductal papilloma is a small growth that occurs inside the duct of the breast near the nipple. Symptoms may include spontaneous, unilateral nipple discharge that may be bloody to clear in color. The mammographic appearance is typically normal. Performing galactography or ductography, a contrast-enhanced procedure, to visualize the ducts can reveal a filling defect that would indicate the presence of an intraductal papilloma. Cannulation of the duct in question can be problematic, however, and these examinations are not always successful. Sonography of the breast may be helpful for this condition. Papillomas are usually removed to exclude ductal carcinoma in situ or papillary cancer.

PAGET DISEASE OF THE NIPPLE

Paget disease of the nipple first appears as a crusty or scaly nipple sore or as a discharge from the nipple. Slightly more than half of patients who have this cancer also have a lump in the breast. Paget disease may be invasive or noninvasive.

Many more pathologic conditions of the breast exist. The aforementioned are simply a few of the most commonly diagnosed conditions.

Mammography Terminology

Certain positioning terminology used in mammography must be understood and used correctly. These terms and their abbreviations are used to identify images and serve as standard nomenclature, as approved by the ACR in October, 1995 (Table 20.1). It is important to use these **terms** and **abbreviations** correctly when applying for ACR accreditation.

Routine And Special Projections

Routine and special projections that are commonly performed in most mammography departments can be found on the following pages.

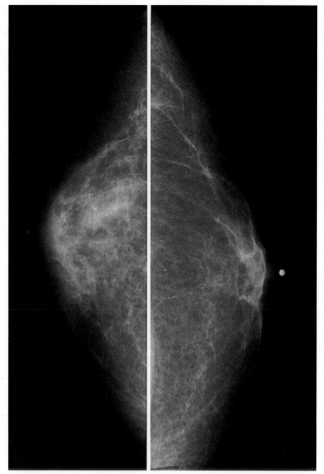

Fig. 20.64 Diffuse gynecomastia in the male breast. (Modified from Ikeda DM: *Breast imaging*, St. Louis, 2005, Mosby.)

TABLE 20.1 MAMMOGRAPHY TERMINOLOGY

ACR NOMENCLATURE	DESCRIPTION
AT	Axillary tail view: Mediolateral 20° to 30° oblique projection
AX	Axillary view: For lymph nodes and other axillary content
CC	Craniocaudal: Basic superior-to-inferior projection
CV	Cleavage view: Double breast compression view (demonstrates breast tissue anterior to sternum and medial aspects of both breasts)
FB	Caudocranial, from below (sometimes in practice also abbreviated as CCFB)
ID	Implant displaced: Eklund method views for augmented breast
LM	Lateromedial projection
LMO[a]	Lateromedial oblique (inferolateral-superomedial): Often used with pacemaker patients (true reverse of MLO)
ML	Mediolateral projection
MLO	Mediolateral oblique (superomedial-inferolateral oblique): Basic oblique
RL[b]	Rolled lateral (superior breast tissue rolled laterally)
RM[b]	Rolled medial (superior breast tissue rolled medially)
SIO[a]	Superolateral-inferomedial oblique: Reverse oblique
TAN	Tangential (also mark image with view [e.g., CC/TAN, MLO/TAN])
XCCL	Exaggerated craniocaudal (laterally): Special CC projection with emphasis on axillary tissue

[a]Image should be marked with any deviation from 0° with *LMO* or *SIO*.
[b]Used as a suffix after projection.
ACR, American College of Radiology.

CRANIOCAUDAL (CC) PROJECTION: MAMMOGRAPHY

Clinical Indications
- Detection or evaluation of calcifications, cysts, carcinomas, or other abnormalities or changes in the breast tissue indicating a possible pathologic condition
- Breasts are imaged separately for comparison.

Technical Factors
- SID—fixed, varies with manufacturer; about 24 inches (60 cm)
- IR size—8 × 10 inches (18 × 24 cm) or 10 × 12 inches (24 × 30 cm), landscape
- Grid
- kVp ranges—analog systems (rare): 23–28; digital systems: 25–45

Shielding Use a waist apron (thyroid shield optional).

Patient Position Erect, if possible

Part Position
- IR height is determined by **lifting the breast** to achieve a 90° angle to the chest wall. The IR is at the level of the **IMF at its upper limits.** (The mammographer should always position from the patient's medial side to ensure that breast tissue is parallel to the IR. Positioning from the lateral aspect of the breast makes tasks more difficult.
- The breast is pulled forward onto the IR centrally with the **nipple in profile whenever possible** (Figs. 20.65 and 20.66).
- The arm on the side that is being imaged is relaxed at the side, and the shoulder is back out of the way.

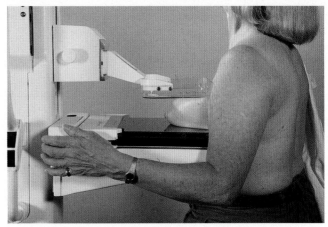

Fig. 20.65 CC projection. (From Long BW, Rollins JH, Smith BJ: *Merrill's atlas of radiographic positioning and procedures,* ed 13, St. Louis, 2016, Mosby.)

- The head is turned away from the side being imaged (facing the technologist).
- Medial tissue of the opposite breast is draped on the corner of the IR.
- Wrinkles and folds on the breast should be smoothed out and compression applied until taut.
- The marker and patient identification information are **always** placed on the **axillary side.**

Positioning Tips

- For patients with a large, protruding abdomen — After placing the patient at the bucky, have the patient take a step backward, keep the feet planted, and then lean forward and place the breast on the IR. This allows all of the breast to reach the IR without blockage from the abdomen.
- Young, small-breasted patients often have tissue that is difficult to image on one projection. To avoid having to do three images (extra dose to the patient), take the first CC image and concentrate on getting the medial tissue; on the second image, make sure the lateral tissue is emphasized. Neither projection should be an exaggerated view. This technique avoids the need to do a straight-on CC and then also having to do both exaggerated views (medial and lateral).

CR

- Perpendicular, centered to the base of the breast, the chest wall edge of the IR; CR not movable

Recommended Collimation Use appropriate cone and collimation.

Respiration Suspend breathing.

NOTE: Position AEC chamber to ensure adequate exposure of the various tissue densities (over the densest part of the breast).

Posterior Nipple Line The posterior nipple line (PNL) is used to evaluate the depth of breast tissue. The PNL is determined by drawing an imaginary line from the nipple to the pectoral muscle or the edge of the image, whichever is the shorter distance. The PNL on a CC projection (Fig. 20.67) should be within about ½ inch (1 cm) of the PNL on an MLO projection (see Fig. 20.71)

Evaluation Criteria

Anatomy Demonstrated • Entire breast tissue should be visualized, including the central, subareolar, and medial breast. • Pectoral muscle should be able to be visualized on 20% to 30% of patients (see Fig. 20.66 and 20.67). • PNL measurement must be within about ½ inch (1 cm) of MLO measurement.

Position and Compression • Nipple is seen in profile. • Tissue thickness is distributed evenly on IR, indicating optimal compression.

NOTE: Nipple marker may be required if nipple cannot be placed in profile.

Collimation and CR • CR and collimation chamber are fixed and are centered correctly if breast tissue is properly centered and visualized on IR.

Exposure • Dense areas are adequately penetrated, resulting in optimal contrast. • Sharp tissue markings indicate **no motion.** • R or L view marker (RCC, LCC) and patient information are correctly placed at axillary side of IR. • **No artifacts** are visible.

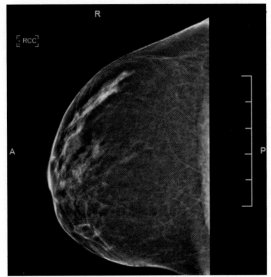

Fig. 20.66 CC projection.

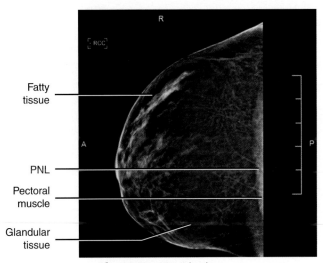

Fig. 20.67 CC projection.

MEDIOLATERAL OBLIQUE (MLO) PROJECTION: MAMMOGRAPHY

SUPEROMEDIAL-INFEROLATERAL OBLIQUE

Clinical Indications

- Detection or evaluation of calcifications, cysts, carcinomas, and other abnormalities or changes in the deep lateral aspect of breast tissue
- Breasts are imaged separately for comparison.

Technical Factors

- SID—fixed, varies with manufacturer; about 24 inches (60 cm)
- IR size—8 × 10 inches (18 × 24 cm) or 10 × 12 inches (24 × 30 cm), landscape
- Grid
- kVp ranges: analog systems (rare): 23–28; digital systems: 25–35

Shielding Use a waist apron (thyroid shield optional).

Patient Position Erect, if possible

Part Position ⊞

- Tube and IR remain at right angles to each other; CR enters the breast **medially,** perpendicular to the patient's pectoral muscle. Proper assessment as to the angle of the pectoral muscle on the patient's chest wall is a must if the image is going to demonstrate the maximum amount of breast tissue. This angle can be properly determined by the technologist using the extended palm along the lateral aspect of the breast and lifting it slightly away from the body and matching the angle of the palm (Fig. 20.68).
- Adjust IR height so that the top of the IR is at the level of the axilla.
- With the patient facing the unit and the feet forward exactly as in the CC view, place the arm of the side being imaged along the top of the IR, in a relaxed state.
- Pull the breast tissue and pectoral muscle **anteriorly** and **medially away from the chest wall.** Assess the angle of the pectoral muscle and adjust the unit accordingly. Push the patient slightly toward the angled IR until the inferolateral aspect of the breast is touching the IR. The nipple should be in profile.
- Apply compression slowly with the **breast held away from the chest wall and up** to prevent sagging and present the region of the IMF (Fig. 20.69).
- The upper edge of the compression device rests under the clavicle, and the lower edge includes the IMF.
- Wrinkles and folds on the breast should be smoothed out and compression applied until taut.
- If necessary, have the patient gently retract the opposite breast with the other hand to prevent superimposition.
- The R or L view marker (RMLO, LMLO) should be placed high near the axilla.

CR

- Perpendicular, centered to the base of the breast, the chest wall edge of the IR; CR not movable

Recommended Collimation Use appropriate cone down paddle and select collimation if applicable.

Respiration Breathing instructions will vary depending on whether conventional or 3D units are used.

NOTE: To show *all* the breast tissue on this projection with a large breast, two images may be needed, one positioned higher to get all of the axillary region and a second positioned lower to include the main part of the breast. If applicable, place AEC chamber to appropriate position to ensure adequate exposure of various tissue densities.

Evaluation Criteria
Anatomy Demonstrated • Entire breast tissue is visible, from the pectoral muscle to level of nipple (Figs. 20.70 and 20.71). • IMF must be seen, and breast must not be drooping.
Position and Compression • Nipple is seen in profile. • Breast is seen to be pulled out and away from chest with even thickness indicating optimal compression.
Collimation and CR • CR and collimation are fixed and are centered correctly if breast tissue is correctly centered and visualized on IR.
Exposure • Dense areas are adequately penetrated, resulting in optimal contrast. • Sharp tissue markings indicate **no motion.** • R or L view marker and patient information are correctly placed at axillary side. • **No artifacts** are visible.

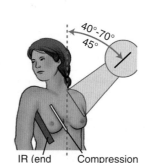

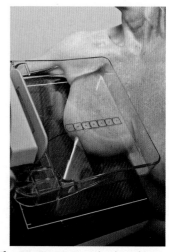

IR (end view) / Compression paddle
Fig. 20.68 MLO projection.

Fig. 20.69 MLO projection. (Note x-ray tube/film unit is angled about 45°; see Fig. 20.71.)

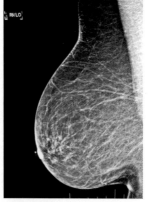

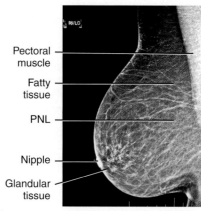

Pectoral muscle
Fatty tissue
PNL
Nipple
Glandular tissue

Fig. 20.70 MLO projection. **Fig. 20.71** MLO projection. PNL should be within 1 cm of PNL of CC projection.

SPECIAL PROJECTIONS (ADDITIONAL VIEWS)

MEDIOLATERAL (ML) PROJECTION: TRUE LATERAL BREAST POSITION

Clinical Indications
- Breast pathologic conditions, especially inflammation or other pathologic changes in the lateral aspect of the breast
- This projection may be requested by the radiologist as an optional projection to confirm an abnormality seen only on MLO.
- Also useful for evaluating air-fluid levels in structures or high concentrations of calcium within a cyst (milk of calcium)

Technical Factors
- SID—fixed, varies with manufacturer; about 24 inches (60 cm)
- IR size—8 × 10 inches (18 × 24 cm) or 10 × 12 inches (24 × 30 cm), landscape
- Grid
- kVp ranges: analog systems (rare): 23–28; digital systems: 25–35

Shielding Use a waist apron (thyroid shield optional).

Patient Position Standing; if not possible, seated

Part Position 🔲
- The tube and IR remain at right angles to each other as **CR is angled 90°** from vertical.
- Adjust the IR height to be centered to midbreast.
- With the patient facing the unit feet forward, place arm of the side being imaged forward and the hand on the bar toward the front (Fig. 20.72).
- Pull the breast tissue and pectoral muscle **anteriorly** and **medially away from the chest wall.** Push the patient slightly toward the IR until the inferolateral aspect of the breast is touching the IR. The nipple should be in profile.
- Apply compression slowly with the **breast held away from the chest wall and up** to prevent sagging. After the paddle has passed the sternum, rotate the patient until the breast is in a true lateral position.
- Wrinkles and folds on the breast should be smoothed out and compression applied until taut.
- Open the IMF by pulling the abdominal tissue down.
- If necessary, have the patient gently retract the opposite breast with the other hand to prevent superimposition.
- The R or L view marker should be placed high and near the axilla.

Positioning Tips
- For the larger patient with extra adipose tissue in the upper arm and back — Once the patient is positioned for an MLO, keep one hand on the breast against the IR and take the other arm and pull back on the posterior tissue from around the back of the patient. This will reduce the likelihood of a skin fold.
- For the upper arm — As you are positioning the arm across the top of the IR, slightly internally roll the arm and pull the fatty tissue (wings) toward the back of the IR. In addition, while applying compression, place your free hand over the dependent shoulder and pull up on the upper breast tissue to reduce the large fold that often appears there.

CR
- Perpendicular, centered to the base of the breast, the chest wall edge of the IR; CR not movable

Recommended Collimation Use appropriate cone and collimation.

Respiration Suspend breathing.

NOTE: Position AEC chamber to appropriate position to ensure adequate exposure of various tissue densities.

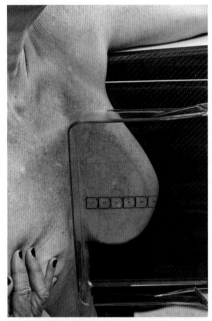

Fig. 20.72 ML projection.

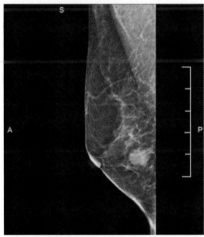

Fig. 20.73 ML projection.

Evaluation Criteria
Anatomy Demonstrated • Lateral view of entire breast tissue includes axillary region, pectoral muscle, and open IMF (Fig. 20.73).
Position and Compression • Nipple is seen in profile; tissue thickness is evenly distributed on IR, indicating optimal compression. • Axillary breast tissue (generally including pectoral muscle) is included, indicating correct centering and IR vertical placement.
Collimation and CR • CR and collimation chamber are fixed and are centered correctly if breast tissue is correctly centered and visualized on IR.
Exposure • Dense areas are adequately penetrated, resulting in optimal contrast. • Sharp tissue markings indicate **no motion.** • R and L view markers and patient information are correctly placed at axillary side of IR. • **No artifacts** are visible.

SPECIAL PROJECTIONS (ADDITIONAL VIEWS)

EXAGGERATED CRANIOCAUDAL (LATERALLY) (XCCL) PROJECTION

Clinical Indications
- Potential breast pathologic condition or change in breast tissue; also emphasizes axillary tissue
- Most frequently requested optional projection when CC projection does not show all axillary tissue or when a lesion is seen on MLO but not on CC

Technical Factors
- SID—fixed, varies with manufacturer; about 24 inches (60 cm)
- IR size—8 × 10 inches (18 × 24 cm) or 10 × 12 inches (24 × 30 cm), landscape
- Grid
- kVp ranges: analog systems (rare): 23–28; digital systems: 25–35

Shielding Use a waist apron (thyroid shield optional)

Patient Position Erect, if possible

Part Position
- Begin as if to do a CC projection, then **rotate the body** away from the IR slightly as needed to include more of the **axillary** aspect of the breast onto the IR.
- Put the patient's hand on the bar toward the front and relax the shoulder (some recommend angling the unit 5° lateromedially).
- The head is turned away from the side that is being imaged (facing the technologist).
- The breast is pulled forward onto the IR, wrinkles and folds should be smoothed out, and compression is applied until taut. The nipple should be in profile (Fig. 20.75).
- The R or L view marker is always placed on the axillary side.

CR
- Perpendicular, centered to the base of the breast, the chest wall edge of the image receptor; CR not movable

Collimation Use appropriate cone and collimation.

Respiration Suspend breathing.

NOTES: If a lesion is deeper or superior, an **AT** view is required.

If a lesion is not found on lateral aspect of breast, a **medially exaggerated craniocaudal** view should be performed.

Position AEC chamber to appropriate position to ensure adequate exposure of various tissue densities.

Evaluation Criteria
Anatomy Demonstrated • Axillary breast tissue, pectoral muscle, and central and subareolar tissues are included (Figs. 20.75 and 20.76).
Position and Compression • Nipple is seen in profile. • Tissue thickness is evenly distributed, indicating optimal compression. • Axillary tissues, including pectoral muscle, are visualized, indicating correct positioning with sufficient body rotation.
Collimation and CR • CR and collimation are fixed and are centered correctly if breast tissue is correctly centered and visualized on IR.
Exposure • Dense areas are adequately penetrated, resulting in optimal contrast. • Sharp tissue markings indicate **no motion.** • R and L markers and patient information are correctly placed at axillary side of IR. • **No artifacts** are visible.

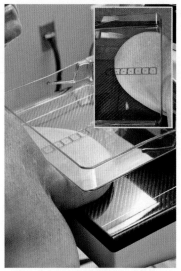

Fig. 20.74 XCCL projection. *Note:* Patient is turned so that axillary tissue is included on the image. Arm and hand are forward for ease in turning the body.

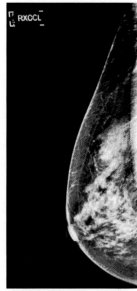

Fig. 20.75 XCCL projection.

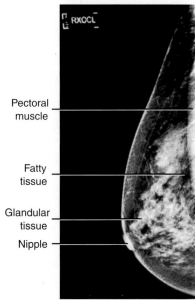

Pectoral muscle

Fatty tissue

Glandular tissue

Nipple

Fig. 20.76 XCCL projection.

SPECIAL PROJECTIONS (ADDITIONAL VIEWS)

IMPLANT DISPLACED (ID) (EKLUND METHOD)[24]

WARNING: Extreme care and precautions must be taken during this ID procedure to prevent rupture of the augmented implant.

Clinical Indications
• Detection and evaluation of breast pathologic condition underlying the implant
• Potential complications of breast augmentation, such as intracapsular or extracapsular leakage of implant

NOTE: It is important for the technologist to explain to the patient that two sets of images must be taken to examine the breasts properly. Both sets of images are taken with the use of standard views. One set is taken with the implants in place and assesses the integrity of the implants. The second set of images includes the displaced views, which allow proper compression of breast tissue for adequate evaluation for the presence of a pathologic change (Figs. 20.78 and 20.79).

Eklund Method[24] The Eklund method of "pinching" the breast (Figs. 20.79 and 20.80) is performed after the standard CC and MLO projections are taken. During this procedure, the implant is pushed posteriorly and superiorly to the chest wall so that the anterior breast tissue can be compressed and visualized in the usual manner (see Fig. 20.78).

Exception The Eklund method can be performed on most patients with implants; however, some implants become encapsulated, and only the routine views with the implant in place can be done. An additional projection, such as the mediolateral or lateromedial view, may be helpful for demonstrating all tissue.

Manual Exposure Techniques For projections done with the implant in place, only **manual exposure techniques should be set** on the generator because the implant prevents the x-rays from reaching the AEC detector. **This causes overexposure of the breast,** and the AEC system possibly may go to maximum backup exposure time.

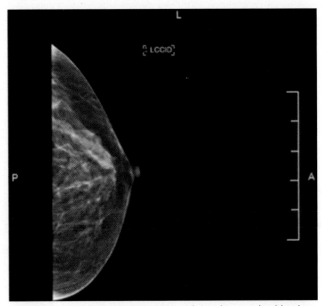

Fig. 20.78 Standard CC projection with implant pushed back (same patient as in Fig. 20.77).

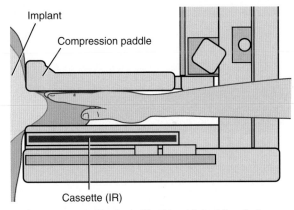

Fig. 20.79 Positioning with Eklund "pinch" technique.

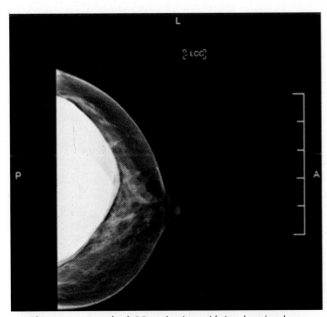

Fig. 20.77 Standard CC projection with implant in place.

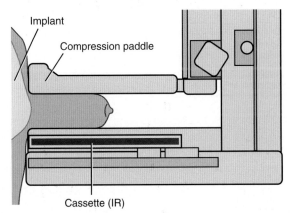

Fig. 20.80 Breast in place for CC projection with implant pushed back.

RADIOGRAPHS FOR CRITIQUE

This section consists of an ideal projection (Image A) along with one or more projections that may demonstrate positioning and/or technical errors. Critique Figs. C20.81 and C20.82. Compare Image A to the other projections and identify the errors. While examining each image, consider the following questions:

1. Is all essential anatomy demonstrated on the image?
2. What positioning errors are present that compromise image quality?

3. Are technical factors optimal?
4. Is there evidence of collimation and are pre-exposure anatomic side markers visible on the image?
5. Do these errors require a repeat exposure?
   Feedback for each set of images is located on the faculty Evolve site.

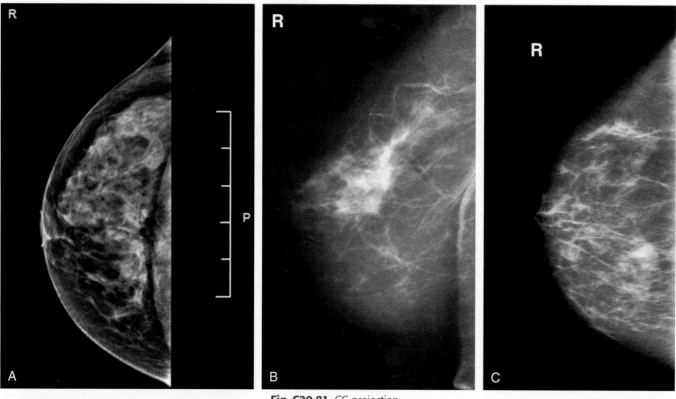

Fig. C20.81 CC projection.

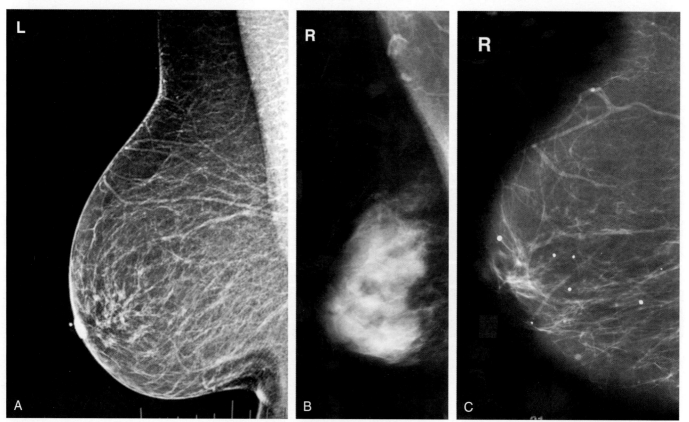

Fig. C20.82 MLO projection.

PART SIX ▪ BONE DENSITOMETRY

Contributor: **Sharon R.Wartenbee**, RTR, BD, CBDT, FASRT

Introduction

Bone densitometry is the use of various technologies to **measure the bone mineral content (BMC) and bone mineral density (BMD) of specific skeletal sites in the body.** According to the National Institutes of Health, osteoporosis is a skeletal disorder characterized by compromised bone strength predisposing to an increased risk of fracture.[25] Bone strength reflects the integration of two main features: bone density and bone quality. In 2014, The National Osteoporosis Foundation (NOF) estimated that 54 million adults over the age of 50 were affected by osteoporosis or low bone mass. With current trends, the NOF expects this number to grow to 72.2 million by the year 2030.[26] Although this disease is considered an "old age" disease, because of certain metabolic conditions, it can strike at any age. The medical, economic, and social costs associated with the health problems of patients with osteoporosis are alarming. Due to an aging population, the cost of care is expected to rise to $25.3 billion by 2025.[27] The importance of early detection and diagnosis has increased overall interest in bone densitometry techniques. Advanced applications of bone densitometry have significantly affected the diagnosis and management of this disease process. However, the need for accuracy of these methods also requires precision by the technologist performing the examination.

HISTORY

Before dedicated bone densitometry methods were developed, standard radiographs of the dorsal and lumbar spine were evaluated for detection of any visible changes in the bone density; this proved to be a very subjective method. A loss of 30% to 50% of trabecular bone may produce the first visible changes on radiographs.[28] Radiographic detection of osteoporosis typically was delayed until late in the course of the disease. Often the fracturing of a bone was the first indicator of the presence of osteoporosis. The measured loss of height or anterior curvature of the thoracic spine, resulting in a "humped" appearance, is usually an indicator of a more advanced stage. Evaluation with dedicated bone densitometry equipment is the best objective method to measure bone mass loss in early stages, before these dramatic symptoms occur and begin to affect the quality of life.

COMPOSITION OF BONE

To understand the underlying principle of bone densitometry, the technologist must have a basic understanding of bone composition and how the osteoporotic process occurs. Bone is a living tissue that is constantly undergoing change to meet the body's metabolic and physiologic needs. Bone matrix is 90% collagen and 10% other proteins. Bone mineral is a combination of calcium and phosphorus (hydroxyapatite). Cortical (compact) bone makes up the shafts of the long bones and the outer envelope of all bones. Cancellous (trabecular) bone makes up the inner parts of the bones of the axial skeleton. Bone cells are osteoclasts, osteoblasts, osteocytes, and lining cells.

Osteoclasts and Osteoblasts

Osteoclasts and osteoblasts are the principal osteocytes (bone cells) responsible for bone remodeling. **Osteoclasts remove bone, causing bone resorption,** whereas **osteoblasts build or replace bone tissue.** The rate at which this process is accomplished contributes to bone density. When we are young and actively growing, osteoblasts build or replace our bone tissue. By the age of 20 years,

the average woman has acquired 98% of her skeletal mass or **peak bone mass.** Determinants of peak bone mass include heredity (sex and race; 75%) and lifestyle factors (e.g., calcium, vitamin D, exercise, smoking; 25%). Building bone mass during childhood and teenage years can be the best defense against osteoporosis in adulthood, but continuing a healthy lifestyle is also important. Typically, by age 35, more bone is removed than replaced, resulting in a gradual decrease in bone. Increasing age causes bones of the skeleton to become thinner and weaker. With loss of bone density, the incidence of fractures of the hip, spine, wrist, and other bones from little or minimal trauma is increased. Early detection through bone densitometry can lead to intervention before associated skeletal fractures occur.

Bone Mineral Content Versus Bone Mineral Density

The BMC is a measurement of the **quantity or mass of bone measured in grams (g).** The BMD is the **ratio of BMC to projected area of the bone,** and the calculated quantity is expressed in units of **g/cm^2**. T-scores and Z-scores, which are used in bone densitometry and are described later in this section, are determined using the quantity **BMD,** sometimes referred to simply as bone density.

Purpose

Bone densitometry is used to do the following:
- Measure BMD
- Detect bone loss
- Establish the diagnosis of osteoporosis
- Assess an individual's risk for fracture
- Assess a patient's response to osteoporosis therapy
- Perform vertebral fracture assessment

Bone densitometry is accomplished through a variety of methods and techniques with the use of ionizing radiation. These methods and techniques are described later in this section.

Clinical Risk Factors and Indications

The Bone Mass Measurement Act of 1998 (formerly called the Balanced Budget Act of 1997) provided Medicare coverage of medically necessary bone densitometry after July 1, 1998. Bone densitometry is indicated for individuals who meet specific medical criteria and individuals considered at risk. Risk factors for low bone mass include the following:
- Female gender
- Advanced age
- Family history
- Ethnicity
- Low body weight (<127 lb)
- Lifestyle

Additional risk factors are as follows:
- Estrogen deficiency
- Nutritional deficiency – calcium or vitamin D deficiencies
- Sedentary lifestyle
- Frequent falls (for varied reasons)
- Alcohol abuse or tobacco use

Specific diseases or conditions are also associated with the development of osteoporosis, such as the following:
- Hormonal – hypogonadism, **hyperparathyroidism**, hyperthyroidism, diabetes mellitus (insulin dependent)
- Rheumatoid arthritis (accompanied by steroid use)

- Gastrointestinal conditions – gastrectomy, intestinal bypass, Crohn disease, celiac sprue
- Medications – anticonvulsants, excessive vitamin A, thyroid hormone, medroxyprogesterone (Depo-Provera), glucocorticoids

BMD AND FRACTURE RISK

Bone strength and bone density are very closely related. Individuals with low BMD also have an increased risk for fragility fracture. Numerous studies have demonstrated that the age-adjusted relative risk for fracture increases approximately twofold for each decrease of 1 standard deviation (SD) in BMD. The use of BMD to predict future fractures is more accurate than the use of serum cholesterol to predict cardiovascular disease. The relationship between fracture risk and BMD is continuous; there is no BMD threshold above which fragility fractures do not occur.

When measured at any site, BMD shows approximately the same fracture risk for each 1 SD decrease in BMD. However, obtaining a BMD of the proximal femur is better for predicting fractures of the hip compared with other measurement sites. The relative risk is 2.7 for each 1 SD decrease in BMD of the hip; this means that a woman whose BMD is 2 SD below the mean for her age is more than seven times (2.7 × 2.7) more likely to have a hip fracture than a woman of the same age whose BMD is equal to the mean. Studies suggest an incidence of fracture risk of 1 in 2 for women and up to 1 in 4 for men age 50 and older due to osteoporosis.[27]

Assessment of Fracture Risk

Fracture risk prediction is enhanced by the combination of BMD and clinical risk factors. Individuals with multiple clinical risk factors have a higher risk for fracture than individuals with fewer clinical risk factors at a given BMD. Individuals with low BMD have a greater risk for fracture than individuals with higher BMD for a given number of clinical risk factors. Patients with low BMD and multiple clinical risk factors are at greatest risk for fracture. Fracture risk should be based on both BMD and the presence of clinical risk factors.

World Health Organization Diagnostic Criteria for Diagnosis of Osteoporosis

With the development of dual-energy x-ray absorptiometry (DXA) units capable of highly precise and accurate measurement of BMD, the paradigm for diagnosing osteoporosis has shifted from the occurrence of a fragility fracture to the risk for sustaining a fragility fracture in the future. This shift in emphasis from the presence of a fracture to the risk for fracture is evident in the internationally agreed-on description of osteoporosis as a **systemic skeletal disease characterized by low bone mass and microarchitectural deterioration of bone tissue, with a consequent increase in bone fragility and susceptibility to fracture.**

Instead of calculating a fracture risk, the World Health Organization (WHO) in 1994 recommended the use of BMD for the diagnosis of osteoporosis. Osteoporosis in postmenopausal white women is defined as a BMD value more than **2.5 SDs** below the average for a young normal population (i.e., a T-score < −2.5). The **T-score** is simply the number of SDs the individual's BMD is from the mean BMD of a young normal population of the same sex and ethnic background.

An individual's T-score is used to classify the individual as normal, osteopenic, or osteoporotic (Table 20.2). **Normal** is defined as a T-score of no less than −1.0; **osteopenia** (preferred term currently is **low bone mass** or **low bone density**) is a T-score less than −1.0 but greater than −2.5; and **osteoporosis** is a T-score of −2.5 or less. An additional classification of **severe osteoporosis** is given to individuals with a T-score of −2.5 or less, with one or more fragility fractures present.

According to the International Society for Clinical Densitometry (ISCD), BMD reporting in premenopausal women or men younger than 50 years should be done in Z-scores rather than T-scores (especially in children). These scores report the expected range for age-appropriate individuals. In this category, a Z-score of −2.0 or less is defined as "below the expected range for age," and a Z-score greater than −2.0 is "within the expected range for age." Osteoporosis cannot be diagnosed in men under age 50 on the basis of BMD alone. However, the WHO diagnostic criteria may also be applied to women in the menopausal transition.[29]

Osteoporosis Management

The FDA has approved the use of several drugs for the treatment and prevention of osteoporosis (Table 20.3). These drugs either (1) inhibit bone resorption (antiresorptive agents) or (2) stimulate bone formation (anabolic agents).

Antiresportic medications include[30]:
- Estrogen
- Selective estrogen receptor modulators (SERMs)
- Bisphosphonates
- RANK ligands
- Calcitonin

Anabolic medications include[30]:
- Parathyroid hormone
- Romosozumab

Estrogen Estrogen replacement therapy has been shown to reduce bone loss, increase bone density in both the spine and the hip, and reduce the risk for hip and spinal fractures in postmenopausal women.

Mode of action Antiresorption.

TABLE 20.2 INDIVIDUAL T-SCORE CLASSIFICATIONS

TERM	T-SCORE	DESCRIPTION
Normal	≥ −1.0	Bone mass of no less than −1.0
Osteopenia (low bone mass)	< −1.0 but > −2.5	Condition of lower than normal bone mass
Osteoporosis	≤ −2.5	Disorder defined by reduction in the amount of bone mass of < −2.5
Severe osteoporosis	≤ −2.5+ fracture	Disorder with reduced bone mass of ≤ −2.5 combined with presence of one or more fragility fractures

TABLE 20.3 OSTEOPOROSIS DRUGS OR AGENTS

TYPE	DRUGS OR AGENTS
Antiresorptive agents (inhibit bone resorption)	Estrogen – estrogen replacement therapy (ERT)
	Selective estrogen receptor modulators (SERMs)
	Raloxifene (Evista)
	Bisphosphonates
	Alendronate (Fosamax)
	Risedronate (Actonel)
	Ibandronate (Boniva)
	Calcitonin (Miacalcin)
Anabolic agents (stimulate bone formation)	Parathyroid hormone
	Teriparatide (Fortéo)
	Abaloparatide (Tymlos)
	Romosozumab (Evenity)

SERMs Raloxifene (Evista) prevents bone loss at the spine, hip, and total body and reduces fractures.

Mode of action Antiresorption.

Bisphosphonates Alendronate (Fosamax), risedronate (Actonel), ibandronate (Boniva) and zoledronic acid (Reclast) reduce bone loss, increase bone density in both the spine and the hip, and reduce the risk for both spine and hip fractures. These medications are most effective in treating postmenopausal women and are most commonly prescribed for all patients in treating and preventing osteoporosis. However, alendronate and risedronate are FDA approved for treatment only in men.

There are infusion versions of ibandronate (Boniva) and zoledronic acid (Reclast). This allows a patient to forego the daily or weekly regimen of pill taking. Intravenous Boniva is taken quarterly, and intravenous Reclast can be taken annually.

Mode of action Antiresorption.

RANKL Ligand (RANKL) RANKL is bound together with RANK to promote osteoclast survival and increased bone absorption. This process creates a monoclonal antibody called *denosumab*. Denosumab is marketed under the brand name Prolia and is FDA approved to treat osteoporosis in postmenopausal women with a high fracture risk.

Mode of action Antiresorption.

Calcitonin Calcitonin (Miacalcin) is a naturally occurring non–sex hormone that is involved in calcium regulation and bone metabolism. It slows bone loss, increases spinal bone density, and relieves pain associated with bone fractures. It reduces the risk for spinal fracture and also may reduce hip fracture risk.

Mode of action Antiresorption.

Parathyroid Hormone The parathyroid hormone 1-34 (PTH 1-34) analog teriparatide (Forteo) and abaloparatide (Tymlos) stimulate bone formation. They are used for treating osteoporosis in men and postmenopausal women who have a high risk of fracture. Foreteo is available as a prefilled multidose subcutaneous injection pen and should not be taken for more than 2 years. Tymlos is also available in a prefilled multidose subcutaneous daily pen. The manufacturer is working on developing a transdermal patch for ease of delivery of the medication..

Mode of action Bone formation.

Romosozumab (Evenity)[31] Romosozumab is a monoclonal antibody that blocks the protein sclerostin and forms new bone without breaking it down. In clinical trials, Evenity substantially increased bone density and prevented fractures more effectively than other available treatments. It is a monthly injection and should only be taken for 1 year. Experts anticipate the drug will be offered to patients at highest risk, such as those with a serious fracture or those who did not respond to other medications.

Mode of action Bone formation.

Contraindications
Bone densitometry is contraindicated if quality control procedures and standardizations are not maintained to ensure accurate results. Anatomic malformations of the anatomic site, such as those exhibited with the spine, also may provide less accurate results; examples include osteophytes, overlying calcifications, compression fractures, and

scoliosis of greater 15 degrees.[32] The presence of a previous fracture or a metallic prosthesis prevents measurement of BMD at the affected anatomic site. Procedures such as vertebral augmentation (vertebroplasty and kyphoplasty) can also affect an accurate measurement of vertebral BMD and should be excluded from the analysis.

As with any radiographic examination, a pregnant patient should not be scanned, and the standards that have been established to prevent inadvertent exposure to the fetus should be maintained. Additionally, the patient should be scheduled at least 1 week after the date of any prior radiographic contrast examination or with administration of any isotopes for a nuclear medicine study.

PATIENT PREPARATION
The patient is instructed to wear loose clothing with no dense objects (e.g., belt, zipper) in the abdominal and pelvic area. Departmental protocol may require the patient to be gowned during the procedure to ensure an artifact-free acquisition.

MAJOR EQUIPMENT, METHODS, AND TECHNIQUES
Several commercial techniques are available to perform bone density using ionizing radiation or ultrasound. The most widely used and versatile device is DXA. Advantages of this type of scanner include a low radiation dose, wide availability, ease of use, short scan time, high-resolution images, good precision, and stable calibration.[32] Central devices measure the spine and hip. These are also capable of measuring the forearm and total body. Peripheral devices are capable of measuring the wrist, heel, and finger. Bone densitometry techniques include the following:

- Radiographic absorptiometry (peripheral densitometry)
- Single-energy x-ray absorptiometry (peripheral densitometry)
- **DXA** (central densitometry)
- Peripheral dual-energy absorptiometry (peripheral densitometry)
- **Quantitative computed tomography (QCT)** (central densitometry)
- Peripheral computed tomography (peripheral densitometry)
- **Quantitative ultrasound (QUS)** (peripheral densitometry)

DXA, QCT, and QUS are performed more commonly, and DXA is the most widely accepted method for measuring bone density. It also remains the superior examination for monitoring the effects of therapy.

Dual-Energy X-Ray Absorptiometry
Dual-energy x-ray absorptiometry *(ab-sorp"-she-om'-a-tre)* is a technique that is commonly used in current practice (Fig. 20.83).

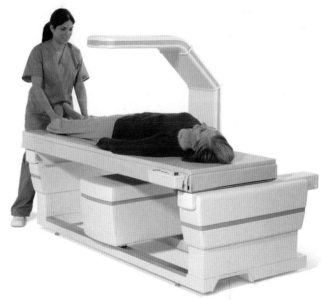

Fig. 20.83 Hologic Horizon DXA system. (Courtesy Hologic, Inc., Bedford, MA.)

There are three DXA equipment manufacturers in the US: Hologic Inc., GE Healthcare Lunar iDXA, and Norland Swissray systems.[32] The physical basis of DXA incorporates the **use of a high and a low x-ray energy beam to determine the areal mass of tissue.** This action may be accomplished through the use of an energy switching system (pulsing) or rare earth filters. Energy switching systems are alternated between a specific high and low kilovoltage. Filters used in conjunction with energy discriminating detector systems separate the x-ray beam into effective high and low energies. Hologic uses an energy switching system and GE/Lunar and Norland Swissray use the rare earth filter system.

The first such systems used a single pencil-beam type of x-ray beam and detector. Most DXA systems use a **fan-beam method** with an **array of detectors.** Such units are faster and, depending on the beam geometry, scanning can be accomplished within a few minutes.

After the scan is completed, the selected site is analyzed, and a bone mineral report is generated. This report typically contains the bone mineral image of the anatomic part scanned and the BMD, which is calculated for all areas scanned. The BMD is calculated as BMD = BMC/Area. These three parameters on the DXA printouts are area in centimeters squared (cm^2), BMC in grams (g), and BMD in g/cm^2. Because BMD reduces the effect of body size, it is the most widely used parameter The BMD is also shown in T-scores and Z-scores on the printout. The information collected is compared with normal databases of bone density to determine the diagnosis. According to the ISCD's Position Statements 2015, it is not possible to "quantitatively" compare BMD or to calculate a least significant change (LSC) between facilities or machines without cross-calibration.[29]

Z-Score and T-Score The two standards used to compare the patient's bone density measurements are the Z-score and the T-score. The **Z-score** standard **compares the patient with an average individual of the same age and sex.** The T-score compares the patient with an average young, healthy individual of the same sex with peak bone mass.[33] These values can facilitate assessment of the presence or extent of osteoporosis risk for future fracture.

Quantitative Computed Tomography

The basis of QCT is related to the attenuation of ionizing radiation as it passes through tissues at the selected site, most often a central site. An **8- to 10-mm slice** is obtained through four separate vertebral bodies, or **20 to 30 continuous 5-mm slices** are obtained over two or three vertebral bodies between T12 and L5.

A calibration standard (phantom) is scanned routinely at the same time for correlation, and image analysis software averages the values from all bones. It allows **3D or volumetric analysis** of data (Fig. 20.84) and cannot be compared to DXA because of the volumetric analysis in the QCT.

Quantitative Ultrasound

Ultrasound has been in existence for more than 40 years, but it has been used for clinical evaluation of BMD only since the late 1990s. QUS is a **nonionizing technique** that is used to assess BMD in **peripheral sites.** The technique offers relatively quick and simple measurements, with no radiation exposure to the patient. QUS is used in peripheral sites with minimal soft tissue covering. The most commonly selected site is the **os calcis** (heel) (Fig. 20.85); however, some systems also measure the finger and tibia. QUS is only recommended as a screening process and should not be used for serial scanning and for monitoring the effects of therapy.

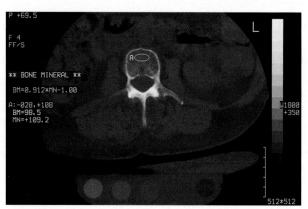

Fig. 20.84 QCT scan through L1 with calibration phantom.

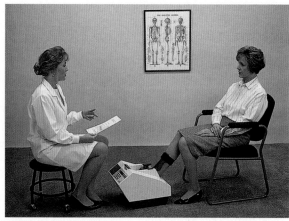

Fig. 20.85 QUS unit assessing os calcis. (Courtesy Hologic, Inc., Bedford, MA.)

RADIATION SAFETY

As with all radiologic examinations, the benefits of the examination should outweigh the risks. The radiation dose that the patient undergoing bone densitometry receives is much lower than the dose used in conventional radiography. The effective dose from a bone density examination of both spine and hip is typically less than 5 μSv (1 rem = 10^4 μSv). Natural background levels are 5 to 8 μSv per day. It has been widely stated that natural background radiation is the equivalent of approximately 200 chest x-rays per year.[34] A BMD examination of 5 μSv would equate to less than one chest x-ray. The dose range for QCT is higher, approximately 30 μSv.[35] DXA examinations offer diagnostic information at a very low risk of radiation compared with the potential benefits.

Technologists should always follow the ALARA principle for both themselves and the patient. However, the most effective radiation safety practice is well-educated, knowledgeable, and conscientious DXA technologists who take pride in their work.

Positioning for DXA

Positioning considerations for DXA are described in greater detail because this is the prevalent densitometric technique used. Standard operating procedures (SOPs) developed by the interpreting clinician and the technologists should be available in the department and should be followed for consistency. It is also important to follow the manufacturer's guidelines for scan acquisition and analysis.

Spine DXA of the lumbar spine is obtained for evaluation of the current status of the spine and most importantly for predicting vertebral fracture risk. The patient is placed in a supine position, with the midsagittal plane aligned with the midline of the table (Fig. 20.86).

The spine should be straight and aligned with the scan field with equal amounts of soft tissue on either side of the spine. The image should be evaluated to ensure an artifact-free acquisition. The region included should be from **T12 to below the iliac crest.** Analysis is to be obtained according to the manufacturer's guidelines from L1 through L4. Any abnormal vertebral body, such as compression fractures and osteophytes, is not considered in the assessment of BMD because this could add falsely to the BMD reading measurement. According to the ISCD Position Statements, BMD should not be made using a single vertebra. If only one evaluable vertebra remains after excluding other vertebrae, diagnosis should be based on a different valid skeletal site. If there is more than a 1.0 T-score difference between a vertebra and the adjacent vertebrae, it is recommended to exclude the vertebrae in question from the analysis.[29]

Hip DXA of the hip is most valuable for predicting future hip fracture. The patient is placed in a supine position, with the midsagittal plane aligned with the midline of the table. The patient's legs are extended, and shoes are removed.

The legs are positioned as for a **true anteroposterior (AP) projection of the hips.** The legs are rotated internally, approximately 15° to 20°, to place the femoral necks parallel to the imaging surface. An immobilizing support device that allows for correct positioning typically is available with the DXA unit. This device aids the patient in retaining this position, ensuring consistency for subsequent studies (Fig. 20.87).

The scan should include the proximal femur, with the midline of the femoral body parallel to the lateral edge of the scan). Depending on the manufacturer, bilateral hips can be scanned simultaneously. Acquisition and analysis should always be attained according to the manufacturer's guidelines (Fig. 20.88).

Forearm The nondominant forearm is routinely scanned because it is expected to have a lower BMD than the dominant forearm. A forearm should *not* be scanned if there is a history of fracture in the wrist, internal hardware, or severe deformity from arthritis. The forearm is scanned under specific conditions, such as spine or hip artifacts, severe

degeneration or arthritis, or severe scoliosis. Obvious patient limitations, including exceeding the weight limit for the table, wheelchair confinement, or inability to lie down because of extreme pain, would also require the forearm scan as a second site. Documented hyperparathyroidism as an existing diagnosis would also indicate the need for a forearm scan **in addition** to the spine and hip (Fig. 20.89). The 33% radius (⅓ radius) of the nondominant forearm is used. Scan acquisition and analysis should be followed according to the manufacturer's guidelines.[29]

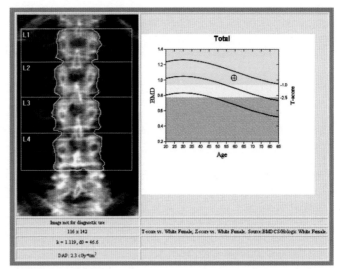

Fig. 20.86 Spine scan. (Courtesy Avera Medical Group McGreevy Clinic, Sioux Falls, SD.)

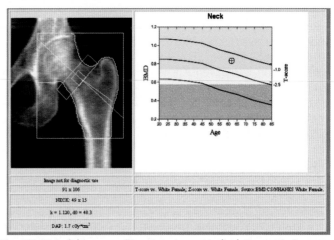

Fig. 20.87 Left hip scan. (Courtesy Avera Medical Group McGreevy Clinic, Sioux Falls, SD.)

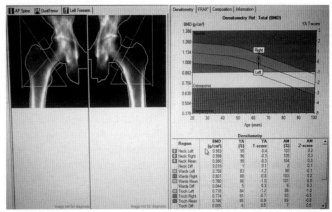

Fig. 20.88 Bilateral hip scan. (Courtesy Pioneer Medical Center, Viborg, SD.)

DXA Precision and Accuracy

Precision, which commonly is referred to as "reproducibility," is the ability of a quantitative measurement technique to reproduce the same numeric result when repeatedly performed in an identical fashion. In a DXA system, reproducibility is the ability to obtain consistent BMD values on repeated measurements of the same patient over a short period of time. To monitor bone loss or the efficacy of treatment, high precision (i.e., small variation in measurements) is essential. Precision determines the LSC in BMD that can be statistically recognized as a real change in BMD that is not due to random errors of measurement.

According to the ISCD's Position Statements, the following precision assessment guidelines should be followed:

- Each DXA facility should determine its precision error and calculate the LSC.
- The precision error supplied by the manufacturer should not be used.
- Every technologist should perform an in vivo precision assessment using patients representative of the clinic's patient population.
- Each technologist should do one complete precision assessment after basic scanning skills have been learned (e.g., manufacturer training) and after having performed approximately 100 patient scans.[29]

To perform a precision assessment:

- Measure 15 patients 3 times or 30 patients 2 times, repositioning the patient after each scan.
- Calculate the root mean square standard deviation for the group. Use the calculator on the ISCD website: https://www.ISCD.org.
- Calculate the LSC for the group at 95% confidence interval.[29]

The minimum acceptable precision for an individual technologist is:

- Lumbar spine: 1.9% (LSC = 5.3%)
- Total hip; 1.8% (LSC = 5%)
- Femoral neck; 2.5% (LSC = 6.9%)

Remediation is required if a technologist's precision is worse than these values. Precision assessment should be considered standard clinical practice. It is not research and may potentially benefit patients. It should not require approval of an institutional review board. Adherence to local and state safety regulations is necessary. Performance of a precision assessment requires the consent of participating patients.[29]

The poorer the precision, the greater the change in BMD required for the change to be recognized as real. Because the rate of change of bone in normal individuals or patients who are being treated is small, **good measurement precision is essential for detecting changes in BMD.** Achieving the best DXA precision requires the technologist to position the patient carefully in a consistent manner for scanning, analyze the scan in a consistent manner, and perform instrument quality control tests routinely in accordance with the manufacturer's protocols.

Accuracy Accuracy is defined as **how well the measured value reflects the true or actual value of the object measured.** Accuracy is the difference between true and measured values compared with the true value of the quantity measured, expressed in percentage points. Typically, the accuracy of a DXA unit is better than 10% and is sufficient for the clinical assessment of fracture risk and the diagnosis of osteoporosis. Scanners made by different manufacturers are calibrated differently, and the BMD of a patient measured with DXA units of different manufacturers may differ by 15%, depending on the skeletal site scanned. Even if identical DXA scanners made by the same manufacturer are used to scan a patient, the measured BMD of the patient may differ by several percentage points.

Cross-calibration techniques can reduce differences between DXA units produced by different manufacturers to less than several percentage points. However, if the goal is to monitor a patient's BMD longitudinally, it is not recommended that follow-up scans be performed with different scanners, (unless cross calibrated) even if they are produced by the same manufacturer. Most clinical situations do not involve comparison of BMD values of the same individual measured on different densitometers. The more common situation is the comparison of two readings of the same individual made at different times with the same DXA unit. In this scenario, the precision of the measurement is more important than accuracy.

Vertebral Fracture Assessment

Vertebral fracture assessment (VFA) is the correct term used to denote densitometric spine imaging, which is performed for the sole purpose of detecting vertebral fractures. VFA does not measure bone density (Fig. 20.90).

According to the ISCD's Position Statements, VFA is indicated when the T-score is −1.0 and one or more of the following is present:

- Age > 70 years in women or > 80 years in men
- Historical height loss > 1.5 inches (> 4 cm)
- Self-reported but undocumented prior vertebral fracture
- Glucocorticoid therapy equivalent to > 5 mg of prednisone or equivalent per day for > 3 months.

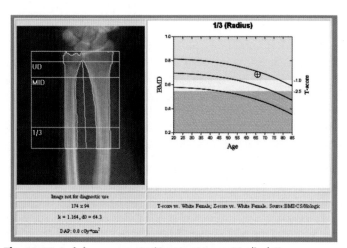

Fig. 20.89 Left forearm scan. (Courtesy Avera Medical Group McGreevy Clinic, Sioux Falls, SD.)

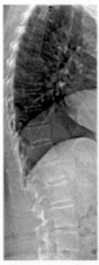

Fig. 20.90 Vertebral fracture assessment scan. (Courtesy Avera Medical Group McGreevy Clinic, Sioux Falls, SD.)

During vertebral fracture assessment, a single-energy or dual-energy scan of the thoracolumbar spine is performed. The scan is performed in the lateral projection, although an AP projection may be taken additionally. The software measures vertebral heights and compares them with reference values. The Genant Visual Semi-quantitative Method is the current clinical technique of choice for classifying vertebral fracture with VFA. As noted earlier, VFA is designed to detect vertebral fracture only and not any other abnormalities (Fig. 20.91).[29]

Fracture Risk Models (FRAX)

The FRAX tool has been developed by the University of Sheffield, UK to evaluate the 10-year probability fracture risk of patients. FRAX is based on individual patient models that incorporate the risks associated with clinic risk factors and the BMD at the femoral neck or the total hip. The use of nonhip sites is not recommended. To estimate the 10-year probability risk of a major osteoporotic fracture, FRAX uses clinical risk factors with the femoral BMD. It is intended to assess fracture risk only and to assist the physician in making treatment decisions for postmenopausal women and men age 50 or older.

Another important fact is that FRAX cannot be used if the patient is on pharmacologic treatment for osteoporosis. Patients who have been off osteoporosis medications for 1 year or more are considered untreated.

All fracture prediction models should be used judiciously in managing patients and should not be replaced by clinical judgment. Most DXA machines have FRAX software installed so that the 10-year fracture will be available on the report.[27] Otherwise, the FRAX tool can be accessed at the following website: https://www.sheffield.ac.uk/FRAX/tool.aspx?country=9.

Summary

Bone densitometry requires a high level of technical expertise if the system's potential is to be realized. Both precision assessment and accuracy are required. Follow-up scans monitoring BMD changes should be performed with the same DXA scanner. BMD results from different machines should not be quantitatively compared unless cross-calibration is performed. Interdevice variability can be ±5% to 7%. Should a new unit be introduced to a facility, cross-calibration needs to be completed. For this reason, previous scans taken from a different facility cannot be directly compared. Patient positioning, the technique used, and scan settings must be consistent with the baseline study to ensure good precision and true diagnostic comparisons. The use of bone densitometry as a diagnostic tool is expected to continue to expand as the technology advances and is complemented by improvements in osteoporosis management.

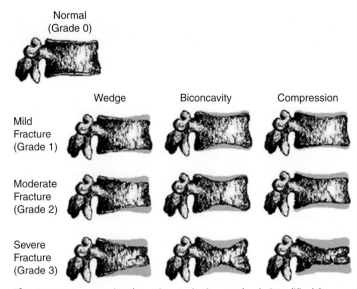

Fig. 20.91 Genant visual semi-quantitative method. (Modified from Griffith JF, Genant HK. *Osteoporosis,* ed 4, Waltham, 2013, Academic Press Elsevier.)

PART SEVEN ▪ MAGNETIC RESONANCE IMAGING (MRI)

Contributor: **Kathryn A. Wissink,** RT(R)(MR)

Introduction

MRI is a noninvasive imaging modality that has the ability to produce high-resolution images without the use of ionizing radiation. MRI uses magnetic fields, radiofrequency pulses, and a computer system to generate cross-sectional slices (views) from any angle; for example, if the body were viewed in the anterior to posterior; head to foot; or left to right direction. MRI generates images with exceptional soft tissue detail that is unmatched by other imaging applications. In addition, MRI is used to evaluate organs, bone, vessels, valves, tendons, ligaments, and cartilage. Clinical examinations include neurologic, body, breast, cardiac, musculoskeletal, and vascular areas. Fig. 20.92 is an example of an MRI 3T system.

Although MRI is lauded for its lack of ionizing radiation, use of the modality is not without some inherent risks. All technologists must be well versed in MRI safety and the potential hazards associated with a strong magnetic field. **MRI safety education is mandatory for all facility personnel who enter the MRI environment (MRI zones). This includes technologists, radiologists, ancillary staff, and emergency responders.** Additionally, an understanding of the physical principles of MRI enables the technologist to perform the examination with optimal image quality.

MAGNETIC RESONANCE IMAGING COMPARISON WITH COMPUTED TOMOGRAPHY

In clinical applications, MRI is often compared with CT because these imaging modalities both acquire cross-sectional images (slices). CT scanners acquire multiple x-rays (ionizing radiation) at various angles and then uses those x-rays to form a 3D image of the organ being examined. A computer measures the intensity all of the various x-rays taken at different angles and synthesizes the images to form a 3D computer model of internal organs[36] (Fig. 20.93).

Although CT does an excellent job demonstrating bony anatomy, with MRI you can visualize soft tissue and anatomic structures that may have been obscured on CT images (Fig. 20.94). Bone attenuates, or weakens, x-ray photons in CT, which may lead to "beam hardening" artifacts that result in streaks and loss of soft tissue detail on the final image. Equipment manufacturers have developed software applications to help eliminate these artifacts; however, artifacts are still at times a consideration for image detail. Because MRI does not share this limitation, exams that may be compromised in CT (e.g., brain posterior fossa or spinal cord) are better demonstrated with MRI. MRI has the ability to acquire image data in all three orientations (axial, sagittal, and coronal) and can reconstruct additional slices and image planes when needed (Figs. 20.95 and 20.96).

There are times when CT is preferred over MRI. MRI examinations are more costly than CT scans. In addition, some patients are unable to enter the MRI scanner due to contraindications, such as

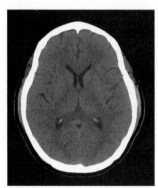

Fig. 20.93 CT axial brain. (Courtesy of Siemens Medical Solutions USA, Inc.)

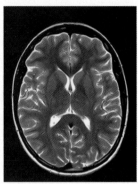

Fig. 20.94 MR T2 axial brain. (Courtesy of Siemens Medical Solutions USA, Inc.)

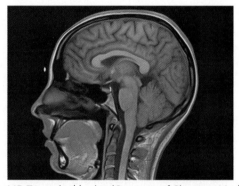

Fig. 20.95 MR T1 sagittal brain. (Courtesy of Siemens Medical Solutions USA, Inc.)

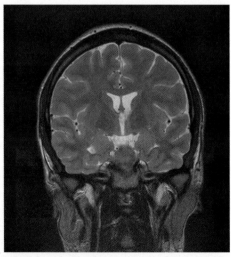

Fig. 20.96 MR T2 coronal brain. (Courtesy of Siemens Medical Solutions USA, Inc.)

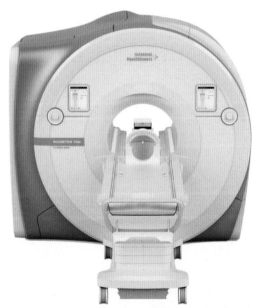

Fig. 20.92 MRI 3T system. (Courtesy of Siemens Medical Solutions USA, Inc.)

MRI-unsafe pacemakers, aneurysm clips, or cochlear implants. All implantable devices that enter the MR environment must be cleared by a licensed medical professional as **"MR conditional,"** and it must be verified that they are safe to be scanned at the specified field strength being used (1.5T, 3T, or 7T). Although CT and MRI have distinct advantages and disadvantages, they both serve the health care provider well in diagnosing pathology, structural anatomy, and trauma.

MRI and CT technologists must have an in-depth knowledge of anatomic structures and cross-sectional anatomy for accurate viewing of images obtained from various orientations (planes). A thorough knowledge of bony landmarks, organs, and vessels enables the technologist to interpret images appropriately to determine whether the slices and the field of view (FoV) are adequately covering the region of interest.

MRI technologists are required to understand how modifying technical parameters affects image quality and the **signal-to-noise ratio (SNR)**. These technical parameters also affect **contrast** and **spatial resolution,** with SNR and spatial resolution maintaining an inverse relationship. Therefore, if the technologist selects factors that increase overall SNR, there is almost always a corresponding decrease in spatial resolution (and vice versa). To attain optimal image quality, the technologist must manipulate various technical parameters to create the appropriate balance between SNR and spatial resolution.

Although CT and conventional radiography use detectors to measure the transmission of the x-ray beam, MRI uses a radiofrequency coil (RF coil). During the MRI exam the radiofrequency is transmitted into the body and the coil acts as an antenna to receive the radiofrequency signal coming from the body. The signal is digitized, and the data is transmitted and processed by a computer that generates the images. The coil or coils used may be a frame that surrounds the body part being examined (e.g., head/neck or foot/ankle coil) (Figs. 20.97 and 20.98)

The patient may also lie directly on the coil (e.g., spine coil), or the coil may wrap around the body part being examined (e.g., wrist and elbow coils). The coil or coils selected depend on the body part being examined. In MRI, various sequences are acquired with different contrasts (weightings) to evaluate anatomy and aid in diagnosing diseases and pathology.

Because no ionizing radiation is used, MRI is currently deemed safer than CT in terms of biologic tissue damage. However, MRI safety considerations must be identified and understood. The basic principles of MRI safety are discussed on the following pages.

PHYSICAL PRINCIPLES OF MRI

In MRI, each body part is typically called an examination (e.g., C-spine, brain, knee), and each examination is composed of numerous pulse sequences. Each pulse sequence is similar to a different projection in an x-ray study. Sequences in MRI vary not only by orientation (projection), but also by contrast weighting. Image contrast is defined as the relative difference in the signal strength between two adjacent tissue types. Contrast is affected by the sequence selected and the combination of acquisition parameters defined. For example, one sequence may demonstrate a fatty lesion as an area with bright signal (T1 weighting), whereas another sequence demonstrates the same fatty lesion with dark, or low, signal (T2 weighting). Comparing the characteristics of fatty lesions on both T1- and T2-weighted images provides the radiologist with more information for an accurate diagnosis.

During each MRI sequence, the MRI scanner deposits energy into the patient using radiofrequency (RF) pulses designed to "excite" hydrogen nuclei. Unlike ionizing radiation, these RF pulses have long wavelengths and low frequencies.

Once the hydrogen nuclei are excited, the scanner uses a **RF coil** to measure the resulting signal produced by these excited nuclei. The electrical signal from the coil is transmitted through an analog-to-digital converter (ADC) and then to a computer, where the raw-data matrix is reconstructed mathematically using a process

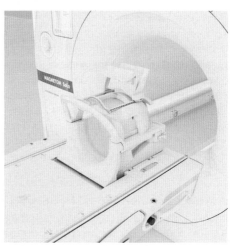

Fig. 20.97 MR head/neck coil. (Courtesy of Siemens Medical Solutions USA, Inc.)

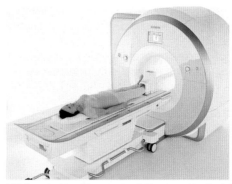

Fig. 20.98 MR foot/ankle. (Courtesy of Siemens Medical Solutions USA, Inc.)

known as **Fourier transform (FT);** this converts the raw data to form the final MR image. The main components of the MRI system include (Fig. 20.99):

- Magnet coil – Generates the magnet field to produce magnetization in the patient
- Radiofrequency system – Aids in generating a signal through excitation
- Gradients – Localization of slices and voxels, encodes the signal and has a key function in the generation of the image
- High-performance computer – Digitizes raw data into MRI images. Software is used to review images and post-processing data.

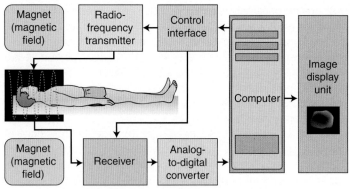

Fig. 20.99 Main components of the MRI system.

Interaction of Nuclei with Magnetic Fields

Clinical MRI uses the hydrogen nuclei (single proton) to produce an image. Hydrogen is found in water molecules and can also be found in bone and fat. MRI depends on the abundance of hydrogen protons, because the hydrogen nuclei provide a strong magnetic field used to generate MRI images.

Nuclei that have an odd number of protons and neutrons are unbalanced. They generate a net nuclear spin or **spin angular momentum,** and consequently are suitable for diagnostic MR imaging. However, hydrogen is only one example of MR-active nuclei present in the human body. Table 20.4 provides a list of MR-active nuclei found in the body suitable for MR clinical and spectroscopy examinations. Theoretically, numerous suitable nuclei exist, yet "clinical" imaging currently is only performed using **hydrogen nuclei** (which contain a single proton and no neutrons).

TABLE 20.4 **NUCLEI USED FOR MR SPECTROSCOPY (MRS)**	
SYMBOL	**NAME**
^{1}H	Hydrogen
^{13}C	Carbon
^{15}N	Nitrogen
^{39}K	Potassium
^{19}F	Fluorine
^{23}Na	Sodium
^{31}P	Phosphorus
^{17}O	Oxygen

Precession

MRI is possible because a magnetic nucleus **precesses** (spins or wobbles) around a strong **static** (unchanging) **magnetic field,** known as **B0.** The phenomenon of precession **occurs whenever a spinning object is acted upon by an external force.** An example of precession is shown in Fig. 20.100. A spinning top, when acted on by the force of gravity, precesses, or wobbles, about the line defined by the direction of gravitational force. In MRI, the proton of a hydrogen nucleus precesses when placed in a strong magnetic field and spins around its axis, giving it angular momentum. The precessional frequency is also referred to as the **Larmor frequency** or *resonance frequency.*

The **rate of precession** of a proton in a magnetic field **increases as the strength of the magnetic field increases.** Hydrogen protons precess at a constant rate of 42.58 MHz/Tesla (known as the **gyromagnetic ratio**).

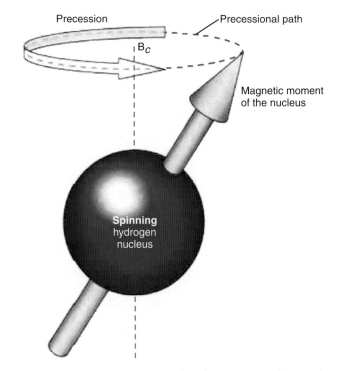

Fig. 20.100 Precession. (From Westbrook C. *MRI at a glance,* ed 3, New Jersey, 2016, Wiley.)

Net Magnetization

Once the patient is placed within the MRI scanner, the precessing hydrogen protons align with or against the main magnetic field (B0). Protons aligned (parallel) with B0 (spin up) are considered low-energy protons because they require less energy to point in the same direction as the main static field. Protons aligned against (antiparallel) to B0 are in the opposing direction of the main static field and are considered high-energy protons (spin down); these protons are not used for imaging. Simply put, it requires much more energy to swim against a current than with it. In clinical scanning, because there are always more protons aligned in the low-energy state, the slice now has a **net magnetization (NM),** which is the sum of all the magnetic moments averaged together.

MRI scanners continue to increase in static field strength (i.e., replacing clinical magnets 1.5T with a 3T and up to 7T). As static field strengths increase, it becomes more difficult for protons to remain in the high-energy state, resulting in a larger number of usable low-energy protons and greater net magnetization. If **net magnetization** increases, more protons are manipulated for imaging. This results in a higher overall signal received by the RF coil and a better image quality.

Resonance

To create an image, the low-energy precessing protons in the net magnetization vector must be pushed away from alignment with B_0. Protons aligned with B0 are said to lie in the **longitudinal plane,** also known as the **z axis.** If an RF pulse with a **matching precessional frequency** is applied to these protons, the protons will shift away from the longitudinal plane and into the **transverse plane (xy axis).** This occurs because the RF pulse has deposited energy into the low-energy protons, causing them to become excited and shift into a higher energy state. This exchange of energy between the low and high energy states at a specific frequency is known as **resonance.**

Resonance occurs only in protons with matching precessional frequencies. This means that for clinical MRI scanners, only hydrogen protons resonate because the RF pulses are emitted from the RF coil tuned to the precessional frequency of hydrogen. Any other protons in the area (e.g., oxygen, carbon, nitrogen) will not resonate because they each have a different precessional frequency.

Relaxation

Before receiving the RF excitation pulse, the hydrogen protons are in alignment with B0 and precessing (spinning at the same frequency) randomly in different phases (different directions). An RF pulse is applied to the precessing nuclei for a very brief period of time. This excitation pulse accomplishes two things: it forces the precessing protons into the transverse plane (x-y plane) and away from B_0, and it forces the protons to precess in phase (same direction). As soon as the RF pulse is turned off, the nuclei begin to return to equilibrium in a process called **relaxation.** As the nuclei relax, the MRI signal received from the precessing nuclei diminishes.

The **rate of relaxation** relays information about normal tissue and pathologic processes within the tissues, because normal tissue and tissue with pathology relax at different rates. The appearance of tissue on the MRI image is dependent on the relaxation rate. Relaxation may be divided into two categories, commonly referred to as **T1** and **T2 relaxation** (Fig. 20.101).

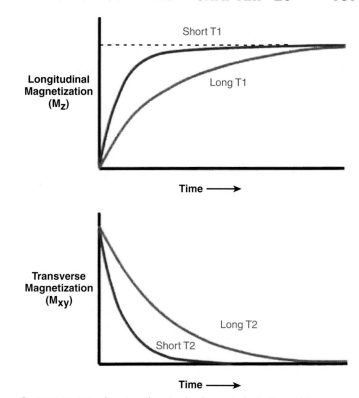

Fig. 20.101 T1 relaxation (longitudinal or spin lattice) and T2 relaxation (transverse or spin-spin). (Courtesy Allen D. Elster, MRIquestions.com.)

T1 Relaxation Following the RF excitation pulse, precessing protons are pushed away from the longitudinal plane and into the transverse plane. This is necessary for the MRI scanner to detect the signal specific to these protons. Precessing protons within the transverse plane create a voltage in the receiver coil, which translates to signal for the MRI image.

As previously noted, the protons will not stay in the transverse plane but will instead relax back into the longitudinal plane due to the dephasing of photons. Protons dephase due to the inherent tissue properties and static magnetic field imperfections caused by the MR magnet. This process is known by many names: **T1 relaxation, longitudinal relaxation, spin lattice relaxation,** or **T1 recovery.** As more protons experience T1 relaxation, the MRI signal decreases in strength. **T1 relaxation** is defined as the time it takes for 63% of the **longitudinal magnetization** to recover in the tissue (37% remains in the transverse plane).

T2 Relaxation At the same time as T1 relaxation, the randomly precessing protons are forced by the RF pulse to precess together, or in phase (phase coherence), to create **transverse magnetization.** The increase in the number of protons precessing in phase subsequently increases the signal received by the receiver coil, resulting in a higher signal and a better image. However, just as with T1 relaxation, once the RF pulse is removed, the protons will lose **phase coherence.** This loss of phase coherence is called **T2 relaxation, spin-spin relaxation, or T2 decay.** Similarly to T1 relaxation, the MRI signal decreases as more protons experience T2 decay and spin out of phase **(phase incoherence).** T2 relaxation is defined as the time it takes for **transverse magnetization** to lose 63% of its original value (37% remains in phase).

The rate of T1 and T2 relaxation changes after exposure to the RF pulse constitutes the primary basis from which the MR image is reconstructed. However, a third factor, **spin density,** also plays a minor role in determining the appearance of the MR image.

Spin Density A stronger signal is received if the **quantity** of hydrogen nuclei that are present in a given volume of tissue is **increased.** The measure of the quantity is called the **proton density,** or **spin density.** Spin density is important because an adequate number of protons is required to produce a signal. For example, the ventilated airways and alveolar spaces within the lungs are rarely imaged in MRI because of the sparse number of hydrogen protons found in air. To image airways with MRI, hyperpolarized gas (xenon or helium) may be introduced to increase the proton density.

Summary

MRI contrast resolution is highly dependent on MRI signal strength received by a an RF coil. A stronger signal results in improved contrast resolution on the final image.

The **strength of the MRI signal** is determined by the number of nuclei per unit volume **(spin density)** and the orientation of the nuclei with respect to the static magnetic field **(T1 relaxation)** and with respect to each other **(T2 relaxation).** Other factors such as flowing blood or the presence of contrast material also play a key role.

MRI is a fundamentally different way of looking at the body compared to other imaging modalities. In radiography, the physical density (grams per milliliter) and atomic number of tissues help to determine the appearance of the image. The rate of recovery of atoms from their interactions with x-rays is not important in radiography. However, the **rate of recovery of nuclei** after the application of radio waves is the most important factor in determining the MR image (Fig. 20.102). High tissue density, such as that seen in dense bone structure, does *not* result in image contrast in MRI. Cortical bone does not produce an MRI signal because the hydrogen nuclei are tightly bound within the bony matrix. As seen in the sagittal head MRI image (Fig. 20.102A), soft tissues such as **gray and white matter** of the brain, the brainstem, and the corpus callosum are clearly visualized due to the response of the nuclei in these tissues.

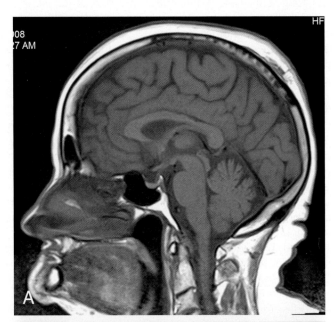

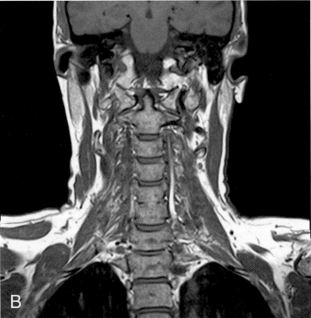

Fig. 20.102 A, Sagittal head MRI (T1-weighted image). B, Coronal C-spine MRI (T1-weighted image). (**A** courtesy NEA Baptist, Jonesboro, AR; **B** courtesy White River Medical Center, Batesville, AR.)

MRI Magnets

The most visible and probably most often discussed component of the MRI system is the magnet. The **magnet is what provides the powerful static** (constant strength) **magnetic field about which the nuclei precess.** There are a variety of MR magnets available, such as permanent, resistive, and superconducting. These all share a common purpose which is to create a very strong magnetic field that is measured in units of **tesla.** Nikola Tesla (1856–1943) was a Serbian-American researcher (born in Croatia) in electromagnetic phenomena. He defined a *tesla (T)* as an SI unit of magnetic flux density equal to 1 weber per square meter (SI unit of measurement). One Wb/m^2 (weber per square meter) is the SI unit measurement of magnetic flux, named after the German physicist Wilhelm Weber (1804–1891). Field strengths most commonly used clinically vary from 0.2 to 7T but can range for research purposes from 0.2T (ultralow field) to 45T (ultrahigh field). In comparison, the magnitude of the earth's magnetic field at its surface ranges between approximately 25,000 and 65,000 nanoteslas (nT) (0.25–0.65 gauss).[37]

The fringe field is the magnetic field measured in gauss (G), that exists outside the magnet's center; the higher the field strength, the larger the fringe field. Depending on the magnet, manufacturer, and other system-specific characteristics, the amount that the fringe field extends around the MRI scanner may vary. Carl F. Gauss (1777–1855) was a German physicist who defined *gauss (G)* as a measurement of magnetic flux density in lines of flux per square centimeter (CGS unit of measurement); 1 T = 10,000 G. 5-gauss line is marked, typically by a line on the floor in the MRI department. The area outside the 5-gauss line is considered safe regarding the levels of the static magnetic field exposure. However, MR safety zones have been established and are enforced for any personnel entering the MR surrounding area and magnet room.

Permanent magnets Ferromagnetic substances are objects that retain magnetism after being exposed to a magnetic field. Such substances (e.g., nickel, cobalt, and aluminum alloys) may be used to produce a **permanent magnet** that can be used for clinical scanning. For use in MRI, permanent magnets are typically low-field magnets with field strengths up to **0.4T.**

Advantages of permanent magnet systems include an open-bore design that requires no cooling and no additional electrical power and has a limited fringe field. Permanent magnets also have lower operating costs compared to the other two types of magnets. Disadvantages include the cost, weight of the magnet, relatively low operational field strengths, inability to turn off the magnetic field, and potential inhomogeneity in the magnetic field.

Resistive magnets **Resistive magnets** work on the principle of electromagnetism and are made out of either aluminum or copper. A magnetic field is created by passage of an electrical current through a coil of wire. Resistive magnets require **large amounts of electrical power** and a cooling mechanism. Electrical power is needed to provide the high currents necessary for the production of high-strength magnetic fields, which must be considered as part of the operating costs.

The high electrical current produces heat that is generated by the resistance of the wire to the flow of electricity. This resistance acts as a type of friction that produces heat and ultimately limits the amount of current that can be produced. Typical resistive MR systems produce magnetic field strengths of up to **0.6T.** The advantage of a resistive magnet is the ability to turn the magnetic field on and off. The disadvantage is the high cost of the electrical power needed for the magnet.

Superconducting magnets The **most common type** of magnet used is the **superconducting magnet.** Superconducting magnets are electromagnets that pass electric current through coils of superconductive wire made of niobium-titanium alloy embedded in copper and cooled by liquid helium (cryogens). Superconductive magnets are designed in the shape of a tunnel and have a homogeneous magnetic field. Superconductive magnets are ramped up to the required field strength, which for diagnostic imaging is most commonly **1.5T, 3T,** or **7T,** and do not then require additional current to maintain the magnetic field.

A significant factor in the cost of superconducting magnets is the low-temperature cooling materials, called **cryogens.** The two cryogens commonly used are **liquid nitrogen** (−196°C) and **liquid helium** (−270°C). Liquid helium is typically used in all superconducting magnets because of its lower temperature. Gaseous helium is a nonrenewable resource mined from noble gases and converted to liquid helium. This is a very expensive process, and only a few helium-rich sites exist in the world. Due to the shortages of liquid helium, clinical magnets are now equipped with "zero boil-off" (ZBO), so that during normal operation of the MR system, the magnet will not lose helium. Future superconductive magnets may not contain cryogens. Gifford-McMahon (G-M) cryocoolers are being developed that can maintain temperatures below 9.4K without using liquid helium.[38]

The advantages of superconductive magnets include higher field strengths, consumption of less electricity, and a larger range of applications. Disadvantages include the use of liquid helium as a coolant and the size of the magnet bore, which may result in claustrophobia for patients.

Flared and short bore design A superconducting short bore magnet with a flared design (70 cm) helps relieve the anxiety and possible claustrophobia for some patients (Fig. 20.103). The outward design and appearance of these systems are similar for the 1.5T and 3T MR systems.

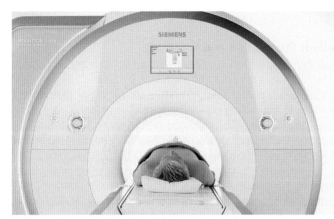

Fig. 20.103 Superconducting short bore magnet with a flared design. (Courtesy of Siemens Medical Solutions USA, Inc.)

Open MRI system An **open bore MRI system** is shown in Fig. 20.104. This is a 0.2T **permanent magnet**. Other manufacturers produce **open resistive** magnets of similar size. An advantage to an open MR magnet is that the design may help patients who are claustrophobic or unable to fit into a traditional closed bore magnet. Disadvantages of these systems are that they only perform basic applications, require longer scan times, and produce lower resolution images.

PATIENTS ASPECTS: CONTRAINDICATIONS, PREPARATION, ANXIETY, AND MONITORING
Contraindications
An MR examination is contraindicated for patients with electronic and electrically conductive metals, implants and some external or implanted medication pumps (used to deliver insulin, chemotherapy, or pain-relieving drugs). For a more comprehensive list see Box 20.2[39–41] Some newer pacemakers and several internal drug infusion pumps may be considered MR conditional and safe to image with MRI. However, before the MRI procedure, if possible, any contraindicated material must be removed prior to entering the MR magnet room. Implants and devices that *cannot* be removed must be researched and deemed MR safe or MR conditional by a qualified medical professional (MRI technologist or MRI radiologist) to ensure it is safe to enter the MR environment. Before the MR examination can be performed, the radiologist must review whether the implant or device is safe to be scanned and provide the final approval.

Although pregnancy in not an absolute contraindication, it is typically preferred not to scan a patient during the first trimester. However, there are no known verified risks regarding performing MR exams on pregnant women or fetuses.[42] If an MRI examination is indicated for a pregnant patient the referring physician and radiologist must determine risk versus benefit. An informed consent should be obtained from the patient and clinically documented. The radiologist must then provide final approval before the patient undergoes the MR scan. A pregnant patient who undergoes an MRI examination is *not* given a contrast agent gadolinium-diethylenetriaminepentaacetic acid (Gd-DTPA), because the safety of the fetus has not been verified.

Finally, alternative imaging methods are occasionally recommended based on contraindications or the clinical condition of the patient. MRI may be unsuitable for patients on ventilators or those in need of heavy monitoring, in addition to patients with multiple intravenous medication needs.

Patient Preparation and Screening
Each person involved in patient scheduling and preparation plays a key role in a successful MRI examination. When the appointment is scheduled, a brief form, brochure, or facility website may be provided to the patient explaining the MR examination. A thorough patient history must be obtained before the MR examination is performed. When patients arrive for the MR exam, they are required to fill out an MRI screening form (Box 20.3).

The screening form has questions regarding the patient's history, implants, prosthetics, surgeries, tattoos/or body piercing, insulin pumps, allergies, and medical conditions. The MRI Technologist reviews the screening form with the patient and includes any additional medical history discovered. The patient is then required to change into scrubs or a patient gown for the procedure. In addition, the patient must remove all metal, analog watches, credit cards, metallic jewelry and electronic devices (e.g., hearing aids, cell phones, and tablets). Body-piercings made of ferromagnetic materials should be removed due to potential jewelry movement, heating, and production of image artifacts. If removal of metallic body-piercing jewelry is impossible, the patient should be informed of the potential risks of leaving the jewelry in place. The technologist should also clear this with the radiologist prior to proceeding with the examination.

When preparing the patient for an MR examination, it may also helpful to explain and review the following:
1. Describe the MRI procedure
2. Importance of removing all metal prior to the exam (ferrous material)
3. Importance of changing into a patient gown or scrubs
4. Lack of ionizing radiation
5. Emphasis on the importance of holding still
6. Explain the noises produced during the MR exam
7. Hearing protection (earplugs)
8. Coil used for the exam and purpose
9. Squeeze ball – alert system to notify the technologists that immediate patient assistance is required
10. Two-way communication and monitoring during the exam
11. Length of examination
12. Inform the patient if contrast will be administered and how

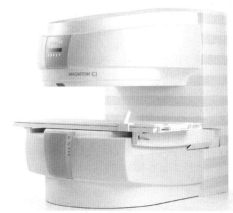

Fig. 20.104 MR open bore system. (Courtesy of Siemens Medical Solutions USA, Inc.)

BOX 20.2 MRI CONTRAINDICATIONS[29,30,37,53]
- Pacemakers (unless certified as MRI safe)
- Defibrillators (unless certified as MRI safe)
- Aneurysm clips (unless certified as MRI safe)
- Metallic fragments in or near the eye
- Cochlear implants
- Starr-Edwards pre–6000 model prosthetic heart valve
- Internal drug infusion pumps
- Internal pain pumps (unless certified as MRI safe)
- Neurostimulators
- Bone growth stimulators
- Ferromagnetic gastrointestinal surgical clips
- Electrically conductive implants and prostheses
- Metallic spirals for contraception (IUDs [intrauterine devices])
- Artificial anus (anus praeter) with magnetic closure
- Transdermal drug patches with metallic backings
- Transdermal or other similar implant (e.g., body piercings and magnetic piercings)
- Bullets and shrapnel
- Silver-embedded microfiber clothing or copper-infused clothing

BOX 20.3 **SAMPLE MRI SCREENING FORM**

MRI Patient Screening Form

PATIENT INFORMATION

Date of Exam	Height _____ Weight _____
Patient Name	Date of Birth
Reason for Exam:	

☒ Yes ☒ No   Previous imaging of body part being scanned today?   Where?   Requested?

PATIENT HISTORY

Do you have any of the following:

☒ Yes ☒ No   **Pacemaker or Defibrillator**
☒ Yes ☒ No   Mechanical Heart Valve
☒ Yes ☒ No   Stents
☒ Yes ☒ No   Vena Cava Umbrella/ IVC Filter
☒ Yes ☒ No   **Neurostimulator**/External Electrodes
☒ Yes ☒ No   Brain, Eye or Ear Surgery
☒ Yes ☒ No   **Brain Aneurysm** Clips
☒ Yes ☒ No   Programmable Shunt
☒ Yes ☒ No   Removable Hearing Aid/**Cochlear Implant**
☒ Yes ☒ No   Removable Dental Work
☒ Yes ☒ No   Infusion Pump
☒ Yes ☒ No   Wound Dressing (i.e. Acticoat 7)
☒ Yes ☒ No   **Breast Tissue Expanders**
☒ Yes ☒ No   Tattoos and/or Body Piercings
☒ Yes ☒ No   Small Bowel **Camera Capsule** Study*
☒ Yes ☒ No   **Metallic Gunshot wound, shrapnel, BB**
☒ Yes ☒ No   **Metal fragments in eyes or body***
☒ Yes ☒ No   **Insulin Pump**

Do you have any of the following Medical Conditions?

☒ Yes ☒ No   Claustrophobia
☒ Yes ☒ No   Diabetic
☒ Yes ☒ No   History of Kidney Disease
☒ Yes ☒ No   Dialysis/Kidney Failure
☒ Yes ☒ No   History of Liver Disease
☒ Yes ☒ No   Iron deficiency treated with Feraheme
☒ Yes ☒ No   Medication Skin Patches
☒ Yes ☒ No   Latex Allergy
☒ Yes ☒ No   Hypertension (High Blood Pressure)
☒ Yes ☒ No   History of Cancer Type_____

Radiation Therapy/Chemo_____

Women: Last Menstrual Period _____
☒ Yes ☒ No   Pregnancy* Weeks

List all medication allergies

*Supervising Radiologist Approval:_____ Date: _____

List all PRIOR Surgeries	**List all Medications currently taking**
1 _____	1 _____
2 _____	2 _____
3 _____	3 _____
4 _____	4 _____
5 _____	5 _____
6 _____	6 _____

******I acknowledge the above information is true and accurate to the best of my knowledge.* Your physician or radiologist may deem it necessary to have an IV injection of a contrast agent containing gadolinium to improve the quality of your MR examination. I understand the use of contrast and have had all my questions answered.**

Patient Signature _____ Date: _____

(Parent or Guardian if patient is a minor or Incapacitated)

TECHNOLOGIST SECTION

☒   **History of previous Gadolinium reaction**

Istat Results_____ GFR_____

☒   Post injection instructions given

☒ Yes ☒ No   Barriers to Learning, Please explain: _____

Contrast Name _____
Amount
Lot _____ Exp
Injection Site _____ No:
Device Used _____
Tech Initials

EXAM:	PID:

Tech Comments: _____

Screening Tech attest information reviewed   Tech Completing Exam

Relieving Patient Anxiety

The aperture or bore of the magnet (gantry) with a patient being positioned on the MRI table is shown in Fig. 20.105. This may be a narrow and confining space, and some patients may experience claustrophobia, become anxious, or becomes emotionally distressed. The MRI technologist must be prepared and take steps to ensure the patient experiences as little anxiety as possible. Steps can be taken to help reduce patient anxiety:

1. Explain the examination.
2. Play music.
3. Provide relaxation techniques (e.g., patient closes eyes and thinks of something pleasant).
4. Use cushions and pads to make the patient comfortable.
5. Move patient slowly into the magnet.
6. Take another person into the room (e.g., family member) to stay during the procedure.

NOTE: Not all facilities allow family and friends into the MRI examination room. This is at the discretion of the facility. All those entering the MR examination room must fill out the MR screening form and must be interviewed by the MR technologists.

7. Provide a squeeze ball, which, when squeezed, sets off an alarm notifying the MR technologists that the patient needs immediate attention.
8. Provide constant communication with the patient in-between sequences to help relieve anxiety.
9. If sedation is to be used, explain this process. The type of sedation and contraindications vary depending on department routines. The patient must be closely monitored if sedated and must be accompanied by a friend or family member who can drive the person home after the MR examination.

PATIENT MONITORING

Talking to the patient may be required throughout the examination (in-between sequences) to reassure the patient during the procedure. If the technologist is speaking to the patient during the examination, it is important to remind them not to talk or move during or in-between pulse sequences. Since this may result in motion artifacts and the pulse sequence may need to be repeated.

Various types of sedation can be used during an MR examination, including oral, intravenous (IV), and general anesthesia.[43] All portable anesthesia machines, monitoring devices, IV poles, and oxygen tanks must be checked to ensure they are MR conditional and safe to enter the MRI examination room.

MRI SAFETY

MRI Safety Zones

The American College of Radiology (ACR) has defined four safety zones within an MRI facility for all personnel who enter or have access to these areas.[44]

- **Zone I:** All areas accessible to the general public (e.g., entrance to the facility).
- **Zone II:** Public area, interface between unregulated zone I and strictly controlled zones III and IV. MR safety screening is performed in this area (e.g., reception area, waiting room, changing room, and/or patient screening area) by the MRI technologists.
- **Zone III:** Area near the magnet room (e.g., MR control area next to the magnet room); all patients must be accompanied by MR personnel or an MRI technologist.
- **Zone IV:** All ferromagnetic objects must be removed that are not considered MR safe or MR conditional (e.g., inside the MR magnet room). All personnel entering zone IV must be accompanied by an MRI technologist.

LEVEL 1 AND LEVEL 2 MR PERSONNEL[54]

Level 1 personnel: Personnel who have passed the minimum MR safety education to ensure their own safety and are now cleared to work within zone III.

Level 2 personnel: MRI personnel with more extensive training in MRI safety and any issues that may arise, such as potential thermal loading or burns and neuromuscular excitation from rapidly changing gradients. The MR medical director is responsible for identifying individuals who qualify as level 2 MR personnel. It is understood that the medical director will have the necessary education and experience in MR safety to qualify as a level 2 MR professional.

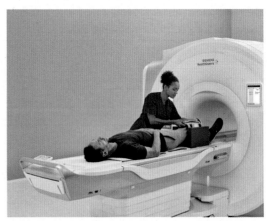

Fig. 20.105 Positioning of patient in MR bore. (Courtesy of Siemens Medical Solutions USA, Inc.)

SAFETY CONSIDERATIONS

Safety is mandatory for all personnel entering the MR environment (e.g., technologist, patient, and medical and ancillary personnel). MR safety concerns are due to the interaction of the magnetic fields with metallic objects and tissues. During the MRI scan, patients and personnel in the immediate area are exposed to the magnetic fields.

Safety concerns associated with MRI that result from the interaction of these magnetic fields with tissues and metallic objects are discussed as follows:

- Projectiles (missile effects)
- Electromechanical implants and devices
- Translational force and torque
- Tissue heating (specific absorption rate [SAR])
- Peripheral nerve stimulation (gradient magnetic fields [time-varying magnetic fields])
- Burns
- Pregnancy
- MRI contrast agents

Projectiles/Missile Effects

Ferrous objects entering the MR room (e.g., keys, patient beds, oxygen tanks) may be strongly attracted to the MR magnet and become projectiles when pulled at a high speed into the magnet bore, causing injury to the patient, MR personnel, and/or the MR magnet. MR safety screening is therefore mandatory for anyone entering the MR scan room (Zone IV), as previously discussed. Every facility has MRI safety warning signs and posters to help prevent unauthorized personnel from entering these restricted areas. Newer door security systems may also be installed that incorporate a detector array that sets off an alarm when a ferrous metal object crosses the sensor (Fig. 20.106).

The fringe field is measured in gauss, and the strength of the fringe field is inversely proportional to the cube of the distance from the bore of the magnet; that is, the danger of ferrous projectiles becomes greater as they move closer to the magnet (Fig. 20.107). If a small ferromagnetic object was released close to the magnet, it could become lethal because it would attain a terminal velocity of 40 miles per hour by the time it reached the center of the magnet.[45] This phenomenon is known as the **missile effect** because of the dangerous speed at which objects may project into the scanner.

In the event of a **code (respiratory or cardiac arrest)**, it is highly recommended to remove the patient from the MR scan room (Zone IV). All emergency responders and ancillary staff must be trained to effectively and safely respond to a code in the MR examination areas (Zone III and Zone IV) to prevent any safety injuries and/or accidents.

As a rule, ferrous patient equipment, such as oxygen tanks, IV pumps, wheelchairs, carts, and patient monitoring equipment, are not allowed inside the 5-G line. However, nonferrous oxygen tanks, wheelchairs, patient gurneys, IV poles, and other equipment have been designed to be used specifically within the MRI examination area.

Electromechanical Implants and Devices

Adverse events are possible if electronic implants or devices enter the magnet room and interact with the static magnetic field or RF field. Newer MR implants and devices are now available and considered **MR conditional** as long as specific requirements are followed; these guidelines are set by the implant/device manufacturer and must be adhered to as directed.

As a general rule, the 5-G line is used as the primary safety line for all foreign (metallic) objects within the MRI suite.

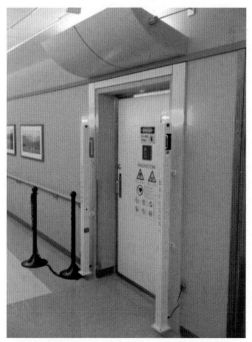

Fig. 20.106 Warning posters and door security.

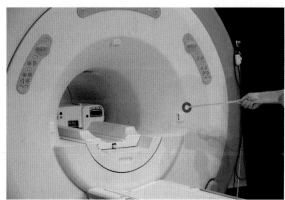

Fig. 20.107 Demonstration of potential hazard of projectiles. A metallic object (ferromagnetic washer) shown in midair suspension as it is strongly attracted toward the magnet. If not securely held back by the rope, it would become a dangerous projectile. (This demonstration is not recommended without adequate precautions and safety measures.)

Translational Force and Torque

Metallic objects (e.g., aneurysm clips, ventriculoperitoneal shunts, and stents) may be located inside or on the patient's body. These are a concern when they are introduced into the static magnetic field because translational and rotational forces on the ferromagnetic object may cause the objects to **torque** (twist), damaging the tissue surrounding a structure.[46]

Caution is recommended for all patients who have had recent placement of surgical clips or stents. All surgically implanted objects or devices should be evaluated for MRI safety. Patients with metallic foreign objects such as bullets and shrapnel and, especially, intraocular metallic objects must be carefully screened. If it is unclear whether a metallic foreign body may be lodged in the eye, screening orbits must be performed using either conventional radiographs (x-rays) or CT. The screening scans must be evaluated and the patient cleared by a radiologist before the MRI procedure can be performed.

Specific Absorption Rate: Tissue Heating

The **Specific Absorption Rate (SAR)** is defined as the rate RF energy is absorbed into the tissues.
- SAR is measured in units of Watts per kilogram (W/kg).
- SAR is specific to the body part and tissue type.
- SAR represents the rate of RF exposure and amount of RF absorbed.

Technologists must be aware of SAR limits and understand how to manipulate technical factors so that SAR limits are not exceeded. According to the FDA, whole-body averaged SAR limits should not exceed 4W/kg for 15 minutes of scanning, or a rise 1°C in the core of the body.[47] The MRI system calculates the SAR based on the information entered by the technologist during patient registration. SAR calculations may also take into consideration the temperature and humidity of the MR magnet room. Although manufacturers' systems may perform the SAR calculations differently, all are required to follow FDA guidelines and the standards set by the International Electrotechnical Commission (IEC).

In addition, IEC has defined three operating modes for MRI systems: **Normal Operating Mode, First Level Controlled Mode,** and Second Level Controlled Mode (Second Level Controlled Mode is used *only* for research and not for clinical imaging).
- **Normal Operating Mode**: This mode is considered safe for all patients, regardless of their medical condition or state, and requires only routine patient monitoring.
- **First Level Controlled Mode**: This mode requires medical supervision and an assessment by a qualified medical practitioner of risk versus benefit. Patients with thermoregulatory impairment (unable to sweat) or who are unable to communicate *should not* be scanned in First Level Controlled Mode.

It is important for technologists to remain in visual and verbal contact at all times with any patient or person in the MRI suite or the magnet bore. If the patient or person in the MRI suite complains of discomfort for any reason, imaging should be stopped immediately and the cause of the discomfort should be assessed before the scan is resumed.

Specific Energy Dose (SED) The SED is the total accumulated amount of energy that is deposited into the body. The SED is measured in joules per kilogram (joules/kg). The SED is specific to the body part and tissue; it represents the "energy" of the RF and the amount of the energy "dose" that goes into the body. The SED is proportional to the change in temperature, or the total temperature rise, in the body. Just like the SAR, the SED is monitored continuously by the MR system. SED calculations are required to follow FDA guidelines and IEC standards.

Peripheral Nerve Stimulation: Gradient Magnetic Fields (Time-Varying Magnetic Fields)

The effect on the body caused by gradient magnetic fields (also known as *time-varying magnetic fields*) is referred to as *peripheral nerve stimulation*. The MRI scanner is equipped with three pairs of gradient coils. These gradients are necessary for **spatial localization** of the MRI signal. Each gradient coil is an electromagnet and produces a small magnetic field when current is applied. Magnetic fields produced by the gradient coils constantly change direction by quickly reversing the electrical current, thereby manipulating the protons' phase and precessional frequency. This gradient reversal creates the "knocking" noise heard when an MR pulse sequence is running.

Biologic effects due to time-varying magnetic fields may include:
- Peripheral nerve stimulation: Temporary stimulation of muscle and nerves (e.g., numbness and tingling in the hands and feet)
- Magnetophosphene: Visual flashes of light caused by induced current stimulating the retina
- Acoustic noise: Noise caused by gradient switching; hearing protection (earplugs or headphones) must be worn by all patients

Patient Burns

Patient burns resulting from MR imaging are uncommon but can occur. The most common burns resulting from MR are due to direct skin contact with the side of the bore, loops in the coil cable, arms and legs crossed, and coil cables coming in direct contact with (pressed tightly against) the skin (Fig. 20.108). MR technologists can place nonconducting pads to provide additional separation between the patient and the side of the bore, electronic elements, and coil cables.

Pregnancy

MRI may be indicated for use in pregnant patients if other forms of diagnostic imaging are inadequate or require exposure to ionizing radiation, such as general radiography or CT.

Although **pregnancy** is not an absolute contraindication, it typically is preferred not to scan a patient during the first trimester. However, no known risks have been verified for performing MR exams on pregnant women or fetuses.[42] If an MRI examination is indicated for a pregnant patient, the referring physician and the radiologist must determine risk versus benefit. If it is determined that the MR examination is required, informed consent *should be* obtained from the patient and clinically documented. The radiologist must then provide final approval before the patient undergoes the MR scan. A pregnant woman who undergoes an MRI examination is not given a contrast agent (Gd-DTPA) because the safety of the fetus has not been verified.

OCCUPATIONAL HAZARDS

To date no long-term biologic adverse effects have been documented for technologists who work in the MRI department. As a precaution, some MRI centers have recommended that technologists who are pregnant should remain outside the scan room when the gradients are pulsing. In addition, sensory effects (vertigo, nausea, dizziness, metallic taste, and visual phosphenes) may occur *only* when in the MR magnet room. These effects are not common for all patients or personnel but are more prevalent with higher field strengths (≥3T). Radiobiologists continue to investigate the possibility and occurrence of adverse effects as a result of electromagnetic fields.

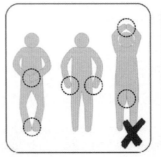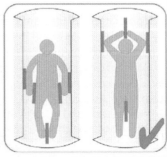

Fig. 20.108 Localized regions of high RF and bore wall contact. (Courtesy of Siemens Medical Solutions USA, Inc.)

CONTRAST AGENTS

Gadolinium (gad or gado)-based contrast agents or MRI contrast is administered only if clinical findings are indicated and when ordered by a physician or radiologist. Most MRI contrast agents used in a clinical setting work by shortening the T1 relaxation time of tissues via interactions with the contrast agent. A popular contrast agent is Gd-DTPA (Magnevist). Gadolinium (gad"-o-lin'-e-um) is a rare element that is metallic and highly magnetic (Fig. 20.109). Various brands of MR contrast agents are commercially available in the U.S. market. They are placed in two different groups: macrocyclic agents and linear agents. Both macrocyclic and linear agents can be either nonionic or ionic (Table 20.5).[48]

The amount (dose) of the MRI contrast is administered using manual intravenous injection or a power injector and is typically followed with a saline flush to ensure all the contrast is administered. The amount of contrast given can be as low as 0.1 mmol per kg of body mass. Guidelines regarding the amount (dose) of contrast can be found on the package insert of the brand of contrast administered. The imaging procedure should be completed within 1 hour of the injection. Patients may experience unusual sensations at the injection site (e.g., burning, itching, and pain) and should be observed during and after the injection for any possible reactions. Gd-DTPA has lower toxicity and causes fewer side effects than iodinated contrast agents.

Gadolinium may be contraindicated for patients who are pregnant, have kidney disease, or have had a previous allergic reaction. Because MRI contrast is excreted through the kidneys, patients who have a severe kidney disease, are at risk for renal insufficiency, or have a history of diabetes or hypertension requiring therapy are usually required to have an estimated glomerular filtration rate (eGFR) test performed prior to the MRI scan. The eGFR test may also be required as part of the standard of care for the MR facility. Each imaging facility has a certain eGFR range deemed safe for contrast medium injections, but the FDA recommends *not* injecting gadolinium-based contrast agents in patients with a GFR <30 mL/min/1.73 m^2.[49]

Gd-DTPA often helps to differentiate primary disease (tumor) from secondary effects (edema). It also helps in the evaluation of metastasis, infection, inflammatory processes, and subacute cerebral infarcts. Gd-DTPA enhances sensitivity in detecting primary and secondary tumors in the brain (Figs. 20.110 and 20.111) and can help to differentiate scarring from recurrent disk disease in the spine postoperatively.

Physiologic Gating and Triggering

MR has the capability of performing physiologic gating/triggering to reduce artifacts resulting from cardiac motion, respiratory artifacts, and pulsatile flow. For example, **triggering**, a type of "prospective gating," is used to acquire static images during a specific time in the cardiac cycle.

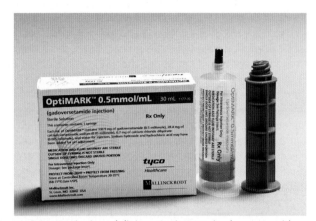

Fig. 20.109 Nonionic gadolinium OptiMARK (gadoversetamide injection). (Courtesy Mallinckrodt, Inc, St. Louis, MO.)

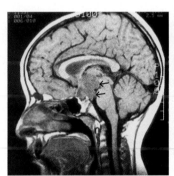 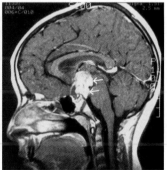

Fig. 20.110 Without contrast agent (T1-weighted image). Pathologic changes appear gray (see arrows).

Fig. 20.111 With contrast agent, Gd-DTPA (T1-weighted image). Pathology appears as bright areas in central brain (see arrows).

TABLE 20.5 MRI CONTRAST AGENTS FDA-APPROVED FOR USE IN THE US[48]			
BRAND NAME	**CHEMICAL NAME**	**STRUCTURE**	**COMMENTS**
Magnevist	Gadopentetate (Gd-DTPA)	Linear ionic	Oldest agent (FDA approved in 1988); below average relaxivity; probable ↑ risk of Nephrogenic Systemic Fibrosis (NSF).
MultiHance	Gadobenate (Gd-BOPTA)	Linear ionic	Highest relaxivity of all extracellular gadolinium agents due to transient protein binding; 3% to 5% hepatocyte uptake; competitive inhibitor for cMOAT drugs (tamoxifen, methotrexate, cisplatin); QT prolongation.
Omniscan	Gadodiamide (Gd-DTPA-BMA)	Linear nonionic	Low thermodynamic stability; disproportionately ↑ risk of NSF; may interfere with serum Ca^{++} measurements; lowest rate of reactions.
Dotarem	Gadoterate (Gd-DOTA)	Macrocyclic Ionic	One of the oldest agents with the market share in Europe, most recent entry (2013) into US market; strongest Gd binding per Keq.
ProHance	Gadoteridol (Gd-HP-DO3A)	Macrocyclic Nonionic	Lowest osmolality and viscosity of all agents; below average relaxivity.
Gadavist	Gadobutrol (Gd-BT-DO3A)	Macrocyclic Nonionic	Highest viscosity due to 1.0M formulation (all others 0.5M); above average relaxivity; marketed as Gadovist outside the US.
Eovist (USA)	Gadoxetrate (Gd-EOB-DTPA)	Linear Ionic	Designed for liver imaging; ~50% uptake by hepatocytes after initial extracellular phase; joint renal and biliary excretion; very high relaxivity due to size and transient protein binding.

cMOAT, Canalicular multispecific organic anion transporter; *Fe,* iron; *NSF,* nephrogenic systemic fibrosis.

MRI TISSUE CONTRAST

MR images are influenced by parameters that determine tissue contrast: T1, T2, and proton density (PD). However, the repetition time (TR) and echo time (TE) are modified to emphasize a particular type of contrast (Table 20.6).[50,51]

MRI PULSE SEQUENCES

An MRI pulse sequence is comprised of RF pulses and magnetic field gradient pulses used in combination with the data acquisition timing to produce MR images. There are a variety of pulse sequences to choose from; however, there are primary pulse sequences that these variations are based on: **Spin Echo (SE)** and **Gradient Echo (GRE).** All other pulse sequences variations are based on **SE and GRE** and are modified by switching the pulsing, gradients applied, RF pulses, adding gradient echo pulses, and modifying additional parameters. Pulse sequences can be acquired as 2D individual slices in a single acquisition or as a 3D volume/slab acquired in a single acquisition. MR vendors also have their own naming conventions for the same pulse sequence (e.g., **Turbo Spin Echo** and **Fast Field Echo**); this is due to patents. MR pulse sequences used for clinical imaging include **Spin Echo (SE), Turbo Spin Echo (TSE)** or **Fast Spin Echo (FSE), Gradient Echo (GRE), Inversion Recovery,** and **Echo Planar Imaging (EPI).**

- *Spin Echo (SE):* Pulse sequence consists of a 90° pulse followed by a 180° refocusing pulse, then the echo is generated. SE contrast weightings include T1, T2 and proton density (PD).[50]

- *Turbo Spin Echo (TSE) or Fast Field Echo (FSE):* Pulse sequence consists of a 90° pulse followed by multiple 180° refocusing pulses (RF); each refocusing pulse generates an echo. All the echoes combined are referred to as an echo train (ET), the total number of 180° RF pulses and echoes is called the *echo train length* (ETL). TSE sequences are faster than the traditional SE sequence. TSE contrast weightings include T1, T2 and PD.[50]

- *Gradient Echo (GRE):* Pulse sequence consists of an RF pulse less than 90° that is applied to partially flip net magnetization into the transverse plane. The gradients have opposed RF pulses that are used to dephase (negative gradients) and rephase (positive gradients) the transverse magnetization. Because there is no refocusing pulse, GRE sequences with long TEs are T2* (T2 star) weighted (due to magnetic susceptibility) instead of T2, as are SE and TSE.[52] There are many variations of GRE, which have been defined in Table 20.7.[51–53]

- *Inversion Recovery:* Pulse sequence is based on an SE sequence. A 180° preparation pulse is applied to null the signal (fat, water, or cerebrospinal fluid [CSF]) defined by the time interval (TI-interval between 180° pulse and the 90° pulse). Once the RF pulse finishes, the spinning nuclei start to relax. Once net magnetization passes the transverse plane (null point for that tissue), then the 90° excitation pulse is applied and the echo is generated. Variations of inversion recovery have been defined in Table 20.8.[53,54]

TABLE 20.6 MRI TISSUE CONTRAST[52,66]

SEQUENCE VARIANT	WEIGHTING	REPETITION TIME (TR)	ECHO TIME (TE)	SIGNAL DIFFERENCES	STRUCTURES
Spin Echo, Turbo Spin Echo, or Fast Field Echo	T1 weighted	Short	Short	Low signal for increased water content; high signal for fat; high signal for MRI contrast agents. Standard sequence used and compared to other sequences.	Anatomic structures; edema, tumor, infarction, inflammation, infection, hemorrhage
Spin Echo, Turbo Spin Echo, or Fast Field Echo	T2 weighted	Long	Long	High signal for increased water content; low signal for fat; low signal for MRI contrast agents. Standard sequence used and compared to other sequences.	Lesions, inflammatory changes; soft tissue and bone disorders
Spin Echo, Turbo Spin Echo, or Fast Field Echo	Proton density (PD) weighted	Long	Short	High signal from meniscus tears.	Anatomic structures; cartilage; joint disease and injury

TABLE 20.7 MR GRADIENT ECHO SEQUENCE VARIATIONS[65–67]

GRADIENT ECHO SEQUENCE	SIEMENS HEALTHINEERS	GE	PHILIPS
Spoiled Gradient Echo (GRE)	FLASH and TurboFLASH	Spoiled GRASS (SPGR); Fast SPGR or Fast GRE	T1-FFE and TFE
Coherent GRE with FID refocusing	FISP	GRASS	FFE
Coherent GRE with Echo refocusing	PSIF	SSFP	T2-FFE
Coherent GRE with balanced FID/echo refocusing	True FISP	FIESTA COSMIC	b-FFE
Coherent balanced GRE with dual excitation	CISS	FIESTA-C	—
Coherent double GRE using combined FID and echoes	DESS	MENSA	—
Spoiled GRE using combined multiple FIDs	MEDIC	MERGE	M-FFE
Ultrafast GRE	TurboFLASH (2D) MPRAGE (3D)	FAST GRE BRAVO (3D)	TFE 3D T1-TFE
Spoiled 3D GRE variants	VIBE	FAME or LAVA-XV	THRIVE
Susceptibility weighted	SWI	SWAN 2.0	SWIp
Arterial spin labeling (ASL)	ASL	ASL	ASL

b-FFE, Balanced fast field echo; *BRAVO,* brain volume imaging; *CISS,* constructive interference in steady state; *COSMIC,* coherent oscillatory state acquisition for the manipulation of imaging contrast; *DESS,* double echo in steady state; *FAME,* fast acquisition with multiphase elliptical fast gradient echo; *FID,* Free induction decay; *FIESTA,* fast imaging employing steady state acquisition; *FIESTA-C,* variation of FIESTA/true FISP sequence; *FISP,* fast imaging with steady state precession; *FLASH,* fast low angle shot; *GRASS,* gradient recall acquisition using steady state; *FFE,* fast field echo; *LAVA-XV,* liver acquisition with volume acceleration; *MEDIC,* multiecho data image combination; *MENSA,* multiecho in steady state acquisition; *MERGE,* multiple echo recombined gradient echo; *M-FFE,* multiple fast field echo; *MPRAGE,* magnetization prepared rapid gradient echo; *PSIF,* reversed FISP; *SSFP,* steady state free precession; *SWAN 2.0,* susceptibility-weighted angiography; *SWI:* susceptibility-weighted imaging; *SWIp,* susceptibility-weighted imaging with phase enhancement; *TFE,* turbo field echo; *THRIVE,* T1-weighted high-resolution isotropic volume examination; *VIBE,* volumetric interpolated breath-hold examination.

- *Echo planar imaging (EPI):* An EPI sequence uses a single echo train to collect data from all of the lines of k-space in one TR period. The phase-encoding gradient and frequency-encoding (readout) gradient are tuned on and off rapidly, allowing k-space to be filled quickly, shortening the acquisition time. There are two types of echo planar sequences: **SE** and **GRE.** These sequences can be acquired as a **single-shot EPI,** in which all lines of k-space are acquired in a single TR, and **multi-shot EPI,** in which all lines of k-space are acquired in two or more TR periods.[50] EPI variations are used for an array of applications, such as **Diffusion-Weighted Imaging (DWI), Diffusion Tensor Imaging (DTI), Diffusion Spectrum Imaging (DSI), fMRI (BOLD), Spectroscopy,** and **Perfusion.** These techniques further described later in this chapter.

MRI EXAMINATIONS

MRI is used to evaluate internal organs, structures, and pathology in various body regions. As previously discussed, images can be acquired in multiple orientations using different pulse sequences and weightings. MR imaging can be performed without a contrast agent, or with and without contrast when clinically indicated. Scan times vary depending on the number of sequences acquired and type of examination performed (e.g., brain, spine, abdomen, breast, cardiac, and musculoskeletal). The goal of MRI is to ensure the safety of personnel and patients and obtain optimal image quality in a reasonable amount of scan time.

Brain and Spine Imaging

MRI is used frequently for brain and spine examinations due to the exceptional detail visualized. The fundamental sequences used are T1, T2, and PD. Additional sequences may be added, depending on the facility's standard protocols as defined by a radiologist and/or clinical indications. For example, a FLAIR sequence is acquired routinely in the brain to suppress CSF to better visualize periventricular hyperintense lesions, such as multiple sclerosis plaques (MS). A 3D, heavily T2-weighted sequence (3D HASTE, 3D TSE) with fat suppression may also be acquired in the spine. This provides a myelogram effect and is clinically used to evaluate spinal cord enlargement, cord atrophy, and cord compression. In addition, if clinically indicated in either the brain or the spine, an intravenous contrast injection may be administered, and a T1-weighted sequence would be acquired pre-contrast and post-contrast for comparison.

- **Brain anatomy visualized** includes grey versus white matter, lobes, cerebellum, sinuses, basal ganglia, ventricles, pons, nerves, orbits, pituitary, internal auditory canal (IAC), and the brainstem; these can all be visualized in detail.
- **MR brain clinical indications** include vascular (ischemic and hemorrhagic stroke, AVM, aneurysm, venous thrombosis), tumor, infection (abscess, cerebritis, encephalitis, meningitis); white matter diseases (MS and other demyelinating disorders), neoplasm, infectious diseases (including diseases associated with acquired immunodeficiency syndrome [AIDS] and herpes), trauma (epidural hematoma, contusion, subdural hematoma), congenital malformations, and hydrocephalus.[48]
- **Spine anatomy visualized** includes nerve roots, spinal cord, intravertebral disc spaces, vertebral body, foramina, facets, CSF, and subcutaneous fat (Fig. 20.112).
- **MR spine clinical indications** include Chiari malformations, congenital spine anomalies, fractures, abscesses, tumor evaluation, syringohydromyelia (syrinx), spondyloarthropathies, rheumatoid arthritis, preoperative and postoperative evaluation, infectious disease (abscess, osteomyelitis, discitis), myelopathy, spinal cord infarct, MS and other white matter diseases, evaluation of the vertebral bodies, and severe scoliosis.

Magnetic resonance angiography (MRA) and *(magnetic resonance venogram (MRV)* procedures are acquired to evaluate arterial and venous circulation in various body parts (e.g., head, neck, chest, abdomen, pelvis, and legs) (Fig. 20.113). MRA enables radiologists to evaluate major arteries, and MRV can be used to evaluate veins. In the brain, an MRA of the circle of Willis has been proven to be valuable clinically in diagnosing aneurysms, occlusions, stenosis, and other anomalies. A brain MRV is clinically used to evaluate venous blood flow.

- **MRA anatomy visualized** includes the circle of Willis (COW) in the brain, carotids (neck); thoracic and abdominal aorta; renal arteries; peripheral arteries (legs); and coronary arteries (heart).

INVERSION RECOVERY	SIEMENS HEALTHINEERS	GE	PHILIPS
TABLE 20.8 **MR INVERSION RECOVERY SEQUENCE VARIATIONS**[65,66]			
Short-Tau IR	TIRM or STIR	STIR	STIR
Long-Tau IR	TIRM, Dark-Fluid	FLAIR	FLAIR
Dual Inversion Recovery (DIR)	DIR SPACE	CUBE DIR	Dual IR-TSE
True IR	TIR, True IR	—	Real IR

DIR SPACE, Double inversion recovery SPACE sequence; *FLAIR,* fluid attenuation inversion recovery; *STIR,* short-tau inversion recovery; *TIR,* true inversion recovery; *TIRM,* turbo inversion recovery magnitude; *TSE,* turbo spin echo.

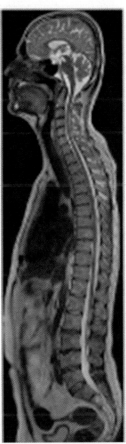

Fig. 20.112 T2 Sagittal head and spine. (Courtesy of Siemens Medical Solutions USA, Inc.)

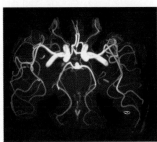

Fig. 20.113 MRA circle of Willis brain (COW). (Courtesy of Siemens Medical Solutions USA, Inc.)

- MRA clinical indications (head and neck) include aneurysms, occlusions, stenosis, obstructions, arteriovenous malformation, dissection of arteries, sinus thrombosis and intracranial venous occlusive disease.
- MRA clinical indications (thorax, abdomen, pelvis, and lower extremities) includes stenosis, aneurysm, cerebral venous thrombosis, aorta dissection, and intracranial hypertension, vascular malformations and vascular anastomoses, and peripheral artery disease.
- MRV anatomy visualized includes venous circulation in the chest, abdomen, pelvis and lower leg (calf).
- MRV clinical indications include vein occlusion, vein stenosis, deep vein thrombosis, pulmonary emboli, peripheral vascular disease, tumor invading a vein, vascular abnormalities, venous thrombosis, and evaluation of postoperative venous sites and bypass grafts.

Musculoskeletal Imaging

MRI musculoskeletal imaging is an unsurpassed technique for evaluating soft tissue, ligaments, tendons, cartilage, and bone in the extremities. MRI is a primary method of evaluating internal derangements of the knee, meniscal abnormalities, avascular necrosis of the hip and other bony regions, soft tissue masses, and bone marrow abnormalities. Musculoskeletal examinations include the knee, shoulder, wrist, elbow, foot, ankle, and long bones (legs and arms) (Figs. 20.114 and 20.115).

For the knee, for example, additional sequences may be included, depending on the facility's standard protocols as defined by a radiologist and/or clinical indications. Additionally, if clinically indicated, an intravenous contrast injection may be administered, and a T1-weighted sequence would be acquired pre-contrast and post-contrast for comparison.

- Musculoskeletal anatomy visualized includes soft tissue, tendons, cartilage, ligaments, meniscus, muscles, labrum, rotator cuff, and bone.
- MR musculoskeletal clinical indications include joint disorders (degenerative arthritis); fractures; osteonecrosis; bone marrow disorders; bone and soft tissue tumors; inflammatory changes; edema (fluid); tears in the meniscus, ligaments, or tendons in the knee; rotator cuff tears in the shoulder; labrum tears in the shoulder and hip; and avascular necrosis in the hip or other bony regions.

Body Imaging: Abdomen and Pelvis

MR body imaging fundamental sequences include T1-weighted, T1-weighted in and opposed-phase, T1-weighted without/with contrast, T2-weighted, and Gradient Echo.. Additionally, 2D and 3D sequences may be added, depending on the facility's standard protocols as defined by a radiologist and/or clinical indications. To reduce breathing motion, breath-hold and/or free-breathing techniques are routinely used; however, some facilities may prefer to use respiratory triggering as a replacement for breath-holds and/or free-breathing. Sequences acquired with respiratory triggering are dependent on the patient breathing, so if the person breathes erratically during the acquisition, the imaging time can increase significantly. If clinically indicated an intravenous contrast injection may also be administered, then a T1 sequence would be acquired pre-contrast and post-contrast for comparison. In some instances, dynamic imaging (pre- and post-contrast with multimeasurements) may also be part of a routine protocol for body examinations to see arterial, venous, and delayed enhancement (e.g., liver) (Figs. 20.116 and 20.117).

- Body anatomy visualized in the abdomen includes liver, kidneys, spleen, pancreas, gallbladder, adrenal glands, large/small bowel, ascending/descending aorta, renal arteries/veins, and biliary tract. In the pelvis, bone, soft tissue, bladder, ovaries, uterus, ureters, rectum, fetus in utero, and the prostate gland.
- MR body clinical indications includes evaluation of tumors, liver diseases (cirrhosis, fatty liver), inflammatory bowel disease (Crohn disease and ulcerative colitis); pelvic floor disease; inflammation of vessels (vasculitis); adrenal lesions, polycystic kidney disease, and renal masses.

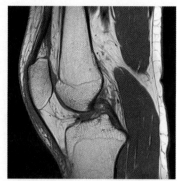

Fig. 20.114 T1 SE sagittal knee. (Courtesy of Siemens Medical Solutions USA, Inc.)

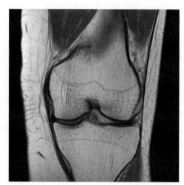

Fig. 20.115 PD TSE coronal. (Courtesy of Siemens Medical Solutions USA, Inc.)

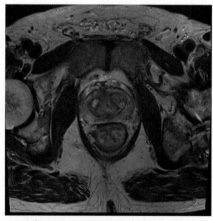

Fig. 20.116 T2 axial prostate. (Courtesy of Siemens Medical Solutions USA, Inc.)

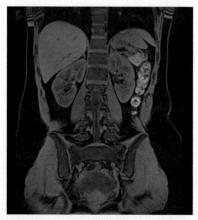

Fig. 20.117 T1 VIBE Dixon coronal abdomen and pelvis. (Courtesy of Siemens Medical Solutions USA, Inc.)

Breast Imaging

Breast MRI is a supplemental exam performed in conjunction with routine screening, mammography and ultrasound for diagnosis and staging of breast cancer. Breast MR is typically performed on patients who have a higher risk of breast cancer (family history, positive **BRCA1** or **BRCA2** gene mutation). Breast MR has the ability to evaluate the breasts bilaterally and the entire breast parenchyma from nipple to chest wall, and from medial to lateral. The ability to see the entire breast also helps to evaluate the size, depth and extent of the cancer, abscess, or other breast anomalies that may be present. Breast MR imaging is always performed using a dedicated breast coil with the patient lying on the coil in the prone position. The optimal timeframe for performing a breast MR exam on a premenopausal woman is 7 to 14 days from the start of menstrual cycle.[56]

Different techniques are used for breast MRI, including dynamic MR breast imaging (Fig. 20.118), axial breast imaging, MR breast biopsy, and MR breast implant evaluation.

- **Dynamic MR breast imaging:** Routine breast MR imaging acquired with multiple measurements and using an intravenous contrast injection. Clinically used to detect and stage breast cancer, evaluate benign lesions, fibrocystic changes, ductal carcinoma in-situ (DCIS), and invasive carcinoma.[48]
- **MR breast biopsy:** Routine breast MR imaging acquired with grid or pillar attached to the breast coil. The grid or pillar is seen on the MR image and used to localize the area of interest (lesion). Once the lesion is localized, a needle is used to remove a tissue sample that is then sent to a lab to be evaluated by a pathologist.
- **MR implant imaging:** These images are acquired to evaluate important information regarding the implant's integrity and any abnormalities and to evaluate breast tissue for pathology.

Because breast MRI has a higher incidence of false positives compared to mammography, mammography is still considered the most effective screening tool for breast cancer. However, performing both mammography and breast MRI can increase breast cancer detection.[48]

Cardiac Imaging

MR cardiac imaging is used to evaluate cardiac anatomic structures and function. MR is also used to evaluate heart values, heart chambers, blood flow through major vessels (coronaries) and structures around the heart (pericardium). This examination is triggered using a technique called an electrocardiogram (ECG). ECG leads are placed on the chest to synchronize the sequence with the heart during the data acquisition. Triggering reduces the motion from the heart so diagnostic images can be obtained. An intravenous contrast injection may also be used if ordered by a physician to evaluate myocardial ischemia, infarction (stress perfusion) and microvascular obstruction (resting perfusion).[57]

Cardiac MR clinically can be used to evaluate cardiovascular disorders such as tumors, infection, coronary artery disease, inflammatory conditions, treatment planning, and the effects of surgical changes (congenital heart disease)[57] (Fig. 20.119).

Diffusion-Weighted Imaging (DWI)

DWI is based on measuring the random (Brownian) motion of water molecules within a voxel of tissue.[58] Diffusion of the water protons in the brain follows a pattern of least resistance along the boundaries/obstacles (cell membranes, nerve fibers, pathology) of the surrounding tissue structure and properties. When pathology is present, the diffusion pattern is disturbed and the amount of diffusion changes in the affected area. The image contrast shows the difference in rate of diffusion between tissues.

The diffusion sequence has the ability to calculate multiple b-values and an Apparent Diffusion Coefficient (ADC) map. The ADC map is acquired to differentiate between T2 shine through and pure diffusion contrast. When an MRI DWI sequence is performed on a patient within (0 to 7 days) of an acute stroke, the DWI image is bright (high signal intensity), and the ADC map is dark (low signal intensity) in the area of the stroke[59] (Figs. 20.120 and 20.121).

MR DWI APPLICATIONS AND CLINICAL INDICATIONS[60]

- **Brain:** Evaluate ischemic stroke, differentiate between acute and chronic stoke, tumor grading, differentiate abscess from necrotic tumors; assess active demyelination, white matter diseases (MS, Alzheimer disease, human immunodeficiency virus [HIV] encephalopathy).

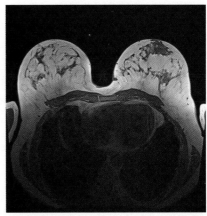

Fig. 20.118 T1 FLASH 3D non-FS axial breast. (Courtesy of Siemens Medical Solutions USA, Inc.)

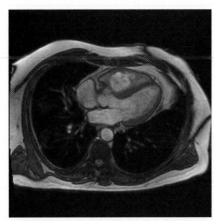

Fig. 20.119 True FISP four-chamber heart. (Courtesy of Siemens Medical Solutions USA, Inc.)

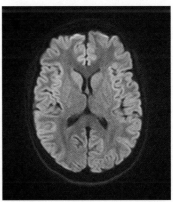

Fig. 20.120 Diffusion trace axial brain. (Courtesy of Siemens Medical Solutions USA, Inc.)

- **Head/neck:** Carcinoma, lymphomas, benign salivary gland tumors, benign cysts, benign from malignant tumors, lymphoma from squamous cell cancer, benign from metastatic lymphadenopathy.
- **Abdomen:** Focal liver lesion detection, diffuse hepatic parenchymal disease (nonalcoholic fatty liver disease) and hepatic fibrosis, differentiate malignant from benign pancreatic lesions, liver metastases, pancreatic adenocarcinoma, and kidney disease.
- **Prostate:** Characterize and grade prostate lesions, tumor detection, local tumor staging, and detection of tumor recurrence after primary treatment.[61]
- **Breast:** Malignant versus benign breast lesions, differential diagnosis between DCIS and invasive breast cancer.
- **Musculoskeletal:** Differentiate acute osteoporotic from malignant compression fractures,

DIFFUSION TENSOR IMAGING (DTI)

DTI is based on an EPI sequence. DTI uses a complete mathematical equation to model 3D anisotropy (Tensor). The tensor image displays the direction and magnitude of anisotropic diffusion. The diffusion tensor sequence acquires six or more diffusion directions to create a relationship between the data acquired and the diffusion gradients used in the pulse sequence. The directional variation in the tendency of the water molecules to diffuse within a voxel is the definition of DTI.

DTI data is also used to trace the 3D path of white matter fiber tracks; this process is called (fiber tracking or tractography) (Fig. 20.122). The preferential diffusion direction implies white matter tract structure.

DTI data sets are post-processed to create additional grey scale maps, color maps, and color fiber tracks (tractography). Tractography is used clinically to determine the outcome of treatment by evaluating the integrity, displacement, or involvement of tumors and/or trauma.

PERFUSION: DYNAMIC SUSCEPTIBILITY CONTRAST (DSC)

Dynamic susceptibility contrast perfusion is a method for measuring the flow of blood in the brain. It requires a rapid injection of contrast (gadolinium), infused into the blood by a power injector and monitored as it passes through the brain's microvasculature. As gadolinium enters the circulation, it induces susceptibility changes due to it paramagnetic properties, resulting in shorter T2* values and significant signal loss, depending on the local concentration. If the blood-brain barrier is disrupted by disease (tumor, infection), the result is T1 shortening and contrast enhancement. DSC perfusion, once acquired, can process various inline perfusion maps in grey scale when loaded into a post-processing algorithm. These perfusion maps can also be processed in color (the availability of inline perfusion maps depends on the MR manufacturer, the perfusion sequence used, and the parameters available). A list of DSC perfusion maps is presented in Table 20.9.[62,63] relCBV, relCBF, relMTT

DSC perfusion clinical indications for brain tumors include tumor vascularity, evaluation of response to therapy, and surgical intervention (stereotactic biopsy). DSC perfusion clinical indications for cerebral ischemia include acute stroke and transient ischemic attack (TIA), vascular stenosis, and vasospasm.

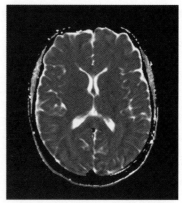

Fig. 20.121 Diffusion ADC axial brain. (Courtesy of Siemens Medical Solutions USA, Inc.)

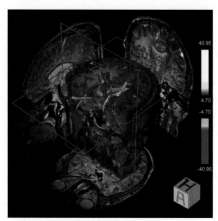

Fig. 20.122 Tractography brain. (Courtesy of Siemens Medical Solutions USA, Inc.)

TABLE 20.9 **DYNAMIC SUSCEPTIBILITY CONTRAST (DSC) PERFUSION MAPS**[57,58]	
DSC PERFUSION MAPS	**DEFINITION**
Global Bolus Plot (GBP)	Validates the quality of the bolus passage and is used to monitor the time course of contrast uptake.
Percentage of Baseline at Peak (PBP) or Percentage Signal Recovery (PSR)	Percentage of MR signal-recovery relative to the pre-contrast baseline image at the end of first pass perfusion.
Time to Peak (TTP)	Time from initial arterial contrast injection to bolus peak, maximum signal loss within the organ of interest.
Cerebral Blood Volume (CBV)	Volume of blood in a given region of brain tissue (measured in milliliters per 100 g of brain tissue)
Cerebral Blood Flow (CBF)	Volume of blood passing through a given region of brain tissue per unit of time (measured in milliliters per minute of 100 g of brain tissue)
Mean Transit Time (MTT)	Average time for a single contrast molecule (not entire bolus) to pass through tissue.

PERFUSION: ARTERIAL SPIN LABELING

Arterial Spin Labeling (ASL), also referred to as **Arterial Spin Tagging**, is a noninvasive MRI perfusion technique that evaluates cerebral blood flow by magnetically labeling inflowing blood. ASL does not rely on an injection of contrast; rather, it uses the blood water content as an endogenous contrast agent for measuring MR perfusion. ASL labeling uses the water molecules circulating in the brain; using an RF pulse, it tracks the blood as it circulates through the brain, capturing a "label" image. A "control" image is then acquired before the blood water is labeled. Then the label and control images are subtracted, and the signal differences directly reflect the tissue perfusion[64] (Fig. 20.123).

ASL supports various techniques, including pulsed arterial spin labeling and pseudo-continuous arterial spin labeling.

- **Pulsed arterial spin labeling (PASL):** Blood water is inverted as it passes through a labeling slab instead of a plane.[64]
- **Pseudo-continuous arterial spin labeling (PCASL):** Blood water is inverted as it flows through the brain in one plane. CASL is characterized by a single long pulse (1 to 3 seconds).[64]

ASL is used instead of MR DSC perfusion when a contrast agent cannot be administered or as a routine perfusion technique. Clinically, ASL, like DSC perfusion, can assess cerebral infarction, acute and chronic stroke, brain tumors, epilepsy, neurodegenerative disease (Alzheimer disease), frontotemporal dementia, and Parkinson disease.[64]

FUNCTIONAL MAGNETIC RESONANCE IMAGING AND BLOOD OXYGENATED LEVEL DEPENDENT

There are two terms typically associated with functional imaging. **Functional Magnetic Resonance Imaging (fMRI)** and **Blood Oxygenated Level Dependent (BOLD).** fMRI is the study of the function of specific neural regions and/or activities of a structure. fMRI displays areas of the brain that are participating in certain motor, sensory, or cognitive activities (e.g., movement of the hand, memory, sense of smell, and visual perception). This activity is measured by detecting changes in the oxygen levels and the increased blood flow to the brain in response to the neural activity. Because the blood flow and neural activation are linked, the areas of the brain that are more active consume more oxygen due to the increased blood flow; these are the areas that display the activation

BOLD is a term used for a functional MRI technique. BOLD uses local changes in blood flow as an indicator of momentary activation of a region of the brain. This technique uses the differences in deoxyhemoglobin that introduce homogeneity into the magnetic field where oxyhemoglobin does not. If an increase of deoxyhemoglobin concentration is seen, there is a decrease in the image intensity.

Prior to the fMRI examination, the patient is instructed in how to perform an exercise or sequence of events (paradigm). Paradigms are designed to increase the neuronal activity in a specific area or region of the brain. The stimulus is performed with a period of activation followed either by a period of rest or by having the patient perform an alternate task (e.g., alternate left- and right-hand finger tapping; Fig. 20.124). The paradigm is then repeated using multiple measurements to increase the BOLD signal, similar to using multiple averages. There are a variety of BOLD stimuli that can be performed by the patient; the stimulus selected depends on the area of the brain and motor cortex being evaluated. BOLD stimuli include motor, sensory (visual and auditory), and cognitive stimuli (Table 20.10). Images are then post-processed to evaluate the area of activation (motor cortex) and the proximity to the pathology for surgical planning.

fMRI allows the clinician to analyze the cerebral organization of functional systems, displays changes in activity due to local brain lesions, and assists in mapping brain function in relation to

intracranial tumors, epileptic foci, or vascular malformations prior to surgery. Presurgical planning for tumor resection is the most widespread use of clinical fMRI. The goal of fMRI is to maximize the resection of pathologic tissue, leave the motor cortex intact, reduce surgical risk, and improve patient outcomes so they result in minimal neurologic deficit.

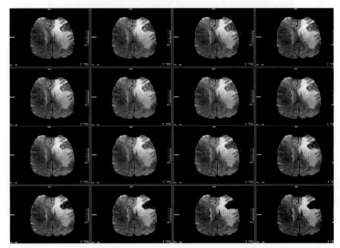

Fig. 20.123 Perfusion dynamic with contrast, showing 1 slice across time. (Courtesy of Siemens Medical Solutions USA, Inc.)

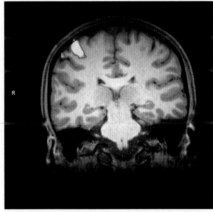

Fig. 20.124 BOLD finger tapping brain. (Courtesy of Siemens Medical Solutions USA, Inc.)

TABLE 20.10	**TYPES FOR STIMULI BOLD TECHNIQUE**	
BOLD STIMULUS	**FUNCTION PERFORMED BY PATIENT**	**CLINICAL APPLICATION**
Motor	Finger tapping, ankle flexing, tongue flexing	Presurgical planning to assess effects of lesion proximity to motor strip
Sensory (auditory)	Rhyming or word generation	Assess and visualize lesions proximity and effect of Broca's area (brain cortex)
Sensory (visual)	Focus on specific images or projections	Assess visual cortex, assist surgeon with minimizing negative surgical effects on vision
Cognitive	Thought and reasoning; learning and repeating pairs of words, memory, and decision making	Assess anatomic areas associated with processes

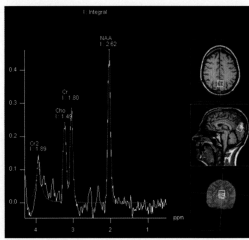

Fig.20.125 SVS 135 brain spectrum. (Courtesy of Siemens Medical Solutions USA, Inc.)

MAGNETIC RESONANCE SPECTROSCOPY

Magnetic Resonance Spectroscopy (MRS) is a diagnostic tool used to collect biochemical information from localized areas of interest. Spectroscopy sequences are acquired in addition to routine clinical imaging to clarify ambiguous findings.

^{1}H (hydrogen) MRS sequences include Single Voxel Spectroscopy (SVS) and 2D or 3D Chemical Shift Imaging (CSI). ^{1}H MRS techniques include Spin Echo (SE) or Point-Resolved Spectroscopy(PRESS) and Stimulated Echo Acquisition Mode (STEAM).

SVS post-processing results include a **single enlarged spectrum with reference images** (sagittal, axial, and coronal) (Fig. 20.125) and a **result table**. **2D** and **3D CSI results** include an **enlarged spectrum** that can be processed at various locations within the Field-of-View (FoV), **reference images, spectral maps, metabolite images, peak information maps, ratio of metabolites,** and a **result table**. Proton spectroscopy is FDA approved for use in the brain, breast, and prostate.

In a **research setting, multi-nuclear spectroscopy** can also be acquired in muscle, the heart, and the liver. Elements other than hydrogen found in the periodic table are evaluated with multi-nuclear spectroscopy. For example, muscle phosphorus (^{31}P) can be evaluated; a special coil tuned to ^{31}P would be used so that data acquired could be viewed and undergo post-processing.

^{1}H MRS spectroscopy is used to reflect the metabolic state of various tissues; show metabolic changes resulting from disease; monitor the effect of therapy; and follow metabolic pathways in biochemical research. Clinical applications for ^{1}H MR brain spectroscopy can include infection, epilepsy, neurodegenerative diseases, hypoxia, stroke, cerebral ischemia, demyelination, developmental delays, intracranial neoplasms, and evidence of other white matter diseases (e.g., MS plaques).

MRI TERMINOLOGY[52,65,66]

5-gauss line: Line that identifies the perimeter surrounding an MRI scanner; the area inside the line experiences static magnetic field strengths greater than 5 G (gauss).The 5-gauss line (outermost line) is the perimeter within which ferromagnetic objects are prohibited.

Artifacts: Signal intensities in an MR image that do not correspond to the spatial distribution of tissue in the image plane. They result from physiologic and system-related effects (e.g., overfolding artifact, distortion artifact, flow artifact, motion artifacts).

B0: Main static magnetic field of an MRI system.[67]

BRCA1 and **BRCA2 genes:** Breast cancer genes that increase a person's chance of developing breast cancer.[65]

Coil: Single or multiple loops of wire designed to produce a magnetic field from current flowing through the wire or to detect a changing magnetic field by voltage induced in the wire.[66]

Cryogen: Cooling agent, such as liquid helium or nitrogen. In MR imaging, cooling agents are used to maintain the superconductivity of the magnet.

Echo time (TE): Time between the middle of the (90°) excitation pulse to the center of the echo. TE determines image contrast and is usually measured in milliseconds (ms).

Flip angle: Defines the angle of the excitation for a pulse sequence. It is the angle to which the net magnetization is rotated relative to the main magnetic field direction via the application of a radiofrequency (RF) excitation pulse at the Larmor frequency.

Fourier transform (FT): Mathematical technique for MR signal to be decomposed into a sum of sine waves of different frequencies, phases, and amplitudes.

Free induction decay (FID): Signal that is induced by the RF excitation of the nuclear spins and that decreases exponentially without external influence at a characteristic time constant T2*.

Fringe field: Magnetic field outside the magnet that does not contribute to imaging; also called a *stray field.*

Coronal plane: Orthogonal plane dividing the body into posterior and anterior parts (i.e., frontal plane).

Gadolinium-DTPA (Gd-DTPA): Contrast agent used in MRI; the update of gadolinium-containing contrast agent reduces the T1 and T2 values of tissues, depending on the concentration. The T1 effect is the more relevant in clinical examinations.

Gating: Physiologically controlled imaging; synchronization of imaging with a time window so that a particular event or signal from among many will be selected and others will be eliminated or discarded. A variety of means for detecting these time windows can be used. (e.g., ECG, peripheral triggering, pulse triggering, respiratory triggering). An MRI technique used to minimize motion.

Gauss (G): Older unit for magnetic field strength. Today, the unit tesla (T) is used (1 tesla = 10,000 gauss).

Gradient coils: Coils used to generate magnetic gradient fields. Gradient coils are operated in pairs in the magnet, at the same current but of opposite polarities. One of the coils increases the static magnetic field a certain amount; the opposite coil reduces it by the same amount, changing the magnetic field overall. The change is the linear gradient. According to the coordinate axes (e.g., x, y, and z).

Gradient-induced magnetic field: Magnetic field that changes in strength in a given direction; it is necessary for selection of a region for imaging (slice selection) and for encoding the location of the MRI signal.

Gyromagnetic ratio: A constant for any given nucleus that relates the nuclear MR frequency and the strength of the external magnetic field. The value of the gyromagnetic ratio for hydrogen (1D) is 42.58 MHz/T).[68]

Hydrogen nuclei: Most abundant atom in the body; used in MRI for clinical scanning.

Image contrast: Contrast in the image is the relative difference in the signal strength between two adjacent tissue types.

Larmor frequency: Frequency at which the nuclear spins precess around the direction of the outer magnetic field (i.e., precessional frequency). The Larmor frequency depends on the type of nucleus and the strength of the magnetic field. At 1.5T, the Larmor frequency of protons is approximately 63 MHz.

Longitudinal magnetization (M_z): Exposing the human body to a strong magnetic field (B0) causes the protons to align in the direction of B0; the preferred energetic status of nuclei is to be parallel with the magnetic field or in the z-direction.[69]

Matrix size: Size of the raw-data matrix; it influences not only the spatial resolution, but also the measurement time and signal-to-noise ratio.

MR conditional: An item that has been demonstrated to pose no known hazards in a specified MR environment with specified conditions of use. Field conditions that define the MR environment include static magnetic field strength, spatial gradient, time rate of change of the magnetic field (dB/dt), RF fields, and Specific Absorption Rate (SAR). Additional conditions, including the specific configuration of the item, may be required.[70]

MR safe: An item that poses no known safety hazards in the MR environment. MR safe items are nonconducting, nonmetallic, and nonmagnetic items.[70]

MR unsafe: An item that is known to pose hazards in all MR environments. MR unsafe items include magnetic items, such as a pair of ferromagnetic scissors.[70]

Net magnetization vector (NMV): In MRI the summation of all the magnetic moments of the individual hydrogen nuclei.[71]

Permanent magnet: Magnet whose magnetic field originates from permanently ferromagnetic materials to generate a magnetic field between two poles of the magnet. There is no requirement for additional electrical power or cooling. Permanent magnets cannot be turned off, even in case of emergency. These magnets are usually low-field magnets (0.4T).[72]

Phase coherence: All protons pointing in the same phase direction. This occurs once the RF pulse is turned off and the spins precess about B0.

Precession: Wobbling motion that occurs when a spinning object is the subject of an external force. In MRI the proton of a hydrogen nucleus spins around its axis, giving it an angular moment.[73]

Proton density (PD): Long repetition time (TR) (reduces T1); short echo time (TE) (minimizes T2). See also *Spin density*.

Pulse sequences: Chronological order of RF pulses and gradient pulses used to excite the volume to be measured, generate the signal, and provide spatial encoding.

Radiofrequency (RF): Portion of the electronic spectrum in which electromagnetic waves can be generated by alternating current fed to an antenna. The RF pulses used in MRI are commonly in the 1 to 100 megahertz range. The primary effect on the human body is energy dissipation in the form of heat, usually on the surface of the body. Energy absorption is an important value for establishing safety thresholds.

Radiofrequency (RF) coil: Used for transmitting RF pulses or receiving MR signals.[66]

Radiofrequency (RF) magnetic fields: Electromagnetic radiation just lower in energy than infrared; RF magnetic fields are applied during pulse sequences.

Radiofrequency (RF) pulse: Burst of RF energy that, at the correct Larmor frequency, rotates the macroscopic magnetization vector by a specific angle, depending on the amplitude and duration of the pulse.[40]

Receiver coil: Coil of the RF receiver; it detects the MRI signal.[66]

Relaxation time: Following excitation, the nuclear spins tend to return to their equilibrium position, in accordance with these time constants, and release excess energy.[66]

Repetition time (TR): Time between two excitation pulses. Within the TR interval, signals may be acquired with one or more echo times or phase encodings (depending on the pulse sequence). TR is one of the measurement parameters that determines contrast. The acquisition time (TA) is directly proportional to TR.

Resistive magnet: Type of magnet that uses the principles of electromagnetism to generate the magnetic field. Typically, large current values and significant cooling of the magnet coils are required. A resistive magnet does not require cryogens, but it needs a constant power supply to maintain a homogeneous magnetic field and can be expensive to maintain. These magnets are usually low-field magnets (0.6T).[72]

Resonance: Exchange of energy between two systems at a specific frequency. In MRI resonance is generated by applying RF pulses at the same frequency as the nuclei precessing. The energy associated with the RF pulses shifts the nuclei from a low to a high energy state.

Sagittal plane: Orthogonal plane dividing the body into left and right parts (i.e., longitudinal plane).

Signal-to-Noise Ratio (SNR or S/N): Relationship between the intensity of signal and noise. The SNR can be improved by increasing the number of averages and the Field-of-View (FoV) and by using smaller bandwidth, a shorter echo time (TE), and thicker slices.

Spatial resolution: Ability to differentiate neighboring tissue structures. The higher the spatial resolution, the better small pathologies may be diagnosed.

Specific Energy Dose (SED) Total accumulated amount of energy that is deposited into the body. The SED is measured in joules per kilogram (joules/kg).

Specific Absorption Rate (SAR): Rate at which RF energy is absorbed into the body and exposed tissues. The SAR is measured in units of Watts per kilogram (W/kg).

Spin angular momentum: An angular spin that is the result of an odd number of protons and neutrons.

Spin density: Density of resonating nuclear spins in a given region; one of the principal determinants of the strength of the MRI signal from that region.[66]

Static magnetic field (B0): Main magnetic field, measured in Tesla. B0 direction runs parallel to the z-axis.

Superconducting magnet: Electromagnets that are partially built from superconducting materials and reach a much higher magnetic field intensity. The coil windings of superconducting magnets are made of wires. Liquid helium is commonly used as a coolant. Superconducting magnets typically exhibit field strengths of greater than 0.5T and operate clinically up to 7T.[72]

Superconductivity: Material characteristic of various alloys that at very low temperatures (close to absolute zero) results in a complete loss of electrical resistance. Electrical current can then flow without loss; that is, the magnet is "always on" without any power supply.

T1 relaxation: Tissue-specific time constant that describes the return of the longitudinal magnetization to equilibrium. After time T1, the longitudinal magnetization grows back to approximately 63% of its end value. Also, a tissue parameter that determines contrast (e.g., spin-lattice, longitudinal relaxation time, or thermal relaxation).

T2 relaxation: Tissue-specific time constant that describes the decay of transverse magnetization in an ideal homogeneous magnetic field. After time T2, transverse magnetization has lost 63% of its original value. Also, a tissue parameter that determines contrast (e.g., spin-spin relaxation or transverse relaxation).

Tesla (T): SI unit for magnetic field strength. Approximately 20,000 times as strong as the earth's magnetic field (1 Tesla = 10,000 gauss); older (CGS) unit; 1T also equals 1 newton/amp-m.[66]

Time-varying (gradient) magnetic field (dB/dt): In MR systems, this type of field provides position-dependent variation in magnetic field strength. The gradients are pulses, and the faster the imaging sequence, the greater the gradient fields change rate.[74]

Torque: Force that causes or tends to cause a body to rotate; vector quantity given by the product of the force and the position vector where the force is applied.[66]

Transverse magnetization: Net magnetization vector located in the transverse plane that is in phase coherence.

Transverse plane: Orthogonal plane dividing the body into superior and inferior parts (i.e., axial plane).

References

Chapter 1

1. *Mosby's medical dictionary*, ed 10, St. Louis, 2016, Elsevier.
2. Drake R, Vogl AW, Mitchell AWM: *Gray's anatomy for students*, ed 3, Elsevier Churchill Livingstone, 2015, p 14.
3. Drake R, Vogl AW, Mitchell AWM: *Gray's anatomy for students*, ed 3, Elsevier Churchill Livingstone, 2015, p 20.
4. *2018 primary certification and registration handbook for radiography*, St. Paul, 2018, American Registry of Radiologic Technologists.
5. Friedrich *Trendelenburg*, a surgeon in Leipzig, 1844–1924.
6. George Ryerson *Fowler*, an American surgeon, 1848–1906.
7. *Merrill's atlas of radiographic positioning and procedures*, vol 1, ed 14, St Louis, 2019, Elsevier, p 73.
8. *Dorland's illustrated medical dictionary*, ed 33, Philadelphia, Elsevier Healthsciences.
9. Frank ED, Ballinger PW, Bontrager KL: Two terms, one meaning, *Radiol Technol* 69:517, 1998.
10. *ARSRT 2018 primary radiography certification handbook, attachment B*, St Paul, 2017, American Registry of Radiologic Technologists.
11. ARRT 2019, September, standards of ethics A. *Code of Ethics*. Retrieved from: https://www.arrt.org/docs/default-source/governing-documents/arrt-standards-of-ethics.pdf?sfvrsn=c79e02fc_18
12. *ASRT curriculum guide in Radiography*, American Society of Radiologic Technologists, 2017.
13. Bushong S: *Radiologic science for technologists*, ed 11, St Louis, 2017, Mosby.
14. Statkiewicz-Sherer MA, Visconti PJ, Ritenour ER, et al.: *Radiation protection in medical radiography*, ed 8, St Louis, 2018, Elsevier.
15. Kuipers G, Velders XL, de Winter RJ, et al.: Evaluation of the occupational doses to interventional radiologists, *Cardiovasc Intervent Radiol* 31:483, 2008.
16. Hedrick WR, Feltes JJ, Starchman DE, et al.: Managing the pregnant radiation worker: a realistic policy for hospitals today, *Radiol Manage* 8:28, 1986.
17. Keriakes JG, Rosenstein M: *Handbook of radiation doses in nuclear medicine and diagnostic x-ray*, Boca Raton, Fla, 1980, CRC Press.
18. ICRP: ICRP statement on tissue reactions/early and late effects of radiation in normal tissues and organs—threshold doses for tissue reactions in a radiation protection context. ICRP Publication 118, *Ann ICRP* 41(1/2), 2012.
19. *ImageWisely Campaign*, 2019. Retrieved at. www.imagewisely.org
20. *ImageGently Alliance 2014*. Retrieved at www.imagegently.org

Chapter 2

1. Drake RL, Vogl AW, Mitchell AWM, editors: *Gray's anatomy for students*, ed 4, Philadelphia, 2019, Elsevier Churchill Livingstone.
2. *Mosby's medical dictionary*, ed 10, St. Louis, 2016, Elsevier.
3. *Dorland's illustrated medical dictionary*, ed 33, Philadelphia, 2019, Saunders.
4. McQuillen-Martensen K: *Radiographic image analysis*, ed 4, St. Louis, 2015, Elsevier Saunders.
5. Eisenberg R, Johnson N: *Comprehensive radiographic pathology*, ed 5, St. Louis, 2012, Mosby Elsevier.
6. Centers for Disease Control and Prevention: What are the risk factors for lung cancer?. http://www.cdc.gov/cancer/lung/basic_info/risk_factors.htm.
7. Berkow R, Beer M, Fletcher A: *The Merck manual of medical information*, Whitehouse Station, NJ, 1997, Merck Research Laboratories.
8. Fremgen B, Frucht S: *Medical terminology: a living language*, ed 7, New York, 2019, Pearson.

Chapter 3

1. *Mosby's medical dictionary*, ed 9, St. Louis, 2013, Elsevier, p 352.
2. Eisenberg RL, Johnson NM: *Comprehensive Radiographic Pathology*, ed 5, St. Louis, 2012, Elsevier Mosby, p 199.
3. *Mosby's medical dictionary*, ed 9, St. Louis, 2013, Elsevier, p 1842.
4. *Mosby's medical dictionary*, ed 9, St. Louis, 2013, Elsevier, p 1843.
5. Eisenberg RL, Johnson NM: *Comprehensive radiographic pathology*, ed 5, St. Louis, 2012, Elsevier Mosby.

Chapter 4

1. Berquist TH: *Imaging of orthopedic trauma and surgery*, Philadelphia, 1986, Saunders.
2. McQuillen-Martensen K: *Radiographic image analysis*, ed 4, St. Louis, 2015, Elsevier Saunders.
3. Griswold R: Elbow fat pads: a radiography perspective, *Radiol Technol* 53:303, 1982.
4. Eisenberg R, Johnson N: *Comprehensive radiographic pathology*, ed 6, St Louis, 2015, Elsevier Mosby.
5. Robert M: The classic: Radiography of the trapeziometacarpal joint. Degenerative changes of this joint, *Clin Orthop Relat Res* 472(4):1095, 2014. [Translated from the French; original publication 1936].
6. Long B, Rafert J: *Orthopedic radiography*, Philadelphia, 1995, Saunders.
7. Lewis S: New angles on the radiographic examination of the hand—II, *Radiogr Today* 54(29), 1988.
8. Folio L: Patient controlled stress radiography of the thumb, *Radiol Technol* 70:465, 1999.
9. Long B, Rafert J: *Orthopedic radiography*, Philadelphia, 1995, Saunders, pp 44–45.
10. Brewerton DA: A Tangential radiographic projection for demonstrating involvement of metacarpal head in rheumatoid arthritis, *Br J Radiol* 40:233, 1967.
11. Rafert JA, Long BW: Technique for diagnosis of scaphoid fractures, *Radiol Technol* 63:16, 1991.
12. Stecher WR: Roentgenography of the carpal navicular bone, *AJR Am J Roentgenol* 37:704, 1937.
13. Bridgman CF: Radiography of the carpal navicular bone, *Med Radiog Photog* 25:104, 1949.
14. Browning PD: Carpal tunnel syndrome imaging, *Medscape*, http://emedicine.medscape.com/article/388525-overview#a5
15. Coyle GF: *Radiographing immobile trauma patients. Unit 7. Special angled views of joints—elbow, knee, ankle*, Denver, 1980, Multi-Media Publishing.

Chapter 5

1. Eisenberg R, Johnson N: *Comprehensive radiographic pathology*, ed 6, St Louis, 2016, Elsevier.
2. Kowalczyk N: *Radiographic pathology for technologists*, ed 6, St Louis, 2018, Elsevier.
3. Manaster BJ: *Handbooks in radiology*, ed 2, Chicago, 1997, Mosby.
4. Rafert JA, Long BW, Hernandez EM, et al.: Axillary shoulder with exaggerated rotation: the Hill-Sachs defect, *Radiol Technol* 62:18, 1990.
5. Clements RW: Adaptation of the technique for radiography of the glenohumeral joint in the lateral position, *Radiol Technol* 51:305, 1979.
6. Ikemoto RY, Nascimento LGP, Bueno RS, et al.: Anterior glenoid rim erosion measured by x-ray exam: a simple way to perform the Bernageua profile view, *Rev Bras Ortop* 45(6):538–542, 2010.

7. Long BW, Rafert JA: *Orthopaedic radiography*, Philadelphia, 1995, Saunders, pp 168–170.
8. Neer II CS: Acromioplasty for the chronic impingement syndrome in the shoulder: a preliminary report, *J Bone Joint Surg Am* 54:41, 1972.
9. Neer II CS: Supraspinatus outlet, *Orthop Trans* 11:234, 1987.
10. Long BW, Rafert JA: *Orthopaedic radiography*, Philadelphia, 1995, Saunders, p 194.
11. Sloth C, Lundgren JS: The apical oblique radiograph in examination of acute shoulder trauma, *Eur J Radiol* 9:147, 1989.
12. Garth Jr WP, Slappey CE, Ochs CW: Roentgenographic demonstration of instability of the shoulder: the apical oblique projection, *J Bone Joint Surg Am* 66:1450, 1984.
13. Simovitch R, Sanders B, Ozbaydar M, et al.: Acromioclavicular joint injuries: diagnosis and management, *J Am Acad Orthop Surg* 17(4):207–219, 2009.
14. Shaffer BS: Painful conditions of the acromioclavicular joint, *J Am Acad Orthop Surg* 7(3):176–188, 1999.

Chapter 6

1. Frank ED, et al.: Mayo Clinic: radiography of the ankle mortise, *Radiol Technol* 62:354, 1991.
2. Manaster BJ: *Handbooks in radiology*, ed 2, St Louis, 1997, Year Book Medical.
3. Keats TE, et al.: Normal axial relationships of the major joints, *Radiology* 87:904, 1966.
4. McQuillen-Martensen K: *Radiographic image analysis*, ed 4, St Louis, 2015, Elsevier Saunders.
5. Martensen KM: Alternate AP knee method assures open joint space, *Radiol Technol* 64:19, 1992.
6. Merchant AC, et al.: Roentgenographic analysis of patellofemoral congruence, *J Bone Joint Surg Am* 56:1391, 1974.
7. Hughston AC: Subluxation of the patella, *J Bone Joint Surg Am* 50:10036, 1968.
8. Manaster BJ: *Handbooks in radiology, skeletal radiology*, ed 4, St Louis, 1989, Year Book Medical.
9. Turner GW, Burns CB: Erect position/tangential projection of the patellofemoral joint, *Radiol Technol* 54:11, 1982.
10. Hobbs DL: Tangential projection of the patella, *Radiol Technol* 77:20, 2005.
11. McQuillen-Martensen K: *Radiographic image analysis*, St Louis, 2015, Elsevier Saunders, p 352.

Chapter 7

1. Drake R, Vogel AW, Mitchell AWM: *Gray's anatomy for students*, ed 3, Philadelphia, 2015, Elsevier, p 441.
2. American Academy of Orthopaedic Surgeons: https://orthoinfo.aaos.org/en/diseases--conditions/pelvic-fractures/.
3. Drake R, Vogel AW, Mitchell AWM: *Gray's anatomy for students*, ed 3, Philadelphia, 2015, Elsevier, p 448.
4. Rossi F, Dragoni S: Acute avulsion fractures of the pelvis in adolescent competitive athletes: prevalence, location and sports distribution of 203 cases collected, *Skeletal Radiol* 30:127–131, 2001.
5. Long BW, Rafert JA: *Orthopaedic radiography*, Philadelphia, 1995, Saunders.
6. Clements RS, Nakayama HK: Radiographic methods in total hip arthroplasty, *Radiol Technol* 51:589–600, 1980.

Chapter 8

1. *Mosby's Dictionary of medicine, nursing & health professions*, ed 10, St. Louis, 2016, Elsevier.

Chapter 9

1. Carucci LR: Imaging obese patients: problems and solutions, *Abdom Imaging* 38(4):630–646, 2013.
2. Martensen-McQuillen K: *Radiographic image analysis*, ed 4, St. Louis, 2015, Elsevier, p 429.
3. Francis C: Method improves consistency in L5-S1 joint space films, *Radiol Technol* 63:302–305, 1992.
4. Frank ED, Stears JG, Gray JE, et al.: Use of the posteroanterior projection: a method of reducing x-ray exposures to radiosensitive organs, *Radiol Technol* 54:343–347, 1983.

Chapter 10

1. Statkiewicz-Sherer MA, Visconti PJ, Ritenour ER, et al.: *Radiation protection in medical radiography*, ed 7, St. Louis, 2014, Elsevier, p 233.

Chapter 11

1. Drake R, Vogel AW, Mitchell AWM: *Gray's anatomy for students*, ed 3, Philadelphia, 2015, Elsevier, p 1125.
2. Drake R, Vogel AW, Mitchell AWM: *Gray's anatomy for students*, ed 3, Philadelphia, 2015, Elsevier, p 842.
3. Standring S: *Gray's anatomy: the anatomical basis of clinical practice*, ed 41, Philadelphia, 2015, Elsevier Churchill Livingstone.
4. *Mosby's medical dictionary*, ed 9, St. Louis, 2013, Elsevier Mosby, p 353.
5. *Mosby's medical dictionary*, ed 9, St. Louis, 2013, Elsevier Mosby, p 1300.
6. Gray H: *Gray's anatomy*, ed 30, Philadelphia, 1985, Lea & Febiger.
7. Martensen-McQuillen K: *Radiographic image analysis*, ed 5, St. Louis, 2019, Elsevier Saunders.

Chapter 12

1. Clemente CD: *Gray's anatomy*, ed 30, Philadelphia, 1985, Lea & Febiger.
2. Eisenberg RL, Johnson NM: *Comprehensive radiographic pathology*, ed 7, St. Louis, 2021, Elsevier.
3. Meschan I: *Synopsis of analysis of roentgen signs in general radiology*, Philadelphia, 1976, Saunders.
4. Ell R: *Handbook of gastrointestinal and genitourinary radiology*, St. Louis, 1992, Mosby.
5. Kowalczyk N: *Radiographic pathology for technologists*, ed 7, St. Louis, 2017, Elsevier.
6. Statkiewicz Sherer MA, Visconti P, Ritenour ER, Welch Haynes K: *Radiation protection in medical radiography*, ed 8, St. Louis, 2017, Elsevier.
7. Martensen McQuillen K: *Radiographic image analysis*, ed 5, St. Louis, 2019, Elsevier.

Chapter 13

1. Drake RL, Vogl W, Mitchell AWM: *Gray's anatomy for students*, ed 4, Philadelphia, 2019, Elsevier.
2. Standring S: *Gray's anatomy: the anatomical basis of clinical practice*, ed 41, Philadelphia, 2015, Elsevier.
3. Ell SR: *Handbook of gastrointestinal and genitourinary radiology*, St. Louis, 1992, Mosby.
4. McLemore LJ: Inflammatory bowel disease, *Radiol Technol* 78:299, 2007.

Chapter 14

1. *Dorland's illustrated medical dictionary*, ed 33, Philadelphia, 2019, Elsevier Saunders.
2. *Webster's new world college dictionary*, ed 5, New York, 2014, Macmillan.
3. Wilmot A, Mehta N, Jha S: The adoption of low-osmolar contrast agents in the United States: historical analysis of health policy and clinical practice, *Am J Roentgenol* 199(5):1049–1053, 2012.
4. Caschera L, Lazzara A, Piergallini L, Ricci D, Tuscano B, Vanzulli A: Iodinated contrast: name, structure, charge, and osmolality, contrast agents in diagnostic imaging: present and future, *Pharmacol Res* 110:65–10075, 2016.
5. American College of Radiology (ACR): ACR manual on contrast media, version 10.3, 2018. www.acr.org/-/media/ACR/Files/Clinical-Resources/Contrast_Media.pdf.
6. Ell SR: *Handbook of gastrointestinal and genitourinary radiology*, St. Louis, 1992, Mosby.
7. Linn-Watson TA: *Radiographic pathology*, ed 2, Philadelphia, 2014, Elsevier Saunders.
8. Eisenberg RL, Johnson NM: *Comprehensive radiographic pathology*, ed 6, St. Louis, 2015, Elsevier Mosby.
9. https://www.stanfordchildrens.org/en/topic/default?id=posterior-urethral-valves--90-P03110.

Chapter 15

1. American Registry of Radiologic Technologist: *Radiography Examination Content specifications*. Retrieved from www.arrt.org/docs/default-source/discipline-documents/radiography/rad-content-specifications.pdf?sfvrsn=6dda01fc_32, 2017.
2. Eisenberg R, Johnson N: *Comprehensive radiographic pathology*, ed 6, St. Louis, 2015, Elsevier Mosby.

3. American College of Radiology: *ACR Appropriateness Criteria®: blunt chest trauma*. Retrieved from https://acsearch.acr.org/list, 2013.
4. American College of Radiology: *ACR Appropriateness Criteria®: blunt abdominal Trauma*. Retrieved from https://acsearch.acr.org/list, 2012.
5. American College of Radiology: *ACR Appropriateness Criteria®: acute hand and wrist trauma*. Retrieved from https://acsearch.acr.org/list, 2013.
6. American College of Radiology: *ACR Appropriateness Criteria®: acute shoulder pain*. Retrieved from https://acsearch.acr.org/list>, 2010.
7. American College of Radiology: *ACR Appropriateness Criteria®: acute trauma to the foot*. Retrieved from https://acsearch.acr.org/list>, 2014.
8. American College of Radiology: *ACR Appropriateness Criteria®: acute trauma to the ankle*. Retrieved from https://acsearch.acr.org/list>, 2014.
9. American College of Radiology: *ACR Appropriateness Criteria®: acute trauma to the knee*. Retrieved from https://acsearch.acr.org/list>, 2014.
10. American College of Radiology: *ACR Appropriateness Criteria®: acute hip pain—suspected hip fracture*. Retrieved from https://acsearch.acr.org/list>, 2013.
11. American College of Radiology: *ACR Appropriateness Criteria®: suspected spine trauma*. Retrieved from https://acsearch.acr.org/list>, 2012.
12. Johnston J, Fauber T: *Essentials of radiographic physics and imaging*, St. Louis, 2012, Elsevier Mosby.
13. American College of Radiology: *ACR Appropriateness Criteria®: Head trauma*. Retrieved from https://acsearch.acr.org/list>, 2012.
14. Medtronic for Healthcare Professionals: O-Arm Surgical Imaging System. Retrieved from http://www.medtronic.com/for-healthcare-professionals/products-therapies/neurological/surgical-navigation-and-imaging/o-arm-surgical-imaging-system/>.
15. Manaster BJ: *Handbook of skeletal radiology: handbooks in radiology*, St. Louis, 1989, Mosby.

Chapter 16

1. Creo A, Schwenk F: Bone age: a handy tool for pediatric providers, *Pediatrics* 140(6):1–11, 2017, https://doi.org/10.1542/peds.2017-1486.
2. Breen M, Tsai A, Stamm A, Kleinman P: Bone age assessment practices in infants and older children among Society for Pediatric Radiology members, *Pediatric Radiology* 46(9):1269–1274, 2016, https://doi.org/10.1007/s00247-016-3618-7.
3. Gilsanz V, Ratib O: *Hand Bone Age*, Germany, 2005, Springer.
4. Greulich WW, Pyle SI: *Radiographic atlas of skeletal development of the hand and wrist*, Stanford (CA), 1959, Stanford University Press.
5. Mansourvar M, Ismail M, Raj R, et al: The applicability of Greulich and Pyle atlas to assess skeletal age for four ethnic groups, *Journal of Forensic and Legal Medicine* 22:26–29, 2014.
6. Chaumoitre K, Saliba-Serre B, Adalian P, Signoli M, Leonetti G, Panuel M: Forensic use of the Greulich and Pyle atlas: prediction intervals and relevance, *European Radiology* 27(3):1032–1043, 2017.
7. Tanner JM, Healy MJR, Goldstein H, Cameron N: *Assessment of skeletal maturity and prediction of adult height (TW3 method)*, London, 2001, W.B. Saunders.
8. Bunch P, Altes T, McIhenny J, Patrie J, Gaskin C: Skeletal development of the hand and wrist: digital bone age companion-a suitable alternative to the Greulich and Pyle atlas for bone age assessment? *Skeletal Radiology* 46:785–793, 2017, https://doi.org/10.1007/s00256-017-2616-7.
9. U.S. Department: of Health and Human Services, Administration for Child and Families, Administration on Children, Youth, and Families, Children's Bureau, 2016. *Child Maltreatment 2016*. Available from https://www.acf.hhs.gov/cb/research-data-technology/statistics-research/child-maltreatment.
10. American College of Radiography: *ACR-SPR practice parameter for the performance and interpretation of skeletal surveys in children*, Practice PARAMETER, 2016. Retrieved from http://www.acr.org/~/media/ACR/Documents/PGTS/guidelines/Skeletal_Surveys.pdf>.
11. www.imagegently.org.
12. Karami, V., Zabihzadeh, M., Shams, N., Gilvand, A. (2017).
13. National Cancer Institute: *Radiation risks and pediatric computed tomography (CT): a guide for health care providers*. Retrieved from http://www.cancer.gov/about-cancer/causes-prevention/risk/radiation/pediatric-ct-scans>, 2012.
14. American College of Radiography: *ACR-SPR Practice Parameters for the performance of pediatric contrast examinati ons of the small bowel*. Retrieved from http://www.acr.org/~/media/ACR/Documents/PGTS/guidelines/Pediatric_contrast_sm_bowel.pdf>, 2013.

Chapter 18

1. Wisely I: Radiation safety in adult medical imaging. Retrieved from http://www.imagewisely.org.
2. American College of Radiology: *Pledge*: Image Wisely: radiation safety in adult medical imaging. Retrieved from http://www.imagewisely.org/Pledge.aspx.
3. McLemore JM: Inflammatory bowel disease, *Radiol Technol* 78:299, 2007.

Chapter 19

1. Tortorici MR, Apfel PJ: *Advanced radiographic and angiographic procedures with an introduction to specialized imaging*, Philadelphia, 1995, FA Davis.
2. American College of Radiology, Society for Pediatric Radiology: *Practice parameter for the performance and interpretation of skeletal surveys in children*, 2016, https://www.acr.org/-/media/ACR/Files/Practice-Parameters/Skeletal-Survey.pdf?la=en.
3. Roberts CC, et al.: ACR Appropriateness Criteria® on metastatic bone disease, *J Am Coll Radiol* vol. 7:400–409, 2010.
4. Chou SS, Kicska GA, Pipavath SN, Reddy GP: Digital tomosynthesis of the chest: current and emerging applications, *Radiographics* 34(2):359–372, 2014, https://doi.org/10.1148/rg.342135057.
5. Machida H, Yuhara T, Mori T, Ueno E, Moribe Y, Sabol JM: Optimizing parameters for flat-panel detector digital tomosynthesis, *Radiographics* 30(2):549–562, 2010, https://doi.org/10.1148/rg.302095097.
6. Ha AS, Lee AY, Hippe DS, Chou SS, Chew FS: Digital tomosynthesis to evaluate fracture healing: prospective comparison with radiography and CT, *Am J Roentgenol* 205(1):136–141, 2015, https://doi.org/10.2214/ajr.14.13833.
7. Kopans DB: Digital breast tomosynthesis from concept to clinical care, *Am J Roentgenol* 202(2):299–308, 2014, https://doi.org/10.2214/ajr.13.11520.

Chapter 20

1. Early PJ, Sodee DB: *Principles and practice of nuclear medicine*, ed 2, St. Louis, 1995, Mosby.
2. Bushong SC: *Radiologic science for the technologist*, ed 7, St. Louis, 2001, Mosby.
3. Weerakkody Y, Pfleger R, et al.: Hybrid imaging. Radiopaedia.org. Retrieved from http://radiopaedia.org/articles/hybrid-imaging.
4. American Cancer Society: Cancer facts and figures 2015. American Cancer Society. Retrieved from http://www.cancer.org/acs/groups/content/@editorial/documents/document/acspc-044552.pdf.
5. American Society for Therapeutic Radiology and Oncology: Fast facts about radiation therapy. Retrieved from https://www.astro.org/News-and-Media/Media-Resources/FAQs/Fast-Facts-About-Radiation-Therapy/Index.aspx.
6. Radiological Society of North America, Inc. Retrieved from http://www.radiologyinfo.org/en/info.cfm?pg=gamma_knife.
7. American Institute for Medical Ultrasound: Prudent clinical use and safety of diagnostic ultrasound. Retrieved from http://www.aium.org/officialStatements/34.
8. Society of Diagnostic Medical Sonography: State Licensure, http://www.sdms.org/advocacy/state-licensure.
9. National Cancer Institute: Cancer Stat Facts: Female Breast Cancer. Retrieved from https://seer.cancer.gov/statfacts/html/breast.html.
10. American Cancer Society: How Common is Breast Cancer?. Retrieved from https://www.cancer.org/cancer/breast-cancer/about/how-common-is-breast-cancer.html.
11. World Cancer Research Fund. Retrieved from http://www.wcrf.org/int/cancer-facts-figures/data-specific-cancers/breast-cancer-statistics.
12. Zehr K: Diagnosis and Treatment of Breast Cancer in Men, *Radiol Technol* 91:51M, 2019.
13. Oeffinger KC, Fontham ETH, Etzioni R, et al.: Breast cancer screening for women at average risk 2015 guideline update from the American Cancer Society, *Journal of American Medicine Association* 314(15), 2015.
14. U.S. Food & Drug Administration: FDA Advances Landmark Policy Changes to Modernize Mammography Services and improve

their Quality. Retrieved from https://www.fda.gov/news-events/press-announcements/fda-advances-landmark-policy-changes-modernize-mammography-services-and-improve-their-quality.

15. Frank ED: Technical aspects of mammography. In Carlton RL, Adler AM, editors: *Principles of radiographic imaging*, ed 3, Albany, NY, 2001, Delmar.

16. Bushong SC: *Radiologic science for the technologist*, ed 11, St. Louis, 2017, Elsevier.

17. Pisano ED, Yaffe MJ, Kuzmiak CM: *Digital mammography*, Philadelphia, 2004, Lippincott Williams & Wilkins.

18. Monreal S: Contrast-Enhanced Digital Mammography, *Radiol Technol* 89:518, 2018.

19. Ikeda DM: *Breast imaging: the requisites*, ed 2, St. Louis, 2011, Elsevier Mosby.

20. Anderson EDC, Muir BB, Walsh JS, et al.: The efficacy of double-reading mammograms in breast screening, *Clin Radiol* 49:248, 1994.

21. Ferrara A: Nuclear imaging in breast cancer, *Radiol Technol* 81:233, 2010.

22. Lee L, Strickland W, Robin A, et al.: *Fundamentals of mammography*, ed 2, Edinburgh, 2003, Churchill Livingstone.

23. Ferrara A: Benign breast disease, *Radiol Technol* 82:447M, 2011.

24. Eklund GW, Busby RC, Miller SH, et al.: Improved imaging of the augmented breast, *AJR Am J Roentgenol* 151:469, 1988.

25. National Institutes of Health: Osteoporosis Overview. https://www.bones.nih.gov/health-info/bone/osteoporosis/overview.

26. The National Osteoporosis Foundation: https://www.nof.org/news/54-million-americans-affected-by-osteoporosis-and-low-bone-mass/.

27. Cosman F, de Beur SJ, LeBoff MS, et al.: Clinician's Guide to Prevention and Treatment of Osteoporosis [published correction appears in Osteoporos Int. 2015 Jul;26(7):2045-7], *Osteoporos Int* 25(10):2359–2381, 2014.

28. Sturtridge W, Lentle B, Hanley DA: The use of bone density measurement in the diagnosis and management of osteoporosis, *Can Med Assoc J* 155(Suppl):924, 1996.

29. International Society for Clinical Densitometry: *Official Position Statements*, http://www.iscd.org.official positions/2015, 2015.

30. Berry, M, ASRT Radiologic Technology, Volume, 90, number 3, January/February 2019.

31. Food and Drug Association: News release. FDA approves new treatment for osteoporosis in postmenopausal women at high risk of fracture, https://www.fda.gov/news-events/press-announcements/fda-approves-new-treatment-osteoporosis-postmenopausal-women-high-risk-fracture.

32. Long,B,Hall Rollings,J, Smith,BJ: Merrill's Atlas of Radiographic Positioning & Procedures,14 ed, Volume Two, Bone Densitometru, pages 466-502.

33. Genant HK, Guglielmi G, Jergas M: *Bone densitometry and osteoporosis*, New York, 1998, Springer.

34. Lewis MK, Blake GM, Fogelman I: Patient dose in dual x-ray absorptiometry, *Osteoporosis Int* 4:11, 1994.

35. Kalender WA: Effective dose values in bone mineral measurements by photon absorptiometry and computed tomography, *Osteoporosis Int* 2:82, 1992.

36. https://www.medicinenet.com/ct_scan_vs_mri/article.htm#how_does_an_mri_magnetic_resonance_imaging_scan_work.

37. https://en.wikipedia.org/wiki/Earth%27s_magnetic_field.

38. http://mriquestions.com/liquid-helium-use.html.

39. Shellock FG, Crues JV: Safety consideration in magnetic resonance imaging, *MRI Decisions* 2:25, 1988.

40. Bushong SC, Clarke G: *Magnetic resonance imaging: physical and biological principles*, ed 4, St. Louis, 2015, Elsevier.

41. http://www.ajnr.org/content/ajnr/early/2012/03/01/ajnr.A2827.full.pdf.

42. https://www.ncbi.nlm.nih.gov/pmc/articles/PMC1479713/.

43. https://www.radiologyinfo.org/en/info.cfm?pg=safety-anesthesia.

44. http://mriquestions.com/acr-safety-zones.html.

45. Shellock FG, Spinazzi A: MRI safety update 2008: part 2, screening patients for MRI, *AJR Am J Roentgenol* 191:1140, 2008.

46. Westbrook C, Kaut Roth C, Talbot J: *MRI in practice*, ed 4, West Sussex, UK, 2011, Wiley-Blackwell.

47. Heiken JP, Brown JJ: *Manual of clinical magnetic resonance imaging*, ed 2, New York, 1991, Raven Press.

48. Zaremba LA: FDA guidelines for magnetic resonance equipment safety. Center for devices and radiological health food and drug Administration. Retrieved from https://www.aapm.org/meetings/02AM/pdf/8356-48054.pdf.

49. https://pubs.rsna.org/doi/full/10.1148/rg.262055063.

50. https://en.wikipedia.org/wiki/MRI_sequence.

51. http://mriquestions.com/commercial-acronyms.html.

52. Siemens Healthineers: MR Acronym Brochures_24-18-11517-01-76

53. http://casemed.case.edu/clerkships/neurology/web%20neurorad/mri%20basics.htm.

54. https://ww5.komen.org/BreastCancer/BreastMRI.html.

55. https://appliedradiology.com/articles/an-overview-of-breast-mri.

56. https://www.ncbi.nlm.nih.gov/pmc/articles/PMC4152773/.

57. https://radiopaedia.org/articles/diffusion-weighted-imaging-1?lang=us.

58. https://radiopaedia.org/articles/diffusion-weighted-mri-in-acute-stroke-1?lang=us.

59. https://www.ncbi.nlm.nih.gov/pmc/articles/PMC6108979/.

60. https://www.ncbi.nlm.nih.gov/pmc/articles/PMC5503962/.

61. http://www.ajnr.org/content/ajnr/36/6/E41.full.pdf.

62. http://mriquestions.com/dsc-curve-analysis.html.

63. https://en.wikipedia.org/wiki/Arterial_spin_labelling.

64. FDA Drug Safety Communication: New warnings for using gadolinium-based contrast agents in patients with kidney dysfunction. U.S. Food and Drug Administration. Retrieved from http://www.fda.gov/Drugs/DrugSafety/ucm223966.htm.

65. *MR Glossary, A dictionary of magnetic resonance*, Siemens Healthcare GmbH, 2015.

66. https://www.nationalbreastcancer.org/what-is-brca.

67. *Dorland's illustrated medical dictionary*, ed 32, Philadelphia, 2012, Elsevier Saunders.

68. https://www.mr-tip.com/serv1.php?type=db1&dbs=Gyromagnetic%20Ratio.

69. MR Physics_Generating and AcquiringSignal Glossary.ver2; Siemens.com/healthineers

70. https://pubs.rsna.org/doi/full/10.1148/radiol.2531091030.

71. https://radiopaedia.org/articles/net-magnetisation-vector?lang=us.

72. https://www.mr-tip.com/serv1.php?type=dev&sub=1.

73. https://www.mr-tip.com/serv1.php?type=db1&dbs=Precession.

74. https://www.sor.org/learning/document-library/safety-magnetic-resonance-imaging/4-time-varying-gradient-magnetic-fields-dbdt.

Additional Resources

Chapter 1

An exposure indicator for digital radiography: *Report of AAPM Task Group 116*, College Park, MD, July 2009, American Association of Physicists in Medicine.

Baxes GA: *Digital image processing*, New York, 1994, John Wiley & Sons.

Carlton R, Adler AM: *Principles of radiographic imaging: an art and a science*, ed 6, New York, 2020, Delmar.

Dreyer KJ, Hirschorn DS, Mehta A, et al.: *PACS picture archiving and communication systems: a guide to the digital revolution*, ed 2, New York, 2005, Springer.

Englebardt SP, Nelson R: *Health care informatics: an interdisciplinary approach*, St Louis, 2002, Mosby.

Huang HK: *PACS: basic principles and applications*, ed 2, Hoboken, NJ, 2010, Wiley.

Papp J: *Quality management in the imaging sciences*, ed 6, St Louis, 2018, Elsevier Mosby.

Shepherd CT: *Radiographic image production and manipulation*, New York, 2003, McGraw-Hill.

Kicken PJ, Bos AJ: Effectiveness of lead aprons in vascular radiology: results of clinical measurements, *Radiology* 197:473, 1995.

Godderidge C: *Pediatric imaging*, Philadelphia, 1995, Saunders.

Chapter 8

Dorland's illustrated medical dictionary, ed 33, Philadelphia, 2019, Elsevier Saunders.

McQuillen Martensen K, *Radiographic image analysis*, ed 5, St. Louis, 2019, Elsevier.

Chapter 10

Drake R, Vogel AW, Mitchell AWM: *Gray's anatomy for students*, ed 4, Philadelphia, 2019, Elsevier Churchill Livingstone.

Martensen KM: *Radiographic image analysis*, ed 4, St. Louis, 2015, Elsevier Saunders.

Chapter 14

Kowalczyk N, Mace JD: *Radiographic pathology for technologists*, ed 7, St. Louis, 2017, Elsevier Mosby.

Mosby's medical dictionary, ed 10, St. Louis, 2016, Elsevier Mosby.

Chapter 17

Alternative Modalities and Procedures

SamAD, 2nd, Morasch MD, Collins J, et al.: Safety of gadolinium contrast angiography in patients with chronic renal insufficiency, *J VascSurg* 38:313, 2003.

Shaw DR, Kessel DO: The current status of the use of carbon dioxide in diagnostic and interventional angiographic procedures, *CardiovascInterventRadiol* 29:323, 2006.

Interventional Angiography

Fourney DR, Schomer DF, Nader R, et al.: Percutaneous vertebroplasty and kyphoplasty for painful vertebral body fractures in cancer patients, *J Neurosurg* (Suppl 1)17, 2003.

Hiwatashi A, Westesson PL: Vertebroplasty for osteoporotic fractures with spinal canal compromise, *AJNR Am J Neuroradiol* 28:690, 2007.

Jost RS, Jost R, Schoch E, et al.: Colorectal stenting: an effective therapy for preoperative and palliative treatment, *CardiovascInterventRadiol* 30:433, 2007.

Levin DC, Rao VM, Parker L, et al.: The changing roles of radiologists, cardiologists, and vascular surgeons in percutaneous peripheral arterial interventions during a recent five-year interval, *J Am CollRadiol* 2(39), 2005.

Liapi E, Geshwind J-F: Transcatheter and ablative therapeutic approaches for solid malignancies, *J ClinOncol* 10:978, 2007.

Chapter 18

Bushong S: *Radiologic science for technologists*, ed 11, St Louis, 2017, Elsevier Mosby.

Carlton R, Adler AM: *Principles of radiographic imaging: an art and a science*, ed 6, New York, 2019, Delmar.

Fricke BL, Donnelly LF, Frush DP, et al.: In-plane bismuth breast shields for pediatric CT: effects on radiation dose and image quality using experimental and clinical data, *AJR Am J Roentgenol* 180:407, 2003.

McLemore JM: Inflammatory bowel disease, *Radiol Technol* 78:299, 2007.

Prokop M, Galanski M: *Spiral and multi-slice computed tomography of the body*, New York, 2003, Thieme.

Schmidt S, Felley C, Meuwly JY, et al.: CT enteroclysis: technique and clinical applications, *Eur Radiol* 16:648, 2006.

Standring S: *Gray's anatomy: the anatomical basis of clinical practice*, ed 41, St. Louis, 2016, Elsevier Churchill Livingstone.

Chapter 20

American Society of Radiologic Technologists (ASRT), www.asrt.org/docs/default-source/practice-standards-published/ps_rt.pdf?sfvrsn=2.

Khan Faiz M, Gibbons John P: *Khan's The Physics of Radiation Therapy*, Lippincott Williams & Wilkins, 2014.

Bushong Stewart C: *Radiologic Science for Technologists: Physics, Biology, and Protection*, Elsevier Health Sciences, 2016.

"Principles of Radiation Therapy." *Clinical Gate*, 13 Mar. 2015, clinicalgate.com/principles-of-radiation-therapy/.

"TomoTherapy Treatment Delivery." *Precise, Innovative Tumor Treatments | Accuray*, 14 Apr. 2018, www.accuray.com/tomotherapy/tomotherapy-treatment-delivery/.

Washington Charles M, Leaver Dennis T: *Principles and Practice of Radiation Therapy*, Elsevier Health Sciences, 2015.

Society of Diagnostic Medical Sonography: SDMS scope of practice and clinical standards for the diagnostic medical sonographer, April 13, 2015. Retrieved from http://www.sdms.org/docs/default-source/Resources/scope-of-practice-and-clinical-standards.pdf?sfvrsn=14>.

Hashemi R, Bradley W, Lisanti C: *MRI: the basics*, ed 2, Philadelphia, 2004, Lippincott Williams & Wilkins.

McRobbie D, Moore E, Graves M, et al.: *MRI: from picture to proton*, ed 2, Cambridge, 2006, Cambridge University Press.

ISCD certification course in clinical bone densitometry for technologists, 2010. Brisbane, Australia.

National Osteoporosis Foundation: What is osteoporosis and what causes it?. https://www.nof.org/patients/what-is-osteoporosis/.

Index

Note: Page numbers followed by f indicate figures, t indicate tables, and b indicate boxes.